# The SAGES Manual of Metabolic and Bariatric Surgery

Omar M. Ghanem • Farah Husain
Judy Y. Chen • Robert B. Lim
Matthew Kroh
Editors

# The SAGES Manual of Metabolic and Bariatric Surgery

Third Edition

SAGES University MASTERS PROGRAM

Springer

*Editors*
Omar M. Ghanem
Department of Surgery
Mayo Clinic
Rochester, MN, USA

Judy Y. Chen
Department of Surgery
University of Washington
Seattle, WA, USA

Matthew Kroh
Surgery
Cleveland Clinic
Cleveland, OH, USA

Farah Husain
Department of Surgery
University of Arizona
Phoenix, AZ, USA

Robert B. Lim
Department of Surgery
Wake Forest University, Atrium Health Carolinas
Charlotte, NC, USA

ISBN 978-3-031-72308-7 ISBN 978-3-031-72309-4 (eBook)
https://doi.org/10.1007/978-3-031-72309-4



This Springer imprint is published by the registered company Springer Nature Switzerland AG
The registered company address is: Gewerbestrasse 11, 6330 Cham, Switzerland

*To my wife and my world, Nadine, whose love and wisdom inspire us all as a family toward distinction and perfection every single day. To my biggest blessings, Yvanna and Yuri, for making me the proudest dad. I would also like to dedicate this book to my colleagues on the SAGES Metabolic and Bariatric Surgery Committee, who contributed to this showpiece manual. To Mrs. Sallie Matthews for her leadership and to the SAGES management team for their support, thank you.*

*Omar M. Ghanem*

*Thank you to my colleagues and friends in the editorial group. It was an honor to work with you. I dedicate this work to my amazing family. Keenan, Parsa, and Cairo, you are always my true north. I love you.*

*Farah Husain*

*If you believe in yourself and have dedication, success is achievable. The price of victory is high, but so are the rewards. I am grateful for my husband and two daughters, whose support drives and inspires me every day.*

*Judy Y. Chen*

*To my mentor, Daniel B. Jones, MD, who took me in and still guides my career in academic medicine.*

*Robert B. Lim*

*To my wife Jean, whose steadfast support and unmatched dedication are the backbone of my career, and to Sophia, Eva, and Carter, who inspire me always. Your strength and encouragement make us possible.*

*Matthew Kroh*

# Preface

"Progress is impossible without change, and those who cannot change their minds cannot change anything," remarked George Bernard Shaw, highlighting the necessity of adaptation and innovation. Metabolic and bariatric surgery as a specialty overall, and this, the third edition of *The SAGES Manual of Metabolic and Bariatric Surgery* embodies this spirit, reflecting the dynamic evolution of technologies, techniques, and data accrual, in the care of patients with severe obesity.

The first edition of the SAGES Manual was a pioneering volume in the field in 2008. With rapid advancements and emerging techniques over the past decade, the second edition provided crucial updates and expanded its scope to include seldom-discussed yet significant topics such as surgical tourism, pregnancy, and innovative pre-market devices. This third edition continues in this tradition of excellence, integrating the latest knowledge and innovations in bariatric surgery.

Severe obesity remains a pressing epidemic, affecting nearly half of the US population and contributing to a high burden of weight-related comorbid diseases. Bariatric surgery has consistently proven effective and durable in treating severe obesity. With technological advancements, particularly in laparoscopic, robotic, and endoluminal techniques, the field has advanced rapidly. Improved data and outcomes have further broadened the spectrum of therapeutic options available to healthcare providers.

The third edition of this manual is designed to present a comprehensive, state-of-the-art approach to current and future bariatric interventions. Significant updates include the rapidly expanding field of endoluminal bariatric procedures, focusing on new devices and theoretical mechanisms. The latest data on innovative laparoscopic approaches to treating obesity, along with long-term outcomes, including expanded surgical procedures and applications of robotics are reviewed. This edition also delves into newer surgical approaches to treat metabolic diseases and obesity, exploring their proposed mechanisms of action and efficacy.

New sections encompass the application of robotic technologies, special circumstances such as transplantation and pregnancy, and the growing roles of telemedicine and social media in bariatric surgery. Each section addresses the evolution of specific treatments available to patients, the initial evaluation and selection of procedures, and future directions for therapy. Uniquely, this text emphasizes both the bariatric and metabolic bases of therapies and outcomes, providing a broader perspective on patient care.

We are thrilled to present the contributions of many founding members of our field alongside those of rising stars. This manual serves as an essential reference for surgeons, obesity medicine specialists, internists, residents, medical students, and allied health members who provide care for patients with obesity. We extend our gratitude to the contributing authors for their expertise and dedication and to Springer Science and SAGES for making this manual a reality. We hope this edition will inspire the next generation to build on the advancements already made and continue to push the boundaries of bariatric surgery.

The Editors.

| | |
|---|---|
| Rochester, MN, USA | Omar M. Ghanem |
| Phoenix, AZ, USA | Farah Husain |
| Seattle, WA, USA | Judy Y. Chen |
| Charlotte, NC, USA | Robert B. Lim |
| Cleveland, OH, USA | Matthew Kroh |

# Contents

# Contributors

**Mujjahid Abbas** Department of Surgery/Bariatric Division, University Hospitals Cleveland Medical Center, Case Western Reserve University School of Medicine, Cleveland, OH, USA

**Barham K. Abu Dayyeh** Mayo Clinic, Rochester, MN, USA

**Andres Acosta** Precision Medicine for Obesity Program, Division of Gastroenterology and Hepatology, Department of Medicine, Mayo Clinic, Rochester, MN, USA

**Pauline Aeschbacher** Department of General Surgery, Bariatric and Metabolic Institute, Cleveland Clinic Florida, Weston, FL, USA

**Eric Ahnfeldt** William Beaumont Army Medical Center, Colorado Springs, CO, USA

**Vance Albaugh** Metamor Institute, Pennington Biomedical Research Center, Louisiana State University, Baton Rouge, LA, USA

Department of Surgery, Louisiana State University Health Sciences Center, New Orleans, LA, USA

**Abdulaziz Karam Ali** Bariatric/MIS Fellow, Department of Surgery, McGill University, Montreal, QC, Canada

**Maria S. Altieri** Department of Surgery, University of Pennsylvania, Philadelphia, PA, USA

**Ali Aminian** Department of General Surgery, Bariatric and Metabolic Institute, Cleveland Clinic, Cleveland, OH, USA

**Diego Anazco** Precision Medicine for Obesity Program, Division of Gastroenterology and Hepatology, Department of Medicine, Mayo Clinic, Rochester, MN, USA

**Amin Andalib** Associate Professor of Surgery, Centre for Bariatric Surgery, Department of Surgery, McGill University, Montreal, QC, Canada

**Abdallah Attia** Division of Minimally Invasive Surgery, Tulane University, New Orleans, LA, USA

**Amanda Belluzzi** Department of Surgery, Mayo Clinic, Rochester, MN, USA

**Joel Brockmeyer** Department of Surgery, D.D. Eisenhower Army Medical Center, Ft. Eisenhower, GA, USA

**Matthew R. Byler** Department of Surgery, University of Virginia, Charlottesville, VA, USA

**Eli Monzon Canales** Division of Laparoendoscopic and Bariatric Surgery, DeWitt Daughtry Family Department of Surgery, University of Miami Miller School of Medicine, Miami, FL, USA

Center for Pediatric Population Health, School of Public Health, The University of Texas Health Science Center at Houston, Dallas, TX, USA

**Felipe Cantú** Department of Surgery, Christus Health System, Hospital Christus Muguerza Reynosa, Reynosa, Mexico

**Felipe J. Cantu Jr** Department of Surgery, Hospital Christus Muguerza, Reynosa, Mexico

Universidad Mexico Americana del Norte UMAN, Reynosa, Tamaulipas, Mexico

**Katherine Carsky** Department of General Surgery, Northwell Health, Lenox Hill Hospital, New York, NY, USA

**Elias Chousleb** Department of Surgery, Jackson North Hospital, Miami, FL, USA

**M. D. Benjamin Clapp** Department of Surgery, Texas Tech Paul Foster School of Medicine, El Paso, TX, USA

**Ricard Corcelles** Cleveland Clinic, Bariatric and Metabolic Institute, Cleveland, OH, USA

Department of Surgery, Cleveland Clinic Lerner College of Medicine, Cleveland, OH, USA

**Jorge Cornejo** Department of General Surgery, Mayo Clinic, Jacksonville, FL, USA

**Florina Corpodean** Metamor Institute, Pennington Biomedical Research Center, Louisiana State University, Baton Rouge, LA, USA

Department of Surgery, Louisiana State University Health Sciences Center, New Orleans, LA, USA

**Lamorna Coyle** Donald and Barbara Zucker School of Medicine at Hofstra/Northwell, Hempstead, NY, USA

**Lillian Craggs-Dino** Advanced Practice Level II Registered Dietitian, Digestive Disease and Surgery Institute, Cleveland Clinic Florida, Weston, FL, USA

**Luke S. Crawford** Division of Minimally Invasive and Elective General Surgery, Department of Surgery, McGovern Medical School at UT Health, Houston, TX, USA

**Nestor de la Cruz-Munoz** Division of Laparoendoscopic and Bariatric Surgery, DeWitt Daughtry Family Department of Surgery, University of Miami Miller School of Medicine, Miami, FL, USA

**Jerry T. Dang, MD, PhD** Digestive Disease Institute, Cleveland Clinic, Cleveland, OH, USA

**Vikrom Dhar** Department of General Surgery, Northwell Health, Lenox Hill Hospital, New York, NY, USA

**Luke K. Dombert** Johns Hopkins University, Baltimore, MD, USA

**W. Troy Donahoo** Division of Internal Medicine, Department of Medicine, University of Florida College of Medicine, Gainesville, FL, USA

Division of Endocrinology, Department of Medicine, University of Florida College of Medicine, Gainesville, FL, USA

**Shaina R. Eckhouse** Division of Minimally Invasive Surgery, Department of Surgery, Duke University School of Medicine, Durham, NC, USA

**Enrique F. Elli** Department of General Surgery, Mayo Clinic, Jacksonville, FL, USA

**Ali Esparham** School of Medicine, Mashhad University of Medical Sciences, Mashhad, Iran

**Maria A. Espinosa** Precision Medicine for Obesity Program, Division of Gastroenterology and Hepatology, Department of Medicine, Mayo Clinic, Rochester, MN, USA

**Lorna A. Evans** Department of General Surgery, Mayo Clinic, Jacksonville, FL, USA

**Sima Fansa** Precision Medicine for Obesity Program, Division of Gastroenterology and Hepatology, Department of Medicine, Mayo Clinic, Rochester, MN, USA

**Fauzi Feris Jassir, MD** Precision Medicine for Obesity Program, Division of Gastroenterology and Hepatology, Department of Medicine, Mayo Clinic, Rochester, MN, USA

Division of General Surgery, Florida Atlantic University, Boca Raton, USA

**George Ferzli** Department of Surgery, New York University Langone Health, New York, NY, USA

**Christine Ren Fielding** Division of Bariatric Surgery, Department of Surgery, NYU Langone Health, New York, NY, USA

**Laura E. Fischer** Department of Surgery, University of Oklahoma Health Science Center, Oklahoma City, OK, USA

**Charlene Franco** SAGES, Los Angeles, CA, USA

**Derek Freitas** Division of Bariatric Surgery, Department of Surgery, NYU Langone Health, New York, NY, USA

**Carlos Galvani** Division of General Surgery, LSU Health, Department of Surgery, New Orleans, LA, USA

**Rachel L. Goldman, MD** Department of Psychiatry, NYU Grossman School of Medicine, New York University, New York, NY, USA

**Alex Morera Grau** Hospital del Mar, Barcelona, Spain

**Victoria J. Grille** Penn State Health Milton S. Hershey Medical Center, Hershey, PA, USA

**Karl Hage** Department of Surgery, Mayo Clinic, Rochester, MN, USA

**Peter T. Hallowell** Department of Surgery, University of Virginia, Charlottesville, VA, USA

**Monique Hassan** Department of Surgery, Baylor College of Medicine, Scott and White Memorial Hospital and Clinic, Temple, TX, USA

**Juan D. Hernandez** Division of General Surgery, Hospital Universitario Fundacion Santa Fe de Bogota, Bogotá, Colombia

Department of Surgery and Anatomy, Universidad de los Andes School of Medicine, Bogotá, Cundinamarca, Colombia

**Charles E. Hill** Department of Surgery, Prisma Health Upstate, Greenville, SC, USA

**Ryan Hill** Department of Surgery, Morehouse School of Surgery, Atlanta, GA, USA

**L. Renee Hilton-Rowe** Center for Obesity and Metabolism, Medical College of Georgia, Augusta, GA, USA

**Juliet Holder-Haynes** Division of Metabolic and Bariatric Surgery, Baylor College of Medicine, Houston, TX, USA

**Mina A. Ibrahim** University Hospitals Parma Medical Center, Parma, OH, USA

Department of Surgery/Bariatric Division, University Hospitals Cleveland Medical Center, Case Western Reserve University School of Medicine, Cleveland, OH, USA

**Mazen Iskandar** Department of Surgery, Baylor Scott and White Medical Center, Waxahachie, TX, USA

**Karimatu Jalloh** Department of Surgery, University of Pennsylvania, Philadelphia, PA, USA

**Mohammad H. Jamal** Department of Surgery, Kuwait University, Kuwait City, Kuwait

**Megan Jenkins** NYU Langone Health, New York, NY, USA

**Crystal N. Johnson-Mann** Division of Gastrointestinal Surgery, Department of Surgery, University of Florida College of Medicine, Gainesville, FL, USA

**Shaneeta Johnson** Department of Surgery, Morehouse School of Medicine and Satcher Health Leadership Institute, Atlanta, GA, USA

**Daniel B. Jones** Department of Surgery, Rutgers New Jersey Medical School, Newark, NJ, USA

**Stephanie Joseph** Department of Surgery, Endeavor Health, Evanston, IL, USA

Detroit Medical Center/Wayne State University School of Medicine, Detroit, MI, USA

**Julia Jurgensen** Department of Metabolic Surgery, Mayo Clinic, Rochester, MN, USA

**Michael Kachmar** Metamor Institute, Pennington Biomedical Research Center, Louisiana State University, Baton Rouge, LA, USA

Department of Surgery, Louisiana State University Health Sciences Center, New Orleans, LA, USA

**Tanyaradzwa M. Kajese** Division of Minimally Invasive and Elective General Surgery, Department of Surgery, McGovern Medical School at UT Health, Houston, TX, USA

**Diana Kantarovich** Department of General Surgery, Northwell Health, Lenox Hill Hospital, New York, NY, USA

**Margaret G. Keane** Johns Hopkins Hospital, Baltimore, MD, USA

**Mai Al Khadem** Department of Surgery/Bariatric Division, University Hospitals Cleveland Medical Center, Case Western Reserve University School of Medicine, Cleveland, OH, USA

**Leena Khaitan** Department of Surgery, University Hospitals Cleveland Medical Center, Cleveland, OH, USA

University Hospitals Parma Medical Center, Parma, OH, USA

**Zhamak Khorgami** Department of Surgery, University of Oklahoma, School of Community Medicine, Tulsa, OK, USA

**Danbee H. Kim** Rutgers New Jersey Medical School, Newark, NJ, USA

**Tammy Kindel** Medical College of Wisconsin, Milwaukee, WI, USA

**Oliver Knoell** Fresno Heart and Surgical Hospital/Community Health Partners, Fresno, CA, USA

University of California-San Francisco-Fresno Medical Education Program, Fresno, CA, USA

**Shanu N. Kothari** Department of Surgery, Prisma Health Upstate, Greenville, SC, USA

**Marina Kurian** NYU Langone Health, New York, NY, USA

**Damien Lazar** Department of Surgery, Icahn School of Medicine at Mount Sinai, Mount Sinai Health System, New York, NY, USA

**Edmund W. Lee** Department of Surgery, Stony Brook University, Stony Brook, NY, USA

**Tiffany C. Lee** Department of Surgery, Oregon Health and Science University, Portland, OR, USA

**Yung Lee, MD, MPH** Department of Surgery, McMaster University, Hamilton, ON, Canada

**S. Julie-Ann Lloyd** Division of Metabolic and Bariatric Surgery, Michael E. DeBakey Department of Surgery, Baylor College of Medicine, Houston, TX, USA

**Ruby D. Lopez Flores** School of Medicine, University of Nevada, Reno, NV, USA

**Victoria Lyo** Department of Surgery, University of California, Davis, Sacramento, CA, USA

Center for Alimentary and Metabolic Sciences, University of California, Davis, Sacramento, CA, USA

**Robert M. MacGregor** Department of Surgery, Washington University School of Medicine, Saint Louis, MO, USA

**Pearl Ma** Fresno Heart and Surgical Hospital/Community Health Partners, Fresno, CA, USA

University of California-San Francisco-Fresno Medical Education Program, Fresno, CA, USA

**Emanuele Lo Menzo** Department of General Surgery, Bariatric and Metabolic Institute, Cleveland Clinic Florida, Weston, FL, USA

**Sarah Messiah** School of Public Health, The University of Texas Health Science Center at Houston (UTHealth), Dallas, TX, USA

**K. Paige Mihalsky** Department of Surgery, University of Oklahoma Health Science Center, Oklahoma City, OK, USA

**Eli Mlaver, MD, MSc** Department of Surgery, Emory University, Atlanta, GA, USA

**Daniel Praise Mowoh** Department of Surgery, University Hospitals Cleveland Medical Center, Cleveland, OH, USA

**Michelle Nessen** Division of Minimally Invasive Surgery, Tulane University, New Orleans, LA, USA

**Abdelrahman Nimeri** Brigham and Women's Hospital, Harvard Medical School, Boston, MA, USA

**Valeria Noguera** Division of Minimally Invasive Surgery, Tulane University, New Orleans, LA, USA

**Thomas O'Hara** Department of General Surgery, D.D. Eisenhower Army Medical Center, Ft. Eisenhower, GA, USA

**Yagnik Pandya** MetroWest Medical Center, Framingham, MA, USA

Boston University School of Medicine, Boston, MA, USA

**Mary Elizabeth Patti** Research Division, Joslin Diabetes Center, Boston, MA, USA

Harvard Medical School, Boston, MA, USA

**Lei Pei** Research Division, Joslin Diabetes Center, Boston, MA, USA

Harvard Medical School, Boston, MA, USA

**D. O. Carl Pesta** McLaren Macomb Bariatric Surgery Institute, Mount Clemens, MI, USA

**Ninoska D. Peterson** Department of Surgery, Bariatric and Metabolic Institute, Cleveland Clinic Lerner College of Medicine of Case Western Reserve University, Cleveland, OH, USA

**Rana C. Pullatt** Foregut and Metabolic Surgery, Department of Surgery, Medical University of South Carolina, Charleston, SC, USA

**Asmaa Al Rashed** Surgery Department, Amiri Hospital, MOH, Kuwait City, Kuwait

**Rachel Reed, MD** Department of Surgery, Emory University, Atlanta, GA, USA

**Jesse Richards** University of Oklahoma Health Sciences Center, Tulsa, OK, USA

**Ann M. Rogers** Penn State Health Milton S. Hershey Medical Center, Hershey, PA, USA

**Raul J. Rosenthal** Department of General Surgery, Bariatric and Metabolic Institute, Cleveland Clinic Florida, Weston, FL, USA

**Mitchell Roslin** Department of General Surgery, Northwell Health, Lenox Hill Hospital, New York, NY, USA

**Jean-Christophe N. Rwigema** Department of Surgery, Endeavor Health, Evanston, IL, USA

University of Florida College of Medicine, Gainesville, FL, USA

**Alex Sanchez** Department of Bariatric Surgery, Orlando Regional Medical Center, Orlando, FL, USA

**Imam N. Sanousi** University of Southern California, Keck School of Medicine, Los Angeles, CA, USA

**Philip Schauer** Metamor Institute, Pennington Biomedical Research Center, Louisiana State University, Baton Rouge, LA, USA

Department of Surgery, Louisiana State University Health Sciences Center, New Orleans, LA, USA

**Ingrid Schmiederer** Cleveland Clinic, Bariatric and Metabolic Institute, Cleveland, OH, USA

**Michael A. Schweitzer** Johns Hopkins University, Baltimore, MD, USA

**S. Scott Davis Jr, MD** Department of Surgery, Emory University, Atlanta, GA, USA

**Meera Shah** Division of Endocrinology, Diabetes and Nutrition, Mayo Clinic College of Medicine, Rochester, MN, USA

**Shinil K. Shah** Division of Minimally Invasive and Elective General Surgery, Department of Surgery, McGovern Medical School at UT Health, Houston, TX, USA

Michael E. DeBakey Institute for Comparative Cardiovascular Science and Biomedical Devices, Texas A&M University, College Station, TX, USA

**Ishna Sharma** Department of Metabolic Surgery, Mayo Clinic, Rochester, MN, USA

**Amy J. Sheer** Division of Internal Medicine, Department of Medicine, University of Florida College of Medicine, Gainesville, FL, USA

**Scott A. Shikora** Department of Surgery, Center for Metabolic and Bariatric Surgery, Brigham and Women's Hospital and Harvard Medical School, Boston, MA, USA

**Ariel Shuchleib** Department of Surgery, Saint Agnes Medical Center, Fresno, CA, USA

**Savannah Smith, MD** Department of Surgery, Emory University, Atlanta, GA, USA

**Konstantinos Spaniolas** Department of Surgery, Stony Brook University, Stony Brook, NY, USA

**Andrea Stroud** Division of Bariatric Surgery, Department of Surgery, Oregon Health and Science University, Portland, OR, USA

**Sarah Suh** Medical College of Wisconsin, Milwaukee, WI, USA

**Samuel Szomstein** Department of General Surgery, Bariatric and Metabolic Institute, Cleveland Clinic Florida, Weston, FL, USA

**Loic Tchokouani** NYU Langone Health, New York, NY, USA

**Andre Teixeira** Department of Bariatric Surgery, Orlando Regional Medical Center, Orlando, FL, USA

**Michael B. Ujiki** Department of Surgery, Endeavor Health, Evanston, IL, USA

**Annie Wang** Department of Surgery, University of California Irvine, Orange, USA

**Erik B. Wilson** Division of Minimally Invasive and Elective General Surgery, Department of Surgery, McGovern Medical School at UT Health, Houston, TX, USA

**Rickesha L. Wilson** Department of General Surgery, Bariatric and Metabolic Institute, Cleveland Clinic, Cleveland, OH, USA

**John Yonge** Department of Surgery, Oregon Health and Science University, Portland, OR, USA

**Linda P. Zhang** Icahn School of Medicine at Mount Sinai, New York, NY, USA

**Theofano Zoumpou** Department of Surgery, Rutgers New Jersey Medical School, Newark, NJ, USA

**Natan Zundel** Department of Surgery, University of Buffalo, NY Jackson North Hospital, Buffalo, NY, USA

JNMC, Miami, FL, USA

# Part I

# Essentials

# What Is the Mastery Program?

# 1

Theofano Zoumpou and Daniel B. Jones

## Introduction

The Society of American Gastrointestinal and Endoscopic Surgeons (SAGES) Masters Program takes a strategic approach to organizing educational resources, shaping them into distinct knowledge blocks [1]. These resources are readily available to surgeons attending the annual SAGES meeting or accessible through the online SAGES University platform (Fig. 1.1).

Currently, the SAGES Masters Program encompasses 13 pathways, including acute care, biliary, bariatrics, colon, foregut, hernia, flexible endoscopy, and robotic surgery. (Fig. 1.2). Each pathway is thoughtfully divided into three progressive levels of targeted performance: competency, proficiency, and mastery (Fig. 1.3). These performance tiers draw inspiration from the Dreyfus model of skill acquisition, which delineates five developmental stages: novice, advanced beginner,

**Fig. 1.1** SAGES Masters Program logo

T. Zoumpou (✉) · D. B. Jones
Department of Surgery, Rutgers New Jersey Medical School, Newark, NJ, USA
e-mail: theo.zoumpou@rutgers.edu; daniel.jones@njms.rutgers.edu



O. M. Ghanem et al. (eds.), *The SAGES Manual of Metabolic and Bariatric Surgery*, https://doi.org/10.1007/978-3-031-72309-4_1

**Fig. 1.2** SAGES Masters Program clinical pathways

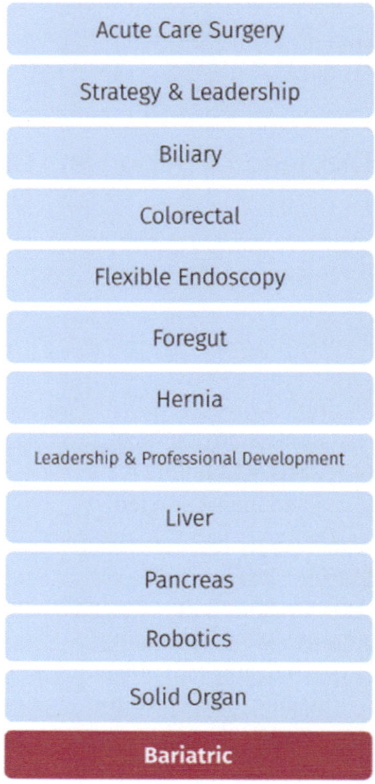


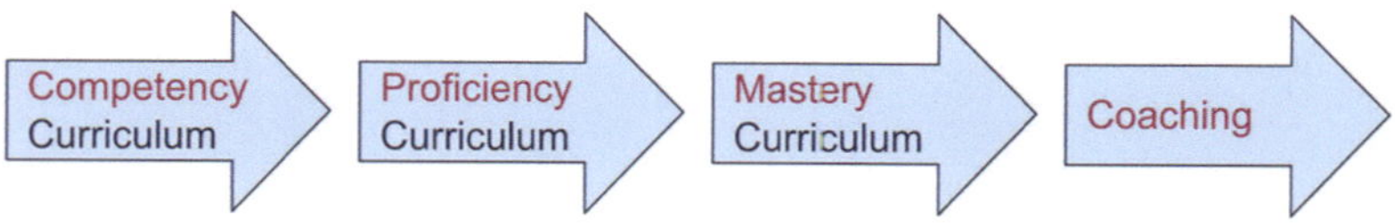


**Fig. 1.3** SAGES Masters Program Progression

competency, proficiency, and expertise [2]. The SAGES Masters Program, however, is rooted in the three more advanced stages of skill acquisition: competency, proficiency, and mastery.

To elaborate, competency signifies the skill level expected of a graduating general surgery chief resident or a minimally invasive surgery fellow. Proficiency, on the other hand, characterizes the capabilities of a surgeon approximately 3 years post-training. Lastly, mastery represents the pinnacle of expertise attainable by seasoned surgeons with several years of practice. For those engaged in the SAGES Masters Program, mastery offers an opportunity to delve deep into their chosen pathway, exploring areas of contention, examining outcomes, embracing best practices, and nurturing the ability to mentor peers. Over time, as members actively engage in coaching and participate in SAGES courses, the aim is for the majority to reach the level of mastery. This iteration of The SAGES Manual of Bariatric Surgery aligns seamlessly with the latest iteration of the SAGES University Masters Program's bariatric surgery pathway.

## Why Engage in the SAGES Masters Program?

The SAGES Masters Program represents a dynamic and transformative approach to postgraduate education, offering enhanced value and a more enjoyable learning experience. In the realm of surgery, after the rigors of residency and fellowship, continuing one's education or transitioning expertise from one focus area to another can be a significant challenge. This underscores the need for innovative avenues for ongoing training.

Traditionally, surgeons have turned to postgraduate courses, industry-sponsored programs, and online resources, such as instructional videos and peer collaboration, to expand their knowledge base. In other words, there is no standardized way to gain or adopt new knowledge once a surgeon is in practice. The SAGES Masters Program, however, introduces a structured curriculum that guides learners from foundational concepts to advanced complexities, seamlessly integrating SAGES' wealth of educational resources. Our goal is for this program to be an accessible, cost-effective, engaging, and valuable means of tracking one's professional growth over time. Ultimately, we aspire to see the SAGES Masters Program evolve into the go-to standard. Each pathway within the curriculum is thoughtfully designed, catering to the principles of adult learning.

Completing the program will enhance surgeons' skills and contribute to optimizing their online professional profiles, reflecting their dedication to continuous improvement and excellence.

## Bariatric Surgery Curriculum

The core of the bariatric surgery curriculum encompasses pivotal elements, including pathway-specific core lectures. Sections will address the evolution of specific treatments available to patients, initial evaluation, preoperative optimization, and selection of procedures for individual patients. Readers will have the opportunity to explore the latest surgical and endoscopic techniques, as well as the medical approaches employed to treat patients, through a comprehensive review of indications, techniques, outcomes, and future directions for therapy. In addition, the manual provides a detailed overview of the discrete roles of different professionals, including physicians, nurses, dieticians, and social workers, in high-quality bariatric surgical care.

Starting in 2018, annual SAGES meeting lectures are categorized into three levels: basic (100), intermediate (200), and advanced (300), allowing attendees to tailor their learning experiences to their specific needs. This classification system also

**Fig. 1.4** The FLS, FUSE, and FES logos

streamlines online access to targeted educational content, ranging from introductory material to advanced topics, including revisional surgery.

Recognizing the need for specialized content at the mastery level, the curriculum introduced 25-minute lectures dedicated to specific subjects. These lectures assume a strong foundation in disease understanding and management, acquired through attendance or viewing of competency- and proficiency-level lectures. Ideally, these mastery-level lectures will also highlight key prerequisite articles from Surgical Endoscopy and other journals, along with relevant SAGES University videos.

To guide learners through the curriculum, the Masters Program offers self-assessment multiple-choice exams for each module. Questions are curated by core lecture speakers and faculty from the SAGES annual meeting. These questions serve as tools for learning assessment, with the criterion set at 80% correct answers. Learners can review incorrect responses, revisit educational content, and retake the exam until they achieve a passing score. The goal is to make sure surgeons have the knowledge as information and treatment patterns change.

The bariatric surgery curriculum of the Masters Program also taps into a wealth of existing SAGES educational resources, including FLS™, FES™, FUSE™, SMART™, top 21 videos, and pearls (Fig. 1.4). These modules are strategically integrated along the curriculum pathway continuum. For example, FLS™ typically falls within the competency curriculum, while the Fundamental Use of Surgical Energy (FUSE™) is a proficiency curriculum requirement. The Fundamentals of Laparoscopic Surgery (FLS™) involves a multiple-choice exam and a skills assessment on a video box trainer, covering tasks such as peg transfer, cutting, intracorporeal and extracorporeal suturing, and knot tying. Since 2010, FLS™ has been a prerequisite for all US general surgery residents seeking eligibility for the American Board of Surgery Qualifying Examinations. The Fundamentals of Endoscopic Surgery (FES™) assesses endoscopic knowledge and technical skills in a simulator, followed by a certifying examination upon module completion. FUSE™, on the other hand, focuses on the safe use of energy devices in the operating room and offers modules and a certifying examination.

The SAGES Surgical Multimodal Accelerated Recovery Trajectory (SMART™) Initiative marries minimally invasive surgical techniques with enhanced recovery pathways (ERPs) for perioperative care to elevate outcomes and patient satisfaction. Resources encompass a website featuring best practices, sample pathways, patient literature, and an implementation timeline. These materials aid surgeons and their surgical teams in the seamless implementation of ERPs. The top 21 videos are meticulously edited recordings showcasing the most frequently performed minimally invasive surgery (MIS) operations and fundamental endoscopy procedures. These cases feature straightforward presentations with high-quality video and clear anatomical visuals. Lastly, pearls offer step-by-step video clips of different operations, with authors presenting various variations for each step. Learners are expected to have a foundational understanding of the procedures covered.

## SAGES Guidelines

The SAGES clinical, practice, and training guidelines, statements, and standards of practice serve as valuable resources for the SAGES Bariatric Masters Program, exemplifying SAGES' pioneering role in promoting excellence in bariatric surgery. Through extensive research, the formulation of guidelines, and the establishment of training standards, SAGES continues to lead the way in defining best practices for surgical procedures. These guidelines are crafted with the full support of the organization and its diverse committees, with the added stamp of approval from the Board of Governors. Each clinical practice guideline is the product of a systematic research, review, and revision process, thoughtfully overseen by the Guidelines Committee and assessed by a suitably diverse team of experts. Regular reviews of these guidelines are scheduled to ensure that the latest relevant developments in medical research, knowledge, and practice are seamlessly incorporated.

## Exploring Facebook™ Groups for Enhanced Surgical Education

Online collaboration through user-generated content offers various platforms, with Facebook™ standing out due to its advanced mobile platform, making it an ideal choice for global professional partnership and daily surgical education. One notable example of this is the SAGES Masters Program Bariatric Facebook™ Group (Fig. 1.5).

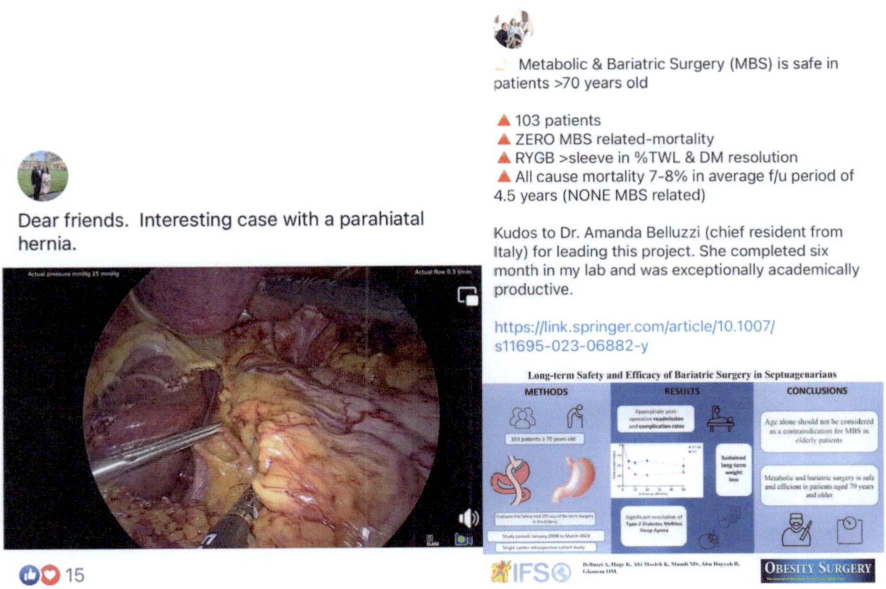


**Fig. 1.5** The SAGES Bariatrics Facebook community

Within the Masters Program, participants will share content, including video clips, imaging, and patient cases, in the closed Facebook™ groups, where fellow participants and SAGES members will provide qualitative feedback. For instance, in the context of the bariatric surgery curriculum, surgeons can submit critical views during a laparoscopic gastric bypass, demonstrating a leak test with methylene blue saline infusion or endoscopic air insufflation. Using the power of crowdsourcing, other surgeons will contribute comments and feedback. It is a secure and safe way to solicit the opinions of other bariatric surgery experts.

These groups serve as a global platform for surgeons and healthcare professionals keen on enhancing outcomes in their respective surgical specialties. Collaboratively, members can share insights, engage in discussions, and post multimedia content related to their chosen fields. By embracing social media in this way, we harness the power of real-time global feedback, potentially leading to improved patient outcomes and a higher standard of care, all while redefining how members of our society interact.

For the initial two levels of the Masters Program, competency, and proficiency, participants will be required to share videos of the anchoring procedures and receive qualitative feedback from their peers. In contrast, for the mastery level, participants will submit a video for evaluation by an expert panel. A standardized video assessment tool will be utilized depending on the specific procedure. A predefined benchmark will also guide the determination of mastery achievement for each procedure.

Upon reaching the mastery level, participants will transition into coaching roles, offering feedback to those in the first two levels. To do this effectively, Masters Program participants must acquire fundamental surgical coaching skills. These skills encompass goal setting, active listening, powerful inquiry, and constructive feedback. Importantly, peer coaching stands apart from traditional education, where there is an expert and a learner; instead, it embraces a "co-learning" model where the coach facilitates the coachee's development through open-ended questions in a non-competitive manner. Mastery of surgical coaching skills is an integral component of the Master's curriculum, fostering a "coaching culture" within the SAGES Masters Program [3].

Recognizing the demand for a structured approach to the education of practicing surgeons, as exemplified by the SAGES Masters Program, is well-founded [4]. Conventional performance feedback tends to wane after formal training, and current methods of Maintenance of Certification (MOC) are deemed suboptimal. Consequently, peer coaching in surgery has gained prominence. SAGES has acknowledged this need and wholeheartedly embraced social media as a vehicle for surgical education. This move aims to provide surgeons worldwide with a free, mobile, and user-friendly platform. Access to the Masters Program groups enables surgeons at all stages of their careers to engage with the Masters Program Curriculum and receive feedback from peers, mentors, and experts. The creation of exclusive surgeon-only private groups specifically for this initiative allows SAGES members posting in these groups to discuss preoperative, intraoperative, and postoperative concerns with their fellow SAGES colleagues and mentors. Additionally, this platform fosters transparent and responsive dialogue on surgical techniques, furthering the pursuit of deliberate, lifelong learning.

## Conclusions

The SAGES Masters Program's bariatric surgery pathway is an exceptional tool for focused and deliberate postgraduate teaching and learning. It is important to note that completion of the curriculum is a requirement for program certification, but it does not guarantee certification of competency, proficiency, or mastery of surgeons. The Masters Program firmly believes in the concept of lifelong learning beyond fellowship and organizes its curriculum from basic principles to more complex content. This innovative and voluntary curriculum promotes confident and deliberate lifelong learning and supports the MOC program. With its comprehensive curriculum, expert insights, and unwavering commitment to the highest standards of practice, this program is not only designed to enhance knowledge and skills but also to instill confidence and competence. We are confident that the knowledge gained here will prove instrumental in your preparation for the American Board of Surgery Metabolic and Bariatric Surgery Focused Practice Designation Exam [5]. May this book serve as your steadfast companion in achieving your aspirations and advancing your expertise in this field of surgery. Best of luck on your educational journey and as you pursue excellence in bariatric surgery.

## References

1. Jones DB, et al. SAGES University MASTERS Program: a structured curriculum for deliberate, lifelong learning. Surg Endosc. 2017;31:4863.
2. Dreyfus SE. The five-stage model of adult skill acquisition. Bull Sci Technol Soc. 2004;24:177–81.
3. Greenberg CC, Ghousseini HN, Pavuluri Quamme SR, Beasley HL, Wiegmann DA. Surgical coaching for individual performance improvement. Ann Surg. 2015;261:32–4.
4. Sachdeva AK. Acquiring skills in new procedures and technology: the challenge and the opportunity. Arch Surg. 2005;140:387–9.
5. https://www.absurgery.org/default.jsp?certfpd_mbs.

# 2 Foundations of Bariatric Surgery

Florina Corpodean, Michael Kachmar, Vance Albaugh, and Philip Schauer

Though the World Health Organization first recognized obesity as a disease in 1948, the vast majority of physicians, payors, politicians, and the public at that time believed that obesity was not a disease but simply a consequence of self-induced poor eating and activity habits. The roots of bariatric surgery and its subsequent remarkable evolution began in the 1950s (Fig. 2.1) when most physicians and surgeons did not consider obesity a treatable condition. Only decades later, did scientific opinion shift toward the adoption of obesity as a disease that is medically or surgically treatable. The early surgical pioneers often met stiff opposition from peers as they forged their way forward to develop safe and effective surgical treatments for obesity.

In 1953 at the University of Minnesota, Richard Varco performed the first known procedure with the intent to cause weight loss in a patient [1]. The operation was a jejunoileal bypass (JIB) with an end-end jejunoileostomy with separate drainage of the bypassed bowel by an ileocecostomy [2, 3]. In 1954, Kremen, also at the University of Minnesota, published the first report of this jejunoileal bypass [4]. Many variations of the JIB were developed over the ensuing decades [5–7]. The end-to-side JIB reported by Payne and DeWind in 1969 included 14 inches of jejunum connected end-side to the ileum 4 inches from the cecum (Fig. 2.2). It along

F. Corpodean · M. Kachmar · V. Albaugh · P. Schauer (✉)
Metamor Institute, Pennington Biomedical Research Center, Louisiana State University, Baton Rouge, LA, USA

Department of Surgery, Louisiana State University Health Sciences Center, New Orleans, LA, USA
e-mail: philip.schauer@pbrc.edu


O. M. Ghanem et al. (eds.), *The SAGES Manual of Metabolic and Bariatric Surgery*, https://doi.org/10.1007/978-3-031-72309-4_2

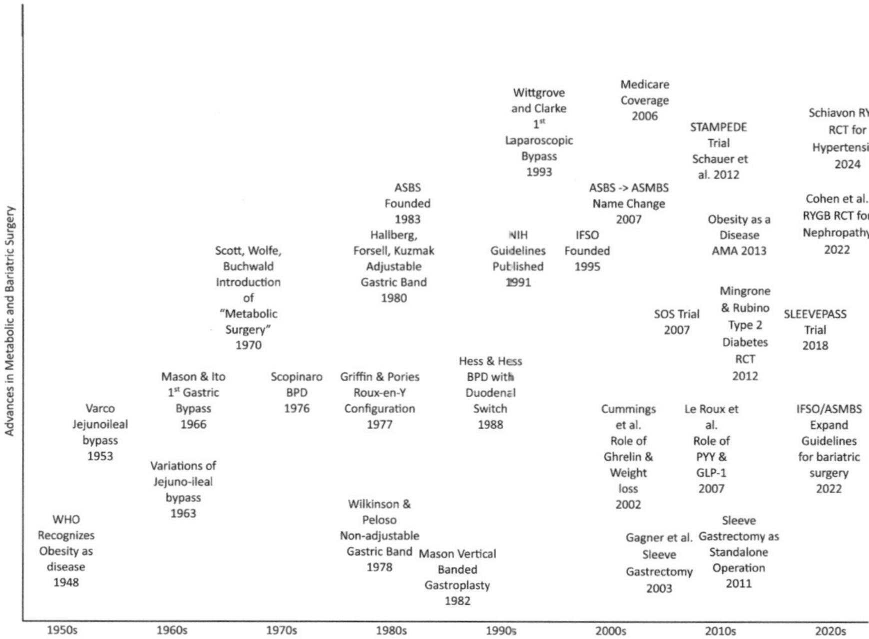


**Fig. 2.1** Noteworthy advancements in the field of metabolic surgery by decade: 1950's–2020's

with the end-to-end jejunoileostomy (40 cm and 4 cm) with ileocecostomy popularized by Buchwald and Varco became two of the more commonly used JIB constructions. While the JIB procedures produced very good weight loss and improvement in dyslipidemia, they were associated with major early and late complications including electrolyte disturbances, vitamin and macronutrient deficiencies, protein malnutrition, diarrhea, kidney stones, and liver failure related to short bowel syndrome and bacterial overgrowth.

A landmark moment occurred on May 10, 1966, when Mason and Ito performed the inaugural gastric bypass operation on a 50-year-old woman grappling with obesity and complications from an incisional hernia [8]. This transformative surgery involved creating an anastomosis between a portion of the gastric fundus and the jejunum, ushering in a new era in weight loss interventions. Notably, advancements by Griffen and Pories et al. in 1977 introduced the Roux-en-Y configuration, aimed at minimizing complications such as bile reflux [9]. Later, surgeons adopted an isolated gastric pouch formed by stapling and dividing the stomach. This approach was further modified by Wittgrove as a totally laparoscopic approach in the early 1990s [9–11] (Fig. 2.3).

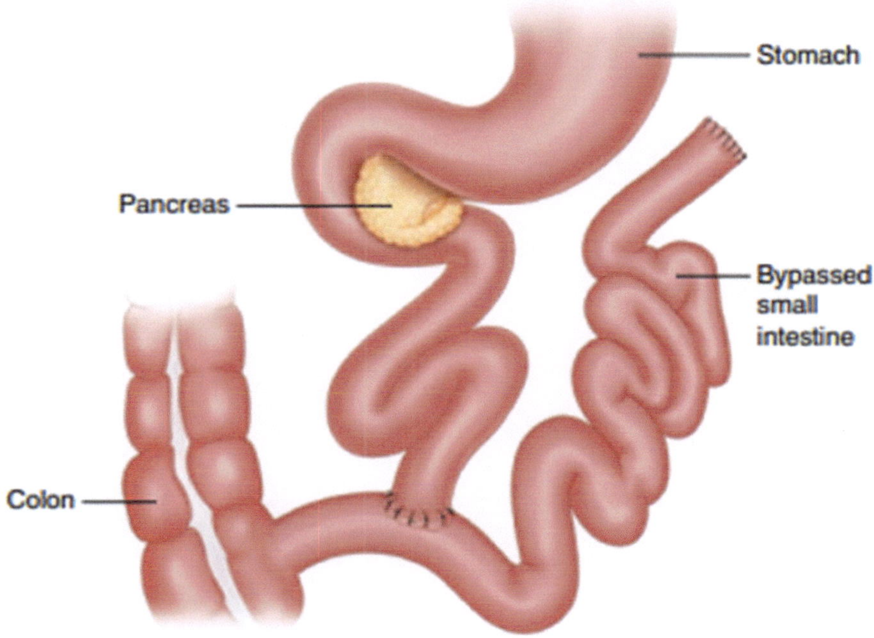


**Fig. 2.2** Jejunoileal Bypass [SAGES Manual of Bariatric Surgery, Fig. 6.1, page 63]

The evolution of bariatric procedures continued with the emergence of alternative procedures like the biliopancreatic diversion, pioneered by Nicola Scopinaro. The intent was to develop an intestinal bypass procedure with less complications than the JIB. Commencing in 1976, Scopinaro and his team conducted numerous biliopancreatic diversions (BPD), characterized by variations like the "ad hoc stomach" or AHS type BPD [12]. This operation featured a gastric pouch of 200–500 mL, along with specific lengths of alimentary limb (200–250 cm) and common channel (50 cm) (Fig. 2.4). Patients undergoing these procedures achieved substantial weight loss, with remarkable results maintained even up to 18 years postoperatively. Though vitamin deficiencies and protein malnutrition were less frequent than seen with JIB, they remained a concerning complication of this procedure. Marginal ulcers were also a common complication. Thus, widespread adoption of the BPD has not occurred.

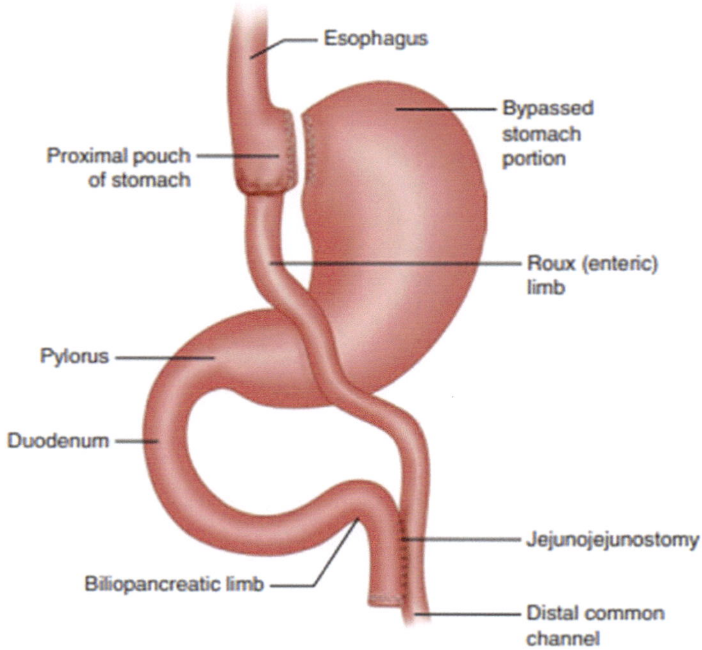


**Fig. 2.3** Roux-en-Y Gastric Bypass [SAGES Manual of Bariatric Surgery, Fig. 6.2, page 65]

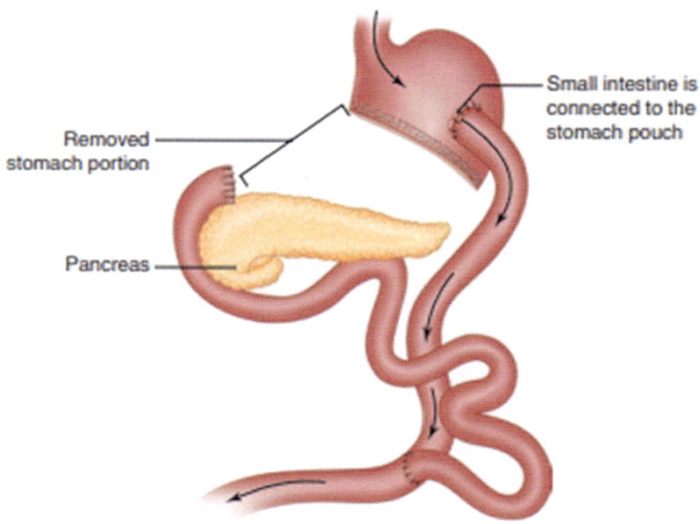


**Fig. 2.4** Biliopancreatic Diversion [SAGES Manual of Bariatric Surgery, Fig. 6.3, page 67]

## Early Advancements in Bariatric Surgery

To enhance the short and long-term safety profile of early bariatric procedures, significant attention in the 1970s and 1980s was directed toward the development of purely "restrictive" techniques that involved either banding or stapling the stomach to reduce food intake. Pioneers like Wilkinson and Peloso introduced the first non-adjustable gastric band in 1978, a concept further elaborated by Holle, Molina, and Oria [13]. This innovation eventually evolved into the adjustable gastric band during the 1980s, spearheaded by Hallberg, Forsell, and Kuzmak, gaining widespread adoption as one of the first laparoscopic bariatric procedures the following decade (Fig. 2.5) [13]. While the adjustable gastric band enjoyed enormous appeal in the late 1990s and early 2000s by the 2010s it lost favor due to poor long-term weight loss, high complication rates, and high revision rates. Bands now represent less than 1% of bariatric operations world-wide.

Concurrently, Printen and Mason pioneered the horizontal gastroplasty, employing a staple line along the lesser curve to create a small gastric pouch linked to the rest of the stomach via a narrow channel [14]. This technique paved the way for the vertical banded gastroplasty, conceptualized by Mason in 1982. Characterized by a 50 mL pouch formed through banding and stapling, this procedure was believed to offer fewer complications by avoiding alterations to intestinal digestion and absorption (Fig. 2.6) [15]. However, its utilization declined due to challenges with revisional operations, weight regain, and erosion of the band along with long-term complications like gastric stenosis and severe gastroesophageal reflux [16]. Variations of gastroplasty, such as the use of a silastic ring introduced by Laws and Piantadosi in 1986, added further complexity [17].

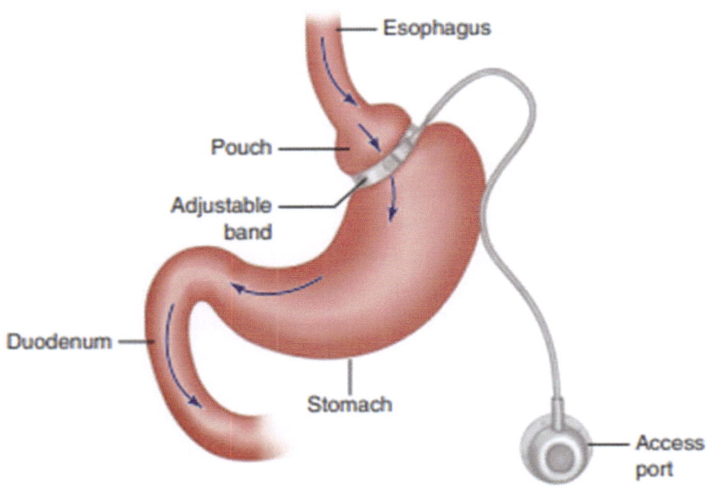


**Fig. 2.5** Adjustable Gastric Band [SAGES Manual of Bariatric Surgery, Fig. 6.7, page 72]

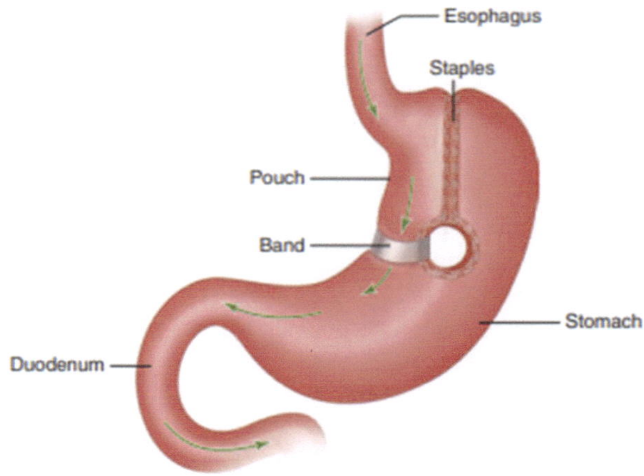


**Fig. 2.6** Vertical Banded Gastroplasty [SAGES Manual of Bariatric Surgery, Fig. 6.6, page 70]

By the early 1990s, substantial advancements had been made in bariatric surgery. The Roux-en-Y gastric bypass (RYGB) emerged as the most commonly performed procedure, with years of refinement resulting in a mortality rate of less than 1% and a morbidity rate of 6%, markedly improving its safety profile [18]. Despite the success of the gastric bypass, research endeavors persisted in optimizing Scopinaro's BPD. The combination of Scopinaro's technique with a sleeve gastrectomy and a duodenal-ileal rather than gastro-ileal anastomosis was pioneered by DeMeester, Hess, and Hess, and the first biliopancreatic diversion with duodenal switch (DS) was performed in May 1988 [19]. The rationale behind this modification was to potentially reduce the incidence of marginal ulceration, based on findings from animal models and patient cases [19], because a duodeno-ileal anastomosis was shown to be less ulcerogenic than a gastro-ileal anastomosis (Fig. 2.7) [20].

## The Laparoscopic Era

Advancements in laparoscopic techniques in the early 1990s revolutionized the landscape of bariatric surgery, expanding the range of procedures available to experienced surgeons (Fig. 2.1). Wittgrove and Clark pioneered the application of minimally invasive surgery to bariatric procedures, publishing their preliminary report in 1993 detailing five laparoscopically performed RYGB operations [21]. While the initial procedure duration varied from 3 to 7.5 h, it significantly decreased with growing expertise. Patients experienced favorable postoperative outcomes, with discharge occurring as early as postoperative day two as opposed to a typical 4–5 day stay for open bariatric operations. By 3 months postoperatively, patients achieved weight loss ranging from 42% to 76% of excess weight [21]. Concurrently, Broadbent and Catona reported successful outcomes of some of the earliest laparoscopically placed gastric bands around the same time [22, 23].

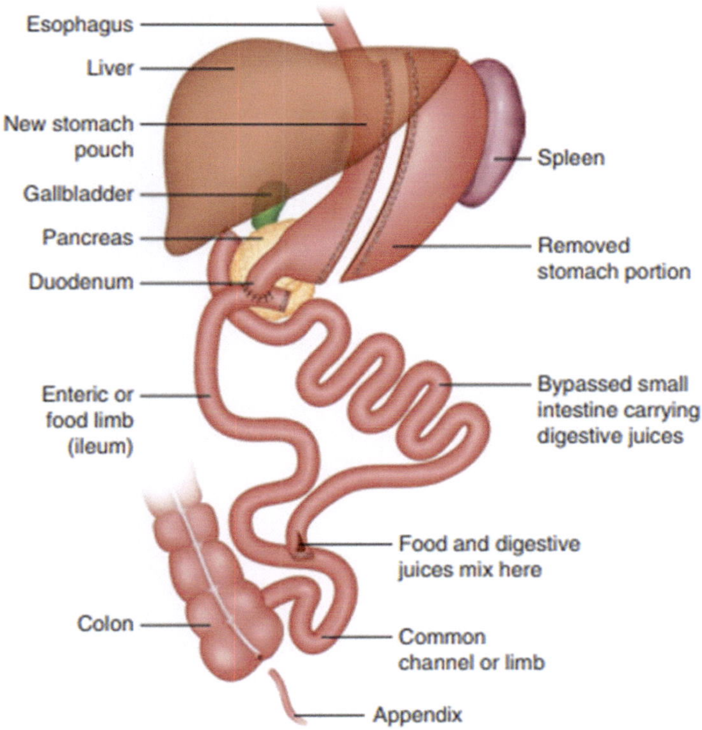


**Fig. 2.7** Duodenal Switch [SAGES Manual of Bariatric Surgery, Fig. 6.4, page 68]

Minimally invasive surgery revolutionized bariatric care, offering complex operations with unprecedented safety levels. Previously, perioperative morbidity and mortality rates following bariatric surgery hovered around 12% and 1% respectively. With the advent of minimally invasive techniques, these rates gradually plummeted to less than 2% and 0.2% respectively [24]. Patients also experienced fewer pulmonary complications, shorter hospital stays, and reduced intraoperative blood loss along with lower rates of incisional hernias and wound complications, translating to substantial cost savings for both patients and healthcare systems [25]. Wittgrove et al., then later Schauer et al., and De Maria et al. demonstrated excellent resolution of weight loss and comorbidities with laparoscopic RYGB, highlighting significant reductions in operative time and complications such as anastomotic leaks [26]. Laparoscopic gastric bypass proved particularly beneficial for patients with severe obesity, a population vulnerable to wound-related and cardiopulmonary complications [27].

As laparoscopic bariatric procedures became increasingly common, numerous studies scrutinizing postoperative outcomes emerged. Podnos et al. observed a shift in complication profiles between laparoscopic and open RYGB, noting fewer wound

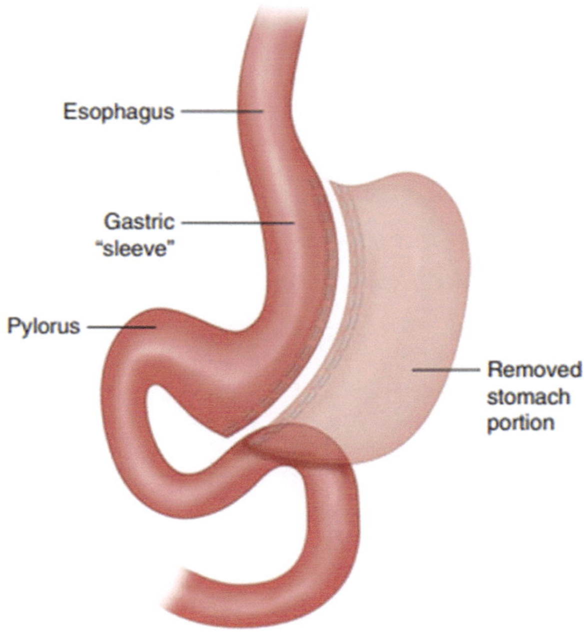


**Fig. 2.8** Sleeve Gastrectomy [SAGES Manual of Bariatric Surgery, Fig. 6.8, page 73]

infections and incisional hernias but an increased incidence of gastrointestinal bleed, stomal stenosis, and bowel obstruction from internal hernia associated with laparoscopic approaches [28]. Similarly, Higa et al. reported higher rates of stomal stenosis at the gastrojejunal anastomosis in laparoscopic gastric bypass patients, mostly amenable to endoscopic dilation therapy [29]. As advanced laparoscopic techniques improved, these related complications reduced in parallel.

Despite the dominance of the RYGB by the mid-1990s and early 2000s, a subset of patients, particularly those with BMI (body mass index) >60, exhibited inadequate weight loss. Ren and Gagner addressed this challenge with laparoscopic BPD-DS, yielding significant weight loss and resolving comorbidities [30]. After Gagner's pioneering work, sleeve gastrectomy emerged as a staged procedure for high-risk patients, eventually garnering recognition as a standalone option for various patient populations, as outlined in the 2011 International consensus guidelines (Fig. 2.8) [31, 32]. The SLEEVEPASS trial in 2018 compared laparoscopic sleeve gastrectomy and laparoscopic RYGB, revealing both procedures to be effective at 5-year weight loss with some advantages of the RYGB [33].

## Shift Toward Metabolic Surgery

While it seems that the shift from pure bariatric procedures to metabolic surgery has gain popularity in the last 15 years, the concept of "metabolic surgery" is not a recent development. As early as 1925, surgeons reported that gastric operations for peptic ulcer surgery or gastric cancer such as gastrojejunostomy, were associated with diabetes resolution and restoration of normal fasting blood sugar [34]. Despite repeated observations of diabetes resolution with other gastric operations over the intervening decades, little attention was paid to gastric operations as potential therapy for metabolic disease. Then, in the late 1960s and early 1970s, surgical investigators such as Buchwald, Varco, Scott, Wolfe and others introduced the concept of "metabolic intestinal surgery," referencing small bowel intestinal bypass procedures and their effects on hyperlipidemia and atherosclerosis [35]. H. William Scott from Vanderbilt was the first to use the term "Metabolic Surgery" in the medical literature [36] while Buchwald and Varco co-edited the first textbook of Metabolic Surgery in 1978 [1]. Two decades later with a focus on glucose metabolism, Pories, in a large landmark study demonstrated that Roux-en-Y gastric bypass (RYGB) achieved resolution of type 2 diabetes in 83% (121 of 146 patients) for a mean follow up of 7.6 years [38]. His study revealed that patients with non-insulin-dependent type 2 diabetes achieved normalization of fasting glucose and insulin and hypertension reduced from 58% to 14% in the study population [38]. His study was the first to show sustained remission of diabetes (> 5 years) in a large sample of patients following an intestinal operation. Many other investigators corroborated these findings that bariatric operations could induce long-term complete diabetes remission [39, 40]. Schauer et al. further validated these findings with the STAMPEDE trial, a randomized controlled study illustrating the superiority of gastric bypass and sleeve gastrectomy over best available medical management for poorly controlled type II diabetes [41]. This trial was one of many original influential studies for the advancement of metabolic surgery [42, 43] (Table 2.1).

**Table 2.1** Most influential original works contributing to the advancement of metabolic surgery

| | Author | Title | Journal | Year | Times Cited |
|---|---|---|---|---|---|
| 1 | Sjöström | Effects of bariatric surgery on mortality in Swedish obese subjects | NEJM | 2007 | 3650 |
| 2 | Sjöström | Lifestyle, diabetes, and cardiovascular risk factors 10 years after bariatric surgery | NEJM | 2004 | 3344 |
| 3 | Adams | Long-term mortality after gastric bypass surgery | NEJM | 2007 | 2039 |
| 4 | Cummings | Plasma ghrelin levels after diet-induced weight loss or gastric bypass surgery | NEJM | 2002 | 2022 |
| 5 | Pories | Who would have thought it? An operation proves to be the most effective therapy for adult-onset diabetes mellitus | Ann Surg | 1995 | 1926 |
| 6 | Schauer | Bariatric surgery versus intensive medical therapy in obese patients with diabetes | NEJM | 2012 | 1702 |
| 7 | Schauer | Bariatric surgery versus intensive medical therapy for diabetes—5-year outcomes | NEJM | 2017 | 1585 |
| 8 | Zhang | Human gut microbiota in obesity and after gastric bypass | Proc Natl Acad Sci USA | 2009 | 1428 |
| 9 | Mingrone | Bariatric surgery versus conventional medical therapy for type 2 diabetes | NEJM | 2012 | 1387 |
| 10 | Schauer | Bariatric surgery versus intensive medical therapy for diabetes—3-year outcomes | NEJM | 2014 | 1201 |

Long-term follow-up studies, spanning 7 to 12 years, consistently demonstrated that individuals undergoing bariatric surgery exhibited superior glycemic control, reduced reliance on diabetes medications, and higher rates of diabetes remission compared to those treated with medical interventions [44]. Mingrone and Sjöström reported comparable results, with improvements in both microvascular and macrovascular complications observed postoperatively [45, 46]. Notably, patients with shorter durations of type II diabetes experienced the highest rates of resolution, underscoring the importance of early surgical intervention [39].

Regarding the choice of procedure, both RYGB and sleeve gastrectomy have demonstrated sustained improvements in glucose homeostasis postoperatively [47]. These findings underscore the efficacy of bariatric surgery as a metabolic intervention, emphasizing its potential to profoundly impact the management of type II diabetes and induce long-term remission. Furthermore these metabolic benefits appear to result in improved life expectancy. In the 2002 POSCH trial, Buchwald et al. were the first to show in a randomized trial that a metabolic operation could reduce mortality compared to controls [37].

## Role of Professional Societies and Accreditation

The American Society of Bariatric Surgery (ASBS) was founded in 1983 and marked a turning point in medical specialization. Dr. Edward Mason, most known for his development of the gastric bypass and vertical banded gastroplasty, initiated an annual course on obesity and its surgical management in the late 1970s. Inspired by the formation of a Japanese obesity society, Dr. Mason transformed his annual course into the inaugural ASBS meeting (1985) first held in Iowa City, IA. The ASBS would later go on to become ASMBS, or American Society for Metabolic and Bariatric Surgery as result of the 2007 Diabetes Surgery Summit, indicating a broader focus on metabolic health and was one of the pivotal events during Schauer's ASMBS presidency [40]. Concurrently, the International Federation of Societies for Obesity and Metabolic Surgery (IFSO), founded in 1995, facilitated global collaboration and knowledge exchange, further advancing bariatric and metabolic surgery worldwide [48].

In 2003, however, the field faced an ethical quandary. A surge in laparoscopic procedures meant that many surgeons, including those with minimal laparoscopic training, were performing procedures on high-risk patients. This led to an increase in reporting of complications by the media, portraying metabolic surgery in a negative light. The ensuing public blame targeted both patients and surgeons, exacerbating bias against patients with obesity.

Recognizing the urgency of the situation, the ASMBS took proactive measures. In addition to its educational initiatives, the society established accreditation standards for surgeons and institutions performing bariatric surgery [49]. This quality initiative became known as the Bariatric Surgery Center of Excellence (BSCOE) [49]. Its foundation aimed to enhance patient safety and improve the overall quality of care. Part of this program included the Bariatric Outcomes Longitudinal Database

(BOLD) program which was implemented in 425 hospitals in the United States as well as 22 countries [18]. The American College of Surgeons (ACS) established its own quality improvement program, called the Bariatric Surgery Center Network (BSCN) [50]. The BSCN and BSCOE joined forces in 2012 and led to the creation of the Metabolic and Bariatric Surgery Surgical Accreditation and Quality Improvement Project (MBSAQIP). MBSAQIP standards were published in 2014 and represent a comprehensive quality program with accreditation standards, data reporting, and certain quality improvement requirements [51].

To meet the growing demand for laparoscopic surgery education, the Fellowship Council was created in 1997. Although initially opposed by organizations such as the ACS and the Accreditation Council for Graduate Medical Education (ACGME), because it was thought that new training programs would diminish learning opportunities for general surgery residents, the Fellowship Council proved a valuable tool for teaching advanced laparoscopy at a number of high-quality programs [52]. The formation of the council allowed for the creation of not only bariatric/metabolic surgery fellowships, but also minimally invasive surgery (MIS), flexible endoscopy, and hepato-pancreato-biliary fellowships. The ASMBS developed a certificate for bariatric surgery fellows with case volume, didactic, and research requirements [53]. Further, for general surgeons wishing to dedicate much of their practice to bariatric surgery, the Focused Practice Designation (FPD) is an exam recognized by the American Board of Surgery (ABS). This designation provides transparent information to patients looking for a surgeon with additional expertise in primary and revisional bariatric surgery, management of bariatric complications and endoscopy [54].

## Scientific and Procedural Advances in Metabolic Surgery

### Improvements in Metabolic Syndrome and the Role of Gut Hormones

Advancements in the understanding and management of metabolic syndrome have been closely tied to the field of bariatric surgery and hormonal weight loss as noted above. This continually expanding field of clinical, translational, and basic science research has generated the most influential publications and the landmark clinical trials within the fields of metabolism and obesity (Table 2.1). These investigations have significantly contributed to the basic understanding of obesity as a disease. Furthermore, while complementing the clinical evidence on the remarkable effects of metabolic surgery, these studies have created a better understanding of the relationships between surgery, hormonal changes, and the improvement of metabolic syndrome. The following is a brief overview of some of the most influential and well cited works that have shaped the thoughts on the complex mechanisms of bariatric surgery, the hormonal changes from surgery, and the implications of metabolic intervention.

Cummings et al. (2002) demonstrated that plasma ghrelin levels significantly decrease after diet-induced weight loss and are profoundly suppressed following RYGB surgery, suggesting a link mechanism between ghrelin suppression and post-surgical weight loss via appetite reduction [55]. Not all studies, though, have demonstrated such marked effects of the RYGB on circulating ghrelin [56]. Rubino et al. (2004) explored the weight independent effects of RYGB on hormonal regulation of glucose metabolism, providing important evidence that early improvements in glucose metabolism following operative intervention are at least partially responsible for the observed metabolic improvements regardless of the amount of weight loss [57]. Le Roux et al. (2007) found that several gut hormones, including ghrelin, peptide YY (PYY), and glucagon-like peptide-1 (GLP-1), act as mediators of both appetite and weight loss after RYGB, further establishing an evidence base for the hormonal basis of the procedure's long-term weight loss success [58]. Karamanakos et al. (2008) compared hormonal changes following RYGB versus the sleeve gastrectomy, noting distinct differences in appetite suppression and levels of ghrelin and peptide YY between the two procedures. This signals a procedure specific magnitude of hormonal modulation following these popular metabolic interventions [59]. Then in 2008, Laferrère et al., demonstrated that RYGB leads to more pronounced changes in glucose and incretin levels in patients with type 2 diabetes compared to a hypocaloric diet, adding to the evidence that the enhancement of glycemic control isn't fully explained by a reduction in caloric intake or weight loss alone [60].

Throughout the 2010s, more evidence added to the understanding of the effects surgery has on metabolism independent of the amount of weight loss. Numerous rodent studies had linked bile acids to increased energy expenditure in rodents [61], with several studies demonstrating intestinal reconfiguration to be associated with marked elevations in bile acids within the blood [62]. Shortly thereafter investigators examined the potential for these effects in humans, with Patti et al. (2009) observing increased serum bile acid levels in patients following gastric bypass, linking these changes in enterohepatic circulation of bile to improvements in glucose and lipid metabolism, suggesting a role for the hormonal effects of bile acids in the postoperative metabolic improvement [63]. These observations were corroborated by Kaplan [64] and Le Roux [65], generating an intense interest in metabolic surgery and its effects on bile acid physiology. Interestingly, this strong metabolic surgery-bile acid link has been demonstrated as early postoperative increases in specific insulin sensitizing bile acids that only come from gut microbiota-dependent metabolism have been observed in humans after RYGB [66].

In a landmark paper in 2014, Ryan et al. identified the Farnesoid X Receptor (FXR), a bile acid receptor, as a primary molecular target for the effects of the sleeve gastrectomy [67]. They noted when FXR was genetically absent, the sleeve gastrectomy was less effective in reducing body weight and mediating glucose improvements. This suggests that alterations in bile acid metabolism and FXR signaling contribute to the metabolic benefits which are believed to occur by augmenting activity of the incretin axis. Albaugh et al. (2019) further established metabolic surgery's contribution of altered intestinal bile acid availability in increasing FXR-GLP-1 axis signaling, emphasizing the complex interplay between gut hormones and metabolic regulation post-surgery [68].

While these highly mechanistic studies have demonstrated broad effects of metabolic surgery on numerous physiologic processes, the findings are generally limited to rodent studies that may or may not be translatable to human physiology. Consequently, surgeons and scientists must continue to work toward understanding which of these observations is conserved between other species and humans, and highly mechanistic studies with human participants are needed to help identify the clinically significant basic science mechanisms underlying these physiologic changes.

Together, these studies offer a glimpse into the physiological pathways through which metabolic and bariatric surgery exert their profound effects on the human body. They underscore the significant role of hormonal changes, in reducing food intake, promoting weight loss, and improving glucose homeostasis following operations like the RYGB and sleeve gastrectomy across both human and rodent models. This body of work also points to contributions from other pathways, including bile acids, gut microbes, leptin, melanocortin, and IGFBP2, to the outcomes of metabolic surgery. Complex knockout genetic studies in rodents have demonstrated that no one hormonal or receptor pathway can abolish the effects of metabolic surgery, arguing for broad effects on physiology overall. Thus, no single mechanism fully explains the surgery's beneficial effects—suggesting a complex interplay between the gut and the rest of the body in regulating body weight than previously appreciated. Despite the advancements documented, much remains to be learned about the nuanced mechanisms underpinning the metabolic improvements of metabolic surgery [69]. One reason that historically restrictive procedures like the gastric band the vertical banded gastroplasty were not successful is their lack of metabolic effects. The sleeve gastrectomy, conversely, was derived as a restrictive procedure but clearly has hormonal and metabolic effects. As such, it is more appropriate to refer to it as a metabolic procedure.

## Procedural Advancements: Endoscopic Approaches

Endoscopic approaches to obesity management have emerged as less invasive alternatives to traditional bariatric operations, offering significant weight loss and metabolic improvements. Techniques such as the gastric balloon, endoscopic sleeve gastroplasty (ESG), and endoscopic duodenal ablation/duodenal liner have been developed, providing a spectrum of options for patients seeking weight loss solutions [70, 71]. The IFSO Worldwide Surveys of 2014 and 2016 detail the prevalence and outcomes of these endoluminal procedures, underscoring their growing role in the obesity treatment landscape [72, 73]. As the field of bariatric endoscopy continues to evolve, these endoscopic approaches signify an advancement in obesity management, promising a future where effective weight loss solutions become more accessible, less invasive, and tailored to individual patient needs. The ongoing research and development in this domain are poised to further refine these techniques, enhancing their safety, efficacy, and applicability,

These scientific and procedural advances highlight the dynamic and evolving landscape of obesity management, emphasizing the critical role of hormonal modulation and innovative endoscopic techniques in addressing this complex disease.

## The Future of Metabolic Surgery

### Obesity as a Disease

While obesity was first recognized in 1948 by the World Health Organization (WHO) as a disease, further recognition has taken over half a century to be recapitulated by many other organizations [74]. While progress has been slow until the recent past, the recognition of obesity as a disease has been pivotal in the way metabolic syndrome (MS) is approached and managed. This acknowledgment has stemmed from a series of significant endorsements and has allowed for a landscape in which the perception and management of obesity have undergone important shifts, particularly with the American Medical Association's (AMA) declaration in 2013 that recognized obesity as a disease with their public health policy H-440.842 [75, 76]. Spurred on by the important evidence highlighted by The Obesity Society (TOS) in its 2008 position statement, the AMA's declaration aimed to alter the medical community's approach toward diagnosing and treating obesity, emphasizing its seriousness and the necessity for a comprehensive treatment paradigm [77]. Despite these intentions, the resolution's impact on many physicians' opinions is limited, with varying perceptions still prevalent about whether obesity should be considered a disease or a risk factor [75].

However, following the AMA's stance, other prominent health organizations—including the World Obesity Federation (WOF) in 2017, The Obesity Society in 2018, the Italian Parliament in 2019, and the European Commission in 2021—made moves to publicly acknowledge the complexities surrounding obesity, underscoring its status as a global health challenge [78–82]. And in an influential move in 2022, six leading organizations in the United States focused on obesity united to confront the obstacles impeding better access to obesity treatments and the reduction of stigma and bias related to the condition. The collaborative included TOS, Obesity Action Coalition (OAC), Obesity Medicine Association (OMA), ASMBS, Stop Obesity Alliance (SOA), and the Academy of Nutrition and Dietetics (AAND) [83, 84]. The acknowledgment from these organizations emphasizes the importance of consensus and unified approaches and strategies in effectively combating obesity.

## New Guidelines and Redefining Obesity

The initial guidelines set by the Panel on CDC in 1991 recognized gastrointestinal surgery as an essential treatment for severe obesity, providing a crucial framework for surgical management and emphasizing patient selection and health benefits [85]. However, over time these recommendations became dated considering advancements in surgical techniques and safety. Instead of promoting access to care, practicing surgeons found the old guidelines as an obstacle to appropriately treating patients with obesity. This, in turn, prompted the ASMBS and IFSO to present an update to the guidelines for the indications for bariatric and metabolic surgery in 2022. Led by Eisenberg et al. [86], these societies incorporated the best research, clinical practice, and technological advancements and considered the complex nature of obesity and overall health, to expand the recommendations for bariatric surgery beyond a simple BMI. The updated guidelines also established the latest in approved surgical techniques and stressed the need for a comprehensive treatment approach—integrating nutritional, psychological, and exercise support. This revision marked a pivotal evolution in the surgical treatment of obesity, aiming to enhance the safety, effectiveness, and reach of metabolic surgery.

Additionally, in 2023 the Lancet Diabetes & Endocrinology Commission on the Definition and Diagnosis of Clinical Obesity embarked on redefining obesity, aiming to align the medical definition more closely with the current understanding of its pathophysiology, risks, and treatment considerations [87]. This redefinition seeks to ensure that obesity is recognized based on its biological and clinical impacts rather than solely on BMI measurements, facilitating more personalized and effective treatment approaches.

## A Look to the Future

The journey toward redefining and managing obesity as a disease is ongoing, with the medical community and health organizations worldwide continuing to evolve their perspectives and approaches in response to this complex health issue. The goal remains to enhance the quality of care for individuals with obesity, improving their health outcomes and quality of life.

## References


1. Wright PD. Metabolic surgery. Henry Buchwald and Richard L. Varco. 235 × 155 mm. pp. 317, with 57 illustrations. 1978. New York: Grune & Stratton. No price given. J Br Surg. 2005(66):447. https://doi.org/10.1002/bjs.1800660639.
2. Buchwald H, Varco RL, Matts JP, Long JM, Fitch LL, Campbell GS, et al. Effect of partial ileal bypass surgery on mortality and morbidity from coronary heart disease in patients with hypercholesterolemia. N Engl J Med. 1990;323:946–55. https://doi.org/10.1056/nejm199010043231404.

3. Buchwald H. The evolution of metabolic/bariatric surgery. Obes Surg. 2014;24:1126–35. https://doi.org/10.1007/s11695-014-1354-3.
4. Kremen AJ, Linner JH, Nelson CH. An experimental evaluation of the nutritional importance of proximal and distal small intestine. Ann Surg. 1954;140:439. https://doi.org/10.1097/00000658-195409000-00018.
5. Lewis LA, Turnbull RB, Page IH. Short-circuiting of the small intestine: effect on concentration of serum cholesterol and lipoproteins. JAMA. 1962;182:77–9. https://doi.org/10.1001/jama.1962.03050400079017b.
6. Payne JH, DeWind LT, Commons RR. Metabolic observations in patients with jejunocolic shunts. Am J Surg. 1963;106:273–89. https://doi.org/10.1016/0002-9610(63)90017-5.
7. Buchwald H, Varco RL. Ileal bypass in lowering high cholesterol levels. Surg Forum. 1964;15:289–91.
8. Mason EE, Ito C. Gastric bypass in obesity. Surg Clin North Am. 1967;47:1345–51. https://doi.org/10.1016/s0039-6109(16)38384-0.
9. Griffen WO, Young VL, Stevenson CC. A prospective comparison of gastric and Jejunoileal bypass procedures for morbid obesity. Ann Surg. 1977;186:500–9. https://doi.org/10.1097/00000658-197710000-00012.
10. Flickinger EG, Pories WJ, Meelheim HD, Sinar DR, Blose IL, Thomas FT. The Greenville gastric bypass. Ann Surg. 1984;199:555–62. https://doi.org/10.1097/00000658-198405000-00010.
11. Aarts EO, Mahawar K. From the knife to the endoscope—a history of bariatric surgery. Curr Obes Rep. 2020;9:348–63. https://doi.org/10.1007/s13679-020-00382-1.
12. Scopinaro N, Adami GF, Marinari GM, Gianetta E, Traverso E, Friedman D, et al. Biliopancreatic diversion. World J Surg. 1998;22:936–46. https://doi.org/10.1007/s002689900497.
13. Steffen R. The history and role of gastric banding. Surg Obes Relat Dis. 2008;4:S7–13. https://doi.org/10.1016/j.soard.2008.04.002.
14. Vest AR, Young JB. Minimally invasive bariatric surgery. New York: Springer; 2014. p. 455–69. https://doi.org/10.1007/978-1-4939-1637-5_49.
15. Mason EE. Vertical banded gastroplasty for obesity. Arch Surg. 1982;117:701–6. https://doi.org/10.1001/archsurg.1982.01380290147026.
16. Greilsamer T, Jacobi D, Krempf M, Boulanger G, Guillouche M, Cariou B, et al. Long-term complications of open mason's vertical banded gastroplasty at a single tertiary center and literature review. Am Surg. 2019;85:1386–90.
17. Shiffman MA. Body contouring, art, science, and clinical practice. Berlin, Heidelberg: Springer; 2010. p. 629–32. https://doi.org/10.1007/978-3-642-02639-3_62.
18. Chousleb E, Rodriguez JA, O'Leary JP. The ASMBS textbook of bariatric surgery. Cham: Springer; 2019. p. 37–46. https://doi.org/10.1007/978-3-030-27021-6_3.
19. Hess DS, Hess DW. Biliopancreatic diversion with a duodenal switch. Obes Surg. 1998;8:267–82. https://doi.org/10.1381/096089298765554476.
20. Trelles N, Gagner M. Updated review of sleeve gastrectomy. Open Gastroenterol J. 2008;2:41–9. https://doi.org/10.2174/1874259900802010041.
21. Wittgrove AC, Clark GW, Tremblay LJ. Laparoscopic gastric bypass, roux-en-Y: preliminary report of five cases. Obes Surg. 1994;4:353–7. https://doi.org/10.1381/096089294765558331.
22. Broadbent R, Tracey M, Harrington P. Laparoscopic gastric banding: a preliminary report. Obes Surg. 1993;3:63–7. https://doi.org/10.1381/096089293765559791.
23. Catona A, Gossenberg M, Manna AL, Mussini G. Laparoscopic gastric banding: preliminary series. Obes Surg. 1993;3:207–9. https://doi.org/10.1381/096089293765559610.
24. Miller MR, Choban PS. Surgical management of obesity. Nutr Clin Pr. 2011;26:526–33. https://doi.org/10.1177/0884533611418336.
25. Nguyen NT, Hinojosa M, Fayad C, Varela E, Wilson SE. Use and outcomes of laparoscopic versus open gastric bypass at academic medical centers. J Am Coll Surg. 2007;205:248–55. https://doi.org/10.1016/j.jamcollsurg.2007.03.011.
26. DeMaria EJ, Sugerman HJ, Kellum JM, Meador JG, Wolfe LG. Results of 281 consecutive total laparoscopic roux-en-Y gastric bypasses to treat morbid obesity. Ann Surg. 2002;235:640–7. https://doi.org/10.1097/00000658-200205000-00005.

27. Schauer PR, Ikramuddin S, Gourash W, Ramanathan R, Luketich J. Outcomes after laparoscopic roux-en-Y gastric bypass for morbid obesity. Ann Surg. 2000;232:515–29. https://doi.org/10.1097/00000658-200010000-00007.
28. Podnos YD, Jimenez JC, Wilson SE, Stevens CM, Nguyen NT. Complications after laparoscopic gastric bypass: a review of 3464 cases. Arch Surg. 2003;138:957–61. https://doi.org/10.1001/archsurg.138.9.957.
29. Higa KD, Boone KB, Ho T. Complications of the laparoscopic roux-en-Y gastric bypass: 1,040 patients - what have we learned? Obes Surg. 2000;10:509–13. https://doi.org/10.1381/096089200321593706.
30. Ren CJ, Patterson E, Gagner M. Early results of laparoscopic biliopancreatic diversion with duodenal switch: a case series of 40 consecutive patients. Obes Surg. 2000;10:514–23. https://doi.org/10.1381/096089200321593715.
31. Tucker ON, Szomstein S, Rosenthal RJ. Indications for sleeve gastrectomy as a primary procedure for weight loss in the morbidly obese. J Gastrointest Surg. 2008;12:662–7. https://doi.org/10.1007/s11605-008-0480-4.
32. Rosenthal RJ, Panel ISGE, Diaz AA, Arvidsson D, Baker RS, Basso N, et al. International sleeve gastrectomy expert panel consensus statement: best practice guidelines based on experience of >12,000 cases. Surg Obes Relat Dis. 2012;8:8–19. https://doi.org/10.1016/j.soard.2011.10.019.
33. Salminen P, Helmiö M, Ovaska J, Juuti A, Leivonen M, Peromaa-Haavisto P, et al. Effect of laparoscopic sleeve gastrectomy vs laparoscopic roux-en-Y gastric bypass on weight loss at 5 years among patients with morbid obesity: the SLEEVEPASS randomized clinical trial. JAMA. 2018;319:241–54. https://doi.org/10.1001/jama.2017.20313.
34. Hanipah ZN, Rubino F, Schauer PR. Remission with an intervention is metabolic surgery the ultimate solution? Endocrinol Metab Clin N Am. 2023;52:65–88. https://doi.org/10.1016/j.ecl.2022.09.002.
35. Starkloff GB, Donovan JF, Ramach KR, Wolfe BM. Metabolic intestinal surgery: its complications and management. Arch Surg. 1975;110:652–7. https://doi.org/10.1001/archsurg.1975.01360110198034.
36. Scott HW. Metabolic surgery for hyperlipidemia and atherosclerosis. Am J Surg. 1972;123:3–12. https://doi.org/10.1016/0002-9610(72)90304-2.
37. Buchwald H, Williams SE, Matts JP, Nguyen PA, Boen JR. Overall mortality in the program on the surgical control of the hyperlipidemias1 1No competing interests declared. J Am Coll Surg. 2002;195:327–31. https://doi.org/10.1016/s1072-7515(02)01275-9.
38. Pories WJ, Swanson MS, MacDonald KG, Long SB, Morris PG, Brown BM, et al. Who would have thought it? An operation proves to be the most effective therapy for adult-onset diabetes mellitus. Ann Surg. 1995;222:339–52. https://doi.org/10.1097/00000658-199509000-00011.
39. Schauer PR, Burguera B, Ikramuddin S, Cottam D, Gourash W, Hamad G, et al. Effect of laparoscopic roux-en Y gastric bypass on type 2 diabetes mellitus. Trans Meet Am Surg Assoc. 2003;121:160–78. https://doi.org/10.1097/01.sla.0000089851.41115.1b.
40. Rubino F, Kaplan LM, Schauer PR, Cummings DE, Delegates DSS. The diabetes surgery summit consensus conference: recommendations for the evaluation and use of gastrointestinal Surgery to treat type 2 diabetes mellitus. Ann Surg. 2010;251:399–405. https://doi.org/10.1097/sla.0b013e3181be34e7.
41. Schauer PR, Kashyap SR, Kathy W, et al. Bariatric surgery versus intensive medical therapy in obese patients with diabetes. N Engl J Med. 2012;366:1567–76. https://doi.org/10.1056/nejmoa1200225.
42. Cohen RV, Pereira TV, Aboud CM, Petry TBZ, Correa JLL, Schiavon CA, et al. Gastric bypass versus best medical treatment for diabetic kidney disease: 5 years follow up of a single-centre open label randomised controlled trial. E Clin Med. 2022;53:101725. https://doi.org/10.1016/j.eclinm.2022.101725.
43. Schiavon CA, Bhatt DL, Ikeoka D, Santucci EV, Santos RN, Damiani LP, et al. Three-year outcomes of bariatric Surgery in patients with obesity and hypertension: a randomized clinical trial. Ann Intern Med. 2020;173:685–93. https://doi.org/10.7326/m19-3781.

44. Courcoulas AP, Patti ME, Hu B, Arterburn DE, Simonson DC, Gourash WF, et al. Long-term outcomes of medical management vs bariatric surgery in type 2 diabetes. JAMA. 2024;331:654–64. https://doi.org/10.1001/jama.2024.0318.
45. Geltrude M, Simona P, Andrea DG, Caterina G, Amerigo I, Laura L, et al. Bariatric surgery versus conventional medical therapy for type 2 diabetes. N Engl J Med. 2012;366:1577–85. https://doi.org/10.1056/nejmoa1200111.
46. Sjöström L, Peltonen M, Jacobson P, Ahlin S, Andersson-Assarsson J, Anveden Å, et al. Association of bariatric surgery with long-term remission of type 2 diabetes and with microvascular and macrovascular complications. JAMA. 2014;311:2297–304. https://doi.org/10.1001/jama.2014.5988.
47. Peterli R, Wölnerhanssen B, Peters T, Devaux N, Kern B, Christoffel-Courtin C, et al. Improvement in glucose metabolism after bariatric surgery: comparison of laparoscopic roux-en-Y gastric bypass and laparoscopic sleeve gastrectomy. Ann Surg. 2009;250:234–41. https://doi.org/10.1097/sla.0b013e3181ae32e3.
48. Deitel M. The International Federation of Obesity: a history for the surgery. Obes Surg. 2001;11:243–4. https://doi.org/10.1381/096089201321336511.
49. Brethauer SA, Chand B, Schauer PR. The SAGES manual, a practical guide to bariatric surgery. New York: Springer; 2008. p. 257–60. https://doi.org/10.1007/978-0-387-69171-8_32.
50. Brahmbhatt RD, Habermann EB, Kellogg TA, Reidt WS, Que FG, Kendrick ML, et al. Factors predicting risk of readmission and reoperation within 30 days of bariatric Surgery: a study using the American College of Surgeons Bariatric Surgery Center Network (ACS BSCN) database. J Surg Res. 2014;186:498. https://doi.org/10.1016/j.jss.2013.11.101.
51. Petrick AT, Gadaleta D. Raising the standard: MBSAQIP: the evolution of 100 years of quality programs. Bariatric Times;2018.
52. Fowler DL, Hogle NJ. The fellowship council: a decade of impact on surgical training. Surg Endosc. 2013;27:3548–54. https://doi.org/10.1007/s00464-013-3007-3.
53. ASMBS. ASMBS Certificate of Acknowledgement of Satisfactory Training: Metabolic and Bariatric Surgery for Fellows 2024.
54. Surgery AB of. Focused Practice Designation in Metabolic and Bariatric Surgery 2024.
55. Cummings DE, Weigle DS, Frayo RS, Breen PA, Ma MK, Dellinger EP, et al. Plasma ghrelin levels after diet-induced weight loss or gastric bypass surgery. N Engl J Med. 2002;346:1623–30. https://doi.org/10.1056/nejmoa012908.
56. Cummings DE. Endocrine mechanisms mediating remission of diabetes after gastric bypass surgery. Int J Obes. 2009;33:S33–40. https://doi.org/10.1038/ijo.2009.15.
57. Rubino F, Gagner M, Gentileschi P, Kini S, Fukuyama S, Feng J, et al. The early effect of the roux-en-Y gastric bypass on hormones involved in body weight regulation and glucose metabolism. Ann Surg. 2004;240:236–42. https://doi.org/10.1097/01.sla.0000133117.12646.48.
58. le Roux CW, Welbourn R, Werling M, Osborne A, Kokkinos A, Laurenius A, et al. Gut hormones as mediators of appetite and weight loss after roux-en-Y gastric bypass. Ann Surg. 2007;246:780–5. https://doi.org/10.1097/sla.0b013e3180caa3e3.
59. Karamanakos SN, Vagenas K, Kalfarentzos F, Alexandrides TK. Weight loss, appetite suppression, and changes in fasting and postprandial ghrelin and peptide-YY levels after roux-en-Y gastric bypass and sleeve gastrectomy. Ann Surg. 2008;247:401–7. https://doi.org/10.1097/sla.0b013e318156f012.
60. Laferrère B, Teixeira J, McGinty J, Tran H, Egger JR, Colarusso A, et al. Effect of weight loss by gastric bypass surgery versus hypocaloric diet on glucose and incretin levels in patients with type 2 diabetes. J Clin Endocrinol Metab. 2008;93:2479–85. https://doi.org/10.1210/jc.2007-2851.
61. Watanabe M, Houten SM, Mataki C, Christoffolete MA, Kim BW, Sato H, et al. Bile acids induce energy expenditure by promoting intracellular thyroid hormone activation. Nature. 2006;439:484–9. https://doi.org/10.1038/nature04330.
62. Culnan DM, Albaugh V, Sun M, Lynch CJ, Lang CH, Cooney RN. Ileal interposition improves glucose tolerance and insulin sensitivity in the obese Zucker rat. Am J Physiol Gastrointest Liver Physiol. 2010;299:G751–60. https://doi.org/10.1152/ajpgi.00525.2009.

63. Patti M, Houten SM, Bianco AC, Bernier R, Larsen PR, Holst JJ, et al. Serum bile acids are higher in humans with prior gastric bypass: potential contribution to improved glucose and lipid metabolism. Obesity. 2009;17:1671–7. https://doi.org/10.1038/oby.2009.102.
64. Ahmad NN, Pfalzer A, Kaplan LM. Roux-en-Y gastric bypass normalizes the blunted post-prandial bile acid excursion associated with obesity. Int J Obes. 2013;37:1553–9. https://doi.org/10.1038/ijo.2013.38.
65. Werling M, Vincent RP, Cross GF, Marschall H-U, Fändriks L, Lönroth H, et al. Enhanced fasting and post-prandial plasma bile acid responses after Roux-en-Y gastric bypass surgery. Scand J Gastroenterol. 2013;48:1257–64. https://doi.org/10.3109/00365521.2013.833647.
66. Albaugh VL, Flynn CR, Cai S, Xiao Y, Tamboli RA, Abumrad NN. Early increases in bile acids post roux-en-Y gastric bypass are driven by insulin-sensitizing, secondary bile acids. J Clin Endocrinol Metab. 2015;100:E1225–33. https://doi.org/10.1210/jc.2015-2467.
67. Ryan KK, Tremaroli V, Clemmensen C, Kovatcheva-Datchary P, Myronovych A, Karns R, et al. FXR is a molecular target for the effects of vertical sleeve gastrectomy. Nature. 2014;509:183–8. https://doi.org/10.1038/nature13135.
68. Albaugh VL, Banan B, Antoun J, Xiong Y, Guo Y, Ping J, et al. Role of bile acids and GLP-1 in mediating the metabolic improvements of bariatric Surgery. Gastroenterology. 2019;156:1041–1051.e4. https://doi.org/10.1053/j.gastro.2018.11.017.
69. Albaugh VL, He Y, Münzberg H, Morrison CD, Yu S, Berthoud H-R. Regulation of body weight: lessons learned from bariatric surgery. Mol Metab. 2023;68:101517. https://doi.org/10.1016/j.molmet.2022.101517.
70. Dayyeh BKA, Bazerbachi F, Vargas EJ, Sharaiha RZ, Thompson CC, Thaemert BC, et al. Endoscopic sleeve gastroplasty for treatment of class 1 and 2 obesity (MERIT): a prospective, multicentre, randomised trial. Lancet. 2022;400:441–51. https://doi.org/10.1016/s0140-6736(22)01280-6.
71. Schouten R, Rijs CS, Bouvy ND, Hameeteman W, Koek GH, Janssen IMC, et al. A multicenter, randomized efficacy study of the EndoBarrier gastrointestinal liner for Presurgical weight loss prior to bariatric Surgery. Ann Surg. 2010;251:236–43. https://doi.org/10.1097/sla.0b013e3181bdfbff.
72. Angrisani L, Santonicola A, Iovino P, Vitiello A, Zundel N, Buchwald H, et al. Bariatric Surgery and Endoluminal procedures: IFSO worldwide survey 2014. Obes Surg. 2017;27:2279–89. https://doi.org/10.1007/s11695-017-2666-x.
73. Angrisani L, Santonicola A, Iovino P, Vitiello A, Higa K, Himpens J, et al. IFSO worldwide survey 2016: primary, Endoluminal, and Revisional procedures. Obes Surg. 2018;28:3783–94. https://doi.org/10.1007/s11695-018-3450-2.
74. James WPT. WHO recognition of the global obesity epidemic. Int J Obes. 2008;32:S120–6. https://doi.org/10.1038/ijo.2008.247.
75. Funk LM, Jolles SA, Voils CI. Obesity as a disease: has the AMA resolution had an impact on how physicians view obesity? Surg Obes Relat Dis. 2016;12:1431–5. https://doi.org/10.1016/j.soard.2016.05.009.
76. Kyle TK, Dhurandhar EJ, Allison DB. Regarding obesity as a disease evolving policies and their implications. Endocrinol Metab Clin N Am. 2016;45:511–20. https://doi.org/10.1016/j.ecl.2016.04.004.
77. Group TO as a DW, Allison DB, Downey M, Atkinson RL, Billington CJ, Bray GA, et al. Obesity as a disease: a white paper on evidence and arguments commissioned by the Council of the Obesity Society. Obesity. 2008;16:1161–77. https://doi.org/10.1038/oby.2008.231.
78. Kopelman P, Finer N. Reply: is obesity a disease? Int J Obes. 2001;25:1405–6. https://doi.org/10.1038/sj.ijo.0801791.
79. Bray GA, Kim KK, JPH W, Federation on behalf of the WO. Obesity: a chronic relapsing progressive disease process. A position statement of the World Obesity Federation. Obes Rev. 2017;18:715–23. https://doi.org/10.1111/obr.12551.
80. Jastreboff AM, Kotz CM, Kahan S, Kelly AS, Heymsfield SB. Obesity as a disease: the Obesity Society 2018 position statement. Obesity. 2019;27:7–9. https://doi.org/10.1002/oby.22378.

81. Serra F, Lenzi A, Pella R, Spinato C, Fatati G, Carruba M, et al. Italy on gaining official parliamentary recognition that obesity is a chronic disease. Eur J Publ Heal. 2020;30(5):ckaa165.322. https://doi.org/10.1093/eurpub/ckaa165.322.
82. Burki T. European Commission classifies obesity as a chronic disease. Lancet Diabetes Endocrinol. 2021;9:418. https://doi.org/10.1016/s2213-8587(21)00145-5.
83. Consensus Statement on Obesity as a Disease - American Society for Metabolic and Bariatric Surgery. n.d.. https://asmbs.org/resources/consensus-statement-on-obesity-as-a-disease/ (accessed March 26, 2024).
84. The Obesity Society - Consensus Statement on Obesity. n.d.. https://www.obesity.org/ (accessed March 26, 2024).
85. Panel CDC. Gastrointestinal Surgery for severe obesity. Ann Intern Med. 1991;115:956–61. https://doi.org/10.7326/0003-4819-115-12-956.
86. Eisenberg D, Shikora SA, Aarts E, Aminian A, Angrisani L, Cohen RV, et al. 2022 American Society of Metabolic and Bariatric Surgery (ASMBS) and International Federation for the Surgery of Obesity and Metabolic Disorders (IFSO) indications for metabolic and bariatric surgery. Obes Surg. 2023;33:3–14. https://doi.org/10.1007/s11695-022-06332-1.
87. Rubino F, Batterham RL, Koch M, Mingrone G, le Roux CW, Farooqi IS, et al. Lancet diabetes & endocrinology commission on the definition and diagnosis of clinical obesity. Lancet Diabetes Endocrinol. 2023;11:226–8. https://doi.org/10.1016/s2213-8587(23)00058-x.

# 3 Obesity Epidemic

Michael A. Schweitzer and Luke K. Dombert

The obesity epidemic pertains to the increasing prevalence of obesity among the global population and has long been a health concern in the Americas. Obesity, defined by the World Health Organization (WHO), involves abnormal or excessive body fat accumulation that may impair health [1]. Various factors contribute to obesity, including genetics, environment, behavior, and metabolic influences. This epidemic has been a significant international health concern for several decades, with prevalence doubling since 1980, with approximately 40% of the global population currently being obese [2]. Obesity remains a substantial challenge for individuals, communities, and healthcare systems.

Over the past few decades, obesity rates have surged in many countries, affecting both developed and developing nations. While numerous studies have sought to identify a single causative factor, increasing urbanization has introduced multiple independent influences. Factors contributing to this surge include changes in diet, reduced physical activity, and societal shifts, such as increased screen time and sedentary work environments [3]. The prevalence of individuals being overweight (BMI >25) had a 50% increase from 1980 to 2015, with obesity (BMI >30) an 80% increase globally [4]. Estimates suggest that if current trends persist without change or challenge, 57.8% of the world's adult population, or 3.3 billion people, will become overweight or obese by 2030 [5].

Obesity is associated with a wide range of severe health problems, including, but not limited to, heart disease, type 2 diabetes, various cancers, sleep apnea, and osteoarthritis. Obesity is an independent risk factor for coronary artery disease, which has increased the rates of myocardial infarction and cardiovascular disease-related deaths [6]. The pathophysiology revolves around elevated blood lipid levels

M. A. Schweitzer · L. K. Dombert (✉)
Johns Hopkins University, Baltimore, MD, USA
e-mail: ldombert@riversidesurg.com



O. M. Ghanem et al. (eds.), *The SAGES Manual of Metabolic and Bariatric Surgery*, https://doi.org/10.1007/978-3-031-72309-4_3

in obese patients with an increase in their non-HDL lipoproteins, which promotes atherosclerosis and serves as a significant risk factor for coronary heart disease. Following the surge in obesity is the closely related diabetic epidemic, referred to as "diabesity," which underscores their close relationship. Excess adipose tissue predisposes patients to insulin resistance and insulin deficiency. It is believed that approximately 90% of type 2 diabetes cases are partially attributed to excess weight [7]. There is substantial evidence that obesity is a risk factor for 13 different types of cancer (endometrial, postmenopausal breast, colorectal, esophageal, renal, meningioma, pancreatic, gastric, liver, multiple myeloma, ovarian, gallbladder, and thyroid). The main molecular pathways associated with tumorigenesis are incompletely defined but are theorized to revolve around the overstimulation of endogenous sex steroids, well-regulated metabolic hormones, insulin dysfunction, and a low-grade chronic inflammatory state [8]. Obesity also negatively affects sleep quality, leading to high rates of insomnia, restless leg syndrome, and sleep-disordered breathing, including primary snoring and obstructive sleep apnea [9]. A significant relationship between osteoarthritis and obesity has long been established. While biomechanical mechanisms were traditionally considered the primary cause, recent research has shed light on the biochemical effects associated with osteoarthritis [10]. The implications of obesity and its associated health issues are costly.

Comorbid conditions experienced by obese individuals not only limit their productivity but also impose a significant economic burden on the healthcare system. On average, an obese patient incurs 32% higher annual healthcare costs compared to a normal-weight patient [11]. In a study of eight countries, it was found that obesity results in an average cost of 1.76% of GDP, when focusing solely on healthcare expenses [12]. This cost is projected to increase to an average of 3.57% of GDP by 2060 [12]. Estimating and assigning value to the lost productivity of obese individuals is more challenging. In the United States alone, obese workers experience a 281% increase in worker's compensation days compared to normal-weight workers, contributing to an estimated national cost of $3.38–11.2 billion annually. This includes reduced lifespans, shortened career times, increased familial support needs, and time off from work.

Obesity-related diseases and all-cause mortality are closely linked to the duration of obesity. Correcting this issue at a young age is crucial, highlighting current trends in childhood obesity. Influences on infant adiposity have been on the rise, with factors such as prematurity, low birth weight, gestational diabetes, excess body mass gain during gestation, and infant formula feeding playing a role. Rapid infant growth during the first 6 months and the first year is associated with subsequent obesity in a person's life course [13]. Only 21% of American school-aged children achieve the recommended 60 min of daily physical activity [14]. In contrast, sedentary screen time has replaced physical activity. While the World Health Organization recommends that children have less than 1 h of screen time per day, recent studies have shown that children have over 7 h of sedentary screen time daily. Despite less physical activity in obese children they are at increased risk of orthopedic fractures in childhood potentially related to alternation in early-stage musculoskeletal maturity [15]. Interventions for childhood obesity are limited compared to those for adults, as children are considered a protected population, making experimental advancements slow. They are highly influenced by stagnant school and community interventions due to lengthy administrative implementation. Behavioral interventions for children include limiting sugar-sweetened beverage consumption, promoting fruit and vegetable intake, reducing screen time, and controlling meal portions. Pharmacologic interventions have been limited, with most studies focusing on children over 12 years old. However, with the development of new medical therapies, this may expand. Surgical intervention is also limited, as only a few centers currently offer adolescent surgery due to concerns about lifelong follow-up and adolescents' ability to adhere to post-operative nutrition and risk management. What is clear that early intervention in childhood obesity does have strong effects in reversing comorbid conditions such as diabetes and other associated medical conditions. Obese children have a three times higher mortality rate before their 30th birthday when compared to normal-weight counterparts [16]. This underlines the importance of early intervention.

Obesity rates vary by socioeconomic status, with disadvantaged communities experiencing higher rates. This is due to increased access to processed, calorie-dense foods compared to healthier options and limited opportunities for physical activity. Hispanics, Blacks, and low socioeconomic populations face higher rates of food insecurity, resulting in poor dietary quality [17]. Children who primarily speak Spanish have higher rates of obesity compared to their peers [14]. There is a growing consideration of obesity as a disadvantaged status, as obese individuals face bias associated with weight discrimination, approaching levels seen with gender and race. All these factors contribute to create the obesity epidemic we see today [14].

Socioeconomic limitations are closely linked to exposure to environmental factors contributing to obesity. A patient's environmental influence can be categorized into three major factors: the built, agroalimentary, and sociocultural environments [17]. The built environment pertains to the physical space surrounding us, with modernizations like elevators, escalators, and electric scooters creating a society where physical exercise is limited, reducing caloric expenditure. The agroalimentary environment relates to the calories consumed, their nature, and how they are ingested. Over time, our world has evolved from hunter-gatherers to fast eaters with easy access to unlimited calories. Sugary beverages maximize caloric absorption, and portion sizes for more complex meals have increased by approximately 30%. Sociocultural environmental factors encompass one's neighborhood, family food culture, and media influences [18]. Low-income neighborhoods have been described as food islands or deserts, indicating the unavailability of nutritious food options with an overabundance of fast-food choices.

Public health efforts differ from clinical approaches to obesity management. They rely on changing environmental parameters for population-wide effects through policy interventions. Programs targeting exercise and dietary habits among youth have demonstrated promising long-term results, particularly in the United States, where the public school system provides 1–2 meals daily. Implementing adult interventions, however, is more challenging. While work-based programs have been tested to parallel school-based programs, their success is limited in comparison. Community-based interventions have been attempted in several studies, with some still ongoing [19]. Implementing such programs is challenging because capturing the entire population is difficult. Interventions have included broadcast media campaigns, initiatives in grocery stores and restaurants promoting healthy choices, and the development of community exercise facilities to encourage physical activity. These initial trials primarily focused on cardiovascular outcomes, with secondary obesity outcomes. Results have been disappointing, with several contributing factors. Public funding is required for these studies, often entailing bureaucratic limitations. Healthy food choice advertisements are consistently overshadowed by privately funded unhealthy advertisements. Public efforts have also explored early interventions to prevent weight gain. The Pound of Prevention study examined multiple groups, with a control group and another group provided with educational resources over 3 years [20]. At the study's conclusion, all groups exhibited weight gain, with no significant difference between the control and intervention groups. However, the treatment group did maintain an interest in weight-related behaviors. In conclusion, public efforts are costly and challenging to implement on a large scale, and the ideal method for intervention remains elusive.

In conclusion, the obesity epidemic is a pressing global health issue with multifaceted implications. Its increasing prevalence, driven by various factors including changes in lifestyle, diet, and socioeconomic disparities, poses a significant challenge to individuals, communities, and healthcare systems. The associated health consequences, economic burden, and long-term impact on childhood obesity underscore the urgency of addressing this epidemic. While public health efforts have aimed to curb its growth, implementing effective, scalable interventions remains a complex task. Obesity's far-reaching consequences demand a comprehensive approach, spanning from early childhood interventions to environmental changes and policy initiatives. Tackling this epidemic requires concerted efforts from healthcare professionals, policymakers, communities, and individuals to promote healthier living and prevent the ongoing expansion of this global health crisis.

**Recommended Text**

"Overweight & Obesity." *Centers for Disease Control and Prevention*, Centers for Disease Control and Prevention, 21 Sept. 2023, www.cdc.gov/obesity/index.html.

Forse, R. Armour, et al. "Epidemiology and Discrimination in Obesity." *The ASMBS Textbook of Bariatric Surgery*, 2nd ed., Springer, Cham, Switzerland, 2020, pp. 3–13.

## References

1. World Health Organization. Obesity and overweight. Fact sheet no 311 January 2015. [cited 2016 20 April 2016]; Available from http://www.who.int/mediacentre/factsheets/fs311/en/.
2. Wong MCS, Huang J, Wang J, et al. Global, regional and time-trend prevalence of central obesity: a systematic review and meta-analysis of 13.2 million subjects. Eur J Epidemiol. 2020;35:673–83. https://doi.org/10.1007/s10654-020-00650-3.

3. Lee A, Cardel M, Donahoo WT. Social and environmental factors influencing obesity. [Updated 2019 Oct 12]. In: Feingold KR, Anawalt B, Blackman MR, et al., editors. Endotext [Internet]. South Dartmouth (MA): MDText.com, Inc.; 2000. Available from: https://www.ncbi.nlm.nih.gov/books/NBK278977/.
4. Chooi YC, Ding C, Magkos F. The epidemiology of obesity. Metabolism. 2019;92:6–10. ISSN 0026-0495. https://doi.org/10.1016/j.metabol.2018.09.005.
5. Kelly T, Yang W, Chen CS, et al. Global burden of obesity in 2005 and projections to 2030. Int J Obes. 2008;32:1431–7. https://doi.org/10.1038/ijo.2008.102.
6. Wilson PWF, D'Agostino RB, Sullivan L, Parise H, Kannel WB. Overweight and obesity as determinants of cardiovascular risk: the Framingham experience. Arch Intern Med. 2002;162(16):1867–72. https://doi.org/10.1001/archinte.162.16.1867.
7. Shalini Verma M, Ejaz Hussain M. Obesity and diabetes: an update. Diabetes Metab Syndr. 2017;11(1):73–9. ISSN 1871-4021. https://doi.org/10.1016/j.dsx.2016.06.017.
8. Friedenreich CM, Ryder-Burbidge C, McNeil J. Physical activity, obesity and sedentary behavior in cancer etiology: epidemiologic evidence and biologic mechanisms. Mol Oncol. 2021;15:790–800. https://doi.org/10.1002/1878-0261.12772.
9. Pennings N, Golden L, Yashi K, Tondt J, Bays HE. Sleep-disordered breathing, sleep apnea, and other obesity-related sleep disorders: an Obesity Medicine Association (OMA). Clinical Practice Statement (CPS) 2022. Obes Pillars. 2022. ISSN 2667-3681;4:100043. https://doi.org/10.1016/j.obpill.2022.100043.
10. Batushansky A, Zhu S, Komaravolu RK, South S, Mehta-D'souza P, Griffin TM. Fundamentals of OA. An initiative of Osteoarthritis and Cartilage. Obesity and metabolic factors in OA. Osteoarthritis Cartilage. 2022;30(4):501–15. ISSN 1063-4584. https://doi.org/10.1016/j.joca.2021.06.013.
11. Yusefzadeh H, Rashidi A, Rahimi B. Economic burden of obesity: a systematic review. Soc Health Behav. 2019;2:7–12.
12. Okunogbe A, Nugent R, Spencer G, et al. Economic impacts of overweight and obesity: current and future estimates for eight countries. BMJ Glob Health. 2021;6:e006351.
13. Larqué E, Labayen I, Flodmark CE, et al. From conception to infancy—early risk factors for childhood obesity. Nat Rev Endocrinol. 2019;15:456–78. https://doi.org/10.1038/s41574-019-0219-1.
14. Batushansky A, Zhu S, Komaravolu RK, South S, Mehta-D'souza P, Griffin TM. Fundamentals of OA. An initiative of Osteoarthritis and Cartilage Obesity and metabolic factors in OA. Osteoarthritis Cartilage. 2022;30(4):501–15. ISSN 1063-4584. https://doi.org/10.1016/j.joca.2021.06.013.
15. Kessler J, Koebnick C, Smith N, Adams A. Childhood obesity is associated with increased risk of most lower extremity fractures. Clin Orthop Relat Res. 2013;471(4):1199–207. https://doi.org/10.1007/s11999-012-2621-z. PMID: 23054515; PMCID: PMC3586019.
16. Marcus C, Danielsson P, Hagman E. Pediatric obesity-long-term consequences and effect of weight loss. J Intern Med. 2022;292(6):870–91. https://doi.org/10.1111/joim.13547. Epub 2022 Aug 5. PMID: 35883220; PMCID: PMC9805112.
17. Anekwe CV, Jarrell AR, Townsend MJ, et al. Socioeconomics of obesity. Curr Obes Rep. 2020;9:272–9. https://doi.org/10.1007/s13679-020-00398-7.
18. Nicolaidis S. Environment and obesity. Metabolism. 2019;100(Supplement):153942. ISSN 0026-0495. https://doi.org/10.1016/j.metabol.2019.07.006.
19. Kathryn M, Schmitz H, Jeffery RW. Public health interventions for the prevention and treatment of obesity. Med Clin North Am. 2000;84(2):491–512., ISSN 0025-7125,. https://doi.org/10.1016/S0025-7125(05)70233-9.
20. Sherwood NE, et al. Predictors of weight gain in the pound of prevention study. Int J Obes. 2000;24(4):395–403.

# Bariatric Surgery Indications in the 2020s

# 4

Charles E. Hill, Scott A. Shikora, and Shanu N. Kothari

## Introduction

Body mass index (BMI) remains the most widely used criteria to screen and stratify patients for consideration of MBS based on the National Institute of Health (NIH) Consensus Development Conference Statement in 1991 [1]. Based on relevant literature from the 1970s and 1980s when vertical banded gastroplasty and Roux-en-Y gastric bypass (RYGB) were the predominant procedures and were primarily performed via laparotomy, the recommendations were as follows:

- BMI ≥ 40 kg/m$^2$.
- BMI ≥ 35 kg/m$^2$ + major comorbidity.
- Documentation of repeated failure of nonsurgical weight loss attempts.
- No history of major psychological disorder.

These guidelines were revisited in 1998, and though no changes were made as the panel did not take into consideration the impact of laparoscopy, national accreditation formats or recently published randomized clinical trials [2]. In 2007, a new panel convened to review the available literature over a prolonged 5-year period, eventually publishing "the NIH has no official medical or surgical position, consensus statement, or guideline regarding the treatment of obesity" and in 2013, deferring any additional guidelines to the American Heart Association, American College

C. E. Hill · S. N. Kothari (✉)
Department of Surgery, Prisma Health Upstate, Greenville, SC, USA
e-mail: shanu.kothari@prismahealth.org

S. A. Shikora
Department of Surgery, Center for Metabolic and Bariatric Surgery, Brigham and Women's Hospital, and Harvard Medical School, Boston, MA, USA



O. M. Ghanem et al. (eds.), *The SAGES Manual of Metabolic and Bariatric Surgery*, https://doi.org/10.1007/978-3-031-72309-4_4

of Cardiology and The Obesity Society [3]. Shortly thereafter, the NIH consensus development program was retired, and the guidelines have not been similarly examined since. Most major health plans adopted the 1991 guidelines as coverage policy despite undergoing no change in over 30 years. This factor has negatively impacted access to care and limited the available treatment options for the increasingly obese population.

Obesity is now recognized as a chronic disease. An improved understanding of the pathophysiology of obesity and the physiologic effects of MBS has led to improvements in the clinical management of obese patients. Similarly, evolving operative techniques and innovations in laparoscopic, endoscopic and robotic approaches have significantly impacted the types of operations performed, now primarily sleeve gastrectomy (SG) and Roux-en-Y gastric bypass (RYGB) in the United States, and greatly improved the outcomes. The establishment of standardized guidelines for outcomes reporting has also significantly impacted the perception and accessibility of metabolic and bariatric surgery (MBS) [4]. A growing body of literature has shown overall weight loss outcomes of greater than 60% excess weight loss that is durable for up to 20 years after surgery and significantly superior to medical therapy alone [5–7]. Improvements in metabolic syndrome and, in some cases, resolution of comorbidities such as hypertension, T2DM, and hypercholesterolemia, are also seen after MBS.:

The outdated 1991 NIH guidelines are no longer supported by the current evidence and fail to address multiple concerns such as the growing population of patients with class I obesity, the significant treatment gap they encounter, and the arbitrary BMI cutoff of 35 kg/m$^2$. BMI has also been shown to discriminate against age, gender, race/ethnicity, fitness and body composition. Over the last 30 years, MBS has also consistently demonstrated to be cost-effective, to improve quality of life, and to reduce the likelihood of developing significant comorbidities in the future. Delaying surgical intervention only serves to diminish its effectiveness. In recognition of these advances, the guidelines for surgery consideration have been revised in a joint statement [8] from the American Society for Metabolic and Bariatric Surgeons (ASMBS) and the International Federation for the Surgery of Obesity and Metabolic Disorders (IFSO) and include::

- BMI $\geq$ 35 kg/m$^2$, regardless of the presence, absence or severity of comorbidities.
- BMI $\geq$ 30 kg/m$^2$ and the presence of metabolic disease.
- BMI thresholds should be adjusted in certain populations, specifically in the Asian population where BMI $\geq$ 25 kg/m$^2$ is considered clinical obesity.
- There is no upper age limit for consideration of MBS.
- Appropriately selected children/adolescents should be considered for MBS.
- MBS should be considered a bridging therapy to other specialty surgery (joint arthroplasty, abdominal wall reconstruction, organ transplantation).

## General Indications

Multiple studies have now shown MBS to be the most effective treatment for obesity, with substantial, long-lasting results across all BMI classes. Studies including patients with class I obesity (BMI 30–34.9 kg/m$^2$) and T2D have repeatedly demonstrated the benefits of MBS in this population, finding significant 5-year weight loss and improvement in comorbidities [9–15]. Randomized trials evaluating MBS vs medical weight management in this cohort found MBS to have exceptional weight reduction and T2D remission over nonsurgical treatments [16–18]. However, medical weight management remains an appropriate treatment strategy for class I obesity, and a trial of nonsurgical therapy is recommended prior to considering MBS in this group.:

There is a substantial body of evidence endorsing the safety and efficacy of MBS in patients with BMI $\geq$ 35 kg/m$^2$ and supports its application in all patients regardless of the presence or absence of obesity-related conditions [9, 10]. Medical therapy alone has proven ineffective at achieving substantial or durable weight loss, and frequently fails to adequately address comorbidities in order to improve overall health in this population. Additionally, even in the absence of obesity-related comorbidities, this excess body weight represents a threat to general health with the risk of developing comorbidities in the future and negatively impacts quality of life. As such, MBS should be strongly considered in all patients with BMI $\geq$ 35 kg/m$^2$ regardless of an associated metabolic syndrome.

## Special Populations

BMI thresholds have long been considered proportionally linked to morbidity risks, though it is recognized that BMI alone is not a perfect predictor of risk. Independent of sex, age, ethnicity and fat distribution, BMI represents a general estimation of obesity and is not necessarily representative across all groups. Truncal and visceral adiposity distribution, independent of BMI, carries a higher risk of metabolic and cardiovascular disease compared to fat distribution primarily in the extremities. Similarly, the prevalence of diabetes and heart disease is higher in the Asian population at lower BMIs compared to the non-Asian population. Adjusting the obesity threshold in this population to BMI of 25–27.5 kg/m$^2$ may help address this discrepancy. Traditional BMI guidelines should not be a barrier to MBS [10, 19–24].

Obesity is rising in prevalence among children and adolescents and carries the same antecedent morbidity and early mortality risks [25]. With durable weight loss and remission of comorbidities, MBS is safe in patients younger than 18 years old and may be considered in children as young as 5 years old as recent studies have shown pubertal development is not affected by MBS [26–28]. Updated guidelines, published by the American Academy of Pediatrics and the ASMBS, include children/adolescents with class II obesity (BMI $\geq$ 120% of the 95th percentile) and a major comorbidity, or those with class III obesity (BMI ≥ 140% of the 95th percentile) alone [29, 30]. In general, though, the preoperative evaluation is more extensive in this population than that of adults.:

MBS has been performed in older populations in recent years including patients ≥70 years old, with similar beneficial results as in the younger cohort and only slightly higher rates of postop complications [31, 32]. Importantly, frailty and cognitive capacity appear to have a greater impact on complication rates than age alone [33, 34]. As such, there is no recommended patient-age limit when considering MBS, but the general risk of surgery should be evaluated in the context of comorbid disease burden as well as general functional status and frailty risk index.

Severe obesity has a significant impact on surgical outcomes outside of MBS and frequently leads to denial for joint replacements, transplant eligibility, and abdominal wall reconstruction efforts. Citing an increased risk of readmissions, wound infections, deep vein thrombosis and operative technical challenges as reasons for ineligibility, the severely obese patient loses access to procedures that may improve their quality of life. Recent case series of patients undergoing MBS prior to total knee and hip arthroplasty, abdominal wall hernia repair, or solid organ transplant have reported promising results. When MBS is performed prior to total arthroplasty or abdominal wall reconstruction, studies have shown decreases in operative time, hospital length of stay and early morbidity [35–39]. Meaningful weight loss after MBS can improve eligibility for renal transplantation by 50% at 5 years and can significantly impact eligibility in liver and heart transplant candidates [40–42]. Based on these results, MBS should be viewed as a potential bridge to these other surgical therapies to improve eligibility and outcomes.:

## Contraindications

While there are no absolute contraindications to MBS, the relative contraindications for general abdominal surgery, such as severe heart failure, unstable angina, active cancer and severe lung disease are still applicable. The medical complexity of obesity requires a comprehensive risk/benefit analysis and evaluation by a multidisciplinary team to determine eligibility. Certain conditions, such as drug and alcohol dependence, psychiatric illness, and impaired intellectual capacity greatly impact MBS outcomes and the patient's ability to comprehend the necessary dietary and lifestyle modifications necessary after surgery, and preoperative evaluation and treatment are essential to address these issues [43–48].:

Specific populations carry a higher risk of morbidity and mortality and should be counseled appropriately. Increasing BMI represents increased disease burden with consequent increasing morbidity and mortality risk, but MBS can be performed safely in patients with BMI > 70 kg/m$^2$ and should be considered in appropriately evaluated patients [49–52]. Liver disease is a well-established obesity-related comorbidity and carries an increased risk of progression to cirrhosis and subsequent hepatic decompensation (94). In patients with compensated cirrhosis and no evidence of portal hypertension, MBS remains a relatively low risk (mortality <1%)

with substantial benefits including preventing the progression of nonalcoholic liver fatty liver disease to cirrhosis and regression of fibrosis in early cirrhosis [53–57]. Revisional MBS is on the rise as primary MBS operations become more common and obesity as a chronic disease requires long-term management and follow-up. Indications for revisional surgery may include weight regain or insufficient weight loss, poor improvement in comorbidities, or complications from the primary surgery. These operations are increasingly complex and carry higher rates of complications than primary interventions, but effectively provide additional weight loss and comorbidity remission in selected patients [58–60].

## Conclusion

The 2022 joint statement from the ASMBS and IFSO is a contemporary, evidence-based guideline that promotes a broader application of metabolic and bariatric surgery (MBS) to enhance the access to care, quality of life and overall health of individuals with obesity. The statement argues that the outdated NIH guidelines from 1991 should be abandoned and no longer practiced or published. National societies and surgeons should actively support the expanded indications and advocate for payors to adopt the new guidelines for coverage policies.:

## References

1. Consensus N. Gastrointestinal surgery for severe obesity. National Institutes of Health Consensus Development Conference Draft Statement. Am J Clin Nutr. 1992;55(2 Suppl):615S–9S.
2. NHLBI Obesity Education Initiative Expert Panel on the Identification, Evaluation, and Treatment of Obesity in Adults (US). Clinical guidelines on the identification, evaluation, and treatment of overweight and obesity in adults: the evidence report. Bethesda, MD: National Institutes of Health, National Heart, Lung, and Blood Institute; 1998.
3. Jensen MD, Ryan DH, Apovian CM, et al. AHA/ACC/TOS guideline for the management of overweight and obesity in adults: a report of the American College of Cardiology/American Heart Association Task Force on Practice Guidelines and The Obesity Society. J Am College Cardiol. 2013;63(25 Part B):2985–3023.
4. Brethauer SA, Kim J, El Chaar M, et al. Standardized outcomes reporting in metabolic and bariatric surgery. Obes Surg. 2015;25:587–606.
5. Maciejewski ML, Arterburn DE, Van Scoyoc L, et al. Bariatric surgery and long-term durability of weight loss. JAMA Surg. 2016;151(11):1046–55.
6. Buchwald H, Avidor Y, Braunwald E, et al. Bariatric surgery: a systematic review and meta-analysis. JAMA. 2004;292(14):1724–37.
7. Arterburn D, Wellman R, Emiliano A, et al. Comparative effectiveness and safety of bariatric procedures for weight loss: a PCORnet cohort study. Ann Intern Med. 2018;169(11):741–50.
8. Eisenberg D, Shikora SA, Aarts E, et al. 2022 American Society of Metabolic and Bariatric Surgery (ASMBS) and International Federation for the Surgery of Obesity and Metabolic Disorders (IFSO) indications for metabolic and bariatric surgery. Springer; 2023.
9. Rubino F, Nathan D, Eckel R. Metabolic surgery in the treatment algorithm for type 2 diabetes: a joint statement by international diabetes organizations. Diab Care. 2016;39:861–77.

10. Aminian A, Chang J, Brethauer SA, Kim JJ. ASMBS updated position statement on bariatric surgery in class I obesity (BMI 30–35 kg/m$^2$). Surg Obes Relat Dis. 2018;14(8):1071–87.
11. Noun R, Slim R, Nasr M, et al. Results of laparoscopic sleeve gastrectomy in 541 consecutive patients with low baseline body mass index (30–35 kg/m$^2$). Obes Surg. 2016;26:2824–8.
12. Varban OA, Bonham AJ, Finks JF, Telem DA, Obeid NR, Ghaferi AA. Is it worth it? Determining the health benefits of sleeve gastrectomy in patients with a body mass index< 35 kg/m$^2$. Surg Obes Relat Dis. 2020;16(2):248–53.
13. Ikramuddin S, Korner J, Lee W-J, et al. Durability of addition of roux-en-Y gastric bypass to lifestyle intervention and medical management in achieving primary treatment goals for uncontrolled type 2 diabetes in mild to moderate obesity: a randomized control trial. Diabetes Care. 2016;39(9):1510–8.
14. Schauer PR, Bhatt DL, Kirwan JP, et al. Bariatric surgery versus intensive medical therapy for diabetes—5-year outcomes. N Engl J Med. 2017;376(7):641–51.
15. Courcoulas AP, Belle SH, Neiberg RH, et al. Three-year outcomes of bariatric surgery vs lifestyle intervention for type 2 diabetes mellitus treatment: a randomized clinical trial. JAMA Surg. 2015;150(10):931–40.
16. O'Brien PE, Brennan L, Laurie C, Brown W. Intensive medical weight loss or laparoscopic adjustable gastric banding in the treatment of mild to moderate obesity: long-term follow-up of a prospective randomised trial. Obes Surg. 2013;23:1345–53.
17. Parikh M, Chung M, Sheth S, et al. Randomized pilot trial of bariatric surgery vs. intensive medical weight management on diabetes remission in type 2 diabetic patients who do NOT meet NIH criteria for surgery and the role of soluble RAGE as a novel biomarker of success. Ann Surg. 2014;260(4):617.
18. Wentworth JM, Playfair J, Laurie C, et al. Multidisciplinary diabetes care with and without bariatric surgery in overweight people: a randomised controlled trial. Lancet Diabetes Endocrinol. 2014;2(7):545–52.
19. Busetto L, Dixon J, De Luca M, Shikora S, Pories W, Angrisani L. Bariatric surgery in class I obesity: a position statement from the International Federation for the Surgery of obesity and metabolic disorders (IFSO). Obes Surg. 2014;24:487–519.
20. Misra A. Ethnic-specific criteria for classification of body mass index: a perspective for Asian Indians and American Diabetes Association position statement. Diabetes Technol Ther. 2015;17(9):667–71.
21. Hsu WC, Araneta MRG, Kanaya AM, Chiang JL, Fujimoto W. BMI cut points to identify at-risk Asian Americans for type 2 diabetes screening. Diabetes Care. 2015;38(1):150.
22. Gill RS, Karmali S, Sharma AM. The potential role of the Edmonton obesity staging system in determining indications for bariatric surgery. Obes Surg. 2011;21:1947–9.
23. Padwal RS, Pajewski NM, Allison DB, Sharma AM. Using the Edmonton obesity staging system to predict mortality in a population-representative cohort of people with overweight and obesity. CMAJ. 2011;183(14):E1059–66.
24. Frattini F, Lavazza M, Rausei S, Rovera F, Boni L, Dionigi G. BMI: the weakness of a milestone in obesity management and treatment. Obes Surg. 2015;25:1940–1.
25. Reilly JJ, Kelly J. Long-term impact of overweight and obesity in childhood and adolescence on morbidity and premature mortality in adulthood: systematic review. Int J Obes. 2011;35(7):891–8.
26. Olbers T, Beamish AJ, Gronowitz E, et al. Laparoscopic Roux-en-Y gastric bypass in adolescents with severe obesity (AMOS): a prospective, 5-year, Swedish nationwide study. Lancet Diab Endocrinol. 2017;5(3):174–83.
27. Inge TH, Jenkins TM, Xanthakos SA, et al. Long-term outcomes of bariatric surgery in adolescents with severe obesity (FABS-5+): a prospective follow-up analysis. Lancet Diab Endocrinol. 2017;5(3):165–73.
28. Alqahtani AR, Elahmedi M, Abdurabu HY, Alqahtani S. Ten-year outcomes of children and adolescents who underwent sleeve gastrectomy: weight loss, comorbidity resolution, adverse events, and growth velocity. J Am Coll Surg. 2021;233(6):657–64.

29. Pratt JS, Browne A, Browne NT, et al. ASMBS pediatric metabolic and bariatric surgery guidelines, 2018. Surg Obes Relat Dis. 2018;14(7):882–901.
30. Armstrong SC, Bolling CF, Michalsky MP, et al. Pediatric metabolic and bariatric surgery: evidence, barriers, and best practices. Pediatrics. 2019;144(6):e20193223.
31. Al-Kurd A, Grinbaum R, Mordechay-Heyn T, et al. Outcomes of sleeve gastrectomy in septuagenarians. Obes Surg. 2018;28:3895–901.
32. Smith ME, Bacal D, Bonham AJ, et al. Perioperative and 1-year outcomes of bariatric surgery in septuagenarians: implications for patient selection. Surg Obes Relat Dis. 2019;15(10):1805–11.
33. Watt J, Tricco AC, Talbot-Hamon C, et al. Identifying older adults at risk of harm following elective surgery: a systematic review and meta-analysis. BMC Med. 2018;16(1):1–14.
34. Gondal AB, Hsu C-H, Zeeshan M, Hamidi M, Joseph B, Ghaderi I. A frailty index and the impact of frailty on postoperative outcomes in older patients after bariatric surgery. Surg Obes Relat Dis. 2019;15(9):1582–8.
35. McLawhorn AS, Levack AE, Lee Y-y, Ge Y, Do H, Dodwell ER. Bariatric surgery improves outcomes after lower extremity arthroplasty in the morbidly obese: a propensity score-matched analysis of a New York statewide database. J Arthroplast. 2018;33(7):2062–2069.e4.
36. Werner BC, Kurkis GM, Gwathmey FW, Browne JA. Bariatric surgery prior to total knee arthroplasty is associated with fewer postoperative complications. J Arthroplast. 2015;30(9):81–5.
37. Li S, Luo X, Sun H, Wang K, Zhang K, Sun X. Does prior bariatric surgery improve outcomes following total joint arthroplasty in the morbidly obese? A meta-analysis. J Arthroplas. 2019;34(3):577–85.
38. Veilleux E, Lutfi R. Obesity and ventral hernia repair: is there success in staging? J Laparoendosc Adv Surg Tech A. 2020;30(8):896–9.
39. Menzo EL, Hinojosa M, Carbonell A, Krpata D, Carter J, Rogers AM. American Society for Metabolic and Bariatric Surgery and American Hernia Society consensus guideline on bariatric surgery and hernia surgery. Surg Obes Relat Dis. 2018;14(9):1221–32.
40. Yemini R, Nesher E, Carmeli I, et al. Bariatric surgery is efficacious and improves access to transplantation for morbidly obese renal transplant candidates. Obes Surg. 2019;29:2373–80.
41. Al-Bahri S, Fakhry TK, Gonzalvo JP, Murr MM. Bariatric surgery as a bridge to renal transplantation in patients with end-stage renal disease. Obes Surg. 2017;27:2951–5.
42. Lee Y, Anvari S, Soon MS, et al. Bariatric surgery as a bridge to heart transplantation in morbidly obese patients: a systematic review and meta-analysis. Cardiol Rev. 2022;30(1):1–7.
43. Mechanick J, Kushner R, Sugerman H, et al. AACE/TOS/ASMBS guidelines: American Association of Clinical Endocrinologists, The Obesity Society, and American Society for Metabolic & Bariatric Surgery Medical Guidelines for Clinical Practice for the perioperative nutritional, metabolic, and nonsurgical support of the bariatric surgery patient. Obesity. 2009;17(1s):S1–70.
44. Rebibo L, Maréchal V, De Lameth I, et al. Compliance with a multidisciplinary team meeting's decision prior to bariatric surgery protects against major postoperative complications. Surg Obes Relat Dis. 2017;13(9):1537–43.
45. Bullen NL, Parmar J, Gilbert J, Clarke M, Cota A, Finlay IG. How effective is the multidisciplinary team approach in bariatric surgery? Obes Surg. 2019;29:3232–8.
46. SAGES Guidelines Committee. SAGES guideline for clinical application of laparoscopic bariatric surgery. Springer; 2008.
47. Kinzl JF, Schrattenecker M, Traweger C, Mattesich M, Fiala M, Biebl W. Psychosocial predictors of weight loss after bariatric surgery. Obes Surg. 2006;16(12):1609–14.
48. Pull CB. Current psychological assessment practices in obesity surgery programs: what to assess and why. Curr Opin Psychiatry. 2010;23(1):30–6.
49. Whitlock G, Lewington S, Sherliker P, et al. Prospective Studies Collaboration: body-mass index and cause-specific mortality in 900 000 adults: collaborative analyses of 57 prospective studies. Lancet. 2009;373(9669):1083–96.
50. Wilkinson KH, Helm M, Lak K, Higgins RM, Gould JC, Kindel TL. The risk of post-operative complications in super-super obesity compared to super obesity in accredited bariatric surgery centers. Obes Surg. 2019;29:2964–71.

51. Stephens DJ, Saunders JK, Belsley S, et al. Short-term outcomes for super-super obese (BMI≥ 60 kg/m²) patients undergoing weight loss surgery at a high-volume bariatric surgery center: laparoscopic adjustable gastric banding, laparoscopic gastric bypass, and open tubular gastric bypass. Surg Obes Relat Dis. 2008;4(3):408–15.
52. Roland JC, Needleman BJ, Muscarella P, Cook CH, Narula VK, Mikami DJ. Laparoscopic Roux-en-Y gastric bypass in patients with body mass index> 70 kg/m². Surg Obes Relat Dis. 2011;7(5):587–91.
53. Aminian A, Al-Kurd A, Wilson R, et al. Association of bariatric surgery with major adverse liver and cardiovascular outcomes in patients with biopsy-proven nonalcoholic steatohepatitis. JAMA. 2021;326(20):2031–42.
54. Patton H, Heimbach J, McCullough A. AGA clinical practice update on bariatric surgery in cirrhosis: expert review. Clin Gastroenterol Hepatol. 2021;19(3):436–45.
55. Ahmed S, Pouwels S, Parmar C, et al. Outcomes of bariatric surgery in patients with liver cirrhosis: a systematic review. Obes Surg. 2021;31:2255–67.
56. Mumtaz K, Lipshultz H, Jalil S, et al. Bariatric surgery in patients with cirrhosis: careful patient and surgery-type selection is key to improving outcomes. Obes Surg. 2020;30:3444–52.
57. Jan A, Narwaria M, Mahawar KK. A systematic review of bariatric surgery in patients with liver cirrhosis. Obes Surg. 2015;25:1518–26.
58. Ma P, Reddy S, Higa KD. Revisional bariatric/metabolic surgery: what dictates its indications? Curr Atheroscler Rep. 2016;18(7):42.
59. Brethauer SA, Kothari S, Sudan R, et al. Systematic review on reoperative bariatric surgery: American society for metabolic and bariatric surgery revision task force. Surg Obes Relat Dis. 2014;10(5):952–72.
60. Lazzati A, Bechet S, Jouma S, Paolino L, Jung C. Revision surgery after sleeve gastrectomy: a nationwide study with 10 years of follow-up. Surg Obes Relat Dis. 2020;16(10):1497–504.

# 5 The Role of the Advanced Practice Provider, Social Worker, and Physical Therapist in the Management of the Bariatric Patient

Julia Jurgensen and Ishna Sharma

## Introduction

An integrated health approach is the key to success for a bariatric patient. A typical bariatric surgery center involves care from advanced providers including nurse practitioners, physician assistants, social workers, as well as physical therapists, in addition to other health care professionals. Advances in the roles of these professionals include the more widespread use of telehealth and remote platforms for patient care. This has been of especially important note after the 2019 COVID pandemic restricted in-person care options [1]. Additionally, the role of self-monitoring tools and devices at home for patients also continues to grow in this field [2]. While the roles of these professionals have been previously established for bariatric surgery, the modalities of care continue to evolve. As more patients undergo bariatric surgery, long-term postoperative considerations such as weight regain also create opportunities for these professionals to further impact patient care and outcomes.

## Introduction of Social Worker

A social worker is a licensed mental health provider who helps patients in a variety of aspects. This includes a patient's behavioral, economic, social, and environmental needs. Social workers, though not mandatory, have traditionally been involved in the preoperative workup of bariatric surgical patients, as they provide a valuable tool in assessing a patient's environmental support, which will be important to their

J. Jurgensen (✉) · I. Sharma
Department of Metabolic Surgery, Mayo Clinic, Rochester, MN, USA
e-mail: jurgensen.julia@mayo.edu


O. M. Ghanem et al. (eds.), *The SAGES Manual of Metabolic and Bariatric Surgery*, https://doi.org/10.1007/978-3-031-72309-4_5

success through their weight management journey. Furthermore, enhanced recovery programs across surgical disciplines typically include a social worker for immediate postoperative support as well [3].

## Preoperative Assessment

The current American Society of Metabolic and Bariatric Surgery (ASMBS) Guidelines for psychosocial evaluation as well as the Metabolic and Bariatric Surgery Accreditation and Quality Improvement Program (MBSAQIP) require a psychosocial evaluation of a bariatric surgery candidate to be performed by a credentialed provider, which includes social workers [4]. A behavioral health specialist in an accredited bariatric center in the United States can be a clinical psychologist, clinical social worker, clinical counselor, psychiatrist, or psychiatric nurse. They typically establish a relationship with the patient preoperatively and continue this relationship both immediately postoperatively as well as during long-term postoperative follow up to provide continuity of care. While patients may want to use their own psychologist, this should be discouraged for the preoperative bariatric evaluation, as they may not know how to perform a comprehensive bariatric evaluation and may not be familiar with counseling a postoperative bariatric patient. While there is currently no standardization beyond this, it is recommended that an individualized patient-centric approach be taken, and involvement of further expertise from psychologists or psychiatrists should be at the behavioral health specialist's discretion. This preoperative discussion should include the following topics.

### Knowledge of Bariatric Surgery

There is a diverse range of understanding of what defines bariatric surgical success, amongst patients as well as amongst healthcare providers [5]. Discussion with a social worker preoperatively provides an opportunity to discuss expectations of the weight management journey, including the surgical component, with the patient. This includes establishing a patient understanding that it is expected for the patient to continue an active role in their journey preoperatively as well as postoperatively. This will likely include a role for attending and participating in postoperative visits, support groups, and self-monitoring. Thankfully, the social elements of a patient's circumstances do not appear to play a large role in patients being dismissed from academic bariatric surgical programs, with the likely explanation that the vast majority of hurdles in this realm can be managed successfully [6].

### Patient Motivation Evaluation

There is a high incidence of comorbid mental health conditions in patients suffering from obesity, including depression, anxiety, negative body image, and negative quality of life [7]. These should be elicited and discussed preoperatively, as management of these conditions, with a plan in place for postoperative continued management, will likely lead to improved overall care for the patient.

### Setting Expectations

Patients have varying expectations from bariatric surgery, and establishing realistic expectations preoperatively is important to overall success. Studies show that when patients are asked about their perceived benefits from surgical intervention, they focus on the psychosocial benefits, rather than the medical changes [8].

### Quality of Life

Patients report concerns with negative quality of life associated with obesity, including social stigma in public, as well as discrimination [8]. They additionally report physical limitations from obesity as a further motivation for surgery [9]. A social worker can help to highlight a patient's specific motivations, and ensure that these are in alignment with realistic expectations from bariatric surgical management. Studies show that these physical limitations do typically improve post-bariatric surgery; however, they do require continued individualized motivation and efforts to sustain [10].

### Support System

The need for social support is well established in successful outcomes for bariatric surgical patients. A preoperative interview with the social worker allows for both assessment of a patient's current support system, as well as an opportunity to highlight the importance of this system in the patient's weight management journey, especially postoperatively. Studies show that high levels of emotional support are protective against weight gain over time, especially in male patients [11]. Patients on extreme ends of the age spectrum, including adolescent patients as well as the elderly, especially benefit from an assessment of available social support [12].

### Environmental and Economic Stressors

There is generally a lack of community, and even a healthcare provider's, understanding of the specific difficulties that come with postoperative bariatric surgical management especially if there is a prevalent bias of surgery as the "easy way out" from obesity [5]. Reviewing this with the patient preoperatively in the setting of a social worker interaction allows for the opportunity to address this with the patient, and educate them on expectations and plans for managing this aspect of post-bariatric surgical care life. Support groups, both preoperatively and postoperatively, are an integral part of this process as well [13]. Furthermore, one part of a bariatric program's time and resource dedication could be for the social worker team to engage in community level initiatives to help combat these biases.

The economic needs of a patient can compound the already harmful effects from the disease of obesity. A social worker evaluation and meeting can help to address these issues and ensure that the patient has reasonable plans in place for postoperative economic management.

### Substance Use and Abuse Screening

The ASMBS position statement of 2021 summarizes extensive data detailing the harmful effects of smoking tobacco for postoperative outcomes for bariatric surgical patients. As such, they recommend smoking cessation completed by 6 weeks prior to a bariatric surgery [14]. The social worker can help to counsel patients on the importance of maintaining smoking cessation both preoperatively and postoperatively, and can serve as a resource for continued efforts.

Marijuana use continues to increase in the United States; however, there is limited data on its safety in bariatric surgery [14]. While marijuana use has not been found to worsen short term outcomes from surgery, more studies are needed for long-term outcomes [15, 16]. Furthermore, effects of marijuana use such as cannabinoid hyperemesis may also need to be taken into consideration when assessing postoperative patient issues. As such, a social worker can help counsel a patient on the role of marijuana use and guide efforts to cessate such use.

Bariatric surgical patients, specifically gastric bypass patients, have been found to have a high risk of developing alcohol use disorder postoperatively [17]. The ASMBS advises alcohol use counseling preoperatively as well as a period of time of abstinence preoperatively [17]. The social worker can aid in the counseling regarding this as well as efforts to cessate from alcohol, and can also promote healthy patterns for alcohol use in the postoperative setting as well.

### Eating Disorders

Bariatric patients may have eating disorders preoperatively, and are also susceptible to developing eating disorders postoperatively [18–20]. Screening for disorders preoperatively by a behavioral health specialist such as a social worker is important to assess appropriateness of a surgical procedure for a patient with an active eating disorder. Furthermore, continued involvement of behavioral health postoperatively provides the opportunity to address any developing disordered eating in the postoperative setting.

## Additional Roles in Postoperative Care

Social workers help patients both immediately following the surgery, in promoting patient wellness, autonomy, family support, and discharge resource planning for setting a safe and secure environment post-hospital stay. They can also be a point of support and communication during the postoperative transition phase for the patient.

### Weight Regain

A minority of bariatric patients experience weight regain, and for these patients it is likely important to provide continued behavioral health and support postoperatively. In addition to barriers such as time restrictions, geographic distance, and financial burdens, bariatric patients may additionally have personal feelings of guilt and embarrassment that further inhibit attempts to reach out for assistance. Perioperative counseling for patients should likely include the guidance to reach back out to the behavioral health provider such as the social worker if a patient notices that they are beginning to regain weight, regardless of the postoperative time frame. Remotely delivered options such as Project HELP have also shown positive results in reversing weight regain [21]. APOLO-Bari is another internet-based program for postoperative bariatric patients which showed similarly positive results for weight loss and weight maintenance [22]. As more patients are undergoing bariatric surgery, weight regain continues to be an important topic of study. It is also important to patients and surgeons to understand that about 20% of patients are either resistant to MBS or susceptible to weight regain, so it is important for patients to follow up with their program to rule out anatomical causes for this and work with their social worker and mental health teams to rule out behavioral and psychological causes of this.

#### Telehealth and Remote Monitoring

Weight maintenance and continued health postoperatively requires long-term monitoring. However, time restrictions, geographic limitations, and financial burden can be significant barriers for patients in access to this monitoring [23]. Remote options including telehealth visits with professionals such as behavioral health specialists may help with these barriers. One survey of bariatric patients shows that an overwhelming majority would be interested in telehealth options for postoperative visits [24]. This became especially important during the 2019 COVID pandemic, with a renewed interest in remote options for perioperative bariatric patient care [25, 26]. Remote options in general may also help with the disparity of access to bariatric care, where patients in rural settings benefit from increased perioperative access to behavioral health and other healthcare professionals, increasing equitable access to specialized care [27, 28]. Furthermore, studies are increasingly finding that telehealth visits are not substandard to in-person visits [29]. The BELLA pilot trial has even found that follow up in mobile applications alone may be beneficial, further reducing the costs associated with healthcare visits for patients; however, more data is needed for long-term bariatric specific outcomes [30]. A different mobile health feasibility study found similarly positive results [31]. Technology in the realm of behavioral health assessment and management continues to be an important area of development.

### Conclusion of the Social Worker

A psychologist or psychiastrist who is knowledgable about bariatric surgery should be involved in a patient's care whenever possible especially in the setting of any pre-existing mental health concerns. There are many nonmedical aspects of a patient's life, including the personal, familial, societal, economic, and environmental factors, that impact their weight and health management journey. A social worker can provide the support, tools, and resources to assist a patient in these realms, and bring better success to their outcomes and experience in the process.

### Introduction of the Advanced Practice Provider

Advanced practice providers (APPs) have a rich history over several decades of providing high-quality and cost-effective patient care. As a result of this history,

APPs have become commonplace in healthcare settings. It is projected that the APP role will see continued growth between now and 2030, as nurse practitioners (NPs) and physician assistants (PAs) are expected to increase in numbers by 50% and 43%, respectively, during that time [32]. The increased utilization of APPs is due to several reasons, including a shift in academic institutions in response to the Accreditation Council of Graduate Medical Education resident duty hours restriction, a reduction in available primary care providers, increased patient safety or quality of care needs, continuity of care needs, and assistance with a reduction in length of stay (LOS) [33, 34].

The presence of APPs has been shown to reduce healthcare costs. These savings are due to several factors, including salary, excellent documentation and reduction in last minute surgical cancellations. APPs' salaries are typically approximately half of a primary care physician's salary. This gap is larger when comparing the APPs' salary to that of a surgeon, which increases the savings when utilizing an APP in a surgeon's practice. Additionally, Kidd, 2023 notes that APPs provide safe, cost-effective care with excellent patient outcomes [35]. Therefore, embedding APPs into a surgical practice can increase patient access while continuing excellent patient care. This is likely due to APPs' ability to decrease the clinical burden of surgical providers. This also allows for more timely and reliable documentation, more availability for consultations while the surgeon is operating, more time to research the medical history while the surgeon is in surgery, all of which results in reducing the last minute cancellation of surgeries [36].

## Nurse Practitioner and Physician Assistant Role

APPs are educated in an advanced setting with either a master's or doctorate degree. NPs have completed a master's or doctoral degree in nursing typically after working as a bedside nurse [34]. Academic NP programmes follow educational standards to ensure the attainment of consistent core competencies at the time of graduation [37]. NP programs focus on specific population foci, such as family medicine, adult geriatric medicine, pediatrics or acute care [35]. In comparison, PAs complete a master's degree in a medical school-based curriculum that is regulated by state medical boards. PAs typically start their schooling after working in the medical field for one to 3 years in a variety of licensed or non-licensed positions [38]. Most PA programs train students to be generalists rather than focusing on a specific population [35]. One of the largest differences between the two professions is that PAs are required to practice in collaboration with a physician, while NP practice requirements vary state to state, with many states' regulations allowing NPs to practice autonomously [34]. Despite these differences in most clinical settings, NPs and PAs perform similar tasks.

NP and PA salaries are similar, according to the US Bureau of Labor Statistics [39]. The average NP salary in 2023 was $124,680, and the average PA salary was $125,270 [39]. The highest salaries for APPs are currently on the West Coast and are higher in the urban setting than in the rural setting [39].

## APPs in the Hospital Setting

According to the AANP, 83.3% of hospital medicine groups reported APP utilization, with 10% of NPs and 41.5% of PAs reporting their main clinical setting in the hospital [40]. Given this high level of utilization, APPs are often seen as a key member of the interdisciplinary team in the hospital and are utilized in numerous roles, including rounding on patients, ordering and interpreting needed testing, completing of discharge paperwork, patient education and assisting in the operating room. The involvement of APPs in hospitalized patients has been shown to increase continuity of patient care as well because APPs do not rotate as often as residents [33].

Studies have shown that increased interdisciplinary care combined with consistent providers has helped improve inpatient patient care and decreases hospital length of stay [33, 41]. Nurses spend the most time with patients, and engagement between the surgical team and nurses is a crucial piece of hospital patient care. Van Soeren et al. found that APPs were seen as approachable by the nursing team, which increased teamwork between the providers and nurses. APPs have been reported to be the "hub, or glue" that keeps interdisciplinary hospital teams together [41]. This is likely due to increased familiarity with the hospital staff, hospital environment and patients in comparison to residents who are frequently changing.

Another essential task that APPs assist with is completion of necessary paperwork, such as discharge paperwork starting immediately after surgery. In the current healthcare environment, streamlining hospital discharge after bariatric surgery is crucial. Additionally, APPs can assist with ensuring that patients receive consistent discharge education. The work that APPs are doing with preparing paperwork, discharge planning and patient education plays a role in length of stay. It has also been noted that the length of stay has been reduced by up to 2 days as a result of utilizing APPs in the hospital setting [34].

## APPs in the Operating Room

APPs can play an important role in the operating room and can play an integral role in the continuity of patient care. APPs can utilize numerous skill sets by combining the surgical first assist role with their traditional role in patient care, both outpatient and inpatient. When APPs are utilized in the operating room, their scope of practice may include roles both in and out of the operating room or isolated to the operating room alone as the surgical first assistant.

Licensure for APPs to work in the operating room differs between the NP and PA. NPs may be required to obtain the registered nurse's first assistant certification to practice as a surgical first assistant. PAs typically enter surgical practice by one of three routes: graduation from a surgically focused PA program, completion of a surgical residency for PAs after graduating from PA school or on-the-job training [42].

## APPs in the Clinic Setting

Utilizing APPs in the clinic setting may be the most valuable utilization of an APP in surgical practice. Given that APPs can work independently in the clinic setting, they are able to treat and diagnose patients pre- and post-surgery, thus increasing the surgeon's ability to focus on the operating room. Kidd et al. noted that the independence of an APP's clinical practice improves clinical capacity, patient satisfaction, workflow optimization and potential downstream revenue improvement [35].

This is due to the APPs' focused clinical time, which is typically longer per patient visit than a surgeon and allows the APP to spend more time educating the patient. Studies have recommended that increased utilization of APPs may positively impact the overall quality of healthcare by creating a patient-centered care system that can decrease the overall cost of healthcare with the lower salary of the APP [43].

An additional long-term postoperative bariatric patient concern that APPs can help with is weight regain. Weight regain after bariatric surgery is common and utilization of the APP in the clinic to assess and manage weight regain can be valuable. Weight regain can be time consuming and challenging to manage for clinicians. APPs often have more focused clinical time to dedicate to this portion of the bariatric surgery practice. Additionally, studies have shown that lower attrition rates in post-surgical clinics are correlated with additional weight loss.

The modality for APP visits is expanding, as telehealth visits are now increasingly offered across healthcare. The use of telehealth for postoperative bariatric surgical patients has been shown to be at least as effective as in-person visits [44]. Therefore, the utilization of APPs and telehealth in the bariatric setting can improve patient access to the bariatric surgery team.

## Conclusion of the Advanced Practice Provider

APPs can be utilized in numerous settings and roles on the bariatric team. They can be utilized in both the clinic and hospital setting including the operating room. They can be utilized pre- and post-surgery to ensure high-quality patient care. In addition, utilization of APPs on the bariatric team is cost effective and can increase revenue by providing high-quality care freeing up the surgeon for the operating room.

## Introduction of the Physical Therapist

Physical therapists (PTs) have a rich history in patient care. The profession was developed in the late 1800s and rapidly advanced during the polio outbreak and World War I [45]. In the decades following the development of the profession, PTs have helped millions of patients with rehabilitation after surgery, injury, and debilitating disease. The literature shows that physical therapy reduces healthcare costs for patients by avoiding surgery and reducing recovery time and/or pharmaceutical costs.

PTs are educated in the advanced setting and require a bachelor's degree followed by a doctorate degree. After degree completion, many PT graduates enroll in a residency or fellowship program prior to beginning formal employment [46].

PTs work in both inpatient and outpatient settings. They can play a crucial role in bariatric surgery before and after surgery. Bariatric surgery patients need physical activity both before and after surgery to reduce surgical complications and increase weight loss success. PTs can assist patients in their physical activity journeys.

## Rationale for PT Involvement

Bariatric surgery is considered an elective procedure, and therefore, attention should be given to maximizing patient health prior to surgery to minimize complications. Numerous studies have shown that a patient's level of pre-surgery physical function is a predictor of postoperative complications and morbidity. Prior to surgery, the primary goal of PT is to reduce the risk of surgery and complications from surgery. Activity has been suggested to increase patient weight loss outcomes and weight maintenance of weight loss long term [47]. The most significant of these complications include pulmonary embolism, postoperative pneumonia and cardiac events.

The role of the PT shifts goals from pre-surgery risk reduction to maximizing weight loss and improving health post-surgery. Post-surgery, patients need to meet ongoing exercise requirements for maximizing weight loss while managing health conditions. PTs have expertise in both areas, and utilization of a PT can help increase the success of bariatric surgery while minimizing surgical risks.

## Initial Evaluation Recommendation

The initial assessment completed by a PT for a patient undergoing bariatric surgery includes a physical assessment of the patient's baseline abilities and the ability to develop long-term exercise goals. This first assessment will guide the PT regarding the length of time needed for therapy and assist with goal setting.

This initial assessment should also include consideration of the patient's weight, BMI, body type, vital signs, pain level, palpation, skin integrity, strengths, weaknesses, posture, endurance, range of motion and functional physical ability [48]. Consideration should be given to recording and tracking the patient's body composition as well. In terms of physical ability assessment, attention should be given to the following [48]:

Ability to walk.
Previous level of activity/fitness.
Gait—ability, coordination disturbance.
Utilization of gait assistant tools.
Fall risk.
Medications with possible effects on patient mobility.
Musculoskeletal limitations.

Mobility getting in and out of a chair/bed.
Pain level related to chronic comorbidities.

Additionally, improving a patient's exercise tolerance with walking can reduce risk postoperatively. Studies have shown an inverse relationship between cardiovascular fitness and complications post-bariatric surgery [49]. ASMBS recommends aerobic and resistance training of 20 min per day, 3–4 days per week before bariatric surgery to improve cardiovascular results, reduce surgical complications and enhance healing postoperatively [50]. Many bariatric surgery patients are unable to meet this recommendation; therefore, an initial evaluation of aerobic ability is crucial. Aerobic ability is commonly tested with the following tests [48, 51].

The six-minute walk test (quantifies aerobic ability).
Timed or untimed stair climb (functional impairment assessment).
Two-minute vital sign recovery assessment (best if patients are unable to tolerate timed testing).
Rate of perceived exertion (evaluates exercise intensity).

## Role of the PT in the Hospital

The most effective way to shorten recovery time after bariatric surgery is movement. This movement starts in the hospital with walking beginning the day of surgery. PTs are important members of the medical team for getting patients out of bed and walking safely. Additionally, PTs are the team members best equipped to assess patients for equipment needs. Common equipment used during hospitalization includes but is not limited to commodes, wheelchairs, transfer equipment, appropriate beds and chairs.

Hospitalization after bariatric surgery is typically between one and 3 days. Involving PTs in the patient's care immediately postoperatively is key to maximizing utilization during the hospital stay. Goals during the hospital stay can include but are not limited to [48]:

Getting out of bed on day zero.
Getting out of bed independently with or without assistive devices.
Adequate respiratory response (oxygen sats appropriate while ambulating).
Independent ambulation with or without assistive devices.

## Long-Term and Postoperative Recommendations

After surgery, the primary goal of the PT is to maximize weight loss while managing conditions such as arthritis, fibromyalgia, osteoporosis and joint pain. ASMBS, the Obesity Society, and the American Association of Clinical Endocrinologists agree that postoperative bariatric surgery patients who perform at least 30 min of exercise per day and follow the recommended post-bariatric diet have a better chance of achieving optimal body weight and improved body composition [52]. Physical therapy can be used to minimize muscle mass loss and improve aerobic function during the rapid weight loss stage after bariatric surgery.

Many post-bariatric surgery patients will need to build up to the recommended 30 min or more of exercise daily [53]. This can be accomplished with a variety of exercises, including walking, swimming, elliptical, and biking (stationary or conventional). Implementing physical therapy and exercise early after bariatric surgery is well known to further weight loss, improve quality of life, and improve mobility and strength [54]. The utilization of self-monitoring physical activity devices can assist patients with meeting this goal and can be reviewed by the PT to determine goals at subsequent visits.

Patients who work with PTs are able to gain the knowledge and confidence that is needed to continue exercising after bariatric surgery. PTs' knowledge in the development of a safe exercise program that includes both aerobic exercise and resistance training is critical to the long-term success of bariatric surgery patients. The long-term goal of surgery and physical therapy should lead to improvement in the functional status and energy levels of the patient. Ultimately, the prognosis of these patients depends on the type of bariatric surgery, the type of exercise program, and the patient's compliance with the diet and exercise regimen that he or she has been given.

### Conclusion of the Physical Therapist

Embedding PTs into the bariatric surgery practice can assist with preparing patients for surgery and reduce surgical complications including pulmonary embolism, postoperative pneumonia and cardiac events. Additionally, utilization of PTs post-surgery can maximize weight loss outcomes and help minimize muscle loss for patients during rapid weight loss. PTs can be utilized in the clinic and hospital setting, therefore involvement of PTs should be early and often in the care of bariatric surgery patients.

## Conclusion

The social worker, APP and PT play critical roles on the bariatric surgery team both pre- and post-surgery. The social worker is an integral member of the behavioral health component of bariatric patient care. The APP role has expanded significantly over the past few decades and their role can be tailored to each bariatric surgery practice. APPs can be utilized in the clinic, hospital and OR setting making them a crucial member of the team and making the team run more efficiently. Physical therapy plays a key role in both the pre-surgery phase preparing patients for surgery, as well as post-surgery to help maximize weight loss without significant muscle loss. All members of the bariatric team play a crucial role in the success of bariatric surgery and should be utilized to their full scope of practice within the team. The ASMBS Integrated Health Track is one resource for continued medical education and certifications available for these professionals [55].

Bariatric patients benefit from the continued involvement of advanced practice providers, behavioral health specialists such as social workers, and physical therapists. The modalities by which these services can be accessed by patients are continuing to evolve.

## References


1. Musella M, Martines G, Berardi G, Picciariello A, Trigiante G, Vitiello A. Lessons from the COVID-19 pandemic: remote coaching in bariatric surgery. Langenbeck's Arch Surg. 2022;407(7):2763–7.
2. van Ede ES, Scheerhoorn J, Bonomi AG, Buise MP, Bouwman RA, Nienhuijs SW. Continuous remote monitoring in post-bariatric surgery patients: development of an early warning protocol. Surg Obes Relat Dis. 2022;18(11):1298–303.
3. Smith TW, Wang X, Singer MA, Godellas CV, Vaince FT. Enhanced recovery after surgery: a clinical review of implementation across multiple surgical subspecialties. Am J Surg. 2020;219(3):530–4.
4. Sogg S, Lauretti J, West-Smith L. Recommendations for the presurgical psychosocial evaluation of bariatric surgery patients. Surg Obes Relat Dis. 2016;12(4):731–49.
5. Sherf-Dagan S, Schechter L, Lapidus R, Sakran N, Goitein D, Raziel A. Perceptions of success in bariatric surgery: a nationwide survey among medical professionals. Obes Surg. 2018;28(1):135–41.
6. Tsuda S, Barrios L, Schneider B, Jones DB. Factors affecting rejection of bariatric patients from an academic weight loss program. Surg Obes Relat Dis. 2009;5(2):199–202.
7. Greenberg I, Perna F, Kaplan M, Sullivan MA. Behavioral and psychological factors in the assessment and treatment of obesity surgery patients. Obes Res. 2005;13(2):244–9.
8. Bocchieri LE, Meana M, Fisher BL. A review of psychosocial outcomes of surgery for morbid obesity. J Psychosom Res. 2002;52(3):155–65.
9. Wee CC, Davis RB, Husky KW, Jones DB, Hame MB. Quality of life among obese patients seeking weight loss surgery: the importance of obesity-related social stigma and functional status. J Gen Intern Med. 2013;28(2):231–8.
10. Kovacs SJ, Courcoulas AP, Rogers RJ, Davis KK, Jakicic JM. Psychosocial factors associated with physical activity in patients who have undergone bariatric surgery. Surg Obes Relat Dis. 2020;16(12):1994–2005.
11. Tymoszuk U, Kumari M, Batterham R, Stafford M. Social support and trajectories of body mass index and waist to hip ratio from mid-adulthood to old age. J Epidemiol Community Health. 2019;73(2):111–6.
12. Cazzo E, Gestic MA, Utrini MP, et al. Bariatric surgery in the elderly: a narrative review. Rev Assoc Med Bras (1992). 2017;63(9):787–92.
13. Bauchowitz AU, Gonder-Frederick LA, Olbrisch ME, Azarbad L, Ryee MY, Woodson M, et al. Psychosocial evaluation of bariatric surgery candidates: a survey of present practices. Psychosom Med. 2005;67(5):825–32.
14. Carter J, Chang J, Birriel TJ, et al. ASMBS position statement on preoperative patient optimization before metabolic and bariatric surgery. Surg Obes Relat Dis. 2021;17(12):1956–76. https://doi.org/10.1016/j.soard.2021.08.024.
15. Shockcor N, Adnan SM, Siegel A, Wise E, Zafar SN, Kligman M. Marijuana use does not affect the outcomes of bariatric surgery. Surg Endosc. 2021;35(3):1264–8.

16. Worrest T, Malibiran CC, Welshans J, Dewey E, Husain F. Marijuana use does not affect weight loss or complication rate after bariatric surgery. Surg Endosc. 2022;36(9):6931–6.
17. Parikh M, Johnson JM, Ballem N. American Society for Metabolic and Bariatric Surgery Clinical Issues Committee. ASMBS position statement on alcohol use before and after bariatric surgery. Surg Obes Relat Dis. 2016;12(2):225–30.
18. Taba JV, Suzuki MO, Nascimento FS, et al. The development of feeding and eating disorders after bariatric surgery: a systematic review and meta-analysis. Nutrients. 2021;13(7):2396.
19. Aylward L, Konsor M, Cox S. Binge eating before and after bariatric surgery. Curr Obes Rep. 2022;11(4):386–94.
20. Sarwer DB, Allison KC, Wadden TA, et al. Psychopathology, disordered eating, and impulsivity as predictors of outcomes of bariatric surgery. Surg Obes Relat Dis. 2019;15(4):650–5.
21. Bradley LE, Forman EM, Kerrigan SG, et al. Project help: a remotely delivered behavioral intervention for weight regain after bariatric surgery. Obes Surg. 2017;27(3):586–98.
22. Conceição EM, Machado PPP, Vaz AR, et al. APOLO-Bari, an internet-based program for longitudinal support of bariatric surgery patients: study protocol for a randomized controlled trial. Trials. 2016;17(1):114.
23. Bradley LE, Thomas JG, Hood MM, Corsica JA, Kelly MC, Sarwer DB. Remote assessments and behavioral interventions in post-bariatric surgery patients. Surg Obes Relat Dis. 2018;14(10):1632–44.
24. Bradley LE, Sarwer DB, Forman EM, Kerrigan SG, Butryn ML, Herbert JD. A survey of bariatric surgery patients' interest in postoperative interventions. Obes Surg. 2016;26(2):332–8.
25. Gualtieri P, Marchetti M, Renzo LD, et al. Impact of COVID-19 on the destiny of bariatric patients. Nutrients. 2022;15(1):163.
26. Hasnain N, Moeed A, Waqar E, Farhan SA, Amreek F. Efficacy of bariatric surgery in COVID-19 patients: an updated systematic review and meta-analysis. Surg Pract Sci. 2022;11:100140.
27. Maurice AP, Punnasseril JEJ, King SE, Dodd BR. Improving access to bariatric surgery for rural and remote patients: experiences from a state-wide bariatric telehealth service in Australia. Obes Surg. 2020;30(11):4401–10.
28. Sudan R, Salter M, Lynch T, Jacobs DO. Bariatric surgery using a network and teleconferencing to serve remote patients in the Veterans Administration Health Care System: feasibility and results. Am J Surg. 2011;202(1):71–6.
29. van Ede ES, Scheerhoorn J, Buise MP, Bouwman RA, Nienhuijs SW. Telemonitoring for perioperative care of outpatient bariatric surgery: preference-based randomized clinical trial. PLoS One. 2023;18(2):e0281992.
30. Yang C, Kessler M, Taebi N, et al. Remote follow-up with a mobile application is equal to traditional outpatient follow-up after bariatric surgery: the Bella pilot trial. Obes Surg. 2023;33(6):1702–9.
31. Wright C, Kelly JT, Byrnes J, et al. A non-randomised feasibility study of a mHealth follow-up program in bariatric surgery. Pilot Feasib Stud. 2023;9(1):176.
32. Mosher A. Nurse practitioner job outlook by state—(2023 updated) retrieved on 09/18/2023. (nursingprocess.org).
33. Collins N, et al. Outcomes of adding acute care nurse practitioners to a Level I trauma service with the goal of decreased length of stay and improved physician and nursing satisfaction. J Trauma Acute Care Surg. 2014;76(2):353–7. https://doi.org/10.1097/TA.0000000000000097. PMID: 24398767.
34. Johal J, Dodd A. Physician extenders on surgical services: a systematic review. Can J Surg. 2017;60(3):172–8. https://doi.org/10.1503/cjs.001516. PMID: 28327274; PMCID: PMC5453759.
35. Kidd VD, Amin A, Bhatia N, Healey D, Fisher C, Rafiq M, Gallegos E, MJA, Munoz K. Optimal use of advanced practice providers at an Academic Medical Center: a first-year retrospective review. Cureus. 2023;15(1):e34475. https://doi.org/10.7759/cureus.34475. PMID: 36733574; PMCID: PMC9889205.

36. Sebach A, Rockelli L, Reddish W, Jarosinkski J, Dolan C. Development of a nurse practitioner–managed preoperative evaluation clinic within a multispecialty orthopedic practice. J Nurse Pract. 2015;11(9):869–77. https://doi.org/10.1016/j.nurpra.2015.06.006.
37. American Academy of Nurse Practitioners. Discussion Paper: Scope of Practice for nurse practitioners. Retrieved from Scope of Practice for Nurse Practitioners (aanp.org) on September 29, 2023; 2022.
38. American Academy of Physician Assistants. Becoming a PA. Retrieved from Become a PA: Getting Your Prerequisites and Certification - AAPA on September 30, 2023.
39. US Bureau of Labor Statistics. Occupational Employment and Wages, May 2022 401171 Nurse Practitioners. Retrieved from Nurse Practitioners (bls.gov) on October 4, 2023. US Bureau of Labor Statistics. (2022). Occupational Employment and Wages, May 2022 29-1071 Physician Assistants. Retrieved from Physician Assistants (bls.gov) on October 4, 2023; 2022.
40. AANP. A state of the nurse practitioner profession. Retrieved from 2020-NP-Sample-Survey-Report.pdf (aanp.org) on October 3, 2023; 2020.
41. Van Soereon M, Hurlock-Chorostecki C, Reeves S. The role of nurse practitioners in hospital settings: implications for interprofessional practice. J Interprof Care. 2011;25:245–51. https://doi.org/10.3109/13561820.2010.539305.
42. American Academy of Surgical Physician Assistants. About Surgical PAs. Retrieved from Surgical PA Profession (aaspa.com) on October 4, 2023.
43. Kippenbrock T, Emory J, Lee P, Odell E, Buron B, Morrison B. A national survey of nurse practitioners' patient satisfaction outcomes. Nurs Outlook. 2019;67(6):707712. https://doi.org/10.1016/j.outlook.2019.04.010.
44. Hlavin C, Ingraham P, Byrd T, et al. Clinical outcomes and hospital utilization among patients undergoing bariatric surgery with telemedicine preoperative care. JAMA Netw Open. 2023;6(2):e2255994. https://doi.org/10.1001/jamanetworkopen.2022.55994.
45. Supplemental Health Care. The history and impact of physical therapy. Retrieved from: The History and Impact of Physical Therapy - Supplemental Health Care (shccares.com) on October 10, 2023; 2017.
46. American Physical Therapy Association. Becoming a PT. Retrieved from Becoming a Physical Therapist | APTA on October 15, 2023; 2023.
47. Santos C, Carvalho M, Oliveira L, Palmeira A, Rodrigues LM, Gregório J. The long-term association between physical activity and weight regain, metabolic risk factors, quality of life and sleep after bariatric surgery. Int J Environ Res Public Health. 2022;19(14):8328. https://doi.org/10.3390/ijerph19148328. PMID: 35886177; PMCID: PMC9321811.
48. Brigham and Women's Hospital. Department of Rehabilitation Services. Physical Therapy Standard of Care: Bariatric Physical Therapy Management of the Bariatric Patient; 2011.
49. Carter J, et al. ASMBS position statement on preoperative patient optimization before metabolic and bariatric surgery. Surg Obes Relat Dis. 2021;17(12):1956–76. https://doi.org/10.1016/j.soard.2021.08.024.
50. King WC, Bond DS. The importance of preoperative and postoperative physical activity counseling in bariatric surgery. Exerc Sport Sci Rev. 2013;41(1):26–35. https://doi.org/10.1097/JES.0b013e31826444e0. PMID: 22710705; PMCID: PMC3529741.
51. Beriault K. Reproducibility of the 6-minute walk test in obese adults. Int J Sports Med. 2009;30(10):725.
52. CORA Development Team. Physical Therapy for Pre- and Post-Bariatric Surgery. Retrieved from Physical Therapy for Pre- and Post-Bariatric Surgery - CORA Physical Therapy on October 15, 2023; 2019.
53. American College of Sports Medicine. Trending Topic | Physical Activity Guidelines. Retrieved from Physical Activity Guidelines Resources (acsm.org) on Oct 21, 2023; 2023.
54. Ren Z, Lu G, Zhang T, et al. Effect of physical exercise on weight loss and physical function following bariatric surgery: a meta-analysis of randomized controlled trials. BMJ Open. 2018;8:e023208. https://doi.org/10.1136/bmjopen-2018-023208.
55. Integrated Health. American Society for Metabolic and Bariatric Surgery. https://asmbs.org/integrated-health. Accessed 30 October 2023.

# The Role of the Registered Dietitian in the Management of the Patient with Metabolic and Bariatric Surgery

6

Lillian Craggs-Dino

## Introduction

Metabolic and bariatric surgery (MBS) is a proven and durable treatment for obesity, but it is not without nutritional risk. Patients who suffer from the disease of obesity also suffer from malnutrition even prior to surgery. This malnutrition can be exacerbated after MBS if not prevented through evidence-based and appropriate nutrition assessment, diagnosis, intervention, and lifelong monitoring by an experienced registered dietitian nutritionist (RDN). The registered dietitian nutritionist is an essential and requisite team member of the interdisciplinary MBS program who can positively affect patient outcomes before, during, and after surgery. RDNs prepare patients preoperatively by optimizing their nutrition status and educating them on their nutritional responsibilities post-operatively. RDNs assess patients, determine their nutritional status, make dietary recommendations to replete nutrients and discuss goals and strategies for health behavior change. RDNs establish trust, rapport, and lifelong relationships with patients and encourage follow-up and support group attendance to maximize outcomes.

## The Registered Dietitian

A Registered Dietitian (RD) is synonymous with a Registered Dietitian Nutritionist (RDN). RDNs are diet, nutrition, and food experts who have graduated from an accredited dietetics program that has a rigorous academic curriculum and

L. Craggs-Dino (✉)
Advanced Practice Level II Registered Dietitian, Digestive Disease and Surgery Institute, Cleveland Clinic Florida, Weston, FL, USA
e-mail: craggsl@ccf.org



O. M. Ghanem et al. (eds.), *The SAGES Manual of Metabolic and Bariatric Surgery*, https://doi.org/10.1007/978-3-031-72309-4_6

supervised practice and training. To be an RDN, one must also successfully pass a national examination. In the United States, there is an optional specialty credential granted by the Commission on Dietetic Registration (CDR) as board-certified in obesity and weight management (CSOWM) which requires additional didactic coursework and board examination. The CDR also offers a certificate of training in obesity for pediatrics and adults as an additional recognition of advanced training in this specialty. RDNs are recognized as credentialed medical professionals and can treat nutrition-related medical conditions.

While dietitians can legally call themselves nutritionists, those individuals who are not credentialed and licensed as registered dietitians cannot claim to be. Those that call themselves "nutritionists" without the credential, may or may not have formal training and education in the field, and they are not credentialed as such. While "nutritionists" can give general nutrition advice, they cannot treat medical conditions through medical nutrition therapy (MNT). MNT is defined as the prevention and treatment of medical conditions such as obesity, malnutrition, diabetes, heart disease, and many other conditions provided by a Registered Dietitian Nutritionist [1]. Therefore, the distinct difference between a Registered Dietitian Nutritionist and just someone calling themselves a "nutritionist" is credentialing, licensure, and scope of practice. MBS programs, whether in a private clinical setting or an academic healthcare organization, hire credentialed RDNs.

RDNs who work in the specialty of metabolic and bariatric surgery (MBS) can work in a variety of settings such as hospitals, clinics, and other healthcare facilities. RDNs can open their own private practices, and enter academia, or industry. They may contract with food and supplement companies and be entrepreneurs of their own. Many RDNs also function as MBS program coordinators, reviewing policy and accreditation standards, and ensuring the program is performing efficiently and effectively. As an interdisciplinary team member, RDNs perform program orientations for patients researching and interested in MBS. RDNs often accompany the surgeon on the patient's first visit to describe the program's requirements. RDNs perform nutrition assessments and education and help navigate patients through the nutritional requirements for the insurance approval process. Without the guidance of the RDN, patients would be unaware of the critical dietary and lifestyle changes necessary for long-term positive outcomes.

RDNs working in the field of MBS have several responsibilities that will be described in this chapter. RDNs:

1. Perform a full nutrition assessment to optimize the patient's nutritional status prior to having surgery. Nutrition assessment and intervention continue throughout the postoperative period to identify and mitigate nutrition complications. RDNs can order and interpret nutrition-related laboratory or other diagnostic services. However, the ordering privileges of RDNs are subject to state laws and regulations, including hospital policies for reimbursement requirements from Medicare, Medicaid, or private payers and Electronic Health Record incentives.
2. Provide ongoing nutrition counseling, education, and support to facilitate lifestyle behavior changes.

3. Give patients guidance for preoperative weight loss or other insurance or program requirements if required.
4. Communicate with the interdisciplinary team.

## Nutrition Assessment and Intervention: Preoperative

Nutrition assessment is defined as a global assessment of both nutritional status and the presence of the potential for illness or the severity of illness because of the fundamental relationship between the two. According to Kesari et al. [1], nutrition assessment is a "detailed, systematic evaluation of a patient's nutritional status conducted by healthcare providers in a team-based setting to diagnose malnutrition and identify underlying pathologies to plan intervention." Nutrition assessment is a systematic method to make decisions on nutritional care, it provides a common language for documentation and communicating the impact of nutrition care, supports patient-centered care and evidenced-based nutrition practice [2, 3].

Obesity is a form of malnutrition and candidates for MBS often present with micronutrient deficiencies, sarcopenic obesity, and inadequate nutritional quality of diet [4]. While there is a consensus on the definition of "malnutrition," it is erroneous to assume that the causes of obesity are solely due to over-nourishment. According to the World Health Organization, malnutrition defines conditions that present as insufficient as well as excess intake of macronutrients and micronutrients [2, 3]. Malnutrition can present as acute, sub-acute, or chronic and may or may not be associated with underlying inflammation [2, 3]. It is well understood that the consequences of malnutrition include higher morbidity and mortality, longer hospital stays, increased costs, and increased patient pain and suffering [1, 2, 3].

Preoperatively, RDNs perform nutrition assessments on surgical candidates for the purpose of optimizing nutritional status to reduce the consequences of malnutrition prior to surgery. Carter et al. [5] describe the purpose of preoperative patient optimization as the management of modifiable risk factors prior to surgery to reduce the risk of peri-operative complications and improve outcomes. There are six domains of optimization: **Nutrition, Medical, Psychosocial, Lifestyle, Education and Support, and Financial**. Within these domains are nine areas of focus to optimize preoperatively, including smoking cessation, nutrition assessment, glycemic control, preoperative weight loss, medical screening, cardiac risk assessment, optimization of obstructive sleep apnea (OSA), physical prehabilitation, and psychosocial optimization [5].

Components of a nutrition assessment include the "ABCDs": A: Anthropometrics; B: Biochemistries; C: Clinical history; and D: Dietary. Figure 6.1 outlines the domains of a nutrition assessment specific to MBS and includes **Food and Nutrition History, Anthropometrics, Biochemistries, Nutrition-Focused Physical Assessment, and Patient History** [1, 2, 3]. In addition to investigating current diet and eating patterns, gathering an understanding of historical attempts and methods used at losing weight provides valuable information. Collecting anthropometrics provides objective and baseline measurements that can be used to assess health

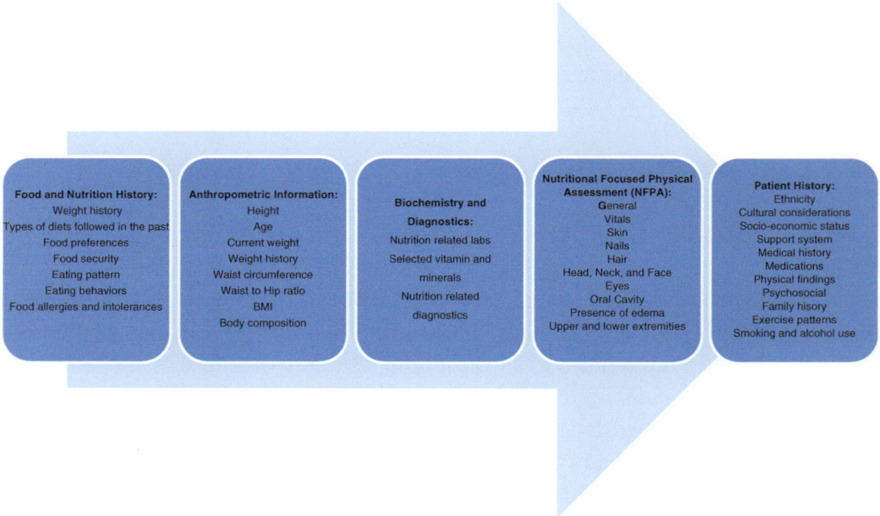


**Fig. 6.1** Components of nutrition assessment specific for MBS [1]

status and encourage goal setting. Healthcare providers are strongly encouraged to consider measuring body composition because collecting a measurement of sole weight without knowing what constitutes it (such as lean body mass versus body fat) does not truly assess the patient's overall health.

Of utmost importance is the correction of vitamin and mineral deficiencies prior to surgery. Due to the nature of MBS, preoperative vitamin and mineral deficiencies are a predictor of postoperative deficiencies [6, 7]. Deficiencies of vitamin D, iron, folate, vitamin B-12, elevated parathyroid hormone, and low transferrin saturation are reported [7]. Literature also cites gender, ethnic, and cultural influences on the prevalence of micronutrient deficiencies in patients who present with obesity [7]. Vitamin and mineral deficiencies can progress to deficiency diseases such as metabolic bone disease, Wernicke's encephalopathy, anemia, and other life-altering and devastating conditions [7, 8, 9].

Prevention of micronutrient deficiencies is the continued focus throughout the patient's weight loss journey and for a lifetime. Currently, there are no published repletion schedules for micronutrient deficiencies in MBS candidates, therefore, a patient-centered approach and individualized intervention after review of pre-op biochemistries is encouraged. Table 6.1 outlines the recommended minimum biochemical testing prior to and post-MBS [8]. In addition, Table 6.2 outlines suggestions for repletion based on the American Dietary Reference Intakes (DRIs) for non-surgical adults [9].

Many MBS programs require patients to follow either a low-calorie diet (LCD, approximately 1000 calories per day) or a very low-calorie diet (VLCD, approximately 800 calories per day) for the purpose of shrinking the size of the liver for

**Table 6.1** Suggested biochemistry labs pre- and post-MBS [8]

| Complete Metabolic Panel (CMP) | Ionized calcium |
|---|---|
| Lipids panel | Zinc (plasma) |
| Thyroid function panel | Thiamin (whole blood, or RBC) |
| A1c | B12 (serum) |
| PTH | MMA*** |
| PT* | Homocysteine (serum) |
| CBC** | Folate (RBC) |
| Copper (serum or plasma) | Vitamin A (plasma retinol) |
| Iron panel | Vitamin E (plasma alpha-tocopherol) |
| 25(OH) D | Vitamin K (phylloquinone) |

*PT = Prothrombin Time, **CBC = Complete Blood Count, ***MMA = Methylmalonic acid

**Table 6.2** Suggested preoperative micronutrient repletion [9]

| Nutrient Supplementation for Patients with WLS and without WLS. | | |
|---|---|---|
| **Nutrients** | | **Non-WLS** |
| | **Dietary reference intake (DRI)** | **Tolerable upper intake level (UL) daily value (DV)** |
| Vit B 1 | 1.2 mg/d 14 years + M | **UL:** None set; no reports of adverse effects from >50 mg B1/d from food or supplements |
| | 1.1 mg/d 19 years + F | **DV: 1.5 mg** |
| Vit B 12 | 2.4 ug/d 14 years + M,F | **UL:** None set; due to its low potential for toxicity |
| | | **DV: 6 ug** |
| Folate | 400 ug/d 19 years + M,F | **UL:** 1000 mcg all ages & pregnancy |
| | | **DV: 400 ug** |
| Calcium | 1000 mg/d 19–70 years M, 19–50 years F | **UL:** 2000–3000 mg /d |
| | 1200 mg 51–70 + years F | **DV:** 1000 mg |
| Vit A | 900 ug/d 14 years + M; 700 ug/d 14 years + F | **UL:** 10,000 IU/d (3000 mcg RAE/d)* retinol |
| | | **DV:** 5000 IU |
| Vit E | 15 mg/d 14 years + M,F | **UL:** 1000 mg/d (1500 IU/d) |
| | | **DV:** 30 mg |
| Vit K | 120 ug/d 19 years + M | **UL:** None set; due to its low potential for toxicity |
| | 90 ug/d 19 years + F | **DV:** 80 ug |
| Vit D | 600 IU/d (15 ug/d) | **UL:** 4000 IU/d (100 ug/d) |
| | 14 years + M,F | **DV:** 400 IU |
| Iron | 8 mg/d 19 years + M | **UL:** 45 mg/d |
| | 8 mg/d 51 years + F | **DV:** 18 mg |
| | 18 mg/d 19–50 years + F | |
| Zinc | 11 mg/d 19 years + M | **UL:** 40 mg/d |
| | 8 mg/d 19 years + F | **DV:** 15 mg |
| Copper | 900 ug/d 19 years + M,F | **UL:** 10,000 mcg/d |
| | | **DV:** 2 mg |

ease and safety of minimally invasive laparoscopic surgery [8]. RDNs educate patients on what foods and liquids are appropriate and strategies to employ for adherence.

## Nutrition Assessment and Intervention: Postoperative

RDNs provide therapeutic continuity after surgery. Research shows patients with MBS favor a long-term relationship with the registered dietitian nutritionist [10]. Patients perceive the RDN as having an integral and positive influence on their long-term success [10]. Patients realize that the RDN helps and guides them with re-learning appropriate eating techniques, making healthy and appropriate food choices, providing strategies for long-term dietary success, and mitigating nutritional deficiencies and challenges [10]. RDNs provide a formative approach to advancing the diet and provide continuing assessment, intervention, monitoring, communication, and support. Figure 6.2 gives an outline of the fundamentals of the post-MBS diet.

While there is no universal and standardized "bariatric diet," suggested dietary progression is based on textural manipulation and progressive inclusion of macronutrients. Prioritizing protein intake is encouraged to reduce the risk and loss of lean body mass during the rapid weight loss period [8]. Typically, 60–80 g/day or 1.0–1.5 g/kg ideal body weight (IBW) of high-quality protein is recommended [8]. Up to 2.0 g/kg may be recommended for more malabsorptive procedures such as the duodenal switch (DS) [8].

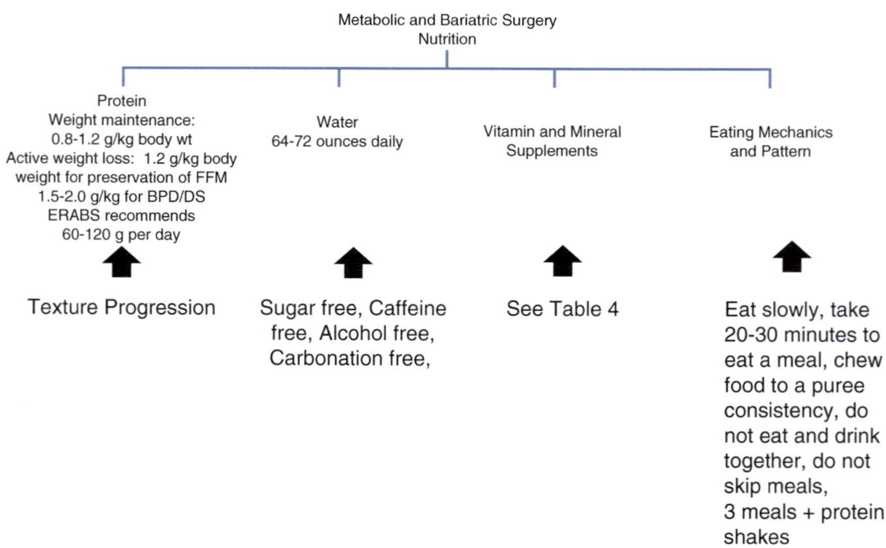


**Fig. 6.2** Fundamentals of the post MBS diet [8]

**Table 6.3** Suggested diet progression post MBS [8]

| Stage | Foods | Duration |
|---|---|---|
| Stage I | Clear liquids, sugar, and caffeine-free | 24 to 48 hours |
| Stage II | A full liquid diet, lactose-free | 10 to14 days |
| Stage III | Mechanically altered or soft foods as recommended by dietitian; assess for textural tolerance; focus on adequate protein intake, hydration, supplements, and proper eating mechanics | Variable |
| Stage IV | A regular diet that incorporates a variety of nutrient-dense foods; focus on adequate protein and caloric intake | Lifelong |

A bariatric diet is typically categorized into phases or stages, starting with a clear liquid diet, followed by a full liquid diet, and then progressing to a pureed or mechanical soft diet and toward the eventual regular diet with some modifications [8]. Table 6.3 gives an example of a typical bariatric diet progression. One reason for manipulating food texture and type, especially in the perioperative period is that food intolerance may be likely and lead to vomiting, nausea, or bezoar formation. Depending on the type of bariatric procedure, tolerance for a variety of foods and textures eventually improves [11]. Including complex, high-fiber carbohydrates is encouraged and may range from 50 to 130 g per day depending on the level of physical activity [8]. Intake of excessively concentrated sweets from juices and simple sugars is discouraged secondary to inducing dumping syndrome and weight recurrence [8]. Intake of unsaturated fats such as omega-3 fatty acids from seafood and monounsaturated fats from nuts, seeds, and whole grains is also encouraged [8]. Some bariatric guidelines suggest a fat intake to fall between 20 and 35% of total calories [8].

RDNs also educate and counsel patients on appropriate eating mechanics and patterns to reduce intolerance. Patients are taught to eat and drink slowly, to chew food to a pureed consistency, to avoid eating and drinking together, to self-monitor, and to avoid problematic foods such as tough meats and foods that cannot be chewed adequately to a pureed consistency. RDNs teach patients about appropriate cooking methods, food products, how to read food labels and recipe modification.

Another critical role of the RDN is to recommend, educate, evaluate, and monitor the adherence and tolerance for vitamin and mineral supplementation. RDNs may have the ability to order nutrition-related laboratory testing and other diagnostics. The revised 2017 Scope of Practice for the RDNs outlines information on how RDNs with ordering privileges can "order and monitor nutrition-related laboratory tests and waived point-of-care laboratory testing." [12] However, for the RDN to be granted ordering privileges, they must meet all organization policies, and federal, and state regulatory qualifications.

Research shows there is a lower rate of deficiency for iron, B12, and vitamin D with better clinical guidance and patient adherence to vitamin and mineral supplementation post-surgery [13]. However, the bad news is vitamin and mineral deficiencies still occur after MBS [13, 14, 15]. Despite good adherence to prescribed supplements, at least one nutritional deficiency is reported in 72.7%, 76.7%, and 93.8% of patients with adjustable gastric band, sleeve gastrectomy, and gastric bypass, respectively [14]. Iron deficiency anemia, neuropathy, and metabolic bone disease are reported across these surgeries. Studies show anemia and metabolic bone disease are reported as high as 40% and 56%, respectively, in patients with the RYGB [15]. Table 6.4 lists the current clinical practice guidelines from several professional international organizations such as the American Society for Metabolic and Bariatric Surgery (ASMBS) [8, 9], the expert consensus from the French Speaking Society of Clinical Nutrition and Metabolism (SFNCM), French Association for the Study and Research on Obesity (AFERO), French Obesity Research Center of Excellence (FORCE), Medical Evaluation Department, Department of Clinical Research Support PARC, and the French and Francophone Society of Obesity Surgery and Metabolic Disorders (SO.FF.CO.MM) [16], the British Obesity and Metabolic Surgery Society (BOMSS) [17], and the Obesity Management Task Force of the European Association for the Study of Obesity [18]. The differences seen between these recommendations for micronutrient intake with MBS underscore the need for improvements in research rigor and interpretation of results. While these guidelines support practitioners with evidence-based practice for decision-making, these recommendations should be utilized within an individualized and patient-centered approach to care with shared decision-making and frequent monitoring to prevent or treat micronutrient deficiency.

## Encouraging Dietary Behavioral Changes through Long-Term Follow-Up, Support Groups, and Nutrition Education

RDNs play an integral role to influence positive patient outcomes. RDNs develop long-term relationships with patients and provide a sense of community by facilitating support groups, they continue to reinforce the patient's nutritional responsibilities post-MBS and prevent the onset of recurrence and relapse toward unhealthy eating habits. According to the Metabolic and Bariatric Surgery Accreditation and Quality Improvement Program (MBSAQIP) [19], accredited MBS programs must provide regularly scheduled, organized support groups. These support groups must be supervised and facilitated by a licensed healthcare provider and made available a minimum of every 2 months [19]. Research shows that those who attend support groups had greater weight loss compared to those who do not attend [20]. In addition, a significant positive association between the number of support group meetings attended and weight loss has also been report [20].

Hameed et al. [21] found that 58% of patients with MBS wanted to attend a support group. Those more likely to attend were those struggling to keep the weight off, to be unhappy with the way they look, or to be experiencing difficulties returning to work [21]. To encourage support group attendance, MBS programs should be aware of what the patient wants and encourage accordingly. Research shows patients want

**Table 6.4** Minimal vitamin and mineral recommendations for MBS [8, 9, 16–18]

| Micronutrient | [16] | [8, 9] | [17] | [18] |
|---|---|---|---|---|
| B1 | 100 mg oral or by perfusion or by intramuscular injection when the patient vomits<br>In the event of suspected Gayet-Wernicke encephalopathy, it is recommended to provide vitamin B1 supplementation by parenteral route (500 mg³×/d) for 3 days, and that it be associated first with magnesium supplementation (magnesium sulfate at 6–8 mmol of magnesium-element over a period of 24 h), and then at 250 mg/d by oral or parenteral route for at least 5 days | ≥12 mg, preferably 50–100 mg | 200–300 mg daily if symptoms of dysphagia, vomiting, poor dietary intake or rapid weight loss | Oral or parenteral thiamine supplementation (50–100 mg/day) should promptly be considered and started in every bariatric patient suffering from persistent vomiting |
| B12 | Oral route at a daily dose of 250 mcg/d to 350 mcg/d or a weekly dose of 1 or 21,000 mcg vials of vitamin B12 Or 1000 mcg by intramuscular injection every 1–3 months, or else 3000 mcg every 6 months | 350–1000 mcg daily, disintegrating OR 1000 mcg monthly injection OR Weekly Nasal Spray | SG, RYGB, BPD/DS, recommended frequency of vitamin B12 IM inj every 3 months | Oral dose of 350–500 μg/day; 1 mg/month intramuscularly, 3 mg every 6 months intramuscularly or 500 μg every week intranasally |
| Folic acid | 400–800 mcg/d | 400–800 mcg OR 800–1000 mcg | 400–800 mcg | Folic acid is usually contained in the multivitamin and mineral supplements routinely used in bariatric patients |

(continued)

**Table 6.4** (continued)

| Micronutrient | [16] | [8, 9] | [17] | [18] |
|---|---|---|---|---|
| Iron | 60–200 mg, oral Intravenous iron supplementation is limited to cases marked by failure and/or intolerance of oral supplementation | Males with no history of anemia: 18 mg<br>Menstruating females and patients who have undergone RYGB, SG, BPD/DS: 45–60 mg | 200 mg ferrous sulfate, 210 mg ferrous fumarate or 300 mg ferrous gluconate daily and twice daily in menstruating women and adjust depending on blood results | Prophylactic empiric iron supplementation is recommended after gastric bypass, biliopancreatic diversion, duodenal switch and sleeve gastrectomy. Iron is usually included in oral multivitamin and mineral preparations with the inclusion of vitamin C, which is able to increase iron absorption |
| Vitamin D | After malabsorptive surgery BPD or BPD-DS, vitamin D supplementation is carried out by the oral route, at a dose of 50,000 IU, 1 or 2 times a week, or else by intramuscular injection (200,000 IU/month)<br>For Roux-en-Y bypass or sleeve gastrectomy, systematic vitamin D supplementation by oral route is recommended either daily (at least 800 IU) | 3000 IU daily to achieve blood levels >30 ng/ml | 2000 and 4000 IU may be required following SG and RYGB and higher following malabsorptive procedures such as BPD/DS | 3000 IU of vitamin D |
| Calcium | 1000–1500 mg/d | 1200–1500 mg/d: RYGB, SG, AGB<br>1800–2400 mg/d: BPD/DS | Ensure good dietary calcium intake, requirements may be higher in individuals who have SG, RYGB or BPD/DS | 1200–2000 mg/day of elemental calcium |

| | | | | |
|---|---|---|---|---|
| Vitamin A | For vitamin A deficiency, supplementation should approximate 50,000 UI a week, it may in some cases be higher | 5000 IU: AGB;<br>5000–10,000 IU: RYGB and SG; and 10,000 IU for BPD/DS | Take a complete MVI/MMI containing U.K. government dietary recommendations for vitamin A<br>BPD/DS: 10000 IU oral daily | Routine supplementation with multivitamins and minerals |
| Vitamin E | Vitamin E insufficiency, supplementation usually ranges from 400 to 500 IU/d | 15 mg and higher if have Hx of deficiency | BPD/DS: 100-IU oral, daily | Routine supplementation with multivitamins and minerals |
| Vitamin K | Vitamin K insufficiency, supplementation consists of 2 mg to 10 mg/week | 90–120 mcg: AGB, RYGB, SG; and 300 mcg for BPD/DS | BPD/DS: 300-µg oral, daily | Routine supplementation with multivitamins and minerals |
| Zinc | If zinc deficiency, supplementation needs to be associated with copper (1 mg of copper for 10 mg of zinc) and not exceed 30 mg/d except in cases of severe malabsorption | 8–11 mg for SG and AGB;<br>8–22 mg for RYGB and 16–22 mg for BPD/DS *add 1 mg cu for every 8–15 mg of zinc | RYGB and SG: 15 mg<br>BPD/DS: 30 mg<br>Add 2 mg cu | Routine supplementation with multivitamins and minerals |

**Table 6.5** Support group topics [22]

| Topic | Topic | Topic |
|---|---|---|
| Back to bariatric basics in time for the new year | Healthy cooking techniques | Mindful eating |
| Carbs are not the enemy! | Healthy eating on a budget | Strategies for a healthy lifestyle |
| Budgeting calories and protein after MBS | Sugar and sugar substitutes, which one and how much | Barriers to weight loss |
| Dining out made simple | Common nutrition issues after surgery | Weight loss reboot |
| Controlling your appetite with portion control | Tips to prevent constipation | Heart healthy bariatric eating |
| Facts about fats | Prebiotics and probiotics | Strategies to get in your proteins |
| Protein shakes and powders | The importance of exercise after MBS | The use of herbs and spices in cooking |
| Recipe exchange | How to use a food diary and apps | Help! My hair is falling out! |
| Everything you need to know about protein | Round table chat: Ask the dietitian | Can I eat this: New product review |
| Healthy hair and skin with weight loss | Is the weight loss honeymoon over? | Meal planning tips for MBS |
| Are you taking your supplements? What could happen if you don't! | How to break the weight loss plateau | Healthy holiday eating |
| Patient testimonies | Weight regain? Don't panic | How much should you be eating? |
| Protein bar or glorified candy bar? | Keep foods safe to eat | Non-scale successes: Let's talk about it |

support groups to provide formal educational sessions in the form of seminars and talks across a range of subject matters related to weight loss, obesity, nutrition, and surgery, and they want moral support from others who have experienced a similar journey [21]. RDNs can facilitate a broad range of interesting topics that will motivate and inform patients. Table 6.5 suggests some topics that RDNs can use in the support groups.

## Conclusion

The Registered Dietitian Nutritionist (RDN) is an essential and requisite team member of the interdisciplinary MBS program. The RDN is a diet and nutrition expert and highly adept in providing a detailed nutrition assessment both preoperatively and post-operatively. Through evidence-based interventions, motivational interviewing, and building long-term relationships, the RDN positively affects patient outcomes by optimizing nutrition status and providing patient-centered and individualized care as the patient with MBS travels through their weight loss and health journey.

## References


1. Kesari A, Noel JY. Nutritional assessment. [Updated 2023 Apr 10]. In: StatPearls [Internet]. Treasure Island, FL: StatPearls Publishing; 2023 Jan. Available from: https://www.ncbi.nlm.nih.gov/books/NBK580496/.
2. Mueller C, Compher C, Ellen DM. American Society for Parenteral and Enteral Nutrition (A.S.P.E.N.) Board of Directors. A.S.P.E.N. clinical guidelines: Nutrition screening, assessment, and intervention in adults. JPEN J Parenter Enteral Nutr. 2011;35(1):16–24. [PubMed].
3. White JV, Guenter P, et al. Consensus Statement: Academy of Nutrition and Dietetics and American Society for Parenteral and Enteral Nutrition: Characteristics Recommended for the Identification and Documentation of Adult Malnutrition (Under-nutrition). JPEN J Parent Ent Nutr. 2012;36:275–83.
4. Sherf Dagan S, Zelber-Sagi S, Webb M, et al. Erratum to: Nutritional status prior to laparoscopic sleeve gastrectomy surgery. Obes Surg. 2017;27:2511. https://doi.org/10.1007/s11695-017-2815-2.
5. Carter J, Chang J, Birriel TJ, Moustarah F, Sogg S, Goodpaster K, Benson-Davies S, Chapmon K, Eisenberg D. ASMBS position statement on preoperative patient optimization before metabolic and bariatric surgery. Surg Obes Relat Dis. 2021;17(12):1956–76. https://doi.org/10.1016/j.soard.2021.08.024. Epub 2021 Sep 3. PMID: 34629296.
6. van der Beek ES, Monpellier VM, Eland I, Tromp E, van Ramshorst B. Nutritional deficiencies in gastric bypass patients; incidence, time of occurrence and implications for post-operative surveillance. Obes Surg. 2015;25(5):818–23. https://doi.org/10.1007/s11695-014-1456-y.
7. Ben-Porat T, Weiss R, Sherf-Dagan S, Nabulsi N, Maayani A, Khalaileh A, Abed S, Brodie R, Harari R, Mintz Y, Pikarsky AJ, Elazary R. Nutritional Deficiencies in Patients with Severe Obesity before Bariatric Surgery: What Should Be the Focus During the Preoperative Assessment? J Acad Nutr Diet. 2020;120(5):874–84. https://doi.org/10.1016/j.jand.2019.10.017. Epub 2019 Dec 28. PMID: 31892499.
8. Mechanick JI, Apovian C, Brethauer S, Garvey WT, Joffe AM, et al. Clinical practice guidelines for the perioperative nutrition, metabolic, and nonsurgical support of patients undergoing bariatric procedures-2019 update: cosponsored by American Association of Clinical Endocrinologists/American College of Endocrinology, The Obesity Society, American Society for Metabolic and Bariatric Surgery, Obesity Medicine Association, and American Society of Anesthesiologists. Surg Obes Relat Dis. 2020;16:175–247.
9. Parrott J, et al. American society for metabolic and bariatric surgery integrated health nutritional guidelines for the surgical weight loss patient 2016 update: micronutrients. 2017;13:727–41.
10. Aarts MA, Sivapalan N, Nikzad SE, Serodio K, Sockalingam S, Conn LG. Optimizing bariatric surgery multidisciplinary follow-up: a focus on patient-centered care. Obes Surg. 2017;27(3):730–6. https://doi.org/10.1007/s11695-016-2354-2.
11. Schweiger C, Weiss R, Keidar A. Effect of different bariatric operations on food tolerance and quality of eating. Obes Surg. 2010;20(10):1393–9. https://doi.org/10.1007/s11695-010-0233-9.
12. Academy of Nutrition and Dietetics Quality Management Committee. Academy of nutrition and dietetics: revised 2017 scope of practice for the registered dietitian nutritionist. J Acad Nutr Diet. 2018;118(1):141–65.
13. Dogan K, Homan J, Aarts EO, de Boer H, van Laarhoven C, Berends FJ. Long-term nutritional status in patients following Roux-en-Y gastric bypass surgery. Clin Nutr. 2018;37(2):612–7. https://doi.org/10.1016/j.clnu.2017.01.022.
14. Lombardo M, Franchi A, Biolcati Rinaldi R, Rizzo G, D'Adamo M, Guglielmi V, Bellia A, Padua E, Caprio M, Sbraccia P. Long-term iron and vitamin B12 deficiency are present after bariatric surgery, despite the widespread use of supplements. Int J Environ Res Public Health. 2021;18(9):4541. https://doi.org/10.3390/ijerph18094541. PMID: 33922904; PMCID: PMC8123142.

15. Montastier E, Chalret du Rieu M, Tuyeras G, Ritz P. Long-term nutritional follow-up post bariatric surgery. Curr Opin Clin Nutr Metab Care. 2018;21(5):388–93. https://doi.org/10.1097/MCO.0000000000000490.
16. Quilliot D, Coupaye M, Ciangura C, Czernichow S, Sallé A, Gaborit B, Alligier M, Nguyen-Thi PL, Dargent J, Msika S, Brunaud L. Recommendations for nutritional care after bariatric surgery: recommendations for best practice and SOFFCO-MM/AFERO/SFNCM/expert consensus. J Visc Surg. 2021;158(1):51–61. https://doi.org/10.1016/j.jviscsurg.2020.10.013. Epub 2021 Jan 9. PMID: 33436155.
17. O'Kane M, Parretti HM, Pinkney J, et al. British Obesity and Metabolic Surgery Society Guidelines on perioperative and postoperative biochemical monitoring and micronutrient replacement for patients undergoing bariatric surgery—2020 update. Obes Rev. 2020;21:e13087. https://doi.org/10.1111/obr.13087.
18. Busetto L, Dicker D, Azran C, et al. Obesity Management Task Force of the European Association for the Study of Obesity Released "Practical Recommendations for the Post-Bariatric Surgery Medical Management". Obes Surg. 2018;28:2117–21.
19. Saber AA, Mackowsky M, Farr M. Metabolic and Bariatric Surgery Accreditation and Quality Improvement Program (MBSAQIP). In: Agrawal S, editor. Obesity, bariatric and metabolic surgery. Cham: Springer; 2023. https://doi.org/10.1007/978-3-030-60596-4_63.
20. Livhits M, Mercado C, Yermilov I, Parikh JA, Dutson E, Mehran A, Ko CY, Shekelle PG, Gibbons MM. Is social support associated with greater weight loss after bariatric surgery?: a systematic review. Obes Rev. 2011;12(2):142–8. https://doi.org/10.1111/j.1467-789X.2010.00720.x. PMID: 20158617.
21. Hameed S, Salem V, Tan TM, Collins A, Shah K, Scholtz S, Ahmed AR, Chahal H. Beyond Weight Loss: Establishing a Postbariatric Surgery Patient Support Group-What Do Patients Want? J Obes. 2018;2018:8419120. https://doi.org/10.1155/2018/8419120.
22. Craggs-Dino L. "Engaging Support Groups". Presented at IFSO, the 25th World Congress, Miami, FL; 2022.

# The Role of the Behavioral Health Provider in the Management of the Patient Seeking Metabolic and Bariatric Surgery

7

Ninoska D. Peterson and Rachel L. Goldman

## Introduction

It has been well-established that obesity is a complex disease that is the result of interactions among biological, environmental, behavioral, and psychological factors. To be effective, strategies to treat obesity should address as many components as possible. Metabolic and bariatric surgery (MBS) is accepted as the most efficient, effective, and durable treatment for obesity, as it produces significant weight loss and both improvements and the prevention, of medical comorbidities [1–5]. However, long-term maintenance of results is not guaranteed. Weight recurrence occurs, and outcomes can depend on individual, behavioral, and psychological factors associated with overall adherence [6, 7].

Behavioral health providers were initially recommended to be part of the bariatric surgery evaluation team in the 1991 National Institutes of Health Consensus Development Conference Statement. The purpose of the entire team was to help select patients who were candidates for bariatric surgery [8]. There have been several updated clinical practice guidelines since that time from the American Association of Clinical Endocrinologists, The Obesity Society, and the American Society for Metabolic & Bariatric Surgery (ASMBS) which states that an assessment of psychological factors should be part of the comprehensive evaluation to assess for surgical risk [9]. Most recently, the ASMBS and the International Federation for the Surgery of Obesity and Metabolic Disorders (IFSO) published a

N. D. Peterson
Department of Surgery, Cleveland Clinic, Bariatric and Metabolic Institute, Cleveland Clinic Lerner College of Medicine of Case Western Reserve University, Cleveland, OH, USA
e-mail: petersn2@ccf.org

R. L. Goldman (✉)
Department of Psychiatry, NYU Grossman School of Medicine, New York, NY, USA



O. M. Ghanem et al. (eds.), *The SAGES Manual of Metabolic and Bariatric Surgery*, https://doi.org/10.1007/978-3-031-72309-4_7

paper on the indications of metabolic and bariatric surgery [10] which states that "the pre-surgical evaluation process is designed to optimize surgical outcomes and implement interventions that can address disordered eating, severe uncontrolled mental illness, or active substance abuse." As such, a psychosocial evaluation is a routine part of the preoperative process in the majority of bariatric surgery programs in the United States and is often required by third-party payers [11]. A recent exploratory study showed that members of the multidisciplinary team viewed the role of the behavioral health provider as identifying contraindications to surgery while behavioral health providers viewed their role as identifying readiness for surgery [12]. In this constantly evolving area of behavioral health in MBS, the role of the behavioral health provider is key in evaluating presurgical patients, but there has also been a shift towards the importance of facilitating psychosocial interventions and long-term management during the pre- and postoperative time period [11–14]. The behavioral health provider should be available postoperatively to address long-term complications and provide continuity of care [13]. It's also important for the bariatric behavioral health provider to have sufficient knowledge of all available obesity treatment options, including surgical, endoscopic procedures, anti-obesity medications (AOM), and lifestyle interventions.

## Qualifications of a Behavioral Health Provider Working Within a Bariatric Surgery Setting

Behavioral health providers come from a number of different educational backgrounds and may be psychiatrists, psychologists, social workers, advanced practice nurses, clinical nurse specialists, licensed mental health counselors, or licensed marriage and family therapists. Behavioral health providers study the mind and behavior, and work with patients throughout the developmental spectrum [15]. Although there is no current standard, those specializing in the field of bariatrics typically have earned a minimum of a master's degree, but many have earned a doctorate degree in clinical or counseling psychology, have completed a clinical internship, and hold a valid license to practice. Many also have additional fellowship training with specialized populations. Behavioral health clinicians can provide initial assessments for mental and behavioral health problems, long-term or short-term therapy, and psychoeducation. Some behavioral health providers, such as psychologists, are also trained to administer and interpret psychological testing or questionnaires and to conduct research. While most behavioral health providers do not prescribe medications, some can be granted the right to prescribe a limited number of psychotropic medications with appropriate training [16].

The current chapter will examine the role of a behavioral health provider in the field of bariatrics. It's important to note that some literature, including previous versions of this book, only referred to psychologists doing this work, but not just psychologists provide these services. The term behavioral health provider, or behavioral health clinician, in this chapter, will be referring to psychologists, therapists, clinical social workers, clinical counselors, psychiatrists, and psychiatric nurses [17]. A

2010 survey of ASMBS members suggested that behavioral health providers in the field of bariatrics should have extensive specialized knowledge and experience in the treatment of obesity and MBS [17]. It's important to ensure that bariatric behavioral health clinicians provide competent, patient-centered care, and ensure that patients seeking MBS receive consistent, high-standard care that meets their needs throughout the pre-and postoperative stages.

## The Presurgical Evaluation

The preoperative psychosocial evaluation serves many purposes, just as the behavioral health provider has many roles. The evaluation can be used to identify patients' strengths and potential challenges, as well as assess for psychosocial contraindications and adherence factors. A guiding question is, "Do the potential benefits of the patient having surgery outweigh the potential risks?" Although the initial purpose was to assess for "suitability," more recent UK guidelines have emphasized the importance of psychological support during the preoperative process and stated that "all patients should have a psychology triage pre-operatively, the intention of which is not to screen out potential candidates but to identify support required to optimise their weight loss and psychological outcomes." [18] The patient and provider can work together to come up with a treatment plan that utilizes the patient's strengths and addresses potential challenges to long-term success [11, 14, 19–21]. Complicated cases will require consultation with the entire multidisciplinary team (i.e., the surgeon, medical providers, dietitians, and nurses) and additional external providers caring for the patient (i.e., psychiatrist, endocrinologist, cardiologist, etc.) [9, 13]. While there are no set standards on how presurgical psychosocial evaluations should be conducted, there is a general consensus regarding the domains that should be addressed, which are beyond the scope of standard psychopathology [11, 20, 22].

The role of the behavioral health provider and the purpose of the presurgical psychosocial evaluation should be clearly explained to the patient, as well as a description of what is going to take place during the appointment. Patients are often anxious about "saying the right thing" in order to "pass" the evaluation and subsequently may engage in positive impression management [23]. The initial evaluation provides the behavioral health provider a chance to establish rapport and develop a relationship with the patient [24]. The typical evaluation involves a semi-structured or structured face-to-face interview, a review of the medical chart, along with possible psychological testing, and/or symptom inventory [11, 14]. Common components of a comprehensive presurgical evaluation include knowledge about bariatric surgery and its risks and benefits, motivations for having surgery, and expectations following surgery, weight and diet history, current and past eating, exercise and lifestyle behaviors, adherence to medications and other medical recommendations, psychiatric history, past and current disordered eating and substance use, as well as current stressors, coping strategies, and social support.

## Knowledge, Motivations, and Expectations

Patient education and knowledge play an important role in MBS, and the information that patients are expected to know is often complex and extensive [25]. These areas are routinely addressed in the initial portions of most evaluations. Patients should be knowledgeable enough to be able to describe the surgical procedure, risks, and benefits of surgery. Additional information can be gathered objectively. For example, Bauchowitz and colleagues [26] developed a measure that assesses knowledge about medical, behavioral, and psychological factors associated with bariatric surgery. Results from a study using this scale suggested that 65% of patients overestimated the degree of weight loss, and only 25% of patients maintained accurate expectations of weight loss. Patients who do not demonstrate adequate knowledge and/or realistic expectations could benefit from other education or intervention.

While motivation for pursuing surgery has not consistently been linked to surgical results, several studies demonstrate that lack of knowledge contributes to unrealistic and inaccurate expectations, which in turn are a key predictor of patient self-efficacy and patient satisfaction. Most patients cite reasons for pursuing MBS that are related to weight loss, improved health, decreased need for medications, improved mobility and fitness, and living longer, along with improvements in body image and self-esteem [27]. Unrealistic motivations (e.g., "so my husband won't leave me," "so I will fit into skinny jeans" or "I will no longer have to think about food and what to eat") and expectations ("I'd like to weigh the same as I did before I had children," "I will no longer be depressed," "I will be pain-free," "or surgery will cure my obesity") provide a degree to which patients presume their lives will drastically change after surgery [20, 26]. Sufficient data suggest that patients seeking surgical [28, 29] and nonsurgical [30] treatments for obesity tend to have unrealistic expectations. These unrealistic expectations may lead patients to accept a greater level of surgical risk. Patients should recognize the contributions of their own behavioral efforts, including lifestyle changes and adherence to postoperative eating and exercise recommendations on long-term results. Therefore, expectations and potential changes in body shape and size, relationships, view of self, etc., also need to be addressed and properly discussed during the preoperative period.

Assessing the domains of knowledge, motivation, and expectations gives the behavioral health provider an idea about a patient's capacity to provide informed consent, and a chance to provide education and correct misinformation [26]. We encourage patients to adopt various measures of success beyond weight loss that encompass improvements in quality of life (i.e., "Non-scale victories"). Examples include changes in clothing size, being able to cross your legs, improvements in fitness, riding on a roller coaster, and getting off of medications [31]. Further, it's important to remind the patient that obesity is a multifactorial complex chronic disease that needs management for the rest of one's life. So, more than one treatment may be necessary for long-term management, and this may include adding AOM after surgery, which does not constitute the patient being a "failure."

## Weight and Diet History

Assessing the patient's weight and diet history is important. Gibbons and colleagues [32] found that patients who sought MBS reported an extensive history of dieting attempts, often beginning in adolescence, but weight loss was never maintained. This area of inquiry includes learning about weight gain trajectories, description of childhood weight/size compared to peers, lowest adult weight, highest adult weight, and factors associated with weight gain and loss over the years (e.g., eating habits, activity level, side effect of medications, pregnancy, smoking cessation, etc.). Any major dieting attempts (e.g., restrictive diets, exercise, medications, etc.) or other obesity treatment, including lifestyle changes or AOM, should also be documented, as this is often required by third-party payers and provides the behavioral health provider with a sense of adherence and challenges faced. Maladaptive weight loss attempts, including vomiting, laxative/diuretic use, starvation, and excessive exercise, should also be assessed and documented. All of this information is helpful and will assist the behavioral health provider in identifying potential issues that could require additional pre- or postoperative intervention.

## Current Eating, Exercise, and Health Habits

The behavioral health provider needs to also assess for maladaptive eating patterns such as skipping meals, emotional factors affecting food choices and eating behaviors, as well as environmental factors (e.g., night shift schedule, responsibility of shopping and cooking) that could be related to poor weight management. Discussion of frequency of eating out at restaurants and eating fast food, favorite/problematic foods, caffeine intake, consumption of high sugar and high caloric beverages, and carbonated beverages also provides an opportunity for education, problem-solving, and potential early interventions. Self-monitoring of food intake (e.g., a food diary) is often recommended as it has consistently been shown to be a key factor in predicting initial weight loss and long-term weight maintenance [33–35]. Food records can be used before and after MBS to help patients learn self-regulation skills when making dietary choices (e.g., timing of eating, portions, and diet quality).

Information should be obtained about current health behaviors, including exercise, sleep, and water intake, as well as adherence to medication regimens, blood glucose monitoring, and CPAP use. Some of this information can be gathered while reviewing medical history, surgical history, current medications, and drug allergies [24]. Many patients take multiple medications, and while they may not remember all the names of their medications, some will provide a list. This shows the ability to problem-solve and adapt, which are positive prognostic indicators for postoperative adherence.

## Past and Current Disordered Eating

A discussion of past and current eating habits, as well as a patient's thoughts surrounding food and eating behaviors, lead to the assessment for diagnosable eating disorders and other problematic eating behaviors found in the *Diagnostic and Statistical Manual-Fifth Edition Text Revision* (DSM-5-TR) [36]. During the clinical interview, it is best to ask questions using diagnostic criteria. It is also helpful to ask open-ended questions to get a better understanding of the patient's eating habits and routines. For instance, instead of asking closed-ended questions such as "Have you ever binged?" or "Are you a binge eater?", the behavioral health provider can ask "Have you ever eaten a large amount of food and felt out of control?" Information can also be corroborated using objective assessment measures.

## Binge Eating Disorder (BED)

Being Eating Disorder was included in the *DSM-5* as a diagnosis, as opposed to only being listed in the Appendix in previous editions of the DSM [37]. Key features include recurrent and persistent intake of an objectively large amount of food, subjective loss of control with eating during a binge episode, and three or more associated symptoms (e.g., eating more rapidly than normal, eating until one is uncomfortably full, eating large amounts when one is not physically hungry, eating alone out of embarrassment, or feeling disgusted, depressed, or guilty after eating). Diagnosable behaviors typically involve distress. The current frequency of binges to be diagnosed also needs to be at least once a week for the past 3 months. Although BED is not limited to patients with obesity, it is the most commonly seen eating disorder among individuals with obesity. BED is more common in patients seeking bariatric surgery than in community samples, but high variability exists in the literature regarding the percentage of patients seeking MBS with BED. Prevalence rates range from 5% to 49% [38–41]. While binge eating disorder is not a contraindication to having bariatric surgery, untreated symptoms (with loss of control as a key predictor) may lead to poorer outcomes. Therefore, this is something that should be addressed prior to surgery if possible. Patients who undergo a four-session group treatment show improvements in eating behaviors and attitudes after this short therapy, and these responders had enhanced surgical outcomes across different bariatric procedures [42].

## Bulimia Nervosa (BN)

Bulimia Nervosa is characterized by (1) recurrent episodes of binge eating (i.e., eating, in a discrete period of time, an amount of food that is definitely larger than what most people would eat during a similar time period and under similar circumstances, accompanied by a sense of lack of control while eating); (2) recurrent compensatory behavior to prevent weight gain (e.g., self-induced vomiting, misuse of laxatives or diuretics, fasting, or excessive exercise); (3) self-evaluation being unduly influenced by body shape and weight concerns; and (4) behaviors occurring at a frequency of once a week for 3 months [36]. Symptoms of BN tend to be rare among bariatric surgery candidates and may be considered a contraindication to these surgical procedures at the time of the evaluation, due to the compensatory behaviors. The lifetime prevalence of BN was reported between 0.0% and 6.8%, while the current prevalence has been reported between 0.0% and 1.0% [40, 41, 43, 44].

## Anorexia Nervosa (AN)

A history of anorexia nervosa is rare in this population but should be evaluated. In evaluating for AN, it's helpful to ask about restrictive dieting to get a better idea of the individual's eating routine and habits as well.

## Night Eating Syndrome (NES)

Night eating syndrome was first identified in 1955 by Stunkard and colleagues [45] as a stress-related eating disorder characterized by a disproportionate consumption of calories at night and/or waking up from sleep to eat, morning anorexia, and insomnia [46]. The relationship between night eating and weight is inconsistent. It is currently classified as an Other Specified Feeding or Eating Disorder (OSFED) in the *DSM-5*. The prevalence of NES ranged from 6% to 64% in patients seeking weight loss treatment and from 8% to 42% for those seeking MBS [47]. Having the comorbidity of NES with obesity has been linked to a poorer prognosis for long-term weight loss and maintenance, especially in MBS patients [48]. A thorough review of a patient's day, including their sleep behaviors and timing of eating is helpful during the preoperative evaluation. Symptoms that should be addressed prior to surgery include general timing of eating and beliefs about eating that are related to sleep.

## Graze Eating

Graze eating is a type of problematic eating behavior that is not a recognized DSM-5 disorder; it is defined as "repetitive, unplanned eating of small amounts of food throughout the day" and is also referred to as nibbling, picking, or unplanned snacking. Approximately 33% of bariatric surgery candidates endorse graze eating, and 32% experience loss of control [49, 50]. Although less research has been done in this area, graze eating has been found to lead to suboptimal weight loss and ultimately can lead to weight reoccurrence [50]. Patients may also engage in graze eating following surgery, as this behavior is easier to engage in compared to binge eating, and it can serve as a maladaptive coping/avoidance strategy [49]. This should not only be assessed preoperatively, but psychoeducation is also important to discuss the possible occurrence and consequences of graze eating postoperatively.

## Other Problematic Eating Behaviors

Another subclinical problematic eating behavior is emotional eating, or eating that occurs in the absence of hunger cues and is influenced by emotions, both positive and negative. Emotional eating is often used to self-soothe or to provide relief from difficult feelings [51]. Patients may refer to this as eating when bored or stressed. Subclinical problematic eating patterns tend to lead to poorer weight loss. Finally, meal skipping, and restrictive eating, should also be addressed, as many patients have an erroneous belief that they will lose weight as a result. In most cases, patterns of meal skipping lead to overconsumption later in the day. Any problematic eating behavior that comes up during the preoperative stage should be properly assessed, discussed, and addressed prior to proceeding with surgery.

## Psychiatric History and Current Mental Health Symptoms

Psychiatric comorbidities are common among bariatric surgery patients, and likely more common than in the general population- particularly mood disorders and binge eating disorder [52]. Prevalence rates of a psychiatric condition in patients preoperatively range from 23% to 68% [9, 39, 40, 52–55]. Accurate prevalence rates are difficult to capture due to social desirability on the patient's end, sample sizes, and differing methods of assessment [23, 39]. There is inconsistent evidence regarding the association between preoperative psychiatric comorbidities and weight loss following bariatric surgery [53, 56, 57]. Fisher and colleagues [58] presented findings from a study of more than 8000 bariatric surgery patients that found no significant differences in changes in weight or BMI in patients with and without preoperative mental illness. However, those with preoperative mental illness had greater use of acute care (specifically ED visits and hospital days) between 3 months after surgery through 2 years of follow-up [58]. These findings support the importance of focusing on ensuring that the patient's mental health is stable and that symptom management is more important than the diagnosis [14], as the functional impact of specific symptoms can vary among individuals with similar diagnoses. It is also important to differentiate between genuine symptoms of depression and those that are secondary to medical conditions (e.g., fatigue, changes in appetite, poor sleep, anhedonia vs limited physical function, etc.)

The following areas should be thoroughly assessed and reviewed in order to provide additional insight into the patient's mood stability and openness to seeking treatment: past and current psychiatric diagnoses, symptom frequency, duration, and impact on current life functioning, as well as family history of mental illness. A patient should also be asked about past and current mental health treatment, including any current or prior therapy with a psychologist, therapist/counselor, social worker, or other mental health provider. Further questions are asked about the concerns addressed in treatment, duration, frequency, modality, and the usefulness of therapy. A signed release of information should be obtained from the patient so the behavioral health provider completing the evaluation can speak to the patient's current provider and receive a summary of treatment notes from at least the past 6 months. This helps provide the evaluator with additional insight in terms of the patient's stability and severity of symptomatology. Further, the provider, patient, and the patient's current mental health provider can work together to create a treatment plan to ensure additional support and appropriate follow-up care, especially for those patients with risk factors.

Information is also gathered about past and current psychotropic medication use. Details about doses, formulations, how often the patient takes PRN medications, frequency of missed doses, and the usefulness of medications for symptom management can also be addressed. Patients and their prescribing providers should be educated about the possible changes in the effectiveness of psychotropic medications after malabsorptive procedures, due to changes in pharmacokinetics. The patient should be encouraged to consult with their physicians or prescribing provider about possibly modifying the formulation or dose postoperatively to achieve similar benefits of symptom management seen before surgery [59, 60]. Similarly, a signed release of information can be obtained from the patient to allow the evaluator to gather additional information from their current providers, and to discuss a follow-up plan postoperatively.

Finally, information about past and current suicidal and homicidal ideation, plan, intent, and attempts is gathered, along with information about self-injurious behaviors and psychiatric hospitalizations. Information regarding dates, duration, reason for admission, and discharge recommendations can provide insight into the nature and severity of psychopathology. The evaluator should request a copy of the discharge summary for any psychiatric hospitalization within the past year.

Depression and obesity have been linked to suicide [61]. Results of the systematic review found that patients undergoing bariatric surgery are four times more likely to commit suicide compared to people in the general population [62]. Patients who have a history of self-harm before surgery (especially in the 2 years preceding surgery) are at an increased risk of post-surgery self-harm, or hospitalization for depression in the first 2 years after surgery. Routine postoperative screenings of depression and suicidal ideation are warranted for this vulnerable subset of patients [63].

Although it is not an absolute contraindication for surgery, a recent psychiatric hospitalization or recent suicidal ideation with, or without, a plan, needs to be thoroughly assessed and discussed with the patient's treatment team, as well as with the bariatric surgery multidisciplinary team. Some bariatric surgery programs prefer patients to be stable for a certain number of months prior to proceeding with surgery.

## Trauma

A brief screening of trauma history is typically conducted, as adverse childhood events are associated with adult obesity [64–66]. A study of bariatric surgery candidates found that 16% of the sample reported a history of sexual abuse [67]. It is important to note that it is not necessary to ask for a detailed account of the abuse or trauma. Basic information and documenting if there is a history of trauma or abuse is enough, and similar to other domains assessed, this should be done in a nonjudgmental and supportive way. Because trauma history can affect the development and maintenance of chronic health conditions, the purpose of this inquiry is to provide perspective on the patient's perceptions of the relationship between abuse and current body weight [68]. Patients with unresolved trauma run the risk of re-experiencing negative feelings. Current trauma and abuse should also be assessed and addressed appropriately. Referral to a mental health provider with expertise in the treatment of trauma is recommended for patients who become distressed when discussing a history of abuse, or if the "experience of a 'barrier weight'" is identified [20, 68].

## Substance Use

It's important that past and current substance use is assessed, including alcohol, nicotine products, and illicit and prescription drugs. In addition to the clinical interview, brief validated screening tools can be used to obtain objective measures to distinguish between abuse and dependence. Guidelines for alcohol consumption from the National Institute of Alcohol Abuse and Alcoholism (NIAA) suggest no more than four standard drinks on an occasion or 14 standard drinks per week for men and no more than three drinks on an occasion or seven standard drinks per week for women. Approximately 2 in 100 people who drink within these limits have alcohol use disorder. Frequency and quantity of alcohol consumption should be assessed to rule out binge drinking [69]. Patients appear to under-report alcohol use during preoperative psychosocial evaluations; phosphatidyl ethanol (PEth) testing measures biomarkers of the presence of alcohol over 2–4 weeks and may be helpful in identifying high-risk drinkers beyond self-report or verifying abstinence [70].

During preoperative appointments, regardless of current and past use, all patients should be educated about the risks of alcohol use with post-MBS anatomy, as they are at increased risk for the development of an Alcohol Use Disorder [71]. There is more data to support changes in physiology driving increased AUD after MBS vs "addiction transfer" (i.e., habit substitution). In particular, after a gastric bypass or sleeve gastrectomy, pharmacokinetic changes occur including increased sensitivity to alcohol, faster absorption, and needing a longer time to become sober [72, 73]. Further information on conducting an alcohol history in the bariatric presurgical patient is presented by Heinberg and colleagues [74].

Frequency, duration, and amounts of past and current nicotine use with cigarettes, cigars, chew, snuff, hookah, vapor, and e-cigarettes should be assessed. Clinical guidelines [75] recommend cessation of tobacco by all patients and state that "Patients who smoke cigarettes should stop as soon as possible, preferably 1 year but at the very least 6 weeks before bariatric procedures." Education about avoiding nicotine after surgery should be provided, given the increased risk of poor wound healing, anastomotic ulcer, and overall impaired health. Information for tobacco cessation and treatment options should be provided in writing.

Active substance abuse is a contraindication for surgery [9, 10]. With the changing landscape of medical, legalized, and recreational cannabis, program guidelines will be dynamic and should evolve with clinical and research knowledge. The preoperative psychosocial evaluations can be helpful in identifying cannabis use versus a Cannabis Use Disorder; information gathered should include frequency of use, route of administration (e.g., smoked, edibles, tinctures), estimated doses, cravings, withdrawal, and tolerance. The focus of education should remain on the safety of surgery and short- and long-term complications. Cannabis use does not appear to put patients at significant risk for short-term medical complications (e.g., 30-day readmissions, 30-day ED visits, surgical site infections) [76–78] or compromised weight loss [77–79]. Patients with Cannabis Use Disorder, however, do appear to be at higher risk for medical complications and longer lengths of stay [80]. Toxicology screening should be ordered for patients who are suspected to be using nicotine and illicit drugs, or misusing prescription drugs. A brief review of legal, social, and occupational problems as a result of substance use should be determined, along with treatment history.

## Stress and Coping

Stress is unavoidable, but chronic and/or acute stress, as well as how an individual copes with stress, can negatively affect a patient's mental health and weight management efforts. Identifying ongoing stress and anticipated, or expected, stressors can be helpful for treatment planning, and can also impact the timing of surgery. Patients should plan ahead for the preoperative requirements and for taking time off after surgery for proper recovery and healing. Current significant life stressors could get in the way of a patient successfully following the postsurgical recommendations and should be discussed with the patient, clinician, and possibly even with the bariatric surgery multidisciplinary team. While not ideal, the recommendation to delay surgery may be made in cases where significant life stressors may actually put a patient at risk for poor surgical outcomes [81]. Discussing the patient's coping mechanisms and how they typically cope with stress is also important, as well as finding alternative coping mechanisms if they typically turn to food during stressful times.

## Family History and Social Support

In addition to general background information that is assessed during a standard psychological evaluation (e.g., marital status, highest education attained, difficulties in school, and employment), information about a patient's support network is key. The decision to have bariatric surgery often affects partners, and other relationships, as well as family members, co-workers, and friends. In some cases, these people can be against bariatric surgery and may even try to sabotage weight loss efforts [81].

Relationship dynamics are complicated both prior to, and post-surgery, and can be impacted positively or negatively. Recent research showed that compared to the general population, adults who are not married and pursue bariatric surgery, are more than twice as likely to get married within 5 years of having surgery. Further, adults who are married and get bariatric surgery, are more than twice as likely to get divorced [82]. Relationships are complex and it's important to remember the different motivating factors for one to pursue MBS in the first place. Many changes occur after surgery, including a change in lifestyle behaviors (such as choosing to be more active and eating at home more) and one partner may not agree with some of these changes. Additional factors such as comparing one's weight to that of a partner or to sociocultural norms can lead to weight competition, weight envy, sabotage, negative weight talk, and disputes over food choices [83]. This may prompt further weight evaluation, body dissatisfaction, and conflict between partners [84]. When positive support between couples is lacking during the preoperative stage, the relationship strain postoperatively is exacerbated. Negative responses from one's partner may be related to anxiety or jealousy. Tension can ensue as the patient may be losing weight, gaining confidence, and engaging in a wider variety of activities, which alters the dynamic of the relationship. For a partner who did not undergo surgery or is not losing weight, insecurity and fear of abandonment can develop [85]. This is why a thorough assessment of current relationships and support is important, as well as a discussion of how relationships may change post-surgery.

Patients can, and should, identify positive sources of support, learn ways to improve adherence to eating recommendations, and discuss their plans and expectations with people in their lives. They often must make changes in their daily routines, including limiting eating out, attending potluck events without overeating, and sometimes cooking separate meals for themselves and their families. This can be difficult if it is not discussed in advance and/or others are not supportive of their decisions. Interventions targeted at helping patients learn stimulus control techniques, how to plan ahead for high-risk situations, addressing concerns and barriers to healthy eating prior to surgery, and communicating their needs to others, can help improve outcomes.

## Psychological Testing

Objective psychological testing is utilized in 50–66% of bariatric surgery programs [11, 19]. Standards for psychological testing in patients seeking MBS do not exist at this time, but common measures typically assess symptoms of mood disorders (e.g., depression and anxiety), eating disorders, cognitive function, and general psychopathology [19, 86–88]. ASMBS guidelines for psychological testing advise consideration of psychometric information, availability of bariatric norms, validity indices to assess the degree of over- or underreporting by the patient, the burden of time and cost for the patient, added value of the assessment measure to information gathered in the clinical interview, and finally the utility of measures related to bariatric surgery outcomes [14]. For a comprehensive review of commonly used measures, the reader is directed to LeMonte [86], Heinberg [87], and Marek and colleagues [88]. Discrepancies between the results of objective measures and the clinical interview should be discussed with the patient. A referral for neuropsychological testing may be indicated to better characterize the etiology and nature of a patient's cognitive deficits if found during brief cognitive screening.

## Psychosocial Reasons for Delay Versus Denial of MBS

Research has not identified standard psychosocial contraindications to bariatric surgery, and studies on predictive outcomes show mixed findings [11, 19]. Differences among study results are likely related to methodological differences in survey instruments. The most common recommendation resulting from psychosocial contraindications is to delay surgery in order to improve a condition (e.g., improve knowledge, referral for treatment for unmanaged/untreated mental illness, address maladaptive eating behaviors or untreated eating disorders, current alcohol or substance use disorder). Studies suggest that bariatric programs do not immediately approve patients due to psychosocial reasons up to 25% of the time [19]. Additional reasons for potential delay include active suicidal ideation, recent suicidal attempts or gestures, recent psychiatric hospitalization, or current purging behaviors. None of these are absolute contraindications but need to be addressed with the multidisciplinary team to determine a feasible treatment plan that would take into consideration the potential risk of delaying surgery versus the medical necessity of MBS. Rates for denial of weight loss surgery (at the time of the evaluation) for psychological reasons range between 2% and 6% [19, 59, 89–91].

## Summary of Evaluation Results

The behavioral health provider should be able to provide a provisional *DSM-5-TR* and/or ICD-10 diagnosis and clinical impression at the end of the evaluation [24]. A summary of the evaluation, identifying the patient's strengths and areas of concern, as well as testing results, treatment requirements, and recommendations should be discussed with the patient. This should then be written and added to the patient's chart, as well as communicated to the members of the multidisciplinary team [11, 14]. Like cardiopulmonary evaluations prior to surgery, these summaries do not "clear" a patient for surgery, rather they estimate the risk of complications in their specialty after or during the surgery.

## The Preoperative Preparation Stage

Information gathered from the presurgical psychosocial evaluation helps to identify the patient's strengths as well as areas of concern and where treatment recommendations can be made that will improve short- and long-term outcomes. The time leading up to surgery, between the time of the evaluation and the surgery date, provides an opportunity for intervention through individual or group counseling. Limited research has been done in this area but some bariatric programs have protocols to provide education for preparing for life after surgery. These may be offered as a one-time education session or as a multiple-session treatment to address specific areas of concern. For example, some bariatric surgery programs offer structured—Cognitive-Behavioral Therapy (CBT)-based group treatment interventions. Other programs offer less structured groups or individual preoperative therapy to address specific concerns, such as emotional eating. Further, many programs offer support groups and patients are recommended to attend, preoperatively. Common session topics of CBT-based treatment groups include the importance of goal setting, self-monitoring, stimulus control, how to identify and challenge negative thought patterns, stress management, relapse prevention skills, managing emotional eating, body image, and education about adjusting to life after surgery.

The aim of additional behavioral health preoperative appointments is to improve problematic behaviors or concerns that have been shown to correlate with poor outcomes. Preoperative weight loss is not always related to long-term outcomes. However, recent studies have associated preoperative weight loss with a number of positive outcomes, including shorter operation times [92] and reduced risk of major complications [93].

## The Postoperative Period

### Postoperative Follow-Up

Patients ideally should attend follow-up appointments after MBS with all members of a multidisciplinary team to address overall adjustment [24]. The focus of the initial postoperative appointments is typically on medical and nutritional concerns. Surgery programs also encourage attendance at support groups as this is associated with improved outcomes [94, 95]. Less well-defined is the role of the behavioral health provider in the postoperative process. This may stem from the erroneous belief from a patient's perspective that the preoperative psychosocial evaluation is a one-time hurdle to surgery, and they only need to return if they are having problems. It is recommended that bariatric programs utilize behavioral and mental health services routinely after surgery even if the patient is doing well. MBS teams should also inform their patients of the availability, role, and importance of continuity of care to improve overall success. In addition to individual postoperative appointments, some programs have shared appointments where patients attend appointments with different providers from the multidisciplinary team at different time points postoperatively (e.g., Shared Medical Appointments with medicine and nutrition). This group format offers additional peer support, accountability, and the benefit of sharing ideas and suggestions.

## Weight Recurrence

Weight recurrence following MBS is the most common reason for patients to return to treatment. A systematic review by Karmali [96] found that postoperative weight recurrence varies according to the duration of follow-up and the type of surgery performed. It's interesting to note though that the literature uses multiple definitions and measures to assess weight recurrence, and therefore the range of weight recurrence shown in the literature is quite varied. Lauti et al. [97] aimed to illustrate how the lack of a standard definition of weight regain (now commonly referred to as weight recurrence) significantly alters reported outcomes. It was also found that weight recurrence varied between 5.7% at 2 years and 75.6% at 6 years depending on the definition employed.

Factors leading to weight recurrence are multifactorial [98]. It's important to remember the chronic nature of the disease and its recurrence despite efforts made by both the patient and their healthcare team. With that being said, adherence to postoperative recommendations is directly associated with maintained weight loss. For patients enrolled in lifestyle interventions, variability in weight loss outcomes appears best accounted for by adherence to their respective diet plans [99, 100]. Data from the Swedish Obese Subjects showed that participants decreased their daily calorie intake from 2800 at baseline to 1500 calories at 6 months after surgery. By 10 years postoperatively, patients increased their intake to 1800–2000 calories [101]. Some weight recurrence is likely related to increased energy intake from factors such as grazing eating [50, 102], increased food urges/cravings [103], and increased snacking [104, 105]. Types of snacks were more likely to be high in calories, such as potato chips, crackers, and high-fat microwave popcorn. Snack foods were also more convenient, required little preparation, and emptied quickly from the gastric pouch of a RYGB.

Patients also experienced changes in food tolerance [106, 107]. In addition to experiencing an increase in pouch size, gastric bypass patients may experience gastrointestinal adaptation, increased food tolerance, and a decrease in the unpleasant symptoms of dumping syndrome. Food tolerance was found to be comparable to controls by 5 years postoperatively [107].

Lack of exercise tends to be the most frequently reported noncompliant behavior post-surgery [104]. Not surprisingly, adherence to exercise has been found to be a strong predictor for weight maintenance [108–110]. Other behaviors related to successful weight maintenance include self-monitoring [35, 98], attendance at support groups [95, 111], adherence to follow-up visits [112], and positive response to binge eating treatment [42]. A multidisciplinary and systematic approach to addressing weight recurrence should focus on lifestyle factors, as well as, psychosocial, medical, and surgical factors [98]. Ongoing research in obesity and obesity treatment continues to support the chronic and serious nature of this disease. Given the complexity of the disease and varied individual responses to treatment, multi-modal therapies should be used to treat this disease in a continuous-care model. As early and as often as possible, all members of the multidisciplinary team should introduce the idea of lifestyle interventions and AOMs before and after MBS.

## Reasons for a Postoperative Referral to a Behavioral Health Provider

Davidson [113] discussed the following topics, in addition to weight recurrence, that warrant a referral to a behavioral health provider specializing in the treatment of obesity:

- Problematic eating behaviors including mindless eating, emotional eating, graze eating, binge eating, night eating, or purging.
- Increased depressive or anxiety symptoms.
- Suicidal thoughts.
- Negative feelings including shame, guilt, fear of failure, or fear of weight recurrence.
- Restrictive eating as a weight control method.
- Poor body image or self-esteem.
- Self-sabotage behaviors.
- Poor treatment compliance or difficulty adhering to the recommended lifestyle changes.
- Difficulties with stress management.
- Reemergence of addictive behaviors including drug use/abuse, alcohol use/abuse, cigarette use, or any nonsubstance-related behavior such as pathological gambling, high-risk sexual behavior, impulsive or compulsive shopping, etc.
- Relationship/support network concerns.
- Intimacy concerns.

Although all of the above could warrant a referral to a behavioral health provider, specifically specializing in the treatment of obesity, there are a few instances where a referral may be imperative. Immediate action for follow-up consultation and treatment would be appropriate for a patient who is presenting with suicidal ideation/intent/plan, increased depressive or anxiety symptoms, reemergence of addictive behaviors, or problematic eating behaviors.

## Summary

Behavioral health providers are considered an essential part of the multidisciplinary team in most bariatric surgery programs. These clinicians should have a thorough understanding of the biological, environmental, behavioral, and psychological contributors and consequences of obesity, treatment options, weight loss after bariatric surgery, and long-term maintenance of treatment effects [14, 24]. This chapter provided an overview of the role of the behavioral health provider in the preoperative psychosocial evaluation, preoperative preparation stage, and postoperative period. While no clear standards currently exist for psychological assessment and treatment of a patient seeking metabolic and bariatric surgery, generally accepted guidelines for assessment and treatment were reviewed. The role of mental health in a surgical process has evolved over the past few decades and will likely continue to progress as additional information is gathered to help optimize long-term medical, psychological, and behavioral outcomes.

## References

1. Buchwald H, Avidor Y, Braunwald E, Jensen MD, Pories W, Fahrbach K, et al. Bariatric surgery: a systematic review and meta-analysis. JAMA. 2004;292(14):1724–37.
2. Courcoulas AP, Christian NJ, Belle SH, Berk PD, Flum DR, Garcia L, et al. Weight change and health outcomes at 3 years after bariatric surgery among individuals with severe obesity. JAMA. 2013;310(22):2416–25.
3. Sjöström L. Review of the key results from the Swedish obese subjects (SOS) trial- a prospective controlled intervention study of bariatric surgery. J Intern Med. 2013;273(3):219–34.
4. Schauer PR, Bhatt DL, Kirwan JP, Wolski K, Aminian A, Brethauer SA, et al. Bariatric surgery versus intensive medical therapy for diabetes- 5-year outcomes. N Engl J Med. 2017;376(7):641–51.
5. Maggard MA, Shugarman LR, Suttorp M, Maglione M, Sugerman HJ, Livingston EH, et al. Meta-analysis: surgical treatment of obesity. Ann Intern Med. 2005;142(7):547–59.
6. Hsu LKG, Benotti PN, Dwyer J, Roberts SB, Saltzman E, Shikora S, et al. Nonsurgical factors that influence the outcome of bariatric surgery: a review. Psychosom Med. 1998;60(3):338–46.
7. Sarwar DB, Wadden TA, Fabricatore AN. Psychosocial and behavioral aspects of bariatric surgery. Obes Res. 2005;13(4):639–48.
8. NIH Consensus Development Conference Panel. Gastrointestinal surgery for severe obesity. Ann Intern Med. 1991;115:956–61.
9. Mechanick JI, Youdim A, Jones DB, Garvey WT, Hurley DL, McMahon MM, et al. Clinical practice guidelines for the perioperative nutritional, metabolic, and nonsurgical support of the bariatric surgery patient—2013 update: cosponsored by American Association of Clinical Endocrinologists, the Obesity Society, and American Society for Metabolic & Bariatric Surgery. Obesity. 2013;21:S1–27.
10. Eisenberg D, Shikora SA, Aarts E, Aminian A, Angrisani L, Cohen RV, et al. 2022 American Society for Metabolic and Bariatric Surgery (ASMBS) and International Federation for the Surgery of Obesity and Metabolic Disorders (IFSO): indications for metabolic and bariatric surgery. Surg Obes Relat Diss. 2022;18(12):1345–56.
11. Bauchowitz AU, Gonder-Frederick LA, Olbrisch ME, Azarbad L, Ryee MY, Woodson M, et al. Psychosocial evaluation of bariatric surgery candidates: a survey of present practices. Psychosom Med. 2005;67(5):825–32.

12. Ratcliffe D, Banting E. What is the role of psychology in bariatric surgery? A survey of the differing views of psychologists, the multidisciplinary team, and patients in the UK. Clin Obes. 2023;29:e12612.
13. Greenberg I, Sogg S, Perna FM. Behavioral and psychological care in weight loss surgery: best practice update. Obesity. 2009;17(5):880–4.
14. Sogg S, Lauretti J, West-Smith L. Recommendations for the presurgical psychosocial evaluation of bariatric surgery patients. Surg Obes Relat Dis. 2016;12:731–49.
15. American Psychological Association (APA). What is APA's definition of a 'psychologist'? [Internet]. 2017. [cited 2017 May 1]. Available from: http://www.apa.org/support/about-apa.aspx.
16. American Psychological Association Practice Organization (APAPO). Prescriptive authority. [Internet] 2017. [cited 2017 May 1].Available from: http://www.apapracticecentral.org/advocacy/authority/prescribing-psychologists.aspx.
17. West-Smith L, Sogg S. Creating a credential for bariatric behavioral health professionals: potential benefits, pitfalls, and provider opinion. Surg Obes Relat Dis. 2010;6(6):695–701.
18. National Institute of Health and Care Excellence. NICE Pathways. Surgery and Other Interventional Procedures for Obese Adults. 2021.
19. Fabricatore AN, Crerand CE, Wadden TA, Sarwer DB, et al. How do mental health professionals evaluate candidates for bariatric surgery? Surv Result Obes Surg. 2006;16:567–73.
20. Sogg S, Mori DL. The Boston interview for gastric bypass: determining the psychological suitability of surgical candidates. Obes Surg. 2004;14(3):370–80.
21. de Zwaan M, Mitchell JE. Chapter 4: Eating disorders and eating behavior pre- and post-bariatric surgery. In: Still C, Sarwar DB, Blankenship J, editors. The ASMBS textbook of bariatric surgery, Integrated health, vol. 2. New York: Springer; 2014. p. 25–32.
22. Heinberg LJ, Ashton K, Windover A. Moving beyond dichotomous psychological evaluation: the Cleveland Clinic behavioral rating system for weight loss surgery. Surg Obes Relat Dis. 2010;6(2):185–90.
23. Rosik CH. Psychiatric symptoms among prospective bariatric surgery patients: rates of prevalence and their relation to social desirability, pursuit of surgery, and follow-up attendance. Obes Surg. 2005;15:677–83.
24. Heinberg LJ, Coughlin JW. The role of behavioral health in bariatric surgery. In: Brethauer SA, Schauer PR, Schirmer BD, editors. Minimally invasive bariatric surgery, vol. Chapter 8. 2nd ed. New York: Springer; 2015. p. 83–92.
25. Gonder-Frederick L, Bauchowitz A, Azarbad L, Bender S, Ryee M, Miller A, et al. Assessment of patient knowledge. In: Rosenthal RJ, Jones DB, editors. Weight loss surgery: a multidisciplinary approach. Edgemont: Matric Medical Communications; 2008.
26. Bauchowitz A, Azarbad L, Day K, Gonder-Frederick L. Evaluation of expectations and knowledge in bariatric surgery patients. Surg Obes Relat Dis. 2007;3(5):554–8.
27. Price HI, Gregory DM, Twells LK. Weight loss expectations of laparoscopic sleeve gastrectomy candidates compared to clinically expected weight loss outcomes 1-year post-surgery. Obes Surg. 2013;23(12):1987–93.
28. Kaly P, Orellana S, Torrella T, Takagishi C, Saff-Koche L, Murr MM. Unrealistic weight loss expectations in candidates for bariatric surgery. Surg Obes Relat Dis. 2008;4(1):6–10.
29. Heinberg LJ, Keating K, Simonelli L. Discrepancy between ideal and realistic goal weights in three bariatric surgery procedures: who is likely to be unrealistic? Obes Surg. 2010;20(2):148–53.
30. Foster GD, Wadden TA, Vogt RA, Brewer G. What is a reasonable weight loss? Patients' expectations and evaluations of obesity treatment outcomes. J Consult Clin Psychol. 1997;65(1):79–85.
31. Huberman WL. The importance of pursuing the patient's definition of success following weight loss surgery: strategies and considerations for the bariatric team. Bariatric. Times. 2013;10(1):14–21.

32. Gibbons LM, Sarwer DB, Crerand CE, Fabricatore AN, Kuehnel RH, Lipchutz PE, et al. Previous weight loss experiences of bariatric surgery candidates: how much have patients dieted prior to surgery? Obesity. 2006;14(Suppl 2):70S–6S.
33. Burke LE, Wang J, Sevick MA. Self-monitoring in weight loss: a systematic review of the literature. J Am Diet Assoc. 2011;111:92–102.
34. Wadden TA, Osei S. The treatment of obesity: an overview. In: Wadden TA, Stunkard AJ, editors. Handbook of obesity treatment. New York: Guilford Press; 2002. p. 229–48.
35. Peterson ND, Middleton KR, Nackers LM, Medina KE, Milsom VA, Perri MG. Dietary self-monitoring and long-term success with weight management. Obesity. 2014;22(9):1962–7.
36. American Psychiatric Association. Diagnostic and statistical manual of mental disorders. 5th ed., text rev. American Psychiatric Publishing; 2022.
37. American Psychiatric Association. Diagnostic and statistical manual of mental disorders. 5th ed. Arlington: American Psychiatric Publishing; 2013.
38. Barbuti M, Brancati GE, Calderone A, Fierabracci P, Salvetti G, Weiss F, Carignani G, Santini F, Perugi G. Prevalence of mood, panic and eating disorders in obese patients referred to bariatric surgery: patterns of comorbidity and relationship with body mass index. Eat Weight Disord. 2022 Apr;27(3):1021–7.
39. Mitchell JE, Selzer F, Kalarchian MA, Devlin MJ, Strain G, Elder KA, et al. Psychopathology prior to surgery in the longitudinal assessment of bariatric Surgery-3 (LABS-3) psychosocial study. Surg Obes Relat Dis. 2012;8(5):533–41.
40. Kalarchian MA, Marcus MD, Levine MD, Soulakova JN, Courcoulas AP, Wisinski MS. Relationship of psychiatric disorders to 6-month outcomes after gastric bypass. Surg Obes Relat Dis. 2008;4:544–9.
41. Mühlhans B, Horbach T, de Zwaan M. Psychiatric disorders in bariatric surgery candidates: a review of the literature and results of a German prebariatric surgery sample. Gen Hosp Psychiatry. 2009;31:414–21.
42. Ashton K, Heinberg L, Windover A, Merrell J. Positive response to binge eating intervention enhances postoperative weight loss. Surg Obes Relat Dis. 2011;7(3):315–20.
43. Mauri M, Rucci P, Calderone A, Santini F, Oppo A, Romano A, e al. Axis I and II disorders and quality of life in bariatric surgery candidates. J Clin Psychiatry. 2008;69(2):295–301.
44. Rosenberger PH, Henderson KE, Grilo CM. Psychiatric disorder comorbidity and association with eating disorders in bariatric surgery patients: a cross-sectional study using structured interview-based diagnosis. J Clin Psychiatry. 2006;67(7):1080–5.
45. Stunkard AJ, Grace WJ, Wolf HG. The night-eating syndrome: a pattern of food intake among certain obese patients. Am J Med. 1955;19(1):78–86.
46. Allison KC, Wadden TA, Sarwer DB, Fabricatore AN, Crerand CE, Gibbons LM, et al. Night eating syndrome and binge eating disorder among persons seeking bariatric surgery: prevalence and related features. Obesity. 2006;14:77S–81S.
47. Allison KC, Lundgren JD, O'Reardon JP, Martino NS, Sarwer DB, Wadden TA, et al. The night eating questionnaire (NEQ): psychometric properties of a measure of severity of the night eating syndrome. Eat Behav. 2008;9(1):62–72.
48. Vander Wal JS. Night eating syndrome: a critical review of the literature. Clin Psychol Rev. 2012;32:49–59. https://doi.org/10.1016/j.cpr.2011.11.001.
49. Goodpaster KP, Marek RJ, Lavery ME, Ashton K, Merrell Rish J, Heinberg LJ. Graze eating among bariatric surgery candidates: prevalence and psychosocial correlates. Surg Obes Relat Dis. 2016;12(5):1091–7.
50. Colles SL, Dixon JB, O'Brien PE. Grazing and loss of control related to eating: two high-risk factors following bariatric surgery. Obesity. 2008;16(3):615–22.
51. Smith M, Segal J, Segal R. Emotional eating: how to recognize and stop emotional eating [Internet]. 2017 [updated 2017 May; cited 2017 May 14]. Available from: https://www.helpguide.org/articles/diets/emotional-eating.htm.
52. Dawes AJ, Maggard-Gibbons M, Maher AR, Booth MJ, Miake-Lye I, Beroes JM, et al. Mental health conditions among patients seeking and undergoing bariatric surgery: a meta-analysis. JAMA. 2016;315:150–63.

53. van Hout GC, Verschure SK, van Heck GL. Psychosocial predictors of success following bariatric surgery. Obes Surg. 2005;15(4):552–60. Review.
54. Livhits M, Mercado C, Yermilov I, et al. Preoperative predictors of weight loss following bariatric surgery: systematic review. Obes Surg. 2012;22(1):70–89.
55. Müller A, Mitchell JE, Sondag C, de Zwaan M. Psychiatric aspects of bariatric surgery. Curr Psychiatry Rep. 2013;15(10):397.
56. Kalarchian MA, Marcus MD, Levine MD, Courcoulas AP, Pilkonis PA, Ringham RM, et al. Psychiatric disorders among bariatric surgery candidates: relationship to obesity and functional health status. Am J Psychiatry. 2007;164(2):328–34.
57. Wimmerlmann CL, Dela F, Mortensen FL. Psychological predictors of weight loss after bariatric surgery: a review of recent research. Obes Res Clin Pract. 2014;8(4):e299–313. https://doi.org/10.1016/j.orcp.2013.09.003. Epub 2013 Oct 13.
58. Fisher D, Coleman KJ, Artervburn DE, Fisher H, Yamamoto A, Young DR, et al. Mental illness in bariatric surgery: a cohort study from the PORTAL network. Obesity. 2017;25(5):850–6.
59. Padwal R, Brocks D, Sharma AM. A systematic review of drug absorption following bariatric surgery and its theoretical implications. Obes Rev Off J Int Assoc Study Obes. 2010;11:41–50.
60. Bland CM, Quidley AM, Love BL, Yeager C, McMichael B, Bookstaver PB. Long-term pharmacotherapy considerations in the bariatric surgery patient. Am J Health Syst Pharm. 2016;73:e469–81.
61. Schneider B, Lukaschek K, Baumert J, Meisinger C, Erazo N, Ladwig KH. Living alone, obesity, and smoking increase risk for suicide independently of depressive mood findings from the population-based MONICA/KORA Augsburg cohort study. J Affect Disord. 2014;152–154:416–21.
62. Wagner B, Klinitzke G, Brähler E, Kersting A. Extreme obesity is associated with suicidal behavior and suicide attempts in adults: results of a population-based representative sample. Depress Anxiety. 2013;30(10):975–81.
63. Lagerros YT, Brandt L, Hedberg J, Sundbom M, Bodén R. Suicide, self-harm, and depression after gastric bypass surgery: a nationwide cohort study. Ann Surg. 2017;265(2):235–43.
64. Alvarez J, Pavao J, Baumrind N, Kimerling R. The relationship between child abuse and adult obesity among California women. Am J Prev Med. 2007;33(1):28–33.
65. Williamson DF, Thompson TJ, Anda RF, Dietz WH, Felitti V. Body weight and obesity in adults and self-reported abuse in childhood. Int J Obes Relat Metab Disord. 2002;26:1075–82.
66. Felitti VJ. Long-term medical consequences of incest, rape, and molestation. South Med J. 1991;84:328–31.
67. Gustafson TB, Gibbons LM, Sarwer DB, Crerand CE, Fabricatore AN, Wadden TA, et al. History of sexual abuse among bariatric surgery candidates. Surg Obes Relat Dis. 2006;2(3):369–76.
68. Gustafson TB, Sarwer DB. Childhood sexual abuse and obesity. Obes Rev. 2004;5(3):129–35.
69. NIH National Institute on Alcohol Abuse and Alcoholism. Alcohol facts and statistics. Statistics. 2017 [Updated 2017 Feb; cited 2017 May 20] Available from: https://pubs.niaaa.nih.gov/publications/AlcoholFacts&Stats/AlcoholFacts&Stats.pdf.
70. Miller-Matero LR, Adkins E, Zohr SJ, et al. Utility of phosphatidylethanol testing as an objective measure of alcohol use during the preoperative evaluation for bariatric surgery. Surg Obes Relat Dis. 2023;19(2):158–64. https://doi.org/10.1016/j.soard.2022.10.025.
71. Ivezaj V, Benoit SC, Davis J, Engel S, Lloret-Linares C, Mitchell JE, et al. Changes in alcohol use after metabolic and bariatric surgery: predictors and mechanisms. Curr Psychiatry Rep. 2019;21(9):85.
72. Blackburn AN, Hajnal A, Leggio L. The gut in the brain: the effects of bariatric surgery on alcohol consumption. Add Biol. 2016;22:1540–53.
73. King WC, Chen JY, Courcoulas AP, Dakin GF, Engel SG, Flum DR, et al. Alcohol and other substance use after bariatric surgery: prospective evidence from a U.S. multicenter cohort study. Surg Obes Relat Dis. 2017;13:1392–402.
74. Heinberg LJ, Ashton K, Coughlin J. Alcohol and bariatric surgery: review and suggested recommendations for assessment and management. Surg Obes Relat Dis. 2012;8(3):357–63.

75. Mechanick JI, Apovian C, Brethauer S, Garvey WT, Joffe AM, Kim J, et al. Clinical practice guidelines for the perioperative nutrition, metabolic, and nonsurgical support of patients undergoing bariatric procedures—2019 update: cosponsored by American Association of Clinical Endocrinologists/American College of Endocrinology, The Obesity Society, American Society for Metabolic & Bariatric Surgery, Obesity Medicine Association, and American Society of Anesthesiologists. Surg Obes Relat Dis. 2020;16:175–247.
76. Diggins A, Heinberg L. Marijuana and bariatric surgery. Curr Psychiatry Rep. 2021;23(2):10. Published 2021 Jan 12.
77. Huang EY, Broderick RC, Li JZ, Serra JL, Ahuja P, Wu S, et al. Weight loss outcomes are not compromised in bariatric patients using cannabis. Surg Endos. 2022;37(3):2194–201.
78. Janes LA, Hammond JW, Bonham AJ, Carlin AM, Ghaferi AA, Varban OA, et al. The effect of marijuana use on short-term outcomes with bariatric surgery. Surg Obes Relat Dis. 2023;19:964–70.
79. Worrest T, Malibiran CC, Welshans J, Dewey E, Husain F. Marijuana use does not affect weight loss or complication rate after bariatric surgery. Surg Endos. 2022;36:6931–6.
80. Shah RM, Patel S, Patel S, Sandhu LK, Chand B. Severe cannabis use is associated with complications and prolonged length of stay in bariatric surgery. Obes Surg. 2023;33:1333–7.
81. Sarwar DB, Allison KC, Bailer BA, Faulconbridge LF. Chapter 1. Psychosocial characteristics of bariatric surgery candidates. In: Still C, Sarwar DB, Blankenship J, editors. The ASMBS textbook of bariatric surgery, Integrated health, vol. 2. New York: Springer; 2014. p. 3–9.
82. King WC, Hinerman AS, White GE. Changes in marital status following roux-en-Y gastric bypass and sleeve castrectomy: a US multicenter prospective cohort study. Ann Surg Open. 2022;3(3):e182.
83. Romo LK, Dailey RM. Weighty dynamics: exploring couples' perceptions of post-weight-loss interaction. Health Commun. 2014;29(2):193–204.
84. Klos LA, Sobal J. Marital status and body weight, weight perception, and weight management among U.S. adults. Eat Behav. 2013;14(4):500–7.
85. Bocchieri LE, Meana M, Fisher BL. Perceived psychosocial outcomes of gastric bypass surgery: a qualitative study. Obes Surg. 2002;12(6):781–8.
86. Le Mont D, Moorehead MK, Parish MS, Reto CS, Ritz SJ. Suggestions for the pre-surgical psychological assessment of bariatric surgery candidates. [updated 2017 May; cited 2017]. Available from:http://www.asbs.org/html/pdf/PsychPreSurgicalAssessment.pdf. Accessed 5 April 2010.
87. HeinbergLJ.Theroleofpsychologicaltestingforbariatric/metabolicsurgerycandidates.Bariatric Times [Internet]. 2013 [updated 2017 May; cited 2017 May 14]. Available from http://bariatric-times.com/the-role-of-psychological-testing-for-bariatricmetabolic-surgery-candidates/.
88. Marek RJ, Heinberg LJ, Lavery M, Merrell Rish J, Ashton K. A review of psychological assessment instruments for use in bariatric surgery evaluations. Psychol Assess. 2016;28(9):1142–57.
89. Walfish S, Vance D, Fabricatore AN. Psychological evaluation of bariatric surgery applicants: procedures and reasons for delay or denial of surgery. Obes Surg. 2007;17(12):1578–83.
90. Tsuda S, Barrios L, Schneider B, Jones DB. Factors affecting rejection of bariatric patients from an academic weight loss program. Surg Obes Relat Dis. 2009;5(2):199–202.
91. Sadhasivam S, Larson CJ, Lambert PJ, Mathiason MA, Kothari SN. Refusals, denials, and patient choice: reasons prospective patients do not undergo bariatric surgery. Surg Obes Relat Dis. 2007;3(5):531–5.
92. Alami RS, Morton JM, Schuster R, Lie J, Sanchez BR, et al. Is there a benefit to preoperative weight loss in gastric bypass patients? A prospective randomized trial. Surg Obes Relat Dis. 2007;3(2):141–5. discussion 145–6.
93. Benotti PN, Still CD, Wood GC, Akmal Y, King H, El Arousy H, et al. Preoperative weight loss before bariatric surgery. Arch Surg. 2009;144(12):1150–5.
94. Compher CW, Hanlon A, Kang Y, Elkin L, Williams NN. Attendance at clinical visits predicts weight loss after gastric bypass surgery. Obes Surg. 2012;22(6):927–34.

95. Kaiser KA, Franks SF, Smith AB. Positive relationship between support group attendance and one-year postoperative weight loss in gastric banding patients. Surg Obes Relat Dis. 2011;7(1):89–93.
96. Karmali S, Brar B, Shi X, Sharma AM, de Gara C, Birch DW. Weight recidivism post-bariatric surgery: a systematic review. Obes Surg. 2013;23(11):1922–33.
97. Lauti M, Lemanu D, Zeng ISL, Su'a B, Hill AG, MacCormick AD. Definition determines weight regain outcomes after sleeve gastrectomy. Surg Obes Rel Dis. 2017;13(7):1123–9.
98. Odom J, Zalesin KC, Washington TL, Miller WW, Hakmeh B, Zaremba DL, et al. Behavioral predictors of weight regain after bariatric surgery. Obes Surg. 2010;20(3):349–56.
99. Pagoto SL, Appelhans BM. A call for an end to the diet debates. JAMA. 2013;310(7):687–8.
100. Sarwer DB, Wadden TA, Moore RH, Baker AW, Gibbons LM, Raper SE, et al. Preoperative eating behavior, postoperative dietary adherence, and weight loss after gastric bypass surgery. Surg Obes Relat Dis. 2008;4(5):640–6.
101. Sjöström L. Bariatric surgery and reduction in morbidity and mortality: experiences from the SOS study. Int J Obes. 2008;32(Suppl 7):S93–7.
102. Kofman MD, Lent MR, Swencionis C. Maladaptive eating patterns, quality of life, and weight outcomes following gastric bypass: results of an Internet survey. Obesity. 2010;18(10):1938–43.
103. Burgmer R, Grigutsch K, Zipfel S, Wolf AM, de Zwaan M, Husemann B, et al. The influence of eating behavior and eating pathology on weight loss after gastric restriction operations. Obes Surg. 2005;15(5):684–91.
104. Elkins G, Whitfield P, Marcus J, Symmonds R, Rodriguez J, Cook T. Noncompliance with behavioral recommendations following bariatric surgery. Obes Surg. 2005;15(4):546–51.
105. Faria SL, de Oliveira KE, Faria OP, Ito KM. Snack-eating patients experience lesser weight loss after Roux-En-Y gastric bypass surgery. Obes Surg. 2009;19(9):1293–6.
106. Ernst B, Thurnheer M, Wilms B, Schultes B. Differential changes in dietary habits after gastric bypass versus gastric banding operations. Obes Surg. 2009;19(3):274–80.
107. Suter M, Calmes JM, Paroz A, Giusti V. A new questionnaire for quick assessment of food tolerance after bariatric surgery. Obes Surg. 2007;17:2–8.
108. Elfhag K, Rössner S. Who succeeds in maintaining weight loss? A conceptual review of factors associated with weight loss maintenance and weight regain. Obes Rev. 2005;6(1):67–85.
109. Jakicic JM, Marcus BH, Lang W, Janney C. Effect of exercise on 24-month weight loss maintenance in overweight women. Arch Intern Med. 2008;168(14):1550–9. discussion 1559-60.
110. Coen PM, Goodpaster BH. A role for exercise after bariatric surgery? Diabetes Obes Metab. 2016;18(1):16–23.
111. Livhits M, Mercado C, Yemilov I, Parikh JH, Dutson E, Mehran A, et al. Is social support associated with greater weight loss after bariatric surgery? A systemtic review. Obe Rev. 2011;12:142–8.
112. Pontiroli AE, Fossati A, Vedani P, Fiorilli M, Folli F, Paganelli M, et al. Post-surgery adherence to scheduled visits and compliance, more than personality disorders, predict outcome of bariatric restrictive surgery in morbidly obese patients. Obes Surg. 2007;17(11):1492–7.
113. Davidson P. Behavioral health—when to refer the postop. Paper presented at: Integrated Health: AACE/TOS/ASMBS Postoperative Recommendations Scientific Session; 2014.

# The Role of the Obesity Medicine Physician in the Management of the Bariatric Patient

# 8

Meera Shah

## Introduction

Obesity is a chronic, complex disease that is best served by a team to comprehensively address the biological, anatomical, social, and psychological aspects of managing weight. In practice, this team consists of a physician with an interest in obesity medicine, a psychologist, a dietitian, an exercise therapist, an endoscopist or surgeon and other members on an ad-hoc basis (e.g. diabetes educator). Although the degree of engagement with each one of these groups varies over time, patients under the care of a 'bariatric team' are better supported longitudinally, and team-based care is widely recognized as best practice for patients with obesity [1, 2].

The obesity medicine physician is uniquely positioned to undertake a comprehensive medical assessment of the patient with obesity and make recommendations based on the magnitude and urgency of weight loss needed to improve health. They are also well-equipped to discuss the differences between treatment options including efficacy, risks and long-term durability, and personalize that decision for the individual patient. The American Board of Obesity Medicine (ABOM) currently offers a certification for qualified physicians interested in further training in Obesity Medicine.

Bariatric surgery has been an effective treatment option for obesity for many years, and its popularity continues to rise as the safety and durability of these procedures are increasingly recognized. In parallel, there have been exciting developments in the field of anti-obesity medications (AOMs) that, similar to bariatric surgery, target physiologic pathways involved in appetite regulation. Hence, for the

M. Shah (✉)
Division of Endocrinology, Diabetes and Nutrition, Mayo Clinic College of Medicine, Rochester, MN, USA
e-mail: shah.meera@mayo.edu



O. M. Ghanem et al. (eds.), *The SAGES Manual of Metabolic and Bariatric Surgery*, https://doi.org/10.1007/978-3-031-72309-4_8

first time in a generation, patients with obesity are now able to make an informed choice amongst various effective treatment modalities for their chronic disease of obesity.

Current practice guidelines in the United States recommend that patients with obesity consider bariatric surgery at BMI ≥ 40 kg/m$^2$ without the presence of comorbidities or BMI ≥ 35 kg/m$^2$ if associated with comorbidities. In China, the BMI criteria is set lower (BMI > 32.5 kg/m$^2$, or BMI > 27.5 kg/m$^2$ with comorbidities) [3]. In India, guidelines recommend consideration of bariatric surgery in patients with BMI of ≥35 kg/m$^2$ without a comorbidity, or BMI of ≥30 kg/m$^2$ if associated with comorbidities; and in patients with elevated waist circumference (≥ 80 cm in females and ≥ 90 cm in males) with type 2 diabetes or another weight-related comorbidity [4]. The heterogeneity of these guidelines highlights important differences in ethnicity and metabolic risk, independent of BMI, which should be taken into consideration when counseling an individual patient on the optimal weight-loss strategy.

Many patients who seek bariatric surgery cite improved health and functionality as their primary goals for pursuing weight loss. A key role of the obesity medicine physician is to set realistic expectations with the patient about what constitutes a 'successful' bariatric surgery, and why. For most patients with metabolic or mechanical complications of obesity, a 20–30% total weight loss as is achieved with sleeve gastrectomy or Roux-en-Y gastric bypass, will result in clinically meaningful health improvements. The goal is not to reach a 'normal' BMI and practically speaking, this rarely happens. More importantly, a 'normal' BMI is not necessary to experience the health benefits afforded by weight-loss surgery. These are important conversations to have with the prospective bariatric surgery patient and one that is ideally done in collaboration with a behavioral psychologist who can facilitate pre-operative optimization of the patient's psychological candidacy.

## The Medical Assessment of the Bariatric Patient

A comprehensive medical history, physical examination, medication review and laboratory testing should be undertaken in all patients seeking treatment for obesity.

A history of longstanding difficulty with weight management with multiple cycles of weight loss and regain may make for a stronger case to pursue bariatric surgery in the appropriate patient. Conversely, a patient with multiple previous abdominal surgeries or poor psychosocial functioning may not be the ideal bariatric surgery candidate and non-surgical weight-loss strategies may be more appropriate.

The physical examination can point to a secondary cause of obesity, such as thyroid dysfunction or hypercortisolism. The current European Society of Endocrinology guidelines recommend screening all patients with obesity for thyroid dysfunction with thyroid-stimulating hormone (TSH) [5]. The guidelines recommend against testing for hypercortisolism except when there is clinical suspicion, such as in patients with hyperglycemia, osteoporosis and wide abdominal striae. Additionally, the physical exam may identify findings suggestive of syndromic or genetic forms of obesity such as Bardet Biedl syndrome and Prader-Willi syndrome, and these patients may require screening for associated pathologies. The physical exam is also an opportunity to assess functional capacity and risk of sarcopenia (loss of muscle mass and function) after weight loss from bariatric surgery. Elderly patients are at particular risk for sarcopenia but other populations such as patients with chronic kidney disease, patients on long-term supraphysiologic glucocorticoid dosing or those with significant inactivity at baseline are also at risk [6]. In patients with barriers to activity, such as those with chronic degenerative joint disease, lymphedema or severe obesity, a formal physical therapy assessment and plan should be implemented prior to surgery to reduce the risk of post-operative frailty.

Reviewing the medication record for weight-promoting medications is a key part of the initial assessment of the patient with obesity. Chief amongst these are medications used to treat psychiatric disease, such as anti-depressants, anti-psychotics and anti-epileptics. Where possible, weight-promoting medications should be substituted for weight-neutral or weight-loss medications, but this should be carefully done under the supervision of the patient's psychiatrist. Anti-hypertensive medications such as beta-blockers (atenolol, metoprolol, nadolol, propranolol) and alpha-blockers are associated with weight gain, while ACE inhibitors, angiotensin receptor blockers (ARBs), certain beta blockers (carvedilol, nebivolol), thiazide diuretics and calcium-channel blockers are weight neutral [7].

Glucocorticoids are a class of medications that can contribute to weight gain and increase peri-operative risk for poor wound healing or anastomotic leak. If unable to discontinue glucocorticoid use, the goal is to reduce glucocorticoid dosing to the lowest dose that controls symptoms, a process that can take several weeks or months to achieve. Similarly, immune suppression with other agents, like adalimumab (Humira) or infliximab (Remicade), should not be a barrier to surgery but should be carefully managed pre- and peri-operatively for optimal short and long-term outcomes [8].

Another important class of medications is that used in the treatment of diabetes. Insulin, sulfonylureas, meglitinides and thiazolidinediones are weight promoting, whereas GLP-1 receptor agonists, SGLT-2 inhibitors, metformin and pramlintide are weight-loss promoting. As with any medication, adjustments should be made gradually and in a supervised manner to minimize adverse disruptions to glycemic control. Table 8.1 summarizes classes of medication associated with weight gain and mechanisms by which they do so, where known.

Laboratory assessment of patients with obesity, including those considering bariatric surgery, should include measures of metabolic function—fasting plasma glucose, hemoglobin A1c, liver function tests and a lipid profile; renal function, complete blood count and thyroid function. There is no role for routinely checking vitamin D status, serum testosterone or female gonadal function, except if indicated clinically.

**Table 8.1** Medications associated with weight gain, and putative mechanisms

| Class of medication associated with weight gain | Examples | Putative mechanism |
|---|---|---|
| Anti-depressants* | Tricyclic anti-depressants, e.g. amitriptyline, doxepin<br>Lithium<br>Mirtazapine<br>SSRI e.g. paroxetine | Increased appetite, increased sedation |
| Anti-psychotics | Olanzapine, clozapine, quetiapine, risperidone | Central appetite and satiety dysregulation |
| Anti-epileptics# | Gabapentin, valproic acid, pregabalin, carbamazepine | Central appetite and satiety dysregulation |
| Alpha-blockers | | |
| Beta-blockers | Atenolol, metoprolol, propranolol | Decrease basal metabolic rate |
| Sulfonylureas | Glipizide, glimepiride | Lipogenesis |
| Insulin | | Lipogenesis |
| Thiazolidinedione | Rosiglitazone, pioglitazone | Stem cell differentiation towards adipocytes |
| Meglitinides | Repaglinide, nateglinide | Lipogenesis |

#Topiramate is associated with weight loss
*Bupropion is associated with weight loss

## Prehabilitation

The aim of medically optimizing patients prior to bariatric surgery is to improve outcomes while minimizing complications.

1. Sleep apnea

   Sleep apnea is highly prevalent and yet often undiagnosed in patients with obesity. Patients with sleep apnea are at elevated risk for peri-operative complications, particularly if sleep apnea is severe [9]. Although there is variation in practice it is reasonable to pre-operatively screen all patients with obesity sleep apnea with a questionnaire such as STOP-BANG or with an overnight pulse oximetry, and abnormal results followed up with a sleep study and appropriate treatment.
2. Glycemic control

   Pre-operative guidelines recommend a target hemoglobin A1c below 8% to minimize post-operative outcomes. Intensification of glycemic management may involve insulin for some patients with diabetes to achieve this goal, with careful monitoring of blood glucose particularly if the patient will be adhering to a pre-operative liquid diet. Studies have also shown benefits to improving peri-operative and immediate post-operative glucose control to decrease complications (see below on Special considerations: postoperative monitoring of patients with type 2 diabetes) [10] [11].

3. Liver function

   Metabolic- dysfunction associated with fatty liver disease is present in approximately 50% of patients with obesity [12]. A high index of clinical suspicion for the presence of this condition is important as some patients will not have abnormal liver function tests. Patients with incidentally discovered liver steatosis on imaging (e.g. CT abdomen) should be referred for further staging to determine the severity of fibrosis.
4. Cardiovascular assessment

   Standard pre-operative guidelines for cardiac risk stratification are applied to patients seeking bariatric surgery.
5. Physical functioning

   Patients who undergo bariatric surgery may benefit from a pre-operative program of supervised exercise to reduce post-operative complications. Older patients, who are at higher risk for post-operative sarcopenia, may have the most benefit from this approach; however, the data in this area is still emerging.
6. Pre-operative weight loss

There is limited evidence that supports pre-operative weight loss in patients with a BMI greater than 45 kg/m$^2$ and a prescribed, short-term low-calorie dietary plan may result in lower post-operative complications in this group [13]. However, the vast majority of published evidence suggests that in general, patients achieving pre-operative weight loss see similar operating times, rates of intraoperative and post-operative complications, and weight loss compared to those who do not achieve significant pre-operative weight loss [14]. The requirement for pre-operative weight should therefore not unnecessarily delay patients' progress towards bariatric surgery.

## Post-Operative Monitoring of Bariatric Surgery Patients

### Nutritional Assessment

Patients who have gone through bariatric surgery should be enrolled in a longitudinal program of monitoring for nutritional deficiencies, weight regain (with associated relapse of weight-related comorbidities), and other rare but potentially serious complications of surgery such as alcohol use disorder, nephrolithiasis, bone loss and hypoglycemia.

Patients who undergo bariatric surgery are at risk of nutritional deficiencies for a number of reasons. Firstly, a high proportion of patients who undergo bariatric surgery have unrecognized nutrient deficiencies pre-operatively, due to the consumption of poor nutritional quality foods. Secondly, anatomical changes that occur as a result of bariatric procedures can make the absorption of certain nutrients more difficult (e.g. iron absorption after gastric bypass). Thirdly, the development of food aversions after bariatric surgery can make the consumption of certain foods more difficult (e.g. dairy products), which in turn reduces the likelihood of consumption of specific nutrients (e.g. calcium and vitamin D).

The prevalence of vitamin and mineral deficiencies is variable and dependent on bariatric surgical type. In general, sleeve gastrectomy is associated with the lowest risk of nutrient deficiencies, and the biliary-pancreatic diversion-duodenal switch is associated with the highest risk. Gastric bypass predisposes to the development of iron and vitamin D deficiencies as these nutrients are most efficiently absorbed in the first portion of the duodenum, which is bypassed at the time of surgery. Iron deficiency can be particularly difficult to manage in women with heavy menstrual blood flow and this aspect of the history should be elicited in those patients. Patients with persistent iron deficiency despite adequate oral supplementation may require parenteral (intravenous) iron several times a year.

The nutritional supplementation regimen and recommended testing guidelines for patients after bariatric surgery are as follows [15, 16].

| Recommended nutritional supplementation | Roux-en-Y gastric bypass | Sleeve gastrectomy | BPD-DS or S-ADI |
|---|---|---|---|
| Vitamin D | > 3000 IU/day | 3000 IU/day | > 3000 IU/day |
| Calcium | 1200–1500 mg/day | 1200–1500 mg/day | 1800–2400 mg/day |
| B12 | Oral 350–500 ug/d SQ/IM 1000 mcg/month | Oral 350–500 ug/d SQ/IM 1000 mcg/month | Oral 350–500 ug/d SQ/IM 1000 mcg/month |
| Multivitamin with minerals | >100–200% RDI | >100% RDI | >100–200% RDI |
| Recommended annual testing | CBC, ferritin, vitamin B12*, 25(OH), vitamin D, 24-hour urine supersaturation for oxalate and calcium excretion | CBC, ferritin, vitamin B12*, 25(OH), vitamin D | CBC, ferritin, vitamin B12*, 25 (OH), vitamin D, vitamin A, copper, zinc, 24-hour urine supersaturation for oxalate and calcium excretion |

*If B12 is administered orally or sublingually

## Screening for Alcohol Use Disorder

The prevalence of alcohol use disorder 2 years after sleeve gastrectomy and gastric bypass is approximately 12–15% [17] and this increases the risk of chronic liver disease in the long term [18]. Anatomical changes after gastric bypass surgery contribute to increased hepatic delivery of alcohol and higher peak blood alcohol concentrations which over time, can predispose to the development of alcohol use disorder. Similar to the gastric bypass, sleeve gastrectomy also predisposes to higher and faster peak blood alcohol levels [17, 19] In addition to changes in alcohol metabolism, changes in brain reward processing after bariatric surgery likely contribute to the switch from mal-adaptive eating to problematic alcohol use [20]. The risk of alcohol use disorder increases over time, and therefore all patients should be screened for alcohol use (and misuse) routinely and longitudinally after bariatric surgery.

## Management of Inadequate Weight Loss, Premature Weight Plateaus and Weight Regain After Bariatric Surgery

Despite excellent overall weight loss and weight maintenance outcomes, bariatric surgery is still associated with clinically significant weight regain in some patients [21]. Beyond its impact on cardiometabolic, biomechanical and mental health complications of obesity, weight regain can also have a significant negative impact on quality of life. The reasons for weight regain are often multiple and complex and a multidisciplinary approach addressing eating behaviors, anatomical changes and physical activity routines is needed to tailor a personalized management plan.

Some patients may be reluctant to seek care for weight regain or inadequate weight loss due to their lived experiences of weight stigma or bias in interacting with the healthcare system [22]. Additionally, attrition to follow-up is generally high after bariatric surgery and both these factors result in a lower likelihood of patients seeking care. Patients should be counseled pre-operatively about the likelihood of weight regain and, importantly, the availability of effective treatment options to manage this condition should it happen.

Pharmacotherapy, behavioral therapy, endoscopy, and surgical therapies are all viable options for patients seeking treatment for inadequate weight loss, premature weight plateaus and post-bariatric surgery weight regain. As with any other weight management modality, a multidisciplinary, patient-centered and individualized approach to weight management tends to be most effective at optimizing weight, health outcomes and quality of life.

## Special Considerations: Post-Operative Monitoring of Patients With Type 2 Diabetes

In patients with type 2 diabetes, improvements in glycemic control are seen in the immediate post-operative period before even any weight loss occurs, primarily due to the significant calorie-restricted post-operative diet. With weight loss, further glycemic improvement occurs and most patients with type 2 diabetes see a maximum improvement in hemoglobin A1c approximately 12 months after surgery [23]. An important part of the post-operative care of patients with type 2 diabetes is adjusting anti-diabetes medication to avoid hypo- and hyperglycemia. The patient is encouraged to regularly monitor blood glucose levels and report back to their care team for advice on medication adjustment. In general, the likelihood of achieving remission of type 2 diabetes after bariatric surgery is worse in patients who achieve less weight loss, have a longer duration of diabetes and those on insulin therapy pre-operatively [24]. Nevertheless, almost all patients with type 2 diabetes experience clinical improvement in glucose control and concurrently, a reduction in the number and/or dose of anti-diabetic agents.

## Conclusion

The obesity medicine physician is an integral part of the multidisciplinary team caring for the bariatric patient. They are well-positioned to address medical comorbidities pre-operatively; and postoperatively, establish a program of longitudinal follow-up to ensure optimal nutrition and weight outcomes, screen for relapse of medical comorbidities, add anti-obesity medications when indicated and assess for repeat endoscopic or surgical interventions. Their role as coordinators of care within the bariatric practice should allow patients to feel more confident in their ability to do well before, immediately after and for many years following bariatric surgery.

## References

1. Sauerland S, Angrisani L, Belachew M, Chevallier JM, Favretti F, Finer N, et al. Obesity surgery: evidence-based guidelines of the European Association for Endoscopic Surgery (EAES). Surg Endosc. 2005;19(2):200–21.
2. NICE. Evidence Review for referral for bariatric surgery. 2023.
3. Jia W. Obesity in China: its characteristics, diagnostic criteria, and implications. Front Med. 2015;9(2):129–33.
4. Bhasker AG, Prasad A, Raj PP, Wadhawan R, Khaitan M, Agarwal AJ, et al. OSSI (obesity and metabolic surgery Society of India) guidelines for patient and procedure selection for bariatric and metabolic surgery. Obes Surg. 2020;30(6):2362–8.
5. Pasquali R, Casanueva F, Haluzik M, van Hulsteijn L, Ledoux S, Monteiro MP, et al. European Society of Endocrinology Clinical Practice Guideline: endocrine work-up in obesity. Eur J Endocrinol. 2020;182(1):G1–G32.
6. Yuan S, Larsson SC. Epidemiology of sarcopenia: prevalence, risk factors, and consequences. Metabolism. 2023;144:155533.
7. Jensen MD. Obesity 2020: from basic mechanisms to clinical pearls. Endocrinol Metab Clin N Am. 2020;49(2):xiii–xiv.
8. Maroun J, Vahibe A, Shah M, Mundi MS, Acosta A, McKenzie TJ, et al. Impact of chronic immunosuppression on short-, mid-, and long-term bariatric surgery outcomes. Obes Surg. 2023;33(1):240–6.
9. Sun X, Yu J, Luo J, Xu S, Yang N, Wang Y. Meta-analysis of the association between obstructive sleep apnea and postoperative complications. Sleep Med. 2022;91:1–11.
10. Basishvili G, Yang J, Nie L, Docimo S Jr, Pryor AD, Spaniolas K. HbA1C is not directly associated with complications of bariatric surgery. Surg Obes Relat Dis. 2021;17(2):271–5.
11. Meister KM, Hufford T, Tu C, Khorgami Z, Schauer PR, Brethauer SA, et al. Clinical significance of perioperative hyperglycemia in bariatric surgery: evidence for better perioperative glucose management. Surg Obes Relat Dis. 2018;14(11):1725–31.
12. Chan KE, Koh TJL, Tang ASP, Quek J, Yong JN, Tay P, et al. Global prevalence and clinical characteristics of metabolic-associated fatty liver disease: a meta-analysis and systematic review of 10 739 607 individuals. J Clin Endocrinol Metab. 2022;107(9):2691–700.
13. Anderin C, Gustafsson UO, Heijbel N, Thorell A. Weight loss before bariatric surgery and postoperative complications: data from the Scandinavian Obesity Registry (SOReg). Ann Surg. 2015;261(5):909–13.
14. Bettini S, Belligoli A, Fabris R, Busetto L. Diet approach before and after bariatric surgery. Rev Endocr Metab Disord. 2020;21(3):297–306.
15. Roust LR, DiBaise JK. Nutrient deficiencies prior to bariatric surgery. Curr Opin Clin Nutr Metab Care. 2017;20(2):138–44.

16. Parrott J, Frank L, Rabena R, Craggs-Dino L, Isom KA, Greiman L. American society for metabolic and bariatric surgery integrated health nutritional guidelines for the surgical weight loss patient 2016 update: micronutrients. Surg Obes Relat Dis. 2017;13(5):727–41.
17. Ibrahim N, Alameddine M, Brennan J, Sessine M, Holliday C, Ghaferi AA. New onset alcohol use disorder following bariatric surgery. Surg Endosc. 2019;33(8):2521–30.
18. Mellinger JL, Shedden K, Winder GS, Fernandez AC, Lee BP, Waljee J, et al. Bariatric surgery and the risk of alcohol-related cirrhosis and alcohol misuse. Liver Int. 2021;41(5):1012–9.
19. Acevedo MB, Eagon JC, Bartholow BD, Klein S, Bucholz KK, Pepino MY. Sleeve gastrectomy surgery: when 2 alcoholic drinks are converted to 4. Surg Obes Relat Dis. 2018;14(3):277–83.
20. Blackburn AN, Hajnal A, Leggio L. The gut in the brain: the effects of bariatric surgery on alcohol consumption. Addict Biol. 2017;22(6):1540–53.
21. King WC, Hinerman AS, Belle SH, Wahed AS, Courcoulas AP. Comparison of the performance of common measures of weight regain after bariatric surgery for association with clinical outcomes. JAMA. 2018;320(15):1560–9.
22. Himmelstein MS, Knepp KA, Phelan SM. The role of weight stigma in weight regain in bariatric surgery. Front Endocrinol. 2022;13:1076696.
23. Schauer PR, Bhatt DL, Kashyap SR. Bariatric surgery or intensive medical therapy for diabetes after 5 years. N Engl J Med. 2017;376(20):1997.
24. Purnell JQ, Dewey EN, Laferrere B, Selzer F, Flum DR, Mitchell JE, et al. Diabetes remission status during seven-year follow-up of the longitudinal assessment of bariatric surgery study. J Clin Endocrinol Metab. 2021;106(3):774–88.

# 9 How to Create a Comprehensive Bariatric Center

M. D. Benjamin Clapp and D. O. Carl Pesta

The concept of a dedicated bariatric center has been refined over the last three decades. Metabolic and bariatric surgery (MBS) has been performed since Varco first described the jejunal ileal bypass in 1953, and the concept that these surgeries require special resources has been part of the history of MBS since the beginning [1]. There was a continuous improvement both in surgical technique and outcomes, but MBS was still held with great skepticism until the turn of the twenty-first century. Prior to that, the MBS patient had higher operative risks and these surgeries were performed through an open laparotomy. Not until the laparoscopic revolution, with its concurrent decrease in surgical morbidity and morbidity, did MBS gain greater acceptance [2]. However, there were still high complication rates and reported mortality rates up to 3.5% [3]. To respond to these high complication and death rates, the American Society of Bariatric Surgeons fostered the concept and development of Centers of Excellence. These were bariatric centers that specialized in the treatment of patients with the disease of obesity. The Surgical Review Corporation was created in 2005 to accredit surgeons and centers as experts in bariatric surgery. This funneling of patients to dedicated bariatric centers dropped morbidity and mortality rates dramatically [4]. In 2012, the American Society of Metabolic and Bariatric Surgeons (ASMBS) and the American College of Surgeons jointly created the Metabolic and Bariatric Surgery Accreditation and Quality Improvement Program (MBSAQIP) to further increase quality and safety for patients with the disease of obesity [5]. There are now over 900 accredited bariatric centers in the United States and Canada, providing safe, life-saving surgery to over 240,000 patients a year.

M. D. Benjamin Clapp (✉)
Associate Clinical Professor of Surgery, Department of Surgery, Texas Tech Paul Foster School of Medicine, El Paso, TX, USA

D. O. Carl Pesta
McLaren Macomb Bariatric Surgery Institute, Mount Clemens, MI, USA



O. M. Ghanem et al. (eds.), *The SAGES Manual of Metabolic and Bariatric Surgery*, https://doi.org/10.1007/978-3-031-72309-4_9

The accreditation process is addressed in another chapter, and all centers must meet minimum standards. This chapter addresses what constitutes not only an accredited center but what constitutes a comprehensive bariatric center. The MBSAQIP Standards Manual defines a comprehensive bariatric center; however, this is a narrow definition that says the "center demonstrates compliance with all applicable MBSAQIP standards and successfully completes a site visit; center performs a minimum of 50 bariatric stapling procedures annually, and the MBS Clinical Reviewer enters data into the MBSAQIP Registry; approved to perform all ASMBS-endorsed procedures; have access to the multidiscipline of behavioral health, nutrition, and physical therapy, and only approved to provide care to patients 18 years of age and older [7]." The definition considered by highly reliable and high-quality organizations is broader and meant to be more encompassing. This distinction not only provides bariatric surgery services but also treats a range of diseases of obesity. This comprehensive treatment still includes services like dietary intervention and surgery, but it also includes anti-obesity medication when appropriate. The patients can be entered into a medical-only pathway, or surgical with a cross-over between the two. In-house nutrition support with registered dietitians who specialize in the treatment of obesity should be included. The comprehensive approach also addresses psychological aspects of obesity, and the mental health specialist can be in-house or outsourced. Comprehensive centers should have their own physical therapy teams to pre-habilitate the patients and focus on intense rehabilitation after surgery. As will be demonstrated in this chapter, the defining characteristic of a comprehensive bariatric center is the focus of a more expanded multidisciplinary approach. Comprehensive centers should be considered the highest standard of MBS care and should be willing to treat complications of MBS even if the primary surgery was not done by them.

## Obtaining Accreditation

Obtaining accreditation in the US follows the pathway of the American College of Surgeons (ACS) format of following established standards as is seen in other specialties such as trauma and cardiovascular surgery. The Standards Manual is available as a PDF download via the ASC website: www.facs.org [6].

There are currently eight types of centers available each with similar yet distinct qualifications (Table 9.1). Depending on whether the center is in the United States, Canada or abroad, the number of cases performed annually, the age of patients treated (adult, adolescent, or both,) and the availability of obesity medicine specialists for adults and/or adolescent patients, determines which type of accreditation the center is eligible for. With the exception of a "Data Collection Center", which is specifically for centers outside of the United States, and cannot be formally accredited, all centers must demonstrate compliance with all applicable MBSAQIP standards, undergo a site visit and have an MBS clinical reviewer complete training and enter data into the MBSAQIP Registry. The remaining differentiating criteria include case volume and the age limits of patients. Low acuity centers must perform

**Table 9.1** Types of accredited centers

| | |
|---|---|
| 1. | Data Collection Center |
| 2. | MBSAQIP Comprehensive Center |
| 3. | MBSAQIP Comprehensive Center with Adolescent Qualifications |
| 4. | MBSAQIP Comprehensive Center with Obesity Medicine Qualifications |
| 5. | MBSAQIP Comprehensive Center with Adolescent and Obesity Medicine Qualifications |
| 6. | MBSAQIP Low Acuity Center |
| 7. | MBSAQIP Adolescent Center |
| 8. | MBSAQIP Ambulatory Surgery Center |

*MBSAQIP* Metabolic and Bariatric Surgery Accreditation and Quality Improvement Program

>25 cases annually, and comprehensive centers >50 cases. Ambulatory Surgery Centers require >25 cases and must follow Ambulatory Surgery Center Patient and Procedure Selection criteria [7].

The process for initial application is outlined in the manual. A center first reviews its eligibility based on its ability to satisfy the criteria set forth. Following this, an application is submitted via the website. Once completed, a pre-review questionnaire is filled out online demonstrating full compliance with standards, and the application fee paid. Fees are set by the American College of Surgeons and are currently around $10,000. A recent survey of centers has found that this can be prohibitively expensive and prevent application in some hospital settings. The MBS clinical reviewer is then trained, and a site visit is arranged and completed. Following this, a determination will be made as to accredit the center or not. If accepted the accreditation is retroactive from the day of the site visit and is maintained for 3 years with compliance reports sent in the second and third year and with the reaccreditation application sent in the third year. For reaccreditation, the center must submit a pre-accreditation questionnaire 6 months prior to the end of the accreditation period and if satisfactory, apply for a site visit and the cycle restarts [7].

## Surgical Options Offered by Comprehensive Centers

Any comprehensive bariatric center should be able to offer the range of common metabolic and bariatric operations that are endorsed by the ASMBS. This includes the sleeve gastrectomy (SG) and Roux-en-Y gastric bypass (RYGB), as well as biliopancreatic diversion with duodenal switch (BPD-DS) and the adjustable gastric band (AGB) [8]. These operations have been performed for decades and make up the large majority of MBS in the United States. Recently, the ASMBS has endorsed two new procedures: the single anastomosis duodenal interposition with sleeve (SADI) and the one anastomosis gastric bypass (OAGB) [9]. Surgeons at a comprehensive bariatric center should be able to manage complications, both surgical and nutritional, of these operations, even if they do not perform them. A comprehensive center should not only perform one procedure, like the SG.

Comprehensive centers should also be able to revise any of the aforementioned metabolic surgeries. Revisions now make up the third most common operation performed, after the SG and RYGB [10]. Revision may take the form of anatomic modifications of the previous operation for technical reasons or as a conversion to another MBS for weight recurrence or reflux. Examples of the first instance would be resizing or revising a gastric pouch in an RYGB, and of the second converting an SG to an RYGB, SADI or DS. Implicit to this is the ability to adequately diagnose and work up any issues that may lead to conversion or revision.

MBSAQIP standards require the availability of endoscopic service at an accredited center, but comprehensive centers should incorporate bariatric endoscopic therapy for obesity as well as MBS complications. These can be performed by surgeons, or by gastroenterologists and a team approach can be helpful. Bariatric endoscopy prior to surgery can modify the operative plan and/or prepare the surgeon for the operation [11]. Therapeutic endoscopy is an integral part of the treatment of complications after MBS, especially when managing strictures and leaks. There are also primary bariatric endoscopic options such as the endoscopic sleeve gastroplasty (ESG) which has shown good outcomes that seem to be durable in the midterm, although the ESG is not yet endorsed by the ASMBS and as such, is not a requirement for a comprehensive center [12]. The same device used to perform this procedure can also be used in a revisional role, such as stoma reduction. The intragastric balloon (IGB) is another primary endoscopic bariatric procedure that can be offered to a patient. The patients choosing a primary endoscopic therapy also have the option of going on to a surgical procedure in the future if necessary.

## Medical Management of Obesity

Complete care of the obese patient requires a team approach and a comprehensive MBS program will have an internist to provide this aspect of medical care. The often-complex comorbidities of a patient considering metabolic surgery require attention preoperatively and postoperatively. Integral to this is a qualified obesity medicine physician (OMP). Most often this is an internal medicine physician with special interest, and more often now, special training in the management of the bariatric patient. The American Board of Obesity Medicine (ABOM), The Obesity Medicine Association (OMA), The Obesity Society and other organizations offer extensive continuing medical education in the management of the disease of obesity. The ABOM now offers a certifying exam designating those who pass the exam as delegates of the American Board of Obesity Medicine to highlight their expertise in the field of obesity medicine.

The OMP can manage patients medically and some patients do not require surgical intervention. This is done with a combination of nutrition, anti-obesity medications (AOM), and lifestyle modifications including exercise and behavior therapy. The newly released medications, such as glucagon-like peptide-1 receptor agonists (GLP1-RA) show promise as an effective method of weight loss; however, they have not yet proven to be as effective as MBS [13]. A multimodal approach combining AOMs with MBS, similar to the multimodal approach in cancer treatment, maybe the preferred management of the disease of obesity in the future.

From a patient access standpoint, the emergence of newer medications has opened the door to physicians speaking to patients about more effective treatments for the disease of obesity. In days past the "eat less, exercise more" mantra was all the untrained physicians had to offer. With more effective medical treatment available, these physicians can begin discussions with their patients about effective obesity treatment. This can lead to a referral to an OMP or bariatric surgeon. The addition of a well-trained OMP to an accredited bariatric program is paramount for creating a comprehensive bariatric center.

## Nutritional Support

Nutritional evaluation and support for MBS patients is one of the most important services that an accredited center can offer. Patients with obesity are often malnourished and undergoing MBS will in some cases increase the level of malnourishment. The Nutrition Committee of the ASMBS Integrated Health Clinical Issues and Guidelines Committee has published recommendations for preoperative evaluation as well as postoperative requirements for micronutrients [14]. All caregivers of MBS patients should be familiar with these recommendations. One of the most important members of the multidisciplinary team is the registered dietitian. They will be able to educate and guide the patient during their journey. The dietitian should have special knowledge about MBS patients and be familiar with the various procedures. They should evaluate every patient prior to surgery but should also follow the patients long term. Optimally there will be a follow-up schedule as well as easy availability on an as-needed basis. Educating the MBS patient about nutrition and micronutrient needs is an ongoing, lifelong endeavor.

Nutritional supplements are an essential part of postoperative care for the MBS patient. All accredited bariatric centers should educate patients about these supplements. The ASMBS guidelines need to be communicated to the patients so they can make informed purchases of supplements. The products of one specific vendor should not be endorsed over another vendor, but the nutritionist and surgeon can help the patients make an informed choice. There is great variability in the quality of supplements, and this is not a well-regulated area. For this reason, many comprehensive centers offer vitamin and protein supplements as a point of sale or in conjunction with a reputable vendor. Even so, the patient should be given enough information to make an informed choice.

## Psychological Support

Psychological aspects of the disease of obesity can interfere with long-term success after bariatric surgery. For this reason, a comprehensive bariatric surgery program should involve specialists in the field of behavioral therapy. The behavioral therapist could be a part of the program or outsourced. This has become more common after the COVID-19 pandemic and the widespread adoption of telemedicine.

The role of the behavioral therapist is multifactorial. In the preoperative phase, the evaluation is used to identify significant psychological contraindications for surgery (e.g., substance abuse, or severe poorly controlled depression.) Additionally, the provider can provide support for the patient as they progress through their treatment or delineate recommended therapy prior to surgical intervention [15].

Screening should include a thorough interview of the patient to evaluate the patient's understanding, coping mechanisms, and support structure after surgery. Additionally, psychometric testing is employed which can give more comprehensive data regarding personality traits and psychopathology that may not be directly obtained through an interview alone [16].

A comprehensive center will not employ behavioral services only in the pre-op period to provide a psychological risk assessment of patients. Instead, they will be employed postoperatively as well as there are several Axis I diseases that MBS patients are at risk for after surgery such as suicide, alcohol dependence, and marital stress.

## Prehabilitation, Recovery and Ongoing Fitness

Patients with the disease of obesity often are compromised from a strength and endurance standpoint. There have been studies that demonstrated the value of prehabilitation in patients before colorectal surgery [17]. Patients who undergo a preoperative program improve their functional capacity. Especially in patients with mobility issues, preoperative evaluation by a physical therapist (PT) can improve outcomes. Early mobilization is essential in the postoperative period and the patient should have an in-house evaluation by PT prior to discharge. Some comprehensive centers employ PT or even physical trainers, but the cost associated with this may be out of reach for most programs.

## Conclusions

In conclusion, the creation of a comprehensive bariatric center provides optimal outcomes for our patients suffering from the disease of obesity and is distinct from the more narrow definition described by the MBSAQIP standards. The centralization of resources not only makes the journey of the patient easier but decreases complication rates in the short and long term. A critical element of a comprehensive bariatric center is a multidisciplinary approach to the complex disease of obesity that provides lifelong care. Comprehensive centers also have higher volumes and can care for higher acuity patients. They are able to perform any of the procedures endorsed by the ASMBS and have an obesity medicine physician to assist with the more challenging management of the more complex obese patients.

## References

1. Buchwald H. The evolution of metabolic/bariatric surgery. Obes Surg. 2014;24(8):1126–35. https://doi.org/10.1007/s11695-014-1354-3. PMID: 25008469.
2. Wittgrove AC, Clark GW, Schubert KR. Laparoscopic gastric bypass, roux-en-Y: technique and results in 75 patients with 3-30 months follow-up. Obes Surg. 1996;6(6):500–4. https://doi.org/10.1381/096089296765556412. PMID: 10729899.
3. Livingston EH, Huerta S, Arthur D, Lee S, De Shields S, Heber D. Male gender is a predictor of morbidity and age a predictor of mortality for patients undergoing gastric bypass surgery. Ann Surg. 2002;236(5):576–82. https://doi.org/10.1097/00000658-200211000-00007. PMID: 12409663; PMCID: PMC1422615.
4. Pratt GM, McLees B, Pories WJ. The ASBS bariatric surgery centers of excellence program: a blueprint for quality improvement. Surg Obes Relat Dis. 2006;2(5):497–503; discussion 503. PMID: 17015199. https://doi.org/10.1016/j.soard.2006.07.004.
5. Clapp B, Harper B, Barrientes A, Wicker E, Alvara C, Tyroch A. The MBSAQIP is going viral! 194 hits and still going strong. Surg Obes Relat Dis. 2020;16(10):1401–6. https://doi.org/10.1016/j.soard.2020.06.006. Epub 2020 Jun 12. PMID: 32682772.
6. Metabolic and Bariatric Surgery Accreditation and Quality Improvement Program. https://www.facs.org/quality-programs/accreditation-and-verification/metabolic-and-bariatric-surgery-accreditation-and-quality-improvement-program/ Accessed 10/2023.
7. Optimal Resources for Metabolic and Bariatric Surgery 2019 Standards—Revised 2019. American Society of Metabolic and Bariatric Surgeons. www.facs.org/mbasqip Accessed 10/2023.
8. Clapp B, Ponce J, DeMaria E, Ghanem O, Hutter M, Kothari S, LaMasters T, Kurian M, English W. American Society for Metabolic and Bariatric Surgery 2020 estimate of metabolic and bariatric procedures performed in the United States. Surg Obes Relat Dis. 2022;18(9):1134–40. https://doi.org/10.1016/j.soard.2022.06.284. Epub 2022 Jun 26. PMID: 35970741.
9. ASMBS Consensus Statements. www.asmbs.org. Accessed 10/2023.
10. Clapp B, Harper B, Dodoo C, Klingsporn W, Barrientes A, Cutshall M, Tyroch A. Trends in revisional bariatric surgery using the MBSAQIP database 2015-2017. Surg Obes Relat Dis. 2020;16(7):908–15. https://doi.org/10.1016/j.soard.2020.03.002. Epub 2020 Apr 3. PMID: 32299713.
11. Parikh M, Liu J, Vieira D, Tzimas D, Horwitz D, Antony A, Saunders JK, Ude-Welcome A, Goodman A. Preoperative endoscopy prior to bariatric surgery: a systematic review and meta-analysis of the literature. Obes Surg. 2016;26(12):2961–6. https://doi.org/10.1007/s11695-016-2232-y. PMID: 27198238.
12. Abu Dayyeh BK, Bazerbachi F, Vargas EJ, Sharaiha RZ, Thompson CC, Thaemert BC, Teixeira AF, Chapman CG, Kumbhari V, Ujiki MB, Ahrens J, Day C, MERIT Study Group, Galvao Neto M, Zundel N, Wilson EB. Endoscopic sleeve gastroplasty for treatment of class 1 and 2 obesity (MERIT): a prospective, multicentre, randomised trial. Lancet. 2022;400(10350):441–51. https://doi.org/10.1016/S0140-6736(22)01280-6. Epub 2022 Jul 28. PMID: 35908555.
13. Sarma S, Palcu P. Weight loss between glucagon-like peptide-1 receptor agonists and bariatric surgery in adults with obesity: a systematic review and meta-analysis. Obesity (Silver Spring). 2022;30(11):2111–21. https://doi.org/10.1002/oby.23563. PMID: 36321278.
14. ASMBS Integrated Health Nutritional Guidelines for the Surgical Weight Loss Patient 2016 Update: Micronutrients. https://asmbs.org/resources/integrated-health-nutritional-guidelines. Accessed 10/2023.

15. Sarwer DB, Heinberg LJ. A review of the psychosocial aspects of clinically severe obesity and bariatric surgery. Am Psychol. 2020;75(2):252–64. https://doi.org/10.1037/amp0000550. PMID: 32052998; PMCID: PMC7027921.
16. Sogg S, Lauretti J, West-Smith L. Recommendations for the presurgical psychosocial evaluation of bariatric surgery patients. Surg Obes Relat Dis. 2016;12(4):731–49. https://doi.org/10.1016/j.soard.2016.02.008. Epub 2016 Feb 12. PMID: 27179400.
17. Bousquet-Dion G, Awasthi R, Loiselle SÈ, Minnella EM, Agnihotram RV, Bergdahl A, Carli F, Scheede-Bergdahl C. Evaluation of supervised multimodal prehabilitation programme in cancer patients undergoing colorectal resection: a randomized control trial. Acta Oncol. 2018;57(6):849–59. https://doi.org/10.1080/0284186X.2017.1423180. Epub 2018 Jan 12. PMID: 29327644.

# MBSAQIP and the Value of Accreditation 10

Eric Ahnfeldt

## Introduction

"Quality Improvement" is a ubiquitous term in the healthcare industry. Even Hippocrates sought to provide his patients with the best quality care available at the time [1]. Over the last two decades physician and hospital reimbursements from payer sources have been tied to participation in various quality improvement programs. The implementation of these programs can be expensive and arduous, requiring more administrative personnel, education, and facility upgrades. Despite being voluntary programs, the fear of ever losing accreditation status, can lead executive officers to link staff bonuses to the maintenance of accreditation. That poses the following question: does participation in these programs lead to better outcomes?

The development of QI programs evolved throughout much of the twentieth century and has become woven within the Western healthcare system. As a result, both the financial basis and the structure of healthcare delivery are now inextricably tied to outcomes-based medicine. However, with their ability to capture vast amounts of patient-specific data, these programs have allowed for large-scale highly-powered risk modeling for morbidity and mortality. In doing so, significant advances have been made, shaping the practice of surgery. The Metabolic and Bariatric Surgery Accreditation and Quality Improvement Program (MBSAQIP) is one of the newer quality improvement programs and has a unique history originating out of multiple societies.

The MBSAQIP's structure and function have led to landmark discoveries and advances in the practice of metabolic surgery. In addition, with its partnership with the American Board of Surgery, it is now actively shaping the education and training for future generations of metabolic and bariatric surgeons.

E. Ahnfeldt (✉)
Evans Army Community Hospital, Colorado Springs, CO, USA
e-mail: eric.p.ahnfeldt.mil@mail.mil



O. M. Ghanem et al. (eds.), *The SAGES Manual of Metabolic and Bariatric Surgery*, https://doi.org/10.1007/978-3-031-72309-4_10

## History

In 1917 The American College of Surgeons (ACS) developed the first Hospital Standardization Conference. The conference focused on improving practices and standardizing processes based on input from surgeons throughout the country [2]. It was out of this conference that the ACS developed the "Minimum Standards for Hospitals" which was published and sent to the fellows of the American College of Surgeons on March 1, 1918 [3–5]. The conference was held annually and was directed by the ACS Hospital Standards Committee. By 1926, the ACS published the first standards manual for hospitals. It is this committee in partnership with the American College of Physicians, the American Hospital Association, the American Medical Association and the Canadian Medical Association that directed the formation of the independent not-for-profit organization in Chicago Illinois known then as the Joint Commission on Accreditation of Hospitals (JCAH) in 1951 [5]. In July of 1965, President Lyndon B Johnson signed the Medicare and Medicaid Act. Within this act, language was adopted deeming hospitals accredited by the JCAH to be in compliance with most Medicare Conditions of Participation, and therefore, eligible to be funded through Medicare and Medicaid programs [6, 7]. Despite these advances, these standards were only agreed upon by expert opinion without any outcomes-based data supporting them. It wasn't until 1996 that the now-renamed Joint Commission on Accreditation of Healthcare Organizations (JCAHO) adopted ORYX measures tying performance measurement to accreditation [8].

Meanwhile, a gap remained between quality healthcare and accreditation. While the original minimum standards targeted the structure of a hospital or system, and while ORYX (JCAHO) and SCIP (Centers for Medicare and Medicaid Services [CMS]) evaluated performance measures, no accrediting organization based its accreditation on outcomes. On December 3, 1985, Congress passed Public Law 99-166 stipulating that the Veteran's Administration (VA) must report its surgical outcomes to congress annually on a risk-adjusted basis to factor in a patient's severity of illness and compare them to national averages. To accomplish this the VA set up the National VA Surgical Risk Study (NVASRS) in 1991 [9]. Using embedded nurses in 44 VA medical centers to collect data, the VA built a database of patients' preoperative risk factors and postoperative outcomes. Utilizing this database, the VA was able to develop risk models for 30-day mortality and morbidity in nine surgical specialties. The outcomes, when applied to these risk-adjusted models, matched the quality of processes and systems in each of the hospitals. Now for the first time, quality care could be compared across multiple medical centers based on outcomes. The data from the study was reported in the Journal of the American College of Surgeons in 1995 [9].

The need for ongoing quality improvement and the VA's requirement to report outcome data to Congress led to the creation of the National Surgical Quality Improvement Program (NSQIP). By 1999 NSQIP was expanded outside the VA. And to date, there are over 700 hospitals participating in the program [10].

As NSQIP gained widespread acceptance, the ACS identified several unique subspecialties that would benefit from having specific accreditation standards. In 2005 the ACS released the first Bariatric Surgery Center Network accreditation standards manual (ACS BSCN). The year prior, the American Society for Metabolic and Bariatric Surgery (ASMBS) published their own standards for Bariatric Surgery Centers of Excellence (BSCOE). Both programs kept the following principles central to their accreditation: the leadership of surgeons, the multidisciplinary approach toward the treatment of obesity, and outcomes reporting to a national registry. In 2006 CMS determined that they would only reimburse for bariatric surgery performed at centers of excellence [11, 12]. By 2011, over 100,000 patients per year were entered into either one of the registries [13].

Both ACS and ASMBS identified the opportunity to develop a stronger more unified quality improvement program by combining their respective programs. In March 2012 the two separate programs were unified into the Metabolic and Bariatric Surgery Accreditation and Quality Improvement Program (MBSAQIP) [13]. As of 2023, MBSAQIP has been used as the major source for driving quality improvement research within the field of metabolic and bariatric surgery. A simple Google Scholar search reveals an average of 40 peer-reviewed articles using MBSAQIP data have been published per month every month for the last 3 years.

## Economics of Accreditation

MBSAQIP evaluates procedural volume, risk-adjusted outcomes, process measures, hospital organization and structure to determine accreditation. As a result, there is a significant investment in not only the small cost of participating in the program but also the much greater cost of hiring additional personnel, training and education, infrastructure or facility upgrades and allocating interdepartmental time toward committee meetings. However, these programs would not have succeeded if there were no return on this investment.

At the time of this publication, the initial fee is $10,000 to join the MBSAQIP with an annual participation fee of $6400 annually. This fee allows access to the MBSAQIP Registry, site visit costs, administrative support for the MBSAQIP central staff, and the plaque issued to centers granted MBSAQIP accreditation [14]. However, many sites do not have the requisite personnel required by the program. It is these employee salaries that constitute much of the annual cost of the program for the institution. Three of the necessary positions that require compensation are the Metabolic and Bariatric Surgery (MBS) Director, the MBS Coordinator, and the MBS Clinical Reviewer. Each of these positions requires a significant time investment into the program. These usually are remunerated as a percentage of a full-time equivalent (FTE) or as an additional portion added to an annual salary. For compliance with the MBSAQIP program, the institution must show documentation of a job description or contract, designating an individual into the position within the program at the institution [15].

Initial capital investment to retrofit facilities and upgrade equipment to provide care and safe facilities for obese patients can be extremely costly depending on the status of existing facilities. But there is a return on investment.

On Monday the fourth of January 1965, a landmark piece of legislation was passed entitled, "The Social Security Amendments of 1965. Within this act was a provision that hospitals accredited by the Joint Commission on Accreditation of Hospitals fulfilled the standard of Medicare Conditions of Participation. And these accredited hospitals were thus entitled to receive payments from Medicare [6–8]. With the passage of this legislation, began a new era in medical economics. Now accreditation was linked to revenue generation. Furthermore, accreditation was now a magnet for Medicare patients, thereby increasing accredited hospital's Medicare patient population and boosting revenue. By 1994, 95% of managed care contracts were made with accredited hospitals and organizations [16, 17]. From 2006–2013, the concern for quality care for bariatric surgery patients was so acute that the Centers for Medicare and Medicaid Services issued a national coverage determination (NCD) limiting reimbursements for bariatric surgery to only those performed at accredited centers. Private insurance coverage followed suit, essentially making accredited centers the only centers that could get reimbursed for doing bariatric surgery [11, 12]. During these years the return on investment justified the cost of accreditation. Accredited bariatric centers now could advertise their status, becoming more popular with patients and referring physicians. Accredited bariatric centers achieved improved success reflected in lower morbidity and mortality that can, at least in part, be attributed to their commitment to the QI process integral to the maintenance of accreditation through MBSAQIP [12].

## Resources

The structure and standards of the MBSAQIP are clearly defined in the ACS/ASMBS joint publication, "Optimal Resources for Metabolic and Bariatric Surgery" published in 2019. There are eight standards by which each participating institution is evaluated. These standards include institutional administrative commitment, program scope and governance, facilities and equipment resources, personnel and services resources, patient care (expectations and protocols), data surveillance and systems, quality improvement, and education both professional and community. As part of standard 2, "Program Scope and Governance", each respective program must have a Metabolic and Bariatric Surgery (MBS) committee, program director, program coordinator, and clinical reviewer. Some specialized centers that offer adolescent metabolic and bariatric surgery must also have an obesity medicine director (OMD). These institutionally supported positions ensure that the programs' standards are integrated into the hospital's systems and practices. They also ensure ongoing education and outcomes-based process improvement initiatives are implemented throughout the institution [15].

Furthermore, through participation in the program, the institution participates with the MBSAQIP Data Registry and is allowed access to the registry. The MBSAQIP Data Registry is the first nationwide metabolic and bariatric surgery outcomes database to produce a comprehensive, risk-adjusted report of aggregate and site-level data. This allows for centers to compare their outcomes against an aggregate data set of >150,000 metabolic & bariatric principal operative procedures. In addition, an ongoing series of risk-adjusted reports are available on a semiannual basis (SAR) to participating centers that maintain a minimum of 80% complete 30-day patient follow-up rate [13].

There are additional institutional resources that are required to maintain accreditation. MBSAQIP requires facilities to have a full line of equipment and furniture for the care of metabolic and bariatric patients. This includes radiology equipment to accommodate larger bariatric patients, blood pressure cuffs and other monitoring devices to provide accurate measurements for larger patients. Additionally, hospital furniture and restrooms must be able to accommodate bariatric patients [15].

Surgeons that are verified through the MBSAQIP and are practicing at an MBSAQIP-accredited center have the opportunity through the American Board of Surgery (ABS) to sit for the ABS-focused practice designation (FPD) examination in metabolic and bariatric surgery. This designation recognizes surgeons that have focused their practice on one particular aspect of a given field within general surgery. These surgeons have additional expertise in the field of metabolic and bariatric surgery and dedicate a significant portion of their practice to the surgical care of patients suffering from obesity. The surgeons who achieve this designation typically perform primary, revisional, and endoscopic bariatric surgery [18].

## Accreditation Process

The accreditation process for the Metabolic and Bariatric Surgery Accreditation and Quality Improvement Program (MBSAQIP) is a rigorous and critical aspect of ensuring the safety and quality of care provided to patients undergoing metabolic and bariatric surgery. MBSAQIP focuses on improving the overall patient experience and outcomes.

The first step in the accreditation process involves hospitals and surgical centers voluntarily applying to become MBSAQIP-accredited. Institutions seeking accreditation must meet specific criteria that encompass facilities, staffing, equipment, and processes. This application typically includes detailed documentation of the institution's practices, as well as a commitment to continuous quality improvement [14].

These surveyors assess whether the institution meets the established standards for patient care, safety, and outcomes. They examine various aspects, such as surgical staff qualifications, surgical volume, and adherence to clinical practice guidelines.

The accreditation process also includes comprehensive data submission. Institutions must submit data on their patients' outcomes and experiences before and after surgery. This data is essential for benchmarking, tracking trends, and identifying areas for improvement. MBSAQIP uses a risk-adjusted outcomes methodology to ensure that accurate comparisons can be made across different facilities.

MBSAQIP accreditation requires ongoing commitment to quality improvement. Accredited institutions must continuously monitor and evaluate their performance, participate in regular case review conferences, and make necessary changes to enhance patient care.

The MPSAQIP accreditation revolves around a 3-year accreditation cycle. It is a comprehensive approach to enhancing patient care. It emphasizes the importance of continuously meeting specific standards, conducting thorough reviews, and improving patient outcomes. It also encourages institutions to be proactive in addressing any issues and maintaining the highest level of care for MBS patients.

During the accreditation process, each of the bariatric surgeons at the evaluated institution has an opportunity to become an MBSAQIP-verified surgeon. This official verification signifies the surgeon's commitment to ongoing quality improvement and commitment to excellence in bariatric surgery [14].

## Outcomes

The relationship between accreditation status and clinical outcomes has been a central question of multiple large studies [19–23]. A large systematic literature review by Hussein et al. in 2021 found a significant positive relationship between accreditation status and clinical outcomes. They concluded that accreditation is one element that complements other quality improvement strategies [24].

In 2013 Kwon et al. performed a retrospective review of the rates of inpatient mortality, 90-day reoperations, complications, readmissions, and total payments at Centers of Excellence (COE) sites vs Non-COE sites around the time of the CMS NCD determination [12]. Using a regression model, his team found that accreditation itself had a significant impact on 90-day complications and reoperation rates.

More recently in 2022, Clapp et al. published a comparative analysis of complication rates from bariatric surgery between the Metabolic and Bariatric Surgery Accreditation and Quality Improvement Program (MBSAQIP) and the National Quality Improvement Program (NSQIP) [25]. This team found a significant increase rate of myocardial infarction, sepsis, organ/space surgical site infections, deep vein thrombosis, urinary tract infections, pulmonary embolism, ventilator dependence >48 hours, and pneumonia in cases found within NSQIP as compared to MBSAQIP. These researchers postulated that "because only 18% of centers reported to both databases, … the other 82% of NSQIP centers are not accredited for bariatric surgery by the ACS. By definition, hospitals reporting to the MBSAQIP are accredited. The increased complications reported in the NSQIP likely reflect the effects of nonaccreditation."

Regarding MBSAQIP specifically, in an article published in September of 2023, Morton et al. evaluated the results of 619 MBSAQIP site surveys over 2 years [26]. They documented the various deficiencies that each site surveyor identified and the corrective actions that each site took in response to the deficiencies. During the study period, deficiencies were present at 149 of the 619 program site surveys. The two most common deficiencies were centered around data collection and institutional collaboration. These deficiencies also had the highest rate of resolution after being identified. Ultimately, 98.9% of the sites were able to gain or maintain their accreditation. While only seven programs were denied accreditation. Thus 142 centers were able to take feedback from MBSAQIP to improve their processes. This study demonstrates the additional benefits of centers' participation in the MBSAQIP.

## DATA/Research

Through participation in MBSAQIP, each center is given access to the Participant Use Data File (PUF). The PUF is a Health Insurance Portability and Accountability Act-compliant data file containing cases submitted to the MBSAQIP Registry. The PUF contains patient-level data that does not identify hospitals, healthcare providers, or patients. Only centers that participate in MBSAQIP have access to this data [14]. It is this PUF that has been the source of over 500 peer-reviewed articles published this year, 2023. Many of these publications are clinical investigations that contribute to our understanding of metabolic and bariatric surgery. In addition, they also contribute to the successful academic growth and promotion of institutions and investigators within those institutions. Participation in the MBSAQIP is a potential indirect source for increased academic funding through ongoing research and publication.

## Impact of MBSAQIP Data

From its inception, MBSAQIP has been a powerful tool ushering in a new chapter in evidence-based, outcomes-focused, quality improvement. Multiple risk calculators have been developed using the registry [27–29]. Highly significant population-based clinical practice guidelines regarding VTE prophylaxis and extended prophylaxis have been established [30]. Evaluation of new procedures such as single-anastomosis duodenoileal bypass with sleeve and new technologies such as the robotic platform can rapidly be assessed for safety, and efficacy [31, 32]. Countless evaluations and studies have been harvested from the MBSAQIP registry focusing on certain patient categories [33, 34], comorbidities [35], and critically important gender and racial disparities [33, 36–41]. The registry has even been utilized to critically analyze itself [42]. In all the MBSAQIP Registry has been the subject of almost 3000 publications. As new technology is developed and artificial intelligence matures into the research sphere of large-scale data analytics, MBSAQIP and its Registry will continue to grow, evolve, and advance. Through this process, the benefits that MBSAQIP accreditation brings to clinicians, patients, researchers and institutions will continue to be apparent.

## References


1. Miles SH. The Hippocratic Oath and the ethics of medicine. Oxford University Press; 2004.
2. Whight J. The American College of Surgeons, minimum standards for hospitals, and the provision of high-quality laboratory services. Arch Pathol Lab Med. 2017;141(5):704–17.
3. Nahrwold DL, Kernahan PJ. A century of surgeons and surgery: the American College of Surgeons 1913–2012. Chicago, IL: American College of Surgeons; 2012.
4. Hornsby JA. Hospitals as they are: the hospital problem of today—what is it? Bull Am Coll Surg. 1917;1:4–11.
5. Roberts JS, Coale JG, Redman RR. A history of the joint commission on accreditation of hospitals. JAMA. 1987;258(7):936–40.

6. US Dept of health, education, and welfare: conditions of participation for hospitals. Social Security Administration, 1966.
7. Social Security Amendments of 1965, 89–97, 89th Cong., 1st Sess. 1965.
8. The Joint Commission History Timeline. https://www.jointcommission.org/-/media/tjc/documents/tjc-history-timeline-through-2022.pdf. Accessed 9.15.2023.
9. Khuri SF, Daley J, Henderson W, Barbour G, Lowry P, Irvin G, Gibbs J, Grover F, Hammermeister K, Stremple JF, et al. The National Veterans Administration Surgical Risk Study: risk adjustment for the comparative assessment of the quality of surgical care. J Am Coll Surg. 1995;180(5):519–31.
10. ACS. About ACS NSQIP; n.d.. https://www.facs.org/quality-programs/data-and-registries/acs-nsqip/about-acs-nsqip/.
11. Blackstone R. Accreditation in metabolic and bariatric surgery: pro versus con. Surg Obes Relat Dis. 2014;10(2):198–202.
12. Kwon S, Wang B, Wong E, Alfonso-Cristancho R, Sullivan SD, Flum DR. The impact of accreditation on safety and cost of bariatric surgery. Surg Obes Relat Dis. 2013;9(5):617–22.
13. American Society for Metabolic and Bariatric Surgery. MBSAQIP | American Society for Metabolic and Bariatric Surgery; n.d.. https://asmbs.org/integrated-health/mbsaqip.
14. ACS. Standards; n.d. https://www.facs.org/quality-programs/accreditation-and-verification/metabolic-and-bariatric-surgery-accreditation-and-quality-improvement-program/standards/.
15. Optimal resources for metabolic and bariatric surgery, 2019 standards. Chicago: American College of Surgeons; 2019. [updated 2019; cited 2019 Jun 15]. Available from: https://www.facs.org//media/files/qualityprograms/bariatric/2019_mbsaqip_standards_manual.ashx?la=en.
16. Viswanathan HN, Salmon JW. Accrediting organizations and quality improvement. Am J Manag Care. 2000;6(10):1117–30.
17. Bergman R. No accreditation, no contract, say most managed care plans. Hosp Health Netw. 1994;68:64.
18. American Board of Surgery. Metabolic and Bariatric Surgery Focused Practice Designation; n.d.. https://www.absurgery.org/default.jsp?certfpd_mbs.
19. Brubakk K, Vist GE, Bukholm G, Barach P, Tjomsland O. A systematic review of hospital accreditation: the challenges of measuring complex intervention effects. BMC Health Serv Res. 2015;15(1):280.
20. Greenfield D, Pawsey M, Hinchcliff R, Moldovan M, Braithwaite J. The standard of healthcare accreditation standards: a review of empirical research underpinning their development and impact. BMC Health Serv Res. 2012;12(1):329.
21. Greenfield D, Braithwaite J. Developing the evidence base for accreditation of health care organisations: a call for transparency and innovation. Qual Saf Health Care. 2009;18(3):162–3.
22. Salim FM, Rahman MH. The impact of joint commission international healthcare accreditation on infection control performance: a study in Dubai hospital. Glob J Bus Soc Sci Rev. 2017;5(1):37–45.
23. de Santé HA. Literature review on the impact of hospital accreditation. Paris: MATRIX Knowledge Group; 2010.
24. Hussein M, Pavlova M. Ghalwash, Groot W, the impact of hospital accreditation on the quality of healthcare: a systematic literature review. BMC Health Serv Res. 2021;21:1057.
25. Clapp B, et al. Does accreditation matter? An analysis of complications of bariatric cases using the metabolic and bariatric surgery accreditation and quality improvement program and National Quality Improvement Program databases. Surg Obes Relat Dis. 2022;18(5):658–65.
26. Morton J, English W, Jones D, Provost D. Lessons learned from the metabolic and bariatric surgery accreditation and quality improvement program site surveys: common deficiencies and corrective actions. Surg Obes Relat Dis. 2023;20(2):1–6.
27. Aminian A, et al. Development of a sleeve gastrectomy risk calculator. Surg Obes Relat Dis. 2015;11(4):758–64.
28. Tewksbury C, et al. Validation and improvement of a highly predictive bariatric surgery mortality risk calculator to include sleeve gastrectomy using MBSAQIP 2015–2017 data. Surg Obes Relat Dis. 2020;16(6):725–31.

29. Grieco A, et al. The Metabolic and Bariatric Surgery Accreditation and Quality Improvement Program bariatric surgical risk/benefit calculator: 30-day risk. Surg Obes Relat Dis. 2021;17(6):1117–24.
30. Imbus JR, et al. Extended postoperative venous thromboembolism prophylaxis after bariatric surgery: a comparison of existing risk-stratification tools and 5-year MBSAQIP analysis. Surg Obes Relat Dis. 2023;19(8):808–16.
31. Nasser H, et al. Comparative analysis of robotic versus laparoscopic revisional bariatric surgery: perioperative outcomes from the MBSAQIP database. Surg Obes Relat Dis. 2020;16(3):397–405.
32. Clapp B, et al. Single-anastomosis duodenoileal bypass with sleeve in the United States: a first comparative safety analysis of the Metabolic and Bariatric Surgery Accreditation and Quality Improvement Program database. Surg Obes Relat Dis. 2023;19(1):11–7.
33. Poliakin L, et al. Outcomes of adolescents compared with young adults after bariatric surgery: an analysis of 227,671 patients using the MBSAQIP data registry. Surg Obes Relat Dis. 2020;16(10):1463–73.
34. Janik MR, et al. Safety of laparoscopic sleeve gastrectomy and Roux-en-Y gastric bypass in elderly patients—analysis of the MBSAQIP. Surg Obes Relat Dis. 2018;14(9):1276–128.
35. Afraz S, et al. Bariatric surgery outcomes in oxygen-dependent patients: analysis of the MBSAQIP database. Surg Obes Relat Dis. 2019;15(9):1571–80.
36. Falvo A, et al. Comparison of short-term outcomes following Roux-en-Y gastric bypass in male and female patients using the MBSAQIP database. Surg Obes Relat Dis. 2020;16(9):1236–41.
37. Edwards MA, et al. Racial disparities in bariatric perioperative outcomes among the elderly. Surg Obes Relat Dis. 2022;18(1):62–70.
38. O'Neill SM, et al. An analysis of readmission trends by urgency and race/ethnicity in the MBSAQIP registry, 2015–2018. Surg Obes Relat Dis. 2022;18(1):11–20.
39. Edwards MA, et al. Outcomes in racial and ethnic minorities after revisional robotic-assisted metabolic and bariatric surgery: an analysis of the MBSAQIP database. Surg Obes Relat Dis. 2020;16(12):1929–37.
40. Corcelles R, Del Gobbo GD, et al. Comment on: Outcomes in racial and ethnic minorities following revisional robotic-assisted metabolic and bariatric surgery: a matched analysis of the MBSAQIP database. Surg Obes Relat Dis. 2020;16(12):1937–8.
41. Sarvepalli S, et al. Outcomes in racial cohorts undergoing robotic-assised revisional metabolic and bariatric surgery: an MBSAQIP matched cohort analysis. Surg Obes Relat Dis. 2020;15(10):S13–4.
42. Clapp B, et al. MBSAQIP database: are the data reliable? Surg Obes Relat Dis. 2024;20(2):160–4.

# Essentials: Preoperative Optimization for Bariatric Surgery

# 11

Victoria J. Grille and Ann M. Rogers

## Introduction

Obesity is a chronic, sometimes recurring medical condition. Although there is no cure for obesity, surgery continues to be the optimal treatment as it provides the best and most durable weight loss, improves comorbidities and reduces overall mortality. The current indications for surgery may be found in the ASMBS/IFSO 2022 updated guidelines [11] and were discussed in Chap. 4 of this book.

## Preoperative Assessment

Preoperative optimization is the management of modifiable risk factors prior to elective surgery, with the goal of reducing the risk of perioperative complications and improving outcomes [4]. All patients being evaluated for MBS should undergo a comprehensive nutritional, medical, psychosocial, and behavioral assessment in order to either identify optimizable risk factors or to deem the patient to be currently ineligible for MBS. This process is essential; patients with poorly managed chronic medical conditions, untreated mental health diagnoses, and poor nutritional status have a higher risk of adverse perioperative complications and poorer outcomes. Literature supports postponing surgery until optimization is achieved as this can reduce complication rates by about 40% [19]. The utilization of a multidisciplinary approach involving a comprehensive MBS team allows for the creation of individualized patient-focused plans to ensure optimization.

V. J. Grille · A. M. Rogers (✉)
Penn State Health Milton S. Hershey Medical Center, Hershey, PA, USA
e-mail: arogers@pennstatehealth.psu.edu



O. M. Ghanem et al. (eds.), *The SAGES Manual of Metabolic and Bariatric Surgery*, https://doi.org/10.1007/978-3-031-72309-4_11

## Medical Evaluation

Obesity is often associated with significant medical comorbidities including cardiovascular disease, obstructive sleep apnea, chronic kidney disease, diabetes, degenerative joint disease, cancers and much more. Measures should be taken to ensure these medical conditions are optimally treated prior to surgery in order to reduce postoperative complications and ensure patient safety in the perioperative period. This task requires a combined approach between primary care physicians, obesity medicine specialists, cardiologists, endocrinologists, pulmonologists, nephrologists and others, depending on the individual's comorbidities. All these consultations are at the surgeon's discretion.

A systematic medication history should be reviewed to identify any medications potentially contributing to weight gain, such as antihypertensives, antidepressants, mood stabilizers, hormone therapy, and others. Some of the common medications that cause weight gain are listed in Table 11.1. [44] If the patient is taking such medications, there should be an attempt to seek an alternative. [4] When considering which procedure a patient should undergo, the patient's comorbidities should be taken into account. Patients with advanced organ insufficiency, chronic steroid use, or uncontrolled hypertension are at increased risk of complications such as leaks for all operations. Therefore, after medical optimization, a shorter procedure with a lower risk profile is often a better choice. In general, the benefits of MBS on patient's comorbidities outweigh the associated risks [42].

MBS has been shown to reduce cardiovascular adverse events, improve glycemic and lipid profiles, and reduce an individual's risk of early death. The surgical treatment of severe obesity when compared to nonsurgical treatment has shown a significant reduction in cardiovascular disease with a 49% lower risk. [12] This risk reduction has shown significant benefits along with an associated low-risk profile.

**Table 11.1** Common medications that contribute to weight gain

| Medication class | |
|---|---|
| Antidepressants | Paxil, amitriptyline, Remeron, Effexor, Cymbalta |
| Type 2 Diabetes mellitus | Insulin, sulfonylureas, Glitazone, |
| Hypertension/ cardiovascular | Beta-blockers |
| Epilepsy/seizure | Gabapentin, Lyrica, Divalproex, Valproic acid |
| Antipsychotics | Clozapine, Zyprexa, Seroquel, Risperdal, lithium, Perphenazine, Ziprasidone |
| Anti-histamines | Zyrtec, Allegra, doxepin, Cyproheptadine |
| Contraception | Injectables |
| Sleep | Ambien |
| Others | Corticosteroids |

[4] Although there are no cardiac risk assessments specific to MBS, patients should still undergo routine cardiac workup based on recommendations from the American College of Cardiology (ACC) and the American Heart Association (AHA) [4].

Similarly, there is evidence that weight loss improves glomerular filtration rate and MBS reduces the risk of progression to end-stage renal disease. Although studies have shown that there is a higher risk of complications after MBS in individuals with advanced kidney disease, the absolute morbidity and mortality rates were low, with the benefits of MBS outweighing the perioperative complication risks. However, it is recommended to intervene early in the progression of chronic kidney disease. [5].

## Cancer Screening

Obesity also increases the risk for malignancies in at least 14 organ systems. The etiology is not fully known, but all patients preparing for bariatric surgery should undergo age-appropriate cancer screening prior to undergoing MBS. [4] Concurrent malignancy is not an absolute contraindication to proceeding with MBS. [15].

## OSA/Pulmonary Function

Obstructive sleep apnea (OSA) is one of the most common comorbidities in patients with severe obesity. The physiologic effects result in intermittent hypoxia and increased carbon dioxide levels, increasing an individual's risk of cardiovascular and pulmonary postoperative complications. Screening for OSA should be mandatory in the preoperative period to identify and adequately treat individuals and reduce complications [8].

A consensus-based expert panel guideline was developed in 2016, recommending screening all patients for OSA before MBS using the STOP-BANG scoring system (Table 11.2), or the Berlin Questionnaire. Patients in the study underwent further pulmonary evaluation to determine if CPAP should be implemented given its ability to decrease hypoxic events and associated pulmonary complications in the perioperative period. It is recommended that patients with a high STOP-BANG score undergo sleep testing. This can be done at home or at a sleep center. Patients diagnosed with OSA on CPAP were also advised preoperatively to bring their own CPAP machine into the hospital for the postoperative period. The EAES strongly recommends the use of CPAP in the perioperative period for MBS patients, who have a higher risk of postoperative pneumonia and reintubation. The use of CPAP was also shown to shorten the length of hospital stay (LOS) [10].

**Table 11.2** STOP–BANG Questionnaire for OSA

| | |
|---|---|
| Snoring | Do you snore loudly (louder than talking or heard through a closed door?) |
| Tired | Do you often feel tired, fatigued or sleepy during the daytime? Do you fall asleep in the daytime? |
| Observed | Has anyone observed you stop breathing or choking or gasping during your sleep? |
| Blood pressure | Do you have, or are you being treated for high blood pressure? |
| BMI | BMI > 35 kg/m$^2$ |
| Age | Age > 50 years |
| Neck | Circumference (measured around Adam's apple) > 43 cm (17 in) for males, > 41 cm (16 in) for females |
| Gender | Male |
| ONE POINT SCORED FOR EACH POSITIVE RESPONSE<br>HIGH RISK >5<br>INTERMEDIATE RISK 3–4<br>LOW RISK <3 | |

Ref. [6]

## Glycemic Control

Perioperative hyperglycemia has been shown to be directly linked to an increased risk for postoperative complications and morbidity. [18] One study retrospectively looked at patients with and without diabetes (T2D) undergoing laparoscopic MBS. Both subsets of patients with perioperative hyperglycemia (glucose ≥126) had a higher rate of infectious complications. The patients with diabetes who had hyperglycemia had higher readmission rates, and the patients without diabetes but with hyperglycemia had prolonged LOS [28]. Another study looked at A1c, perioperative glucose levels and associated complications. Those with elevated A1c ≥ 6.5% and perioperative hyperglycemia had higher rates of complications and a higher A1c level correlated to more difficulty in controlling perioperative hyperglycemia. In this study, patients with a history of coronary artery disease and non-white race were more likely to have a higher A1c. [17] Another retrospective review of preoperative A1c in gastric bypass patients showed worse postoperative glucose control with higher preoperative A1c. These patients also had less postoperative weight loss and fewer diabetic remissions along with increased morbidity [33].

All MBS patients should undergo A1c and fasting blood glucose testing preoperatively, as this is a modifiable risk factor. If these tests are found to be elevated, maximal medical treatment should be initiated along with lifestyle/behavioral/diet modification prior to surgical intervention. Fultang, etc., looked at the preoperative predictors of T2D remission following bariatric surgery as not all patients achieve remission. Those with higher A1c levels and preoperative insulin therapy were predictors of a lower rate of remission. The most significant independent predictors of T2D remission were duration of diabetes and plasma C-peptide concentration. Age and BMI may also play a role, as younger patients and those with a BMI between

40 and 50 kg/m$^2$ seem to be more successful at achieving remission. [13] Although this supports the fact that glycemic control should be optimized prior to MBS, current evidence does not show that delaying surgery in an attempt to decrease A1c levels preoperatively improves complication rates. However, controlling a patient's hyperglycemia preoperatively may improve outcomes. [4].

Per the American Society of Anesthesiologists, patients on daily dosing of glucagon-like-peptide-1 (GLP-1) receptor agonists should be advised to hold their medications on the day of surgery. Any patient who is on weekly dosing of GLP-1 agonists should consider holding these medications 1 week prior to surgery due to the associated gastrointestinal symptoms such as severe nausea, vomiting, and delayed gastric emptying. [20]. SGLT-2 inhibitors should be stopped 3–4 days prior to surgery, in order to avoid the risk of euglycemic ketoacidosis. [34] Consideration should be made to consult an endocrinologist for preoperative management in diabetic patients.

## Nutritional Evaluation

All patients who qualify for MBS should meet with a bariatric-specialized qualified dietician who will perform a full nutritional assessment, including weight history, eating behaviors/patterns, MBS understanding, and surgery expectations, and will provide patient-specific behavioral dietary guidance. [38]. A personalized nutrition plan should be developed before and after surgery as patients have different lifestyles, behaviors, and physiologic, hormonal and genetic responses in terms of weight loss. There is a direct correlation between preoperative and postoperative medical nutrition therapy and behavioral modification that leads to increased physical activity and improved outcomes of MBS [4].

Although patients with severe obesity are, by definition, overweight, they are simultaneously nutritionally deficient, often due to the consumption of energy-rich, but nutrient-depleted foods. Studies have shown that there are specific, obesity-related nutritional deficiencies and that MBS patients should be evaluated by a dietician to determine if any supplementation is necessary. [22] It is estimated that 20–30% of patients planning to undergo MBS are nutrient deficient and it is reported that patients who received preoperative correction of their deficiencies did not develop new micronutrient deficiencies; however, those that did not undergo preoperative correction continued to have deficiencies despite postoperative supplementation. [9].

The most common nutritional deficiencies seen in MBS patients include iron, vitamin B12, ferritin, thiamine, folate, and vitamin D. [32]. Patients need to be educated that these deficiencies can worsen postoperatively so it is imperative that they be optimized preoperatively and continue to be monitored postoperatively. Of note, preoperative anemia has been shown to independently increase the risk of postoperative complications and LOS. Early intervention to optimize deficiencies prior to surgery could prevent many adverse outcomes. [18].

## Functional Status: Prehabilitation

Weak recommendations have been made regarding prehabilitation because there is insufficient supporting data [43]. There is some evidence that it may improve a patient's general fitness and respiratory capacity, as well as reduce admission to rehab facilities postoperatively by reducing functional decline [19]. Studies show that it may help reduce morbidity and hospital length of stay. [3] Part of the reason for this limited data to support prehabilitation/preoperative exercise programs may be due to high rates of non-adherence to such programs. [22] However, more functionally dependent people are the high-risk patients.

There is data identifying some MBS patients as "bariatric surgery resistant," meaning that they do not experience significant weight loss, improvement in cardiac health, or diabetes remission. This leads to the question of possible improved outcomes with a combined approach of preoperative lifestyle and pharmacotherapy interventions, exercise programs, and further cardiometabolic optimization. [16]. There is insufficient evidence that preoperative physical activity has an impact on postoperative weight loss; however, it does show that preoperative physical activity has a direct relationship with postoperative physical activity and quality of life. [30].

## Diet Prior to Surgery: Preoperative Weight Loss and Reduction of Liver Volume

Strong recommendations have been made to support short-term preoperative weight loss with a very low or low-calorie diet prior to bariatric surgery [43]. This regimen is recommended for 2–4 weeks prior to surgery and has been shown to decrease liver volume, as well as improve whole-body insulin sensitivity and glycemic state before surgery. This effect can further predict the success of diabetes resolution postoperatively. This short-term (2–12 weeks) very-low-calorie diet (less than 1200 calories per day) has been shown to result in a 10% preoperative weight loss and a 15–20% reduction in liver volume. [38] There is little evidence to support that a liver-shrinking diet improves postoperative weight loss; however, it has been shown to decrease operative time. Weight loss prior to surgery should be at the surgeon's discretion for safety issues. Preoperative insurance-mandated weight loss, however, has not been shown to correlate with postoperative outcomes in any significant way and should not be supported or enforced. [37] Preoperative weight loss should not affect a patient's ability to have surgery and should not be required by programs to prove adherence.

## Smoking/Alcohol Assessment

All patients should be screened for alcohol and tobacco use. Any patient with an alcohol use disorder should be alcohol-free for at least 1–2 years. [26, 43] Nicotine testing should also be done as smoking is the strongest risk factor for postoperative complications [18] A routine cotinine test can give inaccurate results as levels can take 7–10 days to return to normal after cessation of nicotine or nicotine replacement therapy. [2] An alternative would be to perform carbon monoxide testing, which is only detectable for 24 h after the last cigarette.

There is strong evidence to support that patients who smoke or who are second-hand smokers have a higher incidence of postoperative complications. [39] The NSQIP database was used to look at the 30-day complication rates and readmissions for individuals undergoing laparoscopic sleeve gastrectomy and laparoscopic Roux-en-y gastric bypass in patients who smoked. Such patients had a higher likelihood of death or serious morbidity, readmission, wound and respiratory complications. [45] The effects of smoking - vasoconstriction, vascular dysfunction from increased oxidative stress, impaired angiogenesis, and relative hypoxia and hypercoagulability from increased platelet aggregation—all predispose patients who smoke to the risk of leak. [42] Due to this, it is strongly recommended that patients stop smoking at least 6–8 weeks prior to surgery as it can decrease complication rates by greater than 50%. [4, 25] Patients should be provided with smoking-cessation resources. Studies have shown that there is a high rate of return to smoking for prior tobacco users after MBS. This is more common in younger patients and those who have a shorter duration of abstinence. [14, 21] As gastric bypass patients can develop marginal ulcers, and these are more common in the smoking than the non-smoking population, consideration should be given as to whether patients who have recently quit smoking should be offered gastric bypass. [41].

## Psychosocial Evaluation

A preoperative psychosocial evaluation completed by a qualified behavioral health provider is recommended and is also currently required by many third-party payors before approving MBS [27]. Patients with obesity have a higher prevalence of mental health diagnoses. Although the majority of patients experience and report significant improvements in psychosocial functioning after MBS, untreated psychosocial issues can negatively impact weight loss outcomes, LOS, postoperative complications, and readmission rates. [36].

Preoperative psychological screening serves several purposes including identifying any psychological conditions that would be a contraindication to surgery such as active substance abuse, or severe, poorly controlled depression, evaluating any psychosocial factors that could be contributing to obesity, and helping individuals understand and adapt to the lifestyle/behavioral modifications that they will undergo after MBS. Patients who have severe or untreated bipolar disorder, unstable schizophrenia and psychosis, or intractable bulimia are not currently considered candidates for MBS. [7].

Although current substance use disorder is a contraindication to bariatric surgery, a history of substance use disorder is not. Special considerations need to be made when treating individuals with a history of substance abuse, especially regarding postoperative pain management. Research has not shown that a history of substance abuse predisposes a patient to a higher risk for relapse after MBS; however, there is varied and conflicting evidence that MBS patients may be at increased risk for developing postoperative alcohol use disorder. [40].

## Anesthesia

Some anesthetic agents can negatively impact a patient's postoperative recovery, especially in terms of postoperative nausea and vomiting (PONV). All MBS patients should be evaluated by the anesthesia team preoperatively to determine if they are at risk for PONV, which could increase LOS. The recommendations for the prevention of PONV in MBS are the same as the guidelines for the general surgical population with a polypharmacological approach [26]. However, MBS-specific enhanced recovery protocols exist and are frequently used. [31].

Patients with obesity may have a 30% greater chance of difficult/failed intubation and more difficulty with bag-mask ventilation [29]. Experienced anesthesiologists and specialized equipment should be readily available, as patients with obesity are prone to rapid desaturation. Special positioning for the induction and intubation of patients with obesity, particularly those with sleep apnea, is well-described. [23].

## Imaging/Diagnostics

There is no consensus on what if any, preoperative imaging is required for MBS. Many programs have patients undergo an upper endoscopy or upper gastrointestinal series (UGI) for preoperative planning, but imaging should be determined on an individual basis.

## Estrogen Cessation

Estrogen-containing oral contraceptives and hormone replacement therapy increase the risk of venous thromboembolism (VTE), which is already elevated in patients with obesity. It is recommended that estrogen/hormone replacement therapy (HRT) cessation take place at least 1 month prior to MBS and be continued for at least 1 month postoperatively. Patients should be counseled on alternative forms of birth control during this period [24].

## Venous Thromboembolism Prophylaxis

There is a link between obesity and an increased risk of thrombosis related to upregulation in the tissue factor pathway in obesity and metabolic syndrome [35]. To mitigate the risk for VTE, thromboprophylaxis (both chemical and mechanical) is indicated preoperatively, intraoperatively, and postoperatively, according to the

**Table 11.3** Recommended dosages of LMWH based on BMI

| Enoxaparin–VTE Prophylaxis | |
|---|---|
| BMI 30–39 kg/m$^2$ | Use standard prophylaxis dosing (30 mg every 12 h or 40 mg once daily) |
| BMI ≥ 40 kg/m$^2$ | 40 mg every 12 h (30% increase from standard prophylaxis dose) |
| BMI ≤ 50 kg/m$^2$ | 40 mg every 12 h |
| BMI > 50 kg/m$^2$ | 60 mg every 12 h |

updated ASMBS position statement on VTE prophylaxis. [1] Evidence supports that low molecular weight heparin (LMWH) is more effective than unfractionated heparin (UFH) in preventing VTE in patients with severe obesity. It has been shown to have better bioavailability with a lower risk of heparin-induced thrombocytopenia (HIT) while still minimizing the risk of bleeding. IVC filter placement preoperatively is not recommended in MBS patients as the potential complications outweigh the benefits. [1] Table 11.3 lists the recommended dosages of LMWH in MBS patients based on BMI.

## Environment

Studies on postoperative recovery in colorectal patients have shown that favorable hospital environments, such as those that are well-lit and that promote social interaction, may decrease anxiety and modify patient behavior. However, no such studies exist in the MBS population. [22] Further studies may elucidate these questions.

## Patient Education

Individuals should not undergo MBS without understanding the lifestyle changes, both short-term and long-term, associated with MBS.

Understanding the available procedures, the risks associated, the long-term implications, and the lifestyle modifications that are necessary to sustain health are essential for the success of MBS patients. A multidisciplinary team that the patient can rely on for support, education, and guidance throughout the process is helpful in this regard.

There is no defined optimal timeline/frequency of visits patients should undergo preoperatively to ensure success in and after an MBS program. [30] Factors that prolong a patient's progression through an MBS program are likely to lead to an increased dropout rate, thus limiting access to care.

## Conclusion

Obesity is a chronic, recurring disease. Although MBS continues to be the most effective treatment, it is only intended to be one of the components in a multifaceted treatment process. There is currently no standardized protocol for preoperative optimization for patients undergoing MBS; however, optimization in general can be done and will lead to improved outcomes.

## References


1. Aminian A, Vosburg RW, Altieri MS, Hinojosa MW, Khorgami Z. The American Society for Metabolic and Bariatric Surgery (ASMBS) updated position statement on perioperative venous thromboembolism prophylaxis in bariatric surgery. Surg Obes Relat Dis. 2022;18:165–74. https://doi.org/10.1016/j.soard.2021.10.023.
2. Benowitz NL, Bernert JT, Foulds J, Hecht SS, Jacob P, Jarvis MJ, Joseph A, Oncken C, Piper ME. Biochemical verification of tobacco use and abstinence: 2019 update. Nicotine Tob Res. 2020;22:1086–97. https://doi.org/10.1093/ntr/ntz132.
3. Bloc S, Alfonsi P, Belbachir A, Beaussier M, Bouvet L, Campard S, Campion S, Cazenave L, Diemunsch P, Di Maria S, Dufour G, Fabri S, Fletcher D, Garnier M, Godier A, Grillo P, Huet O, Joosten A, Lasocki S, Le Guen M, Le Saché F, Macquer I, Marquis C, De Montblanc J, Maurice-Szamburski A, Nguyen Y-L, Ruscio L, Zieleskiewicz L, Caillard A, Weiss E. Guidelines on perioperative optimization protocol for the adult patient 2023. Anaesth Crit Care Pain Med. 2023;42:101264. https://doi.org/10.1016/j.accpm.2023.101264.
4. Carter J, Chang J, Birriel TJ, Moustarah F, Sogg S, Goodpaster K, Benson-Davies S, Chapmon K, Eisenberg D. ASMBS position statement on preoperative patient optimization before metabolic and bariatric surgery. Surg Obes Relat Dis. 2021;17:1956–76. https://doi.org/10.1016/j.soard.2021.08.024.
5. Carvalho Silveira F, Martin WP, Maranga G, Le Roux CW, Ren-Fielding CJ. The impact of CKD on perioperative risk and mortality after bariatric surgery. Kidney 360. 2021;2:236–44. https://doi.org/10.34067/KID.0004832020.
6. Chung F, Abdullah HR, Liao P. STOP-Bang questionnaire: a practical approach to screen for obstructive sleep apnea. Chest. 2016;149:631–8. https://doi.org/10.1378/chest.15-0903.
7. De Luca M, Angrisani L, Himpens J, Busetto L, Scopinaro N, Weiner R, Sartori A, Stier C, Lakdawala M, Bhasker AG, Buchwald H, Dixon J, Chiappetta S, Kolberg H-C, Frühbeck G, Sarwer DB, Suter M, Soricelli E, Blüher M, Vilallonga R, Sharma A, Shikora S. Indications for surgery for obesity and weight-related diseases: position statements from the International Federation for the Surgery of Obesity and Metabolic Disorders (IFSO). Obes Surg. 2016;26:1659–96. https://doi.org/10.1007/s11695-016-2271-4.
8. De Raaff CAL, Gorter-Stam MAW, De Vries N, Sinha AC, Jaap Bonjer H, Chung F, Coblijn UK, Dahan A, Van Den Helder RS, Hilgevoord AAJ, Hillman DR, Margarson MP, Mattar SG, Mulier JP, Ravesloot MJL, Reiber BMM, Van Rijswijk A-S, Singh PM, Steenhuis R, Tenhagen M, Vanderveken OM, Verbraecken J, White DP, Van Der Wielen N, Van Wagensveld BA. Perioperative management of obstructive sleep apnea in bariatric surgery: a consensus guideline. Surg Obes Relat Dis. 2017;13:1095–109. https://doi.org/10.1016/j.soard.2017.03.022.
9. Deledda A, Pintus S, Loviselli A, Fosci M, Fantola G, Velluzzi F. Nutritional management in bariatric surgery patients. IJERPH. 2021;18:12049. https://doi.org/10.3390/ijerph182212049.
10. Di Lorenzo N, Antoniou SA, Batterham RL, Busetto L, Godoroja D, Iossa A, Carrano FM, Agresta F, Alarçon I, Azran C, Bouvy N, Balaguè Ponz C, Buza M, Copaescu C, De Luca M, Dicker D, Di Vincenzo A, Felsenreich DM, Francis NK, Fried M, Gonzalo Prats B, Goitein

D, Halford JCG, Herlesova J, Kalogridaki M, Ket H, Morales-Conde S, Piatto G, Prager G, Pruijssers S, Pucci A, Rayman S, Romano E, Sanchez-Cordero S, Vilallonga R, Silecchia G. Clinical practice guidelines of the European Association for Endoscopic Surgery (EAES) on bariatric surgery: update 2020 endorsed by IFSO-EC, EASO and ESPCOP. Surg Endosc. 2020;34:2332–58. https://doi.org/10.1007/s00464-020-07555-y.

11. Eisenberg D, Shikora SA, Aarts E, Aminian A, Angrisani L, Cohen RV, de Luca M, Faria SL, Goodpaster KPS, Haddad A, Himpens JM, Kow L, Kurian M, Loi K, Mahawar K, Nimeri A, O'Kane M, Papasavas PK, Ponce J, Pratt JSA, Rogers AM, Steele KE, Suter M, Kothari SN. 2022 American Society of Metabolic and Bariatric Surgery (ASMBS) and International Federation for the Surgery of Obesity and Metabolic Disorders (IFSO) Indications for Metabolic and Bariatric Surgery. Obes Surg. 2023;33:3–14. https://doi.org/10.1007/s11695-022-06332-1.
12. Elsaid MI, Li Y, Bridges JFP, Brock G, Minacapelli CD, Rustgi VK. Association of bariatric surgery with cardiovascular outcomes in adults with severe obesity and nonalcoholic fatty liver disease. JAMA Netw Open. 2022;5:e2235003. https://doi.org/10.1001/jamanetworkopen.2022.35003.
13. Fultang J, Chinaka U, Rankin J, Bakhshi A, Ali A. Preoperative bariatric surgery predictors of type 2 diabetes remission. J Obes Metab Synd. 2021;30:104–14. https://doi.org/10.7570/jomes20084.
14. García-Rodríguez O, Secades-Villa R, Flórez-Salamanca L, Okuda M, Liu S-M, Blanco C. Probability and predictors of relapse to smoking: results of the National Epidemiologic Survey on Alcohol and Related Conditions (NESARC). Drug Alcohol Depend. 2013;132:479–85. https://doi.org/10.1016/j.drugalcdep.2013.03.008.
15. Ghiassi S, El Chaar M, Aleassa EM, Moustarah F, El Djouzi S, Birriel TJ, Rogers AM. ASMBS position statement on the relationship between obesity and cancer, and the role of bariatric surgery: risk, timing of treatment, effects on disease biology, and qualification for surgery. Surg Obes Relat Dis. 2020;16:713–24. https://doi.org/10.1016/j.soard.2020.03.019.
16. Gilbertson NM, Paisley AS, Kranz S, Weltman A, Kirby JL, Hallowell PT, Malin SK. Bariatric surgery resistance: using preoperative lifestyle medicine and/or pharmacology for metabolic responsiveness. Obes Surg. 2017;27:3281–91. https://doi.org/10.1007/s11695-017-2966-1.
17. Goodenough CJ, Liang MK, Nguyen MT, Nguyen DH, Holihan JL, Alawadi ZM, Roth JS, Wray CJ, Ko TC, Kao LS. Preoperative glycosylated hemoglobin and postoperative glucose together predict major complications after abdominal surgery. J Am Coll Surg. 2015;221:854–861e1. https://doi.org/10.1016/j.jamcollsurg.2015.07.013.
18. Greenberg JA, Zwiep TM, Sadek J, Malcolm JC, Mullen KA, McIsaac DI, Musselman RP, Moloo H. Clinical practice guideline: evidence, recommendations and algorithm for the preoperative optimization of anemia, hyperglycemia and smoking. CJS. 2021;64:E491–509. https://doi.org/10.1503/cjs.011519.
19. Jindal P, Patil V, Pradhan R, Mahajan H, Rani A, Pabba U. Update on preoperative evaluation and optimisation. Indian J Anaesth. 2023;67:39. https://doi.org/10.4103/ija.ija_1041_22.
20. Joshi GP, Abdelmalak BB, Weigel WA, Soriano SG, Harbel MW, Kuo CI, Stricker PA, Domino KB. American Society of Anesthesiologists Consensus-Based Guidance on Preoperative Management of Patients (Adults and Children) on Glucagon-Like peptide-1 (GLP-1) Receptor Agonists. American Society of Anesthesiologists (ASA) Task Force on Preoperative Fasting, 2023.
21. Lee SM, Landry J, Jones PM, Buhrmann O, Morley-Forster P. Long-term quit rates after a perioperative smoking cessation randomized controlled trial. Anesth Analg. 2015;120:582–7. https://doi.org/10.1213/ANE.0000000000000555.
22. Lemanu DP, Srinivasa S, Singh PP, Johannsen S, MacCormick AD, Hill AG. Optimizing perioperative care in bariatric surgery patients. Obes Surg. 2012;22:979–90. https://doi.org/10.1007/s11695-012-0648-6.
23. Liew WJ, Negar A, Singh PA. Airway management in patients suffering from morbid obesity. Saudi J Anaesth. 2022;16:314–21. https://doi.org/10.4103/sja.sja_90_22.
24. Lim R. Bariatric surgery for management of obesity: indications and preoperative preparation - UpToDate [WWW Document]. n.d.. https://www.uptodate.com/contents/bariatric-surgery-for-

management-of-obesity-indications-and-preoperative-preparation#H4256532813. (accessed 10.11.23).
25. Lindström D, Azodi OS, Wladis A, Tønnesen H, Linder S, Nåsell H, Ponzer S, Adami J. Effects of a perioperative smoking cessation intervention on postoperative complications: a randomized trial. Ann Surg. 2008;248:739–45. https://doi.org/10.1097/SLA.0b013e3181889d0d.
26. Marinari G, Foletto M, Nagliati C, Navarra G, Borrelli V, Bruni V, Fantola G, Moroni R, Tritapepe L, Monzani R, Sanna D, Carron M, Cataldo R. Enhanced recovery after bariatric surgery: an Italian consensus statement. Surg Endosc. 2022;36:7171–86. https://doi.org/10.1007/s00464-022-09498-y.
27. Mechanick JI, Youdim A, Jones DB, Garvey WT, Hurley DL, McMahon MM, Heinberg LJ, Kushner R, Adams TD, Shikora S, Dixon JB, Brethauer S. Clinical Practice Guidelines for the Perioperative Nutritional, Metabolic, and Nonsurgical Support of the Bariatric Surgery Patient 2013 Update: Cosponsored by American Association of Clinical Endocrinologists, The Obesity Society, and American Society for Metabolic & Bariatric Surgery. Endocr Pract. 2013;19:337–72. https://doi.org/10.4158/EP12437.GL.
28. Meister KM, Hufford T, Tu C, Khorgami Z, Schauer PR, Brethauer SA, Aminian A. Clinical significance of perioperative hyperglycemia in bariatric surgery: evidence for better perioperative glucose management. Surg Obes Relat Dis. 2018;14:1725–31. https://doi.org/10.1016/j.soard.2018.07.028.
29. Members of the Working Party, Nightingale CE, Margarson MP, Shearer E, Redman JW, Lucas DN, Cousins JM, Fox WTA, Kennedy NJ, Venn PJ, Skues M, Gabbott D, Misra U, Pandit JJ, Popat MT, Griffiths R. Peri-operative management of the obese surgical patient 2015: Association of Anaesthetists of Great Britain and Ireland Society for Obesity and Bariatric Anaesthesia. Anaesthesia. 2015;70:859–76. https://doi.org/10.1111/anae.13101.
30. Moore JM, Haemer MA, Fox CK. Lifestyle and pharmacologic management before and after bariatric surgery. Semin Pediatr Surg. 2020;29:150889. https://doi.org/10.1016/j.sempedsurg.2020.150889.
31. Morton J. The first metabolic and bariatric surgery accreditation and quality improvement program quality initiative: decreasing readmissions through opportunities provided. Surg Obes Relat Dis. 2014;10:377–8. https://doi.org/10.1016/j.soard.2014.02.036.
32. O'Kane M, Parretti HM, Pinkney J, Welbourn R, Hughes CA, Mok J, Walker N, Thomas D, Devin J, Coulman KD, Pinnock G, Batterham RL, Mahawar KK, Sharma M, Blakemore AI, McMillan I, Barth JH. British obesity and metabolic surgery society guidelines on perioperative and postoperative biochemical monitoring and micronutrient replacement for patients undergoing bariatric surgery—2020 update. Obes Rev. 2020;21:e13087. https://doi.org/10.1111/obr.13087.
33. Perna M, Romagnuolo J, Morgan K, Byrne TK, Baker M. Preoperative hemoglobin A1c and postoperative glucose control in outcomes after gastric bypass for obesity. Surg Obes Relat Dis. 2012;8:685–90. https://doi.org/10.1016/j.soard.2011.08.002.
34. Plewa MC, Bryant M, King-Thiele R. Euglycemic diabetic ketoacidosis. In: StatPearls. Treasure Island, FL: StatPearls Publishing; 2023.
35. Samad F, Ruf W. Inflammation, obesity, and thrombosis. Blood. 2013;122:3415–22. https://doi.org/10.1182/blood-2013-05-427708.
36. Sarwer DB, Heinberg LJ. A review of the psychosocial aspects of clinically severe obesity and bariatric surgery. Am Psychol. 2020;75:252–64. https://doi.org/10.1037/amp0000550.
37. Schneider A, Hutcheon DA, Hale A, Ewing JA, Miller M, Scott JD. Postoperative outcomes in bariatric surgical patients participating in an insurance-mandated preoperative weight management program. Surg Obes Relat Dis. 2018;14:623–30. https://doi.org/10.1016/j.soard.2018.01.036.
38. Sherf Dagan S, Goldenshluger A, Globus I, Schweiger C, Kessler Y, Kowen Sandbank G, Ben-Porat T, Sinai T. Nutritional recommendations for adult bariatric surgery patients: clinical practice. Adv Nutr. 2017;8:382–94. https://doi.org/10.3945/an.116.014258.

39. Sørensen LT. Wound healing and infection in surgery: the clinical impact of smoking and smoking cessation: a systematic review and meta-analysis. Arch Surg. 2012;147:373. https://doi.org/10.1001/archsurg.2012.5.
40. Spadola CE, Wagner EF, Varga LM, Syvertsen JL, De La Cruz Munoz NF, Messiah SE. A qualitative examination of increased alcohol use after bariatric surgery among racially/ethnically diverse young adults. Obes Surg. 2018;28:1492–7. https://doi.org/10.1007/s11695-017-3022-x.
41. Spaniolas K, Yang J, Crowley S, Yin D, Docimo S, Bates AT, Pryor AD. Association of long-term anastomotic ulceration after Roux-en-Y gastric bypass with tobacco smoking. JAMA Surg. 2018;153:862–4. https://doi.org/10.1001/jamasurg.2018.1616.
42. Spiro C, Bennet S, Bhatia K. Meta-analysis of patient risk factors associated with post-bariatric surgery leak. Obes Sci Pract. 2023;9:112–26. https://doi.org/10.1002/osp4.628.
43. Stenberg E, Dos Reis Falcão LF, O'Kane M, Liem R, Pournaras DJ, Salminen P, Urman RD, Wadhwa A, Gustafsson UO, Thorell A. Guidelines for perioperative care in bariatric surgery: Enhanced Recovery After Surgery (ERAS) society recommendations: a 2021 update. World J Surg. 2022;46:729–51. https://doi.org/10.1007/s00268-021-06394-9.
44. Verhaegen AA, Van Gaal LF. Drugs that affect body weight, body fat distribution, and metabolism. In: Feingold KR, Anawalt B, Blackman MR, Boyce A, Chrousos G, Corpas E, de Herder WW, Dhatariya K, Dungan K, Hofland J, Kalra S, Kaltsas G, Kapoor N, Koch C, Kopp P, Korbonits M, Kovacs CS, Kuohung W, Laferrère B, Levy M, McGee EA, McLachlan R, New M, Purnell J, Sahay R, Shah AS, Singer F, Sperling MA, Stratakis CA, Trence DL, Wilson DP, editors. Endotext. South Dartmouth, MA: MDText.com, Inc; 2000.
45. Yuce TK, Khorfan R, Soper NJ, Hungness ES, Nagle AP, Teitelbaum EN, Bilimoria KY, Odell DD. Post-operative complications and readmissions associated with smoking following bariatric surgery. J Gastrointest Surg. 2020;24:525–30. https://doi.org/10.1007/s11605-019-04488-3.

# 12 Postoperative Bariatric Care and Enhanced Recovery Pathways

Danbee H. Kim

## Clinical Pathways

Clinical pathways are designed to provide evidence-based structure to routine clinical practice and aim to provide consistency in care and reduce healthcare costs. The American Society of Metabolic and Bariatric Surgeons (ASMBS) and Metabolic and Bariatric Surgery Accreditation and Quality Improvement Program (MBSAQIP), therefore, mandate accredited institutions to follow a bariatric surgery clinical pathway [1]. However, such pathways are not required to be uniform, leading to significant practice gaps nationwide.

A recent study that compared clinical pathways among different practicing bariatric surgeons showed variability in preoperative nutritional and psychological evaluation, venous thromboembolic event prophylaxis, pain management and postoperative laboratory studies [2]. To minimize this variability and promote evidence-based healthcare, ASMBS, in collaboration with several experts, recently developed a perioperative care pathway guideline for laparoscopic sleeve gastrectomy and preoperative care guideline for laparoscopic Roux-en-Y gastric bypass [3, 4]. These guidelines include recommendations on routine or selective laboratory studies, consultations, tests, medications and follow-up intervals. Of note, these guidelines were developed as tools to help institutions develop their own clinical pathways and should be used with caution to state the standard of care. The ultimate clinical judgment on the course of action for each bariatric case and the designing of a care plan is at the discretion of the practicing physician.

D. H. Kim (✉)
Assistant Professor of Surgery, Rutgers New Jersey Medical School, Newark, NJ, USA
e-mail: dhk84@njms.rutgers.edu



O. M. Ghanem et al. (eds.), *The SAGES Manual of Metabolic and Bariatric Surgery*, https://doi.org/10.1007/978-3-031-72309-4_12

## Enhanced Recovery After Surgery

Enhanced recovery after surgery (ERAS) first emerged nearly two decades ago and focuses on fast-tracking the surgical recovery process by maintaining normal physiology throughout the perioperative period. The primary focus of the ERAS protocol is to improve patient outcomes and potentially reduce overall hospital costs by preoperative optimization of patients, minimization of perioperative stress, maintenance of postoperative physiology, and shortening of recovery time after surgery [5]. It subdivides the perioperative period into preadmission, preoperative, intraoperative and postoperative phases, and involves a multidisciplinary team, ranging from nursing staff to physicians, intricately working together to provide a patient-centered multimodal perioperative care.

## Preadmission Phase

The preadmission phase focuses on patient education and optimization through such processes as setting realistic expectations on the impact of changes in the patient's life before and after bariatric surgery. This process should be based on an extensive review of the ERAS pathway at multiple points of contact with the patient, including all preoperative visits, phone conversations and written materials. Patients should be screened for smoking and alcohol use and counseled to stop smoking at least 4 weeks before surgery [6] and cease any alcohol consumption for 1–2 years [7] to minimize complications. It is also recommended that patients lose weight using a low- or very low-calorie diet prior to surgery [8, 9]. This recommendation also applies to patients with diabetes. Prehabilitation is also encouraged [10], although the level of evidence for its effectiveness remains low.

Although the level of evidence is low to moderate, mainly due to the paucity of research for bariatric patients in this area, the ERAS society stresses the importance of thorough review and counseling of patients in the preadmission phase to better prepare them for surgery. Intensive preoperative education was shown to reduce patient anxiety, postoperative pain, length of stay (LOS), and improve self-body image in previous meta-analysis and RCT of patients undergoing visceral surgery [11–13]. The preadmission phase is necessary to improve the patient's overall knowledge, motivation, and risk perception and to ultimately prepare the patient to make well-informed autonomous choices.

## Preoperative Phase

### Pharmacologic Intervention

To minimize stress response and maintain homeostasis in the intra and postoperative period, several pharmacological interventions are suggested. Of note, there is a paucity of studies reporting the effect of these interventions in bariatric surgery. Thus, the recommendations for using such interventions remain weak.

Glucocorticoids have anti-inflammatory properties that in theory reduce postoperative stress responses. Although there are still very few on bariatric surgery, several studies on other gastrointestinal surgeries showed that a single dose of 8 mg dexamethasone upon induction of anesthesia was associated with less postoperative nausea, fewer overall complications, reduced systemic inflammatory response, and postoperative pain and ultimately shortened the length of stay [14–16].

Many bariatric patients are on multiple medications for their obesity-related comorbidities. If a patient is on statins preoperatively, they can safely continue them during the perioperative phase. There is limited literature that supports the initiation of statins on statin-naïve patients for bariatric surgery, and RCTs and meta-analysis on this topic in non-cardiac surgeries show conflicting data as well [17, 18]. Therefore, routine perioperative use of statins in patients undergoing bariatric surgery is not recommended. Beta-blockers are also a common home medication for bariatric patients. The benefit of beta-blockade on postoperative outcomes remains controversial [19, 20]. One study assessed the association of preoperative beta-blocker therapy and postoperative outcomes of laparoscopic Roux-en-Y gastric bypass, and the therapy did not yield results showing improvement in long-term survival nor postoperative complication rates [21]. Therefore, routine administration of beta-blockers in the perioperative period is not recommended, but it can be safely continued if the patient is deemed at high risk of cardiovascular events.

There is no consensus on the management of GLP-1 receptor agonists in the perioperative period. There is a concern about delayed gastric emptying with the use of the medication and that it may increase the aspiration risk during induction of general anesthesia. Most programs will hold the medication 1 week prior to planned surgery. The use of GLP-1 agonists will be discussed in more detail in another chapter.

## Preoperative Fasting

Despite outdated speculations of obese patients being more prone to aspiration pneumonia, bariatric patients have no difference in residual gastric fluid volume and pH, compared to normal-weight patients [22]. Therefore, ERAS strongly recommends patients start fasting for solids at least 6 h and for liquids at least 2 h before the induction of anesthesia. This recommendation also applies to diabetics, although further investigation is necessary to determine safety for those with additional aspiration risk factors such as gastroparesis [23].

## Carbohydrate Loading

Preoperative carbohydrate (CHO) conditioning with iso-osmolar drinks consumed 2–3 h before induction of anesthesia has shown to lessen postoperative insulin resistance and promote maintenance of nitrogen and protein reserve in patients undergoing major surgery [24]. However, there still is insufficient evidence to support its routine use in bariatric surgery. A small RCT study showed slightly shorter LOS in patients who underwent sleeve gastrectomy [25], but another study observed higher postprandial glucose concentrations with longer peak duration [26]. However, there was no increase in overall complication rates or postoperative discomfort in those who received CHO loading. Thus, CHO loading may be used selectively in patients undergoing bariatric surgery, including those with diabetes.

### Postoperative Nausea and Vomiting

Many bariatric patients host a variety of risk factors for postoperative nausea and vomiting: female gender, surgery lasting more than 1 h, and use of opioid analgesia [27, 28]. Restrictive upper gastrointestinal surgeries and a history of acid reflux also increase the likelihood of a patient experiencing postoperative nausea and vomiting. Multiple studies have proven the superiority of multimodal pain control and opioid-sparing strategy in reducing the risk of nausea and vomiting, and both methods are strongly recommended in patients undergoing bariatric surgery [29–32]. A combination of three out of the six following agents can be used to reduce postoperative nausea and vomiting including corticosteroids, butyrophenones, neurokinin-1 receptor antagonists, antihistamines, and anticholinergics.

## Intraoperative Phase

### Fluid Management

The difference in body composition in obese patients compared to those of normal-weight patients poses a challenge in determining and maintaining normovolemia during surgery [33]. As every patient's body composition is unique, goal-directed fluid therapy is the best strategy to optimize cardiac output and improve tissue oxygenation and is also applicable postoperatively [34]. There is insufficient evidence to support the use of colloids over crystalloids [35].

### Anesthesia Management

There is no clear consensus on which specific short-acting anesthetic agents or techniques (intravenous versus inhalation) to use for bariatric patients [30, 36], but propofol is a popular induction agent. Despite the speculation that it is a potential cause of rhabdomyolysis reported in some bariatric cases, propofol has not been shown to directly increase the risk of propofol-related rhabdomyolysis in elective bariatric surgery [37]. Multiple studies have proven the benefits of using multimodal opioid-sparing anesthesia in promoting early postoperative recovery in bariatric patients

[29, 38]. Obese patients are at a higher risk of postoperative respiratory depression due to a high prevalence of sleep apnea. Therefore, it is critical to find a delicate balance between opioid-induced side effects and adequate pain management. Preoperative ultrasound-guided transversus abdominis plane (TAP) block has been shown to decrease pain in the immediate postoperative period but for variable durations (3–24 h) [39–41]. Use of liposomal bupivacaine appears to extend this period to about 72 hours, but whether TAP blocks decrease the overall use of opioids remains undetermined [42–44]. Therefore, a combination of locoregional anesthesia, dexmedtomidine, ketamine, and nonsteroidal anti-inflammatory drugs (NSAIDs) is recommended to promote opioid-sparing, multimodal pain management [45].

## Airway Management

There is a slightly increased risk of difficult intubation in patients with severe obesity (BMI >50) [46]. Careful preparation for potentially difficult cases is important. The use of simple or high-flow nasal cannula during apnea time and video laryngoscopy are some available options [47, 48].

## Ventilation Management

Since lung volume does not increase proportionally to the net body weight of a patient, predicted body weight (PBW), which is based on the patient's height and sex, is the best marker to utilize when calculating tidal volume ($V_T$) [49]. Lung-protective strategies such as setting the tidal volume to the range of 6–8 mg/kg of PBW have shown to reduce pulmonary complications in all patients with healthy lungs, regardless of their BMI [50]. Obese patients are more likely to develop atelectasis and require strategies to promote homogenous ventilation without adversely overdistending the alveoli. Pressure-controlled ventilation (PCV) or volume-controlled ventilation (VCV) with inversed respiratory ratio have been suggested as possible strategies [51, 52].

## Neuromuscular Blockade

Deep neuromuscular blockade (NMB) should generally be employed when performing minimally invasive bariatric surgery [53], but residual NMB prior to post-operative extubation can prolong operative time as well as increase the risk of pulmonary complications [54]. Sugammadex has been shown to reverse deep NMB significantly faster than traditional neostigmine [55]. The generally recommended dose for Sugammadex is 2 mg/kg IBW + 40% [56].

## Surgical Approach, Volume and Experience

Laparoscopic surgery is the gold standard surgical approach in bariatric surgery. Compared to open, laparoscopic surgery is associated with faster recovery, shorter length of stay, and lower infection and hernia rates [57, 58]. Studies show that high-volume centers have improved patient outcomes and acceptable complication rates that meet the national average [59, 60]. Active mentorship and comprehensive fellowship training also appear to help maintain favorable outcomes in these centers [61].

## Drains and Tubes

Studies have failed to show any benefit to routine intra-abdominal drain placement after elective bariatric surgery. There was no difference in the leak, postoperative bleeding, abscess formation, or reoperation rates, and it only induced postoperative discomfort in patients [62, 63]. There also is no evidence to support routine nasogastric decompression postoperatively. Orogastric or nasogastric tubes, if used during surgery, should be removed at the end [64].

# Postoperative Phase

## Oxygenation

Many patients with severe obesity suffer from obstructive sleep apnea (OSA), which is associated with higher cardiopulmonary complication rates, including mortality [65]. The STOP-BANG (Snoring, Tiredness during daytime, Observed apnea, high blood pressure, Body mass index, Age, Neck circumference, Gender) questionnaire can be used during preoperative screening to identify these patients and to better prepare the team for potential postoperative respiratory failure [66].

Patients should be closely monitored in the PACU postoperatively since most of the potentially dangerous hypoxic events occur in the immediate phase. Placing patients in a semi-Fowler or sitting position can help prevent atelectasis [67]. There also should be a low threshold to initiate noninvasive positive airway pressure treatment (CPAP or NIPPV) in patients with hypoxemia [68]. Patients who were using CPAP/BiPAP preoperatively should continue them immediately after surgery [69].

## Venous Thromboprophylaxis

Venous thromboembolism (VTE) is a leading cause of morbidity and mortality after bariatric surgery [70]. Obesity, OSA, use of oral contraception and older age are some of the major risk factors associated with VTE, and therefore put many bariatric patients at moderate to high risk [71]. Bariatric patients should receive mechanical prophylaxis such as intermittent pneumatic leg compression and pharmacologic prophylaxis such as unfractionated heparin or low-molecular-weight-heparin (LMWH) within 24 h postoperatively [72]. Dosage and duration should be individualized. Routine placement of retrievable inferior vena cava filters, even in the highest-risk patient, is not recommended [73].

## Nutrition and Supplementation

Bariatric clear liquid diet should start a couple of hours postoperatively before patients advance to more nourishing fluids such as protein shakes [74]. Patients will typically go home on this diet and continue to carefully introduce more solid foods with the consultation of bariatric nutritionists in the following weeks. Nutritionists will work closely with patients to help educate them and assess appropriate nutritional oral intake. Typically, a minimum of 64 ounces of fluid and 60–80 g/day total protein intake or 1.0–1.5 g/kg ideal body weight (IBW) is recommended [74, 75].

After surgery, patients are at risk of developing multiple nutritional deficiencies of iron, folate, vitamin B12, vitamin D, and trace minerals. Therefore, patients are required to adhere to a life-long vitamin and mineral monitoring and supplementing regimen. Thiamine deficiency can also occur because of accelerated weight loss, poor oral intake, vomiting and diarrhea. It is important to detect thiamine deficiency early as it leads to permanent changes in the brain if missed [76]. Providers should, therefore, have a low threshold to initiate thiamine supplementation if there is suspicion of low thiamine level, even before checking the patient's blood levels.

## Other Postoperative Considerations

After the perioperative period, providers must continue to prevent and manage long-term complications of bariatric surgery. Marginal ulcer is a common long-term complication following Roux-en-Y gastric bypass with an incidence rate ranging from 0.6% to 25% [77]. There is some suggestion that the use of PPIs for 3 months postoperatively may reduce the incidence of marginal ulcers [78]. Since prophylactic use of PPI is safe and relatively cheap, it may be routinely given to patients who underwent Roux-en-Y gastric bypass.

With rapid weight loss, patients who have undergone bariatric surgery are at risk of developing gallstones. Recent RCT showed a reduction in the development of symptomatic gallstone disease only in those without pre-existing gallstones prior to surgery when they received prophylactic ursodeoxycholic acid treatment compared with placebo [79]. Therefore, 500–600 mg of ursodeoxycholic acid for 6 months after surgery is recommended in patients without gallstones at the time of surgery. There was no significant reduction of symptomatic gallstone disease in those with asymptomatic gallstones preoperatively. For patients with symptomatic gallstones, cholecystectomy should be done either before or at the time of surgery [80].

## Conclusion

Postoperative care of bariatric patients poses distinct challenges because it involves individuals who are larger and have significant obesity-related comorbidities. Implementing an evidence-based standardized postoperative care protocol, such as Enhanced Recovery After Surgery (ERAS), through a multidisciplinary team can help ensure consistent care and reduce postoperative complications in these patients. Further research is needed to ensure that all recommendations are supported by strong evidence and thus these guidelines will continue to evolve over time. Ultimately, healthcare institutions should utilize these available guidelines as tools to design clinical pathways that would best fit the institution and its patient population.

## References


1. Metabolic & Bariatric Surgery Accreditation & Quality Improvement Program (MBSAQIP). Standards Manual V2.0. Published 2016. Accessed September 17, 2023. https://www.facs.org/qualityprograms/mbsaqip/standards.
2. Telem DA, Majid SF, Powers K, DeMaria E, Morton J, Jones DB. Assessing national provision of care: variability in bariatric clinical care pathways. Surg Obes Relat Dis. 2017;13(2):281–4. https://doi.org/10.1016/j.soard.2016.08.002.
3. Telem DA, Gould J, Pesta C, et al. American Society for Metabolic and Bariatric Surgery: care pathway for laparoscopic sleeve gastrectomy. Surg Obes Relat Dis. 2017;13(5):742–9. https://doi.org/10.1016/j.soard.2017.01.027.
4. Kindel TL, Ganga RR, Baker JW, et al. American Society for Metabolic and Bariatric Surgery: preoperative care pathway for laparoscopic roux-en-Y gastric bypass. Surg Obes Relat Dis. 2021;17(9):1529–40. https://doi.org/10.1016/j.soard.2021.05.011.
5. Jones DB, Abu-Nuwar MRA, Ku CM, Berk LAS, Trainor LS, Jones SB. Less pain and earlier discharge after implementation of a multidisciplinary enhanced recovery after surgery (ERAS) protocol for laparoscopic sleeve gastrectomy. Surg Endosc. 2020;34(12):5574–82. https://doi.org/10.1007/s00464-019-07358-w.
6. Chow A, Neville A, Kolozsvari N. Smoking in bariatric surgery: a systematic review. Surg Endosc. 2021;35(6):3047–66. https://doi.org/10.1007/s00464-020-07669-3.
7. Egholm JW, Pedersen B, Møller AM, Adami J, Juhl CB, Tønnesen H. Perioperative alcohol cessation intervention for postoperative complications. Cochrane Database Syst Rev. 2018;11(11):CD008343. https://doi.org/10.1002/14651858.CD008343.pub3.
8. Roman M, Monaghan A, Serraino GF, et al. Meta-analysis of the influence of lifestyle changes for preoperative weight loss on surgical outcomes. Br J Surg. 2019;106(3):181–9. https://doi.org/10.1002/bjs.11001.
9. Holderbaum M, Casagrande DS, Sussenbach S, Buss C. Effects of very low calorie diets on liver size and weight loss in the preoperative period of bariatric surgery: a systematic review. Surg Obes Relat Dis. 2018;14(2):237–44. https://doi.org/10.1016/j.soard.2017.09.531.
10. Marc-Hernández A, Ruiz-Tovar J, Aracil A, Guillén S, Moya-Ramón M. Impact of exercise on body composition and cardiometabolic risk factors in patients awaiting bariatric surgery. Obes Surg. 2019;29(12):3891–900. https://doi.org/10.1007/s11695-019-04088-9.
11. van Rooijen S, Carli F, Dalton S, et al. Multimodal prehabilitation in colorectal cancer patients to improve functional capacity and reduce postoperative complications: the first international randomized controlled trial for multimodal prehabilitation. BMC Cancer. 2019;19(1):98. https://doi.org/10.1186/s12885-018-5232-6.

12. Koet LL, Kraima A, Derksen I, et al. Effectiveness of preoperative group education for patients with colorectal cancer: managing expectations. Support Care Cancer. 2021;29(9):5263–71. https://doi.org/10.1007/s00520-021-06072-5.
13. Waller A, Forshaw K, Bryant J, Carey M, Boyes A, Sanson-Fisher R. Preparatory education for cancer patients undergoing surgery: a systematic review of volume and quality of research output over time. Patient Educ Couns. 2015;23:S0738. https://doi.org/10.1016/j.pec.2015.05.008.
14. DREAMS Trial Collaborators and West Midlands Research Collaborative. Dexamethasone versus standard treatment for postoperative nausea and vomiting in gastrointestinal surgery: randomised controlled trial (DREAMS Trial). BMJ. 2017;357:j1455. https://doi.org/10.1136/bmj.j1455.
15. Waldron NH, Jones CA, Gan TJ, Allen TK, Habib AS. Impact of perioperative dexamethasone on postoperative analgesia and side-effects: systematic review and meta-analysis. Br J Anaesth. 2013;110(2):191–200. https://doi.org/10.1093/bja/aes431.
16. McSorley ST, Roxburgh CSD, Horgan PG, McMillan DC. The impact of preoperative dexamethasone on the magnitude of the postoperative systemic inflammatory response and complications following surgery for colorectal cancer. Ann Surg Oncol. 2017;24(8):2104–12. https://doi.org/10.1245/s10434-017-5817-3.
17. Singh PP, Lemanu DP, Soop M, Bissett IP, Harrison J, Hill AG. Perioperative simvastatin therapy in major colorectal surgery: a prospective, double-blind randomized controlled trial. J Am Coll Surg. 2016;223(2):308–320.e1. https://doi.org/10.1016/j.jamcollsurg.2016.04.004.
18. Li H, Lin YL, Diao SL, Ma BX, Liu XL. Does short preoperative statin therapy prevent infectious complications in adults undergoing cardiac or non-cardiac surgery? A meta-analysis of 5 randomized placebo-controlled trials. Saudi Med J. 2016;37(5):492–7. https://doi.org/10.15537/smj.2016.5.13733.
19. Jørgensen ME, Andersson C, Venkatesan S, Sanders RD. Beta-blockers in noncardiac surgery: did observational studies put us back on safe ground? Br J Anaesth. 2018;121(1):16–25. https://doi.org/10.1016/j.bja.2018.02.004.
20. Blessberger H, Kammler J, Domanovits H, et al. Perioperative beta-blockers for preventing surgery-related mortality and morbidity. Cochrane Database Syst Rev. 2018;3(3):CD004476. https://doi.org/10.1002/14651858.CD004476.pub3.
21. Stenberg E, Mohseni S, Cao Y, Näslund E. Limited effect of Beta-blockade on postoperative outcome after laparoscopic gastric bypass surgery. Obes Surg. 2020;30(1):139–45. https://doi.org/10.1007/s11695-019-04108-8.
22. Buchholz V, Berkenstadt H, Goitein D, Dickman R, Bernstine H, Rubin M. Gastric emptying is not prolonged in obese patients. Surg Obes Relat Dis. 2013;9(5):714–7. https://doi.org/10.1016/j.soard.2012.03.008.
23. Bertin E, Schneider N, Abdelli N, et al. Gastric emptying is accelerated in obese type 2 diabetic patients without autonomic neuropathy. Diabetes Metab. 2001;27(3):357–64.
24. Smith MD, McCall J, Plank L, Herbison GP, Soop M, Nygren J. Preoperative carbohydrate treatment for enhancing recovery after elective surgery. Cochrane Database Syst Rev. 2014;2014(8):CD009161. https://doi.org/10.1002/14651858.CD009161.pub2.
25. Pimenta GP, Capellan DA, de Aguilar-Nascimento JE. Sleeve Gastrectomy with or without a multimodal perioperative care. A randomized pilot study. Obes Surg. 2015;25(9):1639–46. https://doi.org/10.1007/s11695-015-1573-2.
26. Albalawi Z, Laffin M, Gramlich L, Senior P, McAlister FA. Enhanced recovery after surgery (ERAS(®)) in individuals with diabetes: a systematic review. World J Surg. 2017;41(8):1927–34. https://doi.org/10.1007/s00268-017-3982-y.
27. Kushner BS, Freeman D, Sparkman J, Salles A, Eagon JC, Eckhouse SR. Assessment of postoperative nausea and vomiting after bariatric surgery using a validated questionnaire. Surg Obes Relat Dis. 2020;16(10):1505–13. https://doi.org/10.1016/j.soard.2020.05.017.
28. Groene P, Eisenlohr J, Zeuzem C, Dudok S, Karcz K, Hofmann-Kiefer K. Postoperative nausea and vomiting in bariatric surgery in comparison to non-bariatric gastric surgery. Wideochir Inne Tech Maloinwazyjne. 2019;14(1):90–5. https://doi.org/10.5114/wiitm.2018.77629.

29. Ziemann-Gimmel P, Hensel P, Koppman J, Marema R. Multimodal analgesia reduces narcotic requirements and antiemetic rescue medication in laparoscopic roux-en-Y gastric bypass surgery. Surg Obes Relat Dis. 2013;9(6):975–80. https://doi.org/10.1016/j.soard.2013.02.003.
30. Riley CL. Anesthesia and enhanced recovery after surgery in bariatric surgery. Anesthesiol Clin. 2022;40(1):119–42. https://doi.org/10.1016/j.anclin.2021.11.006.
31. De Oliveira GSJ, Duncan K, Fitzgerald P, Nader A, Gould RW, McCarthy RJ. Systemic lidocaine to improve quality of recovery after laparoscopic bariatric surgery: a randomized double-blinded placebo-controlled trial. Obes Surg. 2014;24(2):212–8. https://doi.org/10.1007/s11695-013-1077-x.
32. Naeem Z, Chen IL, Pryor AD, Docimo S, Gan TJ, Spaniolas K. Antiemetic prophylaxis and anesthetic approaches to reduce postoperative nausea and vomiting in bariatric surgery patients: a systematic review. Obes Surg. 2020;30(8):3188–200. https://doi.org/10.1007/s11695-020-04683-1.
33. Kabon B, Nagele A, Reddy D, et al. Obesity decreases perioperative tissue oxygenation. Anesthesiology. 2004;100(2):274–80. https://doi.org/10.1097/00000542-200402000-00015.
34. Mühlbacher J, Luf F, Zotti O, Herkner H, Fleischmann E, Kabon B. Effect of intraoperative goal-directed fluid management on tissue oxygen tension in obese patients: a randomized controlled trial. Obes Surg. 2021;31(3):1129–38. https://doi.org/10.1007/s11695-020-05106-x.
35. Reiterer C, Kabon B, Zotti O, Obradovic M, Kurz A, Fleischmann E. Effect of goal-directed crystalloid- versus colloid-based fluid strategy on tissue oxygen tension: a randomised controlled trial. Br J Anaesth. 2019;123(6):768–76. https://doi.org/10.1016/j.bja.2019.08.027.
36. Ahmed MM, Tian C, Lu J, Lee Y. Total intravenous anesthesia versus inhalation anesthesia on postoperative analgesia and nausea and vomiting after bariatric surgery: a systematic review and meta-analysis. Asian J Anesthesiol. 2021;59(4):135–51. https://doi.org/10.6859/aja.202112_59(4).0002.
37. Lehavi A, Sandler O, Mahajna A, Weissman A, Katz YS. Comparison of Rhabdomyolysis markers in patients undergoing bariatric surgery with Propofol and inhalation-based anesthesia. Obes Surg. 2015;25(10):1923–7. https://doi.org/10.1007/s11695-015-1626-6.
38. Hung KC, Chiu CC, Hsu CW, et al. Impact of opioid-free anesthesia on analgesia and recovery following bariatric surgery: a meta-analysis of randomized controlled studies. Obes Surg. 2022;32(9):3113–24. https://doi.org/10.1007/s11695-022-06213-7.
39. Ma N, Duncan JK, Scarfe AJ, Schuhmann S, Cameron AL. Clinical safety and effectiveness of transversus abdominis plane (TAP) block in post-operative analgesia: a systematic review and meta-analysis. J Anesth. 2017;31(3) https://doi.org/10.1007/s00540-017-2323-5.
40. Saber AA, Lee YC, Chandrasekaran A, et al. Efficacy of transversus abdominis plane (TAP) block in pain management after laparoscopic sleeve gastrectomy (LSG): a double-blind randomized controlled trial. Am J Surg. 2019;217(1) https://doi.org/10.1016/j.amjsurg.2018.07.010.
41. Ruiz-Tovar J, Garcia A, Ferrigni C, et al. Laparoscopic-Guided Transversus Abdominis Plane (TAP) Block as Part of Multimodal Analgesia in Laparoscopic Roux-en-Y Gastric Bypass Within an Enhanced Recovery After Surgery (ERAS) Program: a Prospective Randomized Clinical Trial. Obes Surg. 2018;28(11):3374–9. https://doi.org/10.1007/s11695-018-3376-8.
42. Bhakta A, Glotzer O, Ata A, Tafen M, Stain SC, Singh PT. Analgesic efficacy of laparoscopic-guided transverse abdominis plane block using liposomal bupivacaine in bariatric surgery. Am J Surg. 2018;215(4) https://doi.org/10.1016/j.amjsurg.2017.09.006.
43. Robertson TC, Hall K, Bear S, Thompson KJ, Kuwada T, Gersin KS. Transversus abdominis block utilizing liposomal bupivacaine as a non-opioid analgesic for postoperative pain management. Surg Endosc. 2019;33(8) https://doi.org/10.1007/s00464-018-6543-z.
44. Becker E, Hernandez A, Greene H, Gadbois K, Gallus D, Wisbach G. Does liposomal bupivacaine decrease postoperative opioid use in conjunction with an enhanced recovery after bariatric surgery pathway? A prospective, double-blind, randomized controlled trial. Obes Surg. 2023;33(2) https://doi.org/10.1007/s11695-022-06417-x.
45. Sinha A, Jayaraman L, Punhani D. Efficacy of ultrasound-guided transversus abdominis plane block after laparoscopic bariatric surgery: a double blind, randomized, controlled study. Obes Surg. 2013;23(4):548–53. https://doi.org/10.1007/s11695-012-0819-5.

46. Moon TS, Fox PE, Somasundaram A, et al. The influence of morbid obesity on difficult intubation and difficult mask ventilation. J Anesth. 2019;33(1):96–102. https://doi.org/10.1007/s00540-018-2592-7.
47. Wong DT, Dallaire A, Singh KP, et al. High-flow nasal oxygen improves safe apnea time in morbidly obese patients undergoing general anesthesia: a randomized controlled trial. Anesth Analg. 2019;129(4):1130–6. https://doi.org/10.1213/ANE.0000000000003966.
48. Hansel J, Rogers AM, Lewis SR, Cook TM, Smith AF. Videolaryngoscopy versus direct laryngoscopy for adults undergoing tracheal intubation: a Cochrane systematic review and meta-analysis update. Br J Anaesth. 2022;129(4):612–23. https://doi.org/10.1016/j.bja.2022.05.027.
49. De Jong A, Wrigge H, Hedenstierna G, et al. How to ventilate obese patients in the ICU. Intensive Care Med. 2020;46(12):2423–35. https://doi.org/10.1007/s00134-020-06286-x.
50. Rackley CR, MacIntyre NR. Low tidal volumes for everyone? Chest. 2019;156(4):783–91. https://doi.org/10.1016/j.chest.2019.06.007.
51. Bagchi A, Rudolph MI, Ng PY, et al. The association of postoperative pulmonary complications in 109,360 patients with pressure-controlled or volume-controlled ventilation. Anaesthesia. 2017;72(11):1334–43. https://doi.org/10.1111/anae.14039.
52. Charlesworth M, Glossop AJ. Strategies for the prevention of postoperative pulmonary complications. Anaesthesia. 2018;73(8):923–7. https://doi.org/10.1111/anae.14288.
53. Fuchs-Buder T, Schmartz D, Baumann C, et al. Deep neuromuscular blockade improves surgical conditions during gastric bypass surgery for morbid obesity: a randomised controlled trial. Eur J Anaesthesiol. 2019;36(7):486–93. https://doi.org/10.1097/EJA.0000000000000996.
54. Koh WU, Park HS, Kim HJ, Yang HS. Prevention and treatment of residual neuromuscular blockade with doxapram during postoperative recovery. Eur J Anaesthesiol. 2021;38(2):197. https://doi.org/10.1097/EJA.0000000000001338.
55. Badaoui R, Cabaret A, Alami Y, et al. Reversal of neuromuscular blockade by sugammadex in laparoscopic bariatric surgery: in support of dose reduction. Anaesth Crit Care Pain Med. 2016;35(1):25–9. https://doi.org/10.1016/j.accpm.2015.09.003.
56. Llauradó S, Sabaté A, Ferreres E, Camprubí I, Cabrera A. Sugammadex ideal body weight dose adjusted by level of neuromuscular blockade in laparoscopic bariatric surgery. Anesthesiology. 2012;117(1):93–8. https://doi.org/10.1097/ALN.0b013e3182580409.
57. Luján JA, Frutos MD, Hernández Q, et al. Laparoscopic versus open gastric bypass in the treatment of morbid obesity: a randomized prospective study. Ann Surg. 2004;239(4):433–7. https://doi.org/10.1097/01.sla.0000120071.75691.1f.
58. Reoch J, Mottillo S, Shimony A, et al. Safety of laparoscopic vs open bariatric surgery: a systematic review and meta-analysis. Arch Surg. 2011;146(11):1314–22. https://doi.org/10.1001/archsurg.2011.270.
59. Zevin B, Aggarwal R, Grantcharov TP. Volume-outcome association in bariatric surgery: a systematic review. Ann Surg. 2012;256(1):60–71. https://doi.org/10.1097/SLA.0b013e3182554c62.
60. Gero D, Raptis DA, Vleeschouwers W, et al. Defining global benchmarks in bariatric surgery: a retrospective multicenter analysis of minimally invasive roux-en-Y gastric bypass and sleeve Gastrectomy. Ann Surg. 2019;270(5):859–67. https://doi.org/10.1097/SLA.0000000000003512.
61. Kim PS, Telem DA, Altieri MS, et al. Bariatric outcomes are significantly improved in hospitals with fellowship council-accredited bariatric fellowships. J Gastrointest Surg. 2015;19(4):594–7. https://doi.org/10.1007/s11605-015-2758-7.
62. Kavuturu S, Rogers AM, Haluck RS. Routine drain placement in roux-en-Y gastric bypass: an expanded retrospective comparative study of 755 patients and review of the literature. Obes Surg. 2012;22(1):177–81. https://doi.org/10.1007/s11695-011-0560-5.
63. Albanopoulos K, Alevizos L, Linardoutsos D, et al. Routine abdominal drains after laparoscopic sleeve gastrectomy: a retrospective review of 353 patients. Obes Surg. 2011;21(6):687–91. https://doi.org/10.1007/s11695-010-0343-4.

64. Rossetti G, Fei L, Docimo L, et al. Is nasogastric decompression useful in prevention of leaks after laparoscopic sleeve gastrectomy? A randomized trial. J Invest Surg. 2014;27(4):234–9. https://doi.org/10.3109/08941939.2013.875606.
65. Ahlin S, Manco M, Panunzi S, et al. A new sensitive and accurate model to predict moderate to severe obstructive sleep apnea in patients with obesity. Medicine. 2019;98(32):e16687. https://doi.org/10.1097/MD.0000000000016687.
66. Chung F, Abdullah HR, Liao P. STOP-Bang questionnaire: a practical approach to screen for obstructive sleep apnea. Chest. 2016;149(3):631–8. https://doi.org/10.1378/chest.15-0903.
67. Lukachan GA, Yadollahi A, Auckley D, et al. The impact of semi-upright position on severity of sleep disordered breathing in patients with obstructive sleep apnea: a two-arm, prospective, randomized controlled trial. BMC Anesthesiol. 2023;23(1):236. https://doi.org/10.1186/s12871-023-02193-y.
68. de Raaff CAL, Gorter-Stam MAW, de Vries N, et al. Perioperative management of obstructive sleep apnea in bariatric surgery: a consensus guideline. Surg Obes Relat Dis. 2017;13(7):1095–109. https://doi.org/10.1016/j.soard.2017.03.022.
69. de Raaff CAL, Coblijn UK, de Vries N, van Wagensveld BA. Is fear for postoperative cardiopulmonary complications after bariatric surgery in patients with obstructive sleep apnea justified? A systematic review. Am J Surg. 2016;211(4):793–801. https://doi.org/10.1016/j.amjsurg.2015.10.026.
70. Daigle CR, Brethauer SA, Tu C, et al. Which postoperative complications matter most after bariatric surgery? Prioritizing quality improvement efforts to improve national outcomes. Surg Obes Relat Dis. 2018;14(5):652–7. https://doi.org/10.1016/j.soard.2018.01.008.
71. Mabeza RM, Lee C, Verma A, et al. Factors and outcomes associated with venous thromboembolism following bariatric surgery. Am Surg. 2022;88(10):2525–30. https://doi.org/10.1177/00031348221103645.
72. Birkmeyer NJO, Finks JF, Carlin AM, et al. Comparative effectiveness of unfractionated and low-molecular-weight heparin for prevention of venous thromboembolism following bariatric surgery. Arch Surg. 2012;147(11):994–8. https://doi.org/10.1001/archsurg.2012.2298.
73. Rowland SP, Dharmarajah B, Moore HM, et al. Inferior vena cava filters for prevention of venous thromboembolism in obese patients undergoing bariatric surgery: a systematic review. Ann Surg. 2015;261(1):35–45. https://doi.org/10.1097/SLA.0000000000000621.
74. Parrott JM, Craggs-Dino L, Faria SL, O'Kane M. The optimal nutritional Programme for bariatric and metabolic surgery. Curr Obes Rep. 2020;9(3):326–38. https://doi.org/10.1007/s13679-020-00384-z.
75. Karlsson A, Wendel K, Polits S, Gislason H, Hedenbro JL. Preoperative nutrition and postoperative discomfort in an ERAS setting: a randomized study in gastric bypass surgery. Obes Surg. 2016;26(4):743–8. https://doi.org/10.1007/s11695-015-1848-7.
76. Bahardoust M, Eghbali F, Shahmiri SS, et al. B1 vitamin deficiency after bariatric surgery, prevalence, and symptoms: a systematic review and meta-analysis. Obes Surg. 2022;32(9):3104–12. https://doi.org/10.1007/s11695-022-06178-7.
77. Beran A, Shaear M, Al-Mudares S, et al. Predictors of marginal ulcer after gastric bypass: a systematic review and meta-analysis. J Gastrointest Surg. 2023;27(6):1066–77. https://doi.org/10.1007/s11605-023-05619-7.
78. Kang X, Zurita-Macias L, Hong D, Cadeddu M, Anvari M, Gmora S. A comparison of 30-day versus 90-day proton pump inhibitor therapy in prevention of marginal ulcers after laparoscopic Roux-en-Y gastric bypass. Surg Obes Relat Dis. 2016;12(5):1003–7. https://doi.org/10.1016/j.soard.2015.11.010.
79. Haal S, Guman MSS, Boerlage TCC, et al. Ursodeoxycholic acid for the prevention of symptomatic gallstone disease after bariatric surgery (UPGRADE): a multicentre, double-blind, randomised, placebo-controlled superiority trial. Lancet Gastroenterol Hepatol. 2021;6(12):993–1001. https://doi.org/10.1016/S2468-1253(21)00301-0.
80. Elgohary H, El Azawy M, Elbanna M, Elhossainy H, Omar W. Concomitant versus delayed cholecystectomy in bariatric surgery. J Obes. 2021;2021:9957834. https://doi.org/10.1155/2021/9957834.

# Obesity as a Chronic Disease: The Need for Long-Term Follow-Up Postoperatively

13

Jesse Richards

Obesity has been formally recognized as a chronic disease by the American Medical Association since 2013. Metabolic and bariatric surgery (MBS) remains the most effective tool for treating obesity and improving long-term health outcomes from systemic changes in the body's set point. However, it is clear that not all patients are able to achieve an optimal body weight or maintain adequate weight loss after MBS.

Modern surgical techniques are extremely safe. The sleeve gastrectomy (SG) remains the most popular MBS surgical intervention [1], but there is a significant subset of patients who experience weight regain, especially 5–10 years or longer after surgery. The rate of long-term weight regain is significantly lower after a Roux-en-Y gastric bypass (RYGB); however, 10–15% of patients will have a significant level of weight regain in the long term [2]. This weight regain has traditionally been regarded as the patient making conscious choices to fall back into old habits; however, we now understand that the neurohormonal compensatory measures that occur after long-term weight loss from MBS can sometimes overpower the weight loss effect and predispose the patient to weight regain [3].

For this reason, it is vital for patients to be monitored on an ongoing basis after MBS. Typically, this monitoring is associated with a post-op visit for a few months to ensure that patients avoid malnutrition. However, also monitoring for appropriate rates of weight loss to identify early sub-responders and appropriately intervene with multidisciplinary treatment may potentially improve long-term outcomes.

With the rise of more effective and better-tolerated anti-obesity medications (AOM), the incorporation of a multidisciplinary approach to postoperative care is more critical than ever. Patients who have successfully lost weight with MBS may begin to regain beyond what is expected within 12–24 months. Patients should be

J. Richards (✉)
University of Oklahoma Health Sciences Center, Tulsa, OK, USA
e-mail: Jesse-R-Richards@ouhsc.edu



O. M. Ghanem et al. (eds.), *The SAGES Manual of Metabolic and Bariatric Surgery*, https://doi.org/10.1007/978-3-031-72309-4_13

asked about their hunger and if they have an inappropriate increase in hunger, should be considered for an initiation or a resumption of previously effective AOMs.

A large part of the weight plateau and potential regain that occurs after MBS depends on the specific mechanism of action of the surgical procedure. While traditionally the RYGB and the duodenal switch were considered to be primarily malabsorptive procedures, we now understand that the direct delivery of nutrients to the more distal small bowel can potentially increase endogenous production of satiety hormones such as glucagon-like peptide 1 (GLP-1) and gastrointestinal polypeptide, (PYY), which help mitigate rises in ghrelin that can occur with weight loss [4, 5]. The SG does not have marked changes, but due to the surgical removal of the primary ghrelin production area of the stomach, can have radical reductions in hunger [6]. However, over a one to three-year period, the body's ghrelin production can compensate and start to trend back up [7], which may lead to higher rates of increased hunger and weight regain after an SG.

As our understanding of the central nervous system's control of homeostatic energy balance improves, we have come to realize that it is not just the stomach or the intestines that control body weight; instead, it is a balance of both the GI tract and the brain. For this reason, if there is a genetic predisposition towards weight gain, either from polygenic obesity risk or monogenic obesity, there can be poor initial weight loss or a much higher risk of long-term weight regain [8]. What was traditionally considered a "failure" of surgery now helps guide additional secondary workup and testing for alternative causes of obesity and hyperphagia, some of which have targeted medical therapy that is currently FDA-approved. For instance, monogenic obesity from Leptin Receptor, PCSK1, or POMC deficiency with setmelanotide [9]. Additionally, patients with syndromic Bardet–Biedl syndrome (BBS) are also approved for setmelanotide. Additional medical treatments are pending and may be beneficial for a significant portion of patients with hyperphagia from genetic obesity that does not normalize after MBS.

All patients should be monitored at least annually for weight trajectory and potential regain, in addition to malnutrition and malabsorption of vitamins and nutrients. In addition to the aforementioned compensatory issues, medical treatment for comorbidities with severely obesogenic medications (antipsychotics, etc.) can affect long-term hunger and satiety and predispose patients to weight regain. If weight regain does begin, then initiation of medical therapy and follow-up with a dietitian along with a multidisciplinary intervention can prevent the loss of health benefits that occur after MBS.

Because of all the positive changes that occur after MBS, patients may be able to lose significant body weight on lower doses or less medical therapy than they required before surgery. Additionally, evaluations for medical treatment may be beneficial to reduce polypharmacy and avoid medications that might exacerbate post-bariatric surgery malnutrition, or other issues. While it is certainly within the scope of surgeons to provide prescription treatment using AOMs, coordination with medical weight loss specialists (bariatrician or obesity medicine specialists) can be highly helpful. Additionally, patients who have undergone MBS typically understand what is important to focus on as it pertains to nutrition in conjunction with newer, highly effective medical weight loss therapies. This understanding is due to their education and instruction while preparing for the postoperative diet and recovery. Growing evidence has shown that the use of more powerful medications like GLP-1 receptor agonists can help achieve meaningful weight loss after MBS. One retrospective, observational study from Switzerland showed that 6 months of GLP-1 receptor agonist treatment in patients who had gained weight after MBS, caused the patients to lose about 66% of their regained weight. [PMID 36765019]. Existing data from liraglutide and semaglutide therapy after MBS demonstrated 7.3% TBW loss and 9.8% TBW loss respectively. Multiple longer-term prospective randomized trials of semaglutide for poor response post-bariatric surgery should soon provide additional data on long-term combination therapy [10].

It is imperative to understand that even after life-altering interventions such as MBS, obesity remains a chronic disease, one that may sometimes improve or sometimes get worse. Understanding this paradigm may help tailor optimal treatment for patients who will best benefit from a multidisciplinary approach. Patients should be followed up annually after the first-year post-surgical intervention and at minimum monitored by a primary care doctor who can refer them back to a higher level of care if they begin to struggle with worsening obesity in the longer postoperative period.

## References

1. Alsuhibani A, Thompson JR, Wigle PR, Guo JJ, Lin AC, Rao MB, Hincapie AL. Metabolic and bariatric surgery utilization trends in the United States: evidence from 2012 to 2021 National Electronic Medical Records Network. Ann Surg Open. 2023;4(4):e317. https://doi.org/10.1097/AS9.0000000000000317. PMID: 38144499; PMCID: PMC10735086.
2. Noria SF, Shelby RD, Atkins KD, Nguyen NT, Gadde KM. Weight regain after bariatric surgery: scope of the problem, causes, prevention, and treatment. Curr Diab Rep. 2023;23(3):31–42. https://doi.org/10.1007/s11892-023-01498-z. Epub 2023 Feb 8. PMID: 36752995; PMCID: PMC9906605.
3. Sima E, Webb DL, Hellström PM, et al. Non-responders after gastric bypass surgery for morbid obesity: peptide hormones and glucose homeostasis. Obes Surg. 2019;29:4008–17. https://doi.org/10.1007/s11695-019-04089-8.
4. Slouha E, Elkersh EM, Shay A, Ghosh S, Mahmood A, Gorantla VR. Significance of hormone alteration following bariatric surgery. Cureus. 2023;15(11):e49053. https://doi.org/10.7759/cureus.49053. PMID: 38116338; PMCID: PMC10729911.
5. Cummings DE, Weigle DS, Frayo RS, Breen PA, Ma MK, Dellinger EP, Purnell JQ. Plasma ghrelin levels after diet-induced weight loss or gastric bypass surgery. N Engl J Med. 2002;346(21):1623–30. https://doi.org/10.1056/NEJMoa012908.
6. Aukan MI, Skårvold S, Brandsaeter IØ, Rehfeld JF, Holst JJ, Nymo S, Coutinho S, Martins C. Gastrointestinal hormones and appetite ratings after weight loss induced by diet or bariatric surgery. Obesity (Silver Spring). 2023;31(2):399–411. https://doi.org/10.1002/oby.23655. Epub 2022 Dec 19. PMID: 36536482; PMCID: PMC10108040.
7. Bohdjalian A, Langer FB, Shakeri-Leidenmühler S, Gfrerer L, Ludvik B, Zacherl J, Prager G. Sleeve gastrectomy as sole and definitive bariatric procedure: 5-year results for weight loss and ghrelin. Obes Surg. 2010;20(5):535–40. https://doi.org/10.1007/s11695-009-0066-6. Epub 2010 Jan 22. PMID: 20094819.

8. Gantz MG, Driscoll DJ, Miller JL, Duis JB, Butler MG, Gourash L, Forster J, Scheimann AO. Critical review of bariatric surgical outcomes in patients with Prader-Willi syndrome and other hyperphagic disorders. Obesity (Silver Spring). 2022;30(5):973–81. https://doi.org/10.1002/oby.23385. Epub 2022 Apr 13. PMID: 35416416.
9. Clément K, van den Akker E, Argente J, Bahm A, Chung WK, Connors H, De Waele K, Farooqi IS, Gonneau-Lejeune J, Gordon G, Kohlsdorf K, Poitou C, Puder L, Swain J, Stewart M, Yuan G, Wabitsch M, Kühnen P, Setmelanotide POMC and LEPR Phase 3 Trial Investigators. Efficacy and safety of setmelanotide, an MC4R agonist, in individuals with severe obesity due to LEPR or POMC deficiency: single-arm, open-label, multicentre, phase 3 trials. Lancet Diabetes Endocrinol. 2020;8(12):960–70. https://doi.org/10.1016/S2213-8587(20)30364-8. Epub 2020 Oct 30. PMID: 33137293.
10. BARI STEP. Clinicaltrials.gov. n.d.. https://clinicalrials.gov/study/NCT05073835.

# Part II

# Therapies

# Medically Supervised Weight Loss and Effects of Anti-Obesity Medications

# 14

Amy J. Sheer, W. Troy Donahoo, and Crystal N. Johnson-Mann

## What Is the (Brief) History of the Development and Significant Failures of Anti-Obesity Medications?

The first depiction of obesity in human figurines was over 30,000 years ago with the Venus of Hohle Fels in southwestern Germany [1]. However, there have been many representations of obesity throughout history since that time. There are also recordings throughout this time of traditional medicine practices using compounds to treat obesity. However, it is only since the dawn of the twentieth century and the emergence of modern health care, as well as an initial appreciation of the role of biological factors in some forms of obesity, such as Cushing's disease and hypothyroidism, that a focused effort on medical treatment began [2].

Following the observation that hypothyroidism was associated with obesity, thyroid hormone was the first true anti-obesity medication (AOM) used to treat obesity in the early 1900s. However, the use was often limited by the effects on pulse and blood pressure. During World War I, dinitrophenol (DNP) was used for munitions but was also found to cause weight loss in subtoxic doses [3]. The mechanism of

A. J. Sheer
Division of Internal Medicine, Department of Medicine, University of Florida College of Medicine, Gainesville, FL, USA

W. T. Donahoo
Division of Internal Medicine, Department of Medicine, University of Florida College of Medicine, Gainesville, FL, USA

Division of Endocrinology, Department of Medicine, University of Florida College of Medicine, Gainesville, FL, USA

C. N. Johnson-Mann (✉)
Division of Gastrointestinal Surgery, Department of Surgery, University of Florida College of Medicine, Gainesville, FL, USA
e-mail: crystal.johnson-mann@surgery.ufl.edu



O. M. Ghanem et al. (eds.), *The SAGES Manual of Metabolic and Bariatric Surgery*, https://doi.org/10.1007/978-3-031-72309-4_14

DNP causing weight loss is through uncoupling of the electron transport chain, resulting in heat formation rather than energy (adenosine triphosphate or ATP) production, thus stimulating metabolism by as much as 50%. Based on these early reports, scientists evaluated the possibility of using DNP for weight loss, and the initial study, published in 1933, showed approximately 20 pounds of weight loss over 10 weeks and no reported side effects. However, as the use grew, so did reports of severe adverse reactions including deaths from hyperpyrexia [4]. In 1935, the American Medical Association rejected DNP from their "New and Nonofficial Remedies," noting at that time, obesity was a "mild chronic condition" and that the risks of treatment outweighed the benefits [5]. In 1937, the drug manufacturing company Isabella Laboratories sent a letter to the Food and Drug Administration (FDA) arguing that obesity contributed to many diseases (including heart disease and diabetes but also pneumonia and colitis) and that treating obesity was "no longer a fad but a health necessity" [4]. Interestingly, the FDA could not control DNP at that time as it was not seen as a drug used to treat a disease but rather as a cosmetic agent. Moreover, it was not until the 1938 Food, Drugs, and Cosmetics Act that the sale of DNP was finally halted [4]. Thus, the controversy of treating obesity as a disease versus a cosmetic issue and the balance between safety and efficacy dates back to one of the first researched AOMs, DNP. Until very recently, these controversies have persisted..

Thyroid hormone, the only other AOM that increases metabolism, was misused for weight loss despite the known risks of atrial fibrillation, excess bone loss, and thyroid storm that far outweighed the benefits until the 1970s [2]. A primarily anorectic agent, amphetamines, were used from the late 1930s until the 1960s as an AOM until they were banned for use due to their addictive potential [2]. Also, during this time, "Rainbow Pills," which were various combinations of thyroid hormone, laxatives, diuretics, and amphetamines, were used as AOMs [2].

Three additional AOM failures are worth discussing: aminorex, fenfluramine, and lorcaserin. Aminorex, an "amphetamine-like drug," was licensed in Germany, Austria, and Switzerland in 1965 to treat obesity. Over the subsequent 7 years, 20% of users developed primary pulmonary hypertension, leading to its withdrawal in 1972. Fenfluramine, a serotonin reuptake inhibitor and a serotonin agonist via one of its metabolites, was approved by the FDA in 1973 for treating of obesity [2]. Studies in the late 1980s and early 1990s showed fenfluramine's dramatic weight loss effect, specifically when combined with phentermine (discussed below) [6]. Although there were rare cases of pulmonary hypertension with fenfluramine, data showing dramatic weight loss (> 15% at 32 weeks) led to an explosion in the use of the combination "Fen-Phen" until 1997 when a significant association between fenfluramine (and the isomer dexfenfluramine) and valvular heart disease was found, leading to the discontinuation of fenfluramine in 1997 [7]. Lorcaserin, a selective serotonin 5-HT2C receptor agonist, was initially developed and approved by the FDA 2012 for weight management [8]. Despite its efficacy in weight-loss, early safety data raised concerns for valvular heart disease and carcinogenicity in rats. A post-marketing study focused on cardiovascular safety of lorcaserin, known as the CAMELLIA-TIMI 61 trial, conducted from 2014 to 2018, detected a potential signal of increased cancer and cancer-related mortality. Subsequent review by the FDA resulted in the voluntary withdrawal of lorcaserin from the marker in 2020 due to the potential cancer risks [8]. Through these failures, we learned that we could treat obesity through neurohormonal targets; however, given the complexity of regulating energy balance, the often narrow therapeutic dose range, and the high potential for off-target effects, this was not an easy path for drug development [8].

Over the years, there have been an almost innumerous array of dietary supplements and alternative therapies marketed for the treatment of obesity. A recent systematic review of over 20,000 articles found only 315 randomized studies of 14 dietary supplements. Of those, only 16 studies were of high enough quality and showed a significant weight difference, but the difference between supplement(s) and placebo was <5% [9]. This led to a perspective article from the Obesity Society concluding "Health care providers should be aware of the lack of evidence and deficiencies in regulatory oversight of dietary supplements marketed for weight loss. Regulatory authorities should protect consumers by ensuring accurate and safe marketing claims and preventing the promotion of unproven and potentially unsafe products and claims" [10].

## What Are the Older FDA-Approved Anti-Obesity Medications?

Phentermine was approved as an AOM in 1959, and it remains the most often prescribed AOM due to its very low cost. In Florida alone, there were almost 994,000 prescriptions for phentermine in 2022. Although this was a 5% decrease from 2021, likely due to the newer and more effective AOMs, this exemplifies the continued widespread use [11]. Phentermine is a sympathomimetic amine that is weakly related to amphetamine but without any demonstrated addictive properties [12]. Phentermine increases the amount of norepinephrine (and less so increases serotonin and dopamine) in hypothalamic nuclei [13]. Because phentermine was approved so long ago and is generic, there are currently no long-term placebo-controlled trials demonstrating its safety and efficacy. Thus, it remains FDA-approved only for "short-term" use, usually interpreted as less than 3 months. However real-world data of long-term phentermine users have found evidence of sustained efficacy and safety over several years [14]. The efficacy of phentermine is highly variable and can range from <5% to 15% with short-term use and over 10% at 6 months [13]. In appropriate patients without serious cardiovascular or serious psychiatric disease and with close monitoring to ensure at least 5% weight loss by 3 months and no significant increase in blood pressure or pulse, common side effects include dry mouth, constipation, and insomnia (if the medication is taken too late in the day) [13].

The only drug currently approved by the FDA that does not work through a central anorectic mechanism is orlistat, which impairs the absorption of dietary triglyceride by inhibiting gastrointestinal lipase, thus blocking the conversion of triacylglycerol to diacylglycerol and monoacylyglycerol and free fatty acids (only monoacylyglycerol and free fatty acids can be absorbed by the intestine) thus resulting in excretion of energy as fecal triglycerides. Perhaps the strongest support for the use of orlistat came from the XENDOS study, which showed at 4 years, a 37% reduction in risk of diabetes with orlistat compared to placebo and a weight loss of

5% with orlistat compared to 3% with placebo [15]. However, even more telling was the fact that only 50% of the treatment group completed the study and almost 100% in the treatment group had adverse gastrointestinal effects, including steatorrhea and anal leakage [15].

Finally, there are two FDA-approved drug combination AOMs, phentermine/topiramate and naltrexone/bupropion. Phentermine/topiramate, marked under the trade name Qsymia®, was FDA-approved in 2012; however, due to teratogenicity of topiramate, it required a REMS (risk evaluation and modulation strategy) program including registration of providers and close monitoring with frequent pregnancy tests and use of effective contraception [16]. It does appear that prenatal exposure to topiramate was lower with the REMS program than for other AOMs. However, pregnancy testing and the use of contraception were inadequate despite this program [16]. In addition to the side effects of phentermine described above and the risk of birth defects, topiramate's side effects include fatigue, paraesthesias, dizziness, altered taste (especially carbonated beverages), and increased risk of recurrence of calcium nephrolithiasis. Table 14.1 highlights the outcomes and drop-outs seen in key studies of phentermine/topiramate at the highest dose of 15.0 mg phentermine plus 92.0 mg topiramate, and this shows about a 10% weight loss with a higher drop-out weight in placebo than treatment over the first year, due to inadequacy of weight loss.

The combination of a sustained released naltrexone and bupropion, sold in the United States as Contrave®, was approved by the FDA for the treatment of obesity in 2014. The drug needs to be slowly titrated up to a maximal dose of 32 mg naltrexone and 360 mg bupropion, and it is contraindicated in people with a seizure disorder, those needing opioid medications, or those who are pregnant/planning pregnancy. Table 14.2 shows the outcomes of noteworthy completed studies with naltrexone/bupropion with a 5% weight loss in participants with diabetes to a 9%

**Table 14.1** Phentermine/Topiramate

| Study | n in highest dose | Duration | Weight loss | Drop-out (placebo, highest dose) |
|---|---|---|---|---|
| EQUIP [17] | 512 | 56 weeks | 10.9% | 47%, 34% |
| CONQUER [18] | 981 | 56 weeks | 9.8% | 43%, 36% |
| SEQUEL [19] | 295 | 52 week extension of CONQUER | 10.5% | 3.1%, 4.4% |

**Table 14.2** Naltrexone/Bupropion

| Study | n in Highest Dose | Duration | Weight Loss | Drop-out (Placebo, Highest Dose) |
|---|---|---|---|---|
| COR-I [23] | 583 | 56 weeks | 6.1% | 49%, 50% |
| COR-BMOD [21] | 591 | 56 weeks | 9.3% | 42%, 42% |
| COR-II [24] | 101 | 56 weeks | 8.2% | 46%, 46% |
| DM Study [20] | 335 | 56 weeks | 5.0% | 41%, 48% |

weight loss when combined with an intensive behavioral program [20, 21]. Side effects include nausea, vomiting, diarrhea, dizziness, tremors, and dry mouth. Prior to approval, the FDA requested a cardiovascular outcomes trial in 2011, which was ongoing at the time of approval and had randomized 4454 patients to placebo and 4456 patients to naltrexone/bupropion [22]. Unfortunately, the sponsor inappropriately disclosed the confidential 25% interim results, leading to the early termination of the study. The 25% and 50% interim analyses were evaluated and showed that the upper limit of the hazard ratio for major cardiovascular events (MACE) did not exceed 2.0; however, it was not possible to assess noninferiority and thus, the overall cardiovascular safety of naltrexone/bupropion remains unknown [22]. Fortunately, we now have several AOMs that will be discussed next, which not only have cardiovascular safety but also are cardioprotective..

## What Are the Incretin-Based Therapies Currently Approved for Weight Loss, their Mechanism of Action, and their Indications?

Glucagon-like peptide-1 receptor agonists (GLP1ra) and dual receptor agonists are medications utilized in treating type 2 diabetes and obesity. The GLP1ra medications approved for weight loss are high-dose liraglutide (Saxenda), semaglutide (Wegovy), and tirzepatide (Zepbound). Tirzepatide is a combination GLP1ra and glucose-dependent insulinotropic polypeptide analog (GIP). These medications are indicated for patients with a BMI >27% kg/m$^2$ with at least one weight-related comorbid condition (hypertension, dyslipidemia, type 2 diabetes, obstructive sleep apnea, cardiovascular disease) or BMI >30 kg/m$^2$. Table 14.3 highlights the FDA-approved incretin therapies for weight loss.

GLP1 and GIP are incretin-peptide hormones secreted from the small intestines which stimulate insulin secretion after an oral glucose load [25]. The related hormone receptors are in multiple organs, including the brain, pancreas, and gastrointestinal tract. Incretin hormone analog therapies act on hormone receptors to stimulate insulin secretion, inhibit glucagon release, reduce gastric emptying, reduce appetite, and increase satiety [25, 26]. This therapy class has profound effects on gastrointestinal motility, which have been lessened by slow dose titrations

**Table 14.3** FDA-Approved Incretin Therapies for Overweight and Obesity

| Drug | FDA-approved minimum age (years) | Minimum dosage | Maximum dosage | Minimum dose titration interval | Administration | Expected mean change in weight at max dose (%) |
|---|---|---|---|---|---|---|
| Liraglutide | 12 | 0.6 mg | 3 mg | Weekly | Once daily | 8 |
| Semaglutide | 12 | 0.25 mg | 2.4 mg | Monthly | Once weekly | 15 |
| Tirzepatide | 18 | 2.5 mg | 15 mg | Monthly | Once weekly | 20 |

[2, 6]. The mechanism of action is multifactorial, with gut, brain, and systemic improvements in insulin sensitivity each contributing to the total efficacy [26, 27]. The available data suggest that multiple GLP1r positive neuronal pathways contribute to the anorectic effects of this class of medications [27].

## Review the Efficacy, Treatment Schedule, Administration, Dosing, and Complications for Incretin-Based Therapy Currently FDA-Approved for Weight Loss

### Liraglutide

In 2014, liraglutide 3 mg daily subcutaneous injection became the first GLP1ra agonist approved for the treatment of obesity in people greater than 12 years of age. At nearly twice the highest dose used for diabetes, liraglutide 3 mg showed efficacy in decreasing mean body weight by 8.4 kg at 56 weeks [28]. This equated to two-thirds of patients treated with liraglutide achieving >5% body weight reduction and one-third achieving >10% [28]. The reduction in body weight was associated with improved cholesterol, high sensitivity C-reactive protein, blood pressure, insulin resistance, plasminogen activator inhibitor-1, and adiponectin [28]. The adverse events (AE) most frequently reported with liraglutide therapy were nausea, vomiting, diarrhea, and biliary disease. The effectiveness of liraglutide was diminished in people with a BMI greater than 40 $kg/m^2$.

### Semaglutide

In 2021, semaglutide 2.4 mg weekly subcutaneous injection was approved for chronic weight management in people greater than 12 years of age. Semaglutide was evaluated for the treatment of obesity in a series of trials known as the Semaglutide Treatment Effect in People (STEP) with Obesity program [29, 30]. STEP 1 enrolled 1961 people with overweight or obesity and randomized them to lifestyle intervention and a placebo or 2.4 mg semaglutide once weekly, with a trial duration of 68 weeks [30]. The mean weight loss in semaglutide-treated individuals was 16.9% vs. 2.4% in the placebo group [30]. Weight loss of >15% was achieved by 54.8% vs 5% of the semaglutide vs. placebo-treated group. Blood pressure, C-reactive protein, hemoglobin A1c, and fasting lipid levels were lower in people treated with semaglutide. The most common adverse events were nausea, vomiting, and diarrhea, consistent with the well-described profile of this class of medications.

Similar results were seen in the STEP 3 trial. This trial evaluated the effect of semaglutide on weight loss in individuals assigned to an initial low-calorie diet for 8 weeks and 30 sessions of intensive behavioral therapy plus 200 min of physical activity, over 68 weeks [31]. Mean weight loss on semaglutide was 17.6% vs. 5% in the placebo group [31]. The proportion of people with >15% weight loss was 55.8%

vs. 13.2%, and >20% weight loss was 35.7% vs. 3.7% for semaglutide vs. placebo treatment, respectively. Interestingly, when comparing STEP 1 and STEP 3, which included an intensive behavioral component, the percent weight loss was similar, suggesting that while the lifestyle component is important for healthy living, the pathophysiology of weight loss is very complex and largely involuntary.

### Tirzepatide

In 2023, tirzepatide 5 mg, 10 mg, and 15 mg weekly subcutaneous injection were approved for chronic weight management for people 18 years of age and older. Tirzepatide is a single novel molecule that activates receptors for GIP and GLP1. In preclinical models, GIP has been shown to decrease food intake and increase energy expenditure, therefore resulting in weight reductions, and when combined with GLP-1 receptor agonism, it may result in greater effects on markers of metabolic dysregulation such as body weight, glucose, and lipids [32]. The efficacy for tirzepatide in obesity was tested in a series of studies known as the SURMOUNT program. In the SURMOUNT-1 clinical trial, there was a dose-dependent weight loss effect with increasing weight loss and dose increase [33]. Over 72 weeks, the mean percentage change in weight was approximately 15% with a 5 mg weekly dose, 19.5% with a 10 mg dose, 20.9% with a 15 mg dose, and 3.1% with a placebo. Participants taking tirzepatide also achieved an approximately three times greater percent reduction in fat mass versus lean mass (33.9% fat mass reduction compared to a 10.9% lean mass reduction). The overall safety and tolerability profile of tirzepatide was like other incretin-based therapies approved for the treatment of obesity. The most reported adverse events were gastrointestinal-related and generally mild to moderate in severity, usually occurring during the dose-escalation period.

## What Are the Safety Concerns, Side Effects, and Contraindications for Incretin-Based Therapy?

### Side Effects and Contraindications

#### Gastrointestinal Effects

Gastrointestinal (GI) disorders were the most frequently reported adverse effects during clinical trials of incretin-based therapies. Among the reported gastrointestinal symptoms, nausea, vomiting, constipation, and diarrhea were the most common, usually developing in 40–70% of patients, and have been reported in up to 85% of patients [29, 34, 35]. GI side effects arise irrespective of the half-life or route of administration of the chosen GLP-1ra [35]. These side effects are usually transient, typically starting during the dose-escalation period and generally resolving shortly after the maintenance dose is reached, and, in most cases, they are mild to moderate in severity [35, 36]. A recent report summarizing the results of several trials reported that the majority (99.5%) of documented GI AEs in people with obesity on GLP-1 RA treatment were non-serious [35, 36]..

### Gastroparesis

Gastroparesis is delayed gastric emptying that often presents with symptoms including nausea, abdominal pain, or bloating. It is associated with hyperglycemia and can be persistent in people with diabetes. However, incretin mimetics have also been shown to slow gastric emptying. Patients should be monitored for symptoms of gastroparesis. In addition, incretin therapies should be used with caution in patients with known gastroparesis [34]. If patients experience gastroparesis symptoms on an incretin mimetic the dose should be reduced or the medication discontinued, depending on severity of symptoms.

### Acute Gallbladder Disease

There is an increased rate of occurrence of acute gallbladder disease with GLP1ra. This is due to the GLP1 effect of inhibiting gallbladder motility and emptying by suppressing cholecystokinin secretion [37]. Acute gallbladder events were associated with weight reduction. GLP1ra increased the risk of gallbladder disease, especially when used at higher doses for longer duration and when used for weight loss [37]. In clinical trials of tirzepatide, cholelithiasis was reported in 1.1% of tirzepatide-treated patients and 1.0% of placebo-treated patients, cholecystitis was reported in 0.7% of tirzepatide-treated patients and 0.2% of placebo-treated patients, and cholecystectomy was reported in 0.2% of tirzepatide-treated patients and no placebo-treated patients [38].

### Pancreatitis

Avoid use of this class of drug in patients with a history of pancreatitis. Acute pancreatitis, including fatal and nonfatal hemorrhagic or necrotizing pancreatitis, has been observed in patients treated with GLP-1 receptor agonists. As a result, GLP-1ra therapy is generally avoided in patients with a history of acute pancreatitis.

### Medullary Thyroid Cancer and Multiple Endocrine Neoplasia Syndrome Type 2

Incretin medications are generally contraindicated in patients with a personal or family history of medullary thyroid carcinoma (MTC) or multiple endocrine neoplasia syndrome type 2 (MEN-2) due to a potential risk of thyroid C-cell tumors, although thyroid C-cell tumors have only been seen in rodent studies. **Patients should be counseled regarding the potential risk for MTC with the use of incretin therapies and informed of symptoms of thyroid tumors (e.g., a mass in the neck, dysphagia, dyspnea, persistent hoarseness). Routine monitoring of serum calcitonin or using thyroid ultrasound is of uncertain value for early detection of MTC.** Such monitoring may increase the risk of unnecessary procedures, due to the low-test specificity for serum calcitonin and a high background incidence of thyroid disease. Significantly elevated serum calcitonin values may indicate MTC and patients with MTC usually have calcitonin values >50 ng/L. If serum calcitonin is measured and found to be elevated, the patient should be further evaluated [38].

### Allergic Reaction

**Incretin-based therapies should be avoided in patients with a known hypersensitivity to this class of medication or any of the components of the medication. Serious hypersensitivity reactions including anaphylaxis and angioedema have been reported.**

### Acute Kidney Injury

In patients treated with GLP-1 receptor agonists, there have been post-marketing reports of acute kidney injury and worsening of chronic renal failure, which may sometimes require hemodialysis. Some of these events have been reported in patients without a known underlying renal disease. Many of the reported events occurred in patients who had experienced nausea, vomiting, diarrhea, or dehydration. Patients should be monitored closely for adverse effects of these medications and volume depletion, especially if on other medications such as anti-hypertensives and diuretics.

### Hypoglycemia

Incretin therapies lower blood glucose and can cause hypoglycemia in patients with and without type 2 diabetes. There is an increased risk of hypoglycemia in patients treated with GLP1ra in combination with insulin and/or insulin secretagogue (e.g., sulfonylurea). The risk of hypoglycemia may be lowered by a reduction in the dose of insulin secretagogue or insulin.

### Suicidal Behavior and Ideation

Suicidal behavior and ideation have been reported in clinical trials with other chronic weight management products. Postmarking data suggests a possible increase in mental health disorders, including depression and suicidal thoughts, in patients taking GLP1ra.

Patients should be monitored for new or worsening symptoms of mental health disorders. Use with caution in patients with a history of suicide attempts and active suicide ideation.

### Pregnancy

There are no anti-obesity medications that should be used in pregnancy or in patients trying to become pregnant. If unintended pregnancy is recognized, discontinue the use of incretin therapy. Available data with incretin therapies in pregnant patients are insufficient to evaluate for a drug-related risk of major birth defects, miscarriage, or other adverse maternal or fetal outcomes [38].

### Females and Males of Reproductive Potential

Liraglutide and semaglutide did not have a clinically meaningful impact on the absorption and kinetics of oral contraceptive pills. It is recommended that liraglutide and semaglutide be discontinued 8 weeks prior to conception. The use of tirzepatide may reduce the efficacy of oral hormonal contraceptives due to delayed gastric emptying. This delay is the largest after the first dose and diminishes over time. Patients using oral hormonal contraceptives should be advised to switch to a non-oral contraceptive method or add a barrier method for 4 weeks after initiation and each dose increase..

## What Are Special Populations to Consider for Use of AOMs?

### Perioperative Care

Delayed gastric emptying and/or ileus with incretin-based therapy can lead to regurgitation and pulmonary aspiration under anesthesia. Based only on expert opinion, the American Society of Anesthesiologists (ASA) on preoperative management of adults and children using a GLP-1ra recommends that patients hold their daily dose of GLP-1ra on the day of the procedure or their weekly dose 7 days before the procedure, whether they are taking a GLP1ra for diabetes or weight loss [39]. However the rationale behind these recommendations are not fully supported by the literature including the lack of persistent delayed emptying with longer term use of GLP-1RA use and the low incidence of aspiration seen during upper endoscopy in this population [40, 41]. Consider holding the GLP1ra longer if the patient has diabetes or known gastroparesis. There is no evidence about the optimal fasting duration for patients on GLP-1ra, and the new guidelines suggest following the standard ASA fasting guidelines.

There is an unclear relationship between phentermine and anesthesia. Hypotension on induction of anesthesia was the most reported complication in perioperative phentermine use [42]. Phentermine-induced hypotension may be unresponsive to vasopressors that rely on catecholamine release. For this reason, it is recommended to stop phentermine at least 4 days prior to elective surgery [42].

### Children/Adolescents

In June 2022, the FDA approved a phentermine-topiramate combined pill (Qsymia) as an adjunct to a reduced-calorie diet and increased physical activity for chronic weight management in pediatric patients aged 12 years and older with a BMI in the 95th percentile or greater standardized for age and gender. Approval was based on data from a trial that evaluated the efficacy and safety of Qsymia in patients aged 12 to 17 years old [43]. At the end of the study, treatment with Qsymia resulted in a statistically significant decrease in BMI compared with placebo (−4.8% with 7.5 mg/46 mg dose and −7.1% with 15 mg/92 mg dose vs. +3.3% with placebo).

Liraglutide and semaglutide have been approved for the treatment of adolescents with obesity. Liraglutide was approved based on the results of a 56-week-long randomized controlled trial in male and female adolescents 12 years of age and older [44]. End-of-trial weight loss of >5% or >10% was observed in 43.3% and 26.1% of liraglutide-treated subjects, respectively.

Semaglutide was approved for the treatment of adolescents with obesity based on the results of a 68-week study of semaglutide 2.4 mg weekly dose vs. placebo, plus lifestyle interventions [45]. The mean change in BMI at 68 weeks was 16.1% with semaglutide versus 0.6% with placebo. Improvements in cardiometabolic risk factors were greater in the treatment group than with placebo..

Wellbutrin-naltrexone (Contrave) is not approved for use in children under the age of 18 due to an increased risk of suicidal thoughts and behaviors.

Tirzepatide has not been approved in adolescents or people under 18 years of age.

## Metabolic Dysfunction-Associated Steatohepatitis (MASH) and Post-Liver Transplant

The therapeutic potential of GLP1ra, such as liraglutide and semaglutide, for the treatment of MASH has been studied. These studies [46–48] show a significant improvement and, in some cases, complete resolution of MASH. Improvement of fibrosis varied between the studies, with the most recent data showing no significant improvement in fibrosis in patients with MASH-related compensated cirrhosis [48]. However, semaglutide in this patient population did improve cardiometabolic parameters, which likely helps to slow fibrosis progression. Additionally, this class of medications has been shown to be safe and effective for use in controlling hyperglycemia following liver and other solid organ transplant [49].

## Cardiovascular Disease

The use of GLP1ra in the treatment of people at high risk for cardiovascular disease development and individuals with established cardiovascular disease has been studied [50–53]. The results of these trials, which included a substantial proportion of people with overweight or obesity and co-existing type 2 diabetes, strongly suggest that the reduction of cardiovascular events seen with GLP1ra represents a class effect.

Liraglutide (1.8 mg daily dose) reduced the rates of major adverse cardiovascular events (MACE) in people with type 2 diabetes [52, 53]. However, the cardiovascular safety of liraglutide 3 mg daily in people with obesity has not been assessed in a dedicated cardiovascular outcomes trial.

The Semaglutide Effects on Cardiovascular Outcomes in People with Overweight or Obesity (SELECT) trial, is the first trial to evaluate the cardiovascular benefits of an anti-obesity medication in this population [51]. The study concluded that in patients with known cardiovascular disease and overweight or obese but without diabetes, weekly semaglutide 2.4 mg was superior to placebo in reducing the incidence of death from cardiovascular causes, nonfatal myocardial infarction, or nonfatal stroke at almost 40 months by 20%. Semaglutide 2.4 mg was also studied in patients with obesity and heart failure with preserved ejection fraction (HFpEF) [54]. The study found that treatment with semaglutide led to larger reductions in heart failure symptoms and physical limitations, greater improvements in exercise function, and greater weight loss than placebo [54].

## Chronic Kidney Disease, End-Stage Renal Disease, and Renal Transplant

GLP-1ra's are effective and safe antihyperglycemic agents for patients with T2D and chronic kidney disease (CKD) [55]. The GLP1ra data shows favorable kidney outcomes with reduced albuminuria and likely preservation of estimated GFR [55]. The glucose-lowering benefits of GLP-1ras are preserved in advanced CKD and have demonstrated efficacy and safety in large clinical trials down to an estimated GFR of 15 ml/min per 1.73 m [55, 56]..

For patients with end-stage renal disease (ESRD) on dialysis, GLP1ra had modest glycemic and obesity benefits [57]. In retrospective cohort studies of transplant populations, GLP1ra improved glycemic control but had less benefit on obesity [57, 58]. There was a heightened risk for hypoglycemia in people with ESRD, particularly those also using insulin [56]. GI side effects were most common in ESRD and renal transplant patients [57]. Larger studies are needed to assess the benefits of incretin therapies in people with ESRD on dialysis and renal transplant.

## Type-1 Diabetes (T1DM)

Off-label use of incretin mimetics has been reported in patients with type 1 diabetes. Multiple studies have confirmed that GLP1ra plus insulin can improve HbA1c levels in patients with T1DM, better than insulin alone [59, 60]. The combination therapy also led to a significant reduction in weight and total daily insulin requirements. Importantly, there was no increased risk of hypoglycemia or diabetic ketoacidosis (DKA), but these patients should be monitored closely while on combined therapy. Patients who have detectable C-peptide, have overweight obesity, or who cannot achieve glycemic goals without hypoglycemia have been found to benefit the most from combined GLP1ra-insulin therapy. Further studies are warranted to evaluate the effect of incretin mimetics on clinical outcomes in patients with T1DM.

## Obstructive Sleep Apnea

The Effect of Liraglutide in Obese Subjects With Moderate or Severe Obstructive Sleep Apnea: SCALE™—Sleep Apnea trial assessed the effectiveness of liraglutide 3 mg daily vs. placebo, in addition to diet and exercise counseling, in nondiabetic patients with obesity and moderate to severe sleep apnea who were unable to tolerate continuous positive airway pressure [61]. The treatment group demonstrated a mean weight loss of 5.7%, together with a reduction in the apnea-hypopnea index (AHI) and improved hemoglobin A1c. Improvements in OSA endpoints were related to the degree of weight loss at the end of the study, with greater improvement seen with greater weight loss. People with OSA often have comorbid conditions, such as diabetes, metabolic syndrome, and obesity, that predispose them to increased cardiovascular risk [62]. The use of incretin mimetics can target multiple conditions at once, thus potentially reducing polypharmacy, and cost, and improving quality of life [63].

## How Do Social Determinants of Health Affect Access to Care and the Uptake of Treatment for Obesity?

Non-medical factors that impact health are categorized as social determinants of health (SDOH). Understanding how these social determinants affect health outcomes and whether patients can adhere to recommended medical treatments is paramount. The Centers for Disease Control categorizes social determinants into five major categories: economic stability, education access and quality, healthcare access and quality, neighborhood and built environment, and social and community context [64, 65]. Each of these facets can negatively impact access to healthcare and utilization of recommended treatments for obesity..

### Economic Stability

Financial security is paramount to ensuring citizens have stable incomes to support their healthcare needs. In the United States, 11.5% (37.9 million) of Americans live in poverty [66]. Financial instability has a ripple effect on housing stability, which can impact other social determinants of health and negatively impact health outcomes [67]. Financial security, or lack thereof, can either aid our patients as they seek out and utilize healthcare, or prevent access to medications and other recommended treatments for obesity. The barrier to accessing treatment can perpetuate existing health disparities in healthcare overall, but also for the treatment of obesity.

### Education Access and Quality

Higher levels of educational attainment are associated with improved health outcomes and longer lifespans, a finding related to an interplay of multiple social determinants for positive outcomes. However, lower levels of education (e.g., attending lower-performing schools, not attending college) are associated with shorter lifespans and lower quality of health,

Approximately 34% of all Americans aged 25 years or more hold a bachelor's degree or higher [68]. Despite this, according to the Miliken Institute, 88% of Americans have a health literacy level that is inadequate to navigate the healthcare system and promote their individual well-being [69]. This poses a significant barrier for the majority of individuals seeking/receiving healthcare.

## Healthcare Access and Quality

Ninety-two percent of Americans (304 million) were insured as of 2022, with the majority carrying private insurance (65.6%). Of those privately insured, 55% carried employer-based coverage [70]. Lack of insurance precludes access to healthcare and can result in delays in diagnosis, altering the recommended care plan [71]. Lower health literacy negatively impacts access, utilization of healthcare, and health outcomes [72]. In the world of treatment for obesity, insurance barriers prevent patients from accessing all options that are available to them (medical and surgical), contributing to the underutilization of obesity treatment.

## Neighborhood and Built Environment

Over half of Americans do not live within ½ mile of a park, and 40% of households do not live within 1 mile of healthier retailers [73]. In 2022, 44 million Americans lived in food-insecure households [74]. Living in the lower income brackets predisposes individuals to neighborhoods and built environments where health is not promoted but seems out of reach. Scarcity of healthier food options within a reachable distance and food insecurity negatively impact patients and contribute to the disease of obesity with decreased physical activity and intake of more heavily processed foods/beverages given restrictions in access to safe outdoor spaces for exercise and healthy, fresh food..

## Social and Community Context

Social connection with others is key to the human experience. This became most apparent during the height of the COVID-19 pandemic when global social isolation was in effect. Social isolation is associated with negative effects on health and increases risks of anxiety, depression, and suicidality. For older individuals, it increases the risk of premature death from all causes, dementia by 50%, and increases the risk of stroke and heart disease [75].

The contribution of the SDOH to obesity cannot be understated. The perfect storm of food deserts, food insecurity, economic instability, unsafe neighborhoods for outdoor play/activity, lack of access to a recreational space (i.e., a park) within walking distance, zoning for poorly performing schools, lack of access to quality healthcare, and social isolation negatively impact health which can also contribute to the development of obesity. Additional barriers from lack of insurance and/or specific insurance plan limitations that preclude patients from accessing and/or receiving treatment pose significant obstacles in obesity care [76]. Understanding the environment where our patients live and the context in which they can seek care is key to maximizing our ability to facilitate care and advocate for our patients.

## How Do we Best Employ AOMs Based on What we Know?

Over time, it has been well established that the prevalence of obesity in the United States continues to rise, with 42% of adult Americans and 20% of children and adolescents affected [77]. Anti-obesity medications have a range of effects on TBW, which increased with the recent introduction of GLP-1 receptor agonists. But how do we best employ AOMs for treating obesity based on our current knowledge?

As we operate on a mere fraction of patients eligible for bariatric surgery annually, there is room for much-improved access to obesity treatment, whether via medical or surgical therapies, or a combination of both are employed. The first consideration, however, is ensuring patient access to physicians and other clinicians who treat the disease of obesity. Provider, patient, and societal views can negatively impact patient treatment utilization by impairing patient referrals for evaluation for bariatric surgery or precluding the pursuit of it by patients as a viable treatment modality [78–81]. Insurance barriers also impair access and utilization of bariatric surgery, with many individual plans of larger insurance carriers (public and private) without coverage for bariatric surgery. Although 36% of patients nationally are publicly insured, most patients undergoing bariatric surgery are privately insured [82–84]. This is especially relevant as children on Medicaid are more likely to have obesity than their privately insured counterparts [85]. These barriers can also negatively impact the consideration of medical options for obesity treatment and prevent access to obesity medicine care teams and subsequent utilization of anti-obesity medications [86]. With the new class of AOMs, insurance barriers pose more of an issue with many patients unable to obtain GLP-1 receptor agonists for the short or longer term [87].

With this information, determining how to utilize AOMs equitably is the challenge. While AOMs have varying degrees of success with weight loss of 5–10%, the newer classes of GLP-1 receptor agonists and tirzepatide have demonstrated weight loss effects of 15–20% after study durations of 68–72 weeks [88]. With increased weight loss benefits of the new generations of AOMs, existing insurance barriers prevent access to obesity treatment. Medicare excludes coverage for these medications for a diagnosis of obesity without other related diagnoses, and global shortages of GLP-1 agonists have contributed to the issue of limited access [88]. Without insurance coverage, the newer AOMs' average retail costs range from $1000–1600 per month which is economically not feasible for most patients [88]. However, long-term use of these medications is recommended for sustained effects [89]. This continued reframing of obesity as a chronic disease is necessary to optimize long-term care with medication, surgery, or a combination of both.

The optimal use for AOMs may be determined by the obesity phenotype, as discussed by Acosta et al. in their 2021 study evaluating patient weight loss outcomes when AOMs are prescribed based on a particular obesity phenotype. In this study, the authors had the participants complete several validated tests and questionnaires after an 8-hour fasting period to classify obesity phenotypes. Based on the classification of phenotypes (hungry brain, hungry gut, emotional eating, and slow burn), AOMs were prescribed considering these phenotypes. A total of 450 patients were included in this study (excluding those with prior major gastrointestinal surgery or endoscopic interventions for weight loss, unable to afford the prescribed medications or have insurance deny coverage, and active use of FDA-approved AOMs before their first visit for the study). Those in whom AOMs were prescribed based on their obesity phenotype had statistically significant differences in weight over the study period of 1 year compared to the non-phenotype guided group, as well as a significantly lower failure rate (defined as <5% total body weight loss) compared to the non-phenotype guided group [90].

Treatment of the disease of obesity requires long-term management for optimal success and may require a combination of therapies over a patient's lifetime. Bariatric surgery is the gold standard for weight loss but requires lifelong follow-up and close monitoring for nutritional deficiencies, late complications of surgically altered anatomy, and weight regain. Utilization of AOMs for weight loss can result in up to 20% of TBWL (depending on the medication) but requires long-term use for maximal benefit. With consideration of financial/insurance-based barriers patients face in obtaining some of these medications, the recommended best use of AOMs is listed below:

1. in combination with lifestyle interventions (behavioral and physical activity),
2. as an upfront weight loss adjunct for patients with severe obesity who are at high risk for general anesthesia due to extremely high BMIs and/or distribution of excess adipose tissue,
3. as an adjuvant therapy post-bariatric surgery for weight regain as part of a multidisciplinary program.

Ultimately, the most successful use of AOMs for weight loss involves considering external patient factors (e.g., SDOH), obesity phenotypes, and long-term patient goals.

## Summary

The disease of obesity has a long history of existence. Still, serious discussions around the negative health impacts did not occur until the twentieth century with the creation of several medications aimed at treating obesity, as well as the rise of surgical treatment options. Despite the continued worsening prevalence of obesity in the United States, treatment is underutilized for a variety of access, financial, and social reasons. In the last several years, options for medical weight loss with the introduction of new classes of AOMs have greatly increased the total body weight loss that can be attained, but also with the continued evidence that obesity is a chronic disease and requires lifelong management for optimal health outcomes. The best use of AOMs must consider the underlying phenotype of obesity, genetic and medical comorbid conditions, goals for use, and how to ensure equitable access is available for all patients.

## References


1. Conard NJ. A female figurine from the basal Aurignacian of Hohle Fels Cave in southwestern Germany. Nature. 2009;459(7244):248–52.
2. Bray GA, Purnell JQ. An historical review of steps and missteps in the discovery of anti-obesity drugs. In: Feingold KR, Anawalt B, Blackman MR, Boyce A, Chrousos G, Corpas E, et al., editors. Endotext. South Dartmouth, MA: MDText.com, Inc. Copyright © 2000-2024, MDText.com, Inc.; 2000.
3. Cutting WCTM. Actions of Dinitrophenol. Proc Soc Exp Biol Med. 1932;29(9):1268–9.
4. Colman E. Dinitrophenol and obesity: an early twentieth-century regulatory dilemma. Regul Toxicol Pharmacol. 2007;48(2):115–7.
5. Horner WD. Cataract following di-nitrophenol treatment for obesity. Arch Ophthalmol. 1936;16(3):447–61.
6. Weintraub M, Sundaresan PR, Madan M, Schuster B, Balder A, Lasagna L, et al. Long-term weight control study. I (weeks 0 to 34). The enhancement of behavior modification, caloric restriction, and exercise by fenfluramine plus phentermine versus placebo. Clin Pharmacol Ther. 1992;51(5):586–94.
7. Connolly HM, Crary JL, McGoon MD, Hensrud DD, Edwards BS, Edwards WD, et al. Valvular heart disease associated with fenfluramine-phentermine. N Engl J Med. 1997;337(9):581–8.
8. de Andrade Mesquita L, Fagundes Piccoli G, Richter da Natividade G, et al. Is Lorcaserin Really Associated With Increased Risk of Cancer? A Systematic Review and Meta-Analysis. Obesity Reviews: An Official Journal of the International Association for the Study of Obesity. 2021;22(3):e13170. https://doi.org/10.1111/obr.13170.
9. Batsis JA, Apolzan JW, Bagley PJ, Blunt HB, Divan V, Gill S, et al. A systematic review of dietary supplements and alternative therapies for weight loss. Obesity (Silver Spring). 2021;29(7):1102–13.
10. Kidambi S, Batsis JA, Donahoo WT, Jastreboff AM, Kahan S, Saunders KH, et al. Dietary supplements and alternative therapies for obesity: a perspective from the Obesity Society's clinical committee. Obesity (Silver Spring). 2021;29(7):1095–8.
11. Florida Department of Health Division of Medical Quality. Annual Report. Fiscal Year 2020-2021. https://www.floridahealth.gov/statistics-and-data/e-forcse/news-reports/_documents/annual-report-2021.pdf.
12. Hendricks EJ, Srisurapanont M, Schmidt SL, Haggard M, Souter S, Mitchell CL, et al. Addiction potential of phentermine prescribed during long-term treatment of obesity. Int J Obes. 2014;38(2):292–8.
13. Lewis KH, Gudzune KA, Ard JD. Phentermine in the modern era of obesity pharmacotherapy: does it still have a role in treatment? Curr Obes Rep. 2024;
14. Lewis KH, Fischer H, Ard J, Barton L, Bessesen DH, Daley MF, et al. Safety and effectiveness of longer-term phentermine use: clinical outcomes from an electronic health record cohort. Obesity (Silver Spring). 2019;27(4):591–602.
15. Torgerson JS, Hauptman J, Boldrin MN, Sjöström L. XENical in the prevention of diabetes in obese subjects (XENDOS) study: a randomized study of orlistat as an adjunct to lifestyle changes for the prevention of type 2 diabetes in obese patients. Diabetes Care. 2004;27(1):155–61.
16. Sarayani A, Donahoo WT, Hampp C, Brown JD, Winterstein AG. Assessment of the Risk Evaluation and Mitigation Strategy (REMS) for phentermine-Topiramate to prevent exposure during pregnancy. Ann Intern Med. 2023;176(4):443–54.
17. Allison DB, Gadde KM, Garvey WT, Peterson CA, Schwiers ML, Najarian T, et al. Controlled-release phentermine/topiramate in severely obese adults: a randomized controlled trial (EQUIP). Obesity (Silver Spring). 2012;20(2):330–42.
18. Gadde KM, Allison DB, Ryan DH, Peterson CA, Troupin B, Schwiers ML, et al. Effects of low-dose, controlled-release, phentermine plus topiramate combination on weight and associated comorbidities in overweight and obese adults (CONQUER): a randomised, placebo-controlled, phase 3 trial. Lancet. 2011;377(9774):1341–52.

19. Garvey WT, Ryan DH, Look M, Gadde KM, Allison DB, Peterson CA, et al. Two-year sustained weight loss and metabolic benefits with controlled-release phentermine/topiramate in obese and overweight adults (SEQUEL): a randomized, placebo-controlled, phase 3 extension study. Am J Clin Nutr. 2012;95(2):297–308.
20. Hollander P, Gupta AK, Plodkowski R, Greenway F, Bays H, Burns C, et al. Effects of naltrexone sustained-release/bupropion sustained-release combination therapy on body weight and glycemic parameters in overweight and obese patients with type 2 diabetes. Diabetes Care. 2013;36(12):4022–9.
21. Wadden TA, Foreyt JP, Foster GD, Hill JO, Klein S, O'Neil PM, et al. Weight loss with naltrexone SR/bupropion SR combination therapy as an adjunct to behavior modification: the COR-BMOD trial. Obesity (Silver Spring). 2011;19(1):110–20.
22. Nissen SE, Wolski KE, Prcela L, Wadden T, Buse JB, Bakris G, et al. Effect of naltrexone-bupropion on major adverse cardiovascular events in overweight and obese patients with cardiovascular risk factors: a randomized clinical trial. JAMA. 2016;315(10):990–1004.
23. Greenway FL, Fujioka K, Plodkowski RA, Mudaliar S, Guttadauria M, Erickson J, et al. Effect of naltrexone plus bupropion on weight loss in overweight and obese adults (COR-I): a multicentre, randomised, double-blind, placebo-controlled, phase 3 trial. Lancet. 2010;376(9741):595–605.
24. Apovian CM, Aronne L, Rubino D, Still C, Wyatt H, Burns C, et al. A randomized, phase 3 trial of naltrexone SR/bupropion SR on weight and obesity-related risk factors (COR-II). Obesity (Silver Spring). 2013;21(5):935–43.
25. Vilsbøll T, Christensen M, Junker AE, Knop FK, Gluud LL. Effects of glucagon-like peptide-1 receptor agonists on weight loss: systematic review and meta-analyses of randomised controlled trials. BMJ. 2012;344:d7771.
26. Müller TD, Blüher M, Tschöp MH, DiMarchi RD. Anti-obesity drug discovery: advances and challenges. Nat Rev Drug Discov. 2022;21(3):201–23.
27. Drucker DJ. GLP-1 physiology informs the pharmacotherapy of obesity. Mol Metab. 2022;57:101351.
28. Pi-Sunyer X, Astrup A, Fujioka K, Greenway F, Halpern A, Krempf M, et al. A randomized, controlled trial of 3.0 mg of Liraglutide in weight management. N Engl J Med. 2015;373(1):11–22.
29. Kushner RF, Calanna S, Davies M, Dicker D, Garvey WT, Goldman B, et al. Semaglutide 2.4 mg for the treatment of obesity: key elements of the STEP trials 1 to 5. Obesity. 2020;28(6):1050–61.
30. Wilding JPH, Batterham RL, Calanna S, Davies M, Van Gaal LF, Lingvay I, et al. Once-weekly Semaglutide in adults with overweight or obesity. N Engl J Med. 2021;384(11):989–1002.
31. Wadden TA, Bailey TS, Billings LK, Davies M, Frias JP, Koroleva A, et al. Effect of subcutaneous Semaglutide vs placebo as an adjunct to intensive behavioral therapy on body weight in adults with overweight or obesity: the STEP 3 randomized clinical trial. JAMA. 2021;325(14):1403–13.
32. Mathiesen DS, Bagger JI, Bergmann NC, Lund A, Christensen MB, Vilsbøll T, et al. The effects of dual GLP-1/GIP receptor Agonism on glucagon secretion-a review. Int J Mol Sci. 2019;20(17)
33. Jastreboff AM, Aronne LJ, Ahmad NN, Wharton S, Connery L, Alves B, et al. Tirzepatide once weekly for the treatment of obesity. N Engl J Med. 2022;387(3):205–16.
34. Sodhi M, Rezaeianzadeh R, Kezouh A, Etminan M. Risk of gastrointestinal adverse events associated with glucagon-like Peptide-1 receptor agonists for weight loss. JAMA. 2023;330(18):1795–7.
35. Gorgojo-Martínez JJ, Mezquita-Raya P, Carretero-Gómez J, Castro A, Cebrián-Cuenca A, de Torres-Sánchez A, et al. Clinical recommendations to manage gastrointestinal adverse events in patients treated with Glp-1 receptor agonists: a multidisciplinary expert consensus. J Clin Med. 2022;12(1)
36. Wharton S, Calanna S, Davies M, Dicker D, Goldman B, Lingvay I, et al. Gastrointestinal tolerability of once-weekly semaglutide 2.4 mg in adults with overweight or obesity, and the

relationship between gastrointestinal adverse events and weight loss. Diabetes Obes Metab. 2022;24(1):94–105.
37. He L, Wang J, Ping F, Yang N, Huang J, Li Y, et al. Association of Glucagon-like Peptide-1 receptor agonist use with risk of gallbladder and biliary diseases: a systematic review and meta-analysis of randomized clinical trials. JAMA Intern Med. 2022;182(5):513–9.
38. Zepbound (tirzepatide) [package insert]. Eli Lilly and Company. Revised 10/2024. https://uspl.lilly.com/zepbound/zepbound.html#pi.
39. Joshi GP. Anesthetic considerations in adult patients on glucagon-like Peptide-1 receptor agonists: gastrointestinal focus. Anesth Analg. 2024;138(1):216–20.
40. Camilleri M, Carlson P, Dilmaghani S. Prevalence and variations in gastric emptying delay in response to GLP-1 receptor agonist liraglutide. Obesity (Silver Spring). 2024;32(2):232–3.
41. Anazco D, Fansa S, Hurtado MD, Camilleri M, Acosta A. Low incidence of pulmonary aspiration during upper endoscopy in patients prescribed a glucagon-like peptide 1 receptor agonist. Clin Gastroenterol Hepatol. 2023;
42. Lim S, Rogers LK, Tessler O, Mundinger GS, Rogers C, Lau FH. Phentermine: a systematic review for plastic and reconstructive surgeons. Ann Plast Surg. 2018;81(4):503–7.
43. Kelly AS, Bensignor MO, Hsia DS, Shoemaker AH, Shih W, Peterson C, et al. Phentermine/Topiramate for the treatment of adolescent obesity. NEJM Evid. 2022;1(6)
44. Kelly AS, Auerbach P, Barrientos-Perez M, Gies I, Hale PM, Marcus C, et al. A randomized, controlled trial of Liraglutide for adolescents with obesity. N Engl J Med. 2020;382(22):2117–28.
45. Weghuber D, Barrett T, Barrientos-Pérez M, Gies I, Hesse D, Jeppesen OK, et al. Once-weekly Semaglutide in adolescents with obesity. N Engl J Med. 2022;387(24):2245–57.
46. Armstrong MJ, Gaunt P, Aithal GP, Barton D, Hull D, Parker R, et al. Liraglutide safety and efficacy in patients with non-alcoholic steatohepatitis (LEAN): a multicentre, double-blind, randomised, placebo-controlled phase 2 study. Lancet. 2016;387(10019):679–90.
47. Newsome PN, Buchholtz K, Cusi K, Linder M, Okanoue T, Ratziu V, et al. A placebo-controlled trial of subcutaneous Semaglutide in nonalcoholic Steatohepatitis. N Engl J Med. 2021;384(12):1113–24.
48. Loomba R, Abdelmalek MF, Armstrong MJ, Jara M, Kjær MS, Krarup N, et al. Semaglutide 2·4 mg once weekly in patients with non-alcoholic steatohepatitis-related cirrhosis: a randomised, placebo-controlled phase 2 trial. Lancet Gastroenterol Hepatol. 2023;8(6):511–22.
49. Sweiss H, Hall R, Zeilmann D, Escamilla J, Bhayana S, Patel R, et al. Single-center evaluation of Safety & Efficacy of glucagon-like Peptide-1 receptor agonists in solid organ transplantation. Prog Transplant. 2022;32(4):357–62.
50. Sattar N, Lee MMY, Kristensen SL, Branch KRH, Del Prato S, Khurmi NS, et al. Cardiovascular, mortality, and kidney outcomes with GLP-1 receptor agonists in patients with type 2 diabetes: a systematic review and meta-analysis of randomised trials. Lancet Diabetes Endocrinol. 2021;9(10):653–62.
51. Lincoff AM, Brown-Frandsen K, Colhoun HM, Deanfield J, Emerson SS, Esbjerg S, et al. Semaglutide and cardiovascular outcomes in obesity without diabetes. N Engl J Med. 2023;389(24):2221–32.
52. Verma S, Bain SC, Buse JB, Idorn T, Rasmussen S, Ørsted DD, et al. Occurence of first and recurrent major adverse cardiovascular events with Liraglutide treatment among patients with type 2 diabetes and high risk of cardiovascular events: a post hoc analysis of a randomized clinical trial. JAMA Cardiol. 2019;4(12):1214–20.
53. Verma S, Poulter NR, Bhatt DL, Bain SC, Buse JB, Leiter LA, et al. Effects of Liraglutide on cardiovascular outcomes in patients with type 2 diabetes mellitus with or without history of myocardial infarction or stroke. Circulation. 2018;138(25):2884–94.
54. Kosiborod MN, Abildstrøm SZ, Borlaug BA, Butler J, Rasmussen S, Davies M, et al. Semaglutide in patients with heart failure with preserved ejection fraction and obesity. N Engl J Med. 2023;389(12):1069–84.
55. Galindo RJ, Beck RW, Scioscia MF, Umpierrez GE, Tuttle KR. Glycemic monitoring and Management in Advanced Chronic Kidney Disease. Endocr Rev. 2020;41(5):756–74.

56. Long JJ LA, Sudhindran V, Pencovici N, Kukla A, Diwan T. Semaglutide tolerability and efficacy in patients with chronic kidney disease stage 4, 5 and end stage renal disease. 2022.
57. Clemens KK, Ernst J, Khan T, Reichert S, Khan Q, LaPier H, et al. Glucagon-like peptide 1 receptor agonists in end-staged kidney disease and kidney transplantation: a narrative review. Nutr Metab Cardiovasc Dis. 2023;33(6):1111–20.
58. KDIGO. 2020 clinical practice guideline for diabetes Management in Chronic Kidney Disease. Kidney Int. 2020;98(4s):S1–s115.
59. Wang W, Liu H, Xiao S, Liu S, Li X, Yu P. Effects of insulin plus glucagon-like Peptide-1 receptor agonists (GLP-1RAs) in treating type 1 diabetes mellitus: a systematic review and meta-analysis. Diabetes Ther. 2017;8(4):727–38.
60. Guyton J, Jeon M, Brooks A. Glucagon-like peptide 1 receptor agonists in type 1 diabetes mellitus. Am J Health Syst Pharm. 2019;76(21):1739–48.
61. Blackman A, Foster GD, Zammit G, Rosenberg R, Aronne L, Wadden T, et al. Effect of liraglutide 3.0 mg in individuals with obesity and moderate or severe obstructive sleep apnea: the SCALE sleep apnea randomized clinical trial. Int J Obes. 2016;40(8):1310–9.
62. Tuomilehto H, Seppä J, Uusitupa M. Obesity and obstructive sleep apnea--clinical significance of weight loss. Sleep Med Rev. 2013;17(5):321–9.
63. Sultana R, Sissoho F, Kaushik VP, Raji MA. The case for early use of glucagon-like Peptide-1 receptor agonists in obstructive sleep apnea patients with comorbid diabetes and metabolic syndrome. Life (Basel). 2022;12(8)
64. 2023 HP. Social Determinants of Health. Available from: https://health.gov/healthypeople/priority-areas/social-determinants-health.
65. ArtigaSHE.BeyondHealthCare:TheRoleofSocialDeterminantsinPromotingHealthandHealth Equity 2018. Available from: https://www.kff.org/racial-equity-and-health-policy/issue-brief/beyond-health-care-the-role-of-social-determinants-in-promoting-health-and-health-equity/.
66. Shrider EAC, John. Poverty in the United States: 2022: U.S. Census Bureau; 2022. Available from: https://www.census.gov/content/dam/Census/library/publications/2023/demo/p60-280.pdf.
67. Khullar DCDA. Health, Income, & Poverty: Where We Are & What Could Help 2018. Available from: https://www.healthaffairs.org/do/10.1377/hpb20180817.901935/full/.
68. [Census Quick Facts]. Available from: https://www.census.gov/quickfacts/fact/table/US/PST045222.
69. Katherine LCKBS. HEALTH LITERACY IN THE UNITED STATES: Enhancing Assessments and Reducing Disparities: Milken Institute; 2022. Available from: https://milkeninstitute.org/sites/default/files/2022-05/Health_Literacy_United_States_Final_Report.pdf.
70. Keisler-Starkey KB, Lisa N. Lindstrom, Rachel A. Health insurance coverage in the United States: 2022: U.S. Census Bureau; 2022. Available from: https://www.census.gov/content/dam/Census/library/publications/2023/demo/p60-281.pdf.
71. Stahl KA, Dodge D, Olecki EJ, Holguin RP, McLaughlin C, Wong W, et al. Insurance status and travel distance to single treatment facility predictive of mastectomy. J Surg Res. 2022;270:22–30.
72. Berkman ND, Sheridan SL, Donahue KE, Halpern DJ, Crotty K. Low health literacy and health outcomes: an updated systematic review. Ann Intern Med. 2011;155(2):97–107.
73. Why It Matters: Centers for Disease Control and Prevention; Available from: https://www.cdc.gov/obesity/about-obesity/why-it-matters.html.
74. Food Security in the U.S.: U.S. Department of Agricultuure; 2022. Available from: https://www.ers.usda.gov/topics/food-nutrition-assistance/food-security-in-the-u-s/key-statistics-graphics/#foodsecure.
75. Loneliness and Social Isolation Linked to Serious Health Conditions: Centers for Disease Control and Prevention; Available from: https://www.cdc.gov/aging/publications/features/lonely-older-adults.html.
76. Gasoyan H, Halpern MT, Tajeu G, Sarwer DB. Impact of insurance plan design on bariatric surgery utilization. Surg Obes Relat Dis. 2019;15(10):1812–8.

77. Stierman Bea. National Health and Nutrition Examination Survey 2017–March 2020 Prepandemic Data Files Development of Files and Prevalence Estimates for Selected Health Outcomes. 2021.
78. Lynch CS, Chang JC, Ford AF, Ibrahim SA. Obese African-American women's perspectives on weight loss and bariatric surgery. J Gen Intern Med. 2007;22(7):908–14.
79. Dolan P, Afaneh C, Symer M, Dakin GF, Pomp A, Yeo H. Assessment of public attitudes toward weight loss surgery in the United States. JAMA Surg. 2019;154(3):264–6.
80. Chao GF, Diaz A, Ghaferi AA, Dimick JB, Byrnes ME. Understanding racially diverse community member views of obesity stigma and bariatric surgery. Obes Surg. 2022;32(4):1216–26.
81. Johnson-Mann C, Martin AN, Williams MD, Hallowell PT, Schirmer B. Investigating racial disparities in bariatric surgery referrals. Surg Obes Relat Dis. 2019;15(4):615–20.
82. Bhogal SK, Reddigan JI, Rotstein OD, Cohen A, Glockler D, Tricco AC, et al. Inequity to the utilization of bariatric surgery: a systematic review and meta-analysis. Obes Surg. 2015;25(5):888–99.
83. Health Insurance Coverage: Centers for DIsease Control and Prevention; 2023 [FastStats - health insurance coverage]. Available from: https://www.cdc.gov/nchs/fastats/health-insurance.htm.
84. Altieri MS, Yang J, Yin D, Talamini MA, Spaniolas K, Pryor AD. Patients insured by Medicare and Medicaid undergo lower rates of bariatric surgery. Surg Obes Relat Dis. 2019;15(12):2109–14.
85. Williams E BA, Rudowitz R. Obesity rates among children: A closer look at implications for children covered by Medicaid: KFF; 2018. Available from: https://www.kff.org/medicaid/issue-brief/obesity-rates-among-children-a-closer-look-at-implications-for-children-covered-by-medicaid/#:~:text=Children%20with%20Medicaid%20are%20more,children%20with%20private%20insurance%20alone.
86. Stephenson J. Report finds large variation in States' coverage for obesity treatments. JAMA Health Forum. 2022;3(3):e220608.
87. Gasoyan H, Sarwer DB. Addressing insurance-related barriers to novel antiobesity medications: lessons to be learned from bariatric surgery. Obesity (Silver Spring). 2022;30(12):2338–9.
88. Elmaleh-Sachs A, Schwartz JL, Bramante CT, Nicklas JM, Gudzune KA, Jay M. Obesity Management in Adults: a review. JAMA. 2023;330(20):2000–15.
89. Grunvald E, Shah R, Hernaez R, Chandar AK, Pickett-Blakely O, Teigen LM, et al. AGA clinical practice guideline on pharmacological interventions for adults with obesity. Gastroenterology. 2022;163(5):1198–225.
90. Acosta A, Camilleri M, Abu Dayyeh B, Calderon G, Gonzalez D, McRae A, et al. Selection of Antiobesity medications based on phenotypes enhances weight loss: a pragmatic trial in an obesity clinic. Obesity (Silver Spring). 2021;29(4):662–71.

# A Precision Medicine Approach for Obesity Management

# 15

Diego Anazco, Fauzi Feris Jassir, Sima Fansa, Maria A. Espinosa, and Andres Acosta

## Introduction

Obesity is a chronic, complex, and multifactorial disease that is strongly associated with multiple chronic, non-communicable diseases [1]. Obesity does not only result in an increased risk for traditional cardiovascular risk factors, such as type 2 diabetes and hypertension, but excess weight by itself also increases the risk of developing cardiovascular events by 34% [2]. Besides this, there is strong evidence to support a causal relationship between excess adiposity and at least 13 different types of cancer [3].

The epidemic growth of obesity has resulted in an unprecedented burden of obesity-associated comorbidities. A report estimated that by 2030, almost 1 in 2 adults in the United States will have obesity, and almost 1 in 4 adults will have severe obesity (i.e., body mass index ≥35 kg/m$^2$) [4]. In 2016, the total cost of obesity and its associated comorbidities was equivalent to 9.3% of the US gross domestic product [5]. Moreover, a study showed that the global disability-adjusted life years attributable to a high body mass index (BMI) has doubled from 1990 to 2017 to reach 70.7 million in women and 77 million in men, mostly due to an increase in cardiovascular disease, diabetes, kidney disease and cancer [6].

D. Anazco · S. Fansa · M. A. Espinosa · A. Acosta (✉)
Precision Medicine for Obesity Program, Division of Gastroenterology and Hepatology, Department of Medicine, Mayo Clinic, Rochester, MN, USA
e-mail: anazcovillarreal.diego@mayo.edu; fansa.sima@mayo.edu; espinosamonteros.maria@mayo.edu; acosta.andres@mayo.edu

F. Feris Jassir
Precision Medicine for Obesity Program, Division of Gastroenterology and Hepatology, Department of Medicine, Mayo Clinic, Rochester, MN, USA

Division of General Surgery, Florida Atlantic University, Boca Raton, USA
e-mail: fferisjassir@health.fau.edu


O. M. Ghanem et al. (eds.), *The SAGES Manual of Metabolic and Bariatric Surgery*, https://doi.org/10.1007/978-3-031-72309-4_15

As a result, there is an impending need for finding safe and effective weight loss interventions. The main objective of obesity management is inducing a successful transition from a pro-obesogenic to a healthy lifestyle that enables an individual to achieve significant weight loss and prevent weight regain [7]. Lifestyle interventions, including medical nutrition therapy and physical activity, are the cornerstone for obesity management; however, they are often insufficient by themselves to achieve significant and maintained weight loss. Previous evidence from the Look AHEAD (Action for Health in Diabetes) showed that 37.7% of participants with type 2 diabetes and overweight or obesity were able to lose at least 10% of their body weight with intensive lifestyle intervention at 1 year [8], and only 39.3% of participants were able to maintain a total body weight loss (TBWL) of 10%.

Previous literature has suggested that a more prominent weight loss (TBWL >10%) might be associated with greater improvements in cardiovascular risk factors than modest weight loss (TBWL: 5–10%) [9, 10]. Hence, multiple patients with obesity usually require additional therapeutic interventions to lose sufficient weight, including antiobesity medication and bariatric and metabolic procedures. To date, bariatric surgery continues to be the most effective approach to achieve significant weight loss and comorbidity improvement or resolution. An umbrella review identified several beneficial effects of bariatric surgery on cardiovascular disease, cancer incidence and mortality, among others [11]. In spite of significant advancements in the bariatric surgery field resulting in safer procedures with shorter recovery times, this treatment modality remains underutilized in patients with severe obesity, particularly among patients with multiple comorbidities, underinsured or in minorities [12].

Perhaps the biggest challenge in obesity treatment is the significant interindividual variability resulting in heterogenous weight loss outcomes for the same intervention. In that regard, precision medicine emerges as a potential alternative in order to try to minimize heterogeneity in response to different treatment modalities for obesity. In this chapter, we aim to explore potential mechanisms behind the heterogeneity in response to bariatric surgery through a review of the postsurgical metabolic and physiologic adaptations seen after metabolic and bariatric surgery. In addition, we intend to present current evidence supporting the implementation of a precision medicine approach for different weight loss interventions, along with the future directions that might lead to personalized treatment for obesity.

## Physiologic Adaptations After Metabolic and Bariatric Surgery

Obesity results from a dysregulation in energy balance that manifests as excessive storage of adipose tissue which predisposes to multiple comorbidities. Both homeostatic and hedonic pathways interact to regulate food intake. The gut-brain axis tightly regulates the different stages of homeostatic eating behavior. Hunger refers to the drive to eat. Satiation is the process that brings an eating episode to an end and

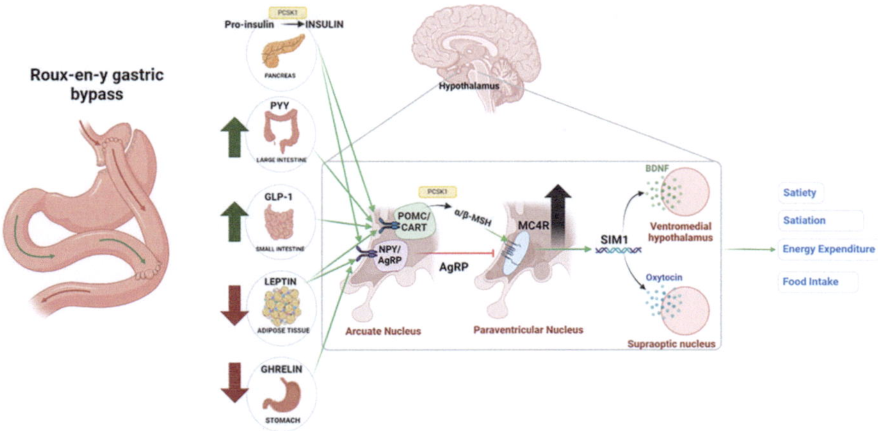


**Fig. 15.1** Hormonal adaptations seen after Roux-en-Y gastric bypass and their effect on central and peripheral mechanisms of energy balance regulation, including the leptin-melanocortin pathway

thus controls the meal size (intrameal inhibition). Postprandial satiety inhibits further eating and increases fullness after a meal has finished (inter-meal inhibition) [13]. These homeostatic processes can be overridden by hedonic or reward-based pathways in order to elicit pleasure or escape negative emotions even in the setting of energy abundance [14, 15]. Bariatric surgery leads to prominent alterations in gut hormones and bile acids [16, 17]. Following bariatric surgery, there is an array of postoperative metabolic and anatomical changes that significantly contribute to weight loss and resolution or improvement of obesity-related comorbidities. The heterogeneity in outcomes after bariatric surgery could be a result of differences in homeostatic adaptations after different bariatric procedures.

Multiple satiety hormones secreted by the gastrointestinal tract (such as glucagon-like peptide-1 (GLP-1), peptide tyrosine tyrosine (PYY), and oxyntomodulin (OXM), among others) reduce food intake through multiple mechanisms including hypothalamic anorexigenic signaling, altered gut motility, and slowing the gastric emptying through the ileal break mechanism [18, 19]. Other gut hormones like ghrelin and cholecystokinin (CCK) also show adaptative postsurgical patterns promoting reduced food intake [20, 21]. In addition, other hormones like vasoactive intestinal polypeptide (VIP), glucagon, amylin, and glucose-dependent insulinotropic polypeptide (GIP) also seem to have an altered secretion pattern following bariatric surgery and while these seem to have a lesser effect on weight loss, they could potentially influence hunger homeostasis (Fig. 15.1).

These hormonal adaptations following bariatric surgery promote a lesser degree of weight loss when compared to bariatric surgery which produces both anatomical alterations and hormonal adaptations [22]. This phenomenon suggests that the hormonal adaptations need to be paired with anatomic alterations (a 30–50 cc gastric pouch with an associated Roux-en-Y gastric bypass (RYGB), resection of the stomach fundus and body creating a sleeve gastric remnant, among others) induced by bariatric surgery to potentiate the weight loss effect which in turn leads to resolution or improvement of obesity-related comorbidities.

## Ghrelin and Leptin

Ghrelin, the orexigenic "hunger hormone," is primarily produced in the stomach. Ghrelin decreases energy expenditure, and lipolysis, increases adipogenesis, and inhibits insulin secretion. Patients with obesity seem to have elevated ghrelin levels, furthermore, after food intake, there seems to be a blunted "ghrelin drop" in this patient population. After sleeve gastrectomy (SG), ghrelin levels decrease due to the removal of a significant portion of the stomach. RYGB also leads to reduced ghrelin secretion [23], likely due to altered gut anatomy and hormonal signaling [24–27]. More importantly, following SG and RYGB this "ghrelin drop" seems to be restored to a certain extent [26–29]. This in turn promotes reduced hunger following a meal, decreased adipogenesis, and increased lipolysis in theory promoting weight loss.

The adipose tissue-derived hormone leptin plays a crucial role in appetite regulation leading to satiety. It is positively correlated with the amount of body fat [30], and it is thought that there is a leptin resistance in patients with obesity [31]. Following SG and RYGB, leptin levels tend to decrease, likely secondary to the weight loss. Duodenal switch surgery (DS) may have a similar effect, although more research is needed [24]. Reduced leptin in the context of continued weight loss suggests that there might be improvement of obesity-induced leptin resistance.

## Glucagon-Like Peptides (GLP), Peptide YY (PYY), and Oxyntomodulin (OXM)

Glucagon-Like Peptide-1 (GLP-1) and Glucagon-Like Peptide-2 (GLP-2) are incretin hormones secreted by intestinal entero-endocrine cells (EEC) that deeply influence glucose homeostasis, gut motility, and hunger homeostasis. GLP-1 influences food intake mainly through two routes, central effects and regulation of gastric motility. Pharmacological blockade of GLP-1 receptors has been shown to increase the activation hunger hunger-related nuclei in the central nervous system (CNS) with visual stimuli [32]. GLP-1 receptor agonists, such as semaglutide, have been associated with significant delays in gastric emptying [33, 34].

SG and RYGB among other bariatric procedures increase postprandial GLP-1 secretion [25], leading to improved glucose control and enhanced insulin sensitivity. DS is likely to have similar effects [24].

PYY is an incretin that is also secreted by entero-endocrine cells at the level of the ileum and colon. It is intimately related to the ileal break mechanism thus slowing gastric emptying and suppressing appetite in a similar fashion to GLP-1. PYY's effects on food intake and energy homeostasis are mainly mediated by $PYY_{3\text{-}36}$. It is intimately related to energy homeostasis and regulates energy expenditure [35]. Both SG and RYGB have been shown to result in increased postprandial PYY levels, promoting early satiety and reduced caloric intake [24–27]. Further characterizing the importance of the postprandial incretin rise following bariatric surgery, an attenuated increase in postprandial GLP-1 and PYY secretion has been related to sub-optimal weight loss outcomes [36].

OXM, derived from proglucagon, is a dual agonist of GLP-1 and glucagon receptors. Its postprandial plasma levels are shown to be increased after SG and RYGB thus contributing to reduced food intake and improved glycemic control [37].

## Cholecystokinin (CCK) and Bile Acids (BA)

CCK, released by the small intestine, regulates gallbladder contraction, pancreatic enzyme secretion, and gastric emptying by relaxing the gastric fundus [38]. Human models have shown that CCK infusions to physiologic and supra-physiologic levels lead to reduced meal sizes [39]. SG and RYGB increase postprandial CCK levels [25, 26], influencing digestion and nutrient absorption. While CCK is unlikely to be the sole agent causing weight loss after bariatric surgery, it does seem to contribute to satiety and decreased food intake due to its influence on hunger homeostasis.

Bariatric surgery alters bile acid secretion and metabolism. RYGB creates an anatomic bypass of the duodenum and proximal jejunum. SG on the other hand decreases meal size inducing caloric restriction while increasing the speed of nutrient delivery into the small bowel [40] with such an impact that delayed gastric emptying is related to poor weight loss outcomes.

Bile acids are ligands to the Takeda G-protein-coupled receptor (TGR-5) which cascades into GLP-1 secretion in gut entero-endocrine cells [41]. TGR-5 has been identified in CNS neurons and astrocytes as well [42]. Following bariatric surgery, there is an increase in postprandial plasma bile acids [43] that is maintained for years as well. Increased gut intraluminal and plasma bile acids increase in turn incretins through TGR-5, thus enhancing lipid and glucose metabolisms. DS is likely to act in a similar way to RYGB with its malabsorptive component secondary to the anatomical alterations further modifying bile acid profiles.

## Obesity, Oxidative Stress, and Bariatric Surgery

Recently, obesity and its relationship to inflammation, oxidative stress and cancer have been in the spotlight of scientific literature due to obesity's nature as a modifiable risk factor. Oxidative stress seems to be a key factor in the development of obesity-related comorbidities like insulin resistance, diabetes, cardiovascular disease, liver disease and cancer [44, 45]. A positive correlation exists between BMI and oxidative stress biomarkers [46]. Known antioxidants have been shown to be decreased in individuals with obesity when compared to those without obesity [47, 48]. Obesity and carcinogenesis share pathophysiological mechanisms like hyperinsulinemia, chronic inflammation, sex hormone metabolism dysfunction, elevated cytokines, and increased oxidative stress [49–53]. In a recent robust meta-analysis and systematic review, the investigators showed Bariatric surgery to be associated with a reduction in the overall incidence of cancer with a risk reduction of 0.62 ($p = 0.002$) [54]. The study portrayed a reduced future incidence of seven different obesity-related cancers in individuals who underwent bariatric surgery: (1) Hepatocellular carcinoma (RR 0.35 $p < 0.00001$), (2) Colorectal cancer (RR 0.63 $p = 0.0002$), (3) Pancreatic cancer (RR 0.52 $p = 0.03$), (4) Gallbladder cancer (RR 0.41 $p = 0.04$), (5) Breast cancer (RR 0.56 $p < 0.00001$), (6) Endometrial cancer (RR 0.38 $p < 0.00001$) and (7) Ovarian cancer (RR 0.45 $p < 0.0001$). They also showed that in patients with obesity who underwent bariatric surgery, there was reduced cancer-related mortality with a risk reduction of 0.51 ($p < 0.00001$) suggesting that bariatric surgery is a sound strategy to prevent cancer and reduce cancer-associated mortality.

## A Precision Medicine Approach to Obesity

Obesity is a complex and heterogeneous condition with a multifactorial etiology driven by the interaction between environmental factors, genetics, and epigenetics [55, 56]. Precision medicine offers a novel framework under which a disease or trait is stratified based on information from specific biological markers (e.g., genomics, metagenomics, transcriptomics, among others), as well as from other clinical, behavioral, and environmental characteristics (Fig. 15.3) [57].

The rapid development of large-scale databases and biobanks, and high-throughput methods for characterizing patients from a multi-omics perspective, have resulted in a rapid advancement in the field of precision medicine [58]. These biological markers can potentially predict an individual's response to a specific therapy, thereby permitting a personalized treatment approach. Ultimately, precision medicine involves the use of all available data to enhance and maximize clinical outcomes.

Current adiposity-based classifications of obesity are tightly correlated with cardiometabolic disease and mortality risk [59]; however, they fail to convey the complexity and multifaceted nature of obesity pathogenesis. As a result, delving into the intricacies of energy regulation in patients with obesity to find specific phenotypes based on measurable parameters of energy balance regulation offers a prominent path to enhance the selection of weight loss interventions. Nonetheless, there are multiple challenges posed by the study of appetite and energy balance regulation in humans, as experimental conditions might not necessarily mimic what occurs in a natural environment [60].

We have previously proposed and validated a standardized protocol for obesity phenotyping to study key parameters of energy balance regulation in a dynamic fashion [61–63]. After overnight fasting, patients undergo resting energy expenditure measurement through indirect calorimetry, body composition analyses by dual-energy X-ray absorptiometry, and blood sampling at fasting and postprandial conditions for hormones and metabolites, alongside with genotyping (Fig. 15.2).

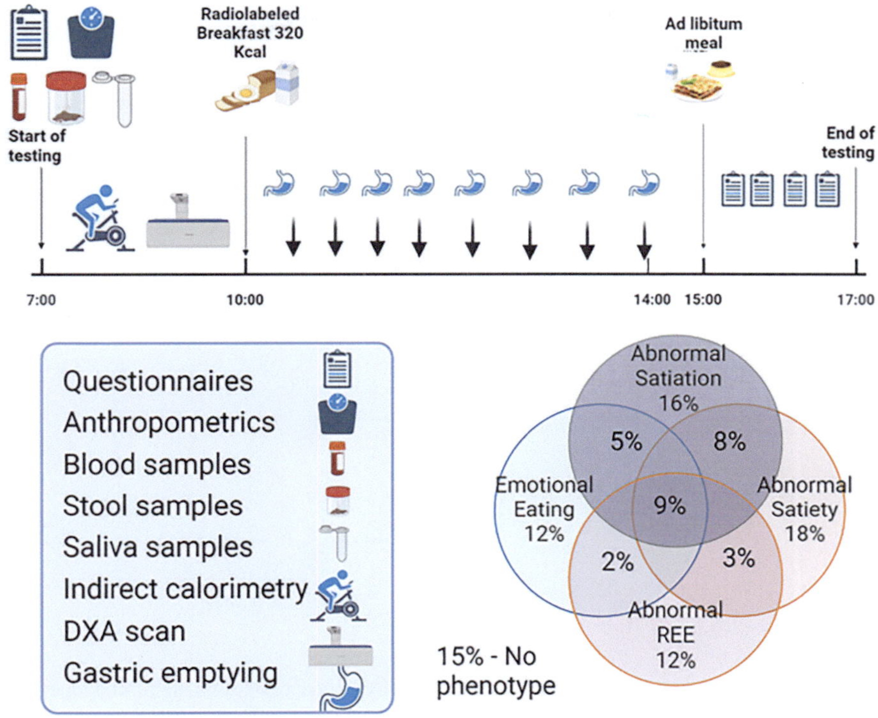


**Fig. 15.2** Standardized protocol for the dynamic study of parameters of energy balance regulation to identify obesity phenotypic traits. Distribution of the obesity phenotypes in a sample of 450 adults with obesity, redrawn from Ref. [61]

After a standardized radiolabeled breakfast, we assess for gastric emptying of solids and liquids through gastric scintigraphy [64]. In addition, participants complete ad libitum meal testing to measure the number of calories needed to achieve satiation with subsequent subjective appetite questionnaires (i.e., visual analogue scale scores). In addition, multiple validated self-administered questionnaires for mood and eating behaviors are gathered through the phenotyping day. As a result, we have proposed a framework for selection of weight loss interventions in patients with obesity based on four actionable obesity phenotypes: abnormal satiation, abnormal postprandial satiety, abnormal energy expenditure and emotional eating [61, 63].

Recent developments in high-throughput profiling for several biological samples have resulted in significant advances within the precision medicine field. The identification of variations among distinct phenotypes across the genome, transcriptome, proteome, metabolome, and microbiome might hold the key to individualize treatment selection in patients with obesity. Further, the integration of information derived from different -omics might help identify specific phenotypes that might benefit the most for specific interventions, resulting in an important shift from the current "one size fits all" paradigm towards a precision medicine approach [57, 65]. For the remainder of the chapter, we will describe existing evidence for the

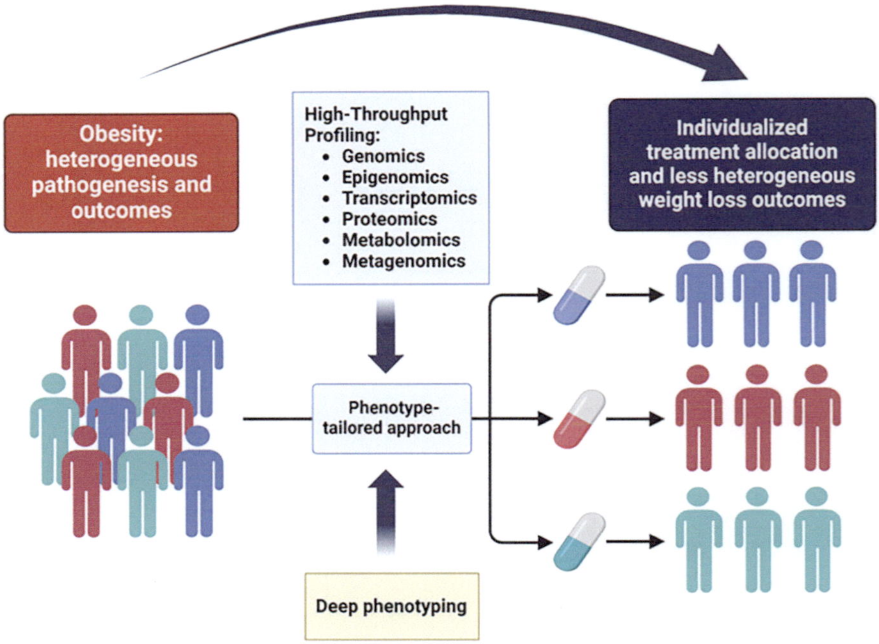


**Fig. 15.3** A precision medicine framework including deep phenotyping and high-throughput profiling technologies for the selection of weight loss interventions in patients with obesity

personalized selection of obesity treatment modalities, including lifestyle interventions, antiobesity medications, endoscopic bariatric and metabolic therapies, and metabolic and bariatric surgery.

## Lifestyle Interventions

There is robust evidence showing the variability in weight loss outcomes of different lifestyle interventions [66]. For instance, a meta-analysis including 48 randomized clinical trials for dietary interventions showed highly variable weight loss outcomes for different interventions and a substantial heterogeneity among studies [67]. Several poorly understood factors, such as genetic factors, differences in neurohormonal mechanisms and physiologic adaptations, and modifications in gut microbiome, as well as differences in adherence and other behavioral factors might contribute to this variability [66].

Some studies have suggested that intensive behavioral sessions and particular diet macronutrient compositions might lead to better weight loss outcomes [68]. Recently, we showed that a phenotype-tailored lifestyle intervention (PLI) led to significantly superior weight loss outcomes at 12 weeks when compared to a standard lifestyle intervention (SLI) (TBWL: 7.4 kg vs. 4.3 kg, $p = 0.004$) [63]. In this study, the PLI consisted of an a priori set of recommendations designed with the intention to improve the altered phenotypic traits observed during baseline obesity phenotyping [63]. This study highlights the importance of a deep comprehension of energy balance regulation to propose mechanistically appropriate interventions for each individual, to counteract the predominant pathophysiologic alterations and improve weight loss outcomes.

The role of genetic factors in determining the response to dietary interventions has been thoroughly studied [69, 70]. Nutrigenetics refers to the discipline that studies the interactions between nutrients and the human genome in relationship to the variation in response to different disease states, including obesity [70]. Particular nutrients might interact with an individual's genetic attributes, resulting in altered regulation of metabolic pathways contributing to either weight gain or weight loss. The role of nutrigenetic-based approaches continues to be studied as certain literature has shown conflicting results. For instance, a study suggested that nutrigenetics-tailored diets led to better long-term BMI reduction [69]. In contrast, a 10-week weight loss intervention study that randomly assigned participants into either a personalized diet group, based on individualized metabolic and genetic information, or a control diet group, showed no significant benefits of a personalized intervention in terms of weight loss outcomes [71]. This field needs to be assessed extensively in order to understand how nutrient-gene interactions might affect interindividual variability in order to minimize heterogeneity.

The interaction between physical activity and genes has been previously assessed. A meta-analysis showed that physical activity may attenuate the weight-gain effect of FTO by 30% [72]. In contrast, a study from the UK Biobank showed a strong gene-environment interaction with self-reported TV watching, highlighting that individuals with a genetic predisposition to obesity might be particularly susceptible to be affected by an obesogenic environment [73].

## Antiobesity Medications

The development of safe and effective long-term antiobesity medications has remained elusive until recently. Incretin-based therapies have transformed the field of obesity medicine, with newer medications being able to induce clinically significant weight loss, while also leading to comorbidity improvement [74] and reduction in cardiovascular mortality [75]. However, even for highly effective antiobesity medications such as semaglutide, up to one-third of patients are not able to achieve a body weight loss of at least 10% after 68 weeks of treatment [76].

As a result, we have proposed that the selection of antiobesity medications based on a framework of actionable and quantitative parameters of energy balance regulation could lead to better weight loss outcomes. In a pragmatic, real-world trial, we showed that phenotype-guided selection of antiobesity medications led to significantly superior weight loss outcomes at 12 months when compared to a non-phenotype-guided, standard of care approach (TBWL: 15.9% vs. 9.0%, difference: −6.9%, $p < 0.001$) [61].

The abnormal satiation phenotype is characterized by an impaired intrameal inhibition resulting in larger meal size and energy intake and is quantified by the number of calories needed to achieve satiation during an ad libitum meal. In a 2-week randomized clinical trial, 24 patients with obesity that underwent obesity phenotyping at baseline and after intervention were randomized to receive either placebo or phentermine-topiramate extended-release (ER, 7.5/46 mg) [62]. In this study, phentermine-topiramate ER led to a significant reduction in the number of calories to achieve satiation during an ad libitum meal (mean difference: 206 kcal) when compared to the placebo group ($p = 0.03$), and there was a correlation between higher energy intake at baseline and weight loss for patients in the treatment group [62]. Semaglutide has also shown a decrease in ad libitum energy intake [77]; however, a study suggested that tirzepatide, a dual GIP and GLP-1 receptor agonist, resulted in numerically larger reductions in ad libitum energy intake when compared to semaglutide (−64.3 kcal, $p = 0.19$) [78]. It is likely that these differences could be due to the action of GIP in the CNS to reduce food intake [79].

The abnormal postprandial satiety phenotype is characterized by an impaired inter-meal inhibition resulting in more frequent return of hunger. We have previously validated the association between gastric emptying of solids and increased postprandial hunger scores [80]. For this phenotype, the selection of GLP-1 receptor agonists, which are known to slow gastric emptying, could potentially restore satiety mechanisms in this subset of patients [33, 81]. In a placebo-controlled randomized clinical trial, liraglutide led to a significant delay in gastric emptying of solids at 5 (median difference: 70 min) and 16 weeks (median difference: 34 min) when compared to placebo, and there was a correlation between gastric emptying of solids half-life at 16 weeks with weight loss in patients assigned to liraglutide ($p = 0.024$) [82].

Currently, the data on whether more potent delaying of gastric emptying is associated with superior weight loss outcomes for semaglutide and tirzepatide is scarce. Additional studies are needed to better understand the mechanisms behind the weight loss induced by these novel medications.

The abnormal energy expenditure phenotype is characterized by lower than expected energy expenditure, and is assessed by the ratio between measured resting energy expenditure through indirect calorimetry [83] and expected resting energy expenditure (i.e., quantified through the Harris-Benedict equation). For this phenotype, we recommended the implementation of a structured physical activity program consisting of resistance training. To date, most antiobesity medications have focused on decreasing energy intake through different mechanisms, rather than increasing resting energy expenditure [84]. Phentermine has shown some secondary effects on energy expenditure [7, 61]. In animal models, tirzepatide led to a slight increase in energy expenditure, which was not evident in animals treated with semaglutide after 7 days [85]; however, further studies are needed to better define which are the most effective interventions among this group.

The emotional eater phenotype is characterized by a strong hedonic or emotional component for eating behaviors, and is often quantified through questionnaires such as the Three Factor Eating Questionnaire (TFEQ-21) [86]. As a complement to a strong behavioral intervention [63], we have suggested that patients with emotional eating might benefit from the combination of bupropion and naltrexone which could potentially modulate appetite, mood, and cravings [7]. In a pooled analysis of four phase 3 clinical trials with naltrexone/bupropion, early responders had significantly lower craving control scores at baseline when compared to non-responders, suggesting the potential for identifying patients that would have better outcomes [87]. Other additional studies have suggested that semaglutide led to improvement in cravings control, which positively correlated with weight loss outcomes at 2 years [88].

Nonetheless, it is likely that other physiologic and behavioral traits of obesity might be associated with heterogeneity in weight loss outcomes to certain antiobesity medications. As a result, a multi-omics-based framework might be necessary to identify potential biologic markers of phenotypic traits for obesity that might permit the personalization of antiobesity medication selection.

## Endoscopic Bariatric and Metabolic Therapies

Endoscopic bariatric and metabolic therapies have been rapidly advancing and represent safe and effective weight loss interventions [89]. These interventions include space-occupying intragastric devices (IGD), aspiration therapy (AT), tissue apposition devices (TAD), duodenal mucosal resurfacing (DMR), incisionless anastomosis devices (IAD), and duodenal-jejunal bypass line (DJBL). These different interventions produce weight loss through distinct mechanisms, and as a result, personalized selection of these endoscopic interventions could enhance effectiveness and tolerability [90].

Space-occupying devices (such as intragastric balloons [IGB] or the transpyloric shuttle [TPS]) can regulate both satiety and satiation through mechanical and hormonal stimuli. A study showed that IGB led to a reduction in ghrelin levels, which positively correlated with weight loss outcomes [91]. In addition, other studies have showed a significant delay in gastric emptying [92–95].

Tissue apposition devices (such as the endoscopic sleeve gastroplasty [ESG] or the Primary Obesity Surgery Endoluminal [POSE]) lead to weight loss through an effect on satiation, both from peripheral hormone signaling and restriction of gastric accommodation [96]. In addition, impairment of gastric emptying and retention of food in the gastric pouch cause increased satiety. The distal plications impair the antral contractions which further delays gastric emptying. In a previous study, it was showed that ESG led to significant delays in gastric emptying when compared to a lifestyle intervention at 3 months (152.3 ± 47.3 vs 89.1 ± 27.9; $p < 0.001$) and 12 months (137 ± 37.4 vs 90.1 ± 23.4; $p < 0.001$). Importantly, the delay in gastric emptying at 3 months was associated with a greater weight loss [97]. However, in a study involving IGB and ESG, IGB led to a greater delay in GE when compared to ESG, while, ESG has a greater impact on satiation than IGB [98].

Aspiration therapy consists of a gastrostomy tube and siphon device in order to aspirate gastric contents from the stomach after meals. About 30% of the ingested amount is aspirated prior to absorption. This accounts for about 80% of the total amount of weight loss experienced by with these intervention, while other potential mechanisms include the need of increased chewing and drinking more water with every meal as shown in various studies [99, 100].

The DJBL bypasses the duodenum, permitting the chyme to pass directly from the stomach to the jejunum. As a result, pancreatic secretions do not mix with the gastric contents separated by the liner. These results in a technique that is similar to a gastric bypass surgery without the permanent alteration in anatomy [101].

DMR consists of hydrothermal ablation of the duodenal mucosa. This procedure has shown promising results for patients with obesity and type 2 diabetes. It has been stipulated that proximal diversion might lead to an increase in incretins, such as GLP-1 and GIP, which might lead to an improvement in abnormal metabolic pathways in patients with obesity and type 2 diabetes [102, 103].

EAD creates an anastomosis that permits the passage of partially undigested food into the distal ileum, increasing the secretion of satiety hormones such ad GLP-1 and PYY in order to enhance weight loss outcomes [104].

Additional studies are needed to better characterize the weight loss mechanisms for different endoscopic bariatric and metabolic therapies; however, based on current knowledge, it is likely that TAD and AT could have a more prominent effect in participants with abnormal satiation, while IGB, EAD or DJBL could be better options for participants with abnormal postprandial satiety.

## Metabolic and Bariatric Surgery

Bariatric surgery remains the most effective intervention for weight loss among patients with obesity, offering long-term weight control compared with lifestyle interventions [105]. Beyond weight loss, its advantages include the improvement of various obesity-associated comorbidities, including type 2 diabetes mellitus, hypertension, and dyslipidemia [105]. Within the realm of bariatric surgeries, sleeve gastrectomy (SG) and Roux-en-y gastric bypass (RYGB) stands out as the most commonly performed interventions in present-day surgical practice, with SG notably surpassing RYGB to become the leading bariatric surgery worldwide in terms of number of surgeries [106].

The outcomes from bariatric surgeries exhibit significant heterogeneity, especially in the long-term after intervention, and complications attributed to the surgery should not be underestimated [107]. Hence, identifying reliable pre-surgical indicators for a risk-benefit assessment before the intervention would be of high value. While numerous studies have demonstrated the significant variability in weight loss outcomes among patients who have undergone bariatric surgery, only a few factors have been associated with superior weight loss outcomes, including young age, male sex, lower preoperative BMI, and absence of type 2 diabetes [105]. However, none of these factors are sufficiently robust to serve as predictive indicators [106]. Understanding the variables influencing weight loss would serve as an initial step in implementing precision medicine within bariatric surgery, leading to not only improved outcomes but also to a decreased rate of complications and a reduction in the need for revisional surgery.

Most recently, the genetic background of individuals has emerged a potentially relevant for bariatric surgery outcomes [108–110]. Weight loss variability following bariatric procedures may be attributed to genetic factors, with a more pronounced impact observed in restrictive/malabsorptive procedures compared to purely restrictive ones [111]. Studies on the impact of genetic makeup on postsurgery weight loss have generated variable results. One study investigated the effects of heterozygous variants in the leptin-melanocortin pathway (LMP) on long-term weight outcomes after RYGB [109]. Carriers had a progressive and significant weight regain in the mid- and long-term after RYGB compared to controls. Another study analyzed the long-term outcomes of LMP genetic variant carriers undergoing SG; results showcased carriers having similar weight loss outcomes than non-carriers when evaluating for total body weight change%, weight loss nadir, and weight regain, suggesting that the weight loss mechanisms induced by SG possibly may bypass an impaired LMP [110].

Moreover, genome-wide-association studies have identified loci in which several single nucleotide polymorphisms (SNPs) are associated with body mass index and waist-hip-ratio [112–114]. These known SNPs have been incorporated into genetic risk scores (GRS), and studies have investigated the predictive ability of those scores regarding weight loss trajectory following surgery [63–65]. A GRS, based on nine BMI-associated SNPs and one WHR-associated SNP, showed a significant association with weight loss at 12-month and 24-month following bariatric surgery [105]. The study also found a positive correlation between excess weight loss percentage (%EWL) at 12 months and %EWL at 24 months, suggesting that individuals who initially respond best to the surgery (those with the highest %EWL at 12 months) are also the most likely to continue improving in the subsequent 12 months. This could prove to be a valuable tool for physicians to adjust recommendations for maintaining sufficient weight loss beyond the first postoperative year. Several studies have evaluated genetic risk scores in post-bariatric surgery weight loss, demonstrating their capability to predict outcomes [115–117]. The development and application of GRS can be considered valuable in the pre-surgical assessment to evaluate the extent to which patients may benefit from bariatric surgery and thus could be utilized to improve weight loss prediction prior to the intervention. With continued refinement, these risk scores hold the potential to help better surgical outcomes and customize therapeutic modalities.

Epigenetics consists of heritable modifications that do not involve changes in the DNA nucleotide sequence [118]. Epigenetic modifications may also explain improvements in metabolism after bariatric surgery. Data suggest that bariatric surgery modifies the DNA methylation profile of specific genes [119]. Establishing the clinical application of epigenetic variations as therapeutic targets may help predict outcomes after bariatric surgery.

Metabolomics involves a detailed examination of metabolites and shows potential to enhance precision medicine practices [120]. Metabolic profiles after MBS show significant changes compared to non-surgical procedures [121, 122].

Metabolomic studies may also help detect biomarkers that predict preoperative metabolic outcomes in bariatric procedures [123]. In parallel, obesity and other chronic diseases are associated with changes in the human microbiota [124]. Bariatric surgery can induce changes in the microbiome [125], with specific taxonomic variations correlating with improved metabolic profiles postsurgery [126].

Despite universally accepted indications for bariatric surgery and the availability of numerous surgical techniques, there are currently no guidelines for implementing a patient-tailored approach when it comes to bariatric surgery [106]. There is significant variability in weight loss response (and weight loss maintenance) following bariatric surgery. It is unlikely that this variability is secondary to variations in technique as there is currently a robust standard of care technique among bariatric surgeons. A good example that portrays this are the effects of variations in pouch size and gastro-jejunostomy (GJ) diameter on weight loss after RYGB. While the pouch should be small (<30 ml) [127] variations among small gastric pouches and GJ diameter don't seem to affect weight loss response [128, 129]. Furthermore, advancing towards the application of precision medicine in the realm of bariatric interventions necessitates a more comprehensive understanding of the factors influencing weight outcomes following these procedures. Machine learning models targeting preoperative factors could serve as a valuable tool in achieving this objective, as they enable a more precise identification of the causal links between determinants of weight gain and weight loss [106].

## Conclusion and Next Steps

The traditional paradigm of trial-and-error for selection weight loss interventions in patients with obesity leads to heterogeneous outcomes and often results in increased medical and financial burden. The selection of weight loss interventions by employing a precision medicine framework might permit the identification of which intervention could potentially benefit a patient the most, enhancing effectiveness and tolerability to the intervention. In addition, such framework could also permit the adequate supply and allocation of weight loss interventions in a more cost-effective manner.

Nonetheless, there is still a long way to go before precision medicine approaches are widely implemented in the clinical management of obesity. There is an impending need for large, multinational collaborative efforts to collect and report data on weight loss outcomes for different interventions in a systematic manner in order to identify which participants could have a better response to a certain intervention. The implementation of large biobanks with deep phenotyping information and outcomes registries will permit the advancement of the precision medicine field in obesity.

Even though the assessment of phenotypic traits of energy balance regulation in obesity offers a prominent path to permit the individualization of weight loss interventions, it is important to recognize that this approach is difficult to implement in a large-scale. As a result, the development of genetic and other -omics based biomarker might help bridge the gap and permit the widespread adoption of a precision medicine framework for selection of weight loss interventions in patients with obesity.

## References


1. Heymsfield SB, Wadden TA. Mechanisms, pathophysiology, and Management of Obesity. N Engl J Med. 2017;376(3):254–66.
2. Limpijankit T, Vathesatogkit P, Matchariyakul D, Wiriyatanakorn S, Siriyotha S, Thakkinstian A, et al. Causal relationship of excess body weight on cardiovascular events through risk factors. Sci Rep. 2022;12(1):5269.
3. Lauby-Secretan B, Scoccianti C, Loomis D, Grosse Y, Bianchini F, Straif K. Body fatness and cancer — viewpoint of the IARC working group. N Engl J Med. 2016;375(8):794–8.
4. Ward ZJ, Bleich SN, Cradock AL, Barrett JL, Giles CM, Flax C, et al. Projected U.S. state-level prevalence of adult obesity and severe obesity. N Engl J Med. 2019;381(25):2440–50.
5. Waters H, Graf M. America's obesity crisis: the health and economic costs of excess weight. Milken Institute; 2018.
6. Dai H, Alsalhe TA, Chalghaf N, Riccò M, Bragazzi NL, Wu J. The global burden of disease attributable to high body mass index in 195 countries and territories, 1990–2017: an analysis of the global burden of disease study. PLoS Med. 2020;17(7):e1003198.
7. Acosta A, Streett S, Kroh MD, Cheskin LJ, Saunders KH, Kurian M, et al. White paper AGA: POWER - practice guide on obesity and weight management, education, and resources. Clin Gastroenterol Hepatol. 2017;15(5):631–49.e10.
8. The Look AHEAD Research Group. Eight-year weight losses with an intensive lifestyle intervention: the look AHEAD study. Obesity (Silver Spring). 2014;22(1):5–13.
9. Wing RR, Lang W, Wadden TA, Safford M, Knowler WC, Bertoni AG, et al. Benefits of modest weight loss in improving cardiovascular risk factors in overweight and obese individuals with type 2 diabetes. Diabetes Care. 2011;34(7):1481–6.
10. Brown JD, Buscemi J, Milsom V, Malcolm R, O'Neil PM. Effects on cardiovascular risk factors of weight losses limited to 5-10. Transl Behav Med. 2016;6(3):339–46.
11. Liao J, Yin Y, Zhong J, Chen Y, Chen Y, Wen Y, et al. Bariatric surgery and health outcomes: an umbrella analysis. Front Endocrinol. 2022;13:1016613.
12. Alvarez R, Bonham AJ, Buda CM, Carlin AM, Ghaferi AA, Varban OA. Factors associated with long wait times for bariatric surgery. Ann Surg. 2019;270(6):1103–9.
13. Blundell J, de Graaf C, Hulshof T, Jebb S, Livingstone B, Lluch A, et al. Appetite control: methodological aspects of the evaluation of foods. Obes Rev. 2010;11(3):251–70.
14. Lutter M, Nestler EJ. Homeostatic and hedonic signals interact in the regulation of food intake. J Nutr. 2009;139(3):629–32.
15. Campos A, Port JD, Acosta A. Integrative hedonic and homeostatic food intake regulation by the central nervous system: insights from neuroimaging. Brain Sci. 2022;12(4):431.
16. Steinert RE, Feinle-Bisset C, Asarian L, Horowitz M, Beglinger C, Geary N. Ghrelin, CCK, GLP-1, and PYY(3-36): secretory controls and physiological roles in eating and Glycemia in health, obesity, and after RYGB. Physiol Rev. 2017;97(1):411–63.
17. Patti ME, Houten SM, Bianco AC, Bernier R, Larsen PR, Holst JJ, et al. Serum bile acids are higher in humans with prior gastric bypass: potential contribution to improved glucose and lipid metabolism. Obesity (Silver Spring). 2009;17(9):1671–7.
18. Chaudhri O, Small C, Bloom S. Gastrointestinal hormones regulating appetite. Philos Trans R Soc Lond Ser B Biol Sci. 2006;361(1471):1187–209.
19. Maljaars PW, Peters HP, Mela DJ, Masclee AA. Ileal brake: a sensible food target for appetite control. A review. Physiol Behav. 2008;95(3):271–81.

20. Sayegh AI. The role of cholecystokinin receptors in the short-term control of food intake. Prog Mol Biol Transl Sci. 2013;114:277–316.
21. De Vriese C, Delporte C. Influence of ghrelin on food intake and energy homeostasis. Curr Opin Clin Nutr Metab Care. 2007;10(5):615–9.
22. Jones B, Sands C, Alexiadou K, Minnion J, Tharakan G, Behary P, et al. The Metabolomic effects of Tripeptide gut hormone infusion compared to Roux-en-Y gastric bypass and caloric restriction. J Clin Endocrinol Metabol. 2021;107(2):e767–e82.
23. Cummings DE, Weigle DS, Frayo RS, Breen PA, Ma MK, Dellinger EP, et al. Plasma ghrelin levels after diet-induced weight loss or gastric bypass surgery. N Engl J Med. 2002;346(21):1623–30.
24. Bharatselvam S, Schwenger K, Ghorbani Y, Fischer S, Jackson T, Okrainec A, et al. A46 METABOLIC OUTCOMES 12-MONTHS POST-BARIATRIC SURGERY: SLEEVE VERSUS ROUX-EN-Y GASTRIC BYPASS. J Can Assoc Gastroenterol. 2024;7(Supplement_1):28–9.
25. Feris F, McRae A, Kellogg TA, McKenzie T, Ghanem O, Acosta A. Mucosal and hormonal adaptations following Roux-en-Y gastric bypass. Surg Obes Relat Dis. 2022;19(1):37–49.
26. Peterli R, Steinert RE, Woelnerhanssen B, Peters T, Christoffel-Courtin C, Gass M, et al. Metabolic and hormonal changes after laparoscopic Roux-en-Y gastric bypass and sleeve gastrectomy: a randomized, prospective trial. Obes Surg. 2012;22(5):740–8.
27. Peterli R, Wölnerhanssen BK, Peters T, Vetter D, Kröll D, Borbély Y, et al. Effect of laparoscopic sleeve Gastrectomy vs laparoscopic Roux-en-Y gastric bypass on weight loss in patients with morbid obesity: the SM-BOSS randomized clinical trial. JAMA. 2018;319(3):255–65.
28. English PJ, Ghatei MA, Malik IA, Bloom SR, Wilding JP. Food fails to suppress ghrelin levels in obese humans. J Clin Endocrinol Metab. 2002;87(6):2984.
29. Erdmann J, Lippl F, Wagenpfeil S, Schusdziarra V. Differential Association of Basal and Postprandial Plasma Ghrelin with Leptin, insulin, and type 2 diabetes. Diabetes. 2005;54(5):1371–8.
30. Kelesidis T, Kelesidis I, Chou S, Mantzoros CS. Narrative review: the role of leptin in human physiology: emerging clinical applications. Ann Intern Med. 2010;152(2):93–100.
31. Obradovic M, Sudar-Milovanovic E, Soskic S, Essack M, Arya S, Stewart AJ, et al. Leptin and obesity: role and clinical implication. Front Endocrinol. 2021;12:585887.
32. ten Kulve JS, Veltman DJ, Gerdes VEA, van Bloemendaal L, Barkhof F, Deacon CF, et al. Elevated postoperative endogenous GLP-1 levels mediate effects of Roux-en-Y gastric bypass on neural Responsivity to food cues. Diabetes Care. 2017;40(11):1522–9.
33. Acosta A, Camilleri M, Burton D, O'Neill J, Eckert D, Carlson P, et al. Exenatide in obesity with accelerated gastric emptying: a randomized, pharmacodynamics study. Physiol Rep. 2015;3(11):e12610.
34. Jensterle M, Ferjan S, Ležaič L, Sočan A, Goričar K, Zaletel K, et al. Semaglutide delays 4-hour gastric emptying in women with polycystic ovary syndrome and obesity. Diabetes Obes Metab. 2023;25(4):975–84.
35. Karra E, Chandarana K, Batterham RL. The role of peptide YY in appetite regulation and obesity. J Physiol. 2009;587(1):19–25.
36. le Roux CW, Welbourn R, Werling M, Osborne A, Kokkinos A, Laurenius A, et al. Gut hormones as mediators of appetite and weight loss after Roux-en-Y gastric bypass. Ann Surg. 2007;246(5):780–5.
37. Laferrère B, Swerdlow N, Bawa B, Arias S, Bose M, Oliván B, et al. Rise of Oxyntomodulin in response to Oral glucose after gastric bypass surgery in patients with type 2 diabetes. J Clin Endocrinol Metabol. 2010;95(8):4072–6.
38. Grider JR. Role of cholecystokinin in the regulation of gastrointestinal motility. J Nutr. 1994;124(8 Suppl):1334s–9s.
39. Ballinger A, McLoughlin L, Medbak S, Clark M. Cholecystokinin is a satiety hormone in humans at physiological post-prandial plasma concentrations. Clin Sci (Lond). 1995;89(4):375–81.

40. Wickremasinghe AC, Johari Y, Laurie C, Shaw K, Playfair J, Beech P, et al. Delayed gastric emptying after sleeve Gastrectomy is associated with poor weight loss. Obes Surg. 2022;32(12):3922–31.
41. Parks DJ, Blanchard SG, Bledsoe RK, Chandra G, Consler TG, Kliewer SA, et al. Bile acids: natural ligands for an orphan nuclear receptor. Science. 1999;284(5418):1365–8.
42. Keitel V, Görg B, Bidmon HJ, Zemtsova I, Spomer L, Zilles K, et al. The bile acid receptor TGR5 (Gpbar-1) acts as a neurosteroid receptor in brain. Glia. 2010;58(15):1794–805.
43. Risstad H, Kristinsson JA, Fagerland MW, le Roux CW, Birkeland KI, Gulseth HL, et al. Bile acid profiles over 5 years after gastric bypass and duodenal switch: results from a randomized clinical trial. Surg Obes Relat Dis. 2017;13(9):1544–53.
44. Jung RT. Obesity as a disease. Br Med Bull. 1997;53(2):307–21.
45. Pi-Sunyer FX. Health implications of obesity. Am J Clin Nutr. 1991;53(6 Suppl):1595s–603s.
46. Vincent HK, Taylor AG. Biomarkers and potential mechanisms of obesity-induced oxidant stress in humans. Int J Obes. 2006;30(3):400–18.
47. Olusi SO. Obesity is an independent risk factor for plasma lipid peroxidation and depletion of erythrocyte cytoprotectic enzymes in humans. Int J Obes Relat Metab Disord. 2002;26(9):1159–64.
48. Ozata M, Mergen M, Oktenli C, Aydin A, Sanisoglu SY, Bolu E, et al. Increased oxidative stress and hypozincemia in male obesity. Clin Biochem. 2002;35(8):627–31.
49. Liu XZ, Pedersen L, Halberg N. Cellular mechanisms linking cancers to obesity. Cell Stress. 2021;5(5):55–72.
50. Dvorak HF. Tumors: wounds that do not heal-redux. Cancer Immunol Res. 2015;3(1):1–11.
51. Balkwill F, Mantovani A. Inflammation and cancer: back to Virchow? Lancet. 2001;357(9255):539–45.
52. Dvorak HF. Tumors: wounds that do not heal. Similarities between tumor stroma generation and wound healing. N Engl J Med. 1986;315(26):1650–9.
53. Karra P, Winn M, Pauleck S, Bulsiewicz-Jacobsen A, Peterson L, Coletta A, et al. Metabolic dysfunction and obesity-related cancer: beyond obesity and metabolic syndrome. Obesity (Silver Spring). 2022;30(7):1323–34.
54. Wilson RB, Lathigara D, Kaushal D. Systematic review and meta-analysis of the impact of bariatric surgery on future cancer risk. Int J Mol Sci. 2023;24(7):6192.
55. Busebee B, Ghusn W, Cifuentes L, Acosta A. Obesity: a review of pathophysiology and classification. Mayo Clin Proc. 2023;98(12):1842–57.
56. Lin X, Li H. Obesity: epidemiology, pathophysiology, and therapeutics. Front Endocrinol. 2021;12:706978.
57. Cifuentes L, Hurtado AM, Eckel-Passow J, Acosta A. Precision medicine for obesity. Dig Dis Interv. 2021;5(3):239–48.
58. Collins FS, Varmus H. A new initiative on precision medicine. N Engl J Med. 2015;372(9):793–5.
59. Bhaskaran K, Dos-Santos-Silva I, Leon DA, Douglas IJ, Smeeth L. Association of BMI with overall and cause-specific mortality: a population-based cohort study of 3·6 million adults in the UK. Lancet Diabetes Endocrinol. 2018;6(12):944–53.
60. Blundell JE, Gillett A. Control of food intake in the obese. Obes Res. 2001;9(S11):263S–70S.
61. Acosta A, Camilleri M, Abu Dayyeh B, Calderon G, Gonzalez D, McRae A, et al. Selection of Antiobesity medications based on phenotypes enhances weight loss: a pragmatic trial in an obesity clinic. Obesity. 2021;29(4):662–71.
62. Acosta A, Camilleri M, Shin A, Vazquez-Roque MI, Iturrino J, Burton D, et al. Quantitative gastrointestinal and psychological traits associated with obesity and response to weight-loss therapy. Gastroenterology. 2015;148(3):537–46.e4.
63. Cifuentes L, Ghusn W, Feris F, Campos A, Sacoto D, De la Rosa A, et al. Phenotype tailored lifestyle intervention on weight loss and cardiometabolic risk factors in adults with obesity: a single-centre, non-randomised, proof-of-concept study. EClinicalMedicine. 2023;58:101923.

64. Vazquez Roque MI, Camilleri M, Stephens DA, Jensen MD, Burton DD, Baxter KL, et al. Gastric sensorimotor functions and hormone profile in normal weight, overweight, and obese people. Gastroenterology. 2006;131(6):1717–24.
65. Woldemariam S, Dorner TE, Wiesinger T, Stein KV. Multi-omics approaches for precision obesity management : potentials and limitations of omics in precision prevention, treatment and risk reduction of obesity. Wien Klin Wochenschr. 2023;135(5–6):113–24.
66. Dent R, McPherson R, Harper ME. Factors affecting weight loss variability in obesity. Metabolism. 2020;113:154388.
67. Johnston BC, Kanters S, Bandayrel K, Wu P, Naji F, Siemieniuk RA, et al. Comparison of weight loss among named diet programs in overweight and obese adults: a meta-analysis. JAMA. 2014;312(9):923–33.
68. Bray GA, Krauss RM, Sacks FM, Qi L. Lessons learned from the POUNDS lost study: genetic, metabolic, and behavioral factors affecting changes in body weight, body composition, and cardiometabolic risk. Curr Obes Rep. 2019;8(3):262–83.
69. Arkadianos I, Valdes AM, Marinos E, Florou A, Gill RD, Grimaldi KA. Improved weight management using genetic information to personalize a calorie controlled diet. Nutr J. 2007;6:29.
70. Barrea L, Annunziata G, Bordoni L, Muscogiuri G, Colao A, Savastano S, et al. Nutrigenetics—personalized nutrition in obesity and cardiovascular diseases. Int J Obes Suppl. 2020;10(1):1–13.
71. Aldubayan MA, Pigsborg K, Gormsen SMO, Serra F, Palou M, Galmés S, et al. A double-blinded, randomized, parallel intervention to evaluate biomarker-based nutrition plans for weight loss: the PREVENTOMICS study. Clin Nutr. 2022;41(8):1834–44.
72. Kilpeläinen TO, Qi L, Brage S, Sharp SJ, Sonestedt E, Demerath E, et al. Physical activity attenuates the influence of FTO variants on obesity risk: a meta-analysis of 218,166 adults and 19,268 children. PLoS Med. 2011;8(11):e1001116.
73. Tyrrell J, Wood AR, Ames RM, Yaghootkar H, Beaumont RN, Jones SE, et al. Gene-obesogenic environment interactions in the UK biobank study. Int J Epidemiol. 2017;46(2):559–75.
74. Volpe S, Lisco G, Fanelli M, Racaniello D, Colaianni V, Triggiani D, et al. Once-weekly subcutaneous semaglutide improves fatty liver disease in patients with type 2 diabetes: a 52-week prospective real-life study. Nutrients. 2022;14(21):4673.
75. Lincoff AM, Brown-Frandsen K, Colhoun HM, Deanfield J, Emerson SS, Esbjerg S, et al. Semaglutide and cardiovascular outcomes in obesity without diabetes. N Engl J Med. 2023;389(24):2221–32.
76. Wilding JPH, Batterham RL, Calanna S, Davies M, Van Gaal LF, Lingvay I, et al. Once-weekly semaglutide in adults with overweight or obesity. N Engl J Med. 2021;384(11):989–1002.
77. Friedrichsen M, Breitschaft A, Tadayon S, Wizert A, Skovgaard D. The effect of semaglutide 2.4 mg once weekly on energy intake, appetite, control of eating, and gastric emptying in adults with obesity. Diabetes Obes Metab. 2021;23(3):754–62.
78. Heise T, DeVries JH, Urva S, Li J, Pratt EJ, Thomas MK, et al. Tirzepatide reduces appetite, energy intake, and fat mass in people with type 2 diabetes. Diabetes Care. 2023;46(5):998–1004.
79. Samms RJ, Coghlan MP, Sloop KW. How may GIP enhance the therapeutic efficacy of GLP-1? Trends Endocrinol Metab. 2020;31(6):410–21.
80. Gonzalez-Izundegui D, Campos A, Calderon G, Ricardo-Silgado ML, Cifuentes L, Decker PA, et al. Association of gastric emptying with postprandial appetite and satiety sensations in obesity. Obesity (Silver Spring). 2021;29(9):1497–507.
81. Halawi H, Khemani D, Eckert D, O'Neill J, Kadouh H, Grothe K, et al. Effects of liraglutide on weight, satiation, and gastric functions in obesity: a randomised, placebo-controlled pilot trial. Lancet Gastroenterol Hepatol. 2017;2(12):890–9.
82. Maselli D, Atieh J, Clark MM, Eckert D, Taylor A, Carlson P, et al. Effects of liraglutide on gastrointestinal functions and weight in obesity: a randomized clinical and pharmacogenomic trial. Obesity. 2022;30(8):1608–20.

83. Cooper JA, Watras AC, O'Brien MJ, Luke A, Dobratz JR, Earthman CP, et al. Assessing validity and reliability of resting metabolic rate in six gas analysis systems. J Am Diet Assoc. 2009;109(1):128–32.
84. Christoffersen BØ, Sanchez-Delgado G, John LM, Ryan DH, Raun K, Ravussin E. Beyond appetite regulation: targeting energy expenditure, fat oxidation, and lean mass preservation for sustainable weight loss. Obesity. 2022;30(4):841–57.
85. Coskun T, Sloop KW, Loghin C, Alsina-Fernandez J, Urva S, Bokvist KB, et al. LY3298176, a novel dual GIP and GLP-1 receptor agonist for the treatment of type 2 diabetes mellitus: from discovery to clinical proof of concept. Mol Metab. 2018;18:3–14.
86. Karlsson J, Persson LO, Sjöström L, Sullivan M. Psychometric properties and factor structure of the Three-Factor Eating Questionnaire (TFEQ) in obese men and women. Results from the Swedish Obese Subjects (SOS) study. Int J Obes Relat Metab Disord. 2000;24(12):1715–25.
87. Dalton M, Finlayson G, Walsh B, Halseth AE, Duarte C, Blundell JE. Early improvement in food cravings are associated with long-term weight loss success in a large clinical sample. Int J Obes. 2017;41(8):1232–6.
88. Wharton S, Batterham RL, Bhatta M, Buscemi S, Christensen LN, Frias JP, et al. Two-year effect of semaglutide 2.4 mg on control of eating in adults with overweight/obesity: STEP 5. Obesity. 2023;31(3):703–15.
89. Saunders KH, Igel LI, Saumoy M, Sharaiha RZ, Aronne LJ. Devices and endoscopic bariatric therapies for obesity. Curr Obes Rep. 2018;7(2):162–71.
90. Lopez-Nava G, Jaruvongvanich V, Storm AC, Maselli DB, Bautista-Castaño I, Vargas EJ, et al. Personalization of endoscopic bariatric and metabolic therapies based on physiology: a prospective feasibility study with a single fluid-filled intragastric balloon. Obes Surg. 2020;30(9):3347–53.
91. Mion F, Napoleon B, Roman S, Malvoisin E, Trepo F, Pujol B, et al. Effects of intragastric balloon on gastric emptying and plasma ghrelin levels in non-morbid obese patients. Obes Surg. 2005;15(4):510–6.
92. Layec S, Val-laillet D, Heresbach D, Malbert C. Gastric tone, volume and emptying after implantation of an intragastric balloon for weight control. Neurogastroenterol Motil. 2010;22(9):1016–e266.
93. Gomez V. Baseline gastric emptying and its change in response to diverse endoscopic bariatric therapies predict weight change after intervention. Obesity. 2016;24(9):1849–53.
94. Su HJ, Kao CH, Chen WC, Chang TT, Lin CY. Effect of intragastric balloon on gastric emptying time in humans for weight control. Clin Nucl Med. 2013;38(11):863–8.
95. Gómez V, Woodman G, Abu Dayyeh BK. Delayed gastric emptying as a proposed mechanism of action during intragastric balloon therapy: results of a prospective study. Obesity (Silver Spring). 2016;24(9):1849–53.
96. Kumar N, Abu Dayyeh BK, Lopez-Nava Breviere G, Galvao Neto MP, Sahdala NP, Shaikh SN, et al. Endoscopic sutured gastroplasty: procedure evolution from first-in-man cases through current technique. Surg Endosc. 2018;32(4):2159–64.
97. Vargas EJ, Rizk M, Gomez-Villa J, Edwards PK, Jaruvongvanich V, Storm AC, et al. Effect of endoscopic sleeve gastroplasty on gastric emptying, motility and hormones: a comparative prospective study. Gut. 2022;72(6):1073–80.
98. Lopez-Nava G, Bautista-Castaño I, Turro R, Vargas EJ, Bazerbachi F, Matar R, et al. 180 Prospective comparison of fluid-filled intragastric balloon and endoscopic gastroplasty on physiologic measures of appetite: insights into mechanism of action and personalization of procedure choice. Gastrointest Endosc. 2019;89(6):AB61.
99. Zhu Y, Hollis JH. Increasing the number of chews before swallowing reduces meal size in normal-weight, overweight, and obese adults. J Acad Nutr Diet. 2014;114(6):926–31.
100. Hollis JH. The effect of mastication on food intake, satiety and body weight. Physiol Behav. 2018;193(Pt B):242–5. https://doi.org/10.1016/j.physbeh.2018.04.027.
101. Ruban A, Ashrafian H, Teare JP. The EndoBarrier: Duodenal-Jejunal bypass liner for diabetes and weight loss. Gastroenterol Res Pract. 2018;2018:7823182.

102. Zervos EE, Agle SC, Warren AJ, Lang CG, Fitzgerald TL, Dar M, et al. Amelioration of insulin requirement in patients undergoing duodenal bypass for reasons other than obesity implicates foregut factors in the pathophysiology of type II diabetes. J Am Coll Surg. 2010;210(5):564–72.
103. Rubino F, Forgione A, Cummings DE, Vix M, Gnuli D, Mingrone G, et al. The mechanism of diabetes control after gastrointestinal bypass surgery reveals a role of the proximal small intestine in the pathophysiology of type 2 diabetes. Ann Surg. 2006;244(5):741.
104. Mehta A, Sharaiha RZ. Bariatric and metabolic endoscopy: impact on obesity and related comorbidities. Ther Adv Gastrointest Endosc. 2021;14:26317745211019156.
105. Katsareli EA, Amerikanou C, Rouskas K, Dimopoulos A, Diamantis T, Alexandrou A, et al. A genetic risk score for the estimation of weight loss after bariatric surgery. Obes Surg. 2020;30(4):1482–90.
106. Pereira SS, Guimarães M, Monteiro MP. Towards precision medicine in bariatric surgery prescription. Rev Endocr Metab Disord. 2023;24(5):961–77.
107. Bandstein M, Voisin S, Nilsson EK, Schultes B, Ernst B, Thurnheer M, et al. A genetic risk score is associated with weight loss following Roux-en Y gastric bypass surgery. Obes Surg. 2016;26(9):2183–9.
108. Anazco D, Ghusn W, Campos A, Cifuentes L, Fansa S, Tama E, et al. Type 2 diabetes remission in patients with heterozygous variants in the leptin-melanocortin pathway after Roux-en-Y gastric bypass: a matched case-control study. Obes Surg. 2023;33(11):3502–9.
109. Campos A, Cifuentes L, Hashem A, Busebee B, Hurtado-Andrade MD, Ricardo-Silgado ML, et al. Effects of heterozygous variants in the leptin-melanocortin pathway on Roux-en-Y gastric bypass outcomes: a 15-year case-control study. Obes Surg. 2022;32(8):2632–40.
110. Feris F, Ghusn W, Campos A, Cifuentes L, De la Rosa A, Sacoto D, et al. The effect of heterozygous gene variants of the leptin-melanocortin pathway on weight loss following sleeve gastrectomy. Obes Surg. 2023;33(7):2246–9.
111. Hagedorn JC, Morton JM. Nature versus nurture: identical twins and bariatric surgery. Obes Surg. 2007;17(6):728–31.
112. Heid IM, Jackson AU, Randall JC, Winkler TW, Qi L, Steinthorsdottir V, et al. Meta-analysis identifies 13 new loci associated with waist-hip ratio and reveals sexual dimorphism in the genetic basis of fat distribution. Nat Genet. 2010;42(11):949–60.
113. Locke AE, Kahali B, Berndt SI, Justice AE, Pers TH, Day FR, et al. Genetic studies of body mass index yield new insights for obesity biology. Nature. 2015;518(7538):197–206.
114. Speliotes EK, Willer CJ, Berndt SI, Monda KL, Thorleifsson G, Jackson AU, et al. Association analyses of 249,796 individuals reveal 18 new loci associated with body mass index. Nat Genet. 2010;42(11):937–48.
115. Gala K, Ghusn W, Fansa S, Abu Dayyeh BK, Ghanem OM, Kellogg T, et al. Effects of heterozygous variants in the leptin-melanocortin pathway on transoral outlet reduction after Roux-en-Y gastric bypass: a case–control study and review of literature. Obes Surg. 2023;33(4):1284–8.
116. Markham A. Setmelanotide: first approval. Drugs. 2021;81(3):397–403.
117. Clément K, Van Den Akker E, Argente J, Bahm A, Chung WK, Connors H, et al. Efficacy and safety of setmelanotide, an MC4R agonist, in individuals with severe obesity due to LEPR or POMC deficiency: single-arm, open-label, multicentre, phase 3 trials. Lancet Diabetes Endocrinol. 2020;8(12):960–70.
118. Wu C-t, Morris JR. Genes, genetics, and epigenetics: a correspondence. Science. 2001;293(5532):1103–5.
119. Morcillo S, Macías-González M, Tinahones FJ. The effect of metabolic and bariatric surgery on DNA methylation patterns. Curr Atheroscler Rep. 2017;19(10):40.
120. Clish CB. Metabolomics: an emerging but powerful tool for precision medicine. Cold Spring Harb Mol Case Stud. 2015;1(1):a000588.
121. Tulipani S, Griffin J, Palau-Rodriguez M, Mora-Cubillos X, Bernal-Lopez RM, Tinahones FJ, et al. Metabolomics-guided insights on bariatric surgery versus behavioral interventions for weight loss. Obesity. 2016;24(12):2451–66.

122. Khoo CM, Muehlbauer MJ, Stevens RD, Pamuklar Z, Chen J, Newgard CB, et al. Postprandial metabolite profiles reveal differential nutrient handling after bariatric surgery compared with matched caloric restriction. Ann Surg. 2014;259(4):687–93.
123. Ha J, Kwon Y, Park S. Metabolomics in bariatric surgery: towards identification of mechanisms and biomarkers of metabolic outcomes. Obes Surg. 2021;31(10):4564–74.
124. Ursell LK, Metcalf JL, Parfrey LW, Knight R. Defining the human microbiome. Nutr Rev. 2012;70:S38–44.
125. Ulker İ, Yildiran H. The effects of bariatric surgery on gut microbiota in patients with obesity: a review of the literature. Biosci Microbiota Food Health. 2019;38(1):3–9.
126. Palleja A, Kashani A, Allin KH, Nielsen T, Zhang C, Li Y, et al. Roux-en-Y gastric bypass surgery of morbidly obese patients induces swift and persistent changes of the individual gut microbiota. Genome Med. 2016;8(1):67.
127. Gao X, Dai S, Wang G, Li W, Song Z, Su Z, et al. Large versus small gastric pouch for Roux-en-Y gastric bypass in individuals with type 2 diabetes and a body mass index $< 35$ kg/m$^2$: six-year outcomes. Front Endocrinol. 2022;13:913062.
128. Athanasiadis DI, Martin A, Kapsampelis P, Monfared S, Stefanidis D. Factors associated with weight regain post-bariatric surgery: a systematic review. Surg Endosc. 2021;35(8):4069–84.
129. Madan AK, Tichansky DS, Phillips JC. Does pouch size matter? Obes Surg. 2007;17(3):317–20.

# The Genetic and Microbial Influences in Obesity and Obesity Management

16

Sarah Suh and Tammy Kindel

## Genetic Influences in Obesity and Obesity Management

The diseases of overweight and obesity are attributed to a complex interaction between lifestyle and environmental factors that interface with an individual's biological and genetic makeup and predisposition for body weight dysregulation. Genetics is a nonmodifiable risk factor in obesity, and this has been demonstrated by twin and adoption studies of adiposity. One of the first studies to explore this in 1997 found that variation in body mass index (BMI) was largely due to heritable genetic differences [1]. Data from more than 25,000 twin pairs and 50,000 biological and adoptive family members in the 1980s and 1990s demonstrated that the weighted mean correlations between genetics and variation in BMI were 0.74 for monozygotic twins, 0.32 for dizygotic twins, 0.25 for siblings, 0.19 for parent-offspring pairs, 0.06 for adoptive relatives, and 0.12 for spouses. Studies published since then have demonstrated that the heritability of obesity is estimated to be 40–80%, with only slightly lower values in twins raised apart compared with those raised together [1–4]. Twin studies have also demonstrated that living in the same home in childhood appears to contribute to very little parallels in BMI; rather, environmental factors that are unique to each person such as individualistic diet and exercise behavior in adolescence appear to play a more dominant role in influencing BMI [3]. Genome-wide association studies (GWAS) have demonstrated at least 500 obesity-associated genetic loci. The genetic influences of obesity include genetic mutations, polymorphisms, and changes in gene expression. This section will focus on the different types of genetic obesity as well as the influence of genetics on weight-loss response.

S. Suh · T. Kindel (✉)
Medical College of Wisconsin, Milwaukee, WI, USA
e-mail: ssuh@mcw.edu; tkindel@mcw.edu



O. M. Ghanem et al. (eds.), *The SAGES Manual of Metabolic and Bariatric Surgery*, https://doi.org/10.1007/978-3-031-72309-4_16

There are three different types of genetic obesity: monogenic, syndromic, and polygenic. **Monogenic obesity** is rare and accounts for less than 5% of obesity [5–7]. It is caused by a mutation in a single gene and is typically associated with hyperphagia and early-onset obesity at the age of three to 5 years. There are several genes that are linked to monogenic obesity as depicted in Table 16.1. The fat mass- and obesity-associated (FTO) gene on chromosome 16 was the first gene identified in GWAS to be linked with obesity. Individuals with single nucleotide polymorphism (SNP) variants in the first intron of FTO have been found to have up to 1.7 times increased risk of obesity in adulthood [8]. The proposed mechanism of this finding is that FTO SNPs increase caloric intake and/or increase energy storage instead of energy utilization. Another hypothesis is that variants in FTO suppress mitochondrial thermogenesis in adipocyte precursor cells which results in a shift from energy-utilizing brown adipose cells to energy-storing white adipose cells [9].

**Table 16.1** Genes associated with monogenic obesity

| Gene | Expressed Protein | Protein Function |
|---|---|---|
| LEP | Leptin | Secreted by white adipocytes and plays a major role in the regulation of energy homeostasis and body weight. |
| LEPR | Leptin receptor | Receptor for leptin hormone. |
| FTO | Fat mass and obesity-associated gene | Unknown exact physiological function however variations in this protein are strongly associated with body mass index, obesity risk, and type two diabetes. |
| PcSK1 | Proprotein convertase subtilisin/kexin enzyme 1 | Protease regulates the secretory pathway in the endoplasmic reticulum of the neuroendocrine system and brain. Mutations are associated with obesity. |
| MC4R | Melanocortin-4 receptor | Membrane-bound receptor that interacts with adrenocorticotrophic hormones. Defects in this gene are a cause of autosomal dominant obesity. |
| POMC | Pro-opiomelanocortin neuropeptide | Encodes a pre-protein that undergoes tissue-specific post-transcriptional processing. Plays an important role in energy metabolism and homeostasis in the anterior pituitary, hypothalamus, and placenta. |
| ASIP | Agouti signaling protein | Regulates lipid metabolism in adipocytes. |
| NTRK2/ TRKB | Neurotrophic tyrosine receptor kinase 2 | Receptor for brain-derived natriuretic factor. Deletions in this gene are strongly associated with morbid obesity. |
| KSR2 | Kinase suppressor of Ras 2 protein | Predicted to enable protein kinase activity within the cytosol and plasma membrane. Positively regulates cold-induced thermogenesis. |
| NPY | Neuropeptide Y | Neuropeptide is widely expressed in the central nervous system and influences stress response, food intake, circadian rhythms, and cardiovascular function. |
| SH2B1 | SH2B adaptor protein 1 | Mediates the activation of various kinases and may function in cytokine and growth factor signaling as well as cellular transformation. |
| ADCY3 | Adenylyl cyclase 3 | Membrane-associated enzyme that catalyzes the formation of the secondary messenger cyclic adenosine monophosphate (cAMP). Widely expressed in the alimentary tract tissue to modulate metabolic balance. |

The leptin-melanocortin pathway in the hypothalamus has also been recognized to play an important role in genetic obesity. Leptin is an appetite-regulating peptide hormone that is produced by adipose cells and therefore proportionally reflects overall adipose storage in the body. Individuals with obesity have an excess of leptin, which leads to leptin resistance with an inadequate satiety response to increased adipose stores. Mutations in the leptin gene, LEP, are rare, autosomal recessive causes of severe, early-onset obesity, hyperphagia, and glucose intolerance. These mutations are known to be loss-of-function mutations causing decreased leptin synthesis, secretion, or failure to bind to the leptin receptor (LEPR) [10–12].

Melanocortin-4 receptor (MC4R) is another widely studied gene and its loss-of-function mutations are associated with early-onset obesity [13]. GWAS has demonstrated that several variants near the MC4R gene are associated with increased BMI in both children and adults [13, 14]. When looking at the influence of genetics on post-operative outcomes, SNPs at the MC4R gene site were also associated with less weight loss at one- and three-year follow-up after a Roux-en-Y gastric bypass procedure [15, 16]. A recent systemic review that evaluated the extent to which genetic variants contribute to weight loss and metabolic outcomes found that SNPs at the adiponectin gene, ADIPOQ, were associated with positive post-operative outcomes in measures of glucose homeostasis and lipid profiles but not with weight loss after surgery [17, 18]. Uncoupled Protein Genes (UCP2) SNPs on the other hand were associated with post-operative weight loss. A limitation of some studies reported in systemic reviews is that they take a candidate gene rather than a genome-wide approach. Ongoing GWAS studies are increasing the speed at which novel genetic associations are being identified.

**Syndromic obesity** is represented by a large variety of phenotypes including developmental delay, intellectual disability, dysmorphic features, and organ system abnormalities which include obesity. Examples include Prader-Willi and Bardet-Biedel syndrome. Prader-Willi syndrome is a neurodegenerative condition that is caused by a deletion in chromosome 15 [19]. The small nuclear ribonucleoprotein (SNRPN) gene is the key genetic component that is missing. The clinical features of Prader-Willi syndrome include behavior problems, delayed development, short stature, hypogonadotropic hypogonadism, and voracious appetite which leads to obesity later in life.

Bardet-Biedel syndrome is an autosomal recessive disorder associated with mutations in greater than 15 different genes. Bardet-Biedel is characterized by obesity and micro-orchidism in men, intellectual disability, retinal dystrophy, polydactyly, renal malformations, polyuria, and polydipsia [20]. Setmelanotide is a melanocortin receptor agonist that is used as a pharmacological treatment for patients at least 6 years of age with Bardet-Biedl syndrome as well as those with mutations in pro-opiomelanocortin (POMC), a deficiency in prohormone convertase, specifically PCSK1, or a deficiency in the leptin receptor to help lose the weight and keep it off [21]. Additional syndromes characterized by obesity and several other abnormalities are summarized in Table 16.2.

**Polygenic obesity** results from the presence of multiple gene variants and polymorphisms that have an additive effect and favor body adiposity. Polygenic obesity is the most common form of obesity, and environmental exposures become a key

**Table 16.2** Clinical features of syndromic obesity

| Syndrome | Gene | Clinical features |
|---|---|---|
| Albright hereditary osteodystrophy (pseudohypoparathyroidism type 1a) | GNAS1 | Short stature, short metacarpals and metatarsals, round facies, delayed dentition, hypocalcemia and/or subcutaneous calcium or bone deposition (osteoma cutis), precocious puberty, mild cognitive deficit. |
| Bardet-Biedl | BBS1–15 | Intellectual disability, hypotonia, retinitis pigmentosa, polydactyly, hypogonadism +/− glucose intolerance, deafness, renal disease. |
| Beckwith-Wiedemann | IGF2 | Hyperinsulinemia, hypoglycemia, hemihypertrophy, intolerance of fasting. |
| Carpenter | RAB23 | Intellectual disability, short stature, brachycephaly, polydactyly, syndactyly of feet, cryptorchidism, umbilical hernia, high-arched palate, hypogonadism in males only. |
| Cohen | COH1 | Intellectual disability, microcephaly, small hands and feet, cryptorchidism, hypotonia and failure to thrive in infancy, prominent central incisors, long and thin fingers/toes. |
| Prader-Willi | NDN, SNRPN | Early growth delay followed by hyperphagia and increased weight gain by 2 to 3 years. Mild to moderate cognitive deficit, microcephaly, short stature, hypotonia, almond-shaped eyes, high-arched palate, narrow hands/feet, delayed puberty (but premature adrenarche). |

**Table 16.3** Features of monogenic and polygenic obesity

| Monogenic obesity | Polygenic obesity |
|---|---|
| Early-onset, severe obesity | Common obesity |
| High genetic contribution | Modest genetic contribution |
| Single mutation in one gene | Hundreds of variants in or near many different genes |
| Rare | Common |
| High penetrance | Low penetrance |
| No environmental influence | The environment has a significant influence |

determinant in the expression of the hundreds of gene variants that could contribute to obesity. Environmental exposures include lifestyle factors such as diet, alcohol, education, exercise, sleep, smoking, and shift work. Studies have demonstrated that consistent physical activity, adequate sleep, and consumption of a healthy diet diminish the risk of obesity in those with FTO SNPs who have a high risk of obesity at baseline [22]. Table 16.3 depicts the key differences in how monogenic versus polygenic obesity is characterized [6, 7].

## Microbial Influences in Obesity and Obesity Management

The gut microbiome is composed of at least 100 trillion microbes that represent approximately 5000 different species [23]. The main species of bacteria include *Prevotella, Ruminococcus, Bacteroidetes,* and *Firmicutes*. In patients with overweight and obesity, the gut microbiome is characterized by reduced diversity and dysfunctional host-gut microbial interactions. The composition of the gut microbiome affects obesity pathogenesis via changes in energy harvest/expenditure, maintenance of gut barrier integrity, and bile acid metabolism.

One of the earliest studies investigating the relationship between the gut microbiome and obesity demonstrated that obesity is linked to changes in the relative abundance of the two dominant phyla of gut microbiota, *Firmicutes* and *Bacteroidetes*, where there was an abundance of *Firmicutes* in the setting of a relative decrease in *Bacteroidetes*. These findings however are not consistent across studies [23–26]. This lack of consistency is due to the complex relationship between diet, microbiota, and obesity development which makes it difficult to design study experiments that isolate the specific role of any one variable and its relationship to the development of obesity or designation as a reflection of the obesity phenotype. With the development of germ-free, "gnotobiotic" mice, however, studies have demonstrated that germ-free mice weigh less than mice with a normal gut microbiome [23]. When germ-free mice received the gut microbiota of obese mice via fecal matter transplantation, they had a significantly greater increase in total body fat compared to those mice that received the gut microbiota of lean mice. These observations have demonstrated a direct relationship between the gut microbiome and adiposity; further, manipulation of the gut microbiota and its downstream metabolic pathways can have a significant effect on host adiposity and metabolism.

Twin studies have demonstrated the influence of genetics, epigenetics, and gut microbial composition [26]. Twins that were dissimilar in BMI revealed a lower proportion of *Bacteroidetes* and a higher proportion of *Actinobacteria* in obese compared with lean twin siblings. Other studies have demonstrated the ability to transfer the lean or obese phenotype via fecal matter transplantation between twins that were discordant for obesity in germ-free mice [27]. Transplanting the lean microbiota to obese mice prevented the development of obesity. This study however was limited by the fact that this effect was specifically found in mice consuming low-fat/high-fiber diets; when the animals consumed high-fat/low-fiber diets, they experienced an increase in BMI and fat mass despite the type of microbiome they received highlighting the important interaction between dietary and gut microbial composition on body mass.

There are several proposed mechanisms to support the link between the gut microbiome and obesity. First, several studies have demonstrated the increase in efficiency of energy harvesting and extraction by the obese gut microbiota compared to the lean gut microbiota. The microbial ceca of obese mice have increased production of short-chain fatty acids (SCFAs), which are utilized for more complex lipogenesis and ultimately adipogenesis throughout the body [28]. Additionally, fecal samples taken from genetically obese mice showed an increase in the relative proportion of *Firmicutes,* which is a major producer of SCFAs. Finally, genetically obese mice were found to have lower fecal energy content compared to their wild-type/lean littermates suggesting the increase in energy harvest/extraction that is capable from the obese gut microbiota. In human studies, there have been significant differences in fecal concentrations of SCFAs between lean, overweight, and obese human subjects. Fecal SCFAs have been reportedly 20% higher in obese individuals than lean individuals [29]. Transplanting fecal microbiota from lean subjects into subjects with obesity however was associated with an increase in butyrate-specific SCFA production, which has been shown to improve glucose metabolism and reduction in adiposity [30]. These diverse aforementioned data highlight the complex interplay between genetics, epigenetics, diet, and gut physiology.

Studies have also demonstrated the ability of the gut microbiome to change carbohydrate and lipid metabolism. When normal mouse microbiota was transplanted into germ-free mice, there was a 60% increase in body fat content and insulin resistance [28]. The germ-free mice were also found to have an increase in triglycerides, and this appeared to be a consequence of increased de novo fatty acid synthesis. The microbiome also appears to have an influence on the ability of bile acids to facilitate the metabolism of dietary fat and the absorption of cholesterol. Bile acids are comprised of cholesterol metabolites and facilitate the absorption of dietary fat and fat-soluble molecules. Up to 10% of the biotransformation of bile acids is facilitated by anaerobic gut microbiota including *Bacteroides, Eubacterium,* and *Clostridium.* Studies have demonstrated that germ-free mice have a larger pool of bile acids, increasing the pool of signaling molecules to activate pathways that improve the glucose and lipid metabolic profile [31].

There is an accumulation of studies that suggest that sleeve gastrectomy is associated with increased diversity and gene richness of the gut microbiota [31–33]. Sleeve gastrectomy appears to shift the structure, diversity, and functional potential of the intestinal microbiome. There appears to be a decreased *Firmicutes/Bacteroidetes* ratio and a shift towards lean microbial phenotypes. Sleeve gastrectomy significantly increases *Proteobacteria, Verrucomicrobia, Bilophilia, Faecalibacterium, Enterococcus,* and *Akkermansia*, which are associated with weight-loss, anti-inflammatory effects, and reduced hedonic eating (Table 16.4) [32–37]. A recent study also revealed pronounced increases in the abundance of *Lactobacillus* spp. in the duodenal epithelium from post-sleeve gastrectomy mice as compared to sham-operated mice [38]. These changes after sleeve gastrectomy may be attributed to changes in anatomy, functional alterations to food transit times, gut pH levels that favor certain bacteria, and corresponding hormone modifications; however, certain studies have found that gut microbial changes occur even when controlling for diet, body weight and caloric intake which may specifically be due to post-surgical gastrointestinal anatomy [39, 40].

In addition to affecting the gut microbiome composition, sleeve gastrectomy is associated with changes to gut microbiome function [41, 42]. The obese gut

**Table 16.4** Interactions between gut microbiota and human health and disease physiology

| Colonic Bacteria | Obese or Lean Phenotype | Associations with Host Health and Disease |
|---|---|---|
| *Firmicutes* | Obese | An increased ratio relative to *Bacteroides* is associated with obesity |
| *Eubacterium*<br>*Ruminococcus* | Obese | Encode primary fermentation enzymes and nutrient transporters, increased levels in obese adults |
| *Alistipes*<br>*Parvimonas*<br>*Fusobacteria* | Obese | Proinflammatory bacteria, increased levels in obese adults |
| *Bacteroides* | Lean | Upregulates gut barrier tight junction protein expression, reduces lipopolysaccharide (LPS) translocation, abundance increases after bariatric surgery |
| *Proteobacteria* | Obese | Decreases mucus production, reported risk factor of gut microbiome dysbiosis, increased in obese adults |
| *Lactobacillus plantarum*<br>*Lactobacillus paracasei* | Lean | Anti-inflammatory bacteria, levels decrease in obese adults |
| *Bifidobacterium* | Lean | Reduces LPS levels and improves intestinal mucosal barrier function, increased in lean adults |
| *Akkermansia muciniphila* | Lean | Modulates gut barrier permeability, levels decrease in adults with obesity and type 2 diabetes mellitus |
| *Faecalibacterium prausnitzii* | Unknown | Blocks NF-κβ activation and inhibits secretions of proinflammatory mediators |
| *Enterococcus* | Unknown | Associated with reduced hunger levels |

Modified from Ref. [37]

microbiome is composed of more lipopolysaccharide (LPS) producing bacteria such as *Prevotella* and *Enterobacter* which cause more metabolic endotoxemia. Patients with obesity therefore experience increased rates of enteric mucus degradation which thins the intestinal barrier and increases gut barrier permeability and pathogen translocation. Post-sleeve gastrectomy microbiota is associated with increased levels of *Bacteroides* and *Bifidobacterium* which are known to reduce LPS levels and improve mucosal barrier function [43]. By maintaining the intestinal barrier, the gut microbiome regulates immune function by preventing excessive translocation of immunostimulatory microbiota and LPS while promoting the uptake of essential nutrients and fluids into the rest of the body. Sleeve gastrectomy has also been shown to re-model the disrupted composition of the gut microbiota and weight gain caused by high-fat diet feeding [44, 45]. Finally, newer evidence is highlighting the role of bacteria in the small intestine, rather than just the large intestine, where sleeve gastrectomy and gastric bypass have resulted in a significant increase in *Lactobacillus* spp., which upregulates hypoxia-inducible factor 2α signaling in the duodenum [38]. The metabolic benefits of this are reported to be reduced weight gain and improved glucose tolerance, particularly in mice that received a high-fat diet.

There is also evidence to suggest a strong link between gut microbiome interactions and bile acid metabolism and regulation [46–48]. Sleeve gastrectomy increases circulating serum bile acid levels, independent of energy restriction in subjects with obesity and in high-fat diet-induced obese mice. Bile acids regulate metabolism by binding to the nuclear receptor, farnesoid-X receptor, also known as FXR. A pivotal study demonstrated that sleeve gastrectomy altered the relative abundances of *Bacteroides* in wild-type mice and there were associated reductions in body weight as well as improved glucose tolerance [49]. These changes however were not observed in FXR knock-out mice, highlighting that bile acids and FXR signaling are closely linked to the presence of specific gut microbiota, and play a crucial role in the beneficial effects of bariatric surgery at the molecular level. Another target of bile acids includes Takeda G-protein-coupled receptor 5 (TGR5), which when knocked out in mice, has demonstrated attenuated metabolic improvements and known favorable shifts in the bile acid pool profiles post-sleeve gastrectomy when compared to wild-type mice [50]. Interestingly however, bacterial species that are known to play an important role in bile acid metabolism did not differ between wild-type and knock-out mice. Finally, Fibroblast Growth Factor 15 (FGF15) is another key regulator of bile acid and FXR activation and has been shown to be upregulated in post-sleeve gastrectomy mice in the terminal ileum. Knock-out models of FGF15 have demonstrated that this receptor is necessary for the metabolic and microbiome responses after sleeve gastrectomy [51].

Roux-en-Y gastric bypass surgery in obese humans and rodents has also induced positive changes in the gut microbiota composition as well as metabolic outcomes [52–55]. Depletion of the gut microbiota for example has been found to reverse the beneficial effects of gastric bypass surgery [56]. Post-gastric bypass mediated gut microbiota transplanted into diet-induced obese rodents appears to reduce adiposity by re-activating energy expenditure from metabolically active brown fat tissue, ultimately leading to improved glucose homeostasis, lipid metabolism, and fatty liver disease. There is also an apparent increase in circulating bile acids after gastric bypass but these findings are not consistent across studies, highlighting the complexity of the nature and impact of gastric bypass anatomy on the intestinal microbiome and its downstream physiologic changes [57–59].

## Conclusion

Obesity is a complex disease that reflects the interactions of inherent genetic variants and environmental factors that influence the gut microbiome.

- Twin studies demonstrate the heritability of obesity.
- There are three different types of genetic obesity: monogenic, polygenic, and syndromic. Monogenic obesity is rare. Polygenic obesity is most common and has multifactorial involvement of genetics and the environment.
- FTO, leptin, and MC4R are recognized to play an important role in genetic obesity.

- Syndromic obesity is represented by a variety of phenotypes including developmental delay, intellectual disability, dysmorphic features, and organ system abnormalities. Prader-Willi and Bardet-Biedel are two syndromes most frequently linked to obesity.
- Obesity-associated gut microbiomes have reduced microbial diversity and dysfunctional host-gut microbiome interactions that impair energy extraction, gut barrier integrity, and bile acid metabolism.
- Bariatric surgery such as sleeve gastrectomy and Roux-en-Y gastric bypass are associated with increased diversity and gene richness of the gut microbiota, promoting weight loss and improvement in metabolic syndrome.

## References


1. Maes HH, Neale MC, Eaves LJ. Genetic and environmental factors in relative body weight and human adiposity. Behav Genet. 1997;27:325–51.
2. Wu Y, Duan H, Tian X, Xu C, Wang W, Jiang W, Pang Z, Zhang D, Tan Q. Genetics of obesity traits: a bivariate genome-wide analysis. Front Genet. 2018;9:179.
3. Macdonald A, Stunkard A. Body-mass indexes of British separated twins. N Engl J Med. 1990;322(21):1530.
4. Stunkard AJ, Harris JR, Pedersen NL, McClearn GE. The body-mass index of twins who have been reared apart. N Engl J Med. 1990;322(21):1483–7.
5. Ranadive SA, Vaisse C. Lessons from extreme human obesity: monogenic disorders. Endocrinol Metab Clin N Am. 2008;37(3):733–8.
6. Massod B, Moorthy M. Causes of obesity: a review. Clin Med. 2023;23(4):284–91.
7. Loos RJF, Yeo GS. The genetics of obesity: from discovery to biology. Nat Rev Genet. 2021;23:120–33.
8. Frayling TM, Timpson NJ, Weedon MN, Zeggini E, Freathy RM, Lindgren CM, Perry JRB, Elliott KS, Lango H, Rayner NW, Shields B, Harries LW, Barrett JC, Ellard S, Groves CJ, Knight B, Patch AM, Ness AR, Ebrahim S, Lawlor DA, Ring SM, Been-Shlomo Y, Jarvelin MR, Sovio U, Bennett AJ, Melzer D, Ferrucci L, Loos RJF, Barroso I, Wareham NJ, Karpe F, Owen KR, Cardon LR, Walker M, Hitman GA, Palmer CAN, Doney ASF, Morris AD, Smith GD, Hattersley AT, McCarthy MI. A common variant in the FTO gene is associated with body mass index and predisposes to childhood and adult obesity. Science. 2007;316:889.
9. Claussnitzer M, Dankel SN, Kim KH, Quon G, Meuleman W, Haugen C, Glunk V, Sousa IS, Beaudry JL, Puviindran V, Abdennur NA, Liu J, Svensson PA, Hsu YH, Drucker DJ, Mellgren G, Gui CC, Hauner H, Kellis M. FTO obesity variant circuitry and adipocyte browning in humans. N Engl J Med. 2015;373:895.
10. Funcke JB, Moepps B, Roos J, Schnurbein J, Verstraete K, Frohlich-Reiterer E, Kohlsdorf K, Nunziata A, Brandt S, Tsirigotaki A, Dansercoer A, Suppan E, Haris B, Debatin KM, Savvides SN, Farooqi IS, Hussain K, Gierschik P, Fischer-Posovszky P, Wabitsch M. Rare antagonistic leptin variants and severe, early-onset obesity. N Engl J Med. 2023;388:2253–61.
11. Funcke JB, von Schnurbein J, Lennerz B, Lahr G, Debain KM, Fischer-Posovszky P, Wabitsch M. Monogenic forms of childhood obesity due to mutations in the leptin gene. Mol Cell Pediatr. 2014;1:3.
12. Rosen CJ. Antagonizing the leptin receptor in obesity. N Engl J Med. 2023;388:2291.
13. van der Meer R, Mohamad SA, Monpellier VM, Liem RSL, Hazebroek EJ, Franks PW, Frayling TM, Janssen IMC, Serlie MJ. Genetic variants associated with weight loss and metabolic outcomes after bariatric surgery: a systematic review. Obes Rev. 2023;24(12):e13626.
14. Farooqi IS, Keogh JM, Yeo GSH, Lank EJ, Cheetham T, O'Rahilly S. Clinical spectrum of obesity and mutations in the melanocortin 4 receptor gene. N Engl J Med. 2003;348(12):1085–95.

15. Lubrano-Berthelier C, Le Stunff C, Bougneres P, Vaisse C. A homozygous null mutation delineates the role of the melanocortin-4 receptor in humans. J Clin Endocrinol Metab. 2004;89:2028.
16. Savastano DM, Tanofsky-Kraff M, Han JC, Ning C, Sorg RA, Roza CA, Wolkoff LE, Anandalingam K, Jefferson-George KS, Figueroa RE, Sanford EL, Brady S, Kozlosky M, Schoeller DA, Yanovski JA. Energy intake and energy expenditure among children with polymorphisms of the melanocortin-3 receptor. Am J Clin Nutr. 2009;90:912.
17. Resende CMM, Durso DF, Borges KBG, Pereira RM, Rodrigues GKD, Rodrigues KF, Silva JLP, Rodrigues EC, Franco GR, Alvarez-Leite JI. The polymorphism rs17782313 near MC4R gene is related with anthropometric changes in women submitted to bariatric surgery over 60 months. Clin Nutr. 2018;37(4):1286–92.
18. Potoczna N, Branson R, Piec KJG, G, Steffen R, Ricklin T, Hoehe MR, Lentes KU, Horber FF. Gene variants and binge eating as predictors of comorbidity and outcome of treatment in severe obesity. J Gastrointest Surg. 2004;8(8):971–82.
19. Butler MG, Hanchett JM, Thompson T. Clinical findings and natural history of Prader-Willi syndrome. In: Butler MG, Lee PDK, Whitman BY, editors. Management of Prader-Willi syndrome. New York: Springer; 2006.
20. Janssen S, Ramaswami G, Davis EE, Hurd T, Airik R, Kasanuki JM, van der Kraak L, Allen SJ, Beales PL, Katsanis N, Otto EA, Hildebrandt F. Mutation analysis in Bardet-Biedl syndrome by DNA pooling and massively parallel resequencing in 105 individuals. Hum Genet. 2011;129:79.
21. Tabuer M. Setmelanotide for controlling weight and hunger in Bardet-Biedel syndrome. Lancet. 2022;10(12):829–30.
22. Tyrrell J, Wood AR, Ames RM, Yaghootkar H, Beaumont RN, Jones SE, Tuke MA, Ruth KS, Freathy RM, Smith GD, Joost S, Guessous I, Murray A, Strachan DP, Kutalik Z, Weedon MN, Frayling TM. Gene-obesogenic environment interactions in the UK Biobank study. Int J Epidemiol. 2017;46:559–75.
23. Turnbaugh PJ, Ley RE, Mahowald MA, Magrini V, Mardis ER, Gordon JI. An obesity-associated gut microbiome with increased capacity for energy harvest. Nature. 2006;444(7122):1027–31.
24. Ley RE, Turnbaugh PJ, Klein S, Gordon JI. Microbial ecology: human gut microbes associated with obesity. Nature. 2006;444(7122):1022–3.
25. Ley RE, Backhed F, Turnbaugh P, Lozupone CA, Knight DRD, Gordon JI. Obesity alters gut microbial ecology. Proc Natl Acad Sci. 2005;102(31):11070–5.
26. Turnbaugh PJ, Hamady M, Yatsunenko T, Cantarel BL, Duncan A, Ley RE, Sogin ML, Jones WJ, Roe BA, Affourtit JP, Egholm M, Henrissat B, Heath AC, Knight R, Gordon JI. A core gut microbiome in obese and lean twins. Nature. 2009;457(7228):480–4.
27. Ridaura VK, Faith JJ, Rey FE, Cheng J, Duncan AE, Kau AL, Griffin NW, Lombard V, Henrissat B, Bain JR, Muehlbauer MJ, Ilkayeva O, Semenkovich CF, Funai K, Hayashi DK, Lyle BJ, Martini MC, Ursell LK, Celemente JC, Treuren WV, Walters WA, Knight R, Newgard CB, Heath AC, Gordon JI. Gut microbiota from twins discordant for obesity modulate metabolism in mice. Science. 2013;341(6150):1241214.
28. Schwiertz A, Taras D, Schafer K, Beijer S, Bos NA, Donus C, Hardt PD. Microbiota and SCFA in lean and overweight healthy subjects. Obesity. 2010;18(1):190–5.
29. Backhed F, Ding H, Wang T, Hooper LV, Koh GY, Nagy A, Semenkovich CF, Gordon JI. The gut microbiota as an environmental factor that regulates fat storage. Proc Natl Acad Sci. 2004;110(44):15718–23.
30. Gao Z, Yin J, Zhang J, Ward RE, Martin RJ, Lefevre M, Cefalu WT, Ye J. Butyrate improves insulin sensitivity and increases energy expenditure in mice. Diabetes. 2009;58(7):1509–17.
31. Swann JR, Want EJ, Geier FM, Spagou K, Wilson ID, Sidaway JE, Nicholson JK, Holmes E. Systemic gut microbial modulation of bile acid metabolism in host tissue compartments. Proc Natl Acad Sci. 2011;108:4523–30.
32. Kellerer T, Brandl B, Buttner J, Lagkouvardos I, Hauner H, Skurk T. Impact of laparoscopic sleeve gastrectomy on gut permeability in morbidly obese subjects. Obes Surg. 2019;29(7):2132–43.

33. Liu R, Hong J, Xu X, Wang W. Gut microbiome and serum metabolome alterations in obesity and after weight-loss intervention. Nat Med. 2017;23(7):859–68.
34. Damms-Machado A, Mitra S, Schollenberger AE, Kramer KM, Meile T, Konigsrainer A, Huson DH, Bischoff SC. Effect of surgical and dietary weight loss therapy for obesity on gut microbiota composition and nutrient absorption. Biomed Res Int. 2015;2015:806248.
35. Sanmiguel CP, Jacob SJ, Gupta A, Ju T, Stains J, Coveleskie K, Lagishetty V, Balioukova A, Chen Y, Dutson E, Mayer EA, Labus JS. Surgically induced changes in gut microbiome and hedonic eating as related to weight loss: preliminary findings in obese women undergoing bariatric surgery. Psychosom Med. 2017;79(8):880–7.
36. Coimbra VOR, Crovesy L, Ribeiro-Alves M, Faller ALK, Mattos F, Rosado EL. Gut microbiota profile in adults undergoing bariatric surgery: a systematic review. Nutrients. 2002;14(23):4979.
37. Brown HN, Barber T, Renshaw D, Farnaud S, Oduro-Donkor D, Turner MC. Associations between the gut microbiome and metabolic, inflammatory, and appetitive effects of sleeve gastrectomy. Obes Rev. 2023;24(9):e13600.
38. Shao Y, Evers SS, Shin JH, Ramakrishnan SK, Bozadijeva-Kramer N, Yao Q, Shah YM, Sandoval DA, Seeley RJ. Vertical sleeve gastrectomy increases duodenal Lactobacillus spp. Richness associated with the activation of intestinal HIF2a signaling and metabolic benefits. Mol Metab. 2022;57:101432.
39. Jahansouz C, Staley C, Bernlohr DA, Sadowsky MJ, Khoruts A, Ikramuddin S. Sleeve gastrectomy drives persistent shifts in the gut microbiome. Surg Obes Relat Dis. 2017;13(6):916–24.
40. Barron M, Atkinson SN, Kirby J, Kindel T. Sleeve gastrectomy prevents hypertension associated with unique shifts in the gut microbiome. Surg Endosc. 2021;35(10):5461–7.
41. Forte N, Fernandez-Rilo AC, Palomba L, di Marzo V, Cristino L. Obesity affects the microbiota-gut-brain axis and the regulation thereof by endocannabinoids and related mediators. Int J Mol Sci. 2020;21(5):1554.
42. Teixeira TFS, Collado MC, Ferreira CLLF, Bressan J, Peluzio M, do CG. Potential mechanisms for the emerging link between obesity and increased intestinal permeability. Nutr Res. 2012;32(9):637–47.
43. Wilbrink J, Bernards N, Mujagic Z, van Avesaat M, Pijls K, Klaassen T, Eljk HV, Nienhuijs S, Stronkhorst A, Wilms E, Troost F, Masclee A. Intestinal barrier function in morbid-obesity: results of a prospective study on the effect of sleeve gastrectomy. Int J Obes. 2020;44:368–76.
44. Shao Y, Shen Q, Hua R, Evers SS, He K, Yao Q. Effects of sleeve gastrectomy on the composition and diurnal oscillation of gut microbiota related to the metabolic improvements. Surg Obes Relat Dis. 2018;14(6):731–9.
45. Munzker J, Haase N, Till A, Sucher R, Haange SB, Nemetshke L, Gnad T, Jager E, Chen J, Riede SJ, Chakaroun R, Massier L, Kovacs P, Ost M, Rolle-Kampczyk U, Jehmlich N, Weiner J, Heiker JT, Kloting N, Seeger G, Morawski M, Keitel V, Pfeifer A, von Bergen M, Heeren J, Krugel U, Fenske WK. Functional changes of the gastric bypass microbiota reactive thermogenic adipose tissue and systemic glucose control via intestinal FXR-TGR5 crosstalk in diet-induced obesity. Microbiome. 2022;10:96.
46. Jahansouz C, Xu H, Hertzel AV, et al. Bile acids increase independently from hypocaloric restriction after bariatric surgery. Ann Surg. 2016;264(6):1022–8.
47. Kindel TL, Krause C, Helm MC, et al. Increased glycine-amidated hyocholic acid correlates to improved early weight loss after sleeve gastrectomy. Surg Endosc. 2018;32(2):805–12.
48. Myoronovych A, Kirby M, Ryan KK, Zhang W, Jha P, Setchell KD, Dexheimer PJ, Aronow B, Seeley RJ, Kohli R. Vertical sleeve gastrectomy reduces hepatic steatosis while increasing serum bile acids in a weight-loss independent manner. Obesity. 2014;22(2):390–400.
49. Ryan KK, Tremaroli V, Clemmensen C, Kovatcheva-Datchary P, Myronovych A, Karns R, Wilson-Perez HE, Sandoval DA, Kohli R, Backhed F, Seeley RJ. FXR is a molecular target for the effects of vertical sleeve gastrectomy. Nature. 2014;590(7499):183–8.
50. McGavigan AK, Garibay D, Henseler ZM, Chen J, Bettaieb A, Haj FG, Ley RE, Chouinard ML, Cummings BP. TGR5 contributes to glucoregulatory improvements after vertical sleeve gastrectomy in mice. Gut. 2017;66(2):226.

51. Bozadjieva-Kramer N, Shin JH, Shao Y, Gutierrez-Aguilar R, Li Z, Heppner KM, Chiang S, Vargo SG, Granger K, Sandoval DA, MacDougald OA, Seeley RJ. Intestinal-derived FGF15 protects against deleterious effects of vertical sleeve gastrectomy in mice. Nat Commun. 2021;12(1):4768.
52. Grassler J, Qin Y, Zhong H, Zhang J, Licinio J, Wong ML, Xu A, Chavakis T, Bornstein AB, Ehrhart-Bornstein M, Lamounier-Zepter V, Lohmann T, Wolf T, Bornstein SR. Metagenomic sequencing of the human gut microbiome before and after bariatric surgery in obese patients with type 2 diabetes: correlation with inflammatory and metabolic parameters. Pharmacogenomics. 2013;13(60):514522.
53. Furet JP, Kong LC, Tap J, Poitou C, Basdevant A, Bouillot JL, Mariat D, Corthier G, Dore J, Henegar C, Rizkalla S, Clement K. Differential adaptation of human gut microbiota to bariatric surgery-induced weight loss: links with metabolic and low-grade inflammation markers. Diabetes. 2010;59(120):3049–57.
54. Liou AP, Pazuik M, Luevano JM Jr, Machineni S, Turnbaugh PJ, Kaplan LM. Conserved shifts in the gut microbiota due to gastric bypass reduce host weight and adiposity. Sci Transl Med. 2013;5(1780):178–88.
55. Li K, Zou J, Li S, Guo J, Shi W, Wang B, Han X, Zhang HW, Zhang P, Miao ZM, Li YS. Farnesoid X receptor contributes to body weight-independent improvements in glycemic control after Roux-en-Y gastric bypass surgery in diet-induced obese mice. Mol Metab. 2020;37:100980.
56. Pournaras DJ, Glicksman C, Vincent RP, Kuganolipava S, Alaghband-Zadeh J, Mahon D, Bekker JHR, Ghatei MA, Bloom SR, Walter JRF, Welbourn R, le Roux CW. The role of bile after Roux-en-Y gastric bypass in promoting weight loss and improving glycemic control. Endocrinology. 2012;153:3613–9.
57. Kohli R, Setchell KD, Kirby M, Myronovych A, Ryan KK, Ibrahim SH, Berger J, Smith K, Toure M, Woods SC, Seeley RJ. A surgical model in male obese rats uncovers protective effects of bile acids post-bariatric surgery. Endocrinology. 2013;154:2341–51.
58. Sayin S, Wahlstrom A, Felin J, Jantti S, Marschall HU, Bamberg K, Angelin B, Hyotylainen T, Oresic M. Backhed FGut microbiota regulates bile acid metabolism by reducing the levels of tauro-beta-muricholic acid, a naturally occurring FXR antagonist. Cell Metab. 2013;17:225–35.
59. De Siqueria CC, Torrinhas RS, Sala P, Pudenzi MA, Angolini CF, Marques da Silva M, Machado NM, Ravacci G, Eberlin MN, Waitzberg DL. Fecal bile acid profile after Roux-en-Y gastric bypass and its association with the remission of type 2 diabetes in obese women: a preliminary study. Clin Nutr. 2019;38:2906–12.

# The Role of Preoperative, Intraoperative, and Postoperative Diagnostic Endoscopy in Bariatric Surgery

17

Yagnik Pandya

Bariatric surgery is increasingly being performed in the United States and internationally since the obesity epidemic. With the new guidelines set forth by the ASMBS/IFSO in 2022, the expected number of bariatric surgeries may rise [1]. Diagnostic endoscopy in the perioperative care of bariatric patients is an invaluable tool in the surgeon's toolbox. This minimally invasive modality not only helps diagnose but also treats various conditions in the perioperative setting. As a bariatric surgeon, it is imperative that one familiarize themselves with the role of endoscopy in this patient population, to be able to better care for their patient. This chapter summarizes the importance of endoscopy in various settings and reviews the role of diagnostic endoscopy in bariatric patients.

## Preoperative Endoscopy

Preoperative evaluation of the foregut anatomy and pathology remains an important aspect of a thorough evaluation of a bariatric patient. While contrast studies like an upper gastrointestinal fluoroscopy (UGI) study can reveal important information, direct visualization of the lumen of the esophagus and stomach is only possible with endoscopy. Debate exists over the routine use of endoscopy in patients seeking metabolic and bariatric surgery (MBS). In 2021, the American Society for Metabolic and Bariatric Surgery (ASMBS) published a position statement on the rationale for the performance of upper gastrointestinal endoscopy before and after metabolic and

Y. Pandya (✉)
Bariatric, General and Cosmetic Surgeon, MetroWest Medical Center, Framingham, MA, USA

Assistant Professor of Surgery, Boston University School of Medicine, Boston, MA, USA
e-mail: yagnik.pandya@mwmc.com


O. M. Ghanem et al. (eds.), *The SAGES Manual of Metabolic and Bariatric Surgery*, https://doi.org/10.1007/978-3-031-72309-4_17

bariatric surgery. The authors looked at over 12,000 patients in 28 studies with symptomatic and asymptomatic patients and found that the average proportions of patients with gastroesophageal reflux disease (GERD), hiatal hernia, erosive esophagitis, and Barrett's esophagus before MBS were 27.3%, 21%, 16.4%, and 2.7%, respectively [2]. According to their recommendation, routine preoperative upper endoscopy in patients seeking bariatric surgery is justifiable and should be done at the surgeon's discretion. Regardless of symptoms of GERD, endoscopy may guide treatment of modifiable conditions such as *H. pylori* infection, duodenal ulcers, etc. It may also lead to the identification of conditions like a hiatal hernia which may be treated during the operation, or identify findings such as a malignancy which may preclude the operation altogether [2].

There is a higher prevalence of GERD in patients with obesity [3]. Increased intra-abdominal pressure from the gravitational forces of the visceral fat, decreased tone of the lower esophageal sphincter (LES), and transient relaxation of the LES are some of the hypothesized mechanisms [4]. Hence, many patients with obesity have symptomatic GERD. Several studies show that the incidence of GERD after sleeve gastrectomy (SG) is higher than after Roux-en-Y gastric bypass (RYGB). [6–8]. Thus, preoperative endoscopy in symptomatic patients may help document the severity of reflux esophagitis and the presence or absence of Barrett's esophagus (Fig. 17.1). This information can be crucial in counselling the patient regarding postoperative reflux symptoms and perhaps influence the choice of operation.

During the preoperative evaluation of a bariatric patient, it is pertinent for the surgeon to recognize the importance of asymptomatic GERD. Kristo et al. showed a 31.1% incidence of GERD in asymptomatic patients undergoing bariatric surgery [5]. In the 2021 ASMBS position statement regarding pre-op esophagogastroduodenoscopy (EGD) in bariatric patients, seven studies reporting the incidence of foregut

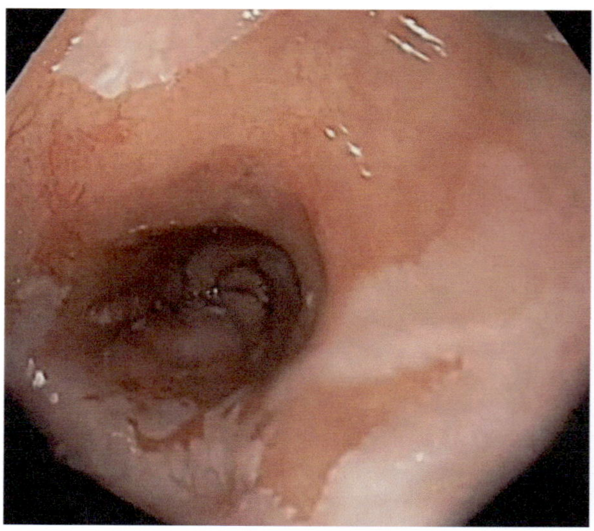

**Fig. 17.1** Barrett's esophagus on white light endoscopy

pathology in asymptomatic patients were analyzed. In 729 asymptomatic patients, hiatal hernia, erosive esophagitis, and Barrett's esophagus were seen in 17%, 16.9%, and 0.7%, respectively [2]. Out of the 25 studies published on this topic, 18 recommended routine use of preoperative EGD in MBS patients. The other seven studies recommended the selective use of EGD.

Bennett et al. [9] examined 48 studies in their meta-analysis and found that 7.8% of all patients undergoing preoperative EGD had a change in their surgical management and 27.5% had a change in medical management due to the endoscopy findings. After removing benign findings, which have a debatable impact on the surgical management of the patient, this number fell to 0.4%. They concluded that in the asymptomatic patient, EGD should be considered optional.

In the meta-analysis by Bennett et al., *H. pylori* infection was one of the commonly reported pathologic findings (36.2%) in eight studies that evaluated it. Some authors believe that eradication of *H. pylori* is important to prevent postoperative marginal ulcers and erosive gastritis [10], but Wolter S et al. did not identify an association between *H. pylori* and postoperative events [11]. Besides, *H. pylori* can be diagnosed and confirmed to be treated by non-endoscopic methods like a stool antigen assay. Also, the incidence of malignancy on routine EGD in their study was only 0.5%. However, the four patients in their study who did have malignancy on preoperative EGD would have had devastating consequences should the condition not have been identified pre-op. Wolter, S. et al. concluded that routine preoperative endoscopy be undertaken in bariatric patients to avoid such risks.

In patients who are scheduled to go a divided procedure like an RYGB or One anastomosis gastric bypass that precludes easy endoscopic access to the remnant stomach and the biliopancreatic limb, surgeons should have a lower threshold for performing preoperative upper endoscopy to evaluate for any incidental pathology. In a study of 523 patients, Schight et al. found that 28% of patients had an abnormality in the future gastric remnant. This did not include *H. pylori* infections. They concluded that routine endoscopic screening before bariatric surgery is not indicated as the number needed to screen to find clinically significant abnormalities was high [12]. Arguably, some rare findings on screening endoscopy could alter the surgical treatment. For example, if gastric intestinal metaplasia is found through endoscopy in a patient being considered for an RYGB, that could potentially alter the surgical plan and the patient may be better suited for a sleeve gastrectomy instead, which allows for ease of future endoscopic surveillance of this condition. The finding of a large hiatal hernia on preoperative EGD (Fig. 17.2) in an otherwise asymptomatic patient allows the surgeon preoperatively to prepare for a concomitant repair.

Preoperative endoscopy in patients getting revisional bariatric surgery is important to evaluate the anatomy of the upper gastrointestinal tract.

It is also important to note that preoperative endoscopy needs to be undertaken extremely carefully in bariatric patients, as a significant number of these patients may have undiagnosed obstructive sleep apnea (if not already diagnosed by then as part of preoperative workup). We routinely perform these in the endoscopy suite or the operating room with an anesthesia team that provides sedation and monitors the

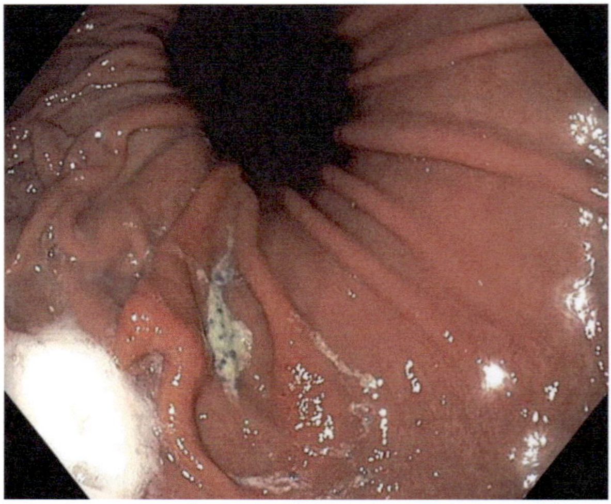

**Fig. 17.2** Large hiatal hernia in an asymptomatic patient

patient. Having said that, McVay T et al. published data that supports endoscopy can be safely performed by non-anesthesia personnel using propofol and adequately trained staff [13].

## Intraoperative Endoscopy

Several surgeons use intra-operative endoscopy for a leak test after the creation of a gastrojejunostomy during a gastric bypass. The air insufflation provided by an endoscope after submerging the anastomosis, helps the surgeon detect the area of air bubbles noted laparoscopically and allows the surgeon to exactly identify the location of the leak (pouch staple line, versus anastomosis, versus staple line of the Roux limb in a side to end anastomosis). However, the data regarding the utility of an intra-operative leak test (endoscopic or non-endoscopic) reveals controversial results. Some studies [14, 15] show the benefit of intra-operative leak testing in bariatric surgery; however, other studies have shown this to not be true [16, 17]. Yolsuriyanwong et al. analyzed the Metabolic and Bariatric Surgery Accreditation and Quality Improvement Program (MBSAQIP) data from 2015 and 2016 (265,309 patients) to evaluate the effect of intra-operative leak test (IOLT) on postoperative leak-related outcomes after primary bariatric surgery and found no evidence of either benefit or harm from IOLT in patients who underwent SG, RYGB and biliopancreatic diversion with duodenal switch (BPDS) [18]. However, an endoscopic leak test was performed only in 27.9% of patients who underwent a leak test. Intraoperative endoscopy for leak testing during SG (Fig. 17.3) appears to be used less frequently. Lufti and Gomberawalla published a case report and a review of 300 SGs in which they utilized intra-operative endoscopy and found it to be beneficial for both leak testing and an educational tool for surgeons to improve their endoscopic skills [19].

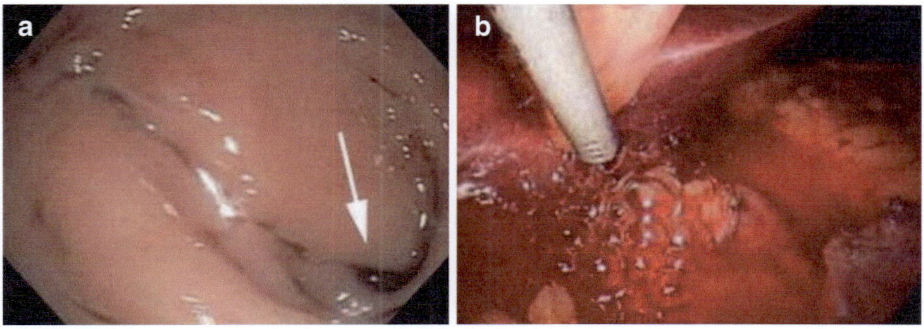


**Fig. 17.3** (**a**) Endoscopic view of a staple line leak (arrow) obtained during on-table endoscopy during a sleeve gastrectomy. (**b**) Laparoscopic view demonstrates bubbles emanating from the sleeve at the distal portion of the staple line

The other benefit of intra-operative endoscopy is to evaluate intraluminal anatomy for bleeding. Staple line bleeding during an SG or an RYGB can be diagnosed and treated at the time of the index operation with endoscopic and/or laparoscopic techniques [19]. Endoscopy in this scenario helps identify the exact bleeding site. Once the site of bleeding is identified endoscopically, the bleeder can be suture ligated laparoscopically while being visualized endoscopically. Some surgeons use the endoscope both as a bougie while fashioning their sleeve and as a tool for evaluating the intraluminal anatomy and the staple line at the end of the procedure without having to intubate the esophagus twice [20, 21]. Another advantage of this maneuver is that the patency of the sleeve can be assessed and areas of narrowing or acute angulation can be visualized. Similarly, in a gastric bypass intraoperative endoscopy can provide valuable information regarding the size of the pouch and patency of anastomosis. It can also provide information on whether the most direct outlet from the anastomosis is the blind afferent limb versus the efferent Roux limb (which can potentially lead to postoperative "candy cane syndrome" [22]). Another theoretical advantage is that intra-operative endoscopy may aid in the accurate identification of the esophagogastric junction in patients undergoing a concurrent hiatal hernia repair at the time of their index bariatric operation. This can be especially helpful in treating large hiatal hernias where one must ascertain that the gastroesophageal (GE) junction has been adequately mobilized and lays in the intra-abdominal position.

## Postoperative Endoscopy

Endoscopy has a proven role in the care of the postoperative bariatric patient [23]. Not only it can help with the diagnosis of various pathologies and conditions in the postoperative setting (marginal ulcer, anastomotic stricture, etc.) but can also help treat them. The role of therapeutic endoscopy is discussed elsewhere in this book.

The incidence of early postoperative bleeding after RYGB is 1–4% [24, 25] and after SG is 0–2.3% [26]. Early postoperative hemorrhage can be diagnosed and treated with endoscopy [27]. For example, for the postoperative patient who underwent an RYGB and developed a drop in the hemoglobin with or without hemodynamic instability, an immediate endoscopy can rule out or rule in an anastomotic bleed. Most of these patients will present with hematemesis but there is a small subset of patients that do not develop hematemesis. Endoscopy in this setting can help diagnose the source. One can evaluate the pouch and the gastrojejunal anastomotic staple line for any active bleeding and/or the presence of a clot which could be a telltale sign of old or ongoing bleeding. Treatment can subsequently be performed with epinephrine injection or clips at the same time [27]. Typically, this is undertaken in the operating room under anesthesia with endotracheal intubation and simultaneous laparoscopy [28]. There are a few reasons for this approach. Firstly, protection of the airway mitigates the risk of aspiration pneumonia. Secondly, the proximal Roux limb can be clamped laparoscopically to avoid bowel dilation which can obscure visualization. Thirdly, should a source not be found endoscopically, one can proceed with laparoscopy to evaluate for other sources of bleeding like intra-abdominal bleeding (if the presentation does not include hematemesis and/or bleeding per rectum), and evaluate the jejunojejunostomy, the remnant stomach, the surgical site, etc.

Similarly, hematemesis after an SG can be effectively evaluated and treated with endoscopy. Endoscopy in this setting helps locate the exact site of intraluminal bleeding and facilitates subsequent therapeutic intervention.

Leaks can be devastating in a bariatric patient. Prompt diagnosis and management are crucial. The mean incidence of an anastomotic/staple line leak after RYGB is reported to be 0.8% and after an SG is 0.7% [29]. Early diagnosis is key to preventing devastating complications. If clinical suspicion of a leak remains high in the postoperative bariatric patient, the next step is an evaluation with either a UGI study or an abdominal CT scan with oral and intravenous contrast. Based on some studies, a CT scan has higher sensitivity and specificity in diagnosing leaks as compared with a UGI study [30]. The role of upper endoscopy as a diagnostic modality in this situation is limited.

Abdominal pain, intolerance to PO intake, refractory nausea and /or vomiting are not uncommon symptoms in the postoperative bariatric patient. An upper endoscopy can help discern the cause in several cases. Postoperative nausea and vomiting can be seen in up to 65% of patients undergoing bariatric surgery [31]. According to a study by Suh et al., patients had twice the increased risk of postoperative nausea and vomiting after SG as compared with RYGB [32]. This can lead to dehydration and malnutrition from PO intolerance. The same study showed increased emergency department visits and prolonged length of hospitalization in these patients with postoperative nausea and vomiting as compared with patients without those symptoms. Etiologies implicated for this occurrence include edema at the staple line causing transient luminal narrowing and release of serotonin from intra-operative manipulation of the stomach. An upper endoscopy can be performed to ascertain easy passage of the endoscope down to the pylorus and help demonstrate patency of the sleeve. Endoscopy in this setting thus rules out kinks and obstruction in the sleeve lumen.

Another etiology of abdominal pain and nausea in postoperative bariatric patients is the presence of a marginal ulcer (Fig. 17.4). The incidence of marginal ulcers after RYGB is reported to be anywhere between 0.6% and 16% [33]. These can present with epigastric pain, nausea, hematemesis melena or a combination of these symptoms. Prompt upper endoscopy can help diagnose the issue and facilitate hemostasis in the event of an actively bleeding ulcer. In our practice, patients are started on an oral proton pump inhibitor and Carafate once the diagnosis is established. A repeat endoscopy can be performed at 3 months to demonstrate healing.

PO intolerance and dysphagia that occur in the late postoperative period (6–8 weeks) can be attributed to either an anastomotic stricture at the gastrojejunal anastomosis after RYGB (Fig. 17.5) or sleeve stenosis after SG. Studies have

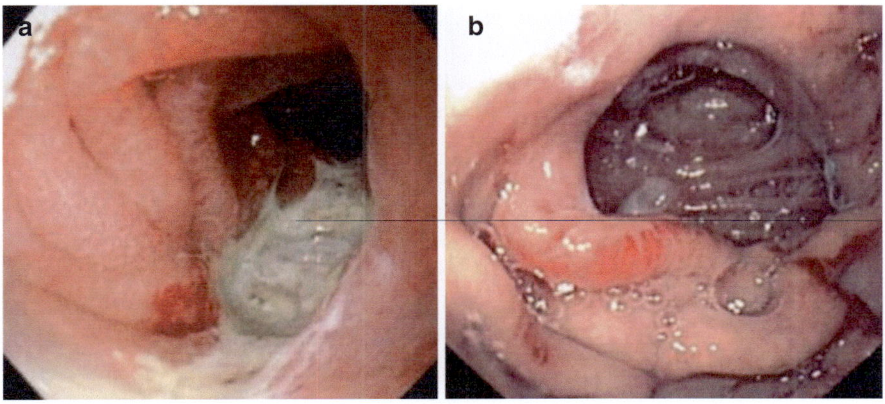


**Fig. 17.4** (**a**) Marginal ulcer; (**b**) Healed marginal ulcer (Photos courtesy of Kevin Reavis, MD)

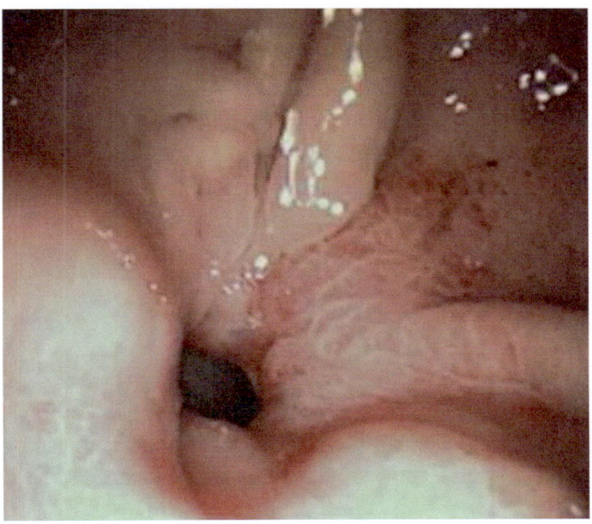

**Fig. 17.5** Anastomotic stricture due to scar formation

reported the incidence of anastomotic strictures to be anywhere between 0.9% and 34% [34, 35]. Ribero Parenti L et al. did a study of 1500 patients and found that 3.4% of patients with a gastrojejunal stricture required endoscopic intervention [36]. An upper endoscopy is the diagnostic modality of choice and allows for balloon dilation in the same setting [37]. A true stenosis or stricture after a sleeve gastrectomy is uncommon. Incidence has been reported to be between 0.69% and 2% [38]. Endoscopy here is a mainstay for diagnosis as well as possible pneumatic dilation in these situations.

Some of the long-term complications of bariatric procedures include GERD and weight gain. In a study of 47 patients with GERD after RYGB, some of the most common findings included a hiatal hernia with pouch herniation into the chest (53.2%), a large-sized pouch (10.6%), abnormal manometry (95.6%, n = 45), or a gastrogastric fistula (4.3%) amongst other rare findings [39]. While the UGI study is one of the first diagnostic modalities, an endoscopy helps quantify the severity of reflux and the presence of Barrett's esophagus which was seen in 14.9% of patients in the study. GERD after SG is a passionately discussed topic amongst the bariatric communities of the world. The ASMBS position statement on the rationale for the performance of upper gastrointestinal endoscopy before and after MBS was published in 2021. They looked at four case series that reported rates of GERD, erosive esophagitis, and de novo Barrett's esophagus after SG [2]. When aggregating data from these case series they found GERD in 67.4%, erosive esophagitis in 38.4%, and de novo Barrett's esophagus in 10.7% of patients. Upper endoscopy remains a cornerstone in the diagnosis of these conditions. They recommended performing EGD in patients ≥3 years. After SG to rule out the presence of Barrett's esophagus. This further emphasizes the role of EGD in postoperative bariatric patients. A subset of patients who undergo SG may benefit from a surveillance endoscopy post-procedure. In a recent 2023 study, questioning the routine utilization of full histopathological examination of sleeve gastrectomy specimens, the authors found an increased rate of gastrointestinal stromal tumors (GIST) and intestinal metaplasia in specimens excised from African American patients and older Hispanic patients [40]. This was the largest series to date that looked at 3543 specimens from SG patients. Most of these specimens were normal (69.6%). However, patients with intestinal metaplasia require surveillance endoscopy every 3 years due to the risk of gastric adenocarcinoma [41], emphasizing the role of diagnostic endoscopy in post-sleeve patients.

Weight gain after bariatric procedures can be multifactorial. Anatomic causes of weight gain can include a large pouch with or without a dilated gastrojejunostomy. Studies have proven the influence of pouch size as well as the size of the gastrojejunal anastomosis on weight gain after gastric bypass [42]. Endoscopy along with a UGI study can be used as a diagnostic modality to evaluate and demonstrate the length and size of the pouch and the diameter of the gastric stoma (Fig. 17.6). Based on this evaluation, the surgeon can further recommend endoscopic therapy versus surgical revision based on the endoscopic findings. A gastrogastric (pouch-gastric) fistula has also been implicated in weight gain after gastric bypass [43]. If the fistula is large enough. Food can preferentially enter the gastric remnant and subsequently

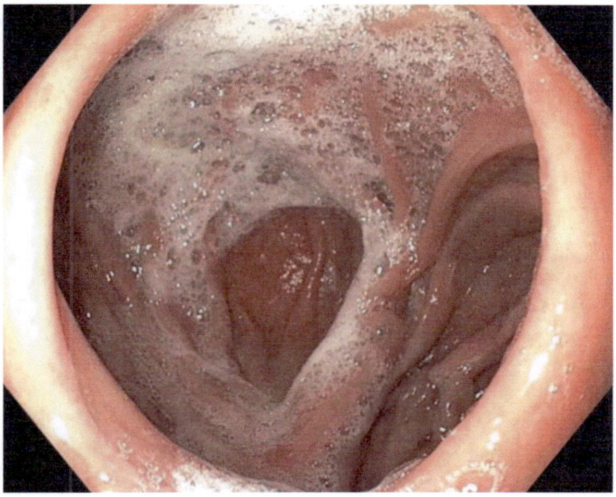

**Fig. 17.6** Dilated gastrojejunal anastomosis

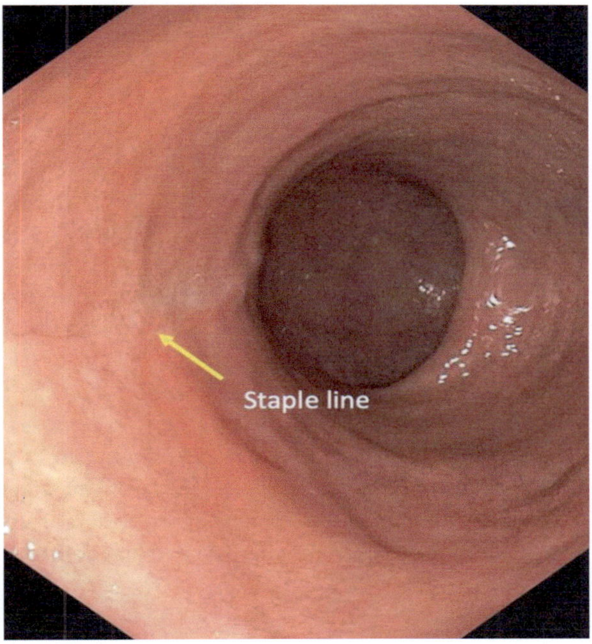


**Fig. 17.7** Endoscopic view of the dilated body of the stomach in sleeve gastrectomy patient with weight regain

the duodenum. This negates the malabsorptive component of the gastric bypass and can cause weight gain. Endoscopy can aid in the diagnosis of this condition and accurately delineate the location (proximal pouch versus close to the GJ anastomosis) of the fistula and association with a concurrent marginal ulcer or a stricture. This information is crucial in planning treatment. In a sleeve patient, weight gain could be attributed to an anatomical reason such as a dilated sleeve (Fig. 17.7) or the presence of a retained fundus [44]. While a UGI study remains the initial diagnostic test of choice, an upper endoscopy can help visualize the intraluminal volume, the

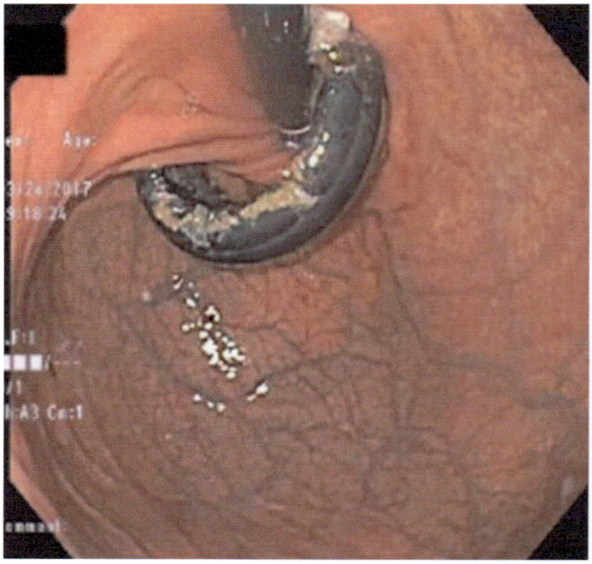

**Fig. 17.8** Endoscopic view of the eroded gastric band

dimensions of the sleeve and the retained fundus, as well as evaluate for reflux esophagitis and Barrett's esophagus in that patient.

Laparoscopic gastric banding for weight loss is not very commonly performed anymore. However, a practicing bariatric surgeon often encounters patients with a gastric band that was placed previously. A systematic review reported the incidence of band erosion to be 1.7% [45]. Patients with erosion can present with early satiety and dysphagia. An UGI study can be inconclusive. Endoscopy is the only test that provides a definitive diagnosis (Fig. 17.8). Endoscopic removal is a viable option in these patients.

Another rare but important diagnosis in which endoscopy plays a crucial role in chronic bleeding from an ulcer/lesion in the bypassed segment of the post gastric bypass anatomy. In this scenario, a gastric remnant or a duodenal ulcer is difficult to diagnose, and one must have a high index of suspicion if the traditional workup is nonrevealing. A double-balloon enteroscopy or a laparoscopic-assisted transgastric endoscopy in the OR can be undertaken to diagnose and treat this pathology [46, 47].

## Conclusion

Upper endoscopy in the bariatric patient is an irreplaceable diagnostic study. It is a relatively low-risk procedure and helps diagnose several conditions that may or may not alter the treatment algorithm in the preoperative patient. The 2021 position statement by the ASMBS has been instrumental in guiding bariatric surgeons regarding the routine use of preoperative endoscopy. Most surgeons agree that symptomatic patients must have an endoscopic evaluation prior to bariatric surgery. Asymptomatic patients must be counselled regarding the possibility of abnormal findings on preoperative EGD, which may need treatment prior to surgery or necessitate tailoring of the approach to the index procedure (for example, repair of a hiatal hernia at the time of bariatric surgery). Intraoperative endoscopy has a critical role in accurately assessing the lumen for the newly constructed postoperative anatomy and the integrity of the anastomosis and staple lines. This can avoid several postoperative complications including bowel obstruction, anastomotic or staple line bleed and leaks. In the postoperative patient, upper endoscopy is an extremely valuable diagnostic and therapeutic tool. It can not only provide accurate intraluminal examination of the patient's anatomy but also diagnose and treat several conditions that affect bariatric surgical patients.

## References


1. Eisenberg D, et al. 2022 American Society for Metabolic and Bariatric Surgery (ASMBS) and International Federation for the Surgery of Obesity and Metabolic Disorders (IFSO): indications for metabolic and bariatric surgery. Surg Obes Relat Dis. 2022;18:1345–56.
2. Campos GM, et al. ASMBS position statement on the rationale for performance of upper gastrointestinal endoscopy before and after metabolic and bariatric surgery. Surg Obes Relat Dis. 2021;17(5):837–47.
3. Jacobson BC, Somers SC, Fuchs CS, et al. Body-mass index and symptoms of gastroesophageal reflux in women. N Engl J Med. 2006;354(22):2340–8.
4. Chang P, Friedenberg F. Obesity and GERD. Gastroenterol Clin N Am. 2014;43(1):161–73.
5. Kristo I, Paireder M, Jomrich G, et al. Silent gastroesophageal reflux disease in patients with morbid obesity prior to primary metabolic surgery. Obes Surg. 2020;30:4885–91.
6. Carter PR, LeBlanc KA, Hausmann MG, Kleinpeter KP, deBarros SN, Jones SM. Association between gastroesophageal reflux disease and laparoscopic sleeve gastrectomy. Surg Obes Relat Dis. 2011;7:569–72.
7. Chiu S, Birch DW, Shi X, Sharma AM, Karmali S. Effect of sleeve gastrectomy on gastroesophageal reflux disease: a systematic review. Surg Obes Relat Dis. 2011;7:510–5.
8. Chuffart E, Sodji M, Dalmay F, Iannelli A, Mathonnet M. Long-term results after sleeve gastrectomy for gastroesophageal reflux disease: a single-center French study. Obes Surg. 2017;27:2890–7.
9. Bennett S, Gostimir M, Shorr R, Mallick R, Mamazza J, Neville A. The role of routine preoperative upper endoscopy in bariatric surgery: a systematic review and meta-analysis. Surg Obes Relat Dis. 2016;12:1116–25.
10. Fernandes SR, et al. The role of routine upper gastrointestinal endoscopy before bariatric surgery. Obes Surg. 2016;26(9):2105–10.
11. Wolter S, Duprée A, Miro J, et al. Upper gastrointestinal endoscopy prior to bariatric surgery-mandatory or expendable? An analysis of 801 cases. Obes Surg. 2017;27:1938–43.
12. Schigt A, Coblijn U, et al. Is esophagogastroduodenoscopy before Roux-en-Y gastric bypass or sleeve gastrectomy mandatory? Surg Obes Relat Dis. 2014;10(3):411–7.
13. McVay T, Fang JC, Taylor L, et al. Safety analysis of bariatric patients undergoing outpatient upper endoscopy with non-anesthesia administered propofol sedation. Obes Surg. 2017;27:1501–7.
14. Valenzuela-Salazar C, Rojano-Rodriguez ME, Romero-Loera S, et al. Intraoperative endoscopy prevents technical defect related leaks in laparoscopic Roux-en-Y gastric bypass: a randomized control trial. Int J Surg. 2018;50:17–21.
15. Al Hadad M, Dehni N, Elamin D, Ibrahim M, Ghabra S, Nimeri A. Intraoperative endoscopy decreases postoperative complications in laparoscopic Roux-en-Y gastric bypass. Obes Surg. 2015;25:1711–5.

16. Sethi M, Zagzag J, Patel K, et al. Intraoperative leak testing has no correlation with leak after laparoscopic sleeve gastrectomy. Surg Endosc. 2016;30:883–91.
17. Bingham J, Kaufman J, Hata K, et al. A multicenter study of routine versus selective intraoperative leak testing for sleeve gastrectomy. Surg Obes Relat Dis. 2017;13:1469–75.
18. Yolsuriyanwong K, et al. Effects of intraoperative leak testing on postoperative leak-related outcomes after primary bariatric surgery: an analysis of the MBSAQIP database. Surg Obes Relat Dis. 2019;15(9):1530–40.
19. Gomberawalla A, Lutfi R. Benefits of intraoperative endoscopy: case report and review of 300 sleeves gastrectomies. Ann Surg Innov Res. 2015;9:13.
20. Frezza EE, Barton A, Herbert H, et al. Laparoscopic sleeve gastrectomy with endoscopic guidance in morbid obesity. Surg Obes Relat Dis. 2008;4(5):575–9. https://doi.org/10.1016/j.soard.2007.12.013.
21. Andreas A, Adamantios M, Antonios A, et al. Laparoscopic sleeve gastrectomy for morbid obesity with intra-operative endoscopy: lessons we learned after 100 consecutive patients. Obes Surg. 2015;25:1223–8.
22. Aryaie AH, Fayezizadeh M, Wen Y, et al. "Candy cane syndrome:" an underappreciated cause of abdominal pain and nausea after Roux-en-Y gastric bypass surgery. Surg Obes Relat Dis. 2017;13:1501–5.
23. Singhal S, Le DL, Duddempudi S, Anand S. The role of endoscopy in bariatrics: past, present, and future. J Laparoendosc Adv Surg Tech A. 2012;22(8):802–11.
24. Nguyen NT, Rivers R, Wolfe BM. Early gastrointestinal hemorrhage after laparoscopic gastric bypass. Obes Surg. 2003;1:62–5.
25. Dick A, Byrne TK, Baker M, Budak A, Morgan K. Gastrointestinal bleeding after gastric bypass surgery: nuisance or catastrophe? Surg Obes Relat Dis. 2010;6(6):643–7.
26. Bransen J, Gilissen LPL, van Rutte PWJ, et al. Costs of leaks and bleeding after sleeve gastrectomies. Obes Surg. 2015;25:1767–71.
27. Jamil LH, Krause KR, Chengelis DL, Jury RP, Jackson CM, Cannon ME, et al. Endoscopic management of early upper gastrointestinal hemorrhage following laparoscopic Roux-En-Y gastric bypass. Am J Gastroenterol. 2008;103(1):86–91.
28. Khan AH, Khaitan L. Management of acute bleeding after bariatric surgery. In: Chand B, editor. Endoscopy in obesity management. Cham: Springer; 2018.
29. Clinical Issues Committee of the American Society for Metabolic and Bariatric Surgery. Updated position statement on the prevention and detection of gastrointestinal leak. May 2015.
30. Bingham J, Shawhan R, et al. Computed tomography scan versus upper gastrointestinal fluoroscopy for diagnosis of staple line leak following bariatric surgery. Am J Surg. 2015;209(5):810–4.
31. Halliday TA, Sundqvist J, Hultin M, Wallden J. Post-operative nausea and vomiting in bariatric surgery patients: an observational study. Acta Anaesthesiol Scand. 2017;61:471–9.
32. Suh S, Helm M, Kindel TL, et al. The impact of nausea on post-operative outcomes in bariatric surgery patients. Surg Endosc. 2020;34:3085–91.
33. Giannopoulos S, et al. Proton pump inhibitor prophylaxis after Roux-en-Y gastric bypass: a national survey of surgeon practices. Surg Obes Relat Dis. 2023;19(4):303–8.
34. Bell RL, Reinhardt KE, Flowers JL. Surgeon-performed endoscopic dilatation of symptomatic gastrojejunal anastomotic strictures following laparoscopic roux-en-Y gastric bypass. Obes Surg. 2003;13:728–33.
35. Dillemans B, Sakran N, Van Cauwenberge S, et al. Standardization of the fully stapled laparoscopic roux-en-Y gastric bypass for obesity reduces early immediate postoperative morbidity and mortality: a single center study on 2606 patients. Obes Surg. 2009;19:1355–64.
36. Ribeiro-Parenti L, Arapis K, et al. Gastrojejunostomy stricture rate: comparison between antecolic and retrocolic laparoscopic Roux-en-Y gastric bypass. Surg Obes Relat Dis. 2015;11(5):1076–84.
37. King NA, Herron DM. Gastrointestinal obstruction after bariatric surgery. In: Nguyen N, Brethauer S, Morton J, Ponce J, Rosenthal R, editors. The ASMBS textbook of bariatric surgery. Cham: Springer; 2020.

38. Lim B, Johnson DC, Davis KA. Early and late complications of bariatric operation. Trauma Surg Acute Care Open. 2018;3(1):e000219.
39. Borbély YJ, et al. Radiologic, endoscopic, and functional patterns in patients with symptomatic gastroesophageal reflux disease after Roux-en-Y gastric bypass. Surg Obes Relat Dis. 2018;14(6):764–8.
40. Yang T, Nyirenda T, Shi M, Petit R, Talishinskiy T. Histopathologic findings in laparoscopic sleeve gastrectomy: is routine full pathologic evaluation indicated? Surg Obes Relat Dis. 2023;19(4):283–8.
41. Banks M, Graham D, Jansen M, et al. British Society of Gastroenterology guidelines on the diagnosis and management of patients at risk of gastric adenocarcinoma. Gut. 2019;68:1545–75.
42. Heneghan HM, Yimcharoen P, Brethauer SA, Kroh M, Chand B. Influence of pouch and stoma size on weight loss after gastric bypass. Surg Obes Rel Dis. 2012;8:408–15.
43. Ribeiro-Parenti L, De Courville G, Daikha A, Arapis K, Chosidow D, Marmuse J-P. Classification, surgical management and outcomes of patients with gastrogastric fistula after Roux-En-Y gastric bypass. Surg Obes Relat Dis. 2017;13(2):243–8.
44. Eid G. Sleeve gastrectomy revision by endoluminal sleeve plication gastroplasty: a small pilot case series. Surg Endosc. 2017;31:4252–5.
45. Egberts K, Brown WA, O'Brien PE. Systematic review of erosion after laparoscopic adjustable gastric banding. Obes Surg. 2011;21:1272–9.
46. Sakai R, Kuga R, Safatle-Ribeiro AV, et al. Is it feasible to reach the bypassed stomach after Roux-en-Y gastric bypass for morbid obesity? The use of double-balloon enteroscope. Endoscopy. 2005;37:566–9.
47. Serrot FJ, Szomstein S, Rosenthal RJ. Postoperative bleeding in the bariatric surgery patient. In: Nguyen N, Brethauer S, Morton J, Ponce J, Rosenthal R, editors. The ASMBS textbook of bariatric surgery. Cham: Springer; 2020.

# Index Endoscopic Bariatric and Metabolic Therapies

# 18

Jean-Christophe N. Rwigema, Stephanie Joseph, and Michael B. Ujiki

## History and Introduction to Endoscopic Bariatric and Metabolic Therapies (EBMTs)

Obesity represents a significant global public health threat. The World Health Organization (WHO) estimates over 650 million adults worldwide have obesity [1]. Long-term randomized trials have shown that bariatric surgery plus medical therapy is superior to intensive medical therapy alone in achieving glycemic control, reducing cardiovascular risk, improving quality of life, and decreasing medication use [2]. Endoscopic bariatric and metabolic therapies (EBMTs), though less effective in achieving weight loss, are a safer and more cost-effective option for patients who fail medical therapy [3].

The use of endoscopic therapies was introduced in 1982 by Nieben and Harboe. Their use of free-floating rubber balloons as artificial bezoars showed promise in short-term weight reduction in a small cohort of patients [4, 5]. Percival built on this concept by using inflated mammary implants that were more resistant to gastric acid as intragastric balloons [5, 6]. In 1985, the Garren-Edwards gastric bubble was approved by the FDA for use in the treatment of obesity but was withdrawn from the market 3 years later due to significant complications and lack of superiority to

J.-C. N. Rwigema (✉)
Department of Surgery, Endeavor Health, Evanston, IL, USA

University of Florida College of Medicine, Gainesville, FL, USA
e-mail: jrwigema@northshore.org

S. Joseph
Department of Surgery, Endeavor Health, Evanston, IL, USA

Detroit Medical Center/Wayne State University School of Medicine, Detroit, MI, USA

M. B. Ujiki
Department of Surgery, Endeavor Health, Evanston, IL, USA


O. M. Ghanem et al. (eds.), *The SAGES Manual of Metabolic and Bariatric Surgery*, https://doi.org/10.1007/978-3-031-72309-4_18

standard therapy [5]. Since then, there have been notable improvements in intragastric balloons and the development of other therapies that have shown to be safe and effective. This chapter will discuss the current restrictive and metabolic EBMTs in use for the treatment of obesity.

## Proposed Molecular Mechanisms of EBMTs

The exact molecular mechanism leading to weight loss after EBMT remains under study and thus, multiple mechanisms have been proposed. Multiple hormonal changes have been described. Ghrelin, which is primarily secreted by the stomach, stimulates appetite and promotes the storage of fat. Bariatric surgeries have been associated with decreased ghrelin levels. A glucose-dependent insulinotropic polypeptide (GIP) and glucagon-like peptide-1 (GLP-1), also known as incretins, are secreted in the duodenum and jejunum, respectively. These hormones contribute to weight loss and improved glycemic control after Bariatric surgery by suppressing glucagon secretion, slowing gastric emptying, and increasing satiety. Additionally, peptide YY, an appetite suppressant that is secreted postprandially in the distal ileum and proximal colon, has been shown to increase after Bariatric surgery. Similar to Bariatric surgery, EBMTs bypass the foregut and accelerate intestinal transit time. This leads to an increase in secondary bile acids that induce the secretion of incretins and ultimately leads to increased insulin levels. Furthermore, obesity leads to alterations in the gut microbiota, which negatively impacts host defenses and the immune system. A decrease in the ratio of *Firmicutes/Bacteroidaceae* bacteria has been observed after EBMTs. The increase in *Bacteroides* also leads to an increase in secondary bile acids [7, 8].

## Restrictive EBMTs

### Intragastric Balloons (IGBs)

FDA status: Reshape, Orbera, Obalon, Spatz FDA-approved.
Elipse pending FDA approval.
Used Internationally.

Intragastric balloons were first established in 1985. This is a non-surgical, reversible procedure that has been shown to achieve effective weight loss while the balloon is in place and sustained post-retrieval. The balloon takes space in the gastric cavity leading to a smaller reservoir for food consumption leading to reduced caloric intake, early satiety, and weight loss [9–11].

#### Contraindications

Preoperative contraindications include patients prone to gastric ulceration, with active ulceration, chronic NSAID, or steroid use, large hiatal hernias, along with patients with premalignant or malignant lesions. Patients with previous bariatric surgery should also refrain from balloon insertion [9–11].

## Technique and Balloon Types

There are several balloon types (Fig. 18.1). The single balloons are placed under conscious sedation or general anesthesia. Upper endoscopy is performed to rule out contraindications. The balloon apparatus is then inserted into the esophagus and gastric lumen. A scope is followed to ensure that the balloon is in the appropriate position and then expanded with about 400-750 cc cc of sterile saline (Each balloon system may have various capacities). Follow-up imaging with X-ray can also be obtained to ensure appropriate positioning. Intragastric balloons are temporary measures and should be taken out 6 months post-procedure [12].

Dual balloon technology is also available. These systems include two balloons that are connected. Inserted in the same fashion as the single balloon then each balloon is expanded under endoscopic visualization [13].

An in-office insertion apparatus that does not require anesthesia or endoscopy is also available. With this system, the patient can swallow the collapsed balloon wrapped in a small capsule and connected to a catheter. The position of the swallowed capsule is confirmed by X-ray prior to filling the balloon through a valved catheter. The valve is made of a biodegradable substance which eventually erodes in the span of 4–6 months allowing the water to spill and the balloon is passed naturally and excreted in the stool [14].

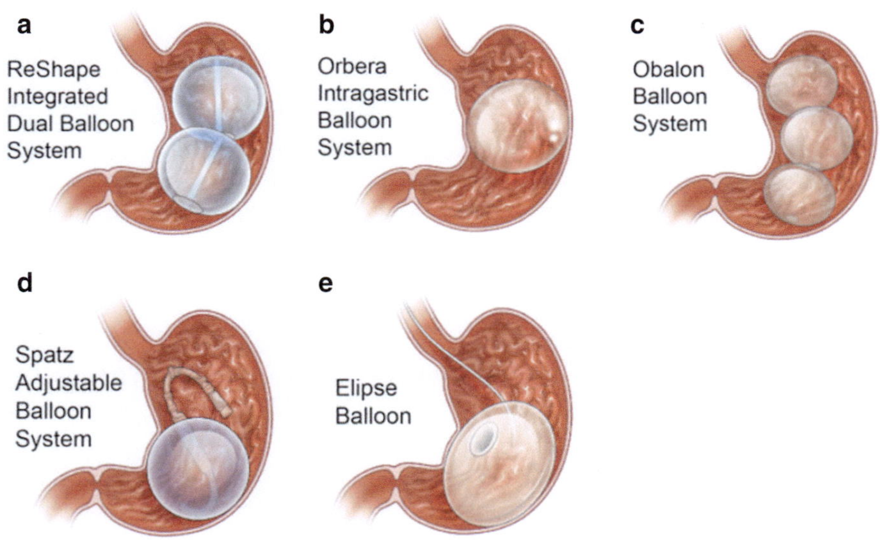


**Fig. 18.1** Types of intragastric balloons

### Retrieval

Intragastric balloons are typically used as a temporary measure. In some cases, the balloon can be placed to induce preprocedural weight loss. Retrieval of the balloon is done under conscious sedation or general anesthesia with endotracheal intubation. The saline or air is removed from the balloon with a catheter mounted with a sharp-tipped suction catheter. After a puncture, the catheter can be placed on suction until deflated. An endoscopic snare or forceps is used to grasp the deflated apparatus and is removed. Specific techniques can differ depending on the balloon type placed. One study showed that the use of a double channel scope along with rat-toothed forceps and a shark polypectomy snare allowed for faster retrieval with less potential for balloon loss and a more comfortable experience for patients under sedation when compared to single instrument retrieval. It can be handy to have a pair of forceps available to pull out the deflated balloon if it drops in the pharynx [15]. Some advocate for balloon removal under general anesthesia so that airway protection can be accomplished during balloon removal.

### Post-Procedure Care and Follow-Up

Patients are placed on Proton Pump Inhibitors to reduce the potential for ulceration. The gastric balloon is not intended for permanent placement and should be removed after 6–12 months.

### Outcomes and Complications

A multi-clinical Brazilian study of 323 patients underwent endoscopic single balloon placement. These patients were followed. At the 6-month mark, there was shown to be an %EWL of 48.3% + −23.3% ($p = 0.74$). This paper showed that in the patients that followed up at 1 (85) year and 2 years (158) post-op weight retention was evident [9].

The Reduce trial was a prospective randomized controlled trial (RCT) for dual intragastric balloon devices. Patients were randomly selected to undergo sham endoscopy or have a dual balloon system in place. At 24 weeks, patients with the balloon device had %EWL of 25.1% compared with diet alone (11.3%) [16]. Dual and single devices are both similar %EWL at the 12-month mark after balloon removal [17].

Patients may complain of nausea, epigastric pain, esophagitis, and gastritis. Although rare, migration of the balloon can cause intestinal obstruction or gastric impaction. A systematic review of 6101 cases showed a mortality rate of 0.05% [18].

## Endoscopic Sleeve Gastroplasty (ESG)

FDA Status: Approved.
Used internationally.

Endoscopic Sleeve Gastroplasty (ESG) is an incisionless procedure that uses an endoscopic stitching device to tubularize the gastric lumen (Fig. 18.4) [19].

## Contraindications

Contraindications to this procedure include gastrectomy, hiatal hernias >5 cm, coagulopathy, preneoplastic lesions, gastric ulceration, or gastritis [20].

## Technique

Key Steps: Box A.

The patient is placed under general anesthesia for this procedure to protect the airway during multiple insertions and removals of the endoscope. It is important that carbon dioxide gas be used for insufflation as the full-thickness suture bites will likely leak into the intraperitoneal space. A single or double-lumen scope is used for an initial survey of the GI tract to ensure that no contraindications to the procedure are present. An esophageal overtube can be placed to protect the esophagus and pharynx from trauma. An endoscopic suturing device is mounted onto a single or double-lumen scope. The suture system is loaded with permanent suture and the tissue helix device is passed through the scope. The initial stitch is positioned just proximal to the incisura at the anterior gastric wall. It is essential that each bite be full thickness as this ensures the integrity of the procedure. The suture pattern, as seen in Fig. 18.2, continues in an "O" or "U" shape and after the last bite is cinched down to narrow the lumen. The suture device is then reloaded, and this pattern continues proximally until reaching the fundus. The fundus is left intact. This pattern continues until the lumen of the stomach is formed into a tubular shape as seen in Fig. 18.3. Upon completion, a final endoscopy is again completed with the single lumen scope to ensure patency and hemostasis [21] (Fig. 18.4).

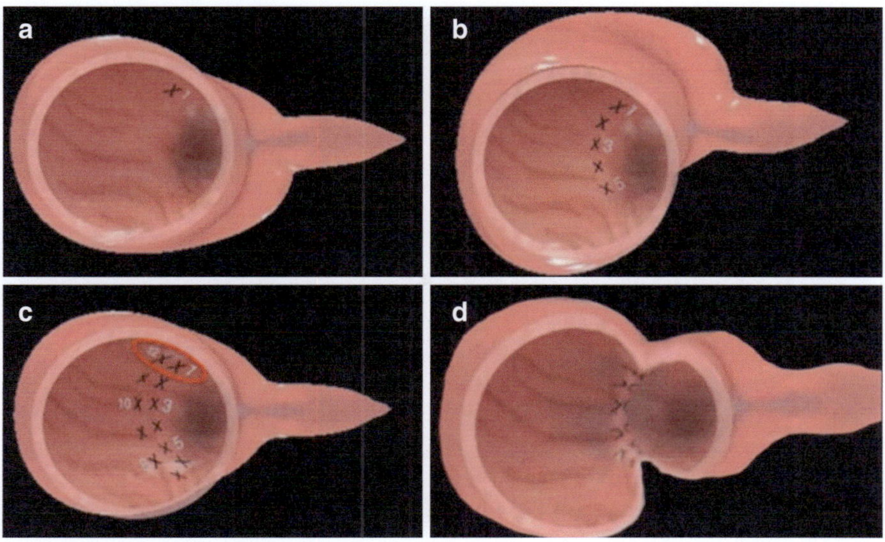


**Fig. 18.2** Suture pattern during ESG

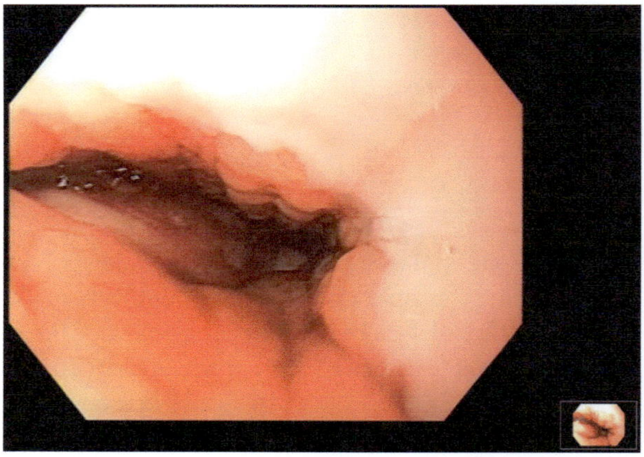

**Fig. 18.3** Endoscopic image of tubularized stomach after ESG

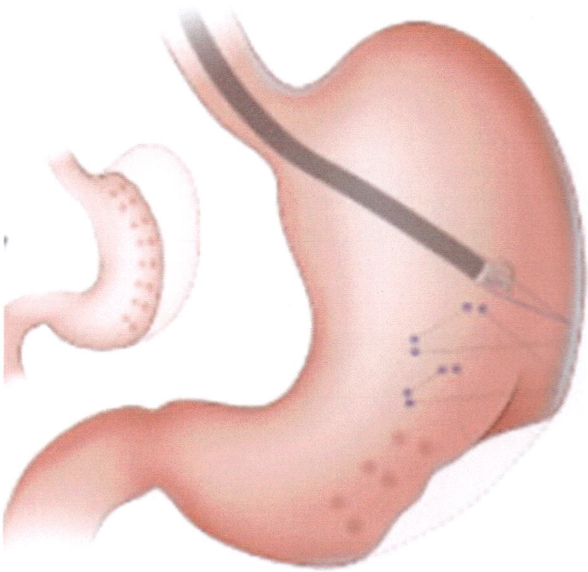

**Fig. 18.4** Stomach after ESG

## Post-Procedure Care and Follow-Up

Patients can be discharged the same day after the procedure. Antiemetics are encouraged in the perioperative period as retching and emesis have been shown to cause suture breakage. Antacids have also been shown to reduce pain and can also be prescribed. Patients are started on a liquid diet and advanced as tolerated as full-thickness bites heal [22].

### Outcomes and Complications

A 2022 multi-institution randomized control trial (MERIT) was conducted to compare ESG with lifestyle modifications alone. The results showed that at 52 weeks Excess Weight Loss (EWL) for ESG was 49.2% compared to 3.2% in the lifestyle modification group. (SD: 32.0%,18.6% $p < 0.0001$). The trial also showed improvement in obesity-related comorbidities in 80% of ESG patients [23].

Few complications have been reported. Nausea and abdominal pain are frequent concerns. Bleeding and leaks have been observed and are frequently managed conservatively. The MERIT trial showed three participants (2%) endured serious adverse events [23].

A systematic review and meta-analysis which included eight studies focused on the efficacy and safety of ESG. The total number of patients in this study was 1722. This study showed at 6 months post-op TBWL was noted to be 15.1% and %EWL was 57.7%. At 18–24 months, TBWL was maintained at 17.2%. Severe adverse events for all patients were noted to be 2.2%. Those events included patients with upper GI bleeding after ESG and eight patients with perigastric leak or fluid collection following the procedure [24].

## Primary Obesity Surgery Endoluminal (POSE)

FDA status: Not approved.
Used internationally.

Primary obesity surgery endoluminal (POSE) procedure uses the Incisionless Operating Platform (IOP®) (USGI Medical, San Clemente, CA, USA) to perform tissue apposition with full-thickness plication thereby reducing gastric volume. This system has four working channels that can accommodate an endoscope and three specialized instruments (g-Prox EZ® Endoscopic Grasper, g-Lix™ Tissue Grasper, and g-Cath™ EZ Suture Anchor Delivery Catheter) [5, 25].

### Technique

General anesthesia is used for this procedure. A standard gastroscopy is performed to aspirate any fluid, as well as to verify for any anatomical irregularities. The shape of the fundus is noted, which may affect the number of suture anchors that will be subsequently placed. The IOP® is inserted transorally and advanced into the stomach. Visualization is achieved with a small-diameter endoscope [26].

Next, suture-anchor plications are placed in the fundus and distal body (Fig. 18.5). To achieve each plication, the target tissue is grasped with the g-Lix™ and pulled and guided into the jaws of the g-Prox®. The g-Prox® jaws are then closed. After insertion of the g-Cath™ system through the g-Prox® lumen, the g-Cath™ needle tip is advanced through the tissue fold and a suture anchor is deployed on each side of the tissue fold to approximate it. The suture anchors are cinched to an appropriate tension. The proximal end of the suture is cut, leaving the cinched anchor pair holding the apposed tissue. Three to four additional plications are placed in the distal

**Fig. 18.5** Stomach after POSE

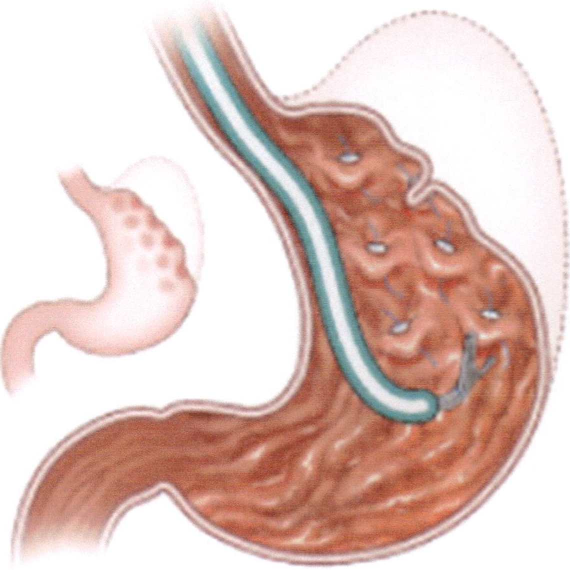

body, creating a tissue ridge near the mouth of the antrum opposite the angular incisure. The IOP® and instruments are removed after this. To conclude the procedure, a gastroscopy is performed to view the plications and ensure hemostasis [26].

## Post-Procedure Care and Follow-Up

Patients can be discharged on the same day or observed overnight. Diet is slowly advanced from liquid to puree, to soft solids, and then full solids by the 6th week.

## Outcomes and Complications

The ESSENTIAL Trial was the first multicenter randomized sham-controlled trial to evaluate the safety and efficacy of the POSE procedure. Three hundred thirty-two subjects were randomized to active (n = 221) or sham treatment groups (n = 111). At 12 months, the mean TBWL was 4.95% in the active and 1.38% in the sham group ($p < 0.0001$). Additionally, improvement in diabetes, defined as a decrease in diabetes medication, occurred in significantly more active than sham subjects at 12 months. The most common complications were pain, nausea, and vomiting. These are typically resolved within 1 week. Thirty-one subjects experienced serious complications with 21 of these occurring in the active group. Of these, one subject required laparoscopy for extra-gastric bleeding and another subject with a hepatic abscess required interventional radiology drainage and antibiotic therapy [27].

Similar to the ESSENTIAL Trial, the MILEPOST Trial was a multicenter randomized trial comparing weight loss and satiety after POSE versus conventional medical therapy. As in the ESSENTIAL trial, the same suture plication technique was utilized during the MILEPOST trial. In both studies, an average of about 13 suture anchors were placed per subject. Forty-four subjects were randomized to treatment (n = 34) or control (n = 10) groups. At 12 months, the mean TBWL was 13% for the treatment group and 5.3% for the control group (p = 0.01). The treatment group showed significant reductions along all satiety parameters at 12 months. No serious device- or procedure-related complications occurred [28]. Though the mean TBWL for the treatment group in the MILEPOST trial (13%) was higher than that observed in the ESSENTIAL trial (4.95%), the MILEPOST trial had a significantly smaller sample size.

## Malabsorptive/Metabolic EBMTs

### Endoluminal Bypass Liners

FDA status: Not approved.
Used internationally.

#### Contraindications

Anatomical variants (short duodenal bulb), peptic ulcer disease.

The duodenal-jejunal bypass sleeve (DJBS), is an endoscopically placed, flexible sleeve that is anchored in the duodenal bulb via a self-expanding nitinol ring with 10 barbs to secure the ring to the muscularis propria. This impermeable fluoropolymer liner spans 60 cm into the small intestine bypassing the duodenum and extending into the proximal jejunum (Fig. 18.6). This device is designed to mimic the excluded biliopancreatic limb of a Roux-en-Y gastric bypass [5, 29, 30].

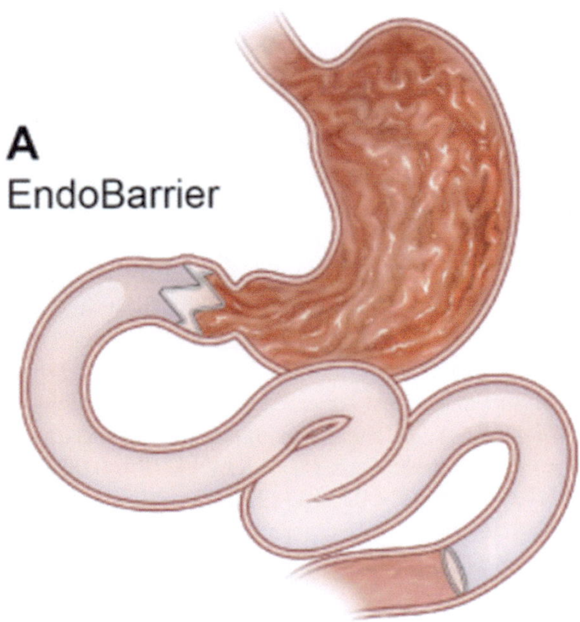


**Fig. 18.6** Stomach and small intestine after DJBS placement

All patients must adhere to a liquid diet for 1 week prior to implantation and 1–2 weeks post-procedure. This facilitates optimal views during endoscopy for implantation of the device and minimizes obstruction of the liner post-procedure. Use of a proton pump inhibitor (PPI) 3 days prior to insertion up to 2 weeks after is recommended to minimize the risk of bleeding from the implant [31].

## Technique

General anesthesia or deep sedation is appropriate. A single dose of broad-spectrum antibiotic (ex, 2 g ceftriaxone) is administered 1–2 hours prior to the procedure. Fluoroscopic imaging is also required for guidance in the insertion or removal of the liner. An endoscopic examination of the upper GI tract is conducted prior to placement to ensure suitability and to detect any anatomical variants or pathology such as peptic ulcer disease [31].

The patient is placed in the left lateral decubitus position. A surveillance endoscopy is performed to rule out contraindications to placement. Once the endoscope is placed in the first part of the duodenum, a guidewire is advanced as distally as possible through the working channel, and the endoscope is then removed. The delivery system, which includes a coaxial catheter system with a capsule containing the sleeve, is advanced over the guidewire until the capsule sits in the pylorus and the distal end sits in the duodenal bulb. The guidewire is subsequently removed. Additional steps outlined in the delivery system are followed to release the device from the capsule. The proximal barbs are anchored in the duodenal bulb and the sleeve is unraveled distal to this with the aid of peristalsis. A gastrografin study is then performed to confirm the proper position of the device and to ensure its patency [31].

## Post-Procedure Care

The patient is usually discharged home the same day following recovery from anesthesia. As discussed above, the patient follows a strict liquid diet for 1–2 weeks following the procedure and continues a PPI for 2 weeks to minimize bleeding.

## Outcomes and Complications

There have been five randomized controlled trials (RCTs) to evaluate the efficacy of endoluminal bypass liners. Jirapinyo et al. conducted a systematic review and meta-analysis assessing the effect of duodenal-jejunal bypass liner (DJBL) on glycemic control in obese patients with Type 2 diabetes mellitus (T2DM). This included the 5 RCTs and nine observational studies. These studies yielded a total of 412 patients. Of these 388 underwent successful placement of DJBL. Reasons for failed implantation included abnormalities such as polyps, sharp angulations, or short duodenal bulb and anesthetic adverse reactions. On average, the device was in place for 8.4 months. At the time of explantation, Hgb A1C decreased by 1.3% ($P < 0.0001$). Fasting insulin decreased by 4.8 mU/L ($P < 0.0001$) and fasting glucose decreased by 44.6 mg/dL ($P < 0.0001$) [32].

Four of the 5 RCTs were included in the subgroup analysis. On average, the device was in place for 4.5 months. At the time of explantation, the DJBL group had a greater decrease in Hgb A1C by 0.9% (P < 0.0001), compared with the control group [32].

At 3 months after device removal, Hgb A1C remained lower than the baseline level by 2.2% (P < 0.0001). This resulted from two studies with 46 patients with an average time of 12.3 months from implantation. At 6 months after device removal, Hgb A1C remained lower than the baseline level by 0.9% (P < 0.0001). This resulted in four studies with 120 patients with an average time of 23.0 months from implantation. There was no significant difference in Hgb A1C compared to baseline level noted from two studies at 12 months after device removal [32].

Ten studies with a total of 352 patients assessed the effect of DJBL on weight loss in patients with obesity and concomitant T2DM. Average weight loss was 11.3 kg (P < 0.0001) at time of explantation corresponding to a BMI reduction of 4.1 kg/m$^2$ (P < 0.0001), and EWL of 36.9% (P < 0.0001). At 6 months after device removal, a TWL of 8% and EWL of 25.5% (P < 0.0001) were noted in two studies with 131 patients. At 12 months after device removal, a TWL of 7.2% and EWL of 27.7% (P < 0.0001) were noted in 2 (80 patients) and 1 (59 patients) studies, respectively [32].

The most common complications reported were abdominal pain, nausea, and vomiting. These occurred most commonly immediately after DJBL implantation. Serious complications occurred in 55 out of 350 DJBL cases (15.7%). These included gastrointestinal bleeding, hypoglycemic events, acute pancreatitis, sleeve migration, severe abdominal pain, liver abscesses, anchor perforation near the pylorus, sleeve obstruction, esophageal perforation during explantation, acute cholecystitis, duodenal fistula, ulceration at the duodenal bulb, and dehydration [32–40].

## Duodenal Mucosal Resurfacing (DMR)

FDA Status: Approved.
Used internationally.

### Contraindications

Absolute contraindications include duodenal or gastric ulcers, duodenitis or gastritis, any premalignant lesions. Varices and telangiectasias and visible structures are also contraindicated. Relative contraindications can include a tortuous duodenum making catheter control difficult [41].

### Technique

The patient can either be placed under general anesthesia or under deep sedation. Initial endoscopy is completed to rule out any contraindications. The catheter is then inserted (Fig. 18.7). It is critical that proper positioning is beyond the duodenal papilla. Applying heat to the papilla can cause harm to the organ. A catheter is inserted between the mucosal and submucosal layers. This layer is lifted with saline circumferentially. The ideal distance of elevations is around 10–12 cm for best results. Once completed, the catheter is replaced by the hydrothermal ablation

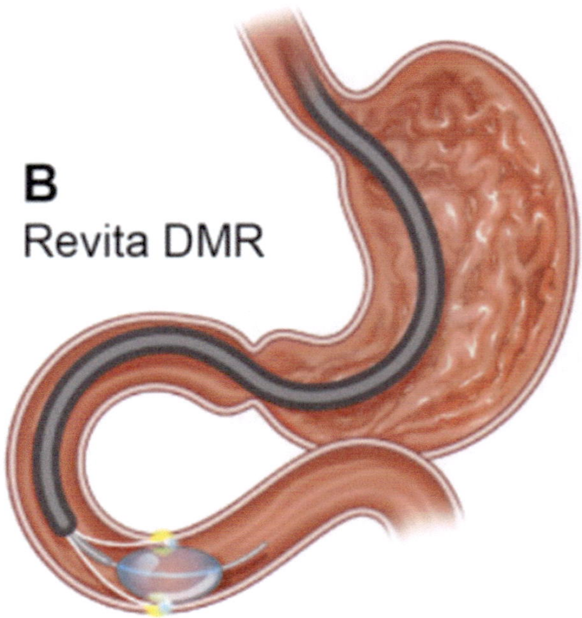


**Fig. 18.7** Ablation during DMR procedure

catheter and the lifted tissue is ablated. Final scope can be done to assure no immediate complications and the patient is awakened [41, 42].

### Post-Procedure Care and Follow-Up

Patients can be admitted for 24-h observation post procedure for monitoring. Once discharged, the initial diet is clear liquids while the mucosa heals. This process can take about 2 weeks. Diet can then be advanced as tolerated.

### Outcomes and Complications

Major complications include duodenal stenosis and injury to the papilla. It is important that only the mucosal layer be lifted, otherwise, stricturing is more likely. Additionally overlapping ablations can cause stricturing.

The REVITA-2 study which was a double blind RCT and other studies have confirmed that DMR influences changes in metabolic processes. Patients experience improvement in metabolic derangements including HbA1c, fasting glucose and liver function tests [43, 44].

## Gastroduodenojejunal Bypass Sleeve

FDA Status: Not approved.
Used internationally.

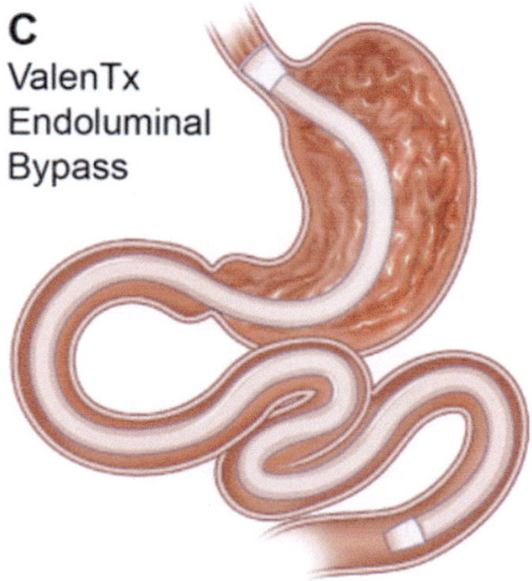


**Fig. 18.8** Stomach and small intestine after GDJBS placement

The gastroduodenojejunal bypass sleeve (GDJBS) is a 120-cm long fluoropolymer sleeve that is anchored at the gastroesophageal junction by endoscopic and laparoscopic techniques. This device extends 120 cm through the stomach into the small intestine creating an endoluminal bypass (Fig. 18.8), which allows food to pass directly from the esophagus into the small bowel avoiding absorption of nutrients in the stomach, duodenum, and jejunum [5, 30, 45, 46].

## Technique

The patient is placed under general anesthesia for the procedure. The procedure begins with placement of the long overtube extending through the pylorus into the duodenal bulb. Through this overtube, the GDJBS is delivered via a delivery catheter to the level of the first portion of the duodenum. Using a toposcopic delivery technique, utilizing computer regulated pressure and flow monitoring, the sleeve, with an attached polyester cuff on the proximal end, is deployed through the pylorus. Proper deployment of the sleeve into the proximal jejunum is aided with fluoroscopy. Once the sleeve is adequately deployed, the delivery catheter is removed, and the long overtube is exchanged for a shorter overtube [46].

The patient is then repositioned from supine to lithotomy for the laparoscopic portion. Appropriate trocars are placed, along with a Nathanson liver retractor. The gastroesophageal junction (GEJ) is dissected circumferentially at the level of the diaphragmatic hiatus and a Penrose drain is placed to assist in manipulation [46].

Endoscopically, the polyester cuff is positioned at the GEJ. The positioning is completed with use of a removable stent, which helps in visualization of the esophageal lumen at the GEJ. The attachment is performed with eight endoscopically delivered, nitinol suture anchors, deployed circumferentially, with the aid of laparoscopic visualization to ensure transmural anchor placement and to avoid any visceral injury. Once the cuff is anchored, the stent is detached and removed through the overtube, via a drawstring at its proximal end. The left and right diaphragmatic crura are then approximated with suture closure laparoscopically. The Penrose drain is removed and the procedure is concluded [46].

### Post-Procedure Care and Follow-Up

The patient is monitored in the hospital for 1 day post-operatively. A gastrografin study is performed on postoperative day 1 to evaluate the sleeve and cuff positions. Once adequate position is ensured, the patient is started on a liquid diet. The patient will be on a full liquid diet for the first 2 weeks, followed by a pureed diet for 2 weeks, and then progressed to a regular diet afterwards.

### Outcomes and Complications

Sandler et al. assessed short-term weight loss and changes in comorbidities in patients who had the GDJBS installed in their single-center prospective trial. The GDJBS was successfully delivered in 22 out of 24 patients and retrieved successfully from all the patients. Of the 22 who underwent successful implantation, five underwent explantation before the end of the 12-week study trial due to odynophagia with the postoperative diet that all resolved after device explantation. The average starting BMI was 42 kg/m$^2$, and the average %EWL was 39.7%. There were seven patients with diabetes and two patients with hypertension, controlled with medications. All these patients were able to stop their medications after device implantation [46].

Sandler et al. followed up these results with another single-center prospective trial, with 13 patients for 1 year. Twelve of the 13 patients had successful implantation of the GDJBS. Of these 12, 2 required early explanation within the first 2 weeks due to dysphagia and odynophagia with associated gastritis. In the 12-month trial, the mean %EWL was 35.9. Six of the 10 remaining patients had fully attached and functional devices during the follow-up period, and achieved a mean %EWL of 54 at the end of the study period. All patients with diabetes had improvements in their fasting glucose levels and were off medications during the study period. Five of the seven patients with hypertension were off medications. No post-explant adverse events were noted [47].

## Endoscopic Anastomosis Devices (Incisionless Magnetic Anastomosis System)

FDA Status: Not Approved in the USA.
Used Internationally.

The Incisionless Magnetic Anastomosis System (IMAS) is a novel technique used to create a dual-path enteral bypass allowing nutrients to flow through native anatomy and the jejuno-ileal anastomosis. The anastomosis is created by

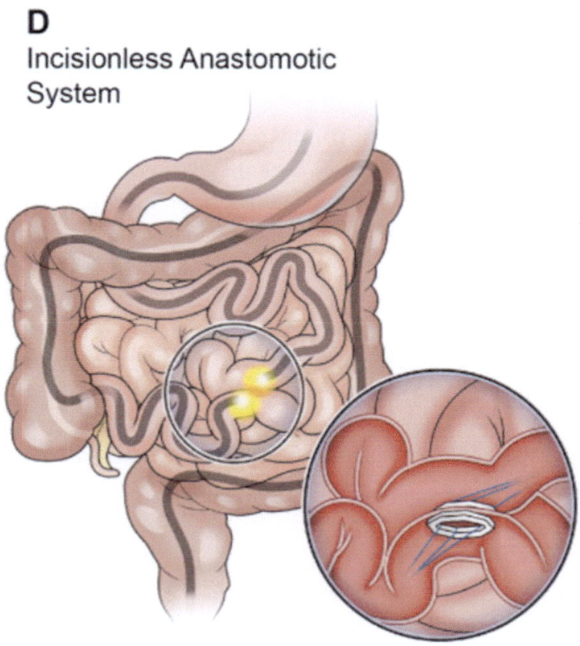


**Fig. 18.9** Placement of IMAS in distal small intestine

simultaneous deployment of self-assembling magnets in the proximal jejunum and ileum. Once the magnets are deployed and couple, they cause necrosis in the tissue sandwiched between them with remodeling of surrounding tissue (Fig. 18.9). This leads to formation of an anastomosis [30].

## Technique

General anesthesia is used for this procedure. A marker is laparoscopically placed in the ileal mesentery 250 cm from the cecum with medium to large clips, and a retrievable metal bowel clamp is placed 10–15 cm distal to the ligament of Treitz. The first magnet is transported via endoscopy to the fourth part of the duodenum and released in the proximal jejunum, where it is attracted to the clamp. The endoscope is retracted to the stomach. A positioning device is used to grasp the magnet, the clamp is removed, and the magnet is directed through the jejunal lumen to the marked ileal position. The second magnet is delivered through the endoscope to the intended magnet fusion site in the first portion of the duodenum and released to self-align with the distal magnet through the intestinal walls. The endoscope and magnet positioning device are withdrawn, and the mesenteric defect is closed with running 2-0 silk suture [48].

## Post-Procedure Care and Follow-Up

Patients can be monitored overnight. Successful magnet placement can be confirmed with abdominal X-ray and fluoroscopically using gastrografin. Patients meet with a nutritionist prior to discharge to discuss diet. In 2–4 weeks, the magnets are expected to be fully fused. Subsequently, they will detach from the duodeno ileal site and be expelled naturally.

### Outcomes and Complications

Machytka et al. [49] conducted the first in-human pilot study to evaluate the technical feasibility and safety of IMAS to create a partial jejunal diversion. Ten patients with obesity and type 2 diabetes, prediabetes, or no diabetes were enrolled. The average total body weight loss was 14.6 and 40.2% EWL at 12 months. A significant reduction in Hgb A1C level was observed in all diabetic (−1.9%) and prediabetic (−1.0%) patients, while reducing or eliminating the use of diabetes medications. No serious complications were noted, but most patients had transient nausea and diarrhea that resolved.

## Conclusion

EBMT is a rapidly evolving field that has yielded promising short-term results. Short-term randomized trials have shown that these techniques provide superior results to medical therapy alone. In addition to their effectiveness in weight loss and comorbidity resolution, there have been promising results in regards to their safety profiles. This has led to their increasing use by surgeons as an alternative to more invasive Bariatric surgical procedures or as an adjunct. Additionally, new techniques, such as endoscopic gastric plication are being studied with encouraging early results. As this field continues to develop, it is important that more randomized trials and long-term studies are performed to assess the long-term efficacy and safety of these techniques and devices. This will likely lead to more of these devices obtaining FDA approval and advancement in the treatment of obesity.

**Box 68.1 Endoscopic Sleeve Gastroplasty Key Steps**

1. Patient positioned: Supine to leftward positioning.
2. General anesthesia induced and endotracheal intubation.
3. Antibiotics administered per guidelines, must cover oral flora.
4. Confirm that $CO_2$ gas is on and that air is off.
5. Initial survey of the GI tract with single lumen scope to rule out contraindications.
6. Esophageal overtube is positioned: Optional, but recommended to reduce pharyngeal trauma.
7. Endoscopic suturing device is mounted onto a double lumen scope.
8. Load suture.
9. Tissue helix is passed through the scope.

10. Initial stitch: Starting at the anterior wall proximal to the incisura.
11. Tissuehelix is pushed into the mucosa and spun to engage tissue: 2 full turns, then pulled away from surrounding organs prior to 1–2 additional turns. A swirling of the tissue will indicate that the tissue is engaged.
12. The tissue is pulled towards the suturing system to ensure gastric tissue is free of surrounding structures.
13. Full-thickness serosa to serosa bite is initiated with suturing system.
14. The needle is then toggled and reloaded onto the suture device ready for the next bite.
15. Bites are taken advancing towards the greater curvature forming an O or U-shaped pattern.
16. Suture anchor is released.
17. Cinch is initiated using the suture cinching device and the suture is anchored and cut.
18. The suturing device is reloaded with a new suture and the process is repeated until the junction between the fundus and proximal body of the stomach is reached.
19. The overtube, if utilized in step 6, is now removed.
20. A final endoscopy is performed to assess the sleeve. The esophagus and oropharynx are also inspected to ensure no tissue trauma.

## References

1. Obesity and overweight. n.d. Retrieved October 19, 2023, from https://www.who.int/news-room/fact-sheets/detail/obesity-and-overweight.
2. Schauer PR, Bhatt DL, Kirwan JP, Wolski K, Aminian A, Brethauer SA, Navaneethan SD, Singh RP, Pothier CE, Nissen SE, Kashyap SR. Bariatric surgery versus intensive medical therapy for diabetes—5-year outcomes. N Engl J Med. 2017;376(7):641–51. https://doi.org/10.1056/NEJMoa1600869.
3. Shahnazarian V, Ramai D, Sarkar A. Endoscopic bariatric therapies for treating obesity: a learning curve for gastroenterologists. Transl Gastroenterol Hepatol. 2019;4:16. 10.21037/tgh.2019.03.01
4. Nieben OG, Harboe H. INTRAGASTRIC balloon as an artificial bezoar for treatment of obesity. Lancet. 1982;319(8265):198–9. https://doi.org/10.1016/S0140-6736(82)90762-0.
5. Štimac D, Klobučar Majanović S, Belančić A. Endoscopic treatment of obesity: from past to future. Dig Dis. 2020;38(2):150–62. https://doi.org/10.1159/000505394.
6. Percival WL. "The balloon diet": a noninvasive treatment for morbid obesity. Preliminary report of 108 patients. Can J Surg. 1984;27(2):135–6.
7. Goyal H, Kopel J, Perisetti A, Mann R, Ali A, Tharian B, Saligram S, Inamdar S. Endobariatric procedures for obesity: clinical indications and available options. Therap Adv Gastroint Endos. 2021;2021:14. Retrieved October 19, 2023, from https://journals.sagepub.com/doi/full/10.1177/2631774520984627#bibr4-2631774520984627.

8. Jirapinyo P, Thompson CC. Endoscopic bariatric and metabolic therapies: surgical analogues and mechanisms of action. Clin Gastroenterol Hepatol. 2017;15(5):619–30. https://doi.org/10.1016/j.cgh.2016.10.021.
9. Sallet JA, Marchesini JB, Paiva DS, Komoto K, Pizani CE, Ribeiro ML, et al. Brazilian multicenter study of the intragastric balloon. Obes Surg. 2004 Aug;14(7):991–8.
10. Crossan K, Sheer AJ. Intragastric balloon. In: StatPearls [Internet]. Treasure Island, FL: StatPearls Publishing; 2022. [cited 2023 Feb 22]. Available from: http://www.ncbi.nlm.nih.gov/books/NBK578184/.
11. Silva LB, Neto MG. Intragastric balloon. Minim Invasive Ther Allied Technol MITAT Off J Soc Minim Invasive Ther. 2022;31(4):505–14.
12. Schapiro M, Benjamin S, Blackburn G, Frank B, Heber D, Kozarek R, et al. Obesity and the gastric balloon: a comprehensive workshop. Gastrointest Endosc. 1987;33(4):323–7.
13. Suchartlikitwong S, Laoveeravat P, Mingbunjerdsuk T, Vutthikraivit W, Ismail A, Islam S, et al. Usefulness of the ReShape intragastric balloon for obesity. Proc Bayl Univ Med Cent. 2019;32(2):192–5.
14. Genco A, Ernesti I, Ienca R, Casella G, Mariani S, Francomano D, et al. Safety and efficacy of a new swallowable intragastric balloon not needing endoscopy: early Italian experience. Obes Surg. 2018;28(2):405–9.
15. Galloro G, Sivero L, Magno L, Diamantis G, Pastore A, Karagiannopulos P, et al. New technique for endoscopic removal of Intragastric balloon placed for treatment of morbid obesity. Obes Surg. 2007;17(5):658–62.
16. Vyas D, Deshpande K, Pandya Y. Advances in endoscopic balloon therapy for weight loss and its limitations. World J Gastroenterol. 2017;23(44):7813–7.
17. Ponce J, Woodman G, Swain J, Wilson E, English W, Ikramuddin S, et al. The REDUCE pivotal trial: a prospective, randomized controlled pivotal trial of a dual intragastric balloon for the treatment of obesity. Surg Obes Relat Dis Off J Am Soc Bariatr Surg. 2015;11(4):874–81.
18. Yorke E, Switzer NJ, Reso A, Shi X, de Gara C, Birch D, et al. Intragastric balloon for management of severe obesity: a systematic review. Obes Surg. 2016;26(9):2248–54.
19. Abu Dayyeh BK, Rajan E, Gostout CJ. Endoscopic sleeve gastroplasty: a potential endoscopic alternative to surgical sleeve gastrectomy for treatment of obesity. Gastrointest Endosc. 2013;78(3):530–5.
20. Lopez-Nava G, Sharaiha RZ, Vargas EJ, Bazerbachi F, Manoel GN, Bautista-Castaño I, et al. Endoscopic sleeve gastroplasty for obesity: a multicenter study of 248 patients with 24 months follow-up. Obes Surg. 2017;27(10):2649–55.
21. Abu Dayyeh BK, Acosta A, Camilleri M, Mundi MS, Rajan E, Topazian MD, et al. Endoscopic sleeve gastroplasty alters gastric physiology and induces loss of body weight in obese individuals. Clin Gastroenterol Hepatol. 2017;15(1):37–43.e1.
22. Lopez-Nava G, Galvao M, Bautista-Castaño I, Fernandez-Corbelle JP, Trell M. Endoscopic sleeve gastroplasty with 1-year follow-up: factors predictive of success. Endosc Int Open. 2016;4(2):E222–7.
23. Abu Dayyeh BK, Bazerbachi F, Vargas EJ, Sharaiha RZ, Thompson CC, Thaemert BC, et al. Endoscopic sleeve gastroplasty for treatment of class 1 and 2 obesity (MERIT): a prospective, multicentre, randomised trial. Lancet. 2022;400(10350):441–51.
24. Hedjoudje A, Abu Dayyeh BK, Cheskin LJ, Adam A, Neto MG, Badurdeen D, et al. Efficacy and safety of endoscopic sleeve Gastroplasty: a systematic review and meta-analysis. Clin Gastroenterol Hepatol. 2020;18(5):1043–1053.e4.
25. Qureshi H, Saeed N, Jovani M. Updates in endoscopic bariatric and metabolic therapies. J Clin Med. 2023;12(3):1126. https://doi.org/10.3390/jcm12031126.
26. Espinós JC, Turró R, Mata A, Cruz M, da Costa M, Villa V, Buchwald JN, Turró J. Early experience with the Incisionless operating platform™ (IOP) for the treatment of obesity. Obes Surg. 2013;23(9):1375–83. https://doi.org/10.1007/s11695-013-0937-8.
27. Sullivan S, Swain JM, Woodman G, Antonetti M, De La Cruz-Muñoz N, Jonnalagadda SS, Ujiki M, Ikramuddin S, Ponce J, Ryou M, Reynoso J, Chhabra R, Sorenson GB, Clarkston WK, Edmundowicz SA, Eagon JC, Mullady DK, Leslie D, Lavin TE, Thompson CC. Randomized sham-controlled trial evaluating efficacy and safety of endoscopic gastric plication for pri-

mary obesity: the ESSENTIAL trial. Obesity. 2017;25(2):294–301. https://doi.org/10.1002/oby.21702.
28. Miller K, Turró R, Greve JW, Bakker CM, Buchwald JN, Espinós JC. MILEPOST multicenter randomized controlled trial: 12-month weight loss and satiety outcomes after pose SM vs medical therapy. Obes Surg. 2017;27(2):310–22. https://doi.org/10.1007/s11695-016-2295-9.
29. Ellsmere JC, Thompson CC, Brugge WR, Chuttani R, Desilets DJ, Rattner DW, Tarnoff ME, Kaplan LM. Endoscopic interventions for weight loss surgery. Obesity. 2009;17(5):929–33. https://doi.org/10.1038/oby.2008.588.
30. Sullivan S, Edmundowicz SA, Thompson CC. Endoscopic bariatric and metabolic therapies: new and emerging technologies. Gastroenterology. 2017;152(7):1791–801. https://doi.org/10.1053/j.gastro.2017.01.044.
31. Ruban A, Ashrafian H, Teare JP. The EndoBarrier: duodenal-Jejunal bypass liner for diabetes and weight loss. Gastroenterol Res Pract. 2018;2018:7823182. https://doi.org/10.1155/2018/7823182.
32. Jirapinyo P, Haas AV, Thompson CC. Effect of the duodenal-Jejunal bypass liner on glycemic control in patients with type 2 diabetes with obesity: a meta-analysis with secondary analysis on weight loss and hormonal changes. Diabetes Care. 2018;41(5):1106–15. https://doi.org/10.2337/dc17-1985.
33. Meek CL, Lewis HB, Reimann F, Gribble FM, Park AJ. The effect of bariatric surgery on gastrointestinal and pancreatic peptide hormones. Peptides. 2016;77:28–37. https://doi.org/10.1016/j.peptides.2015.08.013.
34. Mingrone G, Panunzi S, De Gaetano A, Guidone C, Iaconelli A, Nanni G, Castagneto M, Bornstein S, Rubino F. Bariatric-metabolic surgery versus conventional medical treatment in obese patients with type 2 diabetes: 5 year follow-up of an open-label, single-centre, randomised controlled trial. Lancet. 2015;386(9997):964–73. https://doi.org/10.1016/S0140-6736(15)00075-6.
35. Buse JB, Caprio S, Cefalu WT, Ceriello A, Del Prato S, Inzucchi SE, McLaughlin S, Phillips GL, Robertson RP, Rubino F, Kahn R, Kirkman MS. How do we define cure of diabetes? Diabetes Care. 2009;32(11):2133–5. https://doi.org/10.2337/dc09-9036.
36. Brethauer SA, Aminian A, Romero-Talamás H, Batayyah E, Mackey J, Kennedy L, Kashyap SR, Kirwan JP, Rogula T, Kroh M, Chand B, Schauer PR. Can diabetes be surgically cured? Long-term metabolic effects of bariatric surgery in obese patients with type 2 diabetes mellitus. Ann Surg. 2013;258(4):628–36.; discussion 636-637. https://doi.org/10.1097/SLA.0b013e3182a5034b.
37. Pournaras DJ, Aasheim ET, Søvik TT, Andrews R, Mahon D, Welbourn R, Olbers T, le Roux CW. Effect of the definition of type II diabetes remission in the evaluation of bariatric surgery for metabolic disorders. Br J Surg. 2012;99(1):100–3. https://doi.org/10.1002/bjs.7704.
38. Buchwald H, Avidor Y, Braunwald E, Jensen MD, Pories W, Fahrbach K, Schoelles K. Bariatric surgery: a systematic review and meta-analysis. JAMA. 2004;292(14):1724–37. https://doi.org/10.1001/jama.292.14.1724.
39. American Diabetes Association. Economic costs of diabetes in the U.S. in 2012. Diabetes Care. 2013;36(4):1033–46. https://doi.org/10.2337/dc12-2625.
40. Ogden CL, Carroll MD, Fryar CD, Flegal KM. Prevalence of obesity among adults and youth: United States, 2011–2014. NCHS Data Brief. 2015;219:1–8.
41. Neto MG, Rodriguez L, Becerra P, Mani S, Rothstein R. Hydrothermal duodenal mucosal resurfacing: a novel procedural therapy for metabolic disease. VideoGIE. 2016;1(1):10–1.
42. van Baar ACG, Meiring S, Smeele P, Vriend T, Holleman F, Barlag M, et al. Duodenal mucosal resurfacing combined with glucagon-like peptide-1 receptor agonism to discontinue insulin in type 2 diabetes: a feasibility study. Gastrointest Endosc. 2021 Jul;94(1):111–120.e3.
43. Condello G, Chen CY. Minireview: current status of endoscopic duodenal mucosal resurfacing. Obes Res Clin Pract. 2020 Nov;14(6):504–7.
44. van Baar ACG, Devière J, Hopkins D, Crenier L, Holleman F, Galvão Neto MP, et al. Durable metabolic improvements 2 years after duodenal mucosal resurfacing (DMR) in patients with type 2 diabetes (REVITA-1 study). Diabetes Res Clin Pract. 2022 Feb;1(184):109194.

45. Stimac D, Majanović SK. Endoscopic approaches to obesity. Dig Dis. 2012;30(2):187–95. https://doi.org/10.1159/000336683.
46. Sandler BJ, Rumbaut R, Paul Swain C, Torres G, Morales L, Gonzales L, Schultz S, Talamini M, Horgan S. Human experience with an endoluminal, endoscopic, gastrojejunal bypass sleeve. Surg Endosc. 2011;25(9):3028–33. https://doi.org/10.1007/s00464-011-1665-6.
47. Sandler BJ, Rumbaut R, Swain CP, Torres G, Morales L, Gonzales L, Schultz S, Talamini MA, Jacobsen GR, Horgan S. One-year human experience with a novel endoluminal, endoscopic gastric bypass sleeve for morbid obesity. Surg Endosc. 2015;29(11):3298–303. https://doi.org/10.1007/s00464-015-4081-5.
48. Gagner M, Abuladze D, Koiava L, Buchwald JN, Van Sante N, Krinke T. First-in-human side-to-side magnetic compression duodeno-ileostomy with the magnet anastomosis system. Obes Surg. 2023;33(8):2282–92. https://doi.org/10.1007/s11695-023-06708-x.
49. Machytka E, Bužga M, Zonca P, Lautz DB, Ryou M, Simonson DC, Thompson CC. Partial jejunal diversion using an incisionless magnetic anastomosis system: 1-year interim results in patients with obesity and diabetes. Gastrointest Endosc. 2017;86(5):904–12. https://doi.org/10.1016/j.gie.2017.07.009.

# Adjustable Gastric Banding: Indications and Technique

# 19

Loic Tchokouani, Marina Kurian, and Megan Jenkins

## Introduction

Gastric banding used for the surgical treatment of obesity has undergone many product advancements and technique modifications since its inception in 1978 by Wilkinson and Peloso [1]. Wilkinson and Peloso placed the first gastric band and of note, this band was nonadjustable. It was done via an open technique involving constructing a floppy Nissen fundoplication, and then wrapping the fundoplication with either Dacron, Tacron, or polypropylene mesh. In two different countries concurrently, an adjustable gastric band made of silicone was developed by Kuzmak et al [2] and Foresell et al. [3] Both of these bands were placed via an open approach. The advent and spread of laparoscopy greatly influenced the treatment of obesity. In 1993 Broadbent et al [4] in Australia, and Catona et al [5] in Italy, were the first to implant nonadjustable gastric bands laparoscopically. In 1995, Belachew et al [6] working in Belgium placed the first adjustable gastric band laparoscopically. This was followed by the first workshop held in 1994 in Sweden.

Many brands of adjustable gastric bands have existed however only one currently has FDA approval in the United States: The Lap Band® (Reshape Lifesciences, Irvine, CA). Inamed initially obtained approval in 2001 and the technology was eventually sold to ReShape. The Realize Band® (Ethicon Endo-Surgery, Cincinnati, OH) initially received FDA approval in 2007 but was discontinued by the manufacturer in 2016. Two other bands are used outside of the United States: the Heliogast HAGA® (Helioscopie Vienne, France), and the Midband™ (Mid, Lyon, France) bands.

L. Tchokouani (✉) · M. Kurian · M. Jenkins
NYU Langone Health, New York, NY, USA
e-mail: Loic.Tchokouani@nyulangone.org; Marina.Kurian@nyulangone.org; Megan.Jenkins@nyulangone.org


O. M. Ghanem et al. (eds.), *The SAGES Manual of Metabolic and Bariatric Surgery*, https://doi.org/10.1007/978-3-031-72309-4_19

As the adjustable gastric banding tool evolved via various iterations, the placement technique has as well. Despite the promising results of minimally invasive and minimally anatomy-altering bariatric surgery, there was a noticeable rate of complications with the band procedure. Band erosions, and more frequently band slippages, were seen and required further surgical interventions. The technique described by Broadbent et al [4] involved entering the lesser sac through the lesser omentum, just above the left gastric vessels. A pressure gauge had to be used intraoperatively to make sure the band wasn't too tight. Oftentimes, the band was also inflated intraoperatively. This technique left the patient with a larger pouch, the lesser sac violated close to gastric vessels, variable length of dissection, and a tight band.

Fielding amongst other authors hypothesized the aforementioned features of this first technique directly contributed to the gastric prolapse [7], i.e. band slippages, seen at the rate of 10–15%. Because of this, a new technique, called the pars flaccida technique was developed. [8–13]

## Technique

In the operating room, the patient is placed supine in the reverse Trendelenburg position, with the legs together with no stirrups used. The surgeon stands on the patient's right side, with the monitors at the head of the bed. A split-leg approach can also be used.

The abdomen should be entered in the safest possible way for the surgeon (Veress needle, optiview, cut down). A total of four laparoscopic trocars will be used as well as a liver retractor of the surgeon's choice. Fielding recommends placing trocars in a similar fashion when performing a Nissen fundoplication [13] (See Fig. 19.1). The adjustable gastric band system is primed with sterile saline and inserted into the abdomen in a spot that is easily retrievable later via the 15-mm port. The angle of

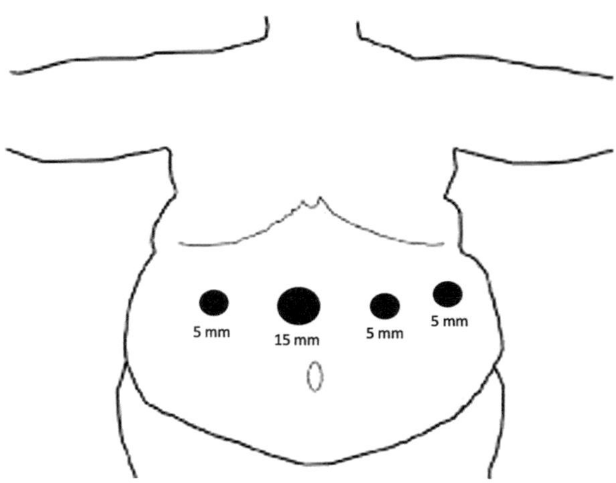


**Fig. 19.1** Suggested placement of trocars

His needs to be explored and the fundus needs to be freed from the diaphragm (See Fig. 19.2). This should be well above the level of the short gastric vessels. This can be done with blunt dissection and/or electrocautery. If an enlarged fat pad is seen, it should be excised as it can disrupt the proper position on the Lap Band.

The pars flaccida is then divided, being mindful of any aberrant left hepatic arteries and the hepatic branch of the vagus nerve (See Fig. 19.3). The nerve should be spared unless the patient has already had a cholecystectomy. The aberrant hepatic artery should also be spared. Once the pars flaccida is incised, the right crus will be visible inferomedially to the caudate lobe of the liver. It is also prudent to note the location of the inferior vena cava which is just to the right and parallel to the right crus.

Once the right crus is identified, the peritoneum just medial to the crus must be incised. The right lateral-most trocar provides the best angle for the next maneuver. A grasper is then placed through the scored peritoneum, medial to the crus, but behind the esophagus. It should be able to emerge into the previously dissected

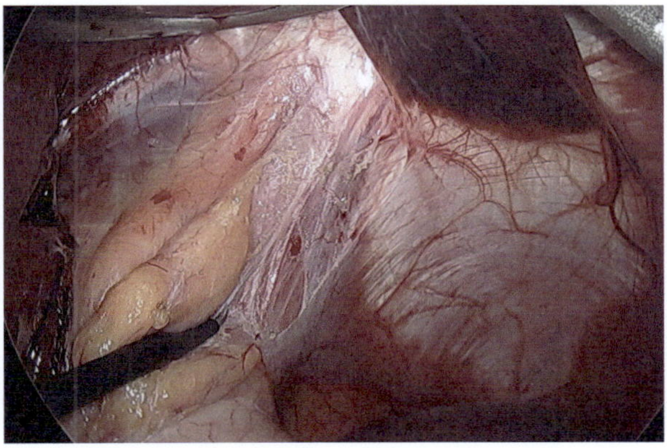

**Fig. 19.2** Dissection of the angle of His

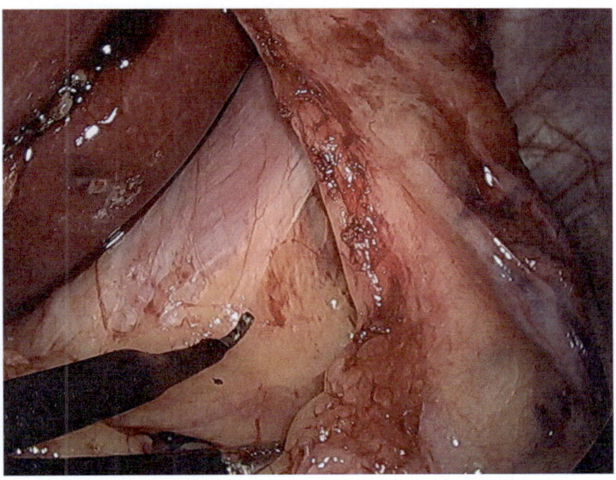

**Fig. 19.3** View after pars flaccida incised and right crus identified

angle of His for a very short distance of about 3–4 cm. Very little force is required to emerge from the right side of the angle of His and if resistance is encountered, a re-examination of the angle taken should be done (See Fig. 19.4).

With the retro-gastric grasper in the proper position, the end tag of the band is handed to the grasper and pulled around the top portion of the stomach (See Fig. 19.5). If the band doesn't easily come around, additional peritoneal attachments may have to be released medial to the crus. Once the band is locked, a 5-mm instrument should be able to pass between the band and stomach. If not, additional fatty tissue between the stomach and the band should be removed.

After appropriately positioning the band and assessing its tightness around the stomach, attention is turned to securing the band in place. We recommend using a permanent 2-0 suture to perform the gastro-gastric plication over the band. The stomach above and below the band are brought together but without undue tension. The suturing should result in having stomach wall covering the band but not covering the buckle as this can contribute to band erosion. This proper suturing helps

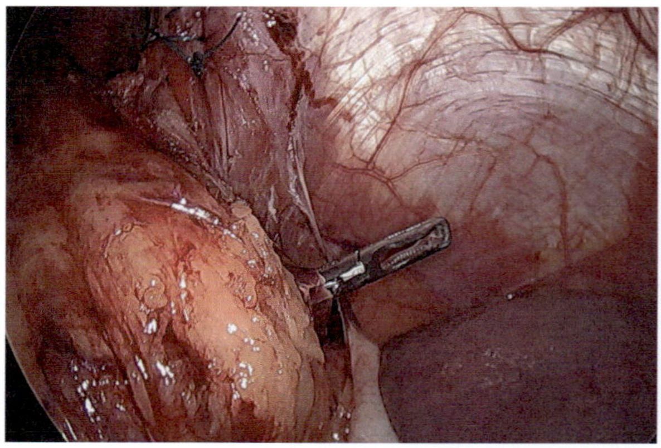

**Fig. 19.4** Posterior dissection

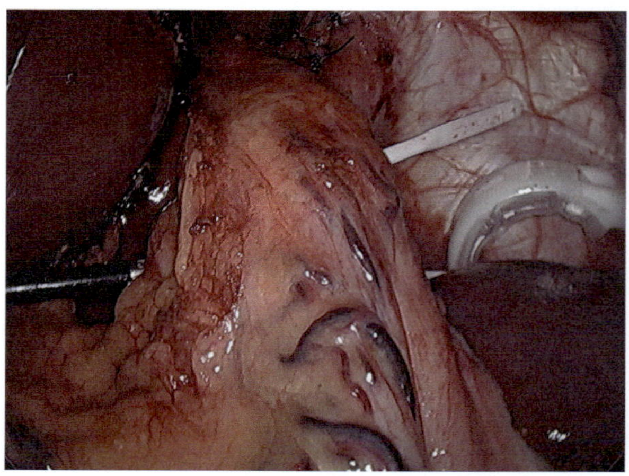

**Fig. 19.5** Band brough through posterior gastric tunnel

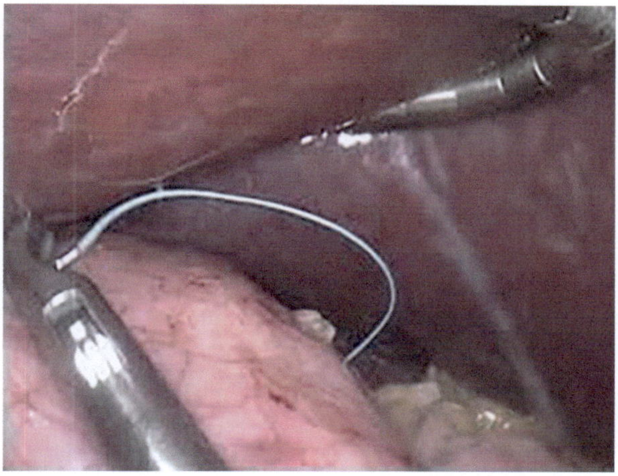

**Fig. 19.6** Gastro-gastric plication over the locked band

prevent herniation of the fundus upward through the band. The suturing should be started as far posterior-lateral as possible and then continued medially to just shy of the lesser curve vessels as this area has been hypothesized as a location of band slippage. Usually, 3–5 running stitches should suffice for the plication (See Fig. 19.6). Some surgeons do a plication below the level of the band to also decrease slippage [14].

Once the band is properly secured, the laparoscopic portion of the procedure is over. The band tubing is now brought out via one of the laparoscopic ports. The port incision is extended lateral and deep down until the rectus sheath is reached. The tubing is then connected to the access port and the port is sutured to the anterior sheath with permanent suture. It is important to verify that the tubing does not enter the abdomen at a right angle but instead at a shallow angle. The band is typically left empty until the first esophagram 4–6 weeks after placement; however, some surgeons may elect to fill the band with 2–3 mL of saline intraoperatively.

## Indications

The indications for adjustable gastric band placement for obesity follow the same guidelines as other bariatric surgeries including the sleeve gastrectomy, the different forms of gastric bypass, the duodenal switches, and revisions for weight gain. The 1991 NIH guidelines were historically used and these included patients with BMI >40, and those with a BMI >35 with other comorbidities associated with obesity (hypertension, sleep apnea, fatty liver disease, diabetes mellitus, etc.) Newer guidelines from the American Society of Metabolic and Bariatric Surgery (ASMBS) and the International Federation of Surgical Obesity and Metabolic Disorders (IFSO) have been released to expand the indications for bariatric surgery. The updated guidelines now recommend bariatric surgery to those patients with BMI >35 regardless of the presence, absence, or severity of obesity-related conditions. Additionally, bariatric surgery should be considered in those patients with a BMI of 30–34.9 and metabolic disease. Even those patients who are unable to achieve substantial and/or durable weight loss or obesity disease-related improvement using non-surgical methods should also be considered candidates for bariatric surgery. Further, ethnic and population differences were considered and bariatric surgery should also be considered for those of Asian descent with a BMI greater than 27.5. Finally, adolescents and select children as well could be candidates for operative intervention [15].

Adjustable gastric band placement represents approximately 1% of bariatric procedures performed. [16] To maximize success with an adjustable gastric band, patient selection and practice structure is paramount. The bariatric practice responsible for the follow-up must continue to maintain the capacity to see their adjustable gastric band patients regularly and even as walk-ins in case of band complications, i.e. slippage or over-adjustment. In concert with a capable practice, patients choosing to receive an adjustable gastric band must be able to continue with frequent and long-term follow-up to ensure short and long-term success. Due to the adjustable nature of the band, the patient must maintain the mentality of continuous follow-up and adjustments. Additionally, expectations must be managed with patients in terms of lifestyle and percentage of excess weight loss. A study by Angrisani et al [17] looking at results for those patients with a BMI >50 who underwent lap-band placement saw a majority of patients that remained with BMIs >35 but did have comorbidity resolution or severity improvement. Angrisani et al [18] also examined outcomes with those patients with a BMI less than or equal to 35. With over 200 patients studied, there was complete resolution of comorbidities with only one patient with a BMI over 30 at 1 year. Additionally, a study by Dixon et al [19] showed more than 76% of the patients successfully achieved the 30% EWL benchmark and even had sustained improvement in generic and weight-specific quality of life, symptoms of depression and the prevalence of binge-eating disorder. The number of subjects with normal fasting triglyceride, high-density lipoprotein cholesterol, plasma glucose and HbA1c increased significantly between baseline and 5 years. Therefore we recommend dedicated pre-operative counseling for all patients undergoing band placement with special expectation discussion with those patients with BMI >50. Patients undergoing adjustable gastric band placement seem to more benefit overall with a lower BMI than those with higher BMIs.

## Band Management

In our practice, band adjustments are performed without the use of imaging, although many bariatric practices utilize fluoroscopy. Adjustments to increase band fluid are offered when patients report increased hunger or larger food intake, while fluid removal is recommended for patients experiencing reflux, night cough, or vomiting. At each visit, a dietary history is taken, and patients are reminded of important behaviors to enhance band outcomes, such as taking small bites, chewing thoroughly, and eating meals slowly. Esophagrams are conducted annually to evaluate esophageal dilation, band positioning, and reflux. Additionally, an esophagram is performed whenever patients exhibit concerning or new symptoms.

## References


1. Wilkinson LH, Peloso OA. Gastric (reservoir) reduction for morbid obesity. Arch Surg. 1981;116(5):602–5. https://doi.org/10.1001/ARCHSURG.1981.01380170082014.
2. Kuzmak LI, Yap IS, McGuire L, Dixon JS, Young MP. Surgery for morbid obesity: using an inflatable gastric band. AORN J. 1990;51(5):1307–24. https://doi.org/10.1016/S0001-2092(07)70154-0.
3. Forsell P, Hallberg D, Hellers G. Gastric banding for morbid obesity: initial experience with a new adjustable band. Obes Surg. 1993;3:369–74. https://doi.org/10.1381/096089293765559052.
4. Broadbent R, Tracey M, Harrington P. Modern surgery: technical innovations laparoscopic gastric banding: a preliminary report. Obes Surg. 1993;3(1):63–7. https://doi.org/10.1381/096089293765559791.
5. Catona A, Gossenberg M, La Manna A, Mussini G. Modern Surgery: Technical Innovations Laparoscopic Gastric Banding: preliminary series. Obes Surg. 1993;3(2):207–9. https://doi.org/10.1381/096089293765559610.
6. Belachew M, Legrand M, Vincent V, et al. Modern surgery: technical innovations laparoscopic placement of adjustable silicone gastric band in the treatment of morbid obesity: how to do it. Obes Surg. 1995;5(1):66–70. https://doi.org/10.1381/096089295765558196.
7. Belachew M, Legrand M, Vincent V, Lismonde M, Le Docte N, Deschamps V. Laparoscopic adjustable gastric banding. World J Surg. 1998;22:955–63.
8. Favretti F, Cadière GB, Segato G, et al. Laparoscopic banding: selection and technique in 830 patients. Obes Surg. 2002;12(3):385–90. https://doi.org/10.1381/096089202321087922.
9. Weiner R, Boekhorn H, Rosenthal R, Wagner D. Surgical endoscopy ultrasound and interventional techniques: a prospective randomized trial of different laparoscopic gastric banding techniques for morbid. Obesity. 2001;15:63–8.
10. Favretti F, Cadiere GB, Segato G, et al. Laparoscopic adjustable silicone gastric-banding (Lap-Band@): how to avoid complications. Obes Surg. 1997;7(4):352–8. https://doi.org/10.1381/096089297765555610.
11. Rubin M, Benchetrit S, Lustigman H, Lelcuk S, Spivak H. Laparoscopic gastric banding with Lap-Band for morbid obesity: two-step technique may improve outcome. Obes Surg. 2001;11(3):315–7. https://doi.org/10.1381/096089201321336674.
12. O'brien PE, Brown WA, Smith A, Mcmurrick PJ, Stephens M. Prospective study of a laparoscopically placed, adjustable gastric band in the treatment of morbid obesity. Br J Surg. 1998;86:113–8. https://academic.oup.com/bjs/article/86/1/113/6269597.
13. Fielding GA, Allen JW. A step-by-step guide to placement of the LAP-BAND adjustable gastric banding system. Am J Surg. 2002;184(6 SUPPL. 2):S26–30. https://doi.org/10.1016/S0002-9610(02)01176-5.
14. Malapan K, Ghinagow A, Se AO, et al. Laparoscopic Adjustable Gastric Banded Plication (LAGBP): the next big thing? Curr Surg Rep. 2013;1(3):142–8. https://doi.org/10.1007/s40137-013-0024-z.
15. Eisenberg D, Shikora SA, Aarts E, et al. 2022 American Society for Metabolic and Bariatric Surgery (ASMBS) and International Federation for the Surgery of Obesity and Metabolic Disorders (IFSO): indications for metabolic and bariatric surgery. Surg Obes Relat Dis. 2022;18(12):1345–56. https://doi.org/10.1016/j.soard.2022.08.013.
16. Metabolic & Bariatric Surgery Fact Sheet 2021; 2021.
17. Angrisani L, Furbetta F, Doldi SB, et al. Results of the Italian multicenter study on 239 super-obese patients treated by adjustable gastric banding. Obes Surg. 2002;12(6):846–50. https://doi.org/10.1381/096089202320995682.
18. Angrisani L, Favretti F, Furbetta F, et al. Italian Group for Lap-Band System®: results of multicenter study on patients with BMI < or =35 kg/m². Obes Surg. 2004;14(3):415–8. https://doi.org/10.1381/096089204322917963.
19. Dixon JB, Eaton LL, Vincent V, Michaelson R. LAP-BAND for BMI 30–40: 5-year health outcomes from the multicenter pivotal study. Int J Obes. 2016;40(2):291–8. https://doi.org/10.1038/ijo.2015.156.

# Sleeve Gastrectomy: Indications and Technique

20

Pauline Aeschbacher, Samuel Szomstein, Emanuele Lo Menzo, and Raul J. Rosenthal

## Introduction

Between 2017 and 2020, obesity was present in 19.7% of children and adolescents and in 41.9% of the adult population [1]. However, during the same period, only 0.2% of the US population underwent metabolic and bariatric procedures [2]. In the search for durable and safe solutions to treat obesity, bariatric surgery has rapidly become popular as the most effective treatment of obesity and related diseases. As its effect becomes more evident, indications for bariatric surgery are expanding. Even though its introduction in bariatric surgery came later, sleeve gastrectomy quickly gained widespread adoption and, by 2013, was by far the most performed bariatric surgery in the United States. Its safety and technical simplicity with minimal anatomical changes are its strengths. Nevertheless, expertise in this surgery, along with knowledge of its potential pitfalls, is mandatory to ensure optimal outcomes.

## The History of Sleeve Gastrectomy

The concept of a vertically shaped gastroplasty for obesity treatment was described in 2001 by Carmichael AR and Johnston D [3–5]. The procedure, named the "Magenstrasse and Mill Procedure," was reported as a safe and more physiological alternative to vertical banded gastroplasty (VBG) and Roux-en-Y gastric bypass (RYGB), providing significant weight loss with potential benefits on insulin

P. Aeschbacher · S. Szomstein · E. L. Menzo · R. J. Rosenthal (✉)
Department of General Surgery and the Bariatric and Metabolic Institute, Cleveland Clinic Florida, Weston, FL, USA
e-mail: pauline.aeschbacher@insel.ch; szomsts@ccf.org; lomenze@ccf.org; rosentr@ccf.org



O. M. Ghanem et al. (eds.), *The SAGES Manual of Metabolic and Bariatric Surgery*, https://doi.org/10.1007/978-3-031-72309-4_20

resistance and cardiovascular risk. However, this procedure only began to gain popularity in the 1990s when Hess and Marceau independently described a tubular-shaped gastroplasty as an alternative restrictive component of the biliopancreatic diversion with duodenal switch (BPD/DS) drastically reducing the rate of marginal ulcer and dumping syndrome [6, 7].

With the goal of finding a safer surgical option for patients with a BMI greater than 60 kg/m$^2$, Regan et al. utilized sleeve gastrectomy as the first step of a two-stage procedure [8]. At this stage, sleeve gastrectomy has demonstrated its effectiveness in achieving initial weight loss, thus allowing for the subsequent confection of either an RYGB or BPD/DS a few months later. In this context, sleeve gastrectomy was found to be effective even if the second procedure was not performed [9, 10]. The concept of sleeve gastrectomy as a stand-alone procedure was supported during the Second International Consensus Summit for Sleeve Gastrectomy in 2009 [11]. In 2012, the American Society for Metabolic and Bariatric Surgery finally recognized sleeve gastrectomy as an "acceptable primary bariatric procedure option." [12] One year later, sleeve gastrectomy became the most performed metabolic and bariatric surgery.

## Mechanism of Action

Two main mechanisms of action account for the substantial weight loss associated with sleeve gastrectomy. First, there is the mechanical restrictive component, which reduces 70–80% of the gastric volume, inherently leading to a lower food intake. Secondly, endocrine changes in the gut and brain hormones—mainly ghrelin, glucagon-like peptide-1 and peptide YY—are responsible for increased satiety, reduced hunger, improved glucose metabolism, and slower intestinal motility (ileal brake).

Sleeve gastrectomy stands out for conserving the usual food route and preserving relevant anatomical structures such as the vagus branches, the pylorus, and a portion of the stomach, especially the antrum. This makes sleeve gastrectomy a more "physiological" option compared to other bariatric procedures.

## Indications

According to ASMBS/IFSO guidelines, metabolic and bariatric surgery should be considered in patients with obesity class II or class I with metabolic diseases, and lower thresholds are considered for the Asian population [13]. Sleeve gastrectomy can be considered for this population alongside RYGB or less common procedures such as adjustable gastric banding, BPD/DS, or one-anastomosis gastric bypass.

A multidisciplinary team assessment and patient compliance along with a good understanding of the long-term implications of bariatric surgery are essential [13].

The technical simplicity and low postoperative morbidity rate of sleeve gastrectomy make it the preferred operation in a high-risk population [14]. Not only patients with BMI greater than 60 kg/m$^2$ but also the elderly population, Child's A and B liver cirrhosis, pre-liver, pre-renal, and pre-cardiac transplant patients benefit from sleeve gastrectomy [15–18]. Sleeve gastrectomy is also the option of choice for patients with Crohn's disease due to the absence of small bowel manipulation and anastomosis [19, 20].

Children and adolescents also benefit from metabolic and bariatric surgery, with better comorbidities resolution than adults [21]. However, data and recommendations on the optimal surgery type are lacking. In the young population, sleeve gastrectomy might offer several advantages over other metabolic and bariatric surgeries, with minimal anatomical changes, remaining options for further surgery in adulthood, and potentially lower risk of malabsorption and vitamin deficiencies (except vitamin B12). Sleeve gastrectomy might also be an alternative to consider for future pregnancies.

Absolute contraindications for sleeve gastrectomy are prohibitive anesthesia risk, advanced oncological disease, and severe uncontrolled psychiatric illness (malignant hyperphagia, acute suicidality).

There is a lot of controversy surrounding GERD and sleeve gastrectomy. Generally, other surgical options such as RYGB should be favored for patients with known GERD unless other factors make sleeve gastrectomy a better option (Crohn's disease, high-risk patients). Usually, uncontrolled GERD, especially in the presence of severe reflux esophagitis and Barrett's esophagus, is considered a relative contraindication. Hiatal hernias without esophagitis are not a contraindication for sleeve gastrectomy, but consideration should be given to repairing the hiatal hernia during the surgery [19, 22].

## Preoperative Planning

Preoperative planning of sleeve gastrectomy follows the steps of a typical bariatric planning process, which include preoperative medical, surgical, psychological anesthetic and nutritional expert assessments [23–25]. A multidisciplinary team contributes to preoperative patient optimization and the reduction of complications [26, 27]. Thorough discussions with the patient are crucial to ensure a good understanding of the potential surgical complications and long-term consequences and implications of bariatric surgery. Patients should also receive counseling regarding the nutritional aspects of sleeve gastrectomy both before and after the surgery, along with access to resources for adequate education and optimal preparation, including multidisciplinary seminars and one-to-one consultations.

Esophagogastroduodenoscopy (EGD) can be useful in the preoperative setting for diagnosing conditions such as GERD with reflux esophagitis and Barrett's esophagus, H-pylori gastritis and, less commonly, benign or malign tumors. However, routine EGD remains controversial [28]. Even though this diagnostic tool may provide crucial information, the advantages of conducting it as a standard procedure do not necessarily outweigh its potential risks and costs. In the United States, it is recommended to perform a preoperative EGD only for symptomatic patients [29]. An upper gastrointestinal contrast series might also be useful for diagnosing hiatal hernias, and abdominal ultrasound can be considered when there are concerns about cholecystolithiasis. Esophageal pH testing and manometry should be reserved for specific cases, such as patients with suspected esophagus dysmotility (e.g., achalasia) or GERD.

Since patients with obesity have a higher risk of obesity-related cancer, standard screening, such as colonoscopy and mammography, should not be neglected in this population [30].

## Technique and Pitfalls

Sleeve gastrectomy involves the vertical removal of a portion of the stomach along the greater curvature. The remaining stomach volume typically ranges between 150 to 200 ml with a functional pylorus and a variable section of the antrum left intact.

The laparoscopic approach is the preferred technique for performing sleeve gastrectomy. Open sleeve gastrectomy is occasionally considered as a concomitant surgery, for example, during liver transplantation or in cases of major adhesions, but should otherwise be avoided.

### Diagnostic Laparoscopy and Trocar Placement

The patient is positioned in supine posture on the operating table with appropriate attachments and pads on pressure points. The surgeon and the camera holder are located on the right side of the patient, while the second assistant and the surgical technician are on the left side (Fig. 20.1a). Alternatively, the surgeon can position himself between the patient's legs as the patient is in a French position (Fig. 20.1b). Typically, the authors access the abdominal cavity under direct visualization by placing a 12-mm optical trocar in the supraumbilical region paramedian left. Following an exploration of the abdominal cavity, two auxiliary 5-mm trocars are

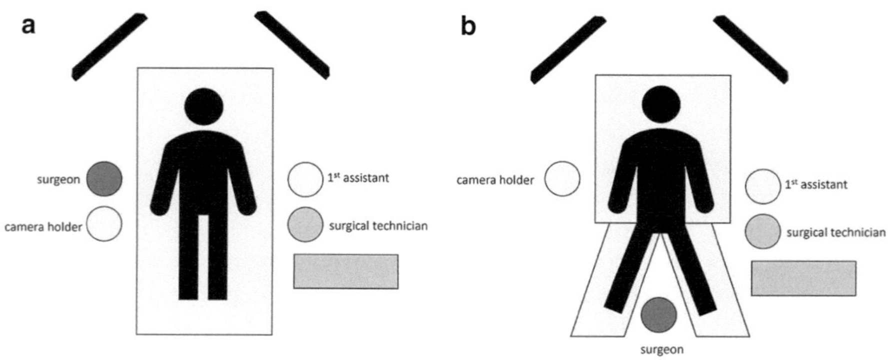


**Fig. 20.1** Surgical setup during a laparoscopic sleeve gastrectomy a) the surgeon stands on the right side of the patient or b) between the patient's legs

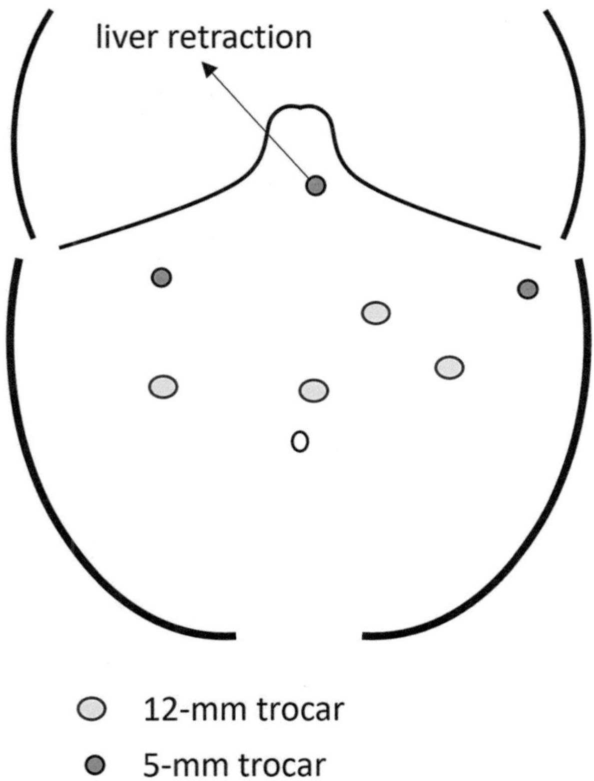


**Fig. 20.2** Trocar position

inserted: one in the subxiphoid region for liver retraction and one below the last rib along the anterior right axillary line for the assistant. The liver is then retracted upward using a "fan-type" retractor. Additional 12-mm trocars are inserted in the right and left upper quadrants, the epigastrium, and a 5-mm trocar in the left paramedian region (Fig. 20.2).

## Pylorus Identification

The pylorus is identified through "palpation" using laparoscopic instruments. Identification of the vein of Mayo at the pyloroduodenal junction might be helpful.

## Mobilization of the Great Curvature

Approximately 6 cm away from the pylorus, the short gastric vessels are divided using an ultrasonic scalpel while lifting the stomach vertically, which provides access to the lesser sac (Fig. 20.3). If the omentum is quite thick, it is advisable to access the lesser sac more superiorly along the greater curvature and then move

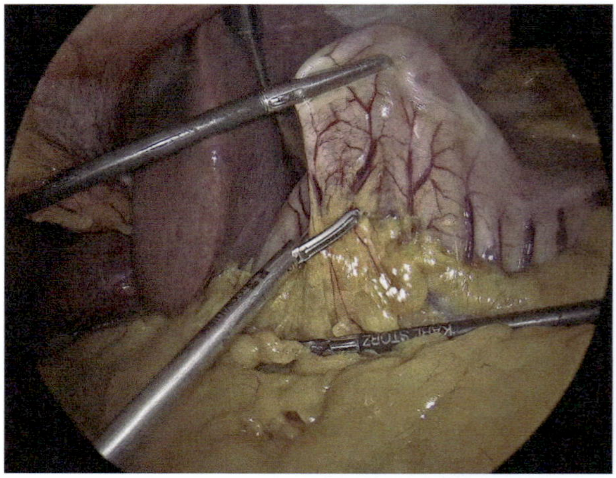

**Fig. 20.3** Dissection of the greater curvature starting 6 cm from the pylorus

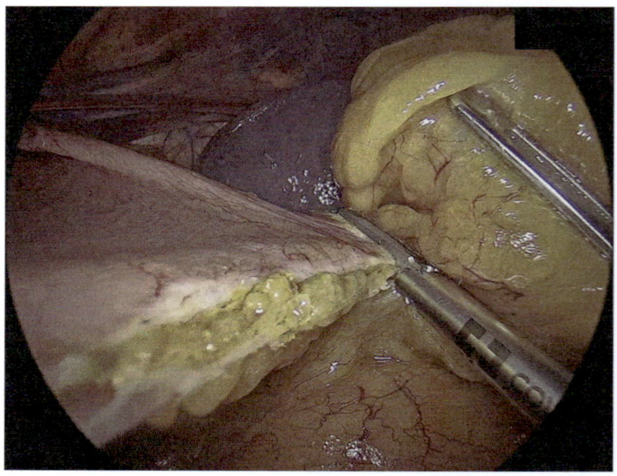

**Fig. 20.4** Dissection of the gastric vessels

more distally toward the pylorus. The remaining short gastric vessels are divided along the greater curvature, close to the stomach. The assistant can provide assistance by holding the major omentum down and carefully stretching the short gastric vessels. Caution should be exercised to avoid causing tears in the spleen capsule due to excessive tension on the short gastric vessel and potential adhesions to the spleen (Fig. 20.4).

Additional posterior gastric adhesions to the pancreas are addressed until a proper visualization of the lesser curvature is achieved (Fig. 20.5).

## Hiatus Evaluation

Discussion on how thoroughly a hiatal hernia should be investigated through intraoperative dissection is still ongoing [31, 32]. The authors recommend an aggressive

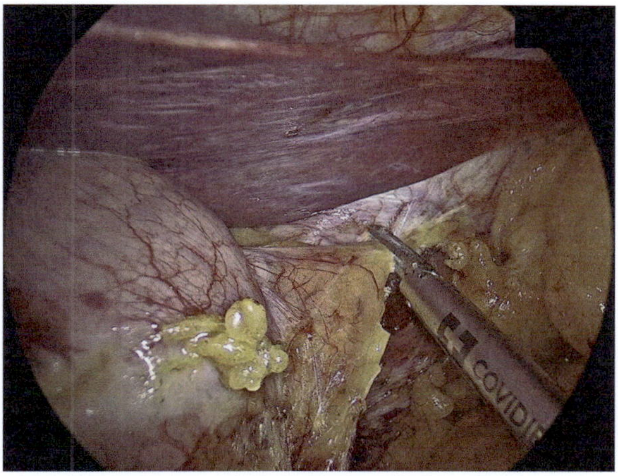

**Fig. 20.5** Mobilization of the posterior gastric adhesions

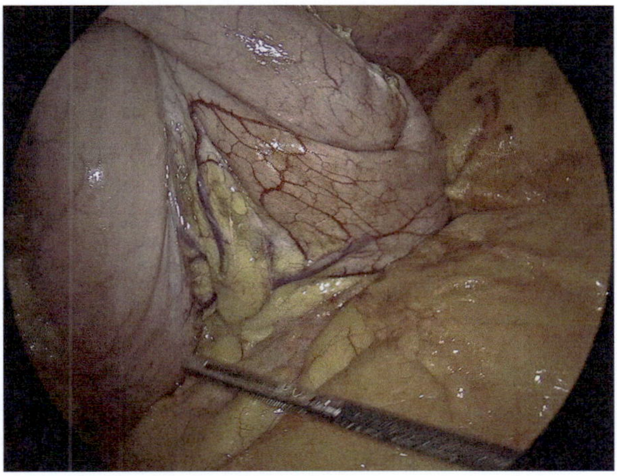

**Fig. 20.6** Exposure of the left crus of the diaphragm

identification of a hiatal hernia, including dissection of the phrenoesophageal membrane and posterior repair if a hernia is present [19, 33, 34].

For the final part of the fundus mobilization at the angle of His, the assistant retracts the upper part of the stomach medially and inferiorly to finally expose the left crus of the diaphragm (Fig. 20.6). The phrenoesophageal membrane is mobilized with care to avoid potential thermal injury to the esophagus. At that stage, the hiatus can be inspected for any possible hiatal hernia, and if relevant, it should be mobilized completely and repaired posteriorly. Usually, the authors prefer to delay the hiatal closure until after completing the sleeve. However, this might not be possible in a bigger hiatal hernia. During the repair, caution should be exercised to preserve the vascularization from the left gastric artery since the gastroepiploic and short gastric vessels were taken down with greater curvature dissection.

## Bougie Insertion

At this stage, an orogastric calibrating bougie is carefully inserted by the anesthesiologist and advanced to the pylorus under direct visual guidance. It is then positioned along the lesser curvature. Assistance with cranial and medial retraction of the fundus might be helpful to guide the bougie past the esophagogastric junction, which is situated posteriorly. The tube can be inserted earlier if the stomach needs to be decompressed during the mobilization of the greater curvature. In our practice, we use a 38 French mercury-weighed Hurst bougie. Various types and sizes of calibrating tubes are described in the literature, with most of the experts routinely using a 36 French bougie. However, there is controversy regarding its impact on postoperative outcomes [35–37].

## Transection of the Stomach

The vertical transection of the stomach is carried out using sequential application of 60-mm linear staplers. The author's practice is to start the stapling at least 6 cm from the pylorus, with the stapler oriented horizontally toward the patient's left shoulder (Fig. 20.7). Once again, there is no consensus for the distance from the pylorus to the transection. However, a distance of 6 cm is associated with less postoperative vomiting, improved gastric emptying, and reduced GERD when compared to 2 cm. Conversely, weight loss tends to be higher with a 2 cm distance [38]. Playing with the articulation of the stapler head and the different trocars helps achieve the optimal angle for staple firing. During this step, it is crucial to respect the incisura angularis to prevent excessive narrowing of the sleeve (Fig. 20.8). The thickness of the stomach decreases as moving cranially; therefore, the closed height of the staple used should be adjusted. Experts recommend not using staples with a

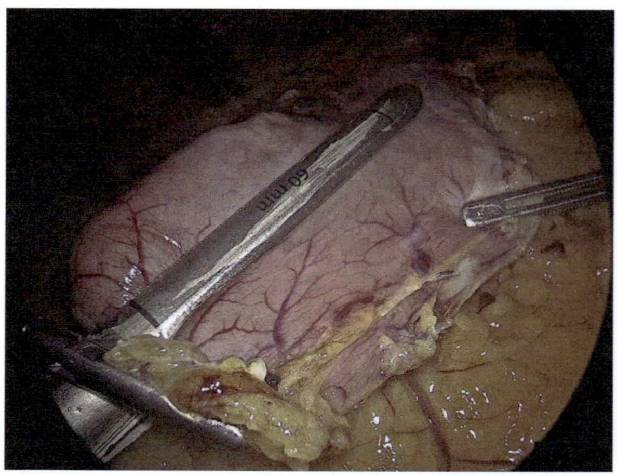

**Fig. 20.7** Confection of the sleeve gastrectomy 6 cm from the pylorus while respecting the incisura angularis with lateral retraction by the assistant

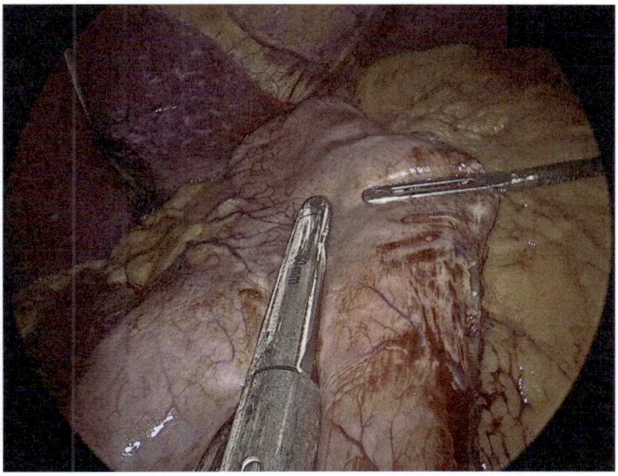

**Fig. 20.8** Visualization of the anterior and posterior aspects of the sleeve before each stapler firing

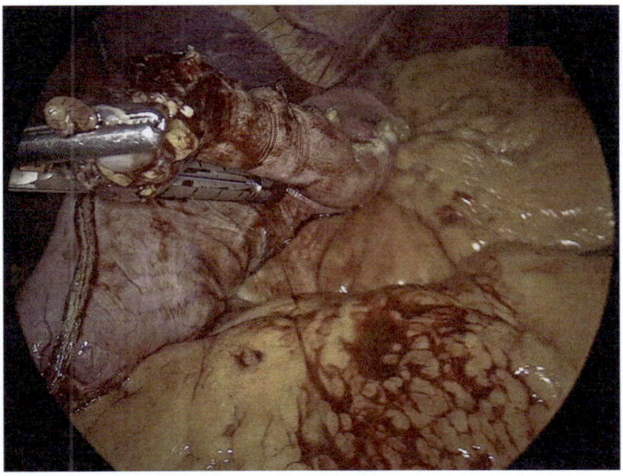

**Fig. 20.9** Last stapler firing at the esophagogastric junction away from the fat pad

closed high smaller than 2.0 mm for the antrum transection and less than 1.5 mm for the rest of the stomach [19].

During stomach transection, it is important to ensure that the lateral retraction by the assistant is not excessive and remains symmetrical in regard to the posterior and anterior walls of the greater curvature. We recommend visualizing both the anterior and posterior aspects of the sleeve before each cartridge is fired (Fig. 20.9). These elements are crucial to prevent excessive narrowing of the sleeve by stapling too close to the bougie and to avoid a spiral twist of the sleeve caused by uneven lateral traction on the stomach's posterior or anterior wall. A twist of the sleeve can lead to distal obstruction with a risk of anastomotic leak. Care should also be taken to prevent stapling the bougie by checking the position of the bougie along the lesser curvature before each firing. When approaching the esophagogastric junction, it is essential to avoid stapling too close to the bougie and instead stay away from the fat pad to prevent ischemia at the superior edge of the sleeve.

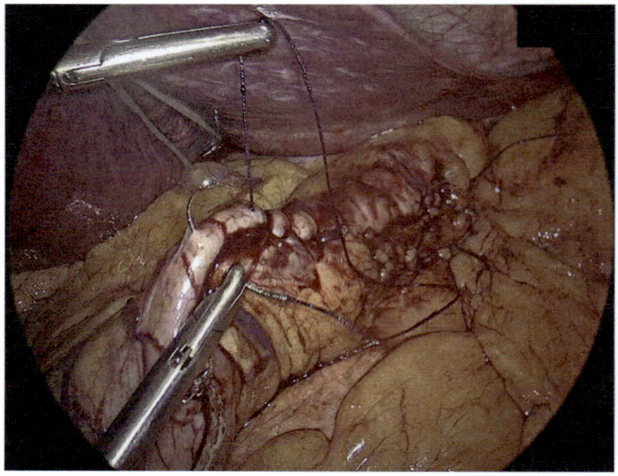

**Fig. 20.10** Imbrication of the staple line with absorbable suture

## Staple Line Reinforcement

Expert opinion and current literature support the use of staple line reinforcement for preventing bleeding events, although no clear effect on leak prevention has been demonstrated [19, 39, 40]. It is our routine practice to reinforce the length of the staple line by imbricating the staple line with absorbable sutures (Fig. 20.10). This reinforcement can also be achieved using absorbable synthetic or biological staple line reinforcement (buttressing) or by oversewing the staple line partially or completely. While overseeing the staple line, it is essential to keep the bougie in place to avoid sleeve stenosis.

## Specimen Extraction and Closure

The procedure concludes with the extraction of the specimen and the closure of port sites. A leak test should be used only selectively as its sensitivity is very low and no significant benefit in preventing anastomotic leaks has been demonstrated when performing it [41, 42].

## Postoperative Care and Complications

There is significant institutional variation in postoperative care. Typically, patients are admitted overnight for observation, especially in the presence of sleep apnea. Same-day surgery is becoming more performed [43]. Individual care in high-risk cases, such as liver cirrhosis, heart failure, or end-stage kidney failure should be managed in collaboration with the appropriate specialty.

Postoperative pain is preferably managed with non-opioid medication such as acetaminophen, especially upon discharge. Loco-regional anesthesia like local anesthetic infiltration and transverse abdominis plan block are recommended strategies to reduce opioid use, thus promoting early recovery [44].

Postoperative nausea is quite common after sleeve gastrectomy, emphasizing the use of non-opioid analgesic medications. It can be controlled with ondansetron, prochlorperazine, or a scopolamine patch.

Complications of sleeve gastrectomy are typically categorized into early and late complications. Frequent early complications specific to sleeve gastrectomy are bleeding, anastomotic leaks, and strictures, while late complications include chronic leaks, strictures, and GERD. We consider the incisura angularis to be the vulnerable point for the development of stenosis, the gastrosplenic ligament for bleeding and the angle of His for leaks (99% of leaks). The management of these complications is addressed in a separate chapter.

## Outcomes

Sleeve gastrectomy leads to significant weight loss with resolution or improvement of hypertension, non-alcoholic steatohepatitis (NASH), type 2 diabetes mellitus (T2DM), and other obesity-related comorbidities and risks. In the STAMPEDE trial, it was found that sleeve gastrectomy and RYGB when combined with intensive medical therapy, were more effective in treating type 2 diabetes mellitus in patients with obesity than intensive therapy alone [45]. Similar positive results were observed in the BRAVES trial for NASH [46].

In comparison to RYGB, sleeve gastrectomy tends to yield lower long-term weight loss and less T2DM remission. However, these potential drawbacks should be considered in light of its lower postoperative morbidity and reoperation risk when compared to RYGB [47, 48].

Sleeve gastrectomy has faced criticism due to an associated weight regain, which is estimated to be around 25%. Weight regain is, unfortunately, a common issue in various bariatric surgeries and should be considered as part of the disease progress rather than being solely attributed to treatment failure.

## Conclusion

Sleeve gastrectomy has emerged as an effective and safe bariatric surgery option for obesity and related diseases, playing a prominent role in modern metabolic and bariatric surgery. It combines mechanical restriction and hormonal changes to promote weight loss. This procedure is suitable for a wide range of patients, including high-risk individuals. Sleeve gastrectomy offers significant weight loss and improvements in associated diseases. While sleeve gastrectomy may appear technically simple, it should not be mistaken for an easy procedure. Underestimating the importance of expertise in the technique and ignoring potential pitfalls can lead to serious complications and impact patients' quality of life. Even with its possible drawbacks, such as weight regain or GERD, it remains a cornerstone in the treatment of obesity with low morbidity and long-term side effects.

## References


1. Stierman B, Afful J, Carroll MD, Chen TC, Davy O, Fink S, et al. National Health and Nutrition Examination Survey 2017–March 2020 prepandemic data files—Development of files and prevalence estimates for selected health outcomes. National Health Statistics Reports; no 158. Hyattsville, MD: National Center for Health Statistics. 2021. https://doi.org/10.15620/cdc:106273.
2. Estimate of Bariatric Surgery Numbers, 2011–2021 | American Society for Metabolic and Bariatric Surgery. Accessed October 18, 2023. https://asmbs.org/resources/estimate-of-bariatric-surgery-numbers.
3. Johnston D, Dachtler J, Sue-Ling HM, King RFGJ, Martin IG. The Magenstrasse and Mill operation for morbid obesity. Obes Surg. 2003;13(1):10–6. https://doi.org/10.1381/096089203321136520.
4. Carmichael AR, Johnston D, King RFGJ, Sue-Ling HM. Effects of the Magenstrasse and Mill operation for obesity on plasma leptin and insulin resistance. Diabetes Obes Metab. 2001;3(2):99–103. https://doi.org/10.1046/J.1463-1326.2001.00129.X.
5. Carmichael AR, Tate G, King RFGJ, Sue-Ling HM, Johnston D. Effects of the Magenstrasse and Mill operation for obesity on plasma plasminogen activator inhibitor type 1, tissue plasminogen activator, fibrinogen and insulin. Pathophysiol Haemost Thromb. 2002;32(1):40–3. https://doi.org/10.1159/000057287.
6. Marceau P, Biron S, Bourque RA, Potvin M, Hould FS, Simard S. Biliopancreatic diversion with a new type of gastrectomy. Obes Surg. 1993;3(1):29–35. https://doi.org/10.1381/096089293765559728.
7. Hess DS, Hess DW. Biliopancreatic diversion with a duodenal switch. Obes Surg. 1998;8(3):267–82. https://doi.org/10.1381/096089298765554476.
8. Regan JP, Inabnet WB, Gagner M, Pomp A. Early experience with two-stage laparoscopic Roux-en-Y gastric bypass as an alternative in the super-super obese patient. Obes Surg. 2003;13(6):861–4. https://doi.org/10.1381/096089203322618669.
9. Roa PE, Kaidar-Person O, Pinto D, Cho M, Szomstein S, Rosenthal RJ. Laparoscopic sleeve gastrectomy as treatment for morbid obesity: technique and short-term outcome. Obes Surg. 2006;16(10):1323–6. https://doi.org/10.1381/096089206778663869.
10. Gagner M, Matteotti R. Laparoscopic biliopancreatic diversion with duodenal switch. Surg Clin North Am. 2005;85(1):141–9. https://doi.org/10.1016/J.SUC.2004.10.003.
11. Gagner M, Deitel M, Kalberer TL, Erickson AL, Crosby RD. The second international consensus summit for sleeve gastrectomy, March 19–21, 2009. Surg Obes Relat Dis. 2009;5(4):476–85. https://doi.org/10.1016/J.SOARD.2009.06.001.
12. ASMBS Clinical Issues Committee. Updated position statement on sleeve gastrectomy as a bariatric procedure. Surg Obes Relat Dis. 2012;8(3):e21-6. https://doi.org/10.1016/J.SOARD.2012.02.001.
13. Eisenberg D, Shikora SA, Aarts E, et al. 2022 American Society for Metabolic and Bariatric Surgery (ASMBS) and International Federation for the Surgery of Obesity and Metabolic Disorders (IFSO): indications for metabolic and bariatric surgery. Surg Obes Relat Dis. 2022;18(12):1345–56. https://doi.org/10.1016/j.soard.2022.08.013.
14. Osland E, Yunus RM, Khan S, Alodat T, Memon B, Memon MA. Postoperative early major and minor complications in laparoscopic vertical sleeve gastrectomy (LVSG) versus laparoscopic roux-en-Y gastric bypass (LRYGB) procedures: a meta-analysis and systematic review. Obes Surg. 2016;26(10):2273–84. https://doi.org/10.1007/S11695-016-2101-8.
15. Sharma I, Nakanishi H, Hage K, et al. Bariatric surgery and left ventricular assist device in patients with heart failure: a systematic review and meta-analysis. Am J Surg. 2023;226(3):340–9. https://doi.org/10.1016/J.AMJSURG.2023.06.014.
16. Hawkins RB, Go K, Raymond SL, Ayzengart A, Friedman J. Laparoscopic sleeve gastrectomy in patients with heart failure and left ventricular assist devices as a bridge to transplant. Surg Obes Relat Dis. 2018;14(9):1269–73. https://doi.org/10.1016/J.SOARD.2018.04.005.

17. Kim Y, Bailey AJ, Morris MC, Kassam AF, Shah SA, Diwan TS. Kidney transplantation after sleeve gastrectomy in the morbidly obese candidate: results of a 2-year experience. Surg Obes Relat Dis. 2020;16(1):10–4. https://doi.org/10.1016/J.SOARD.2019.09.069.
18. Fernando S, Varma J, Dengu F, Menon V, Malik S, O'Callaghan J. Bariatric surgery improves access to renal transplantation and is safe in renal failure as well as after transplantation: a systematic review and meta-analysis. Transplant Rev (Orlando). 2023;37(3):100777. https://doi.org/10.1016/J.TRRE.2023.100777.
19. Rosenthal RJ, et al. International sleeve gastrectomy expert panel consensus statement: best practice guidelines based on experience of >12,000 cases. Surg Obes Relat Dis. 2012;8(1):8–19. https://doi.org/10.1016/J.SOARD.2011.10.019.
20. Garg R, Mohan BP, Ponnada S, et al. Safety and efficacy of bariatric surgery in inflammatory bowel disease patients: a systematic review and meta-analysis. Obes Surg. 2020;30(10):3872–83. https://doi.org/10.1007/S11695-020-04729-4.
21. Chalklin CG, Ryan Harper EG, Beamish AJ. Metabolic and bariatric surgery in adolescents. Curr Obes Rep. 2021;10(2):61–9. https://doi.org/10.1007/S13679-021-00423-3.
22. Hefler J, Dang J, Mocanu V, Switzer N, Birch DW, Karmali S. Concurrent bariatric surgery and paraesophageal hernia repair: an analysis of the Metabolic and Bariatric Surgery Association Quality Improvement Program (MBSAQIP) database. Surg Obes Relat Dis. 2019;15(10):1746–54. https://doi.org/10.1016/J.SOARD.2019.08.025.
23. Mechanick JI, Apovian C, Brethauer S, et al. Clinical practice guidelines for the perioperative nutrition, metabolic, and nonsurgical support of patients undergoing bariatric procedures - 2019 update: cosponsored by the American Association of Clinical Endocrinologists/American College of Endocrinology, the Obesity Society, American Society for Metabolic & Bariatric Surgery, Obesity Medicine Association, and American Society of Anesthesiologists. Surg Obes Relat Dis. 2020;16(2):175–247. https://doi.org/10.1016/J.SOARD.2019.10.025.
24. Carter J, Chang J, Birriel TJ, et al. ASMBS position statement on preoperative patient optimization before metabolic and bariatric surgery. Surg Obes Relat Dis. 2021;17(12):1956–76. https://doi.org/10.1016/J.SOARD.2021.08.024.
25. Sogg S, Lauretti J, West-Smith L. Recommendations for the presurgical psychosocial evaluation of bariatric surgery patients. Surg Obes Relat Dis. 2016;12(4):731–49. https://doi.org/10.1016/J.SOARD.2016.02.008.
26. Bullen NL, Parmar J, Gilbert J, Clarke M, Cota A, Finlay IG. How effective is the multidisciplinary team approach in bariatric surgery? Obes Surg. 2019;29(10):3232–8. https://doi.org/10.1007/S11695-019-03975-5.
27. Rebibo L, Maréchal V, De Lameth I, et al. Compliance with a multidisciplinary team meeting's decision prior to bariatric surgery protects against major postoperative complications. Surg Obes Relat Dis. 2017;13(9):1537–43. https://doi.org/10.1016/J.SOARD.2017.05.026.
28. Kanat BH, Doğan S. Is gastroscopy necessary before bariatric surgery? World J Gastrointest Endosc. 2022;14(1):29–34. https://doi.org/10.4253/WJGE.V14.I1.29.
29. Campos GM, Mazzini GS, Altieri MS, Docimo S, DeMaria EJ, Rogers AM. ASMBS position statement on the rationale for performance of upper gastrointestinal endoscopy before and after metabolic and bariatric surgery. Surg Obes Relat Dis. 2021;17(5):837–47. https://doi.org/10.1016/J.SOARD.2021.03.007.
30. Lunger F, Aeschbacher P, Nett PC, Peros G. The impact of bariatric and metabolic surgery on cancer development. Front Surg. 2022;9:918272. https://doi.org/10.3389/FSURG.2022.918272.
31. Ehlers AP, Chhabra K, Thumma JR, Dimick JB, Varban O. In the eye of the beholder: surgeon variation in intra-operative perceptions of hiatal hernia and reflux outcomes after sleeve gastrectomy. Surg Endosc. 2021;35(6):2537–42. https://doi.org/10.1007/S00464-020-07668-4.
32. Mahawar KK, Carr WRJ, Jennings N, Balupuri S, Small PK. Simultaneous sleeve gastrectomy and hiatus hernia repair: a systematic review. Obes Surg. 2015;25(1):159–66. https://doi.org/10.1007/S11695-014-1470-0.
33. Hider AM, Bonham AJ, Carlin AM, et al. Impact of concurrent hiatal hernia repair during laparoscopic sleeve gastrectomy on patient-reported gastroesophageal reflux symptoms: a state-wide analysis. Surg Obes Relat Dis. 2023;19(6):619–25. https://doi.org/10.1016/J.SOARD.2022.12.021.

34. Ehlers AP, Bonham AJ, Ghaferi AA, Finks JF, Carlin AM, Varban OA. Impact of hiatal hernia repair technique on patient-reported gastroesophageal reflux symptoms following laparoscopic sleeve gastrectomy. Surg Endosc. 2022;36(9):6815–21. https://doi.org/10.1007/S00464-021-08970-5.
35. Haskins IN, Jackson HT, Graham AE, et al. The effect of bougie size and distance from the pylorus on dehydration after laparoscopic sleeve gastrectomy: an analysis of the ACS-MBSAQIP database. Surg Obes Relat Dis. 2019;15(10):1656–61. https://doi.org/10.1016/J.SOARD.2019.08.014.
36. Vu AH, Chiang J, Qian Y, Tursunova N, Nha J, Ferzli G. Do all roads lead to Rome? A retrospective analysis on surgical technique in sleeve gastrectomy. Surg Endosc. 2023;37(10):8064–71. https://doi.org/10.1007/S00464-023-10298-1.
37. Adil MT, Aminian A, Bhasker AG, et al. Perioperative practices concerning sleeve gastrectomy - a survey of 863 surgeons with a cumulative experience of 520,230 procedures. Obes Surg. 2020;30(2):483–92. https://doi.org/10.1007/S11695-019-04195-7.
38. Diab ARF, Kim A, Remmel S, et al. Antral preservation in sleeve Gastrectomy appears to protect against prolonged vomiting and Gastroesophageal reflux disease. A meta-analysis of randomized controlled trials. Obes Surg. 2023;33(12):4103–14. https://doi.org/10.1007/S11695-023-06884-W.
39. Diab ARF, Sher T, Awshah S, et al. Oversewing/suturing of the staple line during sleeve gastrectomy is an effective and affordable staple line reinforcement method: a meta-analysis of randomized controlled trials. Obes Surg. 2023;33(8):2533–45. https://doi.org/10.1007/S11695-023-06672-6/METRICS.
40. Aboueisha MA, Freeman M, Allotey JK, et al. Battle of the buttress: a 5-year propensity-matched analysis of staple-line reinforcement techniques from the MBSAQIP database. Surg Endosc. 2023;37(4):3090–102. https://doi.org/10.1007/S00464-022-09452-Y.
41. Jung JJ, Jackson T, Gordon L, Hutter MM. Intraoperative leak test is associated with the lower postoperative bleed rate in primary sleeve gastrectomy: a propensity-matched analysis of primary and revision bariatric surgery using the MBSAQIP database. Surg Endosc. 2022;36(1):753–63. https://doi.org/10.1007/S00464-020-08264-2.
42. Bingham J, Kaufman J, Hata K, et al. A multicenter study of routine versus selective intraoperative leak testing for sleeve gastrectomy. Surg Obes Relat Dis. 2017;13(9):1469–75. https://doi.org/10.1016/J.SOARD.2017.05.022.
43. Vanetta C, Dreifuss NH, Angeramo CA, et al. Outcomes of same-day discharge sleeve gastrectomy and roux-en-Y gastric bypass: a systematic review and meta-analysis. Surg Obes Relat Dis. 2023;19(3):238–49. https://doi.org/10.1016/J.SOARD.2022.09.004.
44. Ibrahim M, Elnabtity AM, Hegab A, Alnujaidi OA, El Sanea O. Combined opioid free and loco-regional anesthesia enhances the quality of recovery in sleeve gastrectomy done under ERAS protocol: a randomized controlled trial. BMC Anesthesiol. 2022;22(1):29. https://doi.org/10.1186/S12871-021-01561-W.
45. Schauer PR, Bhatt DL, Kirwan JP, et al. Bariatric surgery versus intensive medical therapy for diabetes - 5-year outcomes. N Engl J Med. 2017;376(7):641–51. https://doi.org/10.1056/NEJMOA1600869.
46. Verrastro O, Panunzi S, Castagneto-Gissey L, et al. Bariatric-metabolic surgery versus lifestyle intervention plus best medical care in non-alcoholic steatohepatitis (BRAVES): a multicentre, open-label, randomized trial. Lancet. 2023;401(10390):1786–97. https://doi.org/10.1016/S0140-6736(23)00634-7.
47. Leonard-Murali S, Nasser H, Ivanics T, Shakaroun D, Genaw J. Perioperative outcomes of roux-en-Y gastric bypass and sleeve gastrectomy in patients with diabetes mellitus: an analysis of the Metabolic and Bariatric Surgery Accreditation and Quality Improvement Program (MBSAQIP) database. Obes Surg. 2020;30(1):111–8. https://doi.org/10.1007/S11695-019-04175-X.
48. Li RA, Liu L, Arterburn D, et al. Five-year longitudinal cohort study of reinterventions after sleeve gastrectomy and roux-en-Y gastric bypass. Ann Surg. 2021;273(4):758–65. https://doi.org/10.1097/SLA.0000000000003401.

# Roux-en-Y Gastric Bypass: Indications and Technique

# 21

George Ferzli, Damien Lazar, and Mazen Iskandar

## Introduction

Roux-en-Y gastric bypass is a versatile tool in the bariatric surgeon's armamentarium treating severe obesity and metabolic syndrome. Gastric bypass can be performed via open, laparoscopic, or robotic techniques. The restrictive portion of the surgery is accomplished by the creation of a roughly 30 mL gastric pouch, significantly limiting the gastric capacity to accommodate oral intake, and a Roux, or alimentary, limb bypassing the proximal 75–150 cm of small intestine including the entirety of the duodenum and proximal jejunum to induce malabsorption. The effect of Roux-en-Y gastric bypass goes beyond decreased caloric intake and absorption and includes modulation of glucose homeostasis via changes to the secretion of gastrointestinal hormones. Some incretins such as GLP-1 and PYY are unregulated while others such as glucagon and leptin are downregulated leading to an overall decrease in insulin resistance. These mechanisms explain the immediate effect of gastric bypass on diabetes prior to the achievement of any weight loss.

Ever since its first description by Wittgrove and colleagues in 1994 [1], laparoscopic Roux-en-Y gastric bypass has been the gold standard in weight loss surgery, though both the technical considerations of the procedure itself and the

G. Ferzli (✉)
Department of Surgery, New York University Langone Health, New York, NY, USA
e-mail: George.Ferzli@nyulangone.org

D. Lazar
Department of Surgery, Icahn School of Medicine at Mount Sinai, Mount Sinai Health System, New York, NY, USA
e-mail: Damien.Lazar@mountsinai.org

M. Iskandar
Department of Surgery, Baylor Scott and White Medical Center, Waxahachie, TX, USA
e-mail: Mazen.iskandar@bswhealth.org





O. M. Ghanem et al. (eds.), *The SAGES Manual of Metabolic and Bariatric Surgery*, https://doi.org/10.1007/978-3-031-72309-4_21

perioperative care of post-bypass patients have undergone revision and improvement in the years since [2], with a mortality rate of 2.6% at the turn of the century [3] decreased to less than 0.1% in today's practice [4].

The following chapter is to guide the surgeon through the preoperative evaluation, technical elements, and postoperative care for the performance of a laparoscopic Roux-en-Y gastric bypass, with elements specific to a robotic-assisted Roux-en-Y gastric bypass discussed at the end of the chapter.

## Indications

Guidelines for offering bariatric surgery are provided by different national and international societies, including the American Society for Metabolic and Bariatric Surgery, and the International Federation for the Surgery of Obesity and Metabolic Disorders. As directed by these societies, the indications include the following [5]:

- Body mass index (BMI) ≥35 kg/m$^2$, regardless of presence, absence, or severity of comorbidities
- All nonoperative measures have failed to maintain weight loss for >6 months
- Managed through a specialist obesity service
- Fit enough to survive anesthesia and surgery
- Commits to long-term follow-up

Furthermore, special consideration for offering bariatric surgery should be given to the following groups:

- Individuals with metabolic disease and BMI of 30–34.9 kg/m$^2$.
- Patients of Asian descent in whom a BMI ≥25 kg/m$^2$ suggests clinical obesity, and those with BMI ≥27.5 kg/m$^2$.

While there is a spectrum of bariatric procedures that are appropriate for the patients who meet these criteria, much of the choice between procedures depends on patient preference and existing metabolic syndrome comorbidities. As the Roux-en-Y gastric bypass is the focus of this chapter, it is important to note that severe GERD is an indication for Roux-en-Y gastric bypass over other bariatric procedures both as a primary bariatric procedure and also as a conversion procedure for controlling reflux following sleeve gastrectomy [6].

## Contraindications

There are very few absolute contraindications to bariatric surgery in general and Roux-en-Y gastric bypass in particular. However, absolute contraindications include pregnancy and severe incapacitating systemic diseases including life-threatening end-stage renal disease, unstable coronary artery disease, severe cardiomyopathy or heart failure, cirrhosis, portal hypertension, and/or active cancer; compensated or less severe forms of these diseases may represent only relative contraindications, with the decision to proceed to surgery contingent upon multidisciplinary evaluations and discussions with relevant specialists.

Relative contraindications to Roux-en-Y gastric bypass include large ventral hernias containing bowel, gastric or duodenal pathology such as polyps or adenomas (e.g. FAP) requiring endoscopic surveillance or pre-transplant patients in whom other bariatric procedures such as sleeve gastrectomy may be preferred.

## Technique

While studies have demonstrated that there is significant variability in the technique of performing laparoscopic RYGB [7–9] from positioning to the order and method of enteric anastomosis creation, to stapler types, and even laparoscopic vs robotic platforms, the crucial steps of the procedure are generally agreed upon [10] and will be outlined in this section.

### Patient Positioning (Fig. 21.1) and Immediate Preoperative Procedures

The patient should void prior to entering the operating room. The patient should be positioned supine on the operating table with arms abducted to between 60 and 90°,

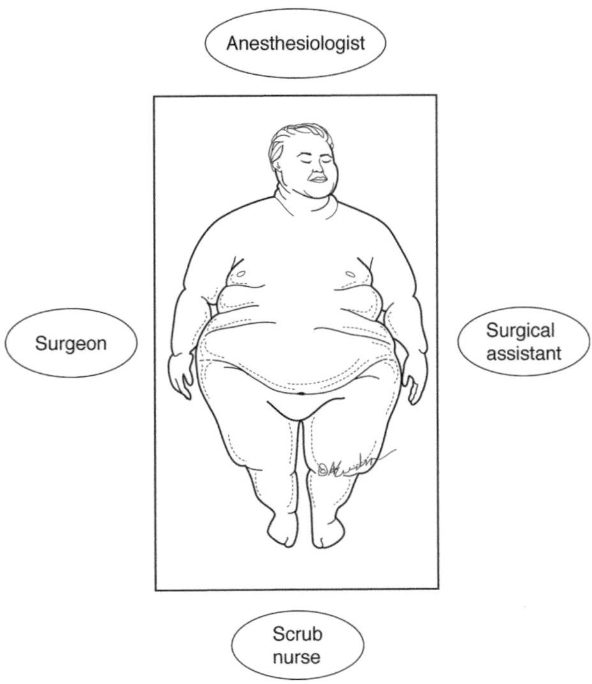


**Fig. 21.1** Patient position

and fully padded and supported. The arms should be secured so that they do not fall out of position if the patient is placed in the reverse Trendelenburg position. If available, a footboard may be placed to facilitate the use of the reverse Trendelenburg position without the patient sliding, and a liver retractor holder may be placed on the patient's right side as high towards the axilla as possible while still allowing access to the holder. The Lloyd Davies position can also be employed with the surgeon standing between the legs.

Intermittent pneumatic compression devices should be placed on the calves bilaterally for mechanical deep vein thrombosis prophylaxis and preoperative antibiotics should be administered. A Foley catheter is not routinely placed for this procedure unless there are additional patient-specific considerations that can be approached on a case-by-case basis. Monitors should be placed bilaterally above each shoulder at a 45-degree angle to the surgeon, who will stand on the patient's right, and to the assistant, who will stand on the patient's left. After induction of anesthesia and following the performance of a surgical time-out, the procedure is ready to commence.

## Abdominal Entry, Establishment of Pneumoperitoneum, and Trocar Placement

Entry to the abdomen can be gained via the preferred method of the primary surgeon, though in patients with severe obesity Veress needle entry performed either over Palmer's point or at the umbilicus, or utilization of an optical viewing trocar over Palmer's point, are generally the preferred technique. Typically, six trocars will

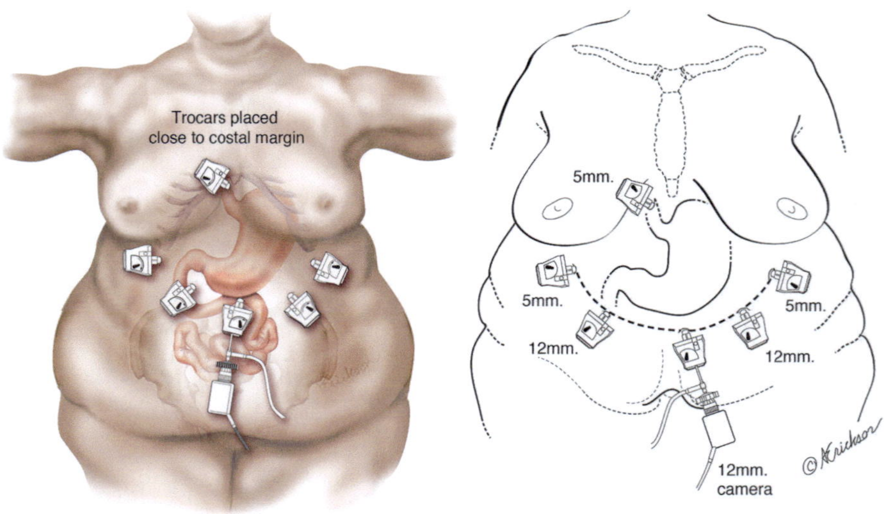


**Fig. 21.2** Laparoscopic trocar placement for RYGB

be used in all (Fig. 21.2), with two or three 12-mm trocars, and three or four 5-mm trocars, placed to triangulate on the stomach and small bowel while maintaining an appropriate distance of at least 15 cm from the target anatomy. The trocars should be extra-long bariatric trocars 10–15 cm in length. After the establishment of pneumoperitoneum to 15 mmHg of $CO_2$, a 5 or 12 mm trocar is placed 16–18 cm below the angle of His and a 30-degree 5 or 10 mm laparoscope is inserted. A 5 mm trocar is inserted just below and to the right of the xiphoid process. This trocar is angled towards the patient's left shoulder so as to come through the falciform. Through this trocar, the left lobe of the liver is retracted anteriorly and cephalad to visualize the angle of His and to determine our approach. Once this is done, the remainder of our trocars are triangulated around the angle of His as follows:

In Fig. 21.2 [11], the three middle trocars are 12 mm ports for a 10 mm camera as well as for suturing and stapling, while the remainder of the trocar's 5 mm ports and the subxiphoid port is either for placement of a liver retractor device or a 5 mm port for an instrument which can be used to retract the left lobe of the liver as needed.

The entire operative field should then be exposed and assessed for any anatomic anomalies, including an evaluation for a hiatal hernia, discussed again during the section on the gastric pouch creation.

Adhesiolysis to ensure unobstructed access to the esophageal hiatus, stomach, transverse colon, and small bowel can be performed as needed at this stage. One can then proceed with the performance of the Roux-en-Y gastric bypass, which can be performed by beginning with the creation of the jejunojejunostomy or the gastric pouch, per the surgeon's preference. This chapter will describe beginning with the creation of the jejunojejunostomy.

## Creation of the Jejunojejunostomy

The greater omentum is swept cephalad to reveal the transverse mesocolon which is retracted superiorly by the assistant with atraumatic graspers. The ligament of Treitz is then identified, keeping in mind its relatively constant anatomic location at the intersection between lines drawn from the left shoulder to the umbilicus and the xiphoid to the left anterior superior iliac spine (Fig. 21.3) [11].

Proceeding distally from the ligament of Treitz, the small bowel is then measured 50 to 150 cm distally by running it in a clockwise fashion, with limb lengths variable by characteristics such as the patient's degree of obesity, risk of nutritional deficiencies, and surgeon preference. The assistant then releases the transverse mesocolon and grasps the small bowel at this distance. An enterotomy is created with hook electrocautery just proximal to the planned transection point in order to facilitate its recognition as the biliopancreatic limb when later creating the jejunojejunostomy. A window in the mesentery is created bluntly and transection of the small bowel is performed using a linear laparoscopic stapler with a 60 mm cartridge of 2.5 mm staples.

The Roux limb is grasped and measured distally 50–150 cm running counterclockwise to identify the location for the jejunojejunal anastomosis. At this point,

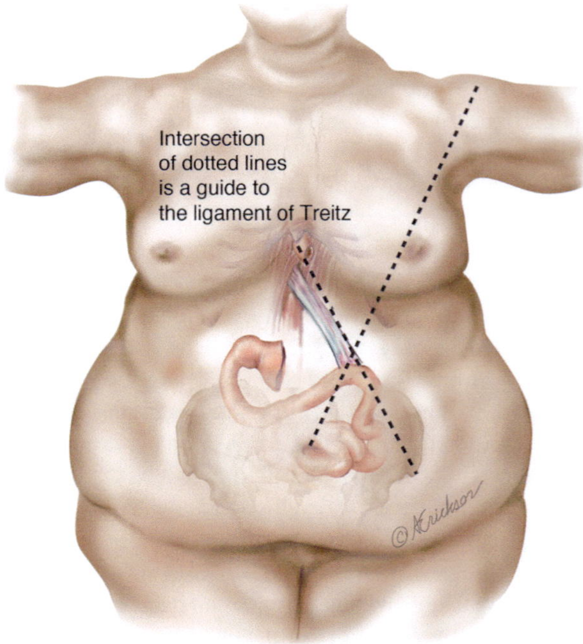


**Fig. 21.3** Landmarks for identification of the ligament of Treitz

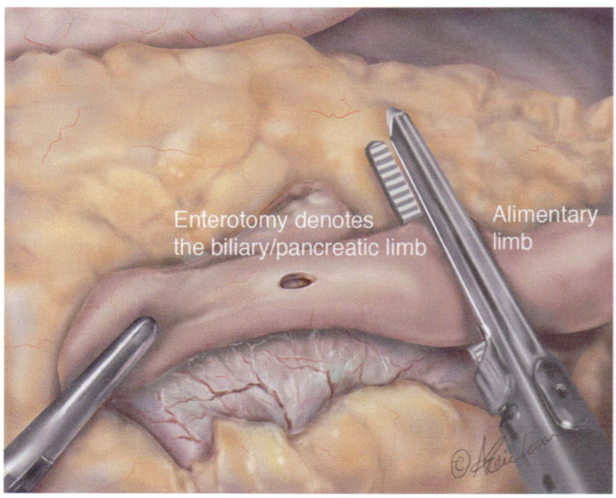


**Fig. 21.4** Enterotomy and stapling across the biliopancreatic limb

the assistant retracts distally and towards the patient's left. The surgeon grasps the bowel proximally and retracts medially in order to create an enterotomy in between (Fig. 21.4). This bowel is brought up to the stapled end of the biliopancreatic limb at the site of the prior enterotomy and a side-to-side stapled jejunojejunostomy is created (Fig. 21.5).

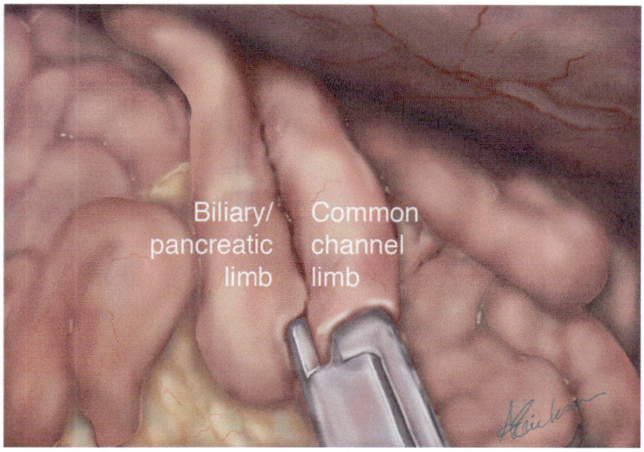


**Fig. 21.5** Feeding the stapler into the bowel

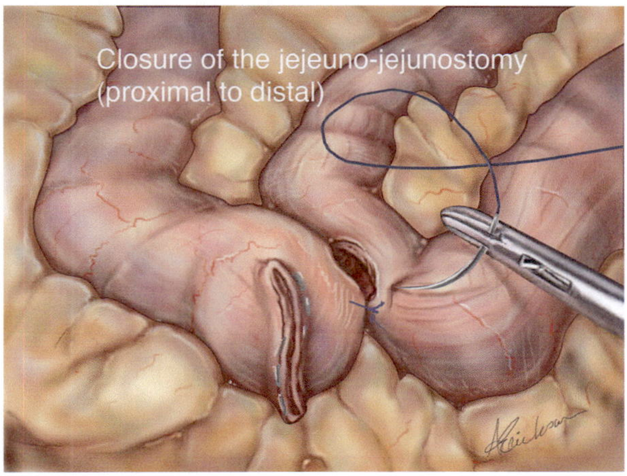


**Fig. 21.6** Closing the enteroenterostomy

The enteroenterostomy is closed with interrupted figure-of-eight 2-0 silk sutures and the mesenteric defect is closed in a similar fashion starting from its root. Alternatively, the enteroenterostomy may be closed in one or two layers using full-thickness absorbable sutures (Fig. 21.6). If two layers are to be used, the first layer is followed by an outer layer of imbricating permanent sutures, either in running or interrupted fashion or the anastomosis may be completed with a second firing of a 60 mm stapler load to extend the anastomosis and then closure of the common enterotomy with a third perpendicular linear stapler firing. Lastly, if preferred, the anastomosis may be created hand-sewn in its entirety with a back row of permanent suture placed prior to the creation of the enterotomy and a full-thickness row of suture placed posteriorly prior to closing the anterior enterotomy.

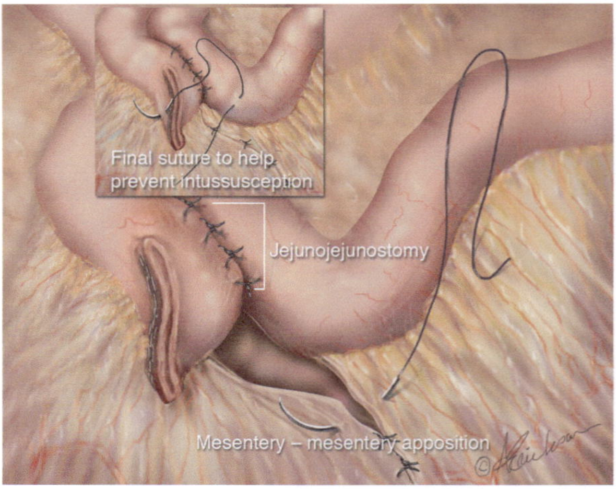


**Fig. 21.7** Closing the mesentery and placing an anti-intussusception stitch

Next, an anti-obstruction Brolin stitch is placed at the staple line of the jejunojejunostomy (Fig. 21.7). Lastly, the mesenteric defect created by the two jejunal limbs is closed with non-absorbable suture in either running or interrupted fashion.

## Evaluation of the Gastroesophageal Junction and Possible Hiatal Hernia Repair

The gastroesophageal junction should be inspected to visualize the Angle of His and Belsey's fat pad and to determine the presence of a hiatal hernia. Traditionally, visualization of the angle of His is obtained via retraction of the left lobe the liver cephalad and anteriorly. The triangular ligament is left in place and the retraction is performed using a fan retractor, a Nathanson retractor, or a laparoscopic grasper inserted through the subxiphoid port, retracting the hepatic lobe from below. A crural stitch to elevate the liver is not advised due to the risk to surrounding structures, such as pericardial tamponade. If using a grasper, ideally, the left side of the right crus just above the GE junction is identified and clamped to maintain retraction (Fig. 21.8). In most cases, this technique may provide sufficient exposure of the angle of His in order to create the gastric pouch.

However, in patients with excessive adiposity and hepatic bulk, adequate exposure may not be possible using this method. An additional adjunct maneuver to improve visualization of the hiatus include placement of the patient in the reverse Trendelenburg position. If these maneuvers still do not allow for sufficient visualization, a mobilization and medial rotation of the left lateral lobe of the liver allows ante-hepatic gastrojejunostomy creation with appropriate visualization of the necessary structures [12].

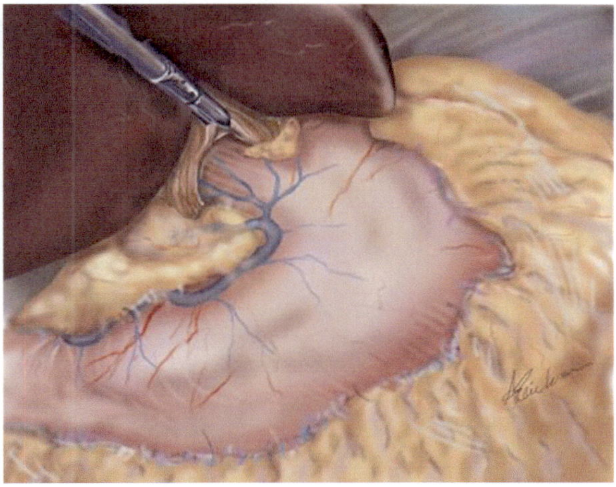

**Fig. 21.8** (**a**) Exposure of the hiatus via retraction of the left hepatic lobe. (**b**) Medial rotation of the left hepatic lobe to expose the hiatus (**c**). A crural stitch to elevate the liver is not advised due to the risk to surrounding structures, such as pericardial tamponade

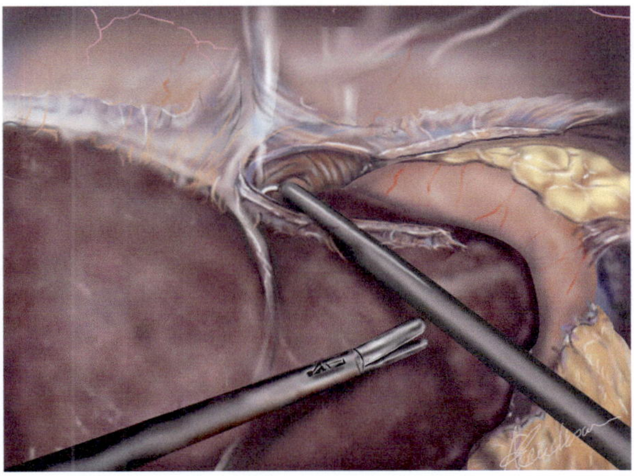

**Fig. 21.9** Clamping the Crus

It is imperative to exercise extreme caution here as the liver can be friable and excessive retraction can result in a large tear of the capsule or even a fracture of the parenchyma. In addition, the left lobe of the liver may become ischemic with the pressure caused by the retractor in which case the retraction must be released periodically. Finally, peak airway pressures must be closely monitored as cephalad retraction may compromise adequate ventilation. Regardless of technique, a bulky liver can prevent satisfactory exposure of the angle of His. In these instances, simply taking down the triangular ligament of the liver and rotating the left lobe of the liver medially may be all that is needed to proceed safely. This can be performed as follows:

The triangular ligament is incised from a lateral to medial direction with an energy source (Figs. 21.9, 21.10). A harmonic scalpel or a ligasure can be used but we prefer hook electrocautery. Care must be taken to avoid injuring the spleen as the

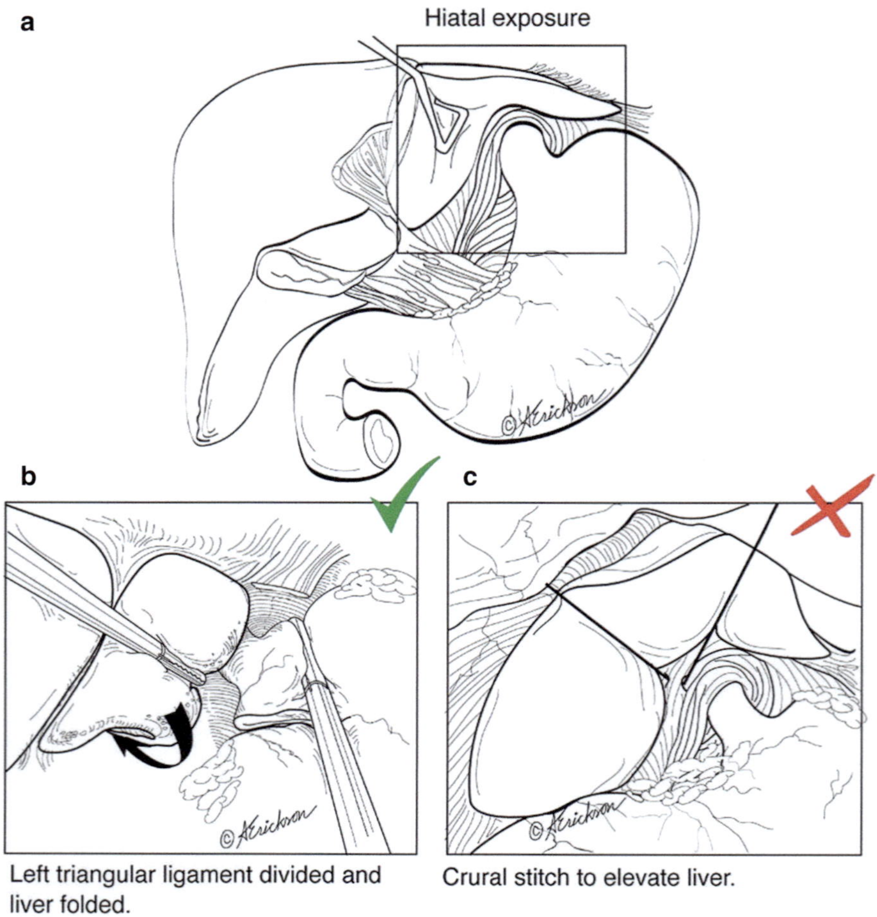


**Fig. 21.10** Incising the triangular ligament and inferior retraction of the left lobe

large left hepatic lobe and the ligament can be wrapped around the upper pole. A key principle when incising the triangular ligament is to stay as close to the liver as possible. A moist sponge can also be placed behind the triangular ligament during its division in order to protect the stomach and the spleen. Once the left lobe is reflected off the spleen, the greater curvature of the stomach is at risk for injury as the incision is carried medially. Again, this can be avoided by staying close to the liver surface. The medial edge of the esophagus signifies the limit of the dissection. Finally, careful attention must be paid to the fat pad of Belsey which must not be encroached as it overlies the GE junction. As long as the liver is not cirrhotic and friable, the left lobe can now be folded inferiorly and medially onto itself. A laparoscopic grasper is then used to maintain retraction by grasping the fatty tissue of the lesser curvature by the pars flaccida.

If present on visual inspection a hiatal hernia repair is performed at this point. The hernia sac is dissected, reduced, and excised. In standard fashion for a hiatal hernia repair, approximately 4–6 cm of intra-abdominal length of esophagus should be obtained and a primary crural repair of the hiatal defect should be performed with permanent suture. In the event of a large hernia defect (greater than 7–8 cm) that cannot be fully closed primarily without tension, the remnant can be used to buttress the hiatus [13].

## Creation of the Gastric Pouch

Prior to creation of the gastric pouch, the anesthesiologist should be asked to advance a 36F calibrating orogastric tube into the stomach, visualized

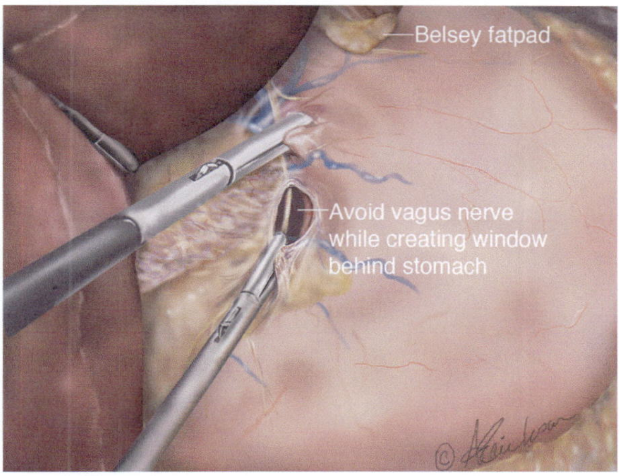


**Fig. 21.11** Preservation of the vagus nerve and replaced left hepatic artery during gastric pouch creation

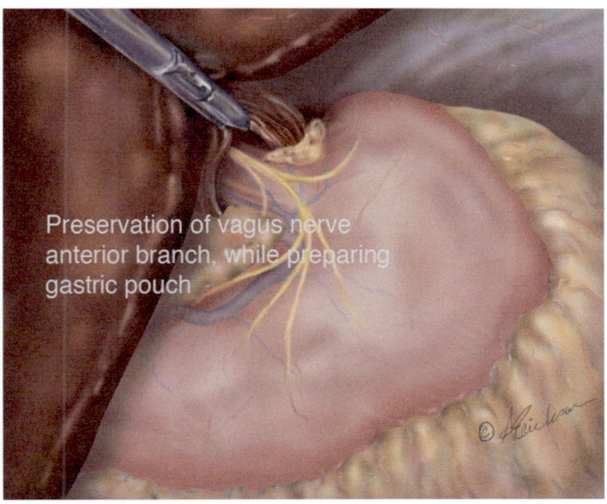


**Fig. 21.12** Preservation of the vagus nerve during gastric pouch creation

laparoscopically by the surgeon, decompress the stomach, remove the tube from suction, and withdraw the tube to the gastroesophageal junction. Dissection of the lesser curvature then begins at the level of the first coronary vein. The authors prefer a perigastric dissection technique over the pars flaccida technique to preserve the right vagus should the need for reversal arise in the future (Fig. 21.11). The avascular connective tissue plane overlying the gastric serosa is peeled away without the need for energy devices. By staying directly on the serosa, we avoid injury to the right vagus nerve and its branches as well as to a replaced left hepatic artery, if present (Fig. 21.12). Dissection of the posterior stomach is performed bluntly with closed graspers, being careful to stay in the correct plane as adhesions are often encountered here. To facilitate this maneuver, the assistant should fan out the stomach by grasping the greater curvature of the stomach at two points.

Dissection proceeds towards the Angle of His. At this point, it is essential to confirm that there is nothing in the stomach or esophagus such as an orogastric tube or temperature probe and, if anything is present, the anesthesiologist is asked to remove it. An endoscopic linear cutting stapler 45 mm load of 3.5 mm staples is introduced from the right upper quadrant trocar and is fired horizontally across the stomach, perpendicular to the esophagus, to create the distal margin of the gastric pouch (Fig. 21.13).

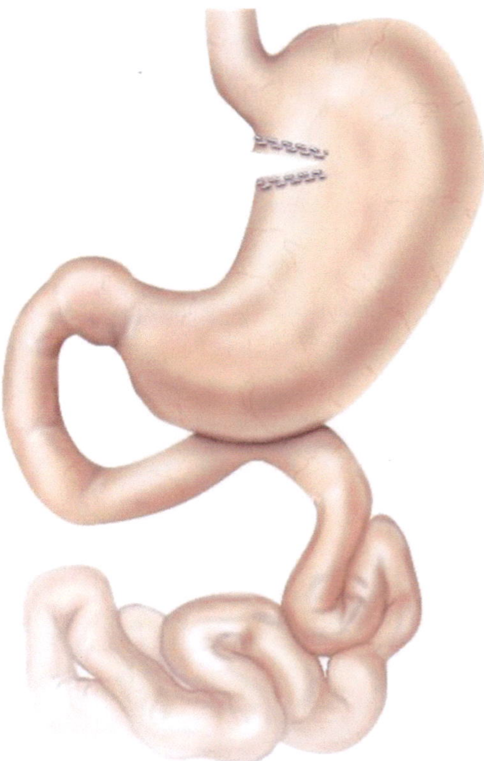

**Fig. 21.13** The first stapler load figured to create the gastric pouch

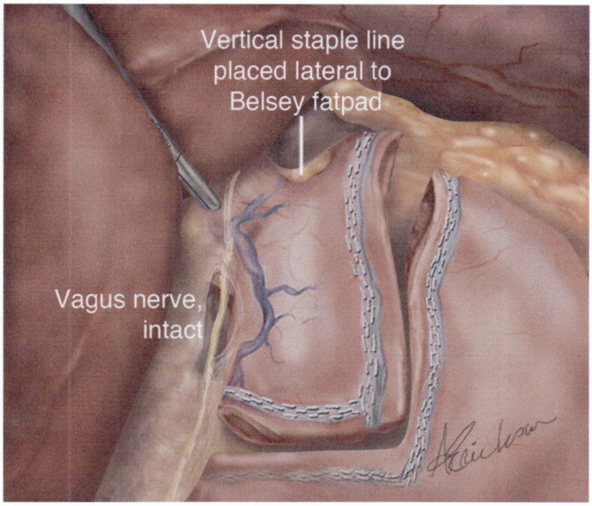


**Fig. 21.14** Completion of the gastric pouch at the angle of His lateral to Belsey's fat pad

The anesthesiologist should then advance the calibrating tube gently to the distal margin of the pouch just created. Traditionally, the gastric pouch is sized by inflating the balloon to 15–30 mL. Alternatively, the balloon may be kept deflated and the diameter of the calibrating tube may be used to guide the lateral staple line, or one can use the terminal branches of the coronary veins, which are fairly constant and serve as an excellent landmark for creating the lateral staple line. The posterior dissection of the stomach is continued cephalad by inserting closed graspers under the lateral edge of the first staple line. Once this space is created, a stapler is introduced from the left upper quadrant port and a second load of staples is fired towards the angle of His, parallel to the calibrating tube and along the edges of the coronary vein branches. Reinforced staples are then used for the remainder of the transection to reduce bleeding and hematoma formation at the staple line, whereas the first two applications are done without reinforcement because the synthetic absorbable film impedes the ability to suture the gastrojejunostomy.

As the angle of His is reached, it is imperative to visualize the upper pole of the spleen which may be adherent to the posterior wall of the stomach. The safest method of dissection here is to open and close the jaws of a blunt grasper to create a window between the stomach and the spleen, being sure to stay lateral to Belsey's fat pad. Once this is accomplished, a final row of staples can be fired to complete the transection (Fig. 21.14). It is important to note that one may intentionally leave a small rim of gastric tissue lateral to Belsey's fat pad in order to ensure that the GE junction is not narrowed. In addition, a pitfall here is to leave a bridge of gastric tissue which will inevitably lead to symptoms similar to a gastrogastric fistula.

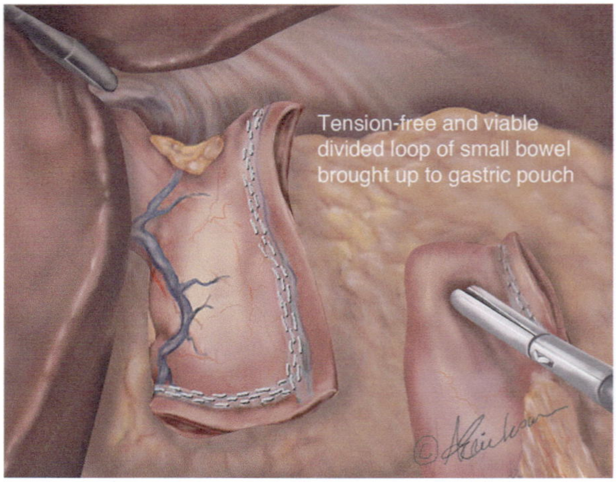


**Fig. 21.15** The Roux (alimentary) limb is brought up to the gastric pouch

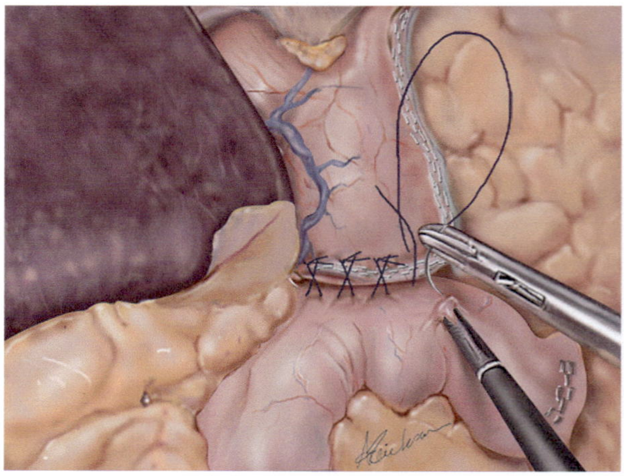

**Fig. 21.16** The posterior layer of the gastrojejunostomy

## Creation of the Gastrojejunostomy

The Roux limb is brought up to the gastric pouch by the assistant and held in place with the staple line facing laterally (Fig. 21.15). This can be done either in an antecolic or retrocolic fashion, though antecolic is more commonly performed, as the latter requires tunneling through the transverse colon mesentery and creates an additional mesenteric defect which must be closed later. If a retrocolic tunnel is to be created, as may be the case if there is insufficient length to bring the limb up without tension in an antecolic fashion, the transverse colon mesentery should be grasped and elevated, exposing the ligament of Treitz. The mesentery can then be incised just to the left of the ligament of Treitz, with dissection proceeding until the lesser sac is entered, at which point the Roux limb can be passed through the tunnel and brought up to the gastric pouch. For an antecolic anastomosis, if there is excessive tension on the limb, the omentum can be divided vertically with either a harmonic scalpel or ligasure device. Division of the mesentery is not recommended as this may compromise the vascularity of the anastomosis.

Many different methods have been described for creation of the gastrojejunostomy. This chapter describes a single layer, ante-gastric, hand-sewn method for anastomosis creation, though the anastomosis can also be created using two layers of suture, or a stapled anastomosis using linear and circular staplers as well, with sutures only for closure of the anterior enterotomy.

Once the Roux limb has been brought cephalad sufficiently for a tension-free anastomosis, it is aligned with the posterior edge of the gastric pouch and a posterior row of 2-0 silk sutures should be placed in either interrupted figure-of-eight or running fashion incorporating the gastric pouch staple line (Fig. 21.16).

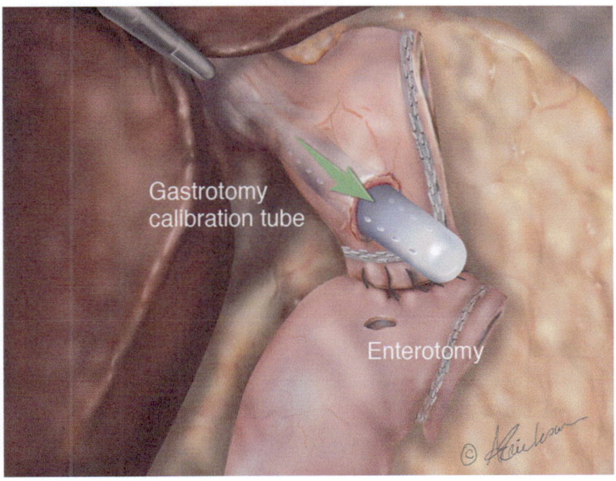


**Fig. 21.17** Calibrating tube pushed through enterotomy to ensure adequate lumen

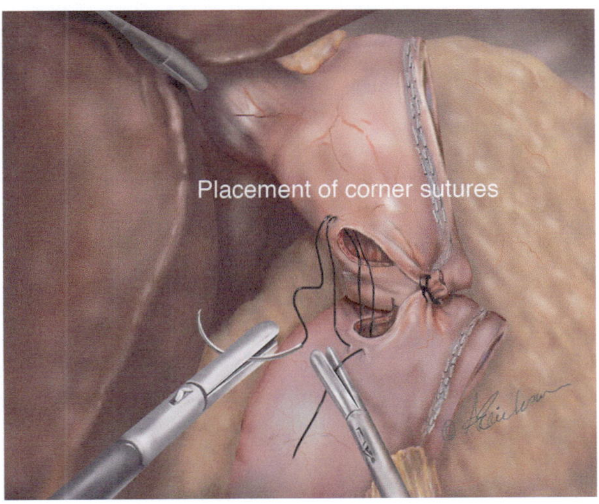


**Fig. 21.18** Corner sutures are placed meticulously

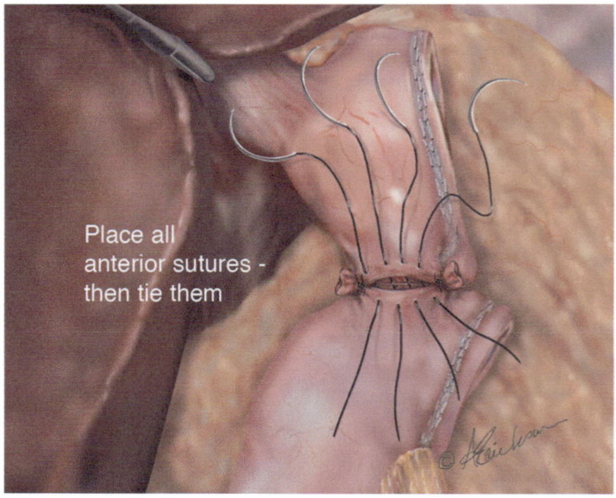


**Fig. 21.19** Tie down sutures after all sutures are placed

The calibrating tube is then pushed in slightly to create a point of tension on the gastric pouch just above the suture line. This minimizes the dispersion of heat as hook electrocautery is used to make a gastrotomy. The calibrating tube is pushed through to ensure an adequately sized lumen and then retracted back (Fig. 21.17). An enterotomy of similar size is created on the Roux limb, also with electrocautery, being careful not to burn the posterior wall.

Next, sutures are placed at the corners (Fig. 21.18). Meticulous technique is used on the corner sutures as these locations are susceptible to leak during intraoperative testing with methylene blue. Begin with the lateral corner by taking a full-thickness outside-in forehand bite of the small bowel from the right sided 10 mm trocar. The serosa of the small bowel can be retracted gently with the left hand in order to ensure that the posterior wall is not incorporated in the stitch, but the mucosa should not be manipulated as bleeding and edema can mask a leak during intraoperative testing. The laparoscopic needle driver is then placed into the left sided 10 mm trocar and a full-thickness bite of the stomach wall is taken in a backhanded fashion from inside-out. This maneuver is repeated to complete the figure-of-eight suture. The right sided corner is then sutured in a mirror-image fashion.

The small bowel is taken backhanded from the left sided trocar and the gastric wall is taken forehanded from the right sided port. Four to five simple sutures are then placed in between without tying in order to safely visualize the back wall. The sutures are grasped upwards on either side of the anastomosis and the calibrating tube is passed into the Roux limb to ensure a patent lumen before tying the sutures.

If desired, another anterior row of imbricating seromuscular sutures can be placed (Fig. 21.19). The anesthesiologist is then asked to manipulate the calibrating tube to ensure that the tube can move without resistance and that it has not been caught by the anastomotic sutures. The gastrojejunostomy is then complete (Fig. 21.20).

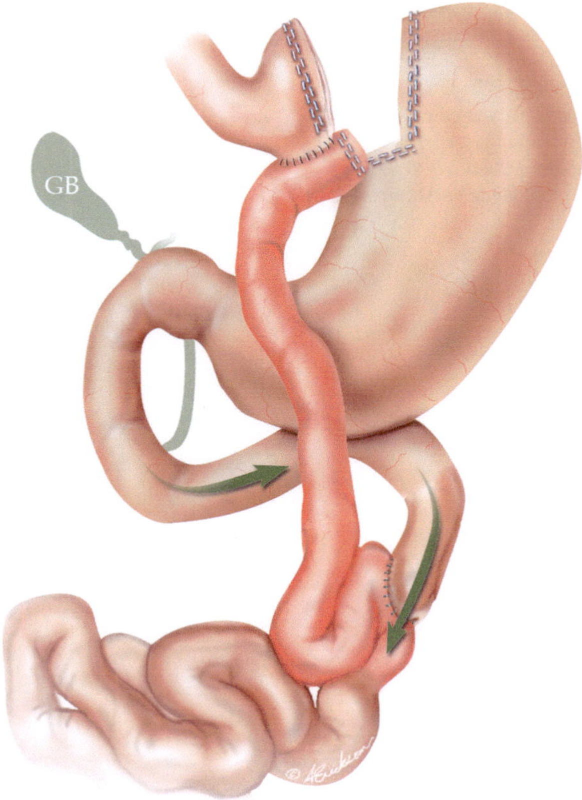


**Fig. 21.20** Anatomy after completion of both anastomoses

## Leak Test

To perform a leak test, the Roux limb is then occluded 10–15 cm distal to the gastrojejunal anastomosis, either with posterior compression or with an atraumatic grasper, and a leak test is performed. This can be performed either with instillation of methylene blue or air via the calibrating tube, or via endoscopy. Both methods will be described here.

Methylene blue leak test via the calibrating tube: The anesthesiologist instills 100–120 mL of methylene blue into the gastric pouch and Roux limb across the anastomosis. Adequate distention of both the gastric pouch and the proximal Roux limb should be visualized as the anterior suture line is carefully inspected. To assess the posterior suture line, the small bowel serosa is gently grasped laterally and medially and rotated in both directions. If a leak is found, it is suture repaired with the lumen distended in order to minimize the risk of catching the opposite wall. The test is repeated until no leak is observed. If no leak is observed, the blue may be suctioned out and the tube removed after being taken off suction.

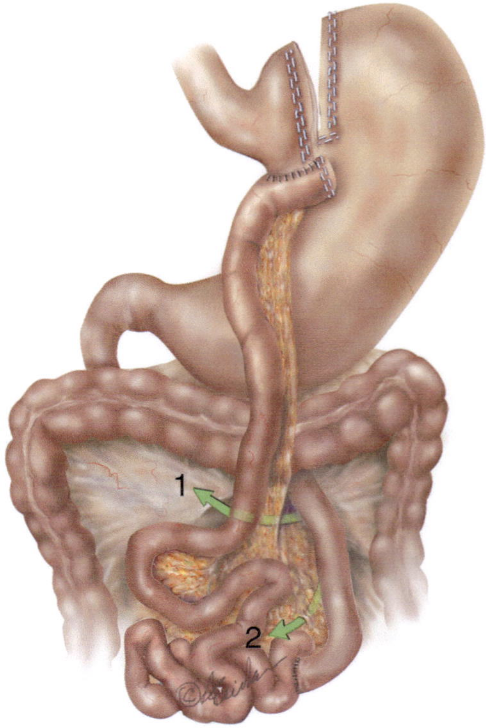


**Fig. 21.21** Mesenteric defects in an antecolic Roux-en-Y gastric bypass. Defect 1 is Peterson's space between the Roux limb and the transverse colon. Defect 2 is at the jejunojejunal anastomosis

Air leak test via the calibrating tube: This test is performed similarly to the endoscopic leak test, however in this instance the anesthesiologist will instill air through the orogastric tube.

Air leak test via endoscopy: an endoscope is inserted slowly via the mouth and through the gastroesophageal junction into the gastric pouch. With the Roux limb occluded, the area surrounding the gastric pouch is laparoscopically irrigated and submerged in water. The gastric pouch is then insufflated endoscopically and the operative field is observed for the presence of bubbles in the water, indicating a leak. The Roux limb and gastric pouch can be gently manipulated during the leak test to increase the accuracy of the test.

## Closure of Mesenteric Defects

Using permanent 2-0 suture, the mesenteric defect between the Roux limb and the transverse colon mesentery, Peterson's space, is closed to prevent internal herniation, as supported in the most recent literature [14] (Fig. 21.21). The defect in the transverse colon mesentery, if in the case of a retrocolic Roux limb (Fig. 21.22), is likewise closed with permanent 2-0 suture, and in the event that the mesenteric

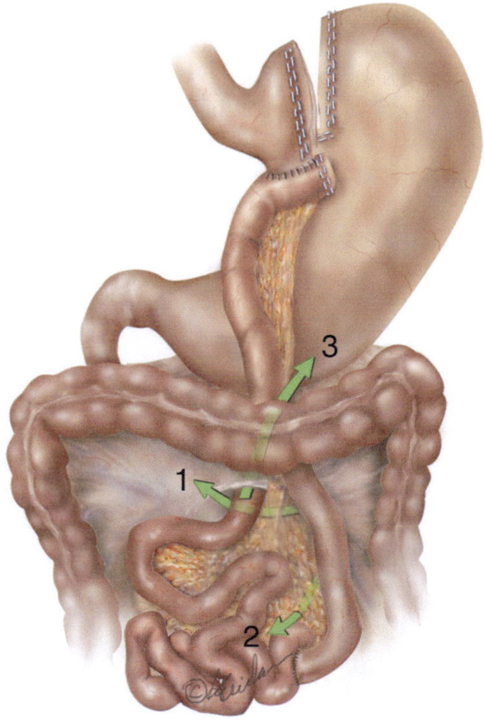


**Fig. 21.22** Mesenteric defects in a retrocolic Roux-en-Y gastric bypass. Defect 1 is Peterson's space between the Roux limb and the transverse colon. Defect 2 is at the jejunojejunal anastomosis. Defect 3 is in the transverse colon mesentery, created by the tunnel for the Roux limb

defect at the jejunojejunostomy was not closed earlier in the procedure, it is closed now.

## Inspection of the Abdomen and Conclusion of the Procedure

After final inspection of the abdomen for bleeding, the liver is allowed to return to its anatomic position. Pneumoperitoneum is evacuated, the trocars are removed, port sites are closed and the procedure is completed.

## Procedure-Specific Complications

In post-laparoscopic RYGB patients, acute postoperative complications include venous thromboembolism, pulmonary embolism, and myocardial infarction. However, abdominal or back pain with fever and tachycardia is an anastomotic leak until proven otherwise. If a leak is suspected clinically, time to diagnosis and treatment is the most important factor in patient survival and so a CT scan with oral contrast should be obtained as soon as possible. A controlled leak can be managed conservatively with continued closed suction drainage as long as the patient remains in stable condition. On the other hand, a sick patient with or without radiographic studies warrants an emergent return to the operating room. If the leak is identified, it can be treated with a buttressed repair, placement of large caliber drains, and placement of a feeding tube distally. In the case where the leak site is not apparent with a methylene blue test, treatment should still consist of drainage and placement of a feeding tube. Controlled leaks may also be managed with endoluminal stenting in the appropriate setting if this therapy is available.

Postoperative bleeding can usually be managed conservatively in stable patients who respond to fluid challenges and blood transfusions. Possible sources include the port sites, anastomoses (less common with the hand sutured technique), and staple lines. Endoscopy may be necessary in cases of persistent gastrointestinal bleeding but this is rare. Also uncommon would be the spleen, liver, omentum, or the mesentery as a source of delayed bleeding. Regardless of the suspected source, unstable patients should be brought back immediately to the operating room.

Internal herniation can occur in an acute or chronic fashion. Usually, it is through the mesenteric defect at the site of the jejunojejunostomy. Patients often present with abdominal or back pain and a CT scan may or may not be helpful as the classic sign of mesenteric swirling is rarely present. In fact, the herniated loop often reduces spontaneously and there may be no abnormal findings on a CT scan. Persistent symptoms without another obvious source warrant a diagnostic laparoscopy. Prevention is the key by meticulously closing this defect during the initial operation. Anastomotic strictures can be managed with repeat endoscopic dilatation. A revision of the anastomosis is rarely required. Marginal ulcer formation is another late complication which may be prevented by promoting smoking cessation, prescribing long-term proton pump inhibitors, and by avoiding the use of NSAIDS in our patients. In addition, all patients are screened for *H. pylori* preoperatively. A new onset ulcer near the anastomotic site should also raise the suspicion of a gastrogastric fistula, particularly if the patient has stopped losing or has begun regaining weight. Diagnosis is confirmed by an upper GI study or endoscopy and the treatment is reoperation if symptoms are refractory to medical or endoscopic therapy. Nutritional and vitamin deficiencies are prevented by prophylactic supplementation and close monitoring of patients' lab tests and weights during their postoperative visits. The most common deficiencies observed are protein, iron, vitamin B12, and vitamin D.

## Additional Considerations; Robotic Platform

The advent of robotic surgery and its increasing utilization in areas with access to this equipment has led to incorporation of the robotic platform into the performance of bariatric surgery. With articulating wrists with 7 degrees of freedom, many surgeons find the technical aspects of intracorporeal suturing required as part of the RYGB procedure less challenging on the robotic platform. While the key steps and flow of the procedure follow the same steps outlined previously in this chapter, there are several important differences outlined here:

1. Robotic port placement: port placement on the robotic platform varies somewhat from the placement as described for the laparoscopic procedure. In the robotic variant, the camera is placed through an 8-mm robotic trocar 20 cm caudad to the xiphoid and 2 cm to the left of the midline. The remaining three trocars are spaced evenly and horizontally across the abdomen approximately 5–8 cm apart, with a 12-mm trocar in the right abdomen and 8-mm trocars in the left mid abdomen and left lateral abdomen. A subxiphoid liver retractor can be placed. An additional laparoscopic assist port may be placed as needed for a bedside assistant to introduce or remove needles, suction, or irrigation as desired.
2. Patient and operating room table positioning. The patients are typically supine with the arms out. Most modern operating rooms are equipped with a table that pairs with the robot allowing adjustment and changes in patient position (e.g., reverse Trendelenburg). Absent this feature, the surgeon must ensure that the table is appropriately positioned prior to docking the robot.
3. Instrumentation: robotic instruments used during the procedure will vary depending on the robotic platform and availability. In general:
   (a) Arm 1 will hold an atraumatic robotic grasper and can be switched out for the stapler for creation of the gastric pouch.
   (b) Arm 2 will hold the 30-degree robotic camera, which will remain in this port for the duration of the surgery.
   (c) Arm 3 will hold a vessel-sealing energy dissecting device for dissection and will be exchanged for a robotic needle driver for portions of the case requiring suturing.
   (d) Arm 4 will hold another atraumatic robotic grasper
4. Technique: Typically, the robotic RNY gastric bypass lends itself better to an omega loop technique rather than a JJ first technique. This has the advantage of keeping most of the work in the LUQ where the functionality of the robot is optimized with the described setup.
5. Leak test: on the robotic platform, the leak test may be formed with indocyanine green given through the calibrating tube rather than methylene blue if preferred by the surgeon.

## References

1. Wittgrove AC, Clark GW, Tremblay LJ. Laparoscopic gastric bypass, Roux-en-Y: preliminary report of five cases. Obes Surg. 1994;4(4):353–7.
2. Lehman Center Weight Loss Surgery Expert Panel. Commonwealth of Massachusetts Betsy Lehman Center for Patient Safety and Medical Error Reduction Expert Panel on weight loss surgery: executive report. Obes Res. 2005;13(2):205–26. https://doi.org/10.1038/oby.2005.30. PMID: 15800277.

3. Morino M, Toppino M, Forestieri P, Angrisani L, Allaix ME, Scopinaro N. Mortality after bariatric surgery: analysis of 13,871 morbidly obese patients from a national registry. Ann Surg. 2007;246(6):1002–7; discussion 1007–9. PMID: 18043102. https://doi.org/10.1097/SLA.0b013e31815c404e.
4. DeMaria EJ, Pate V, Warthen M, Winegar DA. Baseline data from American Society for Metabolic and Bariatric Surgery-designated Bariatric Surgery Centers of Excellence using the bariatric outcomes longitudinal database. Surg Obes Relat Dis. 2010;6(4):347–55. https://doi.org/10.1016/j.soard.2009.11.015. Epub 2010 Jan 4. PMID: 20176512.
5. Eisenberg D, Shikora SA, Aarts E, Aminian A, Angrisani L, Cohen RV, de Luca M, Faria SL, Goodpaster KPS, Haddad A, Himpens JM, Kow L, Kurian M, Loi K, Mahawar K, Nimeri A, O'Kane M, Papasavas PK, Ponce J, Pratt JSA, Rogers AM, Steele KE, Suter M, Kothari SN. 2022 American Society of Metabolic and Bariatric Surgery (ASMBS) and International Federation for the Surgery of Obesity and Metabolic Disorders (IFSO) indications for metabolic and bariatric surgery. Obes Surg. 2023;33(1):3–14. https://doi.org/10.1007/s11695-022-06332-1. Erratum in: Obes Surg 2022 Nov 29;: PMID: 36336720; PMCID: PMC9834364.
6. Strauss AL, Triggs JR, Tewksbury CM, Soriano I, Wernsing DS, Dumon KR, Williams NN, Shao JM. Conversion to Roux-en-Y gastric bypass: a successful means of mitigating reflux after laparoscopic sleeve gastrectomy. Surg Endosc. 2023;37(7):5374–9. https://doi.org/10.1007/s00464-023-10024-x. Epub 2023 Mar 30. PMID: 36997653.
7. Madan AK, Lo Menzo E, Dhawan N, Tichansky DS. Internal hernias and nonclosure of mesenteric defects during laparoscopic Roux-en-Y gastric bypass. Obes Surg. 2009;19(5):549–52. https://doi-org.ezproxy.med.nyu.edu/10.1007/s11695-008-9722-5.
8. Dang JT, Deprato A, Verhoeff K, et al. Variation of laparoscopic Roux-en-Y gastric bypass techniques: a survey of 518 bariatric surgeons. Obes Surg. 2022;32(7):2357–65. https://doi-org.ezproxy.med.nyu.edu/10.1007/s11695-022-06087-9.
9. Vu AH, Chiang J, Qian Y, et al. Do all roads lead to Rome?: a retrospective analysis on surgical technique in Roux-en-Y gastric bypass. Surg Endosc. 2023;37:7254–63. https://doi-org.ezproxy.med.nyu.edu/10.1007/s00464-023-10257-w.
10. Kaijser MA, van Ramshorst GH, Emous M, Veeger NJGM, van Wagensveld BA, Pierie JEN. A Delphi consensus of the crucial steps in gastric bypass and sleeve gastrectomy procedures in the Netherlands. Obes Surg. 2018;28(9):2634–43. https://doi.org/10.1007/s11695-018-3219-7. PMID: 29633151; PMCID: PMC6132743.
11. Ferzli GS, Fingerhut A. Trocar placement for laparoscopic abdominal procedures: a simple standardized method. J Am Coll Surg. 2004;198(1):163–74.
12. Ferzli GS, Edwards ED. Laparoscopic ante-hepatic gastrojejunostomy. Am J Surg. 2008;195(5):708–10.
13. Ferzli G, Liu S, Iskandar M, Fingerhut A. Laparoscopic gastric fundus tamponade: a novel adaptation of the Toupet fundoplication for large paraesophageal hernia repair. Surg Endosc. 2020;34(11):4803–11. https://doi.org/10.1007/s00464-019-07256-1. Epub 2019 Nov 18. PMID: 31741156.
14. Stenberg E, Ottosson J, Magnuson A, Szabo E, Wallén S, Näslund E, Thorell A, Näslund I. Long-term safety and efficacy of closure of mesenteric defects in laparoscopic gastric bypass surgery: a randomized clinical trial. JAMA Surg. 2023;158(7):709–17. https://doi.org/10.1001/jamasurg.2023.1042. PMID: 37163240; PMCID: PMC10173104.

# 22 Robotic Duodenal Switch and SADI-S: Technical Aspects

Andre Teixeira and Alex Sanchez

## Introduction

As the incidence of severe obesity continues to rise within the United States and throughout the world, bariatric surgery offers the most effective and durable solution to combat this ongoing epidemic. While the sleeve gastrectomy and roux-en-y gastric bypass comprise the most popular weight loss options, the biliopancreatic diversion with duodenal switch (BDP/DS or duodenal switch) and single anastomosis duodeno-ileal bypass with sleeve gastrectomy (SADI-S) is the most effective weight loss surgeries available. The duodenal switch and SADI-S offer the greatest magnitude of total body weight (TBWL) and the most significant improvement and resolution of co-morbid conditions, in particular type II diabetes and hyperlipidemia. However, despite their superior weight loss and co-morbidity resolution, duodenal switch operations typically account for less than 5% of the bariatric surgeries performed worldwide. This is likely due to a combination of factors: patient selection, fear of long-term nutritional complications and most importantly, the technical skills required to perform the operation safely. The ability to perform this procedure using the robotic platform eases the technical demands of the operation allowing bariatric surgeons to more freely offer this surgical option [1–5].

The robotic platform has several advantages from a technical standpoint when compared to standard laparoscopy: improved visualization, improved ergonomics, more precise dissection and dexterity of the wristed instruments. These advantages allow surgeons to perform more complex operations in a minimally invasive manner. For the BPD/DS and SADI-S, the 3D visualization and dexterity of the robotic arms give the surgeon more control when dissecting around the duodenum and the

A. Teixeira (✉) · A. Sanchez
Department of Bariatric Surgery, Orlando Regional Medical Center, Orlando, FL, USA
e-mail: andre.teixeira@orlandohealth.com; Alex.sanchez@orlandohealth.com



O. M. Ghanem et al. (eds.), *The SAGES Manual of Metabolic and Bariatric Surgery*, https://doi.org/10.1007/978-3-031-72309-4_22

ability to more easily perform all the anastomoses in a hand-sewn manner. Also, the improved angulation of the robotic stapler, as opposed to the laparoscopic stapler, allows the surgeon to create the sleeve gastrectomy and transect the duodenum with ease. This chapter will be dedicated to the technical aspects involved in performing these two operations using the robotic platform [6–8].

## Biliopancreatic Diversion with Duodenal Switch

### Patient Positioning and Port Placement

The patient is placed in the standard supine position with both arms out at right angles on padded arm boards. A footboard is used and a padded belt is placed across the lower extremities to secure the patient to the table (Fig. 22.1). Peritoneal access is obtained using either a Veress needle followed by an optical trocar or an optical 5 mm laparoscopic trocar in the left mid-abdomen near the mid-clavicular line. A 0° laparoscopic scope is used when accessing the abdominal cavity using either approach and then exchanged for the 30° laparoscopic camera to place the remaining trocars. The trocars are placed in a smile shape across the abdomen: 8 mm right anterior axillary line a few finger breaths below the inferior edge of the liver, 12 mm right mid-clavicular line near the level of the umbilicus, 8 mm supraumbilical midline, 12 mm left mid-clavicular line near the level of the umbilicus and 8 mm left anterior axillary line a few finger breaths beneath the ribs (Fig. 22.2). The liver is then retracted toward the anterior abdominal wall. This can be done several different ways at the discretion of the surgeon, routinely we will place a 5 mm subxyphoid trocar and place a laparoscopic toothed Alice grasper at the superior aspect of the

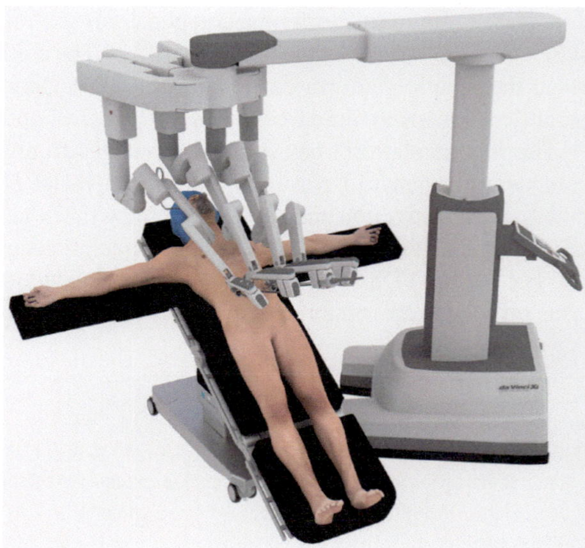

**Fig. 22.1** Patient position

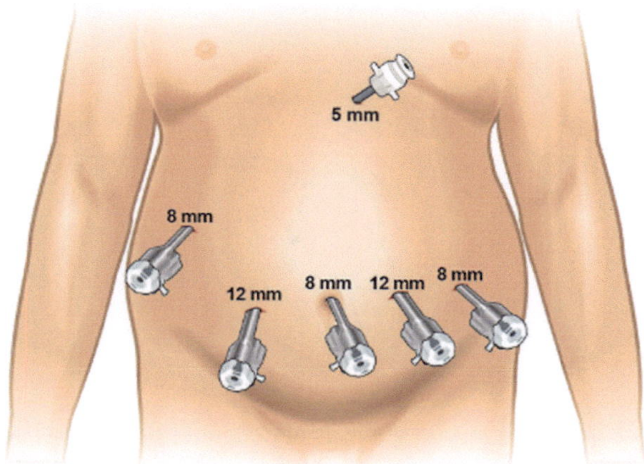


**Fig. 22.2** Robotic port placement

hiatus thus retracting the liver off of the stomach. Alternatively, a full-length 2-0 Ethibond suture placed through the superior aspect of the hiatus and brought out through the abdominal wall on either side of the falciform ligament also works very well.

After the liver has been retracted, I run the bowel laparoscopically starting at the terminal ileum to a point roughly 250–300 cm proximally and a suture is placed in the mesentery to mark this point. The suture is also brought through the superior portion of the greater omentum which prevents the bowel from falling down into the pelvis. This can also be done robotically depending on surgeon preference. A marking pen is used to mark the bowel proximal to the suture in order to ensure no twisting of the mesentery when the bowel is brought up to the duodenum for the anastomosis. Once the suture is placed and bowel marked, the patient is placed in 10–15° reverse Trendelenburg and the robot is brought in from the patient's left side for docking. The instruments used for a duodenal switch from the patient's right to left side are as follows: fenestrated bipolar grasper, assistant trocar/robotic 60 mm (DaVinci) Sureform stapler, 30° robotic camera, vessel sealer/robotic monopolar scissor/large needle driver and tip up grasper or cadiere. After the robot is docked, I begin with the duodenal dissection.

## Duodenal Dissection

Beginning along the greater curvature of the pre-pyloric antrum a plane is created between the antrum anteriorly and the pancreas posteriorly using the vessel sealer and the fenestrated bipolar grasper. The distal antrum is retracted anteriorly using either a cadiere or tip-up grasper. This plane is continued down to the duodenum and a retroduodenal tunnel is created in order to ensure a 1–2 cm cuff of mobilized duodenum. It is important not to be overly aggressive during the retroduodenal dissection which could lead to duodenal stump ischemia and subsequent stump

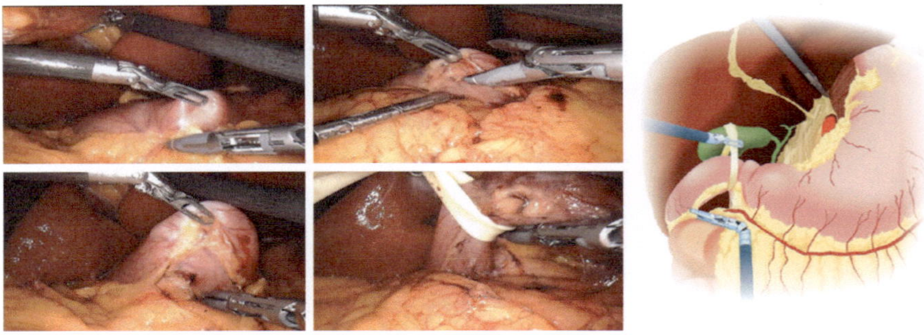

**Fig. 22.3** Duodenum Dissection

blowout or injury to the gastroduodenal artery posterior to the duodenal bulb which could lead to significant hemorrhage. Once the retroduodenal tunnel is completed, a Penrose drain is placed through the tunnel in order to facilitate the placement of the stapler during the transaction of the duodenum. Following the completion of the sleeve gastrectomy, the robotic stapler will be used to transect the duodenum at least 1 cm distal to the pylorus. However, I do not transect the duodenum until after the sleeve gastrectomy portion of the procedure has been completed. It is easiest to bring the stapler in through the left mid-clavicular 12 mm trocar as opposed to the right mid-clavicular site. I prefer to place the anvil side of the stapler through the retroduodenal tunnel given its thinner profile. The previously placed penrose drain is retracted anteriorly to better expose the retroduodenal tunnel and ensure the appropriate placement of the stapling device. Once the stapler has been placed, the Penrose drain is removed to ensure it is not incorporated within the staple line. I prefer to use a white load cartridge but a blue load is perfectly acceptable when transecting the duodenum (Fig. 22.3). I do not routinely oversew or reinforce the staple line of the duodenum.

## Sleeve Gastrectomy

Starting along the greater curvature of the body of the stomach, the lesser sac is entered by dividing the branches of the gastroepiploic arcade using the vessel sealer. The dissection is then carried cephalad along the greater curvature up to the angle of His ensuring that the left crus is clearly identified, no redundant fundus is present posteriorly and no evidence of a hiatal hernia exists. The inferior portion of the greater curvature dissection is then completed ensuring that a few arcade vessels remain between the duodenal dissection plane and the greater curvature dissection to help avoid any ischemic complications as it relates to the duodenoileal anastomosis. After the dissection is completed the calibration tube is advanced into the stomach with the assistance of the anesthesia provider and positioned along the lesser curvature of the stomach with the tip of the calibration tube in the antrum. The calibration tube is then placed on suction to help maintain its position within the stomach. The (DaVinci) Sureform robotic 60 mm stapling device, brought in through the

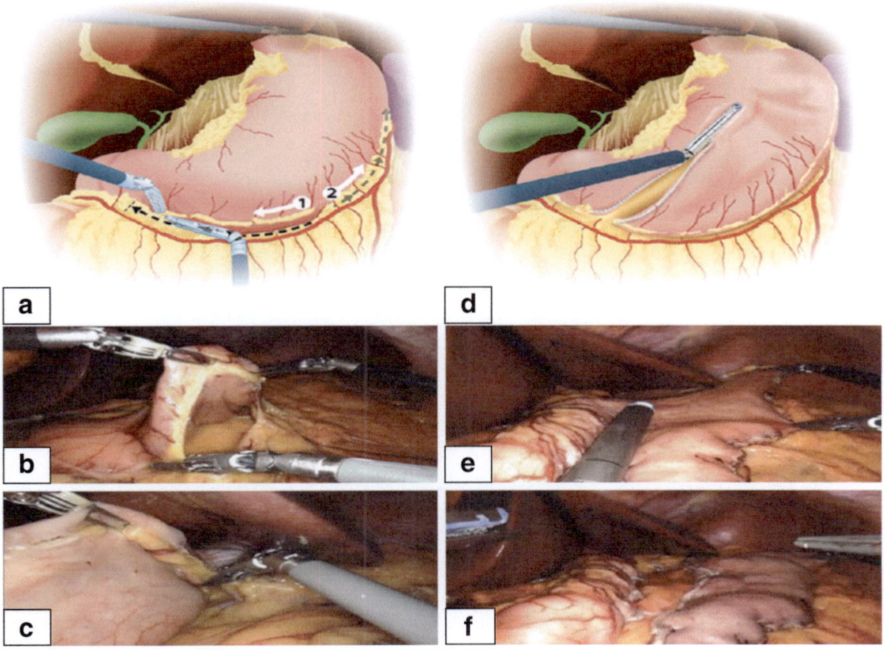


**Fig. 22.4** Sleeve gastrectomy

right mid-clavicular trocar, is used to create the sleeve gastrectomy starting with a green load cartridge at the antrum followed by blue loads for the remainder of the gastric sleeve (Fig. 22.4). It is important to note that the overall size of the sleeve gastrectomy created for a duodenal switch is slightly larger than that made for patients who undergo sleeve gastrectomy alone. This is done to help limit any risk for post-operative dysphagia or oral intolerance.

## Duodenoileostomy

After the sleeve gastrectomy and duodenal transection have been completed the suture used to mark the small bowel is located, the loop of the small bowel is brought up to the duodenum in an antecolic fashion and a posterior suture line is created between the ileum and the duodenum using a suture of your choice, I prefer a 3-0 PDS or Strattifix. For those surgeons who prefer a double-layer anastomosis, this suture will be carried around anteriorly after the inner layer has been completed. Generous enterotomies are created in both the duodenum and ileum using the robotic scissors ensuring that the anastomosis is wide, as to avoid any concerns for anastomotic stricture. The enterotomies are sutured together using a 2-0 or 3-0 suture, commonly Vicryl. The suture used to create the posterior suture line is then brought anteriorly creating a two-layer anastomosis (Fig. 22.5).

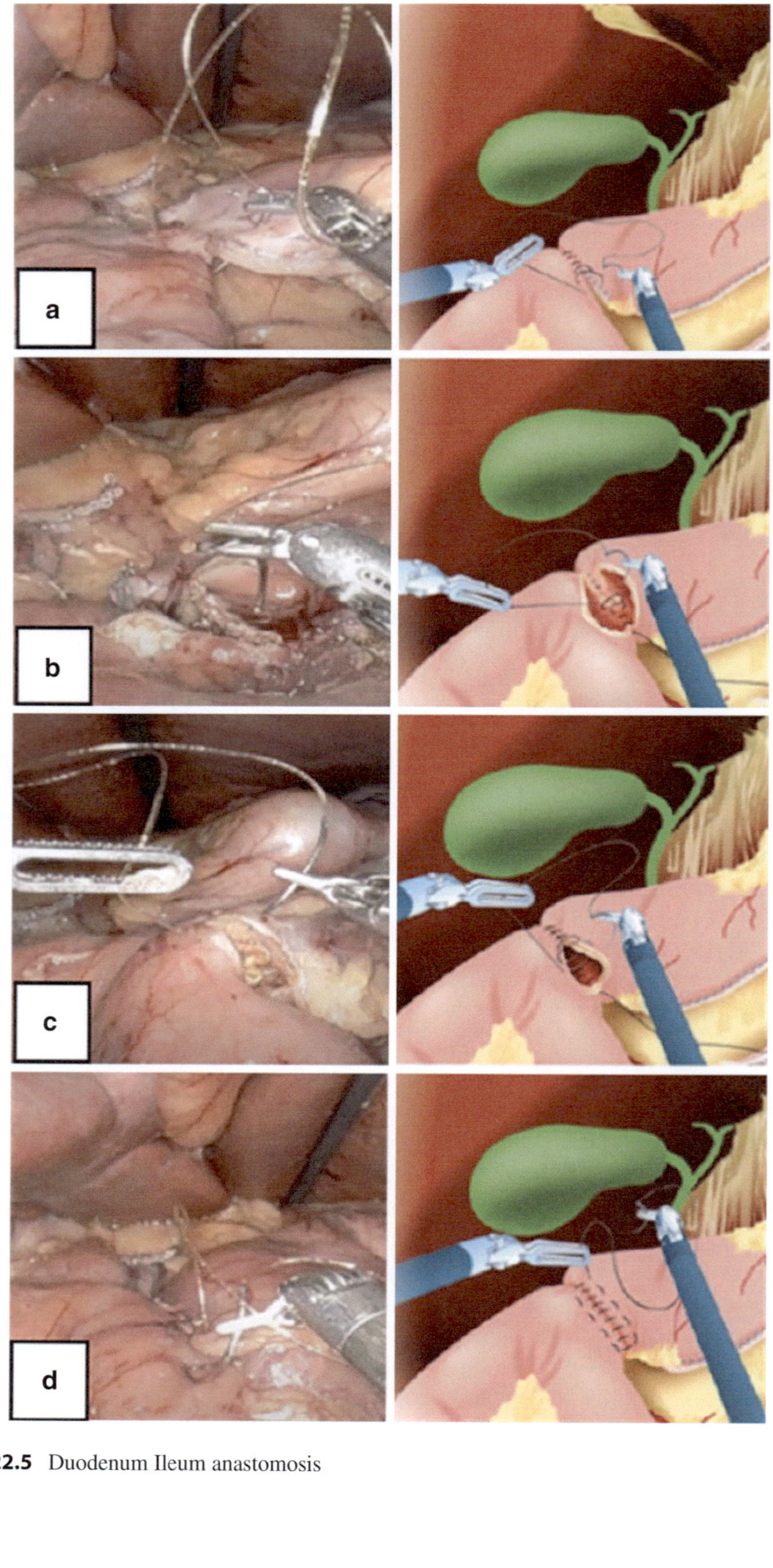


**Fig. 22.5** Duodenum Ileum anastomosis

## Ileoileostomy

After the duodenoileostomy (DI) has been created, attention is then turned to creating the ileoileostomy. This begins by transection of the small bowel just proximal to the DI anastomosis using a white or blue load of the robotic stapler, this will serve as the biliopancreatic (BP) limb of the anastomosis. During this portion of the operation, the robotic stapler is typically brought in through the left mid-clavicular 12 mm trocar. Alternatively, a small window in the small bowel mesentery can be made using the robotic scissors and the stapler brought in via the right mid-clavicular 12 mm trocar. The small bowel is then counted 125 cm distal to the DI anastomosis and sewn to the distal BP limb in order to approximate the bowel loops needed to create the ileoileostomy. The approximated small bowel is then retracted toward the right upper quadrant to allow space for the robotic stapler to enter through the left-sided 12 mm trocar to perform the anastomosis. Enterotomies are created in both the biliopancreatic and roux limbs using robotic scissors. Using a white load of the robotic stapler the anastomosis is created. The common enterotomy is closed in one or two layers depending on surgeon preference. I typically prefer to close the enterotomy in a single layer with a 3-0 PDS or barbed suture in a running fashion (Fig. 22.6). Once the common enterotomy has been closed it is time to address the mesenteric defects.

## Hernia Defects

There are two hernia defects created during this procedure: Peterson's defect made from the antecolic DI anastomosis and the mesenteric defect from the ileoileostomy anastomosis. I do not routinely close the Peterson's defect after a duodenal switch, however, I will close the mesenteric defect. I typically close this defect with a running 3-0 PDS or barbed suture. I bring this suture onto the bowel as well to help avoid any kinking of the ileoileostomy. The use of an absorbable or permanent suture for closure of the mesenteric defect is dependent on surgeon preference.

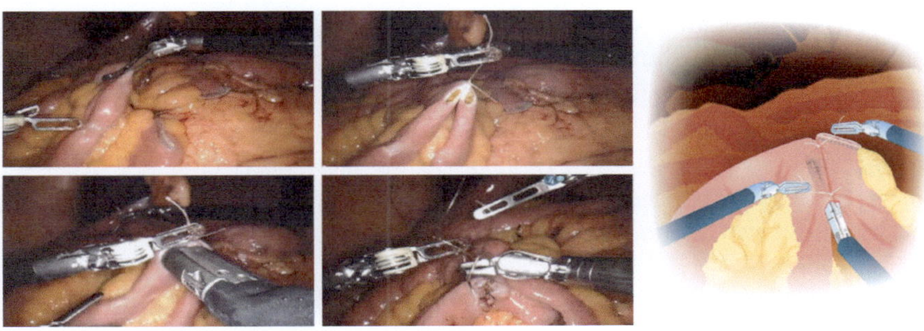

**Fig. 22.6** Ileoileostomy

## Anastomotic/Staple Line Leak Test

I typically test my DI anastomosis and gastric sleeve staple line with a combination of methylene blue dye administered via the calibration tube followed by air insufflation. For those who are concerned about the potential for anaphylaxis to the blue dye, air insufflation with 1 L per minute via the calibration tube is also adequate after the gastric staple line and DI anastomosis have been submerged in saline irrigation. Another option is intra-operative endoscopy and air-insufflation leak test but I find this unnecessary and more time-consuming than the other previously mentioned techniques. Next, I typically place a 19 Fr drain through the right lateral trocar site and place it in the subhepatic space near the duodenal dissection bed in order to monitor for post-operative duodenal stump leak and pancreatic leak. Lipase is sent from the drain on POD2 and the drain is removed prior to discharge if normal.

## Single Anastomosis Duodeno-Ileal Bypass with Sleeve Gastrectomy

The single anastomotic duodenal switch is a simple modification of the traditional switch. It was created in order to limit the risks of macronutrient deficiencies and decrease the technical complexity of the duodenal switch, all while still achieving similar weight loss and resolution of co-morbid conditions when compared to the traditional duodenal switch. The length of the common channel can vary between surgeons but typically is 250–300 cm, as opposed to the traditional duodenal switch which has a common channel of 125–150 cm. The technical aspects of the two procedures are identical with two exceptions: the ileoileostomy is not performed and, therefore, no mesenteric defects need to be closed [9].

## Conclusion

The biliopancreatic diversion with duodenal switch and single anastomosis duodeno-ileal bypass with sleeve gastrectomy are the two most effective bariatric procedures with regard to overall weight loss and resolution of co-morbid conditions. However, these operations are very technically demanding laparoscopically which has contributed to their limited use. The ability to employ the robotic platform to assist in these procedures gives the bariatric surgeon more control over the operation through better visualization, more precise dissection and more ease when performing hand-sewn anastomoses. By approaching these operations in a step-wise manner, these complex bariatric procedures become less daunting and give the surgeon the confidence to offer their patients the full scope of weight loss procedures.

## References

1. Nguyen NT, et al., editors. The ASMBS textbook of bariatric surgery, Bariatric surgery, vol. 1. New York: Springer Science + Business Media; 2015. https://doi.org/10.1007/978-1-4939-1206-3_18.
2. Sjostrom L, Narbro K, Sjostrom CD, Karason K, Larsson B, Wedel H, et al. Effects of bariatric surgery on mortality in Swedish obese subjects. N Engl J Med. 2007;357(8):741–52.
3. Prachard VN, Davee R, Already JC. Duodenal switch provides superior weight loss in the super-obese (BMI>50 kg/m$^2$) compared with gastric bypass. Ann Surg. 2000;10:514–23.
4. Gracia JA, Martinez M, Elia M, Aguilella V, Royo P, Jimenez A, et al. Obesity surgery results depending on technique performed: long-term outcome. Obes Surg. 2009;90:15.
5. Buchwald H, Avidor Y, Braunwald E, et al. Bariatric surgery: a systematic review and meta-analysis. JAMA. 2004;292:1724–37.
6. Van Koughnett JA, Jayaraman S, Eagleson R, Quan D, Wynsberghe AV, Schlachta C. Are there advantages to robotic-assisted surgery over laparoscopy from the surgeon's perspective? J Robot Surg. 2009;3:79–82.
7. Sudan R, Podolsky E. Totally robot-assisted biliary pancreatic diversion with duodenal switch: single dock technique and technical outcomes. Surg Endosc. 2015;29:55–60.
8. Antanavicius G, Katsichtis T, Alswealmeen W, Assali M. Three hundred four robotically assisted biliopancreatic diversion with duodenal switch operations with gradual robotic approach implementation: short-term outcomes, complication profile, and lessons learned. Obes Surg. 2020;30:3961–7.
9. Kallies K, Rogers AM. American Society for Metabolic and Bariatric Surgery updated statement on single-anastomosis duodenal switch. Surg Obes Relat Dis. 2020;16:825–30.

# Single Anastomosis Duodeno-Ileal Bypass with Sleeve Gastrectomy (SADI-S): Indications and Techniques

23

Ingrid Schmiederer, Alex Morera Grau, and Ricard Corcelles

## History of SADI-S

While Roux-en-Y gastric bypass (RYGB) and sleeve gastrectomy (SG) are the most common metabolic procedures currently performed in the United States, new and complex techniques have been developed for greater weight loss efficacy in recent years. The biliopancreatic diversion (BPD) technique was first developed in the 1970s. This demonstrated improved surgical outcomes but also prompted a substantial concern for nutritional deficiencies postoperatively [1–3] Subsequently, in 1988, to help mitigate this complication profile, Dr. Hess and Dr. Hess modified the BPD with the addition of the duodenal switch (BPD-DS) to preserve pyloric and gastric function and to decrease malabsorption with an extended common channel [1, 4]. Still, despite the alterations, the procedure's association with complications, such as diarrhea and malnutrition, hindered its broader implementation.

Therefore, to improve metabolic outcomes and to minimize the anastomotic complications of the BPD-DS) and RYGB procedures, the single anastomosis duodenal-ileal bypass with sleeve gastrectomy (SADI-S) was first described by Dr. Sanchez-Pernaute and Dr. Torres in 2007 [5]. After performing a vertical sleeve gastrectomy, a single duodenal-ileal loop anastomosis is performed, leaving 250–300 cm of the common channel. This new variation, with a single anastomosis

I. Schmiederer
Cleveland Clinic, Bariatric and Metabolic Institute, Cleveland, OH, USA

A. M. Grau
Hospital del Mar, Barcelona, Spain

R. Corcelles (✉)
Cleveland Clinic, Bariatric and Metabolic Institute, Cleveland, OH, USA

Department of Surgery, Cleveland Clinic Lerner College of Medicine, Cleveland, OH, USA
e-mail: corcelr@ccf.org


O. M. Ghanem et al. (eds.), *The SAGES Manual of Metabolic and Bariatric Surgery*, https://doi.org/10.1007/978-3-031-72309-4_23

and preserved pylorus, allows reduced operative time, improves comorbidity resolution, and decreases the rate of associated nutritional deficiencies and surgical complications. [4, 6] As the procedure has become more well-known since 2007, calls for randomized control trials and long-term data have gained momentum.

In 2016, SADI-S was initially deemed 'investigational' as a variant of the BPD-DS) by the American Society for Metabolic and Bariatric Surgery (ASMBS), at a time when the BPD-DS comprised only 0.8% of metabolic and bariatric procedures in the United States [7]. By 2018, the International Federation for the Surgery of Obesity and Metabolic Disorders (IFSO) considered the potential benefits of SADI-S as a recognized metabolic procedure and continued to encourage evaluation for more prospective and comparative evidence [8–10]. Similarly, in an updated statement in 2020, the ASMBS supported the SADI-S—then at 0.25% of metabolic surgical procedures in the United States—but also reinforced that more peer-reviewed data was necessary to fully endorse the procedure as effective and feasible for patients with metabolic comorbidities [7, 11]. Furthermore, the ASMBS pointed out concerns about standardization as it related to technical metrics (e.g., optimal limb lengths, bougie sizes, revision approaches) and outcome-based metrics (weight loss, nutritional standards) [7, 10].

Since then, there have been multiple studies related to the SADI-S and its indications, including a follow-up review of experience with the procedure by Dr. Sanchez-Pernaute et al. at the original institution [6, 12]. Ultimately, available data suggests that SADI-S, as an efficient hypo-absorptive procedure, most benefits patients with higher body mass index (BMI), with more metabolic-associated comorbidities and those who may require revisional surgery after failed previous bariatric operations [5, 13, 14]. In 2021, the IFSO updated its statement to support SADI-S as an operation utilized for significant weight loss with improvement in metabolic health [10].

## Indications and Outcomes

It has been established that the SADI-S procedure is utilized as an effective primary weight loss surgery for patients with higher BMI and metabolic syndromes. One year after the SADI-S, a review of patients performed by Sanchez-Pernaute et al. indicated that the excess weight loss percentage (%EWL) could reach 94.7% and remain steady over 2 years after a SADI-S [5]. Significantly, they found that total weight loss (%TWL) averaged 37% at 5 years in longer-term follow-up. Other studies have confirmed these findings, as Topart et al. found an average %TWL ranging from 32.7 to 41.1% at 1 year [15]. Other studies have reported 80–88% EWL, depending on primary procedures versus revision after SG [16]. In addition to the restrictive nature of the associated sleeve for caloric deficit, the fat malabsorption rate in the SADI-S common channel has been found to be as high as 65%—a percentage that indicates true weightless in patients with severe obesity. [7, 14, 17].

With this weight loss, the metabolic effect of SADI-S in patients with obesity is significant. For patients with diabetes, Sanchez-Pernaute et al. described long-term achievement in controlling diabetes in 70–84% of patients who have undergone

SADI-S [17]. Other studies have also revealed significantly high diabetes remission rates in the context of anti-diabetic medication needs [14] or in HbA1c trends [18]. Compared to 58% of RYGB patients, 88% of SADI-S patients were found to have HbA1c < 6% after 1 year in one prospective cohort study [18]. In a retrospective cohort study between 2013 and 2016 at one institution, Moon et al. found 100% resolution of diabetes at the 2-year follow-up for these patients. For other comorbidities, hyperlipidemia was also significantly resolved at 100%. Hypertension and sleep apnea were resolved at rates close to 50% in the 1-year follow-up period [19].

This technique combines restrictive sleeve gastrectomy with malabsorptive anatomy. Compared to the malabsorption of the RYGB, a SADI-S preserves the pylorus to facilitate satiety and glycemic control. With this multi-factorial approach, authors have also implemented the SADI-S procedure for revision after suboptimal weight regain after a sleeve and as a planned staged procedure for high-risk patients—first the sleeve, followed by time to allow for weight loss and optimization before the scheduled duodeno-ileal bypass operation [13, 14, 16]. This staged process is well-suited for revisional surgery, as the duodeno-ileal anastomosis does not require mobilization of the sleeve the way an RYGB conversion would and it avoids the potential marginal ulceration of a gastro-jejunal anastomosis.

Despite the effectiveness and safety of the SADI-S, one might argue that it is the variations in common channel lengths and sleeve sizing that could account for the spectrum of weight loss. The SADI-S is not fully standardized, as ASMBS suggested in 2020. There is evidence that SADI-S patients with longer sleeves were able to achieve a substantial %EWL with an average of 86% reported at 12 months [18]. For malabsorption, when the common channel is close to 300 cm, the length is found to have correlated with nutritional and metabolic changes with fewer deficiencies [11, 18]. Because weight loss after a SADI-S enhances the quality of life in patients with severe obesity [8], the standardization of this surgical technique and close follow-up for postoperative nutritional support are necessary for the success of SADI-S patients in losing weight and safely resolving comorbidities. As such, this chapter describes surgical technique for the SADI-S that has been successful, as the operation continues to gain utilization in the United States.

## Technique

The SADI-S is a sleeve gastrectomy that is combined with a single anastomosis duodeno-ileostomy and a 200–300 cm common channel. This procedure creates one anastomosis and minimizes mesentery opening.

First, the patient is positioned supine with open arms. In a laparoscopic approach, five incisions are made (Fig. 23.1). In our experience, we use a 5 mm supraumbilical optic trocar, two 12 mm trocars in both flanks, one 5 mm trocar lateral to the left 12 mm trocar, and one 5 mm subxiphoid incision for the liver retractor. If the surgery is performed robotically, we place four trocars following a horizontal supraumbilical line, with one left hand (12 mm) and two right hands (8 mm). To allow for the laparoscopic stapler, a 12 mm right paraumbilical trocar is placed.

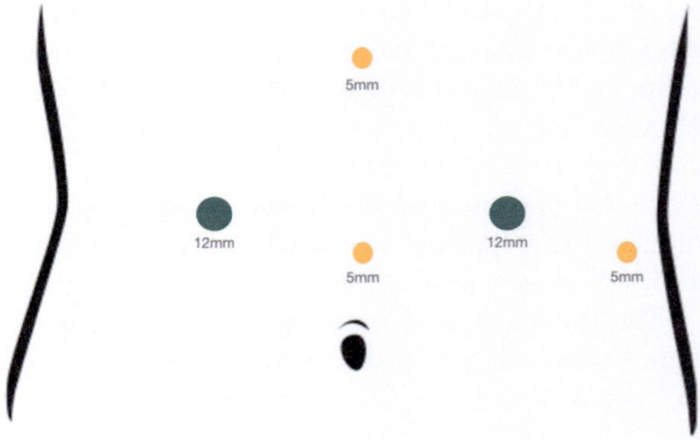


**Fig. 23.1** Laparoscopic Port Placement for SADI-S

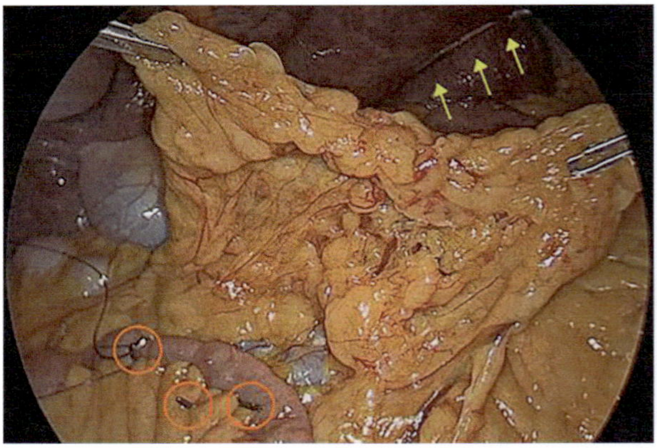

**Fig. 23.2** Placement of Nathanson Retractor (arrows) and Clips for Ileum Measurement (circles)

Whether through a laparoscopic or robotic approach, surgery begins with an inspection of the abdominal cavity. After placing the ports, a subxiphoid liver retractor is placed to expose the relevant anatomy. Our preference is to use a Nathanson liver retractor. Next, the patient is rotated to position with the right side up. The cecum and ileocecal valve are identified. The ileum is traced retrograde to the desired common channel length (this varies between 250 and 300 cm). There, the location for the subsequent duodenal-ileal anastomosis is marked, usually with a PDS suture. It is important to make it clear the orientation of the afferent and efferent limb of the loop, using clips or other markers to prevent misidentification (Fig. 23.2).

The patient is now placed in a reversed Trendelenburg position. In a primary SADI-S, the next step is to perform the sleeve gastrectomy. The gastrocolic ligament is divided from 4–5 cm proximal to the pylorus to the angle of His, using section-ligation devices. Short vessels should be divided up to the left crus to be able to remove the stomach fundus.

The stomach is now divided with an Endo stapler, after placing a bougie, normally between 54 and 40 Fr. To improve the hemostasis of the staple line, reinforced stapler loads can be used, as well as reinforcement with Endo clips or oversewing.

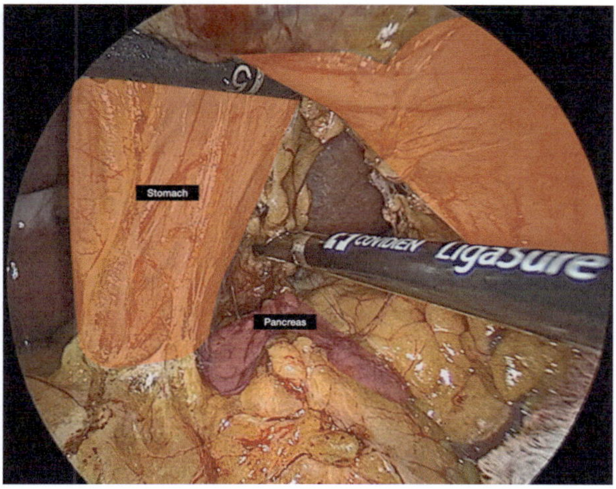


**Fig. 23.3** Retro-gastric and duodenal dissection

In a revision case, the sleeve gastrectomy has already been performed.

Now the procedure continues with the duodenal dissection and transection. There are two equally popular techniques for the dissection of the duodenum. The traditional one starts the dissection 4 cm distal to the pylorus, retracting the duodenum to separate it from the colon, pancreas, and liver. The other method relies on adequate blood supply from the right and left gastric vessels on the lesser curvature. After creating the sleeve, remnant gastroepiploic perforators are divided to dissect the duodenum, normally 3 cm beyond the pylorus. This technique spares vessels from the pancreaticoduodenal arch. As a result, the antrum assumes a linear shape due to the section of gastropancreatic ligaments.

In both approaches, the gastroduodenal artery or the anterior surface of the pancreas will be our distal landmarks for the dissection (Fig. 23.3).

After that, the duodenum is transected with an Endo stapler, with or without reinforcement afterward (Fig. 23.4).

Finally, the marked loop of the ileum is brought up to the duodenal stump in an antecolic manner, and an end-to-side duodeno-ileal anastomosis is fashioned (Figs. 23.5, 23.6, and 23.7).

This anastomosis can be either hand-sewn or stapled, creating a 30-mm anastomosis. In one approach, we create the anastomosis with two posterior and one anterior PDS running sutures. The second technique is to perform a linear-stapled anastomosis using a 30 mm Endo stapler to create a common channel before closing the lateral opening and buttressing the anterior wall with a PDS suture. The type of anastomosis depends on surgeon preference and patient body habitus. In our experience, we typically perform stapled anastomoses in patients with severe abdominal obesity when a hand-sewn technique can be challenging. Drains are not routinely placed.

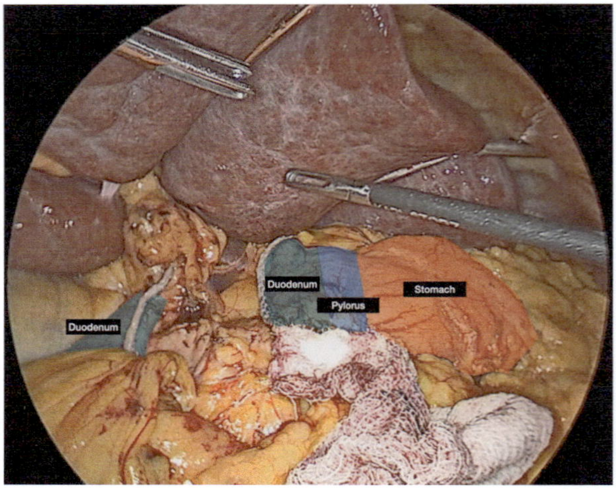


**Fig. 23.4** Reinforced linear staple, transection 3 cm distal to pylorus

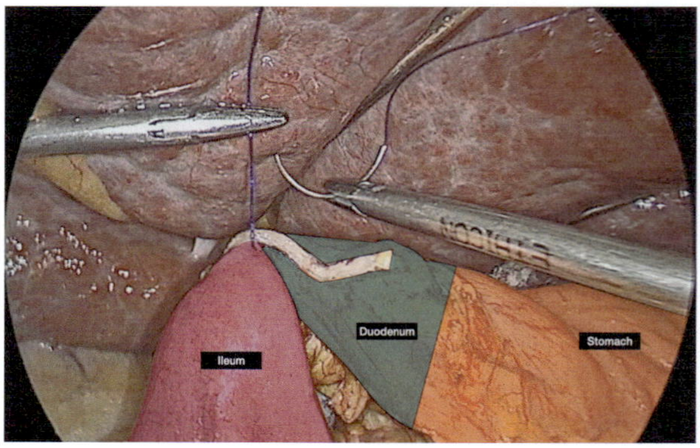


**Fig. 23.5** Anastomosis, incorporating staple line

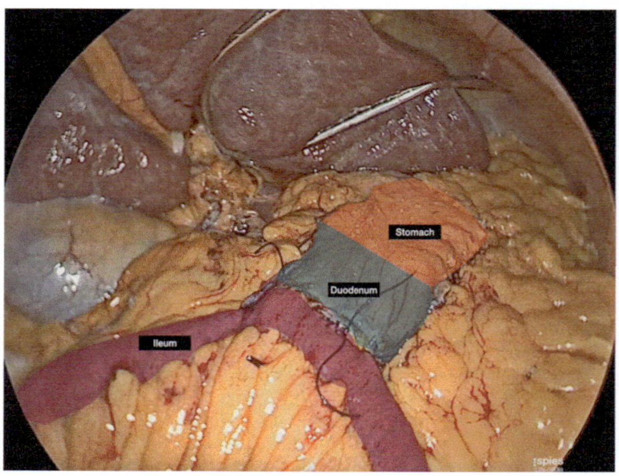


**Fig. 23.6** Final Duodeno-Ileal Anastomosis

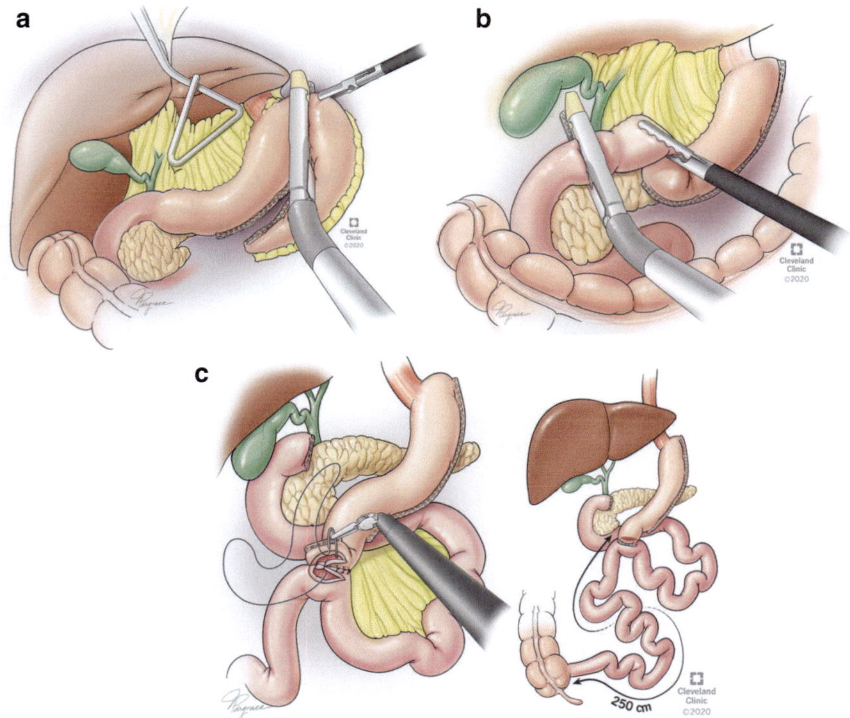


**Fig. 23.7** Overview of SADI-S operative steps. (Reprinted with permission., Cleveland Clinic Foundation ©2024. All Rights Reserved) [20]

## Conclusion

Thus far, the SADI-S has demonstrated promising results for weight loss as a primary procedure and mitigation of weight regain as a revision procedure. In the context of medical comorbidities for patients with obesity, the safe and effective malabsorption of the SADI-S anatomy allows for improvement and potential resolution of diabetes, hyperlipidemia and hypertension, among others. Since its inception in 2007, refinements and approaches to the procedure have continued to evolve as they relate to anatomic considerations, surgical approaches and peri-operative management. The current data and straightforward description of this procedure might serve to encourage surgeons to utilize this technique as an attainable and safe option. An increase in utilization will further allow metabolic surgeons to gather long-term data regarding efficacy and outcomes, which would lead to more precise standardization of this relatively new procedure.

## References


1. Hess DS, Hess DW. Biliopancreatic diversion with a duodenal switch. Obes Surg. 1998;8:267–82.
2. Roth AE, Thornley CJ, Blackstone RP. Outcomes in bariatric and metabolic surgery: an updated 5-year review. Curr Obes Rep. 2020;9(3):380–9.
3. Scopinaro N, Gianetta E, Civalleri D, et al. Bilio-pancreatic bypass for obesity: part II. Initial experience in man. Br J Surg. 1979;66:618–20.
4. Nakanishi H, Matar R, Vahibe A, Abu Dayyeh B, Galvani C, Pullatt R, Davis S, Clapp B, Ghanem O. Single versus double anastomosis duodenal switch in the management of obesity: a meta-analysis and systematic review. Surg Laparosc Endosc Percutan Tech. 2022;32(5):595–605.
5. Sánchez-Pernaute A, Rubio Herrera MA, Pérez-Aguirre ME, et al. Single anastomosis duodeno-ileal bypass with sleeve gastrectomy (SADI-S). One to three-year follow-up. Obes Surg. 2010;20(12):1720–6.
6. Sánchez-Pernaute A, Herrera MÁR, Ferré NP, et al. Long-term results of single-anastomosis duodeno-ileal bypass with sleeve gastrectomy (SADI-S). Obes Surg. 2022;32(3):682–9.
7. Kallies K, Rogers AM. American Society for Metabolic and Bariatric Surgery updated statement on single-anastomosis duodenal switch. Surg Obes Relat Dis. 2020;16:825–30.
8. Admella V, Lazzara C, Sobrino L, et al. Patient-reported outcomes and quality of life after single-anastomosis duodeno-ileal bypass with sleeve gastrectomy (SADI-S): a cross-sectional study with 283 patients from a single institution. Obes Surg. 2023;33:1754–63.
9. Barajas-Gamboa JS, Moon S, Romero-Velez G, et al. Primary single anastomosis duodeno-ileal bypass with sleeve gastrectomy (SADI-S) versus sleeve gastrectomy to SADI conversions: a comparison study of prevalence and safety. Surg Endosc. 2023;37:8682–9.
10. Brown WA, de Leon Ballesteros GP, Ooi G, et al. Single anastomosis duodenal-ileal bypass with sleeve gastrectomy/one anastomosis duodenal switch (SADI-S/OADS) IFSO position statement—update 2020. Obes Surg. 2021;31(1):3–25.
11. Abi Mosleh K, Belluzzi A, Jawhar N, Marrero K, Al-Kordi M, Hage K, Ghanem OM. Single anastomosis duodenoileostomy with sleeve: a comprehensive review of anatomy, surgical technique, and outcomes. Curr Obes Rep. 2024;13(1):121–31. https://doi.org/10.1007/s13679-023-00535-y. Epub ahead of print.
12. Verhoeff K, Mocanu V, Zalasky A, et al. Evaluation of metabolic outcomes following SADI-S: a systematic review and meta-analysis. Obes Surg. 2022;32:1049–63.
13. Pennestrì F, Sessa L, Prioli F, et al. Single anastomosis duodenal-ileal bypass with sleeve gastrectomy (SADI-S): experience from a high-bariatric volume center. Langenbecks Arch Surg. 2022;407:1851–62.
14. Zaveri H, Surve A, Cottam D, et al. Mid-term 4-year outcomes with single anastomosis duodenal-ileal bypass with sleeve gastrectomy surgery at a single US center. Obes Surg. 2018;28:3062–72.
15. Topart P, Becouarn G. The single anastomosis duodenal switch modifications: a review of the current literature on outcomes. Surg Obes Relat Dis. 2017;13(8):1306–12.
16. Liagre A, Martini F, Anduze Y, et al. Efficacy and drawbacks of single-anastomosis duodeno-ileal bypass after sleeve gastrectomy in a Tertiary Referral Bariatric Center. Obes Surg. 2021;31(6):2691–700.
17. Sánchez-Pernaute A, Rubio MÁ, Cabrerizo L, Ramos-Levi A, Pérez-Aguirre E, Torres A. Single-anastomosis duodenoileal bypass with sleeve gastrectomy (SADI-S) for obese diabetic patients. Surg Obes Relat Dis. 2015;11(5):1092–8.
18. Cottam A, Cottam D, Roslin M, et al. A matched cohort analysis of sleeve gastrectomy with and without 300 cm loop duodenal switch with 18-month follow-up. Obes Surg. 2016;26(10):2363–9.

19. Moon RC, Gaskins L, Teixeira AF, Jawad MA. Safety and effectiveness of single-anastomosis duodenal switch procedure: 2-year result from a single US institution. Obes Surg. 2018;28(6):1571–7.
20. Tat C, Del Gobbo GD, Klingler M, Corcelles R. How I do it: robotic single-anastomosis duodeno-ileal bypass with sleeve gastrectomy (SADIS). J Gastrointest Surg. 2020;24(12):2893–5.

# One-Anastomosis Gastric Bypass Technique and Indications

# 24

Asmaa Al Rashed and Mohammad H. Jamal

## Abbreviations

| | |
|---|---|
| %EWL | Excess weight loss |
| ASMBS | The American Society of Metabolic and Bariatric Surgery |
| BMI | Body mass index |
| GERD | Gastroesophageal reflux disease |
| GJ | Gastrojejunostomy |
| IFSO | International Federation for the Surgery of Obesity and Metabolic Disorders |
| MBS | Metabolic and bariatric surgery |
| MBSAQIP | Metabolic and Bariatric Surgery Accreditation and Quality Improvement Program |
| MDT | Multidisciplinary team |
| Mini GB | Mini-gastric bypass |
| MU | Marginal ulcers |
| OAGB | One-anastomosis gastric bypass |
| OFA | Opioid-free anesthesia |
| PE | Pulmonary embolism |
| PPI | Proton pump inhibitor |
| RCT | Randomized controlled trial |
| SADI-S | Anastomosis duodeno-ileal bypass with sleeve gastrectomy |

A. Al Rashed (✉)
Surgery Department, Amiri Hospital, MOH, Kuwait City, Kuwait

M. H. Jamal
Department of Surgery, Kuwait University, Kuwait City, Kuwait
e-mail: Mohammad.Jamal@mail.McGill.ca


O. M. Ghanem et al. (eds.), *The SAGES Manual of Metabolic and Bariatric Surgery*, https://doi.org/10.1007/978-3-031-72309-4_24

## History of One Anastomosis Gastric Bypass

The first one anastomosis gastric bypass (OAGB) was performed in 1997 by Rutledge as a salvage operation for a trauma patient. The first published series followed with 1274 patients that were operated from 1997 to 2001 [1], and it was termed mini-gastric bypass (MGB) which was later changed to one anastomosis gastric bypass (OAGB). The operation described in that series involved creating a long gastric pouch anastomosed in an end-to-side fashion with a loop of jejunum 200 cm from the ligament of Trietz.

The mean excess body weight at one year was reported in that study at 68% and at two years 77% with an overall complication rate of 5.2%. The study did not report on bile reflux but mentioned that six patients had esophagitis postoperatively with one Barrett's esophagus in a patient who had Nissen fundoplication pre-OAGB. In that initial series, only six patients underwent revision due to severe nausea resulting in excessive weight loss. The revision was in the form of only a gastrogastric anastomosis without taking down the gastrojejunal anastomosis.

This was followed up with another publication from the same group, this time with 2410 patients from 1997 to 2004 [2]. The excess body weight loss in one year was 80%, with a complication rate of 5.9% and 0.08% mortality rate. The leak rate was 1.08% and all patients who had a leak were managed surgically. The long-term complications included ulcers in 97 patients (4%) who were treated with medical therapy, but three patients did not respond requiring revision of their surgery. Other long-term complications included iron deficiency anemia (4.9 %). Excessive weight loss with malnutrition occurred in 1.1%. In both papers there was no mention of bile reflux; however, in the later paper, dyspepsia was reported as a long-term complication but managed medically and a revision of the surgery was not required. Of note that in this series the anastomosis was at 180 cm from the ligament of Treitz.

In 2005, two further series were published one from Spain and another from Taiwan [3, 4]. The series from Spain by Carbajo et al., included 209 patients that were operated from 2002 to 2004 [3]. The technique of the surgery was mainly different in the form of the anastomosis that was made in a side-to-side fashion rather than the end of the stomach to the side of jejunum as described in Rutledge's papers. The jejunum was anastomosed 200 cm from the ligament of Trietz. In four of the patients in this series, the MGB was following a restrictive procedure. In 57 patients another operation was added to the MGB in the form of cholecystectomy in 18 patients, ventral hernia repair in 5 patients, and adhesiolysis in 38 patients. The excess body weight loss at one year was 75% and 80% at 2 years.

Two mortalities were reported in this series, one due to massive pulmonary embolism, and one due to pneumonia in a patient who had necrosis of the excluded stomach post OAGB that required a laparotomy for treatment of the necrosis. The leak was observed in 4 patients within 24 h postoperatively and was managed conservatively. Two patients had a laparotomy within the first 24 h postoperatively due to bleeding. In terms of the long-term complications, the authors reported only clinically significant iron deficiency anemia in two patients, and no bile reflux was reported.

The surgery did not gain ground except after further research mainly from groups in South East Asia and India. In 2005, Lee et al. published a randomized controlled trial comparing the OAGB to RYGB [4]. The study recruited 40 patients in each arm and had a minimum follow-up of 2 years. The early complications rate was significantly higher in the RYGB group 20% compared to 7.5% in the OAGB group. All the complications in the OAGB group were minor but in the RYGB group, there were 2 major complications in terms of leak out of the 8 complications. The percentage of excess weight loss was 58.7% and 60.0% at 1 and 2 years, respectively, in the RYGB group, and 64.9% and 64.4% in the OAGB group. The follow-up rate was 100% in both groups with a 2-year minimum follow-up period, only 3 patients from each group developed late complications. Two patients from the OAGB group developed a bleeding marginal ulcer, while one patient in the RYGB group developed bleeding marginal ulcer. All patients who developed late complications did not require reoperation and were treated medically. No patients in the OAGB group develop bile reflux.

Another study by the same group on revisional surgeries for patients who underwent primary OAGB in the same center from January 2001 to December 2009, reported a revisional surgery rate of 1.7% (23 patients) out of 1322 patients who underwent primary OAGB [5]. The most common cause of revision was malnutrition in 9 patients followed by inadequate weight loss in 8 patients. Three patients underwent revisions for bile reflux and three for dissatisfaction. Of note is that the gastrojejunostomy was created with the small bowel at 200 cm distal to the ligament of Trietz.

The metabolic surgery community despite these studies did not accept OAGB as a valid procedure and skepticism continued. Opponents of the procedure demanded further studies, in particular long-term studies to clarify the risks of malignancy in the remnant stomach and bile reflux. A study by Dr. Demaria's group published in 2006 looked at revisional surgeries for OAGB performed in five different hospitals within the same region where OAGB originated [6]. They identified 32 patients with complications post OAGB requiring revisional surgeries. The complications included anastomotic leak in 3 patients, bile reflux in 20, intractable marginal ulcer in 5, malnutrition in 8 and weight regain in 2 patients. Most patients underwent RYGB as the revisional procedure.

The surgery started to gain acceptance outside the USA, with further studies on outcomes and complications getting published. The use of OAGB as a conversional surgery post-sleeve gastrectomy for weight regain became the first option for such indication by our group and we started performing it in 2015. We published one of the first reports coming from the MENA region for OAGB post-sleeve gastrectomy for weight regain, in which 56 patients underwent the procedure. The average weight prior to OAGB was 112 ± 24.6 kg. The minimum weight they have reached is 85 ± 21.3 kg after a duration of 19 ± 9.2 months. Percentage of total weight loss (TWL%) at 1, 3, 6, and 12 months postoperatively was found to be 7.6%, 9.8%, 14.1%, and 28.8%, respectively. TWL% on the last day of follow-up was 24%. In terms of the short-term complications, two patients had marginal ulcers, in which one had a perforation a year after the OAGB and required washout with an omental patch [7]. With further follow-up even after the publication of the study we had to revise 2 patients to RYGB due to bile reflux.

In 2018, IFSO commissioned a task force on OAGB, which performed a systematic review of the literature that included 52 studies of reasonable quality with more than 15 studies having more than 1 year follow-up data on the patients [8]. Four of the studies included were randomized controlled trials. The task force in their position statement and based on the result of the review concluded that OAGB is a recognized metabolic procedure and should no longer be considered investigational. This was the first recognition of OAGB from a professional metabolic surgery organization.

## Patient's Selection, Indications and Contraindications

The OAGB procedure was endorsed by the International Federation for the Surgery of Obesity and Metabolic Disorders (IFSO) in 2018 and the American Society of Metabolic and Bariatric Surgery (ASMBS) in 2022 as a recognized bariatric/metabolic procedure [9, 10]. The indications for the OAGB procedure have been discussed in the literature as a primary MBS and as a secondary/conversional revisional MBS.

### Indications

In an article that used expert-modified Delphi consensus and aimed to generate clinical guidelines for patients' selection in OAGB, a committee of 57 recognized bariatric surgeons from 24 countries created 69 statements. The statements addressed the suitability of OAGB in a variety of clinical conditions [11] to bridge the gap while more long-term evidence emerges about OAGB procedure.

The experts in that article's voting results chose that the OAGB procedure was an acceptable and suitable option in the following cases:

- BMI >70, BMI >60, BMI >50 kg/m$^2$ as a one-stage procedure (91.23%).
- As the second stage of a two-stage bariatric surgery after sleeve gastrectomy for BMI >50 kg/m$^2$ (instead of BPD/DS) (90.91%).
- Weight regains after endoscopic sleeve gastroplasty (98.18%), previous gastric balloon (94.55%), restrictive procedures (90.91%), and Bariclip failure (89%).
- Salvage technique for duodenal perforation during SADI-S and early D-I anastomotic leak in SADI-S (78.18% and 74.55%).
- Low BMI (30–35 kg/m$^2$) with associated metabolic problems (82.46%).
- Patients with medical conditions such as low ejection fraction <30% (87.72%), collagen vascular disease (82.46%), minor thalassemia (81.82%), gallstones (96.36%), nonalcoholic steatohepatitis NASH and cirrhosis child A (81.82%), mild to moderate gastroesophageal reflux disease GERD (A, B) (80.7%), gastro-

paresis (77.19%), esophageal motility disorder (75.44%), chronic renal insufficiency were not on dialysis (74.55%), renal stones (70.91%).
- Stable psychiatric disorders (81.82%).
- Prader-Willi syndrome with BMI >50 (84.2%).
- Patients with subtle drug levels of medications such as lithium or digoxin (75.44%), long-term blood thinners (80.70%), and human immunodeficiency virus HIV on retroviral (77.19%).
- Elderly (age >65 years old) (80.7%).
- Vegetarian and vegan patients (77.19% and 63.16%, respectively).
- Patients with large/giant hiatal hernia with concurrent hiatal hernia repair (71.93%).

## Contraindications

To date, no absolute contraindications have been reported in the literature other than those that preclude laparoscopic surgery and general anesthesia. However, some conditions can be considered relative contraindications based on experts' opinions. As mentioned in the previous article [12], the experts had consensus for disagreement for the suitability of the OAGB procedure predominantly in the following cases:

- Smokers (80.70%)
- Chronic alcoholics (80.70%)
- Children (age 6–13 years) (77.19%)
- Barrett's metaplasia, insulinoma, and intestinal metaplasia of stomach (89.29%, 89.47% and 74.55% respectively)
- Severe GERD (C, D) (75.44%)
- Crohn disease (78.18%)
- Gastric or duodenal ulcers (72.22%)
- NASH and Cirrhosis Child B (70.91%)
- Iron deficiency anemia (70.18%)
- In patients who need OCP (73.68%)
- Leak management from sleeve gastrectomy (77.19%) and mid-sleeve stricture (74.55%)
- Weight regains after RYGB (73.68%)

It is noteworthy to mention that patient selection in OAGB is still a point of discussion among experts and due to the lack of clear scientific evidence, it is important to make a distinction between a clinical guideline that synthesizes available evidence and a consensus statement that represents expert opinion [11] which is level D evidence. Additionally, it is encouraged that patients with obesity need to be evaluated in a comprehensive MDT setting to individualize care and select the best management modality [13].

In revisional bariatric surgery, there are three distinct types of procedures: corrective (re-exploring the anatomy to overcome existing postoperative problems), conversions (rearranging anatomy to perform a different bariatric procedure), and reversals (restoring the original anatomy) [12]. Therefore, it is paramount to clearly document the indications of OAGB procedures in MBS data registries to generate better-quality evidence for future studies.

## Technique with Modifications

The first technique described by Rutledge et al. utilized five laparoscopic ports [1]. One port for the liver retractor, two ports for the assistant surgeon and two for the main surgeon. A large orogastric tube is inserted and a long gastric tube is constructed over the tube using linear staplers. The short gastrics are not divided. The end of the stomach pouch was then anastomosed to a side of the small bowel that is brought antecolic, 200 cm from the ligament of Trietz using staplers to close both the posterior and anterior gastrojejunostomy. This was modified by Dr. Carbajo by adding an antireflux stitch by suturing the afferent limb laterally to the gastric pouch and by performing the gastrojejunostomy in a side-to-side fashion with suturing for closure of the anterior gastrojejunostomy [3]. Our operative technique for the procedure is the following:

The patient is placed on the operative table with both arms out and in a split-leg position. An 11 mm optical trocaris was inserted in the left upper quadrant just off the midline to accommodate the 10 mm camera. It is important that this port visualizes the hiatus and the ligament of Treitz. A 12 mm port for stapling is inserted in the right upper quadrant. Particular attention should be given to this port placement as it should be higher than the stapling port for RYGB, it shouldn't be too medial as entry to the lesser sac will be challenging. A 5 mm port is inserted in the left upper quadrant for the assistant. Another 5 mm port is inserted in the right upper quadrant for the operating surgeon. The assistant surgeon stays in between the patient's leg and the operating surgeon on the patient's right side. A 5 mm liver retractor port is inserted in the epigastrium just below the xiphoid process.

We start by identifying the angle of His and the gastroesophageal (GE) junction by dissecting the GE fat pad and fundal attachment to the left crus. We then start preparing the gastric pouch by identifying the crow's foot on the lesser curvature and then dissecting the gastric serosa just below it from the blood supply to gain access to the posterior stomach. The first stapler should be vertical to divide the gastric antrum 3 cm from the pylorus. We then insert a 36F orogastric tube and staple it all the way to the GE junction to create a long narrow gastric tube. Further dissection of the posterior fundus is usually necessary prior to the last two stapler firings in order to make sure that the pouch is constructed properly. We then suture the staple lines of the gastric pouch and the excluded stomach using 3.00 barbed sutures in a continuous fashion. We then identify the ligament of Trietz and count 180 cm distal to it. We then do an enterotomy in the small bowel and a gastrotomy in the stomach pouch just posterior to the staple line. We use a 5 cm length of the stapler reload to construct the posterior layer of the gastrojejunostomy in a side-to-side fashion. The anterior gastrojejunostomy is sutured with a 3.00 PDS suture in a continuous fashion over the orogastric tube. An antireflux suture is placed at the superolateral angle of the gastrojejunostomy.

A study by Kermansaravi et al. examined the areas of non-consensus in the technique of OAGB and identified various areas of non-consensus in the operative technique that are summarized next [14]. The first transection point from the pylorus at the antrum can vary from 2 to 5 cm. The size of the bougie is variable from 32 to 50 F. The length of the pouch can be from 12 to 18 cm, but it is thought that it should be at least 15 cm to avoid bile reflux. The length of the anastomosis also varies between 25 and 60 mm. Most surgeons prefer an anastomosis to the posterior wall of the stomach but some papers reported an anastomosis to the anterior wall of stomach..

In terms of bowel length, it is thought that biliopancreatic limb BPL longer than 200 cm may result in malabsorption. Some surgeons count the whole bowel length and perform the anastomosis in the middle, some at a point that bypasses 60% of the bowel distal to the ligament of Trietz and some surgeons report the importance of making the common channel at least 400 cm in length. The antireflux stitch is not routinely performed by all surgeons.

Other areas of non-consensus according to the study include the closure of the Petersen defect in which most surgeons do not repair the Petersen defect and according to a survey by MAHAWER et al. only 18% of surgeons close it [15].

## Early Complications

Early complications (occurring within 30 days postoperatively) include anastomotic leak, staple line leak, bleeding, hematoma formation and thromboembolic events.

A study on 2678 patients who had OAGB as a primary or conversional procedure in eight Italian centers showed an intraoperative complications rate of 0.5% and early complications rate of 3.1% [16]. Early complications occurred in 74 out of 2251 (3.2%) who had primary OAGB and in 10 out of 427 (2.3%) patients who had revisional OAGB. Bleeding occurred in 21 patients (0.8%), of which 20 patients needed an operative exploration. Endoluminal bleeding occurred in 25 patients (0.9%) in which 2 patients required surgery and 9 required endoscopic exploration. Five patients developed an anastomotic leak (0.1%), seven patients had a gastric pouch leak (0.26%), six patients had small bowel injury/perforation (0.2%) and one patient had a gastric remnant leak (0.03%). Anastomotic stenosis developed in 5 patients (0.2%). Two patients developed intraabdominal abscesses (0.07%) and two had a pulmonary embolism (0.07%).

In the YOMEGA RCT, the early complications rate in the 117 patients in the OAGB arm was 3.4% [17]. There was one case of peritonitis, one anastomotic stenosis, one wall haematoma, and one haematoma of the gastrojejunal anastomosis. All patients were treated conservatively except in the case of peritonitis.

In a UK study involving seven bariatric units, 925 cases of OAGB performed from 2010 to 2018 were reviewed retrospectively [18]. The majority of patients had OAGB as a primary procedure 913 (98.7%). Early complications were low and included bleeding requiring surgical exploration in 3 [0.3%] patients and one patient developing gastrojejunal anastomosis narrowing (0.1%).

Leak in OAGB in particular when compared to other metabolic procedures is potentially involved with a more severe form of peritonitis due to the presence of bile at the leak site as opposed to leak from sleeve gastrectomy where the pylorus prevents the bile from entering the stomach and RYGB where bile is excluded from the anastomosis. Therefore, surgeons tend to operate early on OAGB leaks to convert the OAGB to RYGB or to perform simple repair and washout especially if the leak is from the gastrojejunal anastomosis.

A metanalysis and systematic review of 46 published studies that included 44318 OAGB cases found 410 leaks reported which gives a leak rate of 1% [19]. All leaks occurred within 6 weeks and no leaks reported after 6 weeks. Acute leaks identified within 7 days of surgery occurred in 33% of patients and the rest identified within 1–6 weeks. CT with or without oral contrast was the most used diagnostic method, followed by diagnostic laparoscopy and upper GI series. Out of the 410 leaks, detailed management was mentioned in 198 patients only. Surgery was the treatment strategy in 123 patients (62.1%) out of the 198 leak patients. The most common surgical strategy utilised was diagnostic laparoscopy and peritoneal washout with or without T-tube placement in 61 patients (30.8%). Conversion to RYGB was performed for leak management in 19 (9.6%) patients. Repair of the anastomosis with drainage performed in 14 (7.1%) patients. No details were given for the type of surgery in 312 (16.2%) of patients and reversal of OAGB to normal anatomy was utilised in one patient.

Non-surgical management in the form of endoscopic therapy was utilised in 33(16.7%) and medical therapy with antibiotics and parenteral nutrition in 27 (13.6%) of patients. Percutaneous tube insertion was performed in 9 (4.6%) of patients..

A retrospective review at a single private clinic in France of 2780 OAGB cases performed by a single surgeon between May 2010 to December 2017, identified 46 patients with leaks (1.7%) [20]. Out of the 2780 patients, 2454 patients underwent primary OAGB and 326 underwent OAGB as a revisional procedure. Leak rate was higher in revisional procedures at 4% (13 of 326 cases). Leak rate in primary OAGB was 1.3% (33 of 2454 cases).

The majority of patients had leak from the gastric pouch 27 patients (59%), 6 from the gastrojejunostomy (13%) and 13 patients had leaks without an identification of the site of leakage (28%). Surgical management was performed in all patients with anastomotic leakage, in 19% of patients with gastric pouch leak and only in 15% with leak of undetermined site. Most of the patients who underwent surgical management had drain placement or T-tube placement and only one patient underwent conversion to RYGB. All leak patients were discharged and no mortality was observed in this cohort.

## Long-term Complications and Considerations

### Bile Reflux

Bile reflux has been reported after OAGB. Musella et al. found about 4% rate for bile reflux in OAGB and a statistical correlation, with pouches shorter than 9 cm [16]. In a study by Chevallier et al., patients underwent upper GI endoscopy and biopsies after OAGB and were found to have foveolar hyperplasia which is a sign of bile reflex in about 17% at 2 years and 4.6% at 4 years without any dysplasia or metaplasia [21]. The initial conservative management for bile reflux is with probiotics and avoiding triggering food such high fat or high-volume meals can be helpful and addition of PPI in case of marginal ulcers. However, if the symptoms were intractable and severe, surgical management with conversion to RYGB is often effective [22].

### GERD

GERD has been reported after MBS and OAGB. In a systematic review and meta-analysis to investigate the incidence of new-onset GERD, reflux change, esophagitis, Barrett's esophagus, and revision due to reflux, gastritis, and marginal ulcer post OAGB by Ali Esparham et al. was published in September 2023. It found that the rate of new-onset reflux after OAGB is 6% in 87 studies with 27,775 patients. The new-onset reflux rate was significantly higher than RYGB but not different from sleeve gastrectomy. The pooled random effects analysis of 44 studies showed that 2% of patients with OAGB were converted to RYGB due to severe reflux. The rate of esophagitis and Barrett's esophagus was 15% and 1%, respectively [23]. Interestingly, complete remission of GERD was reported in 92% of cases after OAGB in long-term follow-up study of 1200 patients as reported by Carbajo et al. [24]..

### Marginal Ulcers (MU)

In any gastric bypass operation, the risk of marginal ulcer at the gastrojejunostomy (GJ) site is often present as this has been attributed to continuous acid secretion by the gastric pouch that causes erosions at the GJ site. A large gastric pouch can result in excessive acid load in contact with the jejunum mucosa that can induces ulcer at the jejunal side of the anastomosis. Therefore, creating a narrow but long pouch and prescribing a PPI after OAGB procedure should reduce MU incidence [22]. OAGB is thought to have a protective effect as the presence of bile at the GJ level can act as a buffer to avoid the constant injury of the epithelium [25].

In a systematic review and meta-analysis of marginal ulcers following OAGB (32 studies with total of 8868 patients, 228 had MU) were analyzed by Lee et al., and found the incidence of MU to be 2.59% (95% CI 1.89–3.52). It was reported that 89.7% were treated conservatively with PPIs, while 10.3% had surgery to treat MU. The researcher concluded that marginal ulcer is an uncommon complication following OAGB and larger, well-designed studies reporting on risk factors, investigation, and management are warranted [26]..

## Bowel Function

Gastrointestinal side effects are frequently reported after MBS. Carina Rossoni et al. conducted a cross-sectional, descriptive, and analytical study that aimed to analyze the bowel function of 114 patients who underwent OAGB with up to 5-year follow-up. They divided the follow-up period to 3 times periods were 1–6 months (T1), 6–12 months (T2), and 1–5 years (T3). The T1 group had more severe symptoms/nausea than the T2 group. The T2 group had a significantly lower defecation frequency than the T1 and T3 groups. As for the occurrence of diarrhea, associations were not found in the considered groups. The T3 group had a greater severity of constipation associated with greater difficulty in consuming red meat, white meat, rice, vegetables, and salads. The study concluded that gastrointestinal symptoms are prevalent in the first postoperative months. However, diarrhea was not common [27].

## Malnutrition

Malnutrition refers to deficiencies, excesses, or imbalances in a person's intake of energy and or nutrients [28]. One of the potential serious long-term side effects or complications of OAGB is malnutrition, and hence lifelong supplements and close follow-up with dietitians is important for OAGB patients.

In a systematic review that was conducted by Nanda Bandlamudi et al., looking at malnutrition following OAGB, 50 studies involving 49,991 patients were included. In-hospital treatment for severe malnutrition was needed for 0.9% ($n = 446$) of patients. Biliopancreatic limb (BPL) length was 150 cm in 1.1% patients, >150 cm in 33.9%, and not reported in 65% patients. Revision of OAGB to normal anatomy was done in 28.2%, to sleeve gastrectomy in 10.3%, RYGB in 9.2%, and shortening of BPL length in 3.8% patients. Eight (0.02%) deaths were reported, while 33.8% of patients responded to treatment; 2.2% did not respond and no report in 63.9% of patients. The study suggested that standardization of the OAGB technique along with robust prospective data collection is required to understand this serious complication [29].

## Conclusion and OAGB Outcome

### Efficacy and Safety

The OAGB procedure has been performed for over 25 years and was recognized more recently by many MBS organizations worldwide as a bariatric/metabolic procedure due to its established safety and efficacy [8–10].

In a systematic review conducted by Balamurugan et al. and published in May 2023, that compared the efficacy and safety between of (RYGB), (OAGB) and (SADI-S) from 2002 to 2022 and has included 18 eligible studies with a total of 62,833 patients (majority had RYGB 87.80%, OAGB 10.85%, SADI-S 1.35%). The weight loss outcomes were greatest with SADI-S (% EWL ± SD, 73.5 ± 2.24 at 5 years) and OAGB (% EWL ± SD 75.84 at 5 years and %TWL 29.2 at 10 years), while lower in RYGB (% EWL ± SD 65.47 ± 5.92 at 5 years and %TWL 26.7 at 10 years). In terms of comorbidities resolution, the analysis showed that SADI-S offered better resolution of diabetes whereas hypertension and dyslipidemia resolution were better with OAGB. While early complications were higher with SADI-S (mean 11.8%), OAGB (8.12%), RYGB (mean 8.06%); the late complications were more frequent with RYGB (48.94%), then SADI-S (22.9%) and the lowest with OAGB (12.39%). The mortality was reported (mean ± SD) in RYGB to be 0.07% ± 0.11 in 11 studies, OAGB 0.09% ± 0.18 in 8 studies, and SADI-S 0.2% ± 0.28 in 3 studies. The systematic review concluded that both SADI-S and OAGB are as effective as RYGB for weight loss, but OAGB offers lesser complications [30].

As we witness the rise of OAGB, it is noteworthy to continue to learn from the long-term outcome of the procedure as well as from the patients' reported outcome. Standardizing the surgical technique of the OAGB operation, comprehensive assessment and patient's selection, and accurate documentation of acute and long-term complication in MBS registries should continue to help in generating better evidence-based medicine for the management of our patients.

## References

1. Rutledge R. The mini-gastric bypass: experience with the first 1274 cases. Obes Surg. 2001;11:276–80. https://doi.org/10.1381/096089201321336584.
2. Rutledge R, Walsh TR. Continued excellent results with the mini-gastric bypass: six-year study in 2410 patients. Obes Surg. 2005;15:1304–8. https://doi.org/10.1381/096089205774512663.
3. Carbajo M, García-Caballero M, Toledano M, Osorio D, García-Lanza C, Carmona JA. One-anastomosis gastric bypass by laparoscopy: results of the first 209 patients. Obes Surg. 2005;15:398–404. https://doi.org/10.1381/0960892053576677.
4. Lee W-J, Yu P-J, Wang W, Chen T-C, Wei P-L, Huang M-T. Laparoscopic Roux-en-Y versus mini-gastric bypass for the treatment of morbid obesity: a prospective randomized controlled clinical trial. Ann Surg. 2005;242:20–8. https://doi.org/10.1097/01.sla.0000167762.46568.98.
5. Lee W-J, Lee Y-C, Ser K-H, Chen S-C, Chen J-C, Su Y-H. Revisional surgery for laparoscopic minigastric bypass. Surg Obes Relat Dis. 2011;7:486–91. https://doi.org/10.1016/j.soard.2010.10.012.

6. Johnson WH, Fernanadez AZ, Farrell TM, MacDonald KG, Grant JP, McMahon RL, et al. Surgical revision of loop ("mini") gastric bypass procedure: multicenter review of complications and conversions to Roux-en-Y gastric bypass. Surg Obes Relat Dis. 2007;3:37–41. https://doi.org/10.1016/j.soard.2006.09.012.
7. Jamal MH, Elabd R, AlMutairi R, Albraheem A, Alhaj A, Alkhayat H, et al. The safety and efficacy of one anastomosis gastric bypass as a revision for sleeve gastrectomy. Obes Surg. 2020;30:2280–4. https://doi.org/10.1007/s11695-020-04484-6.
8. De Luca M, Tie T, Ooi G, Higa K, Himpens J, Carbajo M-A, et al. Mini gastric bypass-one anastomosis gastric bypass (MGB-OAGB)-IFSO position statement. Obes Surg. 2018;28:1188–206. https://doi.org/10.1007/s11695-018-3182-3.
9. De Luca M, Piatto G, Merola G, et al. IFSO update position statement on one-anastomosis gastric bypass (OAGB). Obes Surg. 2021;31(7):3251–78.
10. ASMBS endorsed procedures and FDA approved devices. American Society for Metabolic and Bariatric Surgery website.
11. Kermansaravi M, Parmar C, Chiappetta S, Shahabi S, Abbass A, Abbas SI, Abouzeid M, Antozzi L, Asghar ST, Bashir A, Bhandari M, Billy H, Caina D, Campos FJ, Carbajo MA, Chevallier JM, Jazi AHD, de Gordejuela AGR, Haddad A, ElFawal MH, Himpens J, Inam A, Kassir R, Kasama K, Khan A, Kow L, Kular KS, Lakdawala M, Layani LA, Lee WJ, Luque-de-León E, Loi K, Mahawar K, Mahdy T, Musella M, Nimeri A, González JCO, Pazouki A, Poghosyan T, Prager G, Prasad A, Ramos AC, Rheinwalt K, Ribeiro R, Ruiz-Úcar E, Rutledge R, Shabbir A, Shikora S, Singhal R, Taha O, Talebpour M, Verboonen JS, Wang C, Weiner R, Yang W, Vilallonga R, De Luca M. Patient selection in one anastomosis/mini gastric bypass—an expert modified Delphi consensus. Obes Surg. 2022;32(8):2512–24. https://doi.org/10.1007/s11695-022-06124-7. Epub 2022 Jun 15. PMID: 35704259.
12. Khalaj A, Barzin M, Ebadinejad A, Mahdavi M, Ebrahimi N, Valizadeh M, Hosseinpanah F. Revisional bariatric surgery due to complications: indications and outcomes. Obes Surg. 2023;33(11):3463–71. https://doi.org/10.1007/s11695-023-06832-8. Epub 2023 Sep 28. PMID: 37770774.
13. 2022 American Society of Metabolic and Bariatric Surgery (ASMBS) and International Federation for the Surgery of Obesity and Metabolic Disorders (IFSO): indications for metabolic and bariatric surgery. 2022;33:3–14.
14. Kermansaravi M, DavarpanahJazi AH, ShahabiShahmiri S, Carbajo M, Vitiello A, Parmar CD, et al. Areas of non-consensus around one anastomosis/mini gastric bypass (OAGB/MGB): a narrative review. Obes Surg. 2021;31:2453–63. https://doi.org/10.1007/s11695-021-05276-2.
15. Mahawar KK, Kular KS, Parmar C, Van Den Bossche M, Graham Y, Carr WRJ, et al. Perioperative practices concerning one anastomosis (mini) gastric bypass: a survey of 210 surgeons. Obes Surg. 2018;28:204–11. https://doi.org/10.1007/s11695-017-2831-2.
16. Musella M, Susa A, Manno E, De Luca M, Greco F, Raffaelli M, et al. Complications following the mini/one anastomosis gastric bypass (MGB/OAGB): a multi-institutional survey on 2678 patients with a mid-term (5 years) follow-up. Obes Surg. 2017;27:2956–67. https://doi.org/10.1007/s11695-017-2726-2.
17. Robert M, Espalieu P, Pelascini E, Caiazzo R, Sterkers A, Khamphommala L, et al. Efficacy and safety of one anastomosis gastric bypass versus Roux-en-Y gastric bypass for obesity (YOMEGA): a multicentre, randomised, open-label, non-inferiority trial. Lancet. 2019;393:1299–309. https://doi.org/10.1016/S0140-6736(19)30475-1.
18. Hussain A, Van Den Bossche M, Kerrigan DD, Alhamdani A, Parmar C, Javed S, et al. Retrospective cohort study of 925 OAGB procedures. The UK MGB/OAGB Collaborative Group. Int J Surg. 2019;69:13–8. https://doi.org/10.1016/j.ijsu.2019.07.003.
19. Kermansaravi M, Kassir R, Valizadeh R, Parmar C, Davarpanah Jazi AH, Shahmiri SS, et al. Management of leaks following one-anastomosis gastric bypass: an updated systematic review and meta-analysis of 44 318 patients. Int J Surg. 2023;109:1497–508. https://doi.org/10.1097/JS9.0000000000000346.

20. Liagre A, Queralto M, Juglard G, Anduze Y, Iannelli A, Martini F. Multidisciplinary management of leaks after one-anastomosis gastric bypass in a single-center series of 2780 consecutive patients. Obes Surg. 2019;29:1452–61. https://doi.org/10.1007/s11695-019-03754-2.
21. Chevallier JM, Trelles N, Arienzo R, Zinzindohoue F. Endoscopic findings after laparoscopic omega gastric bypass. In: Obesity surgery. New York: Springer; 2011.
22. Solouki A, Kermansaravi M, Davarpanah Jazi AH, Kabir A, Farsani TM, Pazouki A. One-anastomosis gastric bypass as an alternative procedure of choice in morbidly obese patients. J Res Med Sci. 2018;23:84. https://doi.org/10.4103/jrms.JRMS_386_18. PMID: 30294352; PMCID: PMC6161487.
23. Esparham A, Ahmadyar S, Zandbaf T, Dalili A, Rezapanah A, Rutledge R, Khorgami Z. Does one-anastomosis gastric bypass expose patients to gastroesophageal reflux: a systematic review and meta-analysis. Obes Surg. 2023;33(12):4080–102. https://doi.org/10.1007/s11695-023-06866-y. Epub 2023 Oct 25. PMID: 37880462.
24. Carbajo MA, Luque-de-León E, Jiménez JM, et al. Laparoscopic one-anastomosis gastric bypass: technique, results, and long-term follow-up in 1200 patients. Obes Surg. 2017;27(5):1153–67.
25. Aleman R, Lo Menzo E, Szomstein S, Rosenthal RJ. Efficiency and risks of one-anastomosis gastric bypass. Ann Transl Med. 2020;8(Suppl 1):S7. https://doi.org/10.21037/atm.2020.02.03. PMID: 32309411; PMCID: PMC7154323.
26. Lee S, Supparamaniam S, Varghese C, et al. Marginal ulcers following one-anastomosis gastric bypass: a systematic review and meta-analysis. Obes Surg. 2023;33:2884–97. https://doi.org/10.1007/s11695-023-06762-5.
27. Rossoni C, Bragança R, Santos Z, et al. OAGB bowel function in patients with up to 5 years follow-up: updated outcomes. Obes Surg. 2024;34(1):141–9. https://doi.org/10.1007/s11695-023-06917-4.
28. Malnutrition Q&A. 2020. WHO website: Malnutrition (who.int).
29. Bandlamudi N, Holt G, Graham Y, O'Kane M, Singhal R, Parmar C, Sakran N, Mahawar K, Pouwels S, Potluri S, Madhok B. Malnutrition following one-anastomosis gastric bypass: a systematic review. Obes Surg. 2023;33(12):4137–46. https://doi.org/10.1007/s11695-023-06907-6. Epub 2023 Nov 2. PMID: 37917389.
30. Balamurugan G, Leo SJ, Sivagnanam ST, Balaji Prasad S, Ravindra C, Rengan V, Arora E, Bindal V. Comparison of efficacy and safety between Roux-en-Y gastric bypass (RYGB) vs one anastomosis gastric bypass (OAGB) vs single anastomosis duodeno-ileal bypass with sleeve gastrectomy (SADI-S): a systematic review of bariatric and metabolic surgery. Obes Surg. 2023;33(7):2194–209. https://doi.org/10.1007/s11695-023-06602-6. Epub 2023 May 4. PMID: 37140720.

# Comparative Outcomes in Metabolic Surgery: Weight Loss

# 25

Annie Wang and Victoria Lyo

## Measurements of Postoperative Weight Loss and Definitions of Success

To have a common understanding of weight loss after bariatric surgery, it is important to begin with standardized terminology. At the beginning of the twentieth century, insurance companies used weight as a surrogate for overall health when enrolling patients [1]. To this end, the Metropolitan Life Insurance Company published actuarial data for **ideal body weight (IBW)**, which then became the basis for defining underweight, normal, overweight, and obesity classifications. Several groups have attempted to generate formulae to approximate this number [2] and this inconsistency in IBW calculation can lead to variability in weight loss outcomes [3]. In 2015, the American Society of Metabolic and Bariatric Surgery (ASMBS) published outcomes reporting standards, in which IBW is defined as the weight that corresponds to a **body mass index (BMI)** of 25 kg/m$^2$ [4]. BMI is a measure of weight as a function of height; it is calculated as follows:

$$\text{BMI} = \frac{\text{weight}(\text{kg})}{\left[\text{height}(\text{m})\right]^2} = \frac{\text{weight}(\text{lb})}{\left[\text{height}(\text{in})\right]^2} \times 703$$

A frequently reported measure of weight loss is **excess weight loss (EWL)**, expressed as a percentage:

A. Wang
Department of Surgery, University of California Irvine, Orange, USA
e-mail: anniw18@hs.uci.edu

V. Lyo (✉)
Department of Surgery, University of California, Davis, Sacramento, CA, USA

Center for Alimentary and Metabolic Sciences, University of California, Davis, Sacramento, CA, USA
e-mail: vlyo@ucdavis.edu



O. M. Ghanem et al. (eds.), *The SAGES Manual of Metabolic and Bariatric Surgery*, https://doi.org/10.1007/978-3-031-72309-4_25

$$\%\text{EWL} = \frac{(\text{initial weight}) - (\text{postoperative weight})}{(\text{initial weight}) - \text{IBW}} \times 100\%$$

EWL allows for the comparison of individuals with varying initial weights and varying excess body weight; for this reason, this was the previous standard weight loss metric in the literature. However, when compared to other weight loss metrics, EWL is consistently more error-sensitive and strongly associated with preoperative BMI across multiple studies [5, 6].

Another metric for weight loss is **excess BMI loss (EBMIL)**:

$$\%\text{EBMIL} = \frac{(\text{initial BMI}) - (\text{postoperative BMI})}{(\text{initial BMI}) - 25} \times 100\%$$

Similar to EWL, the EBMIL measure is also highly dependent on initial BMI, leading to variable and inconsistent data in the literature.

Total weight loss (TWL), reported as a percentage, is more commonly used and is the current standard measure of weight loss in bariatric surgery literature [5]. TWL has several advantages as a measure of weight loss: it is easy to measure and calculate, it does not rely upon IBW, and it is easily interpreted by physicians and patients [5]. Given the recent changes in reporting standards, this chapter will report both EWL and TWL where available.

$$\%\text{TWL} = \frac{(\text{initial weight}) - (\text{postoperative weight})}{\text{initial weight}} \times 100\%$$

## Markers of Weight Loss Success and Prediction Models

Successful weight loss after bariatric surgery was previously defined as greater than or equal to 50% EWL [6]. However, given the strong association between preoperative weight and IBW, this definition does not serve as a precise marker of weight loss. The use of TWL percentile charts, similar to pediatric growth charts, has therefore been recommended to assess postoperative weight loss progress [7, 8] (Fig. 25.1).

The Metabolic and Bariatric Surgery Accreditation and Quality Improvement Program (MBSAQIP) data have been used to develop a Bariatric Surgical Risk/Benefit Calculator to estimate one-year weight outcomes after various bariatric operations, available at https://riskcalculator.facs.org/bariatric/index.jsp [9]. More recently, Saux et al. have developed a machine learning-based model for predicting 5-year weight loss trajectories after three common bariatric surgeries [10]. The model is accessible as a web-based prediction tool Stratification of Obesity Phenotypes to Optimize Future Therapy (SOPHIA), available at https://bariatric-weight-trajectory-prediction.univ-lille.fr/ [11].

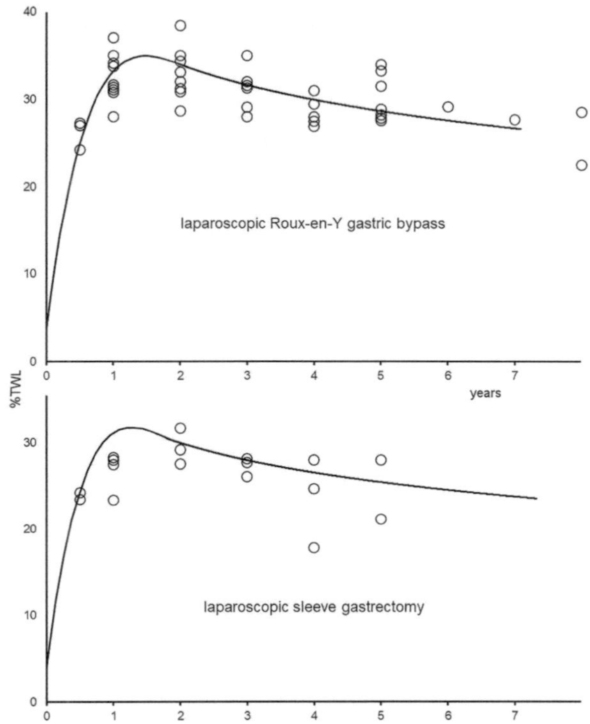


**Fig. 25.1** Total weight loss percentile graphs after laparoscopic Roux-en-Y gastric bypass and after laparoscopic vertical sleeve gastrectomy

## Weight Loss Outcomes After Primary Bariatric Surgery

In the United States, approximately 252,000 primary bariatric procedures are performed annually. Of these operations in 2020, 61% are vertical sleeve gastrectomy (VSG) procedures, 17% are Roux-en-Y gastric bypass (RYGB) procedures, <2% are adjustable gastric banding (AGB) operations and <2% are biliopancreatic diversion duodenal switch (BPD-DS) operations [12]. RYGB was considered the gold standard bariatric surgery, particularly after the laparoscopic technique was described in 1994. AGB became widely popular in the 2000s until VSG was established as a viable primary bariatric operation. It then became more popular, overtaking AGB and RYGB in 2010 and 2013, respectively [13, 14], but there is debate as to whether a gold standard exists today. Several landmark randomized controlled trials have compared weight loss after these operations in different permutations, which we will review in this chapter.

## Earlier Operations: Adjustable Gastric Band and Roux-en-Y Gastric Bypass

AGB was first performed in 1986 [15] and the laparoscopic technique was first described in 1992 [16]. It gained early popularity due to technical ease and a low early complication rate. Due to its popularity, earlier studies of metabolic effects of surgical weight loss focused on AGB compared to medical weight loss. In 2008, Dixon et al. published in *JAMA* a randomized controlled trial comparing type 2 diabetes remission between patients with BMI between 30 and 40 kg/m$^2$ who underwent either conventional diabetes and weight loss therapy ($n = 26$) and those who underwent AGB surgery ($n = 29$) [17]. The secondary outcome measure in this trial was weight loss and, at a 2-year follow-up, the AGB group demonstrated 20% TWL, compared to 1.4% TWL in the control group ($p < 0.001$), which was similar to the results of the Swedish Obese Subjects Study, a prospective controlled trial of 4047 subjects with BMI >34 kg/m$^2$ (males) or BMI >38 kg/m$^2$ (females) who underwent conventional medical treatment versus either AGB, RYGB, and VSG [18]. The 156 patients who underwent AGB had 13.2% TWL compared to the control group, who had a 1.6 ± 12% increase at the 10-year follow-up. In this same study, 10-year weight loss outcomes after RYGB were 25% ($n = 34$).

As AGB gained popularity, several randomized controlled trials compared it to RYGB. A 2009 randomized controlled trial in 250 patients was performed and weight loss outcomes at 4 years were examined. In this study, patients were randomized to RYGB ($n = 111$, 30 mL gastric pouch, 30 cm biliopancreatic limb, 75–100 cm Roux limb) and AGB ($n = 86$) [19]. While the starting mean BMI was higher in the RYGB group (47.5 vs 45.5 kg/m$^2$, $p < 0.01$), the RYGB group achieved an EWL of 68%, compared to 45±% in the AGB group ($p < 0.05$). Similarly, another randomized controlled trial performed in Italy found 66.6% EWL in the RYGB group (30 mL gastric pouch, 40–60 cm biliopancreatic limb, 100–150 cm Roux limb), compared to 47.5% EWL in the AGB group at 5-year follow-up [20].

The AGB began to lose favor because of its variable long-term weight loss results and long-term complications of slippage and erosion became apparent [21]. In the Longitudinal Assessment of Bariatric Surgery (LABS) 7-year follow-up multicenter observational cohort study, almost one-third of the AGB group ($n = 610$) required surgical revision or reversal, compared to <1% of the RYGB group ($n = 1738$) [22]. AGB comprised 55,932 cases in 2011 in the United States, and by 2021, this number declined to 1121 cases [14].

## Vertical Sleeve Gastrectomy

VSG historically was performed as the first stage of a two-staged procedure for BPD-DS in high-risk patients with extreme BMIs, first described in 2005 [23]. As significant weight loss after VSG became apparent, often surgeons and patients were foregoing the planned second stage. In 2009, a prospective study of 135 patients demonstrated EWL 38.6% and 49.4% at six-month and 1-year follow-up, respectively, when VSG was performed as primary standalone bariatric surgery [24]. By 2012, VSG gained increasing acceptance and was recognized by the ASMBS as a primary bariatric operation [25]. At this time, RYGB was the most widespread operation, after taking over from AGB.

Due to the increasing adoption of VSG, several key studies specifically compared outcomes between VSG and RYGB. The Swiss Multicenter Bypass or Sleeve Study (SM-BOSS) was a prospective randomized controlled trial demonstrated EBMIL of 72.3%, 70.9%, and 61.1% in the VSG group (35 Fr bougie) compared to 76.6%, 73.8%, and 68.3% in the RYGB group (50 cm biliopancreatic limb, 150 cm Roux limb) at 1, 3, and 5 years follow-up, respectively [26–28]. The Sleeve versus Bypass (SLEEVEPASS) randomized controlled trial demonstrated a divergence in weight loss outcomes between the two groups with greater weight loss in the RYGB group, starting at the 5-year follow-up. The VSG group (33–35 Fr bougie) had EWL of 49%, 47% and 43.5%, compared to the RYGB group (small gastric pouch, 50–80 cm biliopancreatic limb, 150 cm Roux limb) which had EWL of 57%, 55% and 51.9% at 5, 7 and 10-year follow-up, respectively [29–31]. Another long-term Dutch multicenter study demonstrated similar weight loss outcomes 7 years after RYGB (median 27% TWL) versus VSG (median 27% TWL); the longitudinal data was then used to create surgery-specific bariatric weight loss charts (Fig. 25.1) [7].

## Biliopancreatic Diversion and Duodenal Switch

First performed in humans in 1976, BPD-DS includes a reduced gastric volume for temporary acute weight loss with rapid gastric emptying via a wide gastroenterostomy into a distal ileal segment. The long-term weight loss mechanism is thought to be secondary to a delayed meeting of food with digestive juices from the biliopancreatic limb [32]. As RYGB long-term data accumulated, insufficient weight loss and diabetes recurrence have been noted in patients with BMI >50; therefore, the more malabsorptive BPD-DS was revisited in the 2010s as an alternative metabolic operation for this population [33, 34].

An Italian randomized controlled trial of type 2 diabetic patients who underwent medical therapy, RYGB (laparoscopic, 30 mL gastric pouch, 75 cm biliopancreatic limb, 100 cm Roux limb) or BPD-DS (open approach, 60% distal gastrectomy with 300 mL resultant gastric pouch, 200 cm alimentary limb, 50 cm common limb) found 10-year TWL of 4.2% for the medical therapy group, 28.0% for the RYGB group and 29.2% for the BPD-DS group [35]. A randomized controlled trial comparing BPD-DS (laparoscopic, 36 F sleeve gastrectomy, 150 cm alimentary limb, 100 cm common limb) to RYGB (laparoscopic, small gastric pouch, 120 cm Roux limb, 50 cm biliopancreatic limb) for patients with BMI >50 demonstrated 37.5 ± 12.2% TWL in BPD-DS group ($n = 18$) and 22.8 ± 14.8% TWL in the RYGB group ($n = 16$) [33].

A 2014 Cochrane meta-analysis of randomized controlled trials with 2-year follow-up comparing bariatric surgery with non-surgical interventions reaffirmed these findings [36]. RYGB achieved greater weight and BMI reduction compared to

AGB. RYGB had greater weight and BMI decline compared to VSG, though the difference was small. BPD-DS resulted in greater weight loss compared to RYGB. Another meta-analysis of randomized controlled trials and observational studies in 2014 had similar findings [37].

## One-Anastomosis Gastric Bypass

Initially described by Rutledge in 2001 and an alternative surgical technique described by Carbajo et al. in 2005, the one-anastomosis gastric bypass (OAGB) is a small gastric pouch that is anastomosed to a jejunal loop 200 cm distal to the ligament of Treitz [38, 39]. More recently, the one-anastomosis gastric bypass (OAGB) has risen in popularity and the multicenter, randomized controlled non-inferiority YOMEGA trial compared outcomes between OAGB and RYGB in patients with BMI > 40 or BMI > 35 with comorbidities [40]. At 2 years of follow-ups, the OAGB group ($n$ = 129, 200 cm biliopancreatic limb) had a mean of 35.4% TWL compared to 37.1% TWL in the RYGB group ($n$ = 124, 50 cm biliopancreatic limb, 150 cm Roux limb). As a novel procedure, the early data demonstrates improved weight loss compared to VSG and AGB, improved metabolic profile, with overall low incidence of perioperative complications. As such, the International Federation for the Surgery of Obesity (IFSO) 2021 Position Statement accepts the OAGB as a mainstream and safe primary bariatric operation [41].

A summary of weight loss outcomes from landmark papers reported in the literature for primary operations is listed in Table 25.1.

**Table 25.1** Weight loss outcomes based on operation type

| Primary operation | Short term (<2 years) | Mid-term (5–10 years) | Long term (>10 years) |
|---|---|---|---|
| *Malabsorptive procedures* | | | |
| RYGB | 72–74% EWL [37]<br>31–37% TWL [40] | 45–52% EWL [29] | 55–65% EWL [42, 43]<br>28% TWL [22] |
| OAGB | 51–75% EWL [44, 45]<br>24–35% TWL [44, 45] | 65–77% EWL [46–48]<br>30.7% TWL [47] | – |
| BPD-DS | 65–82% EWL [49] | 80.5% EWL [50]<br>42.1% TWL [50] | 62–80% EWL [42] |
| SADI-S | 80–87% EWL [44, 51]<br>28–52% TWL [44, 51, 52] | 69–96% EWL [50, 52]<br>36–40% TWL [50, 52] | 80.4% EWL [52]<br>34% TWL [52] |

(continued)

**Table 25.1** (continued)

| Primary operation | Short term (<2 years) | Mid-term (5–10 years) | Long term (>10 years) |
|---|---|---|---|
| *Restrictive procedures* | | | |
| AGB | 30–53% EWL [37, 53] 28% TWL [54] | 30–42% EWL [37, 53] | 17–55% EWL [42, 43, 53] 15–21% TWL [22, 54] |
| VSG | 57–78% EWL [37, 49, 55] | 57–84% EWL [29, 49, 55] | 40–57% EWL [49, 56] |
| *Endoscopic* | | | |
| Intragastric balloon | 26–27% EWL [57, 58] 11–14% TWL [57, 58] | – | – |
| Aspiration therapy | 32% EWL [59] 12% TWL [59] | – | – |
| Duodenal jejunal bypass sleeve (DJBS) EndoBarrier®[a] | 12.6–35.3% EWL [58, 60] | – | – |
| Incisionless magnetic anastomosis system (IAS) | 40.2% EWL [61] 14.6% TWL [61] | – | – |
| Endoscopic sleeve gastrectomy (ESG) | 15% TWL [62] | – | – |
| Primary obesity surgery endoluminal (POSE) | 16–45% EWL [63–65] 5–15% TWL [63–65] | – | – |

[a] DJBS EndoBarrier® (GI Dynamics Inc., Lexington MA) is not currently Food and Drug Administration (FDA) approved for use in the United States

## References

1. Komaroff M. For researchers on obesity: historical review of extra body weight definitions. J Obes. 2016;2016:2460285.
2. Kammerer MR, Porter MM, Beekley AC, Tichansky DS. Ideal body weight calculation in the bariatric surgical population. J Gastrointest Surg. 2015;19(10):1758–62.
3. Montero PN, Stefanidis D, Norton HJ, Gersin K, Kuwada T. Reported excess weight loss after bariatric surgery could vary significantly depending on calculation method: a plea for standardization. Surg Obes Relat Dis. 2011;7(4):531–4.
4. Brethauer SA, Kim J, El Chaar M, Papasavas P, Eisenberg D, Rogers A, et al. Standardized outcomes reporting in metabolic and bariatric surgery. Obes Surg. 2015;25(4):587–606.
5. van de Laar AW, Emous M, Hazebroek EJ, Boerma EJ, Faneyte IF, Nienhuijs SW. Reporting weight loss 2021: position statement of the Dutch Society for Metabolic and Bariatric Surgery (DSMBS). Obes Surg. 2021;31(10):4607–11.
6. Diamantis T, Apostolou KG, Alexandrou A, Griniatsos J, Felekouras E, Tsigris C. Review of long-term weight loss results after laparoscopic sleeve gastrectomy. Surg Obes Relat Dis. 2014;10(1):177–83.

7. van de Laar AW, Nienhuijs SW, Apers JA, van Rijswijk AS, de Zoete JP, Gadiot RP. The Dutch bariatric weight loss chart: a multicenter tool to assess weight outcome up to 7 years after sleeve gastrectomy and laparoscopic Roux-en-Y gastric bypass. Surg Obes Relat Dis. 2019;15(2):200–10.
8. van de Laar AW, Acherman YI. Weight loss percentile charts of large representative series: a benchmark defining sufficient weight loss challenging current criteria for success of bariatric surgery. Obes Surg. 2014;24(5):727–34.
9. Grieco A, Huffman KM, Cohen ME, Hall BL, Morton JM, Ko CY. The metabolic and bariatric surgery accreditation and quality improvement program bariatric surgical risk/benefit calculator: 1-year weight. Surg Obes Relat Dis. 2023;19(7):690–6.
10. Saux P, Bauvin P, Raverdy V, Teigny J, Verkindt H, Soumphonphakdy T, et al. Development and validation of an interpretable machine learning-based calculator for predicting 5-year weight trajectories after bariatric surgery: a multinational retrospective cohort SOPHIA study. Lancet Digit Health. 2023;5(10):e692–702.
11. Saux P, Bauvin PB, Raverdy V, Teigny J, Verkindt H, Soumphonphakdy T, et al. Stratification of obesity phenotypes to optimize future therapy (SOPHIA) bariatric weight trajectory prediction. 2023. https://bariatric-weight-trajectory-prediction.univ-lille.fr/.
12. Arterburn DE, Telem DA, Kushner RF, Courcoulas AP. Benefits and risks of bariatric surgery in adults: a review. JAMA. 2020;324(9):879–87.
13. Lo Menzo E, Szomstein S, Rosenthal RJ. Changing trends in bariatric surgery. Scand J Surg. 2015;104(1):18–23.
14. American Society for Metabolic and Bariatric Surgery. Estimate of bariatric surgery numbers, 2011–2021; 2022 [cited 2023]. https://asmbs.org/resources/estimate-of-bariatric-surgery-numbers.
15. Favretti F, Segato G, De Marchi F, De Luca M, Lise M, Cadiere GB, et al. An adjustable silicone gastric band for laparoscopic treatment of morbid obesity—technique and results. Surg Technol Int. 2002;10:109–14.
16. Broadbent R. First successful laproscopic gastric band. Obes Surg. 2001;11(6):778.
17. Dixon JB, O'Brien PE, Playfair J, Chapman L, Schachter LM, Skinner S, et al. Adjustable gastric banding and conventional therapy for type 2 diabetes: a randomized controlled trial. JAMA. 2008;299(3):316–23.
18. Sjöström L, Lindroos AK, Peltonen M, Torgerson J, Bouchard C, Carlsson B, et al. Lifestyle, diabetes, and cardiovascular risk factors 10 years after bariatric surgery. N Engl J Med. 2004;351(26):2683–93.
19. Nguyen NT, Slone JA, Nguyen XM, Hartman JS, Hoyt DB. A prospective randomized trial of laparoscopic gastric bypass versus laparoscopic adjustable gastric banding for the treatment of morbid obesity: outcomes, quality of life, and costs. Ann Surg. 2009;250(4):631–41.
20. Angrisani L, Lorenzo M, Borrelli V. Laparoscopic adjustable gastric banding versus Roux-en-Y gastric bypass: 5-year results of a prospective randomized trial. Surg Obes Relat Dis. 2007;3(2):127–32; discussion 32–3.
21. Snyder B, Wilson T, Mehta S, Bajwa K, Robinson E, Worley T, et al. Past, present, and future: critical analysis of use of gastric bands in obese patients. Diabetes Metab Syndr Obes. 2010;3:55–65.
22. Courcoulas AP, King WC, Belle SH, Berk P, Flum DR, Garcia L, et al. Seven-year weight trajectories and health outcomes in the longitudinal assessment of bariatric surgery (LABS) study. JAMA Surg. 2018;153(5):427–34.
23. Mognol P, Chosidow D, Marmuse JP. Laparoscopic sleeve gastrectomy as an initial bariatric operation for high-risk patients: initial results in 10 patients. Obes Surg. 2005;15(7):1030–3.
24. Fuks D, Verhaeghe P, Brehant O, Sabbagh C, Dumont F, Riboulot M, et al. Results of laparoscopic sleeve gastrectomy: a prospective study in 135 patients with morbid obesity. Surgery. 2009;145(1):106–13.
25. ASMBS Clinical Issues Committee. Updated position statement on sleeve gastrectomy as a bariatric procedure. Surg Obes Relat Dis. 2012;8(3):e21–6.

26. Peterli R, Borbély Y, Kern B, Gass M, Peters T, Thurnheer M, et al. Early results of the Swiss multicentre bypass or sleeve study (SM-BOSS): a prospective randomized trial comparing laparoscopic sleeve gastrectomy and Roux-en-Y gastric bypass. Ann Surg. 2013;258(5):690–4; discussion 5.
27. Peterli R, Wölnerhanssen BK, Vetter D, Nett P, Gass M, Borbély Y, et al. Laparoscopic sleeve gastrectomy versus Roux-Y-gastric bypass for morbid obesity-3-year outcomes of the prospective randomized Swiss multicenter bypass or sleeve study (SM-BOSS). Ann Surg. 2017;265(3):466–73.
28. Peterli R, Wölnerhanssen BK, Peters T, Vetter D, Kröll D, Borbély Y, et al. Effect of laparoscopic sleeve gastrectomy vs laparoscopic Roux-en-Y gastric bypass on weight loss in patients with morbid obesity: the SM-BOSS randomized clinical trial. JAMA. 2018;319(3):255–65.
29. Salminen P, Helmiö M, Ovaska J, Juuti A, Leivonen M, Peromaa-Haavisto P, et al. Effect of laparoscopic sleeve gastrectomy vs laparoscopic Roux-en-Y gastric bypass on weight loss at 5 years among patients with morbid obesity: the SLEEVEPASS randomized clinical trial. JAMA. 2018;319(3):241–54.
30. Grönroos S, Helmiö M, Juuti A, Tiusanen R, Hurme S, Löyttyniemi E, et al. Effect of laparoscopic sleeve gastrectomy vs Roux-en-Y gastric bypass on weight loss and quality of life at 7 years in patients with morbid obesity: the SLEEVEPASS randomized clinical trial. JAMA Surg. 2021;156(2):137–46.
31. Salminen P, Grönroos S, Helmiö M, Hurme S, Juuti A, Juusela R, et al. Effect of laparoscopic sleeve gastrectomy vs Roux-en-Y gastric bypass on weight loss, comorbidities, and reflux at 10 years in adult patients with obesity: the SLEEVEPASS randomized clinical trial. JAMA Surg. 2022;157(8):656–66.
32. Scopinaro N. Biliopancreatic diversion: mechanisms of action and long-term results. Obes Surg. 2006;16(6):683–9.
33. Möller F, Hedberg J, Skogar M, Sundbom M. Long-term follow-up 15 years after duodenal switch or gastric bypass for super obesity: a randomized controlled trial. Obes Surg. 2023;33(10):2981–90.
34. Mingrone G, Panunzi S, De Gaetano A, Guidone C, Iaconelli A, Leccesi L, et al. Bariatric surgery versus conventional medical therapy for type 2 diabetes. N Engl J Med. 2012;366(17):1577–85.
35. Mingrone G, Panunzi S, De Gaetano A, Guidone C, Iaconelli A, Capristo E, et al. Metabolic surgery versus conventional medical therapy in patients with type 2 diabetes: 10-year follow-up of an open-label, single-centre, randomised controlled trial. Lancet. 2021;397(10271):293–304.
36. Colquitt JL, Pickett K, Loveman E, Frampton GK. Surgery for weight loss in adults. Cochrane Database Syst Rev. 2014;2014(8):CD003641.
37. Chang SH, Stoll CR, Song J, Varela JE, Eagon CJ, Colditz GA. The effectiveness and risks of bariatric surgery: an updated systematic review and meta-analysis, 2003-2012. JAMA Surg. 2014;149(3):275–87.
38. Carbajo M, García-Caballero M, Toledano M, Osorio D, García-Lanza C, Carmona JA. One-anastomosis gastric bypass by laparoscopy: results of the first 209 patients. Obes Surg. 2005;15(3):398–404.
39. Rutledge R. The mini-gastric bypass: experience with the first 1,274 cases. Obes Surg. 2001;11(3):276–80.
40. Robert M, Espalieu P, Pelascini E, Caiazzo R, Sterkers A, Khamphommala L, et al. Efficacy and safety of one anastomosis gastric bypass versus Roux-en-Y gastric bypass for obesity (YOMEGA): a multicentre, randomised, open-label, non-inferiority trial. Lancet. 2019;393(10178):1299–309.
41. De Luca M, Piatto G, Merola G, Himpens J, Chevallier JM, Carbajo MA, et al. IFSO update position statement on one anastomosis gastric bypass (OAGB). Obes Surg. 2021;31(7):3251–78.
42. O'Brien PE, Hindle A, Brennan L, Skinner S, Burton P, Smith A, et al. Long-term outcomes after bariatric surgery: a systematic review and meta-analysis of weight loss at 10 or more years for all bariatric procedures and a single-centre review of 20-year outcomes after adjustable gastric banding. Obes Surg. 2019;29(1):3–14.

43. O'Brien PE, MacDonald L, Anderson M, Brennan L, Brown WA. Long-term outcomes after bariatric surgery: fifteen-year follow-up of adjustable gastric banding and a systematic review of the bariatric surgical literature. Ann Surg. 2013;257(1):87–94.
44. Mahdy T, Gado W, Alwahidi A, Schou C, Emile SH. Sleeve gastrectomy, one-anastomosis gastric bypass (OAGB), and single anastomosis sleeve Ileal (SASI) bypass in treatment of morbid obesity: a retrospective cohort study. Obes Surg. 2021;31(4):1579–89.
45. Mustafa A, Rizkallah NNH, Samuel N, Balupuri S. Laparoscopic Roux-En-Y gastric bypass versus one anastomosis (loop) gastric bypass for obesity: a prospective comparative study of weight loss and complications. Ann Med Surg (Lond). 2020;55:143–7.
46. Level L, Rojas A, Piñango S, Avariano Y. One anastomosis gastric bypass vs. Roux-en-Y gastric bypass: a 5-year follow-up prospective randomized trial. Langenbecks Arch Surg. 2021;406(1):171–9.
47. Dayan D, Bendayan A, Nizri E, Abu-Abeid S, Lahat G, Abu-Abeid A. One anastomosis gastric bypass compared with sleeve gastrectomy in elderly patients: safety and long-term outcomes. Obes Surg. 2023;33(2):570–6.
48. Jain M, Tantia O, Goyal G, Chaudhuri T, Khanna S, Poddar A, et al. LSG vs MGB-OAGB: 5-year follow-up data and comparative outcome of the two procedures over long term-results of a randomised control trial. Obes Surg. 2021;31(3):1223–32.
49. Azagury D, Papasavas P, Hamdallah I, Gagner M, Kim J. ASMBS position statement on medium- and long-term durability of weight loss and diabetic outcomes after conventional stapled bariatric procedures. Surg Obes Relat Dis. 2018;14(10):1425–41.
50. Gebellí JP, Lazzara C, de Gordejuela AGR, Nora M, Pereira AM, Sánchez-Pernaute A, et al. Duodenal switch vs. single-anastomosis duodenal switch (SADI-S) for the treatment of grade IV obesity: 5-year outcomes of a multicenter prospective cohort comparative study. Obes Surg. 2022;32(12):3839–46.
51. Andalib A, Bouchard P, Alamri H, Bougie A, Demyttenaere S, Court O. Single anastomosis duodeno-ileal bypass with sleeve gastrectomy (SADI-S): short-term outcomes from a prospective cohort study. Surg Obes Relat Dis. 2021;17(2):414–24.
52. Sánchez-Pernaute A, Herrera MR, Ferré NP, Rodríguez CS, Marcuello C, Pañella C, et al. Long-term results of single-anastomosis duodeno-ileal bypass with sleeve gastrectomy (SADI-S). Obes Surg. 2022;32(3):682–9.
53. Khoraki J, Moraes MG, Neto APF, Funk LM, Greenberg JA, Campos GM. Long-term outcomes of laparoscopic adjustable gastric banding. Am J Surg. 2018;215(1):97–103.
54. Froylich D, Abramovich-Segal T, Pascal G, Haskins I, Appel B, Kafri N, et al. Long-term (over 10 years) retrospective follow-up of laparoscopic adjustable gastric banding. Obes Surg. 2018;28(4):976–80.
55. Huang BW, Shahul SS, Ong MKH, Fisher OM, Chan DL, Talbot ML. Medium term outcomes of revision laparoscopic sleeve gastrectomy after gastric banding: a propensity score matched study. Obes Surg. 2023;33(7):2005–15.
56. Golzarand M, Toolabi K, Farid R. The bariatric surgery and weight losing: a meta-analysis in the long- and very long-term effects of laparoscopic adjustable gastric banding, laparoscopic Roux-en-Y gastric bypass and laparoscopic sleeve gastrectomy on weight loss in adults. Surg Endosc. 2017;31(11):4331–45.
57. Crea N, Pata G, Della Casa D, Minelli L, Maifredi G, Di Betta E, et al. Improvement of metabolic syndrome following intragastric balloon: 1 year follow-up analysis. Obes Surg. 2009;19(8):1084–8.
58. Abu Dayyeh BK, Kumar N, Edmundowicz SA, Jonnalagadda S, Larsen M, Sullivan S, et al. ASGE bariatric endoscopy task force systematic review and meta-analysis assessing the ASGE PIVI thresholds for adopting endoscopic bariatric therapies. Gastrointest Endosc. 2015;82(3):425–38.e5.
59. Thompson CC, Abu Dayyeh BK, Kushner R, Sullivan S, Schorr AB, Amaro A, et al. Percutaneous gastrostomy device for the treatment of class II and class III obesity: results of a randomized controlled trial. Am J Gastroenterol. 2017;112(3):447–57.

60. Rohde U, Hedbäck N, Gluud LL, Vilsbøll T, Knop FK. Effect of the EndoBarrier gastrointestinal liner on obesity and type 2 diabetes: a systematic review and meta-analysis. Diabetes Obes Metab. 2016;18(3):300–5.
61. Machytka E, Bužga M, Zonca P, Lautz DB, Ryou M, Simonson DC, et al. Partial jejunal diversion using an incisionless magnetic anastomosis system: 1-year interim results in patients with obesity and diabetes. Gastrointest Endosc. 2017;86(5):904–12.
62. Alqahtani A, Al-Darwish A, Mahmoud AE, Alqahtani YA, Elahmedi M. Short-term outcomes of endoscopic sleeve gastroplasty in 1000 consecutive patients. Gastrointest Endosc. 2019;89(6):1132–8.
63. Sullivan S, Swain JM, Woodman G, Antonetti M, De La Cruz-Muñoz N, Jonnalagadda SS, et al. Randomized sham-controlled trial evaluating efficacy and safety of endoscopic gastric plication for primary obesity: the ESSENTIAL trial. Obesity (Silver Spring). 2017;25(2):294–301.
64. López-Nava G, Bautista-Castaño I, Jimenez A, de Grado T, Fernandez-Corbelle JP. The primary obesity surgery endolumenal (POSE) procedure: one-year patient weight loss and safety outcomes. Surg Obes Relat Dis. 2015;11(4):861–5.
65. Miller K, Turró R, Greve JW, Bakker CM, Buchwald JN, Espinós JC. MILEPOST multicenter randomized controlled trial: 12-month weight loss and satiety outcomes after pose. Obes Surg. 2017;27(2):310–22.

# 26 Comparative Outcomes in Metabolic Surgery: Diabetes and Cardiovascular Health

Tiffany C. Lee, Ruby D. Lopez Flores, John Yonge, and Andrea Stroud

## Diabetes Outcomes After Metabolic Surgery

### Introduction

Diabetes mellitus remains a major public health problem in the United States, with 13% of the adult population diagnosed with diabetes in 2018 [1]. Approximately 30–53% of diabetes cases are thought to be attributable to obesity. As diabetes is a chronic disease, it may relapse or remit depending on many factors, including lifestyle changes, pharmaceuticals, and even metabolic surgery. As such, improvement or potentially remission of diabetes may be one of the most important indications for metabolic surgery.

### Physiologic Impact of Metabolic Surgery on Diabetes

The mechanism of action behind the effects of metabolic surgery on diabetes remission remains unclear and likely multifactorial. Historically, diabetes remission was thought to be due to associated weight loss following metabolic surgery, resulting in

T. C. Lee · J. Yonge
Department of Surgery, Oregon Health and Science University, Portland, OR, USA
e-mail: leetiff@ohsu.edu; yonge@ohsu.edu

R. D. Lopez Flores
School of Medicine, University of Nevada, Reno, NV, USA
e-mail: rlopezflores@med.unr.edu

A. Stroud (✉)
Division of Bariatric Surgery, Department of Surgery, Oregon Health and Science University, Portland, OR, USA
e-mail: strouda@ohsu.edu


O. M. Ghanem et al. (eds.), *The SAGES Manual of Metabolic and Bariatric Surgery*, https://doi.org/10.1007/978-3-031-72309-4_26

increased insulin sensitivity [2]. However, patients often have improvements in their hyperglycemia resulting in cessation of anti-hyperglycemic medications in the days to weeks following surgery, much sooner than any significant weight loss has occurred. Therefore, weight loss is not the sole etiology for diabetes improvement. More recent research has proposed the impact of alterations in gut hormones as a potential mediator in the impact of metabolic surgery on diabetes remission. Ghrelin, a gastrointestinal hormone involved in appetite regulation and produced primarily in the stomach, has been demonstrated to decrease insulin sensitivity and secretion [3]. The decrease in ghrelin levels postoperatively has therefore been thought to promote insulin function, resulting in better glucose homeostasis. Glucagon-like peptide 1 (GLP-1) has also been shown to stimulate insulin secretion, as well as increase proliferation and decrease apoptosis of pancreatic beta cells [4]. As GLP-1 secretion is enhanced in patients following RYGB and BPD, this has become a reasonable candidate in the mechanism of diabetes remission, particularly in light of the effectiveness of GLP-1 agonist medications. However, there may be other less well-defined physiologic changes in other hormones, bile acid metabolism, or gut microbiota that contribute to the impact of metabolic surgery on diabetes and this remains an area of ongoing research.

## Clinical Impact of Metabolic Surgery on Pre-existing Diabetes

Multiple cohort studies and several randomized controlled trials have compared metabolic surgery to medical management for diabetes management. One of the first randomized controlled trials to primarily study diabetes in the metabolic surgery population was the STAMPEDE trial, which accrued patients between 2007 and 2011 [5]. In this single center, three-armed study, the investigators compared intensive medical therapy versus RYGB versus SG with the primary end-point of hemoglobin A1c (HgbA1c) $\leq$ 6.0% at 12 months. They demonstrated that 12% of the medical therapy group (5/41, mean HgbA1c 7.5 ± 1.8%) achieved the primary end-point, compared to 42% (21/50, mean HgbA1c 6.4 ± 0.9%) of the RYGB group and 37% (18/49, mean HgbA1c 6.6 ± 1.0%) of the SG group. Both surgery groups were significantly more effective at achieving diabetes remission, as well as decreasing the number of diabetes medications, compared to the medical therapy group.

In another single center, randomized controlled trial conducted in Italy between 2009 and 2011, the investigators compared conventional medical therapy versus RYGB versus BPD, with the primary end-point of fasting glucose <100 mg/dL and HgbA1c < 6.5% at 2 years [6]. The results showed the rate of diabetes remission to be none in the medical therapy group, compared to 75% (15/20) of the RYGB group and 95% (19/20) in the BPD group. The average HgbA1c was significantly lower in the RYGB group (6.35 ± 1.42%) and BPD group (4.95 ± 0.49%) compared to the medical therapy group (8.65 ± 1.45%), demonstrating that even if patients were not able to achieve complete diabetes remission, they were still achieving better diabetes control with surgery compared to medical therapy.

Systematic reviews of the literature have summarized the existing evidence for bariatric surgery in diabetes control, despite significant heterogeneity in definition of diabetes remission (including complete versus partial). Gloy et al. included four randomized controlled trials which evaluated diabetes outcomes and found that overall, metabolic surgery led to higher remission rate of diabetes (relative risk 22.1 [95% confidence interval (CI) 3.2–154.3], for complete remission, 5.3 [95% CI 1.8–15.8] in conservative analysis) [7]. Sheng et al. [8] included one randomized controlled trial and nine cohort studies and performed a meta-analysis included over 3000 patients with diabetes, which demonstrated relative rate of diabetes remission to be 5.90 (95% CI 3.75–9.28) for those underwent metabolic surgery compared to medical management.

Given the literature demonstrating the positive impact of metabolic surgery on diabetes management, the International Diabetes Organizations stated in its 2016 guidelines that metabolic surgery is recommended for (a) patients with class III obesity (BMI $\geq$ 40 kg/m$^2$) and diabetes as well as (b) patients with class II obesity (BMI 35.0–39.9 kg/m$^2$) with inadequately controlled hyperglycemia despite lifestyle and optimal medical therapy [9]. A prediction model created by Aminian et al. [10] can be used to calculate the predicted 10-year risks of end-organ complications (all-cause mortality, coronary artery events, heart failure, and nephropathy) of diabetes with and without metabolic surgery. The input variables for the model include risk factors for developing diabetes complications including patient demographics, medical history, clinical data (including HgbA1c, blood pressure, creatinine and triglycerides), and current medications (including insulin, other diabetes medications, lipid-lowering medications, anti-hypertensives, aspirin and warfarin). This risk calculator may be beneficial in counseling patients who are considering surgery. Additionally, the same group developed a procedure selection model to identify which patients, based on the severity of their diabetes, may benefit more from RYGB versus SG [11]. This externally validated model may use to guide clinical decisions regarding recommendations for type of metabolic surgery.

## Clinical Impact of Metabolic Surgery on Diabetes Prevention

Given the beneficial impact that metabolic surgery can have on pre-existing diabetes, it is reasonable to investigate whether metabolic surgery can prevent the onset of diabetes. To this end, the Swedish Obese Subjects (SOS) study, which enrolled over 4000 patients from 1987 to 2001, found that during follow-up of 15 years, the patients who had undergone metabolic surgery (AGB, VBG, or RYGB) had a hazard ratio (HR) for developing diabetes of 0.17 (95% CI 0.13–0.21, $p < 0.001$) compared to the non-surgical control group [12]. A post-hoc analysis of the SOS study also demonstrated that metabolic surgery reduced the incidence of microvascular diabetic complications (retinopathy, diabetic kidney disease, neuropathy) by 44% (HR 0.56, CI 0.48–0.66), with the greatest effect seen in patients with pre-diabetes [13]. They concluded that one microvascular event was prevented for every 22 individuals who underwent surgery over 10 years. This suggests that metabolic surgery can potentially prevent both development and complications of diabetes.

## Long-term Diabetic Outcomes Following Metabolic Surgery

Diabetes is a chronic disease which may recur over time following initial improvement or remission after metabolic surgery. Factors which may be associated with diabetes recurrence include longer duration of diabetes or insulin use preoperatively, use of multiple diabetes medications, lower excess weight loss postoperatively, and weight regain [14]. Subsequent follow-up in the STAMPEDE trial for patients that had diabetes remission (HgbA1c < 6.0%) at 1 year after surgery found that the relapse rate by 3 years was 38% in the RYGB group and 46% in the SG group [5]. By 5 years, only 22.4% of RYGB patients and 14.9% of SG patients sustained remission. However, none of the medical therapy group had diabetes remission at 5 years, indicating metabolic surgery provides superior diabetic outcomes. Adams et al. [15] found in their prospective observational study that patients undergoing RYGB, the rate of diabetes remission (fasting blood glucose <126 mg/dL, HgbA1c < 6.5%, or use of any antidiabetic medication) was 75% at 2 years, 62% at 6 years, and 51% at 12 years. The odds ratio (OR) for incidence of diabetes was 0.08 (95% CI 0.03–0.24) for the surgery group compared to patients that did not undergo surgery. In the SOS study, patients undergoing metabolic surgery (AGB, VBG, RYGB) had OR for diabetes remission (based on fasting glucose levels) of 8.42 (95% CI 5.68–12.5, $p < 0.001$) compared to non-surgical patients [16]. The OR decreased to 3.45 (95% CI 1.64–7.28) at 10 years. These and other studies demonstrate that despite the rate of diabetes remission decreasing over time, the overall rate for patients undergoing metabolic surgery is significantly improved compared to patients managed medically.

## Revisional Surgical Options for Treatment of Persistent or Recurrent Diabetes

The role of revisional surgery in the treatment and management of diabetes is not clearly defined. The majority of studies in revisional metabolic surgery have not sought to investigate this question. Regardless, a review including 30 studies demonstrated that 14–38% of patients had diabetes at time of revisional bariatric surgery, which may result in improvement of diabetes in 65–100% of patients, depending on the type of primary and revisional operation [14]. The definition of diabetes improvement and remission varied across the different studies, from discontinuation/reduction of antidiabetic medications to HgbA1c < 6–6.5% to normal fasting blood glucose without medications. Conversion to RYGB resulted in improvement of diabetes in 79% of patients with prior VBG, 72% with prior AGB, and 62% with prior SG. Revision of RYGB including pouch revision also resulted in significant diabetes improvement in 79% of patients, whereas creation of more distal bypass resulted in diabetes improvement in all 11 patients. Whether these results would be seen in revisional surgery independent of weight control is unclear, as many revision procedures are performed for inadequate weight loss or significant weight regain, not primarily for diabetes treatment. In patients with adequate weight loss but persistent or recurrent diabetes following primary metabolic surgery, pharmacologic therapy may be preferred.

### Summary

In summary, metabolic surgery can play a significant role in the management of diabetes in patients with obesity. The literature clearly shows that metabolic surgery is superior to medical management alone, resulting in higher rates of diabetes improvement and remission, particularly in the short-term. It is important for patients to understand that metabolic surgery is not necessarily a cure for diabetes, and extent and duration of diabetes improvement is dependent on multiple factors, including severity of pre-existing diabetes, surgical procedure type, and degree of weight loss. Patients remain at risk for diabetes recurrence in the long term and should continue to be monitored, particularly if they experience weight regain or recurrence of other medical comorbidities.

## Hypertension and Hyperlipidemia Outcomes After Metabolic Surgery

### Introduction

Early studies in metabolic surgery emphasized improved long-term glycemic outcomes. Current research efforts have shifted to investigating the secondary benefits of metabolic surgery and the pathways influencing these changes. Specifically, the influence of metabolic surgery on hypertension and hyperlipidemia remain at the forefront of these investigations. Hypertension, as defined by the European guidelines as an office systolic measurement ≥140 mmHg or a diastolic ≥80 mmHg [17] or by AHA guidelines as a systolic reading ≥130 mmHg or diastolic reading ≥80 mmHg [18], and hyperlipidemia (elevated total cholesterol or elevated low density lipoprotein above 130 mg/dL) are leading causes of morbidity [19] with a population prevalence of 40% for hypertension and 62% [20] for hyperlipidemia for individuals with obesity [21].

### Influence of Lifestyle on Hypertension and Hyperlipidemia

Non-surgical control of hypertension includes patient modifiable factors and medical therapy. Exercise and weight loss have shown a 1 mmHg reduction in BP for every 1 kg reduction in weight [22]. This linear correlation suggests the underlying cause for obesity-induced hypertension to be linked to adipocyte accumulation. The adipocyte initiates the cascade of events ultimately influencing arterial stiffness, renal absorption of sodium and increased sympathetic nervous system activity [21]. Trials involving intensive lifestyle modifications, as detailed in the Look AHEAD trial, which emphasized reduced sodium intake with exercise, demonstrated improvements in modifiable risk factors. However, a significant long-term reduction in cardiovascular morbidity and mortality was not observed when compared to control patients undergoing standard education [23]. Therefore, the interplay between obesity and hypertension is more complex than carbohydrate ingestion, and simple reduction in adipocyte volume does not fully address the multitude of pathways feeding into the obesity-induced hypertensive state.

Genetic factors impacting metabolism lead to obesity and have a secondary impact on hypertension. Pro-inflammatory cytokine release secondary to insulin resistance and visceral fat storage leads to arterial hypertension and medication-resistant hypertension [24]. Insulin directly leads to increased renal retention of sodium causing volume overload and propagating hypertension [21, 25]. These interactions are still being investigated, but metabolic surgery attacks the fundamental building blocks of hypertension. Utilizing metabolic surgery to achieve a dual goal of weight reduction and physiologic alterations to reduce systemic inflammation and sodium retention stands to hold significant therapeutic value for control of hypertension [26, 27]. Finally, while medical management does treat the elevated BP or lipid panel, if the patient continues to have obesity, a lifetime of medication consumption is mandatory to counteract the physiology of the pathologically hypertrophied adipocyte.

Medication dependence was highlighted by Bramlage et al. in the analysis of the Hypertension and Diabetes Risk Screening and Awareness (HYDRA) study [28]. The authors demonstrated that individuals with a BMI $\geq 40$ had an OR of 5.3 (95% CI 3.1–8.9) for the use of four or more medications to control hypertension compared to normal weight individuals [29]. At lower obesity classes, hypertension remained highly prevalent with insufficient control of hypertension when compared to individuals without obesity [29].

## Physiologic Impact of Metabolic Surgery on Hypertension

Historical teaching fundamentally categorized metabolic surgery as either restrictive or malabsorptive. Hybrid procedures utilized elements of both; however, decades of hormone level studies have begun to elucidate the complex interplay of GI hormones, microbiota, food preferences and systemic inflammation hold over the true mechanism for sustained weight loss. Secondary and systemic influences of metabolic surgery include alterations in the renin-angiotensin-aldosterone cycle, sympathetic nervous system activation, endothelial function, natural vasodilators, and an alteration in pro-inflammatory cytokines [21, 30]. Specifically, reductions in vasoconstrictors including angiotensin-II and increases in vasodilators including atrial natriuretic peptide and nitric oxide after RYGB promote reductions in blood pressure [21, 31, 32]. These secondary influences of metabolic surgery on obesity reinforce that direct weight loss is not the sole predictor for a reduction in hypertension [32].

## Clinical Impact of Metabolic Surgery on Hypertension

Despite variability in surgical technique, patient demographics and randomized data, numerous studies and reviews have demonstrated a reduction in hypertension following metabolic surgery [33–38]. A meta-analysis by Ricci et al. demonstrated a relative risk (RR) reduction of 0.52 (95% CI 0.42–0.64, $p < 0.0001$) for hypertension after RYGB, BPD, or AGB [35]. There appears to be a strong influence on hypertension, particularly with BPD; Valera-Mora et al. [37] demonstrated that 96% had a reduction in blood pressure to within the normal range after BPD. The impact of SG on hypertension appears to be within the range of the previously mentioned metabolic surgeries. At one-year follow-up, Sarkhosh et al. [36] reported a 58% resolution in hypertension, while at 5.35 years follow-up Graham et al. [33] reported a 62% resolution in hypertension. These reviews demonstrate the ongoing positive impact metabolic surgery has on hypertension management. Two recent randomized controlled trials have compared RYGB head-to-head with SG, including the SM-BOSS trial which showed no difference in hypertension remission rates between RYGB and SG [39]. On the other hand, the SLEEVEPASS trial showed a 29% remission rate of hypertension after SG, but significantly higher hypertension remission rate after RYGB, 51% ($p = 0.02$) after 5-year follow-up [40].

The GATEWAY (Gastric Bypass to Treat Obese Patients With Steady Hypertension) trial randomized 100 patients to either RYGB and medical therapy or medical therapy alone with follow-up at 12 months [41]. The primary end-point of ≥30% reduction of anti-hypertensive meds overwhelmingly favored patients receiving metabolic surgery versus medical therapy alone (83.7% versus 12.8%, $p < 0.001$). Secondary end-points of hypertension remission was only noted in patients undergoing RYGB and absent in patient receiving medical therapy alone (45.8% versus 0%) [41]. At 3-year follow-up, these results were confirmed by demonstrating that 35% of patients in the metabolic surgery group were able to sustain a blood pressure of <140/90 compared to only 2% in the medical therapy alone group [42].

## Clinical Impact of Metabolic Surgery on Hyperlipidemia

In their systematic review, Buchwald et al. [43] demonstrated early improvement in dyslipidemia across all metabolic procedures; however, BPD and RYGB produced the most substantial improvements in dyslipidemia (99.1% and 93.6%). AGB, RYGB and BPD were further analyzed in a meta-analysis by Ricci et al. [35], which demonstrated a RR reduction of 0.39 (95% CI 0.27–0.56, $p < 0.001$) for dyslipidemia after these procedures. A systemic review of 26 studies by Al Khalifa et al.

[44] reported an 83.5% rate of either improvement or resolution and a 54% complete resolution rate for dyslipidemia for patients undergoing SG. The outcome variability for complete resolution versus improvement was limited by data available in the included studies. Clinical improvement of dyslipidemia after SG was further demonstrated in the 5-year analysis of the SLEEVEPASS trial with no significant difference between SG and RYGB procedures for this secondary outcome (47% vs 60%, $p = 0.15$) [40]. Interestingly, despite evidence of restrictive procedures, such as the AGB, leading to a reduction in hyperlipidemia, malabsorptive procedures hold a physiological advantage in regards to lipid metabolism. As demonstrated by Benetti et al. [45], independent of weight loss, glucose metabolism and insulin resistance, BPD significantly lowered LDL values compared to patients undergoing AGB. In fact, the authors postulated and showed a slight increase in LDL after AGB, secondary to no change in cholesterol absorption and a mild increase in hepatic catabolism of cholesterol [45]. Intestinal bypass surgery leads to a primary reduction in overall cholesterol uptake and in combination with an increase in hepatic catabolism of cholesterol, a significant reduction in LDL [45]. This mechanism is not present with purely restrictive (AGB) procedures accounting for the diminished impact on hyperlipidemia management in the postoperative period.

### Summary

In summary, metabolic surgery has a dual function for the reduction of obesity-related comorbidities including hypertension and dyslipidemia. The mechanism appears to involve both malabsorption and endocrine alterations that have a cascading influence leading to a reduction in systemic inflammation and local vasodilators. There is strong data supporting the use of metabolic surgery for the control of obesity and obesity-related comorbidities. The expanding influence of medication-induced weight loss holds an uncertain potential as these medications do not lead to surgical malabsorption, a clear precipitant for overall reduction in obesity-related comorbidities.

## Coronary Artery Disease, Myocardial Infarction, and Congestive Heart Failure Outcomes After Metabolic Surgery

### Introduction

Cardiovascular disease (CVD) is one of the major sources of morbidity and mortality in patients with comorbid obesity and type II diabetes mellitus. An "obesity paradox" has been described in the literature which finds that those with higher BMI have an association with lower mortality [46–48]. It is important to note that this paradox is described after a myocardial infarction (MI) has already occurred. However, metabolic surgery appears to play a role in the *prevention* of cardiovascular events. Adams et al. [49] conducted a retrospective cohort study evaluating the long-term mortality of patients who had RYGB compared to matched controls. Of note, while overall death rates were lower among surgical patients (52%, $p < 0.001$) the number one cause of mortality in both groups was CVD with 9.7 per 10,000-person year in the surgery group and 104 per 10,000-person year in the non-surgical control group [49]. This elucidates the critical role that CVD plays in the mortality of individuals with obesity. While the positive effects of metabolic surgery on excess weight and diabetes control have been studied in small randomized controlled trials, there have been fewer studies focusing on long-term cardiovascular outcomes [50–54]. The pathophysiology of obesity-related CVD is thought to be due to altered adipose tissue function, which develops in genetically and environmentally predisposed individuals due to caloric excess [55]. This altered adipose tissue leads to metabolic dysfunction contributing to hypertension, diabetes, and dyslipidemias, which then serve as known risk factors for cardiovascular and coronary disease events.

## Clinical Impact of Metabolic Surgery on Major Cardiovascular Events

Intervention with metabolic surgery has a demonstrated clinical impact on major cardiovascular events. Aminian et al. [50] conducted a retrospective, observational, matched-cohort study of 13,722 patients (2287 surgical patients and 11,435 matched controls) and found that metabolic surgery was significantly associated with a lower risk of major adverse cardiovascular events (HR = 0.61). The primary end-points in the study included coronary artery events (unstable angina, MI, or coronary intervention), heart failure, and atrial fibrillation [50]. Noubani et al. [56] conducted a retrospective analysis of the New York State Statewide Planning and Research Cooperative System (SPARCS), in patients with obesity, those with a history of metabolic surgery had a reduced risk of future coronary revascularization (HR = 0.46, 95% CI 0.42–0.50, $p < 0.0001$), percutaneous coronary intervention (HR = 0.45, 95% CI 0.41–0.49, $p < 0.0001$) and coronary artery bypass grafting (HR = 0.49, 95% CI 0.42–0.56, $p < 0.0001$). The SOS observed a 32% (HR = 0.68, 95% CI 0.54–0.85, $p = 0.001$) reduction in macrovascular complications for patients with diabetes when comparing the surgical group (31.7 per 1000 person-years, 95% CI, 27.0–37.2) to non-surgical controls (44.2 per 1000 person-years, 95% CI, 37.5–52.1), with a median follow-up time of 10 years [54]. These studies demonstrate the positive impact that metabolic surgery can have on decreasing the risk for cardiovascular events with sustainable long-term results.

## Clinical Impact of Metabolic Surgery on Congestive Heart Failure

In congestive heart failure (CHF), it has been demonstrated that excess body weight is associated with greater cardiac hypertrophy, abnormal myocardial energetics, heightened pericardial restraint, and hemodynamic congestion, which is strongly linked to volume expansion and alterations in venous capacitance [57]. This suggests that weight loss can lead to better outcomes for heart failure patients. Datta et al. [58] conducted a literature review of metabolic surgery and its effects on CHF. The authors included seven small, mostly retrospective studies, which showed there was a significant improvement in left ventricular ejection fraction in patients who underwent metabolic surgery [58]. Sorimachi et al. [57] similarly saw benefits to cardiac tissue remodeling observing a reduction in epicardial adipose thickness by 14% ($p < 0.0001$) following metabolic surgery. This study compared echocardiography results of patients before and >180 days following metabolic surgery [57]. This method of comparison demonstrates the direct effects of surgical intervention on cardiac tissue remodeling as patients served as their own comparison.

A few cohort studies have investigated the role of metabolic surgery in patients with CHF and have found positive outcomes following surgical intervention. Benotti et al. [55] conducted a retrospective longitudinal cohort study demonstrating that RYGB patients had reduced risk of major cardiovascular events (HR = 0.58, 95% CI 0.42–0.82, $p = 0.0018$) and reduced risk of development of CHF (HR = 0.38, 95% CI 0.22–0.64, $p = 0.0003$). Improvement in CHF appeared to be the primary driver of the overall composite cardiovascular risk reduction. This study did not see a significant difference in the occurrence of MI between RYGB and control groups, which suggests that the association between BMI and MI may not be as strong as that with CHF [59]. Sundström et al. further demonstrated that RYGB decreases the incidence of new heart failure development compared to intensive lifestyle modification by almost 50% (HR 0.54, 95% CI 0.36–0.82) [60].

## Cardiovascular Outcomes for Patients with Diabetes After Metabolic Surgery

Cardiovascular disease is the leading cause of death for patients with type 2 diabetes. Given the improvement in diabetes and glucose control after metabolic surgery, there is an anticipated benefit for cardiovascular outcomes, including both microvascular and macrovascular disease, in this specific patient population. In the SOS study, with a mean follow-up of 10 years, patients with diabetes who underwent metabolic surgery had decreased risk of developing microvascular disease compared to non-surgical therapy (HR 0.44, 95% CI 0.34–0.56, $p < 0.001$) [54]. In a retrospective matched-cohort study of individuals with diabetes, including 5301 patients who underwent metabolic surgery (76% RYGB, 17% SG, 7% AGB) and

14,934 matched controls, surgery was associated with 40% lower composite risk of macrovascular events at 5 years (2.1% surgical group vs 4.3% control group; HR 0.60, 95% CI 0.42–0.86) [61]. The composite end-point included CAD (MI, unstable angina, percutaneous coronary intervention, or coronary artery bypass grafting) or cerebrovascular events (ischemic stroke, hemorrhagic stroke, carotid stenting, carotid endarterectomy), while there was a 36% decreased risk of CAD, there was no statistically significant difference for cerebrovascular events.

## Summary

Overall, cardiovascular outcomes should be considered as a whole when assessing the effects of metabolic surgery. It is well documented in the literature that metabolic surgery improves all-cause mortality and there is specific emphasis on the benefits for cardiovascular health. While the topic of MI remains controversial, more studies are needed to discover the true effects of metabolic surgery on long-term outcomes. On the other hand, metabolic surgery has been documented to be beneficial to patients with CAD and CHF which results in sustainable long-term health outcomes.

## Stroke Outcomes After Metabolic Surgery

Isolated hypertension holds an attributable stroke risk of 25–50% [62]. Independent analysis on stroke risk reduction after metabolic surgery is limited, but the available data support risk reduction following surgery. [63] reviewed the Mariner database for the incidence of ischemic stroke in patients with obesity (BMI >34) following RYGB and SG against non-surgical control patients with obesity at 1 year, adjusted for comorbidities. Metabolic surgery was associated with a significant risk reduction in all-cause ischemic stroke at 1 year (OR 0.54; 95% CI s0.47–0.61), 3 years (OR 0.96; 95% CI 0.92–1.00) and 5 years (OR 0.78; 95% CI 0.65–0.90) compared to the non-surgical cohort [63]. Importantly, this study isolated ischemic stroke events as the outcome instead of using a typical composite outcome for all cerebrovascular insults, which includes MI, stroke and cardiovascular mortality. Composite results are traditionally utilized when the outcome of interest is rare; however, the Mariner claims database analyzed over 70,000 bariatric surgery patients matched with over 1.3 million non-surgical patients with obesity. Similarly, in the SOS study, the secondary end-point of all-cause stroke was reduced for patients undergoing metabolic surgery (HR 0.66, 95% CI 0.49–0.9, $p = 0.08$) [64]. The SOS database impacted further meta-analyses evaluating stroke as a composite and independent outcome after metabolic surgery, favoring an all-cause decrease in cardiovascular events in the postoperative period [65, 66].

## Conclusion

Medical comorbidities such as diabetes, hypertension, hyperlipidemia, and cardiovascular events are major contributors to morbidity and mortality in patients with obesity. Metabolic surgery has been demonstrated to have a significant benefit not only on weight loss but also on these comorbidities and their complications when compared to medical therapy alone. However, these conditions are chronic diseases that may be at risk for relapse over time despite initial improvement or remission following metabolic surgery. Therefore, continued monitoring long-term along with persistent lifestyle modification is needed to optimize the beneficial effects of metabolic surgery.

## References

1. Cameron NA, Petito LC, McCabe M, Allen NB, O'Brien MJ, Carnethon MR, Khan SS. Quantifying the sex-race/ethnicity-specific burden of obesity on incident diabetes mellitus in the United States, 2001 to 2016: MESA and NHANES. J Am Heart Assoc. 2021;10:e018799. https://doi.org/10.1161/JAHA.120.018799.
2. Cummings DE, Overduin J, Shannon MH, Foster-Schubert KE. Hormonal mechanisms of weight loss and diabetes resolution after bariatric surgery. Surg Obes Relat Dis. 2005;1:358–68. https://doi.org/10.1016/j.soard.2005.03.208.
3. Broglio F, Arvat E, Benso A, Gottero C, Muccioli G, Papotti M, van der Lely AJ, Deghenghi R, Ghigo E. Ghrelin, a natural GH secretagogue produced by the stomach, induces hyperglycemia and reduces insulin secretion in humans. J Clin Endocrinol Metab. 2001;86:5083–6. https://doi.org/10.1210/jcem.86.10.8098.
4. Drucker DJ. Glucagon-like peptide-1 and the islet β-cell: augmentation of cell proliferation and inhibition of apoptosis. Endocrinology. 2003;144:5145–8. https://doi.org/10.1210/en.2003-1147.
5. Schauer PR, Kashyap SR, Wolski K, Brethauer SA, Kirwan JP, Pothier CE, Thomas S, Abood B, Nissen SE, Bhatt DL. Bariatric surgery versus intensive medical therapy in obese patients with diabetes. N Engl J Med. 2012;366:1567–76. https://doi.org/10.1056/NEJMoa1200225.
6. Mingrone G, Panunzi S, De Gaetano A, Guidone C, Iaconelli A, Leccesi L, Nanni G, Pomp A, Castagneto M, Ghirlanda G, Rubino F. Bariatric surgery versus conventional medical therapy for type 2 diabetes. N Engl J Med. 2012;366:1577–85. https://doi.org/10.1056/NEJMoa1200111.
7. Gloy VL, Briel M, Bhatt DL, Kashyap SR, Schauer PR, Mingrone G, Bucher HC, Nordmann AJ. Bariatric surgery versus non-surgical treatment for obesity: a systematic review and meta-analysis of randomised controlled trials. BMJ. 2013;347:f5934. https://doi.org/10.1136/bmj.f5934.
8. Sheng B, Truong K, Spitler H, Zhang L, Tong X, Chen L. The long-term effects of bariatric surgery on type 2 diabetes remission, microvascular and macrovascular complications, and mortality: a systematic review and meta-analysis. Obes Surg. 2017;27:2724–32. https://doi.org/10.1007/s11695-017-2866-4.
9. Rubino F, Nathan DM, Eckel RH, Schauer PR, Alberti KGMM, Zimmet PZ, Del Prato S, Ji L, Sadikot SM, Herman WH, Amiel SA, Kaplan LM, Taroncher-Oldenburg G, Cummings DE, Delegates of the 2nd Diabetes Surgery Summit. Metabolic surgery in the treatment algorithm for type 2 diabetes: a joint statement by International Diabetes Organizations. Diabetes Care. 2016;39:861–77. https://doi.org/10.2337/dc16-0236.
10. Aminian A, Zajichek A, Arterburn DE, Wolski KE, Brethauer SA, Schauer PR, Nissen SE, Kattan MW. Predicting 10-year risk of end-organ complications of type 2 diabetes with and

without metabolic surgery: a machine learning approach. Diabetes Care. 2020;43:852–9. https://doi.org/10.2337/dc19-2057.

11. Aminian A, Brethauer SA, Andalib A, Nowacki AS, Jimenez A, Corcelles R, Hanipah ZN, Punchai S, Bhatt DL, Kashyap SR, Burguera B, Lacy AM, Vidal J, Schauer PR. Individualized metabolic surgery score: procedure selection based on diabetes severity. Ann Surg. 2017;266:650–7. https://doi.org/10.1097/SLA.0000000000002407.
12. Carlsson LMS, Peltonen M, Ahlin S, Anveden Å, Bouchard C, Carlsson B, Jacobson P, Lönroth H, Maglio C, Näslund I, Pirazzi C, Romeo S, Sjöholm K, Sjöström E, Wedel H, Svensson P-A, Sjöström L. Bariatric surgery and prevention of type 2 diabetes in Swedish obese subjects. N Engl J Med. 2012;367:695–704. https://doi.org/10.1056/NEJMoa1112082.
13. Carlsson LMS, Sjöholm K, Karlsson C, Jacobson P, Andersson-Assarsson JC, Svensson P-A, Larsson I, Hjorth S, Neovius M, Taube M, Carlsson B, Peltonen M. Long-term incidence of microvascular disease after bariatric surgery or usual care in patients with obesity, stratified by baseline glycaemic status: a post-hoc analysis of participants from the Swedish obese subjects study. Lancet Diabetes Endocrinol. 2017;5:271–9. https://doi.org/10.1016/S2213-8587(17)30061-X.
14. Yan J, Cohen R, Aminian A. Reoperative bariatric surgery for treatment of type 2 diabetes mellitus. Surg Obes Relat Dis. 2017;13:1412–21. https://doi.org/10.1016/j.soard.2017.04.019.
15. Adams TD, Davidson LE, Litwin SE, Kim J, Kolotkin RL, Nanjee MN, Gutierrez JM, Frogley SJ, Ibele AR, Brinton EA, Hopkins PN, McKinlay R, Simper SC, Hunt SC. Weight and metabolic outcomes 12 years after gastric bypass. N Engl J Med. 2017;377:1143–55. https://doi.org/10.1056/NEJMoa1700459.
16. Sjöström L, Lindroos A-K, Peltonen M, Torgerson J, Bouchard C, Carlsson B, Dahlgren S, Larsson B, Narbro K, Sjöström CD, Sullivan M, Wedel H. Lifestyle, diabetes, and cardiovascular risk factors 10 years after bariatric surgery. N Engl J Med. 2004;351:2683–93. https://doi.org/10.1056/NEJMoa035622.
17. Williams B, Mancia G, Spiering W, Agabiti Rosei E, Azizi M, Burnier M, Clement DL, Coca A, de Simone G, Dominiczak A, Kahan T, Mahfoud F, Redon J, Ruilope L, Zanchetti A, Kerins M, Kjeldsen SE, Kreutz R, Laurent S, Lip GYH, McManus R, Narkiewicz K, Ruschitzka F, Schmieder RE, Shlyakhto E, Tsioufis C, Aboyans V, Desormais I, ESC Scientific Document Group. 2018 ESC/ESH guidelines for the management of arterial hypertension. Eur Heart J. 2018;39:3021–104. https://doi.org/10.1093/eurheartj/ehy339.
18. Whelton PK, Carey RM, Aronow WS, Casey DE, Collins KJ, Dennison Himmelfarb C, DePalma SM, Gidding S, Jamerson KA, Jones DW, MacLaughlin EJ, Muntner P, Ovbiagele B, Smith SC, Spencer CC, Stafford RS, Taler SJ, Thomas RJ, Williams KA, Williamson JD, Wright JT. 2017 ACC/AHA/AAPA/ABC/ACPM/AGS/APhA/ASH/ASPC/NMA/PCNA guideline for the prevention, detection, evaluation, and management of high blood pressure in adults: executive summary: a report of the American College of Cardiology/American Heart Association task force on clinical practice guidelines. Hypertension. 2018;71:1269–324. https://doi.org/10.1161/HYP.0000000000000066.
19. Schauer PR, Burguera B, Ikramuddin S, Cottam D, Gourash W, Hamad G, Eid GM, Mattar S, Ramanathan R, Barinas-Mitchel E, Harsha Rao R, Kuller L, Kelley D. Effect of laparoscopic Roux-En Y gastric bypass on type 2 diabetes mellitus. Ann Surg. 2003;238:467–85. https://doi.org/10.1097/01.sla.0000089851.41115.1b.
20. Bays HE, Toth PP, Kris-Etherton PM, Abate N, Aronne LJ, Brown WV, Gonzalez-Campoy JM, Jones SR, Kumar R, Forge RL, Samuel VT. Obesity, adiposity, and dyslipidemia: a consensus statement from the National Lipid Association. J Clin Lipidol. 2013;7:304–83. https://doi.org/10.1016/j.jacl.2013.04.001.
21. Leggio M, Lombardi M, Caldarone E, Severi P, D'Emidio S, Armeni M, Bravi V, Bendini MG, Mazza A. The relationship between obesity and hypertension: an updated comprehensive overview on vicious twins. Hypertens Res. 2017;40:947–63. https://doi.org/10.1038/hr.2017.75.
22. Neter JE, Stam BE, Kok FJ, Grobbee DE, Geleijnse JM. Influence of weight reduction on blood pressure. Hypertension. 2003;42:878–84. https://doi.org/10.1161/01.HYP.0000094221.86888.AE.

23. Look AHEAD Research Group, et al. Cardiovascular effects of intensive lifestyle intervention in type 2 diabetes. N Engl J Med. 2013;369:145–54. https://doi.org/10.1056/NEJMoa1212914.
24. Schmidt FM, Weschenfelder J, Sander C, Minkwitz J, Thormann J, Chittka T, Mergl R, Kirkby KC, Faßhauer M, Stumvoll M, Holdt LM, Teupser D, Hegerl U, Himmerich H. Inflammatory cytokines in general and central obesity and modulating effects of physical activity. PLoS One. 2015;10:e0121971. https://doi.org/10.1371/journal.pone.0121971.
25. Landsberg L, Aronne LJ, Beilin LJ, Burke V, Igel LI, Lloyd-Jones D, Sowers J. Obesity-related hypertension: pathogenesis, cardiovascular risk, and treatment. J Clin Hypertens (Greenwich). 2012;15:14–33. https://doi.org/10.1111/jch.12049.
26. Kotchen TA. Obesity-related hypertension: epidemiology, pathophysiology, and clinical management. Am J Hypertens. 2010;23:1170–8. https://doi.org/10.1038/ajh.2010.172.
27. Kotsis V, Stabouli S, Papakatsika S, Rizos Z, Parati G. Mechanisms of obesity-induced hypertension. Hypertens Res. 2010;33:386–93. https://doi.org/10.1038/hr.2010.9.
28. Sharma AM, Wittchen H-U, Kirch W, Pittrow D, Ritz E, Göke B, Lehnert H, Tschöpe D, Krause P, Höfler M, Pfister H, Bramlage P, Unger T. High prevalence and poor control of hypertension in primary care: cross-sectional study. J Hypertens. 2004;22:479.
29. Bramlage P, Pittrow D, Wittchen H-U, Kirch W, Boehler S, Lehnert H, Hoefler M, Unger T, Sharma AM. Hypertension in overweight and obese primary care patients is highly prevalent and poorly controlled. Am J Hypertens. 2004;17:904–10. https://doi.org/10.1016/j.amjhyper.2004.05.017.
30. Biobaku F, Ghanim H, Monte SV, Caruana JA, Dandona P. Bariatric surgery: remission of inflammation, cardiometabolic benefits, and common adverse effects. J Endocr Soc. 2020;4:bvaa049. https://doi.org/10.1210/jendso/bvaa049.
31. Ghanim H, Monte S, Caruana J, Green K, Abuaysheh S, Dandona P. Decreases in neprilysin and vasoconstrictors and increases in vasodilators following bariatric surgery. Diabetes Obes Metab. 2018;20:2029–33. https://doi.org/10.1111/dom.13320.
32. Huby A-C, Antonova G, Groenendyk J, Gomez-Sanchez CE, Bollag WB, Filosa JA, de Chantemèle EJB. Adipocyte-derived hormone leptin is a direct regulator of aldosterone secretion, which promotes endothelial dysfunction and cardiac fibrosis. Circulation. 2015;132:2134–45. https://doi.org/10.1161/CIRCULATIONAHA.115.018226.
33. Graham C, Switzer N, Reso A, Armstrong C, Church N, Mitchell P, Debru E, Gill R. Sleeve gastrectomy and hypertension: a systematic review of long-term outcomes. Surg Endosc. 2019;33:3001–7. https://doi.org/10.1007/s00464-018-6566-5.
34. Pareek M, Bhatt DL, Schiavon CA, Schauer PR. Metabolic surgery for hypertension in patients with obesity. Circ Res. 2019;124:1009–24. https://doi.org/10.1161/CIRCRESAHA.118.313320.
35. Ricci C, Gaeta M, Rausa E, Macchitella Y, Bonavina L. Early impact of bariatric surgery on type II diabetes, hypertension, and hyperlipidemia: a systematic review, meta-analysis and meta-regression on 6,587 patients. Obes Surg. 2014;24:522–8. https://doi.org/10.1007/s11695-013-1121-x.
36. Sarkhosh K, Birch DW, Shi X, Gill RS, Karmali S. The impact of sleeve gastrectomy on hypertension: a systematic review. In: Database of abstracts of reviews of effects (DARE): quality-assessed reviews [internet]. Centre for Reviews and Dissemination (UK); 2012.
37. Valera-Mora ME, Simeoni B, Gagliardi L, Scarfone A, Nanni G, Castagneto M, Manco M, Mingrone G, Ferrannini E. Predictors of weight loss and reversal of comorbidities in malabsorptive bariatric surgery. Am J Clin Nutr. 2005;81:1292–7. https://doi.org/10.1093/ajcn/81.6.1292.
38. Wilhelm SM, Young J, Kale-Pradhan PB. Effect of bariatric surgery on hypertension: a meta-analysis. Ann Pharmacother. 2014;48:674–82. https://doi.org/10.1177/1060028014529260.
39. Peterli R, Wölnerhanssen BK, Peters T, Vetter D, Kröll D, Borbély Y, Schultes B, Beglinger C, Drewe J, Schiesser M, Nett P, Bueter M. Effect of laparoscopic sleeve gastrectomy vs laparoscopic Roux-en-Y gastric bypass on weight loss in patients with morbid obesity. JAMA. 2018;319:255–65. https://doi.org/10.1001/jama.2017.20897.

40. Salminen P, Helmiö M, Ovaska J, Juuti A, Leivonen M, Peromaa-Haavisto P, Hurme S, Soinio M, Nuutila P, Victorzon M. Effect of laparoscopic sleeve gastrectomy vs laparoscopic Roux-en-Y gastric bypass on weight loss at 5 years among patients with morbid obesity: the SLEEVEPASS randomized clinical trial. JAMA. 2018;319:241–54. https://doi.org/10.1001/jama.2017.20313.
41. Schiavon CA, Bersch-Ferreira AC, Santucci EV, Oliveira JD, Torreglosa CR, Bueno PT, Frayha JC, Santos RN, Damiani LP, Noujaim PM, Halpern H, Monteiro FLJ, Cohen RV, Uchoa CH, de Souza MG, Amodeo C, Bortolotto L, Ikeoka D, Drager LF, Cavalcanti AB, Berwanger O. Effects of bariatric surgery in obese patients with hypertension. Circulation. 2018;137:1132–42. https://doi.org/10.1161/CIRCULATIONAHA.117.032130.
42. Schiavon CA, Bhatt DL, Ikeoka D, Santucci EV, Santos RN, Damiani LP, Oliveira JD, Machado RHV, Halpern H, Monteiro FLJ, Noujaim PM, Cohen RV, de Souza MG, Amodeo C, Bortolotto LA, Berwanger O, Cavalcanti AB, Drager LF. Three-year outcomes of bariatric surgery in patients with obesity and hypertension: a randomized clinical trial. Ann Intern Med. 2020;173:685–93. https://doi.org/10.7326/M19-3781.
43. Buchwald H, Avidor Y, Braunwald E, Jensen MD, Pories W, Fahrbach K, Schoelles K. Bariatric surgery: a systematic review and meta-analysis. JAMA. 2004;292:1724–37. https://doi.org/10.1001/jama.292.14.1724.
44. Al Khalifa K, Al Ansari A, Alsayed AR, Violato C. The impact of sleeve gastrectomy on hyperlipidemia: a systematic review. J Obes. 2013;2013:643530. https://doi.org/10.1155/2013/643530.
45. Benetti A, Del Puppo M, Crosignani A, Veronelli A, Masci E, Frigè F, Micheletto G, Panizzo V, Pontiroli AE. Cholesterol metabolism after bariatric surgery in grade 3 obesity. Diabetes Care. 2013;36:1443–7. https://doi.org/10.2337/dc12-1737.
46. Elbaz-Greener G, Rozen G, Carasso S, Kusniec F, Marai I, Sud M, Strauss B, Smart FW, Planer D, Amir O. The relationship between body mass index and in-hospital mortality in the contemporary era of an acute myocardial infarction management. Vasc Health Risk Manag. 2021;17:551–9. https://doi.org/10.2147/VHRM.S315248.
47. Kim D-W, Her S-H, Park HW, Park M-W, Chang K, Chung WS, Seung KB, Ahn TH, Jeong MH, Rha S-W, Kim H-S, Gwon HC, Seong IW, Hwang KK, Chae SC, Kim K-B, Kim YJ, Cha KS, Oh SK, Chae JK. Association between body mass index and 1-year outcome after acute myocardial infarction. PLoS One. 2019;14:e0217525. https://doi.org/10.1371/journal.pone.0217525.
48. Lee SN, Moon D, Jo MS, Yoo K-D. Associations between body mass index and clinical outcomes in acute myocardial infarction supported with extracorporeal membrane oxygenation. Acta Cardiol Sin. 2020;36:448–55. https://doi.org/10.6515/ACS.202009_36(5).20200519B.
49. Adams TD, Gress RE, Smith SC, Halverson RC, Simper SC, Rosamond WD, LaMonte MJ, Stroup AM, Hunt SC. Long-term mortality after gastric bypass surgery. N Engl J Med. 2007;357:753–61. https://doi.org/10.1056/NEJMoa066603.
50. Aminian A, Zajichek A, Arterburn DE, Wolski KE, Brethauer SA, Schauer PR, Kattan MW, Nissen SE. Association of metabolic surgery with major adverse cardiovascular outcomes in patients with type 2 diabetes and obesity. JAMA. 2019;322:1271–82. https://doi.org/10.1001/jama.2019.14231.
51. Courcoulas AP, Gallagher JW, Neiberg RH, Eagleton EB, DeLany JP, Lang W, Punchai S, Gourash W, Jakicic JM. Bariatric surgery vs lifestyle intervention for diabetes treatment: 5-year outcomes from a randomized trial. J Clin Endocrinol Metab. 2020;105:866–76. https://doi.org/10.1210/clinem/dgaa006.
52. Johnson BL, Blackhurst DW, Latham BB, Cull DL, Bour ES, Oliver TL, Williams B, Taylor SM, Scott JD. Bariatric surgery is associated with a reduction in major macrovascular and microvascular complications in moderately to severely obese patients with type 2 diabetes mellitus. J Am Coll Surg. 2013;216:545–56; discussion 556-558. https://doi.org/10.1016/j.jamcollsurg.2012.12.019.
53. Mingrone G, Panunzi S, De Gaetano A, Guidone C, Iaconelli A, Capristo E, Chamseddine G, Bornstein SR, Rubino F. Metabolic surgery versus conventional medical therapy in patients

with type 2 diabetes: 10-year follow-up of an open-label, single-centre, randomised controlled trial. Lancet. 2021;397:293–304. https://doi.org/10.1016/S0140-6736(20)32649-0.

54. Sjöström L, Peltonen M, Jacobson P, Ahlin S, Andersson-Assarsson J, Anveden Å, Bouchard C, Carlsson B, Karason K, Lönroth H, Näslund I, Sjöström E, Taube M, Wedel H, Svensson P-A, Sjöholm K, Carlsson LMS. Association of bariatric surgery with long-term remission of type 2 diabetes and with microvascular and macrovascular complications. JAMA. 2014;311:2297–304. https://doi.org/10.1001/jama.2014.5988.
55. Benotti PN, Wood GC, Carey DJ, Mehra VC, Mirshahi T, Lent MR, Petrick AT, Still C, Gerhard GS, Hirsch AG. Gastric bypass surgery produces a durable reduction in cardiovascular disease risk factors and reduces the long-term risks of congestive heart failure. J Am Heart Assoc. 2017;6:e005126. https://doi.org/10.1161/JAHA.116.005126.
56. Noubani M, Zhang X, Yang J, Powers K, Spaniolas K, Pryor AD. The impact of bariatric surgery on the risk of coronary revascularization. Surg Obes Relat Dis. 2022;18:610–9. https://doi.org/10.1016/j.soard.2022.01.013.
57. Sorimachi H, Obokata M, Omote K, Reddy YNV, Takahashi N, Koepp KE, Ng ACT, Rider OJ, Borlaug BA. Long-term changes in cardiac structure and function following bariatric surgery. J Am Coll Cardiol. 2022;80:1501–12. https://doi.org/10.1016/j.jacc.2022.08.738.
58. Datta T, Lee AJ, Cain R, McCarey M, Whellan DJ. Weighing in on heart failure: the potential impact of bariatric surgery. Heart Fail Rev. 2022;27:755–66. https://doi.org/10.1007/s10741-021-10078-w.
59. Bucholz EM, Rathore SS, Reid KJ, Jones PG, Chan PS, Rich MW, Spertus JA, Krumholz HM. Body mass index and mortality in acute myocardial infarction patients. Am J Med. 2012;125:796. https://doi.org/10.1016/j.amjmed.2012.01.018.
60. Sundström J, Bruze G, Ottosson J, Marcus C, Näslund I, Neovius M. Weight loss and heart failure. Circulation. 2017;135:1577–85. https://doi.org/10.1161/CIRCULATIONAHA.116.025629.
61. Fisher DP, Johnson E, Haneuse S, Arterburn D, Coleman KJ, O'Connor PJ, O'Brien R, Bogart A, Theis MK, Anau J, Schroeder EB, Sidney S. Association between bariatric surgery and macrovascular disease outcomes in patients with type 2 diabetes and severe obesity. JAMA. 2018;320:1570–82. https://doi.org/10.1001/jama.2018.14619.
62. Gorelick PB, Whelton PK, Sorond F, Carey RM. Blood pressure management in stroke: viewpoint. Hypertension. 2020;76:1688–95. https://doi.org/10.1161/HYPERTENSIONAHA.120.14653.
63. Williams MD, Kim S, Sarran M, Khalid SI, Becerra AZ, Torquati A, Omotosho P. The effect of bariatric surgery on ischemic stroke risk. Surg Obes Relat Dis. 2021;17:1949–55. https://doi.org/10.1016/j.soard.2021.09.006.
64. Sjöström L, Peltonen M, Jacobson P, Sjöström CD, Karason K, Wedel H, Ahlin S, Anveden Å, Bengtsson C, Bergmark G, Bouchard C, Carlsson B, Dahlgren S, Karlsson J, Lindroos A-K, Lönroth H, Narbro K, Näslund I, Olbers T, Svensson P-A, Carlsson LMS. Bariatric surgery and long-term cardiovascular events. JAMA. 2012;307:56–65. https://doi.org/10.1001/jama.2011.1914.
65. Cardoso L, Rodrigues D, Gomes L, Carrilho F. Short- and long-term mortality after bariatric surgery: a systematic review and meta-analysis. Diabetes Obes Metab. 2017;19:1223–32. https://doi.org/10.1111/dom.12922.
66. Zhou X, Yu J, Li L, Gloy VL, Nordmann A, Tiboni M, Li Y, Sun X. Effects of bariatric surgery on mortality, cardiovascular events, and cancer outcomes in obese patients: systematic review and meta-analysis. Obes Surg. 2016;26:2590–601. https://doi.org/10.1007/s11695-016-2144-x.
67. Estimate of Bariatric Surgery Numbers, 2011–2021 [WWW Document]. American Society for Metabolic and Bariatric Surgery; 2022. https://asmbs.org/resources/estimate-of-bariatric-surgery-numbers. Accessed 29 Oct 2023.

# Part III

# Complications

# Adjustable Gastric Band Associated Complications

# 27

Derek Freitas and Christine Ren Fielding

## Introduction

Adjustable gastric banding (AGB) historically was one of the most common primary bariatric procedures during the early to mid-2000s [1, 2]. However, rates of AGB subsequently declined with a concomitant rise in the laparoscopic sleeve gastrectomy (LSG) [2]. Although less popular in recent years, AGB continues to be an available surgical treatment in properly selected individuals [1, 3]. Additionally, there are still tens of thousands of patients living with an AGB.

Due to its unique nature and implantation of a foreign body, AGB entails its own set of complications that differ significantly from other bariatric procedures such as LSG and Roux-en-Y gastric bypass (RYGB). Although early data showed very low complication rates, later data has shown rates closer to 10–20% in the short term. Longer-term reviews have demonstrated the need for revisional surgery is upwards of 20–40% of patients over 10–15 years [1, 4]. Notably, data are skewed, with earlier studies showing higher complication and reintervention rates but this decreasing in more recent years even over the long term as surgical techniques have improved [1].

Given the large number of patients with an AGB in place, there is a high chance of being called upon to manage complications related to the procedure. This chapter will review the most common complications of AGB including their diagnosis and management. Most complications can be divided into early and late presentations. Early complications typically occur within days to weeks after surgery and include common general surgical complications as well as those unique to AGB. Late complications occur weeks, months, years, or even decades later. Some complications

D. Freitas · C. R. Fielding (✉)
Division of Bariatric Surgery, Department of Surgery, NYU Langone Health, New York, NY, USA
e-mail: Christine.Ren-Fielding@nyulangone.org



O. M. Ghanem et al. (eds.), *The SAGES Manual of Metabolic and Bariatric Surgery*, https://doi.org/10.1007/978-3-031-72309-4_27

**Table 27.1** AGB-related complications during early and late periods

| Early complications | Late complications |
|---|---|
| Esophageal or gastric perforation | Device leak and malfunction<br>– Band, tubing, port |
| Deep venous thrombosis | Band erosion |
| Gastric obstruction | Esophageal or gastric pouch dilation |
| Band infection | Esophageal dysmotility/pseudoachalasia |
| Malpositioned band | Slippage and gastric prolapse |
| | Bowel obstruction |

such as band infection or prolapse can occur in the early or late period. While not exhaustive, Table 27.1 lists some of the most common AGB-specific complications in each period.

## Early Complications

Early complications typically occur in the immediate postoperative period. Often, but not always, they are related to a technical error or missed injury, but may also include other complications such as venous thromboembolism (VTE). Management varies based on the complication but there should be a low threshold for additional workup in the immediate postoperative period as some early complications can cause significant morbidity or even mortality.

### Gastric/Esophageal Perforation

Gastric and esophageal perforation is an extremely rare complication occurring in less than one percent of patients but can be devastating if unrecognized [5]. Typically, the perforation occurs during the posterior dissection to create a tunnel in order to pass the band around the stomach [6]. If recognized intraoperatively, the perforation can be repaired. However, if missed, it can lead to further complications and possible mortality. There should be a suspicion for this complication in any AGB patient presenting with significant abdominal pain, chest pain (particularly if there was mediastinal dissection), fevers, and/or persistent tachycardia in the immediate postoperative period. Any clinical suspicion warrants immediate investigation, and there should be a low threshold for performing an esophagram [7]. Gastrografin should be used as the initial contrast agent. If no leak is demonstrated, then thin barium should be administered given the higher sensitivity for detecting contrast extravasation [7, 8]. A computerized tomography (CT) scan is a valid alternative especially if the differential diagnosis includes pulmonary embolism or other viscous injury. In such instances, a CT scan of the chest, abdomen, and pelvis can be a more prudent strategy for radiographic investigation. Negative imaging does not fully rule out a perforation, and if clinical suspicion remains high, operative exploration is prudent.

## Gastric Obstruction

Acute gastric obstruction is rare in AGB but has several etiologies including band malposition, improper band size, or postoperative edema [6]. Patients will present with acute intolerance to oral intake including potentially their own saliva. Esophagram is the diagnostic test of choice and will demonstrate a lack of contrast passing beyond the level of the band [7, 8]. The esophagram may demonstrate malpositioning of the band. If postoperative edema is the suspected etiology of the obstruction, a trial of non-operative management with nothing per os (NPO), intravenous fluids, and intravenous steroids can be attempted until the edema resolves. Band malpositioning or improper sizing requires operative intervention to correct the band position, remove the perigastric fat pad, or upsize the band. If these efforts fail, the band should be removed.

## Venous Thromboembolism

Patients undergoing bariatric surgery are at moderate-to-high risk of developing VTE [9]. While the rates of VTE). appear to be lower in AGB than LSG and RYGB, the overall rate remains higher than the general population [9, 10]. Therefore, VTE should be on the differential in any patient undergoing AGB who presents with tachycardia, shortness of breath, chest pain, calf pain or swelling, or other concerning signs or symptoms. Importantly the elevated risk appears to extend well beyond the immediate operative period so VTE should remain a consideration several weeks or months after surgery [10]. Standard management includes therapeutic anticoagulation when able, with or without placement of an inferior vena cava filter, or additional interventions as dictated by guidelines [11].

## Band Infection

Band infection may occur in the early postoperative period but may be a late complication as well. The subcutaneous access port may become infected, but it remains a rare complication (<0.5%) [3, 6]. Early infection may occur due to inadvertent breaks in sterile technique during the index operation or simply bacterial colonization despite optimal sterile conditions. Patients may present with abdominal pain, fevers, erythema, induration, fluctuance, or even frank purulent drainage from their access port site. Treatment can be attempted with antibiotics, but if unsuccessful, may require temporary explantation of the affected component or removal of the entire system [6]. Band infections occurring further out from the surgery may be related to contamination during port access but should raise the concern for occult gastric erosion where the infection propagates from the band component back towards the access port.

## Late Complications

While late complications can run the gamut from band erosions, gastric prolapse, and esophageal/pouch issues, the most common tend to be related to port/tubing issues which carry low morbidity and are straightforward to address [3, 4, 12]. If not corrected, device-related complications may lead to weight regain. AGB patients should be followed routinely as an outpatient, not only to monitor weight loss trends and make adjustments to the band as necessary but also to identify some of the potential complications discussed below.

## Gastric Prolapse and Band Slippage

Gastric prolapse, also known as band slippage, occurs when a portion of the stomach fundus or body herniates through the aperture of the band causing the band to "slip" out of normal alignment. If minimal, symptoms of band slippage may be silent and incidentally found in imaging studies. More often, slippage presents with varying symptoms ranging from reflux, food intolerance, abdominal pain, and even complete obstruction [13]. The most common symptom is nocturnal reflux in the form of volume reflux, regurgitation, or cough.

Gastric prolapse can occur in one of three ways: anteriorly, posteriorly, or concentrically creating an asymmetric gastric pouch in the case of anterior or posterior prolapse (see Fig. 27.1) [8]. When posterior prolapse occurs, the posterior portion of the stomach herniates through the band aperture. This was more common in the earlier days of AGB when the "peri-gastric" technique of band placement was employed, but evolution to the standard of the "pars flacida technique" led to significant reductions in posterior prolapse [14, 15]. Anterior prolapse is now the most common variant and occurs when the greater curvature of the stomach, typically the fundus, herniates through the band. The risk of prolapse can be reduced by applying a gastro-gastric stitch which plicates and approximates the greater curve of the stomach below the band to the cardia above the band [13, 16].

An initial abdominal x-ray (AXR) can be used to demonstrate a slipped gastric band; however, esophagram remains the gold standard as not only can multiple views be taken, but the use of oral contrast can evaluate gastric pouch anatomy and emptying [7]. Normal band positioning on anterior-posterior films should show the lateral aspect of the band higher than the medial aspect under the left hemidiaphragm, thus giving a diagonal appearance of the band with the exact angle between the vertical axis of the spinal column and the long axis of the band being no greater than 60° ("Phi angle" Fig. 27.2) [8]. Deviations from this linear diagonal orientation should raise concern for band slippage. Additionally, non-concentric gastric herniation through the band orifice may push the posterior or anterior aspect of the band out of the horizontal plane creating an "O" configuration on anterior-posterior views (Fig. 27.2) [8].

Initial management involves emptying the band completely. This may relieve obstructive symptoms, and the slippage may self-resolve [14]. If band deflation

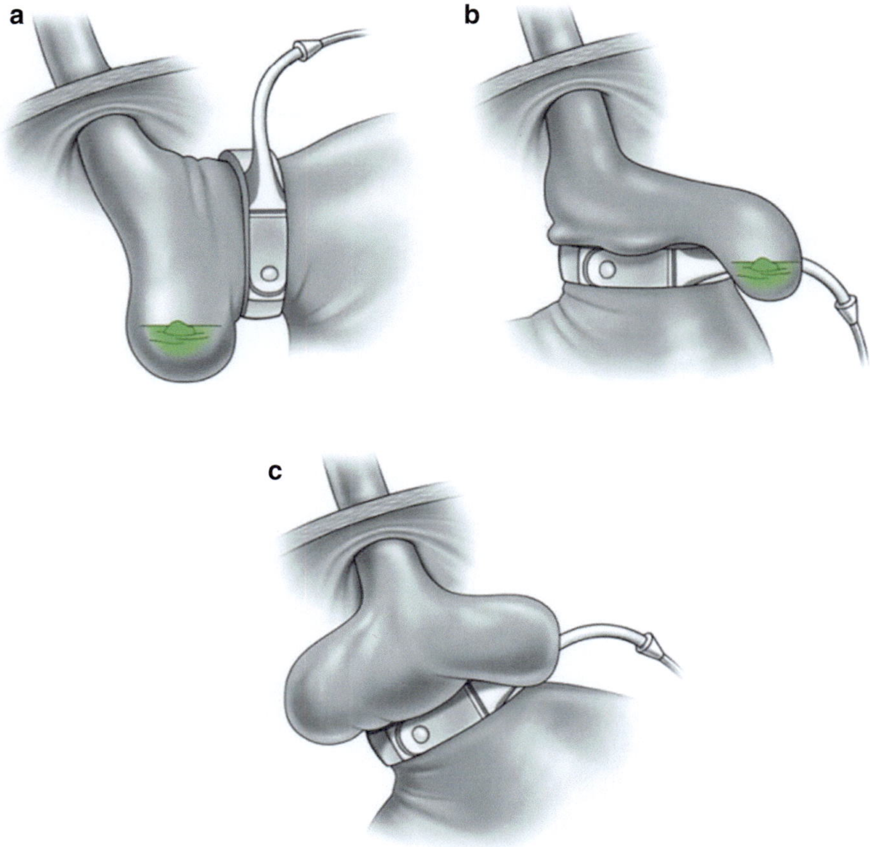


**Fig. 27.1** Three types of gastric prolapse: (**a**) posterior prolapse, (**b**) anterior prolapse, (**c**) concentric prolapse. (*Reprinted with permission from the ASMBS Textbook of Bariatric Surgery: Second Edition. Chapter—Gastric Banding Complications: Management*)

does not relieve symptoms, operative intervention is indicated in order to prevent complications of prolonged prolapse such as gastric volvulus, ischemia, and/or necrosis [7, 14].

If deflation is successful, a follow-up esophagram should be obtained 1–2 weeks later to reevaluate band positioning, gastric pouch size, and passage of contrast [8]. If the band slippage has resolved and the prolapsed stomach reduced, it may be possible to slowly fill the band. However, if band slippage persists or symptoms recur, surgical intervention is indicated and includes: band unlocking, repositioning/revision, or band removal.

Band revision with repositioning is typically performed for patients who have done well with their weight loss and who are not interested in pursuing an alternative bariatric operation if the band is removed [17]. This is performed laparoscopically and may require removal and replacement of the gastric band to avoid stoma

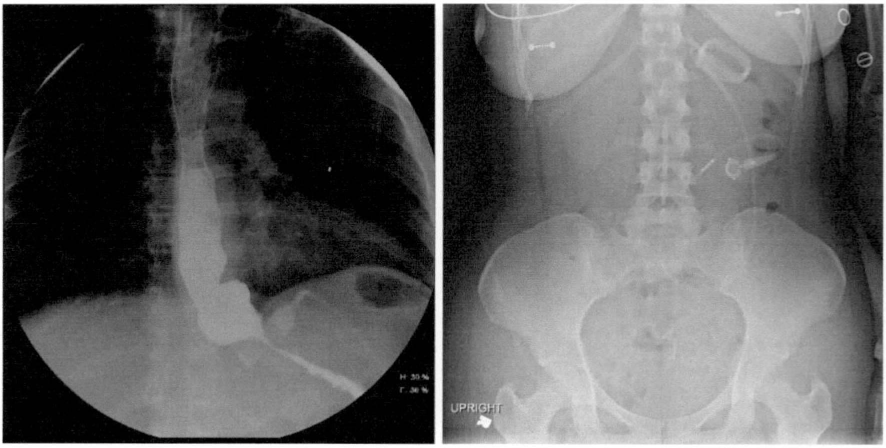


**Fig. 27.2** Left panel shows an esophagram with a normally positioned gastric band. Right panel demonstrates an abdominal x-ray with a slipped gastric band in an "O" configuration and an aberrant angle from the vertical axis of the spine

obstruction if the gastric pouch is dilated. In certain circumstances, the gastric pouch may be significantly dilated and inflamed so the band cannot be rebuckled. In this case, a two-stage approach can be applied by unlocking the band and then returning six or more weeks later to revise the band after allowing inflammation to subside. This technique can also be useful in pregnant patients. Patients who have not had successful weight loss are best served by band removal and evaluation for an alternative bariatric procedure.

## Band Erosion

Band erosion involves the gastric component of the band slowly eroding through the wall of the stomach until it migrates into the gastric lumen (Fig. 27.3). Rarely the band can erode into nearby structures such as the liver, major arteries, or the chest with potentially catastrophic consequences (Fig. 27.4) [18, 19]. Erosion occurs with an incidence of around 0.1–2% with higher early erosion rates inversely correlated with surgeon experience [20, 21]. It also appears to be correlated with undiagnosed gastric prolapse or chronic overtightening of the band [6, 22, 23]. Band erosion is typically a delayed complication occurring two or more years after surgery, and it is usually insidious and rarely results in free perforation into the abdomen. It may initially present with a port infection as the infection spreads from the eroded band along the tubing to the subcutaneous port, but it can present with loss of appetite control, hunger, and weight gain [6]. Patients often lose the effectiveness of the band's appetite control mechanism and start regaining weight.

Endoscopy is the diagnostic gold standard for band erosion; however, imaging studies do have a role. An esophagram may show tracking of contrast

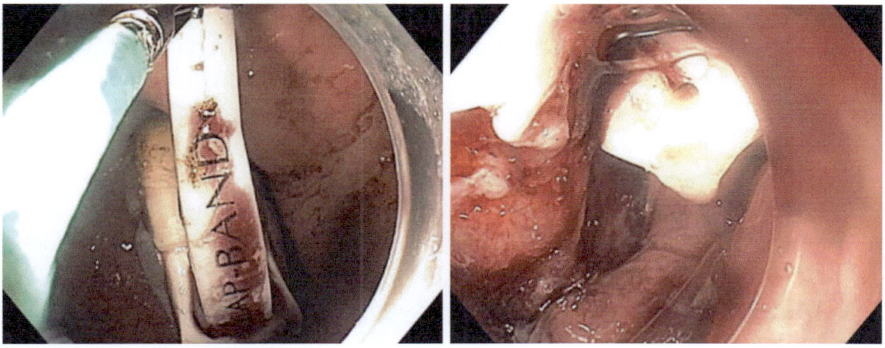


**Fig. 27.3** Upper endoscopy images showing erosion of a gastric band into the lumen of the stomach

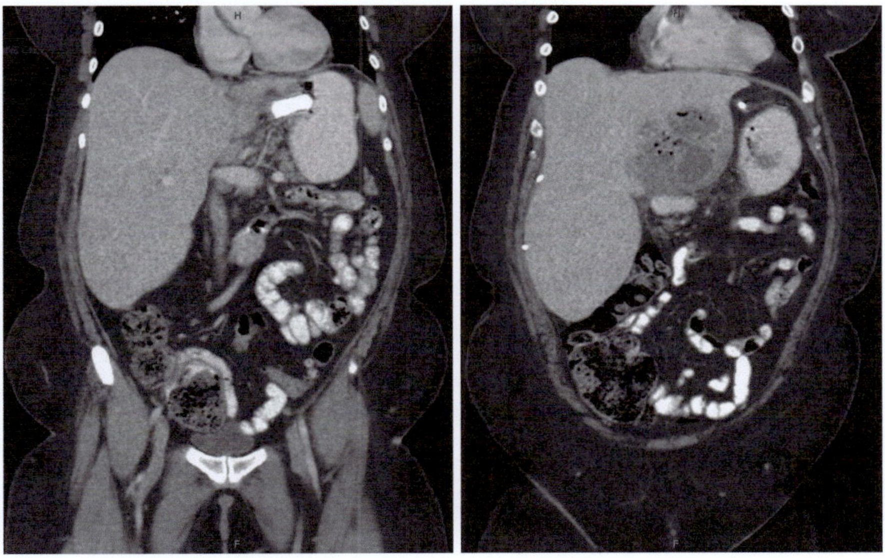

**Fig. 27.4** Abdominal CT scan of a band erosion. The left panel demonstrates air tracking around the band with an apparent intraluminal aspect of the lateral portion of the band. The right panel shows an associated large hepatic abscess

extraluminally outside of and around the band component [7]. Overt leaks into the peritoneal cavity have not been described because erosions tend to be contained. Concern for band erosion may also be discovered on a CT scan with findings such as air around the band, peri-band abscess, surrounding peritoneal fluid, or other findings (Fig. 27.4) [7]. Any of the imaging findings above should prompt upper endoscopy. Even with negative imaging findings, if clinical suspicion of erosion remains, patients should undergo endoscopy.

Band erosion necessitates the removal of the band system. This can be performed laparoscopically or robotically, creating a gastrotomy to remove the band, followed by suture closure of the gastrotomy [21, 24]. Endoscopic removal has become an option if the majority of the band is within the gastric lumen. This technique is being utilized more often but requires a trained endoscopist or surgeon with advanced endoscopic skills, and specific equipment [20, 23]. The access port can be removed under local or general anesthesia. Failure to remove the band endoscopically would require reverting back to surgical removal. Simultaneous conversion to a different bariatric operation during the removal of the eroded gastric band is not recommended.

## Esophageal and Pouch Complications

Over time, AGB can lead to various complications related to the esophagus and gastric pouch. These complications may be due to chronic overtightening of the band but also due to other variables such as changes in esophageal motility and patient compliance with dietary and behavioral modification. The mechanism of the AGB works by providing appetite control and satiety by compressing around the upper stomach and early stimulation of stretch receptors. However, this in turn creates increased resistance to esophageal peristalsis and the subsequent potential for esophageal complications. The two most common symptoms are reflux and dysphagia.

Reflux or dysphagia may be an initial sign of an overtightened band. If the band is too tight, an esophagram will demonstrate an overly narrowed band stoma with or without a dilated gastric pouch and/or esophagus and slowed passage of contrast through the band (Fig. 27.5) [7, 8]. Overtightening, even when it does not cause overt clinical signs and symptoms such as reflux, may cause esophageal dilation in upwards of 60–70% of patients [25, 26]. The amount of dilation can be minimal to severe. If not addressed, patients may develop pseudoachalasia with impaired esophageal motility [27]. Removing all fluid from the band is the first step, which is usually corrective. However, if symptoms persist and manometry confirms pseudoachalasia, band removal is indicated.

Esophageal dilation is not always caused by an overtightened band and may be related to other causes of esophageal dysmotility. Patients with AGB are susceptible to developing regurgitant esophagitis [26, 28]. This is more common if they do not adopt the necessary behavioral and dietary changes. Issues related to dietary compliance on imaging are likely to show normal band positioning and stoma size but with concentric dilation of the pouch or esophageal dilation [7]. Pouch dilation due to poor diet compliance requires proper dietary and behavioral counseling and management. Even with proper initial dietary compliance, if there is slow dilation of the gastric pouch over time, the patient may be able to progressively eat more leading to further pouch dilation and regurgitant esophagitis. Therefore, workup for potential gastric pouch or esophageal issues requires a thorough imaging assessment as well as detailed dietary and behavioral history.

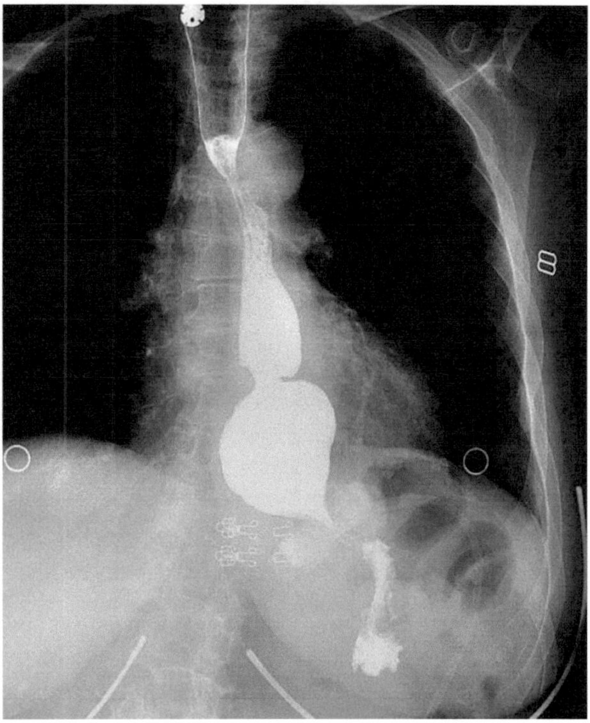

**Fig. 27.5** Esophagram demonstrating an overtightened band with pouch dilation. A hiatal hernia is also present

Reflux esophagitis can also be caused by a hiatal hernia which may not have been recognized or repaired at the initial AGB surgery. On esophagram, a hiatal hernia will often appear as a gastric pouch dilation extending into the mediastinum (Fig. 27.5) and should be repaired. Furthermore, pill esophagitis can be caused by swallowing large or caustic tablets/capsules such as vitamin supplements or doxycycline [29, 30]. Patients should be counseled to avoid large pills after AGB, can be treated with temporary band loosening plus sulcrafate.

## Device Malfunctions

Malfunctions and leaks of the port, tubing, and band are the most common late complications and are typically benign. The incidence ranges between 10 and 20% earlier on with some studies reporting rates closer to 30–40% one to two decades out from surgery [1, 4, 31–33]. A common malfunction is a leak in the gastric band system, which can occur at any part of the device or from complete disconnection of the tubing from the access port. Access port migration can also occur and lead to the inability to tighten or loosen the band system.

The access port is the most common site of device malfunction and the easiest to correct. Aside from port infections, which can occur at any time point, other issues can arise. The most common complication is a leak which often occurs where the port connects to the rest of the band system [31, 33]. Leakage of the saline used to fill the band at this site can occur due to holes in the tubing, loosening of the tubing connection to the port, or full disconnection of the tubing from the port. Holes in the non-membranous portion of the port, tubing adjacent to the port, or at the connector between the port and tubing can occur for a variety of reasons such as iatrogenic damage during port access attempts, external compression of the tubing component, or even chronic wear and tear. Leaks can also occur at other points in the system such as the intra-abdominal tubing or at the band itself.

Regardless of where the leak is, patients often present with weight gain due to increased hunger and the ability to tolerate more food as the band loosens. A device leak can be confirmed by accessing the port and attempting to aspirate all the fluid in the system. If notably less fluid is returned than was previously documented, this is concerning for a leak. This process can be repeated if results are equivocal with a known exact amount placed into the band and aspirated at a later date to assess for a discrepancy. Additionally, sometimes serous colored fluid or air bubbles may even be aspirated. If there is a suspected leak it is important to determine where the leak is in the system as this dictates the intervention needed [33]. An abdominal X-ray may demonstrate an obvious issue such as a tubing disconnect [7]. Water-soluble contrast injection into the port can be performed under fluoroscopy in an attempt to identify the leak location, but this is not always definitive [7].

The location of a leak is best identified intraoperatively by injecting methylene blue solution into the access port while visualizing the tubing entry site into the abdomen under laparoscopy. The dye may be visualized leaking immediately from the tubing/port entry site in the abdominal wall or from a deeper component in the system (Fig. 27.6). Leaks at the port or the port/tubing connection can be repaired by opening the port pocket and addressing the underlying issue (e.g., replacing a leaking port, reconnecting disconnected tubing, trimming broken tubing back to normal tubing and reconnecting it to the port). Leaks deeper in the system require the replacement of the entire band. Care should be taken with leaks in the tubing

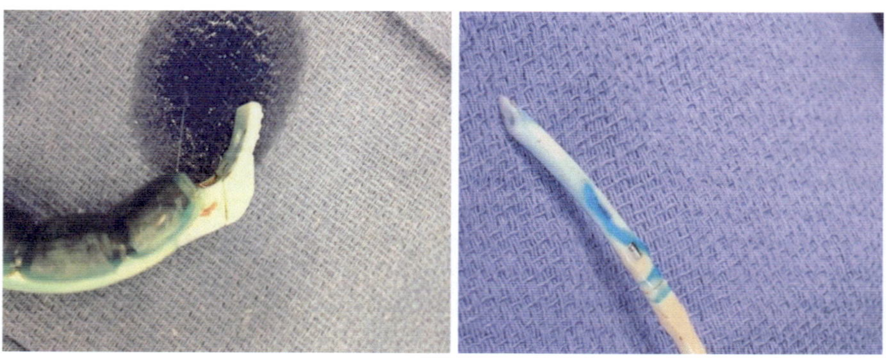

**Fig. 27.6** Example of methylene blue leaking from different band components after removal. The left panel shows methylene blue leaking from the balloon component of a gastric band. The right panel shows leakage from the tubing at the metal connector

especially if the leak is not immediately adjacent to the port. The band system is often constructed of a single silicone mold, and therefore leaks in the tubing further away from the access port site may be indicative of a loss of durability and integrity in the band system material as a whole. This could predispose to future leaks even if the portion of the leaking tubing is trimmed back and reconnected to the access port. Consequently, complete exchange of the system should be considered in such instances.

Another potential device malfunction is displacement of the port making access to the band system difficult or impossible (Fig. 27.7). Ports are rarely initially malpositioned, but as patients lose weight and as the port forms a capsule, it may move. It is recommended to secure ports to the underlying fascia at multiple spots during initial placement in order to minimize this complication. If a port does migrate, fluoroscopy may be a useful tool to aid in accessing it using manual manipulation [7]. If the port remains difficult to access or has entirely flipped over, surgical revision is necessary. Sometimes the port may be well positioned, but kinking of the tubing can prevent the filling or emptying of the band and requires surgical revision [31].

## Miscellaneous Complications

Most late complications will be related to band slippage, erosion, or system leaks but other complications may be encountered. One of the rarer complications is intestinal obstruction related to or caused by the band tubing. Reports in the literature document obstruction related to bowel twisting around the tubing or the tubing strangulating the bowel [31, 34, 35]. Bowel obstructions may also occur from postoperative adhesions. Similarly, patients can develop an incisional hernia at the port tubing entry site which can lead to incarceration or strangulation of the bowel or can develop incisional hernias at any of the laparoscopic port sites [33]. It is important

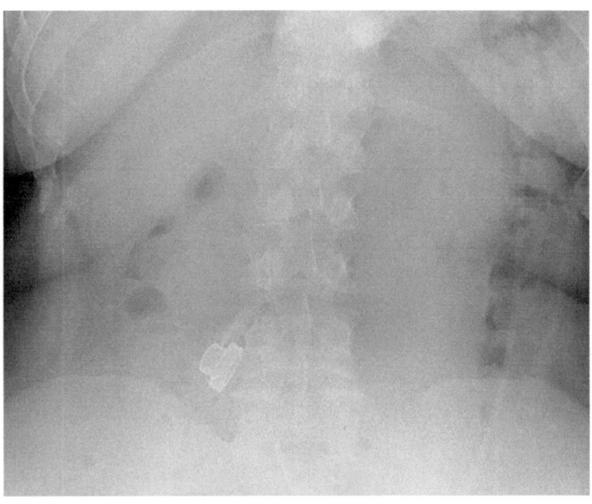

**Fig. 27.7** Abdominal x-ray demonstrating a partially flipped subcutaneous access port

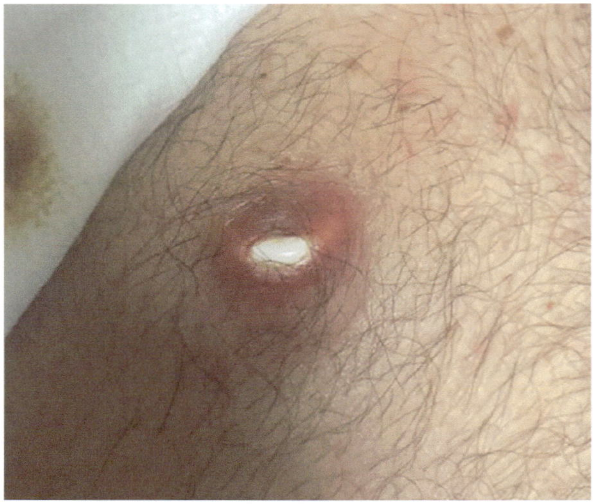

**Fig. 27.8** Subcutaneous access port eroding through the skin

to utilize abdominal CT imaging to evaluate AGB patients presenting with abdominal pain. Other miscellaneous complications can include port prominence causing discomfort, erosion of the port through the skin (Fig. 27.8), or chronic pain from the port or tubing [31]. This may require surgical intervention to revise or remove the affected component.

## Conclusion

Despite adjustable gastric banding being performed in far fewer numbers today, there are a significant number of patients with an existing AGB, and it remains an indicated procedure in properly selected individuals. AGB carries a specific set of potential complications relative to other bariatric surgical procedures. Removal or revision of the band to address related complications is not without its own risks and some retrospective data has shown increased rates of 30-day complications of removal relative to placement [36]. AGB represents a unique bariatric procedure with the introduction of a semi-permanent foreign object into the body. There can be a myriad of complications with varying presentations, workups, and methods of management. Therefore, there should be a committed schedule of follow-up of these patients and a low threshold to pursue further workup in patients presenting with abnormal symptoms.

## References

1. O'Brien PE, MacDonald L, Anderson M, Brennan L, Brown WA. Long-term outcomes after bariatric surgery: fifteen-year follow-up of adjustable gastric banding and a systematic review of the bariatric surgical literature. Ann Surg. 2013;257(1):87–94.

2. Lazzati A. Epidemiology of the surgical management of obesity. J Visc Surg. 2023;160(2s):S3–s6.
3. Parikh MS, Fielding GA, Ren CJ. U.S. experience with 749 laparoscopic adjustable gastric bands: intermediate outcomes. Surg Endosc. 2005;19(12):1631–5.
4. Furbetta N, Gragnani F, Flauti G, Guidi F, Furbetta F. Laparoscopic adjustable gastric banding on 3566 patients up to 20-year follow-up: long-term results of a standardized technique. Surg Obes Relat Dis. 2019;15(3):409–16.
5. Chapman AE, Kiroff G, Game P, Foster B, O'Brien P, Ham J, et al. Laparoscopic adjustable gastric banding in the treatment of obesity: a systematic literature review. Surgery. 2004;135(3):326–51.
6. Snow JM, Severson PA. Complications of adjustable gastric banding. Surg Clin North Am. 2011;91(6):1249–64, ix.
7. Carucci LR, Turner MA, Szucs RA. Adjustable laparoscopic gastric banding for morbid obesity: imaging assessment and complications. Radiol Clin North Am. 2007;45(2):261–74.
8. Levine MS, Carucci LR. Imaging of bariatric surgery: normal anatomy and postoperative complications. Radiology. 2014;270(2):327–41.
9. ASMBS updated position statement on prophylactic measures to reduce the risk of venous thromboembolism in bariatric surgery patients. Surg Obes Relat Dis. 2013;9(4):493–497.
10. Steele KE, Schweitzer MA, Prokopowicz G, Shore AD, Eaton LC, Lidor AO, et al. The long-term risk of venous thromboembolism following bariatric surgery. Obes Surg. 2011;21(9):1371–6.
11. Stevens SM, Woller SC, Kreuziger LB, Bounameaux H, Doerschug K, Geersing GJ, et al. Antithrombotic therapy for VTE disease: second update of the CHEST guideline and expert panel report. Chest. 2021;160(6):e545–608.
12. Carelli AM, Youn HA, Kurian MS, Ren CJ, Fielding GA. Safety of the laparoscopic adjustable gastric band: 7-year data from a U.S. center of excellence. Surg Endosc. 2010;24(8):1819–23.
13. Szewczyk T, Janczak P, Jezierska N, Jurałowicz P. Slippage-a significant problem following gastric banding-a single centre experience. Obes Surg. 2017;27(10):2637–42.
14. Chevallier JM, Zinzindohoué F, Douard R, Blanche JP, Berta JL, Altman JJ, et al. Complications after laparoscopic adjustable gastric banding for morbid obesity: experience with 1,000 patients over 7 years. Obes Surg. 2004;14(3):407–14.
15. O'Brien PE, Dixon JB, Laurie C, Anderson M. A prospective randomized trial of placement of the laparoscopic adjustable gastric band: comparison of the perigastric and pars flaccida pathways. Obes Surg. 2005;15(6):820–6.
16. Le Coq B, Frering V, Ghunaim M, Campan P, Dabrowski A, Mulliez E, et al. Impact of surgical technique on long-term complication rate after laparoscopic adjustable gastric banding (LAGB): results of a single-blinded randomized controlled trial (ANOSEAN study). Ann Surg. 2016;264(5):738–44.
17. Beitner MM, Ren-Fielding CJ, Kurian MS, Schwack BF, Skandarajah AR, Thomson BN, et al. Sustained weight loss after gastric banding revision for pouch-related problems. Ann Surg. 2014;260(1):81–6.
18. Iqbal M, Manjunath S, Seenath M, Khan A. Massive upper gastrointestinal hemorrhage: an unusual presentation after laparoscopic adjustable gastric banding due to erosion into the celiac axis. Obes Surg. 2008;18(6):759–60.
19. Adekunle AD, Nyahoda TS, Koury E, Chahla E. Esophago-pleural fistula complicating a laparoscopic adjustable gastric band. Case Rep Gastroenterol. 2022;16(3):607–11.
20. Di Lorenzo N, Lorenzo M, Furbetta F, Favretti F, Giardiello C, Boschi S, et al. Intragastric gastric band migration: erosion: an analysis of multicenter experience on 177 patients. Surg Endosc. 2013;27(4):1151–7.
21. Egberts K, Brown WA, O'Brien PE. Systematic review of erosion after laparoscopic adjustable gastric banding. Obes Surg. 2011;21(8):1272–9.
22. Singhal R, Bryant C, Kitchen M, Khan KS, Deeks J, Guo B, et al. Band slippage and erosion after laparoscopic gastric banding: a meta-analysis. Surg Endosc. 2010;24(12):2980–6.
23. Manos T, Nedelcu A, Noel P, Zulian V, Danan M, Vilallonga R, et al. Endoscopic gastric band removal. J Clin Med. 2023;12(2):617.

24. Brown WA, Egberts KJ, Franke-Richard D, Thodiyil P, Anderson ML, O'Brien PE. Erosions after laparoscopic adjustable gastric banding: diagnosis and management. Ann Surg. 2013;257(6):1047–52.
25. de Jong JR, Tiethof C, van Ramshorst B, Gooszen HG, Smout AJ. Esophageal dilation after laparoscopic adjustable gastric banding: a more systematic approach is needed. Surg Endosc. 2009;23(12):2802–8.
26. Naef M, Mouton WG, Naef U, van der Weg B, Maddern GJ, Wagner HE. Esophageal dysmotility disorders after laparoscopic gastric banding—an underestimated complication. Ann Surg. 2011;253(2):285–90.
27. Khan A, Ren-Fielding C, Traube M. Potentially reversible pseudoachalasia after laparoscopic adjustable gastric banding. J Clin Gastroenterol. 2011;45(9):775–9.
28. Chen RY, Burton PR, Ooi GJ, Laurie C, Smith AI, Crosthwaite G, et al. The physiology and pathophysiology of gastroesophageal reflux in patients with laparoscopic adjustable gastric band. Obes Surg. 2017;27(9):2434–43.
29. Boltin D, Niv Y. Doxycycline-induced pill esophagitis. Endoscopy. 2014;46 Suppl 1 UCTN:E350.
30. Amendola MA, Spera TD. Doxycycline-induced esophagitis. JAMA. 1985;253(7):1009–11.
31. Lattuada E, Zappa MA, Mozzi E, Antonini I, Boati P, Roviaro GC. Injection port and connecting tube complications after laparoscopic adjustable gastric banding. Obes Surg. 2010;20(4):410–4.
32. Suter M, Calmes JM, Paroz A, Giusti V. A 10-year experience with laparoscopic gastric banding for morbid obesity: high long-term complication and failure rates. Obes Surg. 2006;16(7):829–35.
33. Keidar A, Carmon E, Szold A, Abu-Abeid S. Port complications following laparoscopic adjustable gastric banding for morbid obesity. Obes Surg. 2005;15(3):361–5.
34. Sharma K, Arfan S, Thota SSP, Agbasi C, Khan L, Naqvi L, et al. Small bowel obstruction secondary to laparoscopic adjustable gastric band connecting tube intertwinement within the mesentery: a case report. Cureus. 2023;15(6):e39945.
35. Michiels S, Engelholm JL. Bowel obstruction by sigmoid strangulation as complication after laparoscopic adjustable gastric banding. Acta Chir Belg. 2024;124:307.
36. Jackson TD, Saleh F, Quereshy FA, Sockalingam S, Urbach D, Okrainec A. Short-term morbidity associated with removal and revision of the laparoscopic adjustable gastric band. Surg Obes Relat Dis. 2014;10(6):1110–5.

# 28 Venous Thromboembolism

Ali Esparham and Zhamak Khorgami

## Introduction

Venous thromboembolism (VTE), comprising deep vein thrombosis (DVT) and pulmonary embolism (PE), is a potential complication after bariatric surgery and can contribute to mortality. Despite advancements in surgical techniques and the implementation of preventive protocols, VTE occurs in this population, reported in 0.2–3% of older series [1]. However, the reported incidence is lower in recent series. A systematic review of 19 studies conducted between 2000 and 2010 showed 0.5% PE after laparoscopic bariatric surgery [2]. Another report from the Michigan Bariatric Surgery Collaborative reported 0.33% VTE based on registry from 2006 to 2011 [3]. According to data extracted from the Metabolic and Bariatric Surgery Accreditation and Quality Improvement Program (MBSAQIP) database from 2015 to 2017, the occurrence of DVT was 0.2% for both laparoscopic sleeve gastrectomy (SG) and laparoscopic Roux-en-Y gastric bypass (RYGB) while the incidence of PE was 0.1% following SG and 0.2% following RYGB [4]. Mabeza et al. used the Nationwide Readmissions Database 2016–2018 and reported 0.55% VTE in patients undergoing bariatric surgery [5].

VTE after bariatric surgery is associated with extended length of hospital stay, increased hospitalization costs, unplanned readmission, and mortality [5, 6]. A study using the Bariatric Outcomes Longitudinal Database (BOLD) from 2008 to 2012 revealed that PE within 30 days of bariatric surgery is a significant

A. Esparham
School of Medicine, Mashhad University of Medical Sciences, Mashhad, Iran

Z. Khorgami (✉)
Department of Surgery, University of Oklahoma, School of Community Medicine, Tulsa, OK, USA
e-mail: zhamak-khorgami@ouhsc.edu



O. M. Ghanem et al. (eds.), *The SAGES Manual of Metabolic and Bariatric Surgery*, https://doi.org/10.1007/978-3-031-72309-4_28

independent predictor of one-year mortality (adjusted odds ratios of 34.5 for RYGB and 252 for SG) [7]. Based on another study using MBSAQIP 2015 to 2019, PE can increase the risk of 30-day mortality by 51-fold (5.6% mortality compared to a baseline of 0.1%) [8]. Appropriate prophylaxis can reduce the incidence of VTE after bariatric surgery [9]. An analysis of the MBSAQIP database suggests that interventions aimed at reducing VTE after bariatric surgery can significantly decrease the readmission rate and mortality [10].

## Pathophysiology

The three main described pathogenesis of VTE are venous stasis, endothelial injury, and hypercoagulable state (Virchow triad). In most patients with VTE, several underlying factors for thrombosis can be identified. The heightened risk of VTE in obese individuals is attributed not only to clinical factors like immobility and venous stasis but also to the establishment of a chronic inflammatory state by adipose tissue, disrupting metabolic homeostasis, and impaired fibrinolysis [11, 12]. Adipose tissue contributes to this risk by releasing inflammatory cytokines, leading to the recruitment of pro-inflammatory M1 macrophages. This process results in the secretion of TNF-alpha and IL-6, activating prothrombotic signaling pathways in vascular cells and inhibiting fibrinolysis through increased expression of plasminogen activator inhibitor-1 [11]. Moreover, the bariatric surgery procedure itself amplifies intrabdominal pressure, inducing oxidative stress and endothelial dysfunction [13]. These multifaceted mechanisms contribute to the complex interplay between obesity, inflammation, and surgical interventions and increase the susceptibility to VTE [14]. Metabolic syndrome and obesity-related comorbidities (including atherosclerosis, dyslipidemia, hypertension, heart failure, obstructive sleep apnea, diabetes mellitus, and polycystic ovary syndrome) can be other predisposing factors for VTE in patients with morbid obesity [15–17].

## Clinical Presentation

Common clinical manifestations of DVT include leg pain (80–90%), swelling (80%), and localized tenderness upon palpation (75–85%). The involved leg can be warm, with erythema, and with prominent collateral superficial veins [18]. Signs and symptoms are usually unilateral, limited to the calf in distal DVT, or involving the entire leg in proximal DVT. A significant difference in calf circumference is a valuable finding but Homans' sign (calf pain with foot dorsiflexion) is not a reliable sign to assess for DVT. Phlegmasia cerulea dolens is characterized by severe pain, edema, and cyanosis of the lower extremity due to extensive venous thrombosis and can ultimately cause arterial ischemia. Additionally, 30–60% of individuals with symptomatic proximal DVT may have a concurrent silent PE [19].

PE presents with a diverse range of symptoms, spanning from asymptomatic patients to severe manifestations such as shock or sudden death. A proportion of patients, even those with substantial PE, may have only mild or nonspecific symptoms or remain asymptomatic. The most common respiratory symptoms in patients with PE are dyspnea (at rest or with exertion), pleuritic chest pain, cough, orthopnea, wheezing, and hemoptysis. Possible signs are tachypnea, tachycardia, rales, jugular venous distension, and fever. Some patients may present with arrhythmias (e.g., atrial fibrillation), presyncope or syncope, or hemodynamic instability [20, 21]. The majority of patients with PE have been found to have DVT (71%), mostly in the proximal lower extremity, and may have related signs and symptoms [22].

There are clinical assessment tools to assess the likelihood of VTE upon presentation (Table 28.1). Wells score for DVT is one of the tools for assessing clinical probability in this context. This scoring system categorizes a patient's likelihood of having DVT as either likely or unlikely [27, 28]. Various scoring systems have been

**Table 28.1** Clinical tools to assess the likelihood of venous thromboembolism

| Clinical model | Criteria |
|---|---|
| Wells criteria for DVT [23] | Malignancy with treatment within 6 months or palliative care<br>Paralysis, paresis, or recent cast immobilization of the lower extremities<br>Recently bedridden for ≥3 days, or major surgery in the previous 4 weeks<br>Localized tenderness along the distribution of the deep venous system<br>Entire leg swelling<br>Calf swelling >3 cm larger than the other extremity (measured 10 cm below tibial tuberosity)<br>Pitting edema greater in the symptomatic leg<br>Collateral superficial veins (non-varicose)<br>Previous DVT<br>An alternative diagnosis is less likely than DVT |
| Wells criteria for PE [24] | Clinical signs and symptoms of DVT<br>An alternative diagnosis is less likely than PE<br>Heart rate > 100 beats/min<br>Surgery in the previous 4 weeks or immobilization for at least 3 days<br>Previous PE or DVT<br>Hemoptysis<br>Malignancy with treatment within 6 months or palliative care |
| Geneva score model for PE [25] | Age > 65 years<br>Previous DVT or PE<br>Surgery with general anesthesia or lower extremity fracture within 1 month<br>Active malignant condition<br>Unilateral lower limb pain<br>Hemoptysis<br>Heart rate ≥ 75 beats/min<br>Pain on lower limb palpation and unilateral edema |
| YEARs algorithm for PE [26] | Clinical signs of DVT<br>Hemoptysis<br>PE is the most likely diagnosis<br>D-dimer |

*DVT* Deep vein thrombosis, *PE* Pulmonary embolism

developed to assess the clinical probability of PE. These include the Wells score for PE, the revised Geneva score, and the YEARS algorithm [25, 26, 29–31]. These tools stratify the patient's likelihood of having PE into categories such as likely or unlikely, or low, moderate, and high risk.

## Diagnostic Tests

D-dimer testing serves as a valuable tool to assess the likelihood of VTE. The risk of VTE is low with a normal D-dimer concentration, but an elevated D-dimer is not always associated with the presence of VTE. False-negative test results may occur, especially following the initiation of anticoagulation. As a recommended practice, high-sensitivity D-dimer testing is advised for patients deemed to have a non-high (low or moderate) clinical pretest probability. Conversely, individuals assessed with a high clinical suspicion are recommended to undergo imaging without D-dimer testing [18, 32]. However, D-dimer is elevated after intraabdominal surgeries (25 ± 14 days) and may not be useful in patients with recent bariatric surgery [33].

Patients with clinical suspicion of having DVT should undergo imaging. Compression Ultrasonography (CUS) with Doppler is the primary and most employed imaging test for individuals with a suspected DVT [34, 35]. Whole leg CUS is needed to evaluate for both proximal and distal DVT.

Patients with a likely or high probability of PE need to be evaluated by imaging. Ventilation–perfusion scintigraphy and computed tomography (CT) pulmonary angiography (CTPA) stand out as validated imaging modalities for diagnosing PE, with similar diagnostic accuracy [34]. However, CTPA can be performed in conjunction with CT abdomen and pelvis to assess for both intrabdominal and pulmonary causes of respiratory compromise in the early postoperative period.

## Risk Factors of VTE in Bariatric Surgery Patients

The risk factors associated with VTE following bariatric surgery can be classified into three main categories: demographic, comorbidities, and operative factors. Demographic risk factors for VTE include male gender, older age, higher body mass index (BMI), and black race. Operative factors include operative duration ≥3 h, open surgical procedures, reoperations, bleeding with a need for transfusion, more complex procedures (duodenal switch > RYGB >SG), and postoperative hospital stay ≥3 days. Additionally, comorbidities that elevate the risk of VTE include a history of DVT or PE, congestive heart failure, dyspnea at rest, obstructive sleep apnea, cardiac arrhythmias, immobility, neurologic disorders, paraplegia, venous stasis disease, and advanced-stage chronic kidney disease. Inherited thrombophilia (e.g., factor V Leiden and prothrombin gene mutation, and Protein C, Protein S, and antithrombin defects) is a known risk factor for VTE. Postmenopausal hormonal therapy and estrogen-progestin contraceptives are other risk factors for VTE [1, 4, 5, 36, 37].

## Predicting Models for VTE

There have been recent initiatives aimed at creating predictive tools for the early identification of individual patients susceptible to VTE. The Caprini Score was introduced by Joseph Caprini in 2005 to predict VTE in surgical patients which divides patients into very low, low, moderate, and high risk based on 20 weighted risk factors such as weight, sex, congenital and acquired thrombophilia, history of prior VTE, comorbidities, and type of procedure. Although several studies validated this scoring model, the Caprini model is not specific for bariatric surgery and all the patients who underwent bariatric surgery will be at least moderate risk based on this model [38–41]. Further studies developed risk calculators for VTE in patients with bariatric surgery (Table 28.2). Finks et al. used the Michigan Bariatric Surgery

**Table 28.2** Criteria in risk calculator models for venous thromboembolism after bariatric surgery

| Clinical | Criteria |
|---|---|
| Finks et al. [3] | Previous VTE<br>Male sex<br>Operative time >3 h<br>BMI category<br>Age category<br>Procedure type (duodenal switch>open gastric bypass>laparoscopic gastric bypass > sleeve gastrectomy) |
| Aminian et al. [6] | Male sex<br>Age ≥ 60 years<br>BMI ≥ 50 kg/m$^2$<br>Paraplegia<br>CHF<br>Reoperation<br>Dyspnea at rest<br>Operation >3 h<br>Non-gastric bypass surgery<br>Hospital stay ≥3 days |
| BariClot [37] | Previous VTE<br>Male sex<br>Black race<br>Poor preoperative functional status<br>Higher BMI<br>Longer operative time |
| Nudel et al. [42][a] | Preoperative BMI<br>Age<br>Weight<br>Height<br>Hematocrit<br>Albumin<br>Preoperative BMI change<br>History of DVT<br>History of PE<br>First assist training<br>Race<br>Hypertension |

*VTE* venous thromboembolism, *DVT* deep vein thrombosis, *PE* pulmonary embolism
[a] Predictors with higher importance based on gradient boosting machine model

Collaborative Registry and found that older age, male sex, higher BMI, length of procedure, prior history of VTE, and procedure type were the significant predicting factors of VTE in patients who underwent bariatric surgery [3]. Aminian et al. created a VTE risk calculator using the American College of Surgeons–National Surgical Quality Improvement Program (ACS-NSQIP) which consisted of gender, age, BMI, paraplegia, congestive heart failure, reoperation, dyspnea at rest, operation time, non-gastric bypass surgery, and length of hospital stay. Through their modeling (known as the Cleveland Clinic Calculator), it was determined that nearly 2.5% of patients had a predicted post-discharge VTE risk exceeding 1%, classifying them as "very high risk." The recommendation was to extend thromboprophylaxis for 4 weeks in such cases. Additionally, the group established a cutoff of 0.4% for patients categorized as "high risk," advocating for 2 weeks of extended thromboprophylaxis. This tool is easy to use and has specific recommendations and is widely adopted by healthcare practices seeking guidelines on extended thromboprophylaxis recommendations [6]. Dang et al. developed the BariClot risk calculator utilizing the MBSAQIP database, demonstrating superior efficacy when compared to both the Caprini and Finks calculators. Moreover, Nudel et al. designed a machine-learning approach for predicting VTE after bariatric surgery using gradient boosting machines, artificial neural networks, and logistic regression. Their models showed moderate discriminative ability for predicting VTE with area under the curves (AUC) between 0.6 and 0.7 [42].

## Prophylaxis

VTE prophylaxis after bariatric surgery has been emphasized by different societies, guidelines, and statements [1, 43]. Both mechanical and pharmacologic prophylaxis are considered in this group of patients with moderate to high risk of VTE. An individualized approach to assess risk factors of both VTE and bleeding is needed for each patient to select the best practice. Many bariatric programs implement protocols in their practices to consider these recommendations. The American Society for Metabolic and Bariatric Surgery (ASMBS) Research Committee performed a survey to assess the differences in clinical practice in VTE prophylaxis. This study showed both mechanical and chemical prophylaxis were used by most practices (97%); however, there are variations in VTE prophylaxis in different practices [44].

### Mechanical Prophylaxis

Mechanical prophylaxis options encompass early ambulation, intermittent pneumatic compression, venous foot pumps, and graduated compression stockings. These devices function to optimize blood flow in the deep veins of the lower extremities and prevent venous stasis. These devices are used as complementary measures alongside pharmacoprophylaxis; however, the use of mechanical prophylaxis alone has been reported, exploring both efficacy and bleeding complications. A retrospective single-center study compared early ambulation and sequential compression devices (SCD) versus Lovenox 40 mg twice daily and SCDs. This study showed lower bleeding and VTE rates in mechanical-only prophylaxis; however, the study has many limitations as patients were different in the two cohorts [45]. Another study showed that calf-length SCDs placed before surgery along with early and frequent ambulation can result in a low rate of 30-day VTE and bleeding (DVT: 0.3%, PE: 0.1%, bleeding 0.7%), suggesting the use of mechanical prophylaxis alone can be considered in patients with no major risk factors for VTE [46]. While these studies focused on symptomatic VTE, the incidence of silent DVT is reported to be higher with mechanical-only prophylaxis (6%) compared to combined mechanical and pharmacologic prophylaxis (0%) [47].

The American College of Chest Physicians Evidence-Based Clinical Practice Guidelines recommends either pharmacologic or mechanical prophylaxis for moderate-risk patients. Low-risk bariatric patients may fall in this category; however, many patients with morbid obesity undergoing bariatric procedures also have other VTE risk factors. The ASMBS position statement recommends considering a combination of mechanical and pharmacologic VTE prophylaxis in the majority of bariatric patients [36].

## Pharmacoprophylaxis

Pharmacologic VTE prophylaxis with LMWH or low-dose unfractionated heparin is considered in bariatric surgery patients unless they are at high risk for bleeding complications. If at high risk of bleeding, mechanical prophylaxis is recommended until the bleeding risk subsides, at which point pharmacologic prophylaxis may be initiated [43]. The type of medication, dose, timing of the first dose, frequency in the hospital, and extended prophylaxis after discharge are still under debate. Based on a recent survey of the ASMBS members, most surgeons (82%) consider the first dose of anticoagulation given before surgery and continue the medication during hospital admission. Most surgeons (>80%) consider extended VTE chemoprophylaxis in all or selective patients [44].

Lovenox (enoxaparin) remains the most frequently prescribed medication for pharmacoprophylaxis [44, 48]. Despite the lower cost of unfractionated heparin, there is a discernible shift towards favoring LMWH for prophylaxis [14]. This preference is attributed to the specific binding of LMWH to antithrombin III, enabling better bioavailability through easier subcutaneous absorption which is especially important in patients with severe obesity. Moreover, LMWHs exhibit a longer half-life compared to unfractionated heparin and need less frequent injections. Additionally, LMWH-treated patients are less prone to heparin-induced thrombocytopenia and osteoporosis [40, 49, 50]. The Michigan collaborative investigated three prophylactic regimens and showed LMWH is more effective than unfractionated heparin in VTE chemoprophylaxis in bariatric surgery without an associated increase in bleeding complications [51]. The European Society of Anesthesiology

VTE Guideline Task Force recommends the use of LMWH over unfractionated heparin for perioperative VTE chemoprophylaxis [52].

Giving the first dose of pharmacoprophylaxis before the surgery has been shown to decrease the risk of VTE without significant risk of bleeding [53]. The most effective dosing regimen for postoperative LMWH administration remains uncertain. Additionally, it has been established that dosing modifications should be considered in the presence of renal insufficiency, especially when creatinine clearance is <30 mL/min, owing to the renal excretion of LMWH.

Standardized dosing schedules may underestimate the required dosage in patients with severe obesity, possibly resulting in under-dosing [1]. A 2017 French survey of obesity-specialized care centers showed half of the centers adjusted the dose of LMWH according to total body weight [54]. In a study of patients who received 10 days of weight-adjusted LMWH after bariatric surgery, trough level 6 days after surgery revealed either undetectable Anti-factor Xa activity (AFXa) levels or levels within the lowest detection range. This supports the safety of weight-based higher doses of LMWH after bariatric surgery [55]. Randomized controlled trials have compared different dosages of anticoagulants with no discernible differences in terms of VTE events [56, 57]. Several studies have investigated dose stratification based on BMI, demonstrating the safety and effectiveness of such regimens [58, 59]. In a prospective cohort study, comparing enoxaparin 40 mg every 12 h for BMI ≤50 kg/m$^2$ and 60 mg every 12 h for BMI >50 kg/m$^2$, indicated efficacy of higher doses without more bleeding risk [58].

AFXa has been studied as a measure to adjust the dosing of anticoagulants. The CHEST guidelines suggest monitoring of AFXa for LMWH when the total weight surpasses 150 kg [43]. However, some researchers question the effectiveness of tracking AFXa levels in correlation with VTE or bleeding in the obese population, given the absence of randomized controlled trials [60, 61]. Measuring AFXa at the time of peak plasma concentration (4 h after subcutaneous injection) has been shown to yield the most accurate correlation with clinical effects. While target AFXa levels for LMWHs are not firmly established, some studies have proposed peak concentrations of 0.2–0.4 IU/mL for effective VTE prophylaxis [58, 62, 63].

Rivaroxaban (Xarelto) has been studied for VTE prophylaxis for bariatric surgery. Rivaroxaban, a direct oral anticoagulant (DOAC), inhibits Factor Xa and has a high oral bioavailability (maximum plasma levels within 2–4 h). In a recent randomized controlled trial by Kröll et al., 269 patients received 10 mg of oral Rivaroxaban per day either for 7 days or 28 days. There was only one thromboembolic event (0.4%). Major or clinically relevant bleeding occured in 1.9% of patients with an addition of 3.7% clinically nonsignificant bleeding events. The study concluded that once daily dosing of 10 mg Rivaroxaban is safe and effective as both short- and long-term prophylaxis after bariatric surgery [64]. Another prospective cohort study showed no clinical or radiological signs of thromboembolic events in 110 patients who received extended prophylaxis with Rivaroxaban and with only 0.9% minor bleeding complications [65]. Further research will be needed to explore the role of DOACs in VTE prophylaxis after bariatric surgery.

A prospective, double-blind randomized controlled trial compared enoxaparin 40 mg subcutaneously twice daily with Fondaparinux sodium 5 mg once daily. Fondaparinux demonstrated a higher incidence of adequate AFXa levels compared to enoxaparin (74% vs. 32%). DVT (evaluated by MR venography) and bleeding complication rates were similar in the two groups. This study suggests Fondaparinux can be equally effective in reducing the risk of DVT while more likely to achieve prophylactic AFXa levels [66].

## Extended Pharmacoprophylaxis

Approximately 70–83% of VTE events after bariatric surgery occur after discharge. Patients who experienced a post-discharge VTE had a significantly increased mortality rate [36, 67]. A study by the French National Health Insurance Database showed not receiving post-discharge pharmacoprophylaxis is an independent predictor for VTE within 90 days after bariatric surgery [68]. While earlier studies showed lower utilization of post-discharge pharmacoprophylaxis following laparoscopic bariatric procedures, a recent survey by the ASMBS showed 87% of the ASMBS members use extended chemoprophylaxis in all or selective patients [44, 48]. The efficacy of this practice has been shown in different studies. A single-center comparison of in-hospital-only versus 10-day enoxaparin (30 mg subcutaneously every 12 h) demonstrated a significantly lower 30-day VTE rate in extended prophylaxis (no VTE vs 4.5%) [69]. Meanwhile, post-discharge administration of pharmacoprophylaxis has been shown to be safe with no significant bleeding risk [55, 70].

When considering extended pharmacoprophylaxis, risk calculators may help to predict the level of VTE risk after bariatric surgery. Table 28.2 shows some bariatric-specific models and their criteria. Individualized clinical decision-making is needed to consider patient's risk factors for VTE, risk of bleeding, available medications, and cost. There is no clear guideline regarding the selection, dosage, and duration of chemoprophylaxis for these patients following bariatric surgery [14, 71, 72].

LMWH has been shown to be an effective agent with minimal clinically relevant bleeding complications and proves to be a cost-effective medication for extended thromboprophylaxis [73]. The duration of extended prophylaxis has been different in various studies. Depending on the estimated VTE risk, some studies have recommended extended pharmacoprophylaxis for 2–4 weeks post-discharge. Higher doses may be considered for patients with higher BMI. Several studies have demonstrated the efficacy of BMI-stratified higher doses of enoxaparin (40–60 mg subcutaneously daily or every 12 h) with a low risk of clinically important bleeding [58, 59, 74].

There are concerns with fixed prophylactic doses of anticoagulants in patients with severe obesity, particularly in those with a weight exceeding 150 kg [75]. Studies have investigated adjusting enoxaparin discharge doses based on serum AFXa levels, measured either serially or after a specific dose (e.g., the second dose).

These studies suggest that, without AFXa measurement, 15–30% of patients may receive suboptimal discharge doses [58, 63].

## Monitoring of Pharmacoprophylaxis

Routine monitoring of pharmacoprophylaxis is not commonly conducted in most patients using LMWH. However, mounting evidence suggests that adjustments in LMWH dosing are likely required, particularly in patients with higher weight. LMWH exerts its action on Factor Xa, while unfractionated heparin acts on both Factor II and Xa. Monitoring LMWH involves checking AFXa activity levels to evaluate the therapeutic effect. Peak AFXa levels are typically achieved 3–5 h after LMWH administration. Clearly defined therapeutic peak levels of AFXa range from 0.6–1.0 IU/mL for twice daily dosing and 1.0–2.0 IU/mL for once daily dosing. However, high-level evidence for target peak levels in prophylactic dosing is not as well-established, with generally accepted ranges falling between 0.2 and 0.5 IU/mL [76]. Measuring AFXa may be more critical in patients with higher wight. A study showed that standard chemoprophylaxis dose may be associated with suboptimal AFXa levels in two-thirds of patients with lean body weight >80 kg [77].

## Inferior Vena Cava Filter

Temporary inferior vena cava (IVC) filters have been considered in bariatric surgery in a limited group of patients. The previous literature suggested benefits from prophylactic IVC filter in patients with a high risk of VTE including patients with BMIs >55 kg/m$^2$, history of VTE, immobility, venous stasis, pulmonary hypertension, obesity hypoventilation syndrome, and hypercoagulable states [78, 79]. However, contrasting reports highlight a concern with device-related complications [80, 81]. Further studies showed the use of IVC filters may be associated with a higher incidence of DVT and increased mortality [67, 82]. An MBSAQIP analysis for the years 2015–2016 revealed a low (<1%) utilization of IVC filters in bariatric surgery and found no significant difference in perioperative PE incidence when compared to patients without IVC filter placement [83].

Patients who underwent IVC filter placement have more readmission and reintervention, mainly for filter retrieval. A nationwide observational study showed higher rates of lower extremity and caval DVT in bariatric surgery patients undergoing prophylactic IVC filter placement [84]. Meantime, complications associated with insertion and removal of IVC filter and particular technical challenges in patients with severe obesity should be considered [85]. Other associated complications include device fracture, migration, and IVC penetration [86].

Current guidelines do not recommend IVC filters for primary VTE prevention in bariatric surgery. Based on the ASMBS statement on VTE, prophylactic IVC filter should be considered in combination with other methods, only in selected very high-risk patients when the risk of VTE is higher than device complications [1]. The

American College of Chest Physicians advises against the use of IVC filters for primary VTE prevention in abdominal and pelvic surgery [43]. The latest European guidelines suggest this modality only in rare cases with a very high risk of PE or when there is a contraindication for prolonged pharmacological prophylaxis due to the risk of bleeding [87].

## Portomesenteric Venous Thrombosis

Portomesenteric venous thrombosis (PMVT) refers to a partial or whole thrombosis of the portal venous system in the intrahepatic or extrahepatic venous tract or affecting the splenic or superior mesenteric veins. Ascites, esophageal varices, gastroesophageal bleeding, bowel infarction, and subsequent mortality are among the outcomes that may result from PMVT [88–90]. Although PMVT is an uncommon complication reported in 0.3% of bariatric surgeries, more cases have been reported in recent series [90–92]. The majority of literature indicates that PMVT incidence is higher following SG [90, 93].

Clinical presentation of PMVT is nonspecific and can present days or weeks after surgery. This can present as abdominal pain, nausea, vomiting, leukocytosis, and fever [94–97]. The severity of these symptoms correlates with the extent of mesenteric venous thrombosis and the degree of bowel ischemia. In some cases, symptoms can progress rapidly to septic shock and organ failure [98, 99]. Doppler mesenteric ultrasound and a CT scan with IV contrast can be helpful to diagnose PMVT [100]. As the preferred initial diagnostic modality, a CT scan with IV contrast boasts a sensitivity of 90% [100, 101]. If the initial imaging is not diagnostic and PMVT is suspected, repeat imaging may be needed to further evaluate for this condition.

Treatment options for PMVT span from administration of therapeutic anticoagulation to surgical interventions (bowel resection and liver transplantation). Close monitoring and serial exams of these patients are needed to assess response to treatment, rule out other possible diagnoses (e.g., leak), and evaluate for possible need for surgical exploration and bowel resection. The complexity of treatment modalities is related to the degree of vascular involvement, and the severity of ischemic damage to organs such as the bowel, spleen, or liver [99].

## Treatment

In the case of proximal DVT, anticoagulant therapy is advised for 3 months [102]. Treatment for proximal DVT can be initiated with unfractionated heparin or LMWH and be continued with vitamin K antagonists or DOACs. The decision among these agents typically relies on clinician expertise, considering factors like bleeding risks, patient comorbidities, preferences, cost, and convenience. Thrombolytic therapy is generally not recommended except in cases where patients present with massive iliofemoral or femoral DVT, coupled with a high risk of limb gangrene. The risk of bleeding from recent surgery should be considered in this condition [102, 103].

Isolated distal DVT is identified when a thrombus forms below the popliteal vein without extending to the proximal veins. Although the existing literature is controversial for the treatment of isolated distal DVT, if patients exhibit acute symptoms, possess high-risk features for recurrence and extension, and do not have a bleeding risk, anticoagulation is recommended [102]. Patients with severe obesity who underwent bariatric surgery should be considered with a higher risk of clot extension to the proximal vein and may need treatment like proximal DVT.

For the treatment of PE in patients with stable hemodynamic status, anticoagulation stands as the cornerstone of treatment for patients with a confirmed diagnosis of PE and is recommended for all individuals suspected of the disease, provided there is no active bleeding, even before a formal diagnosis of PE is established. The landscape of anticoagulation for PE has undergone significant evolution in recent years with the introduction of DOACs. In numerous large randomized clinical trials, DOACs have demonstrated comparable efficacy and safety profiles to traditional anticoagulants in patients with acute PE [103–107]. Treatment of PE in patients with unstable hemodynamic status may necessitate interventions beyond anticoagulation. These include systemic thrombolysis, catheter-directed therapy, and embolectomy. Following thrombolysis, anticoagulation should be initiated once the patient achieves stability and without any bleeding complications [103, 108].

## References


1. Aminian A, Vosburg RW, Altieri MS, Hinojosa MW, Khorgami Z. The American Society for Metabolic and Bariatric Surgery (ASMBS) updated position statement on perioperative venous thromboembolism prophylaxis in bariatric surgery. Surg Obes Relat Dis. 2022;18(2):165–74. https://doi.org/10.1016/j.soard.2021.10.023.
2. Becattini C, Agnelli G, Manina G, Noya G, Rondelli F. Venous thromboembolism after laparoscopic bariatric surgery for morbid obesity: clinical burden and prevention. Surg Obes Relat Dis. 2012;8(1):108–15. https://doi.org/10.1016/j.soard.2011.09.005.
3. Finks JF, English WJ, Carlin AM, et al. Predicting risk for venous thromboembolism with bariatric surgery: results from the Michigan Bariatric Surgery Collaborative. Ann Surg. 2012;255(6):1100–4. https://doi.org/10.1097/SLA.0b013e31825659d4.
4. Gambhir S, Inaba CS, Alizadeh RF, et al. Venous thromboembolism risk for the contemporary bariatric surgeon. Surg Endosc. 2020;34(8):3521–6. https://doi.org/10.1007/s00464-019-07134-w.
5. Mabeza RM, Lee C, Verma A, et al. Factors and outcomes associated with venous thromboembolism following bariatric surgery. Am Surg. 2022;88(10):2525–30. https://doi.org/10.1177/00031348221103645.
6. Aminian A, Andalib A, Khorgami Z, et al. Who should get extended thromboprophylaxis after bariatric surgery?: a risk assessment tool to guide indications for post-discharge pharmacoprophylaxis. Ann Surg. 2017;265(1):143–50. https://doi.org/10.1097/sla.0000000000001686.
7. Inaba CS, Koh CY, Sujatha-Bhaskar S, et al. One-year mortality after contemporary laparoscopic bariatric surgery: an analysis of the bariatric outcomes longitudinal database. J Am Coll Surg. 2018;226(6):1166–74. https://doi.org/10.1016/j.jamcollsurg.2018.02.013.

8. Wesley Vosburg R, Druar NM, Kim JJ. Factors associated with increased risk for pulmonary embolism after metabolic and bariatric surgery: analysis of nearly one million patients. Obes Surg. 2022;32(7):2433–7. https://doi.org/10.1007/s11695-022-06102-z.
9. Edwards MA, Spaulding A, Brennan E, Elli EF. Risk stratified venous thromboembolism prophylaxis in bariatric patients using a Caprini assessment: practice patterns and opportunities for improvement. Surg Obes Relat Dis. 2024;20(3):221–34. https://doi.org/10.1016/j.soard.2023.09.018.
10. Daigle CR, Brethauer SA, Tu C, et al. Which postoperative complications matter most after bariatric surgery? Prioritizing quality improvement efforts to improve national outcomes. Surg Obes Relat Dis. 2018;14(5):652–7. https://doi.org/10.1016/j.soard.2018.01.008.
11. Lentz SR. Thrombosis in the setting of obesity or inflammatory bowel disease. Blood. 2016;128(20):2388–94. https://doi.org/10.1182/blood-2016-05-716720.
12. Blokhin IO, Lentz SR. Mechanisms of thrombosis in obesity. Curr Opin Hematol. 2013;20(5):437–44. https://doi.org/10.1097/MOH.0b013e3283634443.
13. Holländer SW, Sifft A, Hess S, Klingen HJ, Djalali P, Birk D. Identifying the bariatric patient at risk for pulmonary embolism: prospective clinical trial using duplex sonography and blood screening. Obes Surg. 2015;25(11):2011–7. https://doi.org/10.1007/s11695-015-1649-z.
14. Hamadi R, Marlow CF, Nassereddine S, Taher A, Finianos A. Bariatric venous thromboembolism prophylaxis: an update on the literature. Expert Rev Hematol. 2019;12(9):763–71. https://doi.org/10.1080/17474086.2019.1634542.
15. Stewart LK, Kline JA. Metabolic syndrome increases risk of venous thromboembolism recurrence after acute deep vein thrombosis. Blood Adv. 2020;4(1):127–35. https://doi.org/10.1182/bloodadvances.2019000561.
16. Gariani K, Hugon-Rodin J, Philippe J, Righini M, Blondon M. Association between polycystic ovary syndrome and venous thromboembolism: a systematic review and meta-analysis. Thromb Res. 2020;185:102–8. https://doi.org/10.1016/j.thromres.2019.11.019.
17. Lippi G, Mattiuzzi C, Franchini M. Sleep apnea and venous thromboembolism. A systematic review. Thromb Haemost. 2015;114(5):958–63. https://doi.org/10.1160/th15-03-0188.
18. Khan F, Tritschler T, Kahn SR, Rodger MA. Venous thromboembolism. Lancet. 2021;398(10294):64–77. https://doi.org/10.1016/s0140-6736(20)32658-1.
19. Stein PD, Matta F, Musani MH, Diaczok B. Silent pulmonary embolism in patients with deep venous thrombosis: a systematic review. Am J Med. 2010;123(5):426–31. https://doi.org/10.1016/j.amjmed.2009.09.037.
20. Liesching T, O'Brien A. Significance of a syncopal event. Pulmonary embolism. Postgrad Med. 2002;111(1):19–20. https://doi.org/10.3810/pgm.2002.01.1096.
21. Castelli R, Tarsia P, Tantardini C, Pantaleo G, Guariglia A, Porro F. Syncope in patients with pulmonary embolism: comparison between patients with syncope as the presenting symptom of pulmonary embolism and patients with pulmonary embolism without syncope. Vasc Med. 2003;8(4):257–61. https://doi.org/10.1191/1358863x03vm510oa.
22. Hirmerova J, Seidlerova J, Chudacek Z. The prevalence of concomitant deep vein thrombosis, symptomatic or asymptomatic, proximal or distal, in patients with symptomatic pulmonary embolism. Clin Appl Thromb Hemost. 2018;24(8):1352–7. https://doi.org/10.1177/1076029618779143.
23. Modi S, Deisler R, Gozel K, et al. Wells criteria for DVT is a reliable clinical tool to assess the risk of deep venous thrombosis in trauma patients. World J Emerg Surg. 2016;11:24. https://doi.org/10.1186/s13017-016-0078-1.
24. Wolf SJ, McCubbin TR, Feldhaus KM, Faragher JP, Adcock DM. Prospective validation of Wells criteria in the evaluation of patients with suspected pulmonary embolism. Ann Emerg Med. 2004;44(5):503–10. https://doi.org/10.1016/j.annemergmed.2004.04.002.
25. Klok FA, Mos IC, Nijkeuter M, et al. Simplification of the revised Geneva score for assessing clinical probability of pulmonary embolism. Arch Intern Med. 2008;168(19):2131–6. https://doi.org/10.1001/archinte.168.19.2131.

26. van der Hulle T, Cheung WY, Kooij S, et al. Simplified diagnostic management of suspected pulmonary embolism (the YEARS study): a prospective, multicentre, cohort study. Lancet. 2017;390(10091):289–97. https://doi.org/10.1016/s0140-6736(17)30885-1.
27. Wells PS, Anderson DR, Bormanis J, et al. Value of assessment of pretest probability of deep-vein thrombosis in clinical management. Lancet. 1997;350(9094):1795–8. https://doi.org/10.1016/s0140-6736(97)08140-3.
28. Wells PS, Anderson DR, Rodger M, et al. Evaluation of D-dimer in the diagnosis of suspected deep-vein thrombosis. N Engl J Med. 2003;349(13):1227–35. https://doi.org/10.1056/NEJMoa023153.
29. Wells PS, Anderson DR, Rodger M, et al. Derivation of a simple clinical model to categorize patients probability of pulmonary embolism: increasing the models utility with the SimpliRED D-dimer. Thromb Haemost. 2000;83(3):416–20.
30. Gibson NS, Sohne M, Kruip MJ, et al. Further validation and simplification of the Wells clinical decision rule in pulmonary embolism. Thromb Haemost. 2008;99(1):229–34. https://doi.org/10.1160/th07-05-0321.
31. Le Gal G, Righini M, Roy PM, et al. Prediction of pulmonary embolism in the emergency department: the revised Geneva score. Ann Intern Med. 2006;144(3):165–71. https://doi.org/10.7326/0003-4819-144-3-200602070-00004.
32. Couturaud F, Kearon C, Bates SM, Ginsberg JS. Decrease in sensitivity of D-dimer for acute venous thromboembolism after starting anticoagulant therapy. Blood Coagul Fibrinolysis. 2002;13(3):241–6. https://doi.org/10.1097/00001721-200204000-00010.
33. Dindo D, Breitenstein S, Hahnloser D, et al. Kinetics of D-dimer after general surgery. Blood Coagul Fibrinolysis. 2009;20(5):347–52. https://doi.org/10.1097/MBC.0b013e32832a5fe6.
34. Lim W, Le Gal G, Bates SM, et al. American Society of Hematology 2018 guidelines for management of venous thromboembolism: diagnosis of venous thromboembolism. Blood Adv. 2018;2(22):3226–56. https://doi.org/10.1182/bloodadvances.2018024828.
35. Mazzolai L, Aboyans V, Ageno W, et al. Diagnosis and management of acute deep vein thrombosis: a joint consensus document from the European Society of Cardiology working groups of aorta and peripheral vascular diseases and pulmonary circulation and right ventricular function. Eur Heart J. 2018;39(47):4208–18. https://doi.org/10.1093/eurheartj/ehx003.
36. Aminian A, Andalib A, Khorgami Z, et al. Who should get extended thromboprophylaxis after bariatric surgery? Ann Surg. 2017;265(1):143–50.
37. Dang JT, Switzer N, Delisle M, et al. Predicting venous thromboembolism following laparoscopic bariatric surgery: development of the BariClot tool using the MBSAQIP database. Surg Endosc. 2019;33:821–31.
38. Holbrook A, Schulman S, Witt DM, et al. Evidence-based management of anticoagulant therapy: antithrombotic therapy and prevention of thrombosis, 9th ed: American College of Chest Physicians evidence-based clinical practice guidelines. Chest. 2012;141(2 Suppl):e152S–84S. https://doi.org/10.1378/chest.11-2295.
39. Afshari A, Ageno W, Ahmed A, et al. European guidelines on perioperative venous thromboembolism prophylaxis: executive summary. Eur J Anaesthesiol. 2018;35(2):77–83. https://doi.org/10.1097/eja.0000000000000729.
40. Caprini JA. Thrombosis risk assessment as a guide to quality patient care. Dis Mon. 2005;51(2–3):70–8. https://doi.org/10.1016/j.disamonth.2005.02.003.
41. O'Connor K, Garcia Whitlock AE, Tewksbury C, Williams NN, Dumon KR. Risk factors for postdischarge venous thromboembolism among bariatric surgery patients and the evolving approach to extended thromboprophylaxis with enoxaparin. Surg Obes Relat Dis. 2021;17(6):1218–25. https://doi.org/10.1016/j.soard.2021.02.023.
42. Nudel J, Bishara AM, de Geus SWL, et al. Development and validation of machine learning models to predict gastrointestinal leak and venous thromboembolism after weight loss surgery: an analysis of the MBSAQIP database. Surg Endosc. 2021;35(1):182–91. https://doi.org/10.1007/s00464-020-07378-x.
43. Gould MK, Garcia DA, Wren SM, et al. Prevention of VTE in nonorthopedic surgical patients: antithrombotic therapy and prevention of thrombosis, 9th ed: American College

of Chest Physicians evidence-based clinical practice guidelines. Chest. 2012;141(2 Suppl):e227S–77S. https://doi.org/10.1378/chest.11-2297.
44. Giannopoulos S, Kalantar Motamedi SM, Athanasiadis DI, et al. Venous thromboembolism (VTE) prophylaxis after bariatric surgery: a national survey of MBSAQIP director practices. Surg Obes Relat Dis. 2023;19(8):799–807. https://doi.org/10.1016/j.soard.2022.12.038.
45. Frantzides CT, Welle SN, Ruff TM, Frantzides AT. Routine anticoagulation for venous thromboembolism prevention following laparoscopic gastric bypass. JSLS. 2012;16(1):33–7. https://doi.org/10.4293/108680812x13291597716906.
46. Clements RH, Yellumahanthi K, Ballem N, Wesley M, Bland KI. Pharmacologic prophylaxis against venous thromboembolic complications is not mandatory for all laparoscopic Roux-en-Y gastric bypass procedures. J Am Coll Surg. 2009;208(5):917–21; discussion 921–3. https://doi.org/10.1016/j.jamcollsurg.2009.01.034.
47. Ahmad KS, Zayed ME, Faheem MH, Essa MS. Incidence of silent deep venous thrombosis after laparoscopic bariatric surgery in patients who received combined mechanical and chemical thromboprophylaxis compared to patients who received mechanical thromboprophylaxis only. Surg Innov. 2021;28(1):144–50. https://doi.org/10.1177/1553350620965812.
48. Clark LN, Helm MC, Gould JC. Practice patterns regarding post-discharge chemoprophylaxis for venous thromboembolism following bariatric surgery in the United States. Surg Obes Relat Dis. 2019;15(5):703–7. https://doi.org/10.1016/j.soard.2019.02.017.
49. Abildgaard A, Madsen SA, Hvas AM. Dosage of anticoagulants in obesity: recommendations based on a systematic review. Semin Thromb Hemost. 2020;46(8):932–69. https://doi.org/10.1055/s-0040-1718405.
50. Brunetti L, Wassef A, Sadek R, et al. Anticoagulant activity of enoxaparin and unfractionated heparin for venous thromboembolism prophylaxis in obese patients undergoing sleeve gastrectomy. Surg Obes Relat Dis. 2019;15(3):363–73. https://doi.org/10.1016/j.soard.2018.12.014.
51. Birkmeyer NJ, Finks JF, Carlin AM, et al. Comparative effectiveness of unfractionated and low-molecular-weight heparin for prevention of venous thromboembolism following bariatric surgery. Arch Surg. 2012;147(11):994–8. https://doi.org/10.1001/archsurg.2012.2298.
52. Venclauskas L, Maleckas A, Arcelus JI. European guidelines on perioperative venous thromboembolism prophylaxis: surgery in the obese patient. Eur J Anaesthesiol. 2018;35(2):147–53. https://doi.org/10.1097/eja.0000000000000703.
53. Abdelsalam AM, ElAnsary A, Salman MA, Nassef SA, Elfergany HM, Aisha HAA. Adding a preoperative dose of LMWH may decrease VTE following bariatric surgery. World J Surg. 2021;45(1):126–31. https://doi.org/10.1007/s00268-020-05782-x.
54. Moulin PA, Dutour A, Ancel P, et al. Perioperative thromboprophylaxis in severely obese patients undergoing bariatric surgery: insights from a French national survey. Surg Obes Relat Dis. 2017;13(2):320–6. https://doi.org/10.1016/j.soard.2016.08.497.
55. Tseng EK, Kolesar E, Handa P, et al. Weight-adjusted tinzaparin for the prevention of venous thromboembolism after bariatric surgery. J Thromb Haemost. 2018;16(10):2008–15. https://doi.org/10.1111/jth.14263.
56. Imberti D, Baldini E, Pierfranceschi MG, et al. Prophylaxis of venous thromboembolism with low molecular weight heparin in bariatric surgery: a prospective, randomised pilot study evaluating two doses of parnaparin (BAFLUX study). Obes Surg. 2014;24(2):284–91. https://doi.org/10.1007/s11695-013-1105-x.
57. Kalfarentzos F, Stavropoulou F, Yarmenitis S, et al. Prophylaxis of venous thromboembolism using two different doses of low-molecular-weight heparin (nadroparin) in bariatric surgery: a prospective randomized trial. Obes Surg. 2001;11(6):670–6. https://doi.org/10.1381/09608920160558588.
58. Borkgren-Okonek MJ, Hart RW, Pantano JE, et al. Enoxaparin thromboprophylaxis in gastric bypass patients: extended duration, dose stratification, and antifactor Xa activity. Surg Obes Relat Dis. 2008;4(5):625–31. https://doi.org/10.1016/j.soard.2007.11.010.
59. Singh K, Podolsky ER, Um S, et al. Evaluating the safety and efficacy of BMI-based preoperative administration of low-molecular-weight heparin in morbidly obese patients undergoing

Roux-en-Y gastric bypass surgery. Obes Surg. 2012;22(1):47–51. https://doi.org/10.1007/s11695-011-0397-y.
60. Paige JT, Gouda BP, Gaitor-Stampley V, et al. No correlation between anti-factor Xa levels, low-molecular-weight heparin, and bleeding after gastric bypass. Surg Obes Relat Dis. 2007;3(4):469–75. https://doi.org/10.1016/j.soard.2006.12.012.
61. Egan G, Ensom MH. Measuring anti-factor xa activity to monitor low-molecular-weight heparin in obesity: a critical review. Can J Hosp Pharm. 2015;68(1):33–47. https://doi.org/10.4212/cjhp.v68i1.1423.
62. Ojo P, Asiyanbola B, Valin E, Reinhold R. Post discharge prophylactic anticoagulation in gastric bypass patient-how safe? Obes Surg. 2008;18(7):791–6. https://doi.org/10.1007/s11695-007-9382-x.
63. Karas LA, Nor Hanipah Z, Cetin D, et al. Assessment of empiric body mass index-based thromboprophylactic dosing of enoxaparin after bariatric surgery: evidence for dosage adjustment using anti-factor Xa in high-risk patients. Surg Obes Relat Dis. 2021;17(1):153–60. https://doi.org/10.1016/j.soard.2020.08.016.
64. Kröll D, Nett PC, Rommers N, et al. Efficacy and safety of rivaroxaban for postoperative thromboprophylaxis in patients after bariatric surgery: a randomized clinical trial. JAMA Netw Open. 2023;6(5):e2315241. https://doi.org/10.1001/jamanetworkopen.2023.15241.
65. Tyselskyi V, Tryliskyy Y, Poylin V, Kebkalo A. Prolonged thromboprophylaxis with rivaroxaban after bariatric interventions: single centre experience. Pol Przegl Chir. 2023;95(4):1–5. doi:10.5604/01.3001.0016.2729.
66. Steele KE, Canner J, Prokopowicz G, et al. The EFFORT trial: preoperative enoxaparin versus postoperative fondaparinux for thromboprophylaxis in bariatric surgical patients: a randomized double-blind pilot trial. Surg Obes Relat Dis. 2015;11(3):672–83. https://doi.org/10.1016/j.soard.2014.10.003.
67. Winegar DA, Sherif B, Pate V, DeMaria EJ. Venous thromboembolism after bariatric surgery performed by Bariatric Surgery Center of Excellence Participants: analysis of the Bariatric Outcomes Longitudinal Database. Surg Obes Relat Dis. 2011;7(2):181–8. https://doi.org/10.1016/j.soard.2010.12.008.
68. Thereaux J, Lesuffleur T, Czernichow S, et al. To what extent does posthospital discharge chemoprophylaxis prevent venous thromboembolism after bariatric surgery?: results from a nationwide cohort of more than 110,000 patients. Ann Surg. 2018;267(4):727–33. https://doi.org/10.1097/sla.0000000000002285.
69. Raftopoulos I, Martindale C, Cronin A, Steinberg J. The effect of extended post-discharge chemical thromboprophylaxis on venous thromboembolism rates after bariatric surgery: a prospective comparison trial. Surg Endosc. 2008;22(11):2384–91. https://doi.org/10.1007/s00464-008-0031-9.
70. Muñoz-Atienza V, Gil-Rendo A, Amo-Salas M, Núñez-Guerrero P, Martín-Fernández J. Extended use of bemiparin as thromboprophylaxis during bariatric surgery: results of anti-factor Xa activity measurements. Surg Obes Relat Dis. 2018;14(3):354–60. https://doi.org/10.1016/j.soard.2017.12.004.
71. Stein PD, Goldman J. Obesity and thromboembolic disease. Clin Chest Med. 2009;30(3):489–93, viii. https://doi.org/10.1016/j.ccm.2009.05.006.
72. Stein PD, Matta F, Goldman J. Obesity and pulmonary embolism: the mounting evidence of risk and the mortality paradox. Thromb Res. 2011;128(6):518–23. https://doi.org/10.1016/j.thromres.2011.10.019.
73. Huo MH, Muntz J. Extended thromboprophylaxis with low-molecular-weight heparins after hospital discharge in high-risk surgical and medical patients: a review. Clin Ther. 2009;31(6):1129–41. https://doi.org/10.1016/j.clinthera.2009.06.002.
74. Scholten DJ, Hoedema RM, Scholten SE. A comparison of two different prophylactic dose regimens of low molecular weight heparin in bariatric surgery. Obes Surg. 2002;12(1):19–24. https://doi.org/10.1381/096089202321144522.
75. Stier C, Koschker AC, Stier R, Sosnierz A, Chiappetta S. Are we missing treatment standards for thromboprophylaxis of the obese and super-obese patient population? A prospective

systematic cohort study. Obes Surg. 2020;30(5):1704–11. https://doi.org/10.1007/s11695-020-04383-w.
76. Wei MY, Ward SM. The anti-factor Xa range for low molecular weight heparin thromboprophylaxis. Hematol Rep. 2015;7(4):5844. https://doi.org/10.4081/hr.2015.5844.
77. Schijns W, Deenen MJ, Aarts EO, et al. The effect of obesity on anti-Xa concentrations in bariatric patients. Obes Surg. 2018;28(7):1997–2005. https://doi.org/10.1007/s11695-018-3130-2.
78. Obeid FN, Bowling WM, Fike JS, Durant JA. Efficacy of prophylactic inferior vena cava filter placement in bariatric surgery. Surg Obes Relat Dis. 2007;3(6):606–8; discussion 609–10. https://doi.org/10.1016/j.soard.2007.08.005.
79. Trigilio-Black CM, Ringley CD, McBride CL, et al. Inferior vena cava filter placement for pulmonary embolism risk reduction in super morbidly obese undergoing bariatric surgery. Surg Obes Relat Dis. 2007;3(4):461–4. https://doi.org/10.1016/j.soard.2007.03.243.
80. Birkmeyer NJ, Share D, Baser O, et al. Preoperative placement of inferior vena cava filters and outcomes after gastric bypass surgery. Ann Surg. 2010;252(2):313–8. https://doi.org/10.1097/SLA.0b013e3181e61e4f.
81. Li W, Gorecki P, Semaan E, Briggs W, Tortolani AJ, D'Ayala M. Concurrent prophylactic placement of inferior vena cava filter in gastric bypass and adjustable banding operations in the Bariatric Outcomes Longitudinal Database. J Vasc Surg. 2012;55(6):1690–5. https://doi.org/10.1016/j.jvs.2011.12.056.
82. Birkmeyer NJ, Finks JF, English WJ, et al. Risks and benefits of prophylactic inferior vena cava filters in patients undergoing bariatric surgery. J Hosp Med. 2013;8(4):173–7. https://doi.org/10.1002/jhm.2013.
83. Haskins IN, Rivas L, Ju T, et al. The association of IVC filter placement with the incidence of postoperative pulmonary embolism following laparoscopic bariatric surgery: an analysis of the metabolic and bariatric surgery accreditation and quality improvement project. Surg Obes Relat Dis. 2019;15(1):109–15. https://doi.org/10.1016/j.soard.2018.10.008.
84. Reddy S, Zack CJ, Lakhter V, et al. Prophylactic inferior vena cava filters prior to bariatric surgery: insights from the national inpatient sample. JACC Cardiovasc Interv. 2019;12(12):1153–60. https://doi.org/10.1016/j.jcin.2019.04.011.
85. Schuster R, Hagedorn JC, Curet MJ, Morton JM. Retrievable inferior vena cava filters may be safely applied in gastric bypass surgery. Surg Endosc. 2007;21(12):2277–9. https://doi.org/10.1007/s00464-007-9370-1.
86. Ayad MT, Gillespie DL. Long-term complications of inferior vena cava filters. J Vasc Surg Venous Lymphat Disord. 2019;7(1):139–44. https://doi.org/10.1016/j.jvsv.2018.01.022.
87. Comes RF, Mismetti P, Afshari A. European guidelines on perioperative venous thromboembolism prophylaxis: inferior vena cava filters. Eur J Anaesthesiol. 2018;35(2):108–11. https://doi.org/10.1097/eja.0000000000000730.
88. Tan SBM, Greenslade J, Martin D, Talbot M, Loi K, Hopkins G. Portomesenteric vein thrombosis in sleeve gastrectomy: a 10-year review. Surg Obes Relat Dis. 2018;14(3):271–5. https://doi.org/10.1016/j.soard.2017.12.010.
89. Carrano FM, Weiner S, Elshafei M, et al. Portomesenteric vein thrombosis after bariatric surgery: an online survey. J Clin Med. 2021;10(17):4024. https://doi.org/10.3390/jcm10174024.
90. Goitein D, Matter I, Raziel A, et al. Portomesenteric thrombosis following laparoscopic bariatric surgery: incidence, patterns of clinical presentation, and etiology in a bariatric patient population. JAMA Surg. 2013;148(4):340–6. https://doi.org/10.1001/jamasurg.2013.1053.
91. James AW, Rabl C, Westphalen AC, Fogarty PF, Posselt AM, Campos GM. Portomesenteric venous thrombosis after laparoscopic surgery: a systematic literature review. Arch Surg. 2009;144(6):520–6. https://doi.org/10.1001/archsurg.2009.81.
92. Salinas J, Barros D, Salgado N, et al. Portomesenteric vein thrombosis after laparoscopic sleeve gastrectomy. Surg Endosc. 2014;28(4):1083–9. https://doi.org/10.1007/s00464-013-3055-8.
93. Luo L, Li H, Wu Y, et al. Portal venous system thrombosis after bariatric surgery: a systematic review and meta-analysis. Surgery. 2021;170(2):363–72. https://doi.org/10.1016/j.surg.2021.03.005.

94. Sheen CL, Lamparelli H, Milne A, Green I, Ramage JK. Clinical features, diagnosis and outcome of acute portal vein thrombosis. QJM. 2000;93(8):531–4. https://doi.org/10.1093/qjmed/93.8.531.
95. Gertsch P, Matthews J, Lerut J, Luder P, Blumgart LH. Acute thrombosis of the splanchnic veins. Arch Surg. 1993;128(3):341–5. https://doi.org/10.1001/archsurg.1993.01420150101018.
96. Kairaluoma MI, Karkola P, Heikkinen D, Huttunen R, Mokka RE, Larmi TK. Mesenteric infarction. Am J Surg. 1977;133(2):188–93. https://doi.org/10.1016/0002-9610(77)90078-2.
97. Bradbury MS, Kavanagh PV, Chen MY, Weber TM, Bechtold RE. Noninvasive assessment of portomesenteric venous thrombosis: current concepts and imaging strategies. J Comput Assist Tomogr. 2002;26(3):392–404. https://doi.org/10.1097/00004728-200205000-00014.
98. Moon RC, Ghanem M, Teixeira AF, et al. Assessing risk factors, presentation, and management of portomesenteric vein thrombosis after sleeve gastrectomy: a multicenter case-control study. Surg Obes Relat Dis. 2018;14(4):478–83. https://doi.org/10.1016/j.soard.2017.10.013.
99. Godoroja-Diarto D, Copaescu C, Rusu E, Constantin A. The role of thromboprophylaxis in patients with portal vein thrombosis: a life-threatening complication after laparoscopic sleeve gastrectomy following 8 years of experience in a Bariatric Center of Excellence. Diagnostics (Basel). 2022;13(1):43. https://doi.org/10.3390/diagnostics13010043.
100. Delhom E, Aufort S, Shrembi V, Lonjon J, Bruel JM, Gallix B. [Acute mesenteric ischemia: value of cross-sectional imaging]. J Radiol. 2011;92(12):1060–71. Ischémie aiguë du mésentère : apports de l'imagerie en coupes. https://doi.org/10.1016/j.jradio.2011.03.029.
101. Sarin SK, Sollano JD, Chawla YK, et al. Consensus on extra-hepatic portal vein obstruction. Liver Int. 2006;26(5):512–9. https://doi.org/10.1111/j.1478-3231.2006.01269.x.
102. Kearon C, Akl EA, Ornelas J, et al. Antithrombotic therapy for VTE disease: CHEST guideline and expert panel report. Chest. 2016;149(2):315–52. https://doi.org/10.1016/j.chest.2015.11.026.
103. Hong J, Ahn SY, Lee YJ, et al. Updated recommendations for the treatment of venous thromboembolism. Blood Res. 2021;56(1):6–16. https://doi.org/10.5045/br.2021.2020083.
104. Büller HR, Prins MH, Lensin AW, et al. Oral rivaroxaban for the treatment of symptomatic pulmonary embolism. N Engl J Med. 2012;366(14):1287–97. https://doi.org/10.1056/NEJMoa1113572.
105. Büller HR, Décousus H, Grosso MA, et al. Edoxaban versus warfarin for the treatment of symptomatic venous thromboembolism. N Engl J Med. 2013;369(15):1406–15. https://doi.org/10.1056/NEJMoa1306638.
106. Schulman S, Kearon C, Kakkar AK, et al. Dabigatran versus warfarin in the treatment of acute venous thromboembolism. N Engl J Med. 2009;361(24):2342–52. https://doi.org/10.1056/NEJMoa0906598.
107. Schulman S, Kakkar AK, Goldhaber SZ, et al. Treatment of acute venous thromboembolism with dabigatran or warfarin and pooled analysis. Circulation. 2014;129(7):764–72. https://doi.org/10.1161/circulationaha.113.004450.
108. Chatterjee S, Chakraborty A, Weinberg I, et al. Thrombolysis for pulmonary embolism and risk of all-cause mortality, major bleeding, and intracranial hemorrhage: a meta-analysis. JAMA. 2014;311(23):2414–21. https://doi.org/10.1001/jama.2014.5990.

# 29 Postoperative Bleeding After Sleeve Gastrectomy

Monique Hassan

## Introduction

The vertical sleeve gastrectomy or sleeve gastrectomy was first performed in 1990 as the first of a two-stage operation for biliopancreatic diversion with duodenal switch (BPD-DS) [1, 2]. The first laparoscopic sleeve gastrectomy (LSG) was performed in 1999 [3]. The original indication for a vertical sleeve gastrectomy was in patients with super obesity (BMI > 60) to induce weight loss to more safely undergo the second stage of the BPD-DS [2, 4]. While following these patients, it was noted that they were having excellent reductions in excess body weight, and in 2008, the indications for laparoscopic sleeve gastrectomy (LSG) were published [5]. The LSG has gained worldwide acceptance and has become the most common weight-loss procedure in the United States [6]. When compared to other weight-loss surgeries, LSG is considered effective and technically easy as it does not require an anastomosis and can be performed using minimally invasive techniques with relatively less morbidity [7–10].

## Technique of LSG

There are many described approaches to performing LSG. The American Society for Metabolic and Bariatric Surgery (ASMBS) describes LSG using the following steps. The procedure starts by dividing the small branches of the gastroepiploic arcade and opening the lesser sac. Dissection is carried out along the greater curve,

M. Hassan (✉)
Department of Surgery, Baylor College of Medicine, Scott and White Memorial Hospital and Clinic, Temple, TX, USA
e-mail: Monique.Hassan@BSWHealth.org



O. M. Ghanem et al. (eds.), *The SAGES Manual of Metabolic and Bariatric Surgery*, https://doi.org/10.1007/978-3-031-72309-4_29

dividing the branches of both gastroepiploic arteries until short gastric vessels are divided using an advanced energy device. The remainder of the gastrocolic ligament (without gastroepiploic vessels transection) is divided distally up to 2 cm proximal to the pylorus. The stomach is lifted to expose its posterior aspect, and all lesser sac attachments are freed. The gastrophrenic ligament is divided, and the angle of His is exposed to determine the presence of a hiatal hernia, adding the full exposure of the left crus to complete the dissection. Prior to the creation of the sleeve, a 34- to 40-Fr bougie is introduced into the stomach to guide the stapling and maintain an adequate lumen of the gastric sleeve. Stapling is performed using sequential firings of a laparoscopic or robotic stapler to create a sleeve that is in a straight line from the gastroesophageal junction. The bougie is removed, and the staple line integrity and hemostasis are assessed [11].

## Overview

Although LSG is considered safe, it carries a risk of complication, as with any surgery. Brethauer et al., who performed a systematic review of LSG outcomes, reported that the complication rate among 36 studies (2570 patients) ranged from 0 to 23.8% [7]. Studies with >100 patients reported a major postoperative complication rate from 0 to 14%. The overall 30-day mortality rate was 0.19%. The overall rate of major complication rates was low, including leaks (2.2%), bleeding requiring reoperation or transfusion (1.2%), and strictures requiring endoscopic or surgical intervention (0.6%) [12]. Postoperative hemorrhage is one of the most common early complications occurring both intraluminal and intra-abdominal (i.e., from the staple line, omentum, port sites, or damage to the liver or spleen). The reported incidence of hemorrhagic complications after sleeve gastrectomy is between 1 and 6% postoperatively [13]. Major postoperative bleeding is defined by the International Society on Thrombosis and Hemostasis as an event leading to a drop of hemoglobin > 2 g/dL and (1) operative revision or radiological intervention for bleeding control or requiring (2) the postoperative transfusion of $\geq$2 red blood cell packs [14]. Major postoperative bleeding is linked to longer hospitalization, major complications (such as sepsis and organ failure), reoperation, and mortality [15]. Therefore, there is a need for preventive strategies due to the severe consequences of early postoperative hemorrhage.

## Causes of Bleeding

Bleeding can occur during the greater curvature vessels' division or gastric stapling. The stomach is supplied by a rich network of submucosal plexus derived from the left and right gastric arteries, gastroepiploic vessels, and short gastric arteries. The division of the short gastric vessels during the mobilization of the gastric fundus in proximity to the splenic upper pole particularly exposes one to the risk of hemorrhage. Incomplete hemostasis after surgical dissection may also cause hemorrhage

[16]. Common sites of bleeding include the trocar insertion site, the short gastric vessels, the liver or spleen, and the omental vessels that have been divided during the dissection of the greater curvature [12, 17, 18].

The LSG is the longest staple line of any bariatric surgical procedure and, therefore, the most common site of bleeding [19]. The incidence of staple line hemorrhage has been reported to be 0–8.7% [12, 17]. Bleeding can occur when dividing the transverse branches of the lesser curvature arteries during the stapling [20, 21]. The mechanism for staple line bleeding is submucosal blood vessel damage, which occurs from vessel transection at tissue edges or with vessel penetration during stapling [16, 22]. Laparoscopic or robotic staplers have become vital in performing sleeve gastrectomy; however, they can be associated with bleeding. The thickness of the gastric wall differs in various parts of the stomach, and this can be underappreciated on visualization. It is thickest at the antrum and progressively thinner towards the fundus [20, 23]. Staple line bleeding can be attributed to inadequate compression due to a staple height that is too large compared with tissue thickness or vessels. Therefore, a single staple height cannot effectively approximate the entire length of the gastric wall's various thicknesses [23]. An expert knowledge of staple heights from the respective equipment manufacturers is required. The selection of the appropriate staple height must be balanced between the risk of leak and bleeding.

## Clinical Presentation

Postoperative hemorrhage after LSG can manifest as intraluminal or extraluminal (intra-abdominal) bleeding. Therefore, interventions required to achieve hemostasis depend on the source of bleeding. The initial evaluation of a patient with suspected clinically significant postoperative hemorrhage is to assess the severity of the bleeding, detect the bleeding source, and recognize the presence of conditions that could affect management. Physical examination is a crucial piece in assessing the extent of postoperative hemorrhage. Mild to moderate hypovolemia, defined as <15% loss of blood volume, usually manifests as resting tachycardia, while blood loss >15% or >40% presents as orthostatic and supine hypotension [16, 24]. In addition, diffuse abdominal tenderness with hypoactive bowel sounds, abdominal distension, tachycardia, rapid fall of hematocrit, and oliguria should prompt consideration of extraluminal blood loss [16, 18, 20, 25]. In a review by Sabry et al., the researchers identified 80 cases of postoperative hemorrhage within the first 6 h out of 1500 patients after laparoscopic sleeve gastrectomy. They found that the vast majority were extraluminal (95%) and presented with tachycardia (>100 b/m), hypotension (<90/60 mmHg), increase in the drainage volume (>100 cc/h), and abdominal pain. In the extraluminal group, the most common bleeding source was the suture/staple line (71%), followed by the omentum (11%), trocar insertion sites (8%), short gastric blood vessels (5%), and pancreatic adhesions (5%) [26].

Intraluminal bleeding may present as an upper gastrointestinal bleed with symptoms such as hematemesis, hematochezia, or melena in addition to hypotension and tachycardia [26]. Unlike laparoscopic Roux-en-Y gastric bypass (LRYGB), in which intraluminal bleeding is relatively common from the anastomosis, intraluminal hemorrhage from the staple line is extremely rare after LSG [18, 27]. Occasionally, the mucosa of the oropharynx, esophagus, or the lesser curvature of the stomach may be damaged during the placement of the bougie and result in early postoperative intraluminal bleeding [16].

## Management Strategies

When bleeding is suspected or identified, conservative management, including stopping anticoagulation and appropriate fluid or blood resuscitation, may be sufficient in many cases [12, 28, 29]. The management strategy for bleeding after LSG is similar to that of other general abdominal surgeries. When bleeding is suspected, the patient should be placed in a monitored unit and have nothing per mouth, and supplemental oxygen by nasal cannula should be administered. Adequate IV access should be established with two large caliber (≥18 gauge) peripheral intravenous catheters or a central venous line, if necessary, for administering fluid or blood products. Laboratory tests, including CBC, serum chemistries, liver tests, and coagulation panel, should be obtained [16, 20, 25, 26]. Multidetector computed tomography (MDCT) is the first-line imaging test for diagnosing postoperative hemorrhage after LSG [30, 31]. MDCT is the most readily available and least invasive test, which also provides detailed vascular mapping and can differentiate active bleeding from hematoma or between intraluminal and extraluminal bleeding [31].

## Extraluminal Bleeding

### Stable Patient

Conservative management can be attempted in stable patients without evidence of active bleeding on imaging. The majority (>80%) of acute postoperative bleeding will be resolved with conservative management, without the need for another procedure or reoperation [25].

### Unstable Patient

Bleeding complications requiring reoperation occur less than 2% of the time after LSG [32]. Hemodynamically unstable patients, as well as those who fail to respond to supportive treatment, have persistent bleeding, or clinical deterioration, require immediate reoperation [16]. Immediate surgical exploration facilitates a diagnosis and allows evacuation of the clot and surgical control of the source of bleeding. Sabry et al. found that hemostasis was achieved with sutures and clips in all patients with bleeding from the suture line. For the other bleeding sites, cauterization, clips, and ligation of the bleeding points were successfully performed. All cases were identified and treated early, as they presented within the first 6 h of surgery. This early management decreased infection rates, length of stay, need for blood transfusion, and faster patient recovery [26].

Surgical evacuation of the hematoma may also simplify the postoperative course, as spontaneous hematoma resorption is more prolonged and may need monitoring. Aboueisha et al. conducted a propensity-matched analysis using the MBSAQIP database, including 513,354 LSG cases. They demonstrated that bleeding after LSG was significantly associated with an increased incidence of leaks (4.4% vs. 0.3%), along with higher morbidity. These results suggest early re-exploration in postoperative bleeding could prevent delayed complications such as leak or abscess [18, 33].

For patients with active extraluminal bleeding, CT scan is the best tool to diagnose bleeding, locate the artery that is the source of bleeding, and help determine the therapeutic strategy [31]. The use of MDCT offers the opportunity for endovascular interventions. Interventional radiology expertise must be available for endovascular intervention and is analogous to managing acute abdominal or gastrointestinal bleeding [20, 31, 34]. If intra-abdominal bleeding is due to the staple line, endovascular techniques are unlikely to be successful, and surgical hemostasis may be indicated. Clinical judgment must be made considering the stability of the patient and available resources.

## Intraluminal Bleeding

Postoperative intraluminal bleeding after LSG is rare, unlike after LRYGB, due to the anastomotic staple lines that are present. Sabry et al. found that only 5% of postoperative bleeding occurred due to intraluminal sources. All patients were treated supportively with fluid resuscitation and monitored closely with lab tests, and these interventions were adequate to manage all intraluminal hemorrhage cases [26]. Aside from clinical signs, upper endoscopy can be an excellent diagnostic and therapeutic modality for managing intraluminal hemorrhage. Upper endoscopy can be done without delay at the bedside with the patient in the intensive care unit (ICU) to diagnose and manage intraluminal bleeding [25]. However, multiple anatomic reasons make the endoscopic management of persistent intraluminal bleeding after LSG difficult. The staple line in the sleeve gastrectomy is everted. Therefore, the staple line will not readily lend itself to endoscopic bleeding control maneuvers. Furthermore, a narrow sleeve may limit endoscopic actions other than evacuating the intraluminal hematoma. A combined approach is recommended to guide emergency laparoscopy for precise localization and management of intraluminal bleeding after LSG [27].

## Prevention

### Preoperative Patient Factors

Although the LSG is safe, even in high-risk patients, higher BMI and comorbidities such as liver disease (non-alcoholic fatty liver), coagulopathy, and hypertension, are independent risk factors for major postoperative bleeding. Comorbidities should be carefully evaluated and optimized preoperatively when possible [15].

Using risk calculators may allow for estimating the risk of postoperative adverse events, improve surgical decision-making, and informed patient consent. In addition, identifying modifiable preoperative factors associated with increased risk of postsurgical adverse events such as hemorrhage would be a considerable benefit [19, 35, 36]. Based on the "sleeve bleed calculator," the authors concluded that the protective factors for hemorrhagic complications were no history of obstructive sleep apnea and no history of hypertension. At the same time, a low level of expertise in bariatric surgery was associated with a higher risk of hemorrhagic complications [19].

### Anticoagulation

Venous thromboembolism (VTE) is a significant cause of morbidity and mortality after bariatric surgery. The use of preoperative low molecular weight heparins (LMWH) for the prevention of venous thromboembolism is considered a significant risk factor for increased postoperative LSG bleeding. In a review of 781 patients, Zeni et al. found that adding preoperative LMWH administration did not significantly decrease the rate of VTE; however, it significantly increased the rate of postoperative bleeding and length of stay [37]. Conversely, a randomized, double-blinded study of 198 consecutive bariatric surgery patients demonstrated that once daily fondaparinux postoperatively was much more likely to produce target prophylactic anti-factor Xa levels than twice-daily enoxaparin in patients undergoing bariatric surgery. Bleeding complications were 5% in the enoxaparin group compared to 3% in the fondaparinux group, which was not a statistically significant increase in postoperative bleeding [38, 39]. Several other studies have examined various regimens for preoperative chemoprophylaxis and have determined that it does not increase rates of bleeding [39–41]. In addition, Neilson et al. found that patients who receive postoperative blood transfusion for the management of perioperative bleeding are at a significantly increased risk for VTE. The etiology of VTE in those who are transfused is likely multifactorial and possibly related to withholding chemoprophylaxis and the potential of a hypercoagulable state induced by the transfusion. Therefore, the authors recommend consideration should be given to reinitiating chemoprophylaxis when safe, extending treatment after discharge, and screening ultrasound in patients who suffer postoperative hemorrhage [42].

## Tranexamic Acid

Tranexamic acid (TXA), a synthetic derivative of the amino acid lysine, is a potent antifibrinolytic drug. It prevents the binding of plasminogen to the surface of fibrin and reduces the activation of fibrin, resulting in inhibition of fibrinolysis [43]. Due to these recognized properties, there has been an increased interest in using TXA to reduce bleeding. Giving TXA at induction may be a simple and economical option for effectively reducing staple line bleeds, leading to a significant decrease in operating times. In a study including LSG patients, the group treated with prophylactic TXA intraoperatively required significantly fewer stitches to stop the bleeding and had lower blood loss and shorter operation duration than the control group. However, no difference in the morbidity and mortality of the patients was detected [44]. Several studies showed the positive effects of TXA to reduce perioperative hemorrhage [45, 46]. In a recent study, the use of tranexamic acid was statistically found to reduce intraoperative bleeding volume, leading to fewer postoperative complications and reducing the length of hospital stay. Thus, tranexamic acid can be an important adjunct for preventing bleeding in the stapling line of patients undergoing LSG [47]. Tranexamic acid administration may be effective in reducing the reoperation rate for bleeding complications after LSG.

## Intraoperative Factors

Adaptations in surgical techniques may provide benefits in reducing postoperative bleeding after LSG. All of these described methods have demonstrated mixed success in reliably reducing bleeding [12, 20, 21]. Surgical principles such as staying close to the serosa of the stomach and elevation of the stomach anteriorly may allow for minimizing intraoperative bleeding during the dissection of the stomach [48]. If bleeding occurs, mechanical compression should be attempted first, as this reduces bleeding in most cases and helps identify the vessel that may be coagulated or controlled with a surgical clip. Staple line bleeding control with monopolar cautery during LSG has also been demonstrated to be a feasible, simple, inexpensive, and relatively safe method [49, 50]. Several energy devices are available for use during the performance of LSG, and there has been no clear evidence that one may be more hemostatic than the other and should be selected based on surgeon comfort level [19, 48, 51].

The development of new stapler technology and designs that improve staple line formation and integrity have efficiently reduced postoperative hemorrhage and reoperation rates. The type of stapler and the cartridge height have been cited as crucial factors for staple line bleeding. If the closed staple height is too high, it may inadequately compress the tissues and result in bleeding [23, 45, 52]. During the stapling stage in LSG, it has been suggested that waiting between compression and firing can help reduce postoperative bleeding [15, 53]. Innovation in surgical stapling technology has evolved from manual to powered staplers. A study comparing manual and powered staplers demonstrated that using powered staplers was associated with a lower rate of bleeding/transfusion vs manual staplers in the real-world setting [54].

Several techniques have been recommended to reinforce the staple line to mitigate the risk of bleeding, such as suturing or oversewing, buttressing, clipping, or gluing. A 2013 consensus summit on sleeve gastrectomy determined that 79% of respondent surgeons reinforce the staple line, and of these surgeons, 57% buttress the staple line and 43% oversew it [55]. A meta-analysis published by Shikora et al. revealed that the incidence of bleeding was dependent on the reinforcement method. In 33 studies where a running suture was used for reinforcement, the bleeding rate was 2.41%, while in 25 studies without staple reinforcement, the bleeding rate was 4.94% [13, 19]. In a recent meta-analysis by Aiofi et al., oversewing was associated with a significantly reduced risk of postoperative bleeding compared to no reinforcement. At the same time, no significant differences were found in the comparison to other treatments [56]. However, Choi et al. did not find any significant benefit for staple line suture oversewing, reasoning that suture oversewing could potentially increase the risk of bleeding because of tissue tearing at the point of stitch penetration [57]. Simon et al. found no conclusive evidence that staple line reinforcement reduced staple line leakage or hemorrhage [58].

A recent study of over 1161 patients who underwent LSG from 2005 to 2019 found no significant bleeding or pRBC transfusion rate between different energy devices used intraoperatively to ligate the greater curve vessels. There was no significant difference between staple brands, staple height, use of reinforced staples, or staple line reinforcement with suture and clips. Surgeons used various techniques to oversew the staple line including complete suturing of the staple line, selective suturing of areas concerning for bleeding, selective clip placement, or not oversewing the staple line. Between these techniques, there was no increase in bleeding or transfusion rate [59].

Various technical modifications, such as applying hemostatic agents on staple lines, have also been described to decrease the incidence of postoperative bleeding [60]. A recent meta-analysis including 2136 LSG patients from nine randomized controlled trials showed a tendency toward less bleeding with fibrin sealant application compared to no reinforcement [18, 61]. However, the hemostatic role of sealants was not evident in that meta-analysis of trials with larger samples [18, 62].

Some investigators have suggested that increasing the systolic blood pressure beyond the normal range (>140 mmHg) in cooperation with anesthesiologists and simultaneously decreasing the intra-abdominal pressure below 10 mmHg at the end of surgery can help detect silent bleeding during surgery. Several studies reported that after adopting this intraoperative protocol, all silent bleeding was detected and adequately controlled during surgery, and there were no postoperative bleeding events after surgery [63, 64]. In addition, Sroka et al. also demonstrated that routine elevation of systolic blood pressure and over-suturing of the staple line minimized the incidence of hemorrhagic events down to 0% with reasonable prolongation of the procedure in their randomized controlled trial [18, 65].

## Special Populations

Management of postoperative hemorrhage after LSG in Jehovah's Witness (JW) patients demands specialized considerations. Many JW patients will not accept transfusions of whole blood, red blood cells, white blood cells, platelets, or plasma. This is based on an interpretation of Bible passages prohibiting blood consumption [66, 67]. Several treatment options are available to mitigate this risk without transfusion of exogenous blood products. These include optimizing preoperative hemoglobin with the use of erythropoietin, utilizing fibrin glue/staple line reinforcement to minimize/control staple line bleeding, and intraoperative use of cell saver devices which recirculate the patient's lost blood in the event of unexpected intraoperative or postoperative blood loss [68]. It is important to note that not all JW patients have the same beliefs when it comes to surgical treatment and the use of biological factors; therefore, having a preapproved individualized plan for how best to manage unexpected bleeding allows for effective postoperative management without infringing upon a patient's religious beliefs [66, 68].

## Chronic Anticoagulated Patient

Bariatric surgery can be safely performed in patients on therapeutic anticoagulation, though this population is at greater risk for bleeding complications in the perioperative period. Meticulous hemostasis in the operating room is critical to preventing bleeding complications. A case control series at a single center compared 15 patients on chronic anticoagulation who underwent sleeve gastrectomy to 30 patients undergoing sleeve gastrectomy not on chronic anticoagulation. One bleeding event occurred in each group, demonstrating no significant difference in bleeding outcomes [69]. In a recent retrospective analysis of 64 patients who underwent bariatric surgery on therapeutic anticoagulation before and after the operation, four patients developed postoperative hemorrhage. Anticoagulation was restarted 24 h after the operation in all four cases, with resumption of the home dose of warfarin and the bridging LMWH in patients being therapeutically bridged. Bleeding became evident 48 h after the operation in two cases and 72 h after the operation in two cases. One patient required reoperation and blood transfusion to control bleeding. The other three patients were managed conservatively with cessation of anticoagulation. Two of these three conservatively managed patients were transfused with an average of 1.5 units of blood [70].

## Conclusion

LSG is an effective metabolic and bariatric procedure rapidly gaining in popularity. Therefore, the number of patients undergoing this procedure will continue to rise. A basic understanding of bleeding complications and available treatment options is essential for all practicing surgeons. Managing postoperative bleeding requires clinical judgment based on the patient's presentation. Bleeding may stop spontaneously or require hemostasis by operative or endovascular means. CT scan can be used to locate the source of bleeding to guide clinical management, possibly avoiding the need for reoperation. Hemodynamically unstable patients or cases of persistent bleeding from the staple line require operative intervention for definitive hemostasis.

## References


1. Marceau P, Biron S, St Georges R, Duclos M, Potvin M, Bourque RA. Biliopancreatic diversion with gastrectomy as surgical treatment of morbid obesity. Obes Surg. 1991;1(4):381–7.
2. Krawczykowski D. The sleeve gastrectomy. In: Karcz WK, Thomusch O, editors. Principles of metabolic surgery [internet]. Berlin, Heidelberg: Springer; 2012 [cited 2024 Feb 19]. p. 201–215. https://doi.org/10.1007/978-3-642-02411-5_18.
3. Seeras K, Sankararaman S, Lopez PP. Sleeve gastrectomy. In: StatPearls [Internet]. Treasure Island: StatPearls Publishing; 2024 [cited 2024 Feb 19]. http://www.ncbi.nlm.nih.gov/books/NBK519035/.
4. Topart P, Becouarn G, Ritz P. Should biliopancreatic diversion with duodenal switch be done as single-stage procedure in patients with BMI > or = 50 kg/m2? Surg Obes Relat Dis. 2010;6(1):59–63.
5. Bellanger DE, Greenway FL. Laparoscopic sleeve gastrectomy, 529 cases without a leak: short-term results and technical considerations. Obes Surg. 2011;21(2):146–50.
6. ASMBS. American Society for Metabolic and Bariatric Surgery. Estimate of bariatric surgery numbers, 2011–2021. 2022 [cited 2023 Nov 26]. https://asmbs.org/resources/estimate-of-bariatric-surgery-numbers.
7. Brethauer SA, Hammel JP, Schauer PR. Systematic review of sleeve gastrectomy as staging and primary bariatric procedure. Surg Obes Relat Dis. 2009;5(4):469–75.
8. Paluszkiewicz R, Kalinowski P, Wróblewski T, Bartoszewicz Z, Białobrzeska-Paluszkiewicz J, Ziarkiewicz-Wróblewska B, et al. Prospective randomized clinical trial of laparoscopic sleeve gastrectomy versus open Roux-en-Y gastric bypass for the management of patients with morbid obesity. Wideochir Inne Tech Maloinwazyjne. 2012;7(4):225–32.
9. Schauer PR, Bhatt DL, Kirwan JP, Wolski K, Brethauer SA, Navaneethan SD, et al. Bariatric surgery versus intensive medical therapy for diabetes—3-year outcomes. N Engl J Med. 2014;370(21):2002–13.
10. Kheirvari M, Dadkhah Nikroo N, Jaafarinejad H, Farsimadan M, Eshghjoo S, Hosseini S, et al. The advantages and disadvantages of sleeve gastrectomy; clinical laboratory to bedside review. Heliyon. 2020;6(2):e03496.
11. Zundel N, Hernandez JD, Gagner M. Laparoscopic sleeve gastrectomy: technique and outcomes. In: Nguyen NT, Blackstone RP, Morton JM, Ponce J, Rosenthal RJ, editors. New York: Springer New York; 2015 [cited 2024 Feb 24]. p. 205–10. http://link.springer.com/10.1007/978-1-4939-1206-3_17.
12. Brethauer SA, Schauer PR, Schirmer BD, editors. Minimally invasive bariatric surgery. 2nd ed. New York: Springer; 2015.
13. Shikora SA, Mahoney CB. Clinical benefit of gastric staple line reinforcement (SLR) in gastrointestinal surgery: a meta-analysis. Obes Surg. 2015;25(7):1133–41.
14. Schulman S, Angerås U, Bergqvist D, Eriksson B, Lassen MR, Fisher W, et al. Definition of major bleeding in clinical investigations of antihemostatic medicinal products in surgical patients. J Thromb Haemost. 2010;8(1):202–4.
15. Kollmann L, Gruber M, Lock JF, Germer CT, Seyfried F. Clinical management of major postoperative bleeding after bariatric surgery. Obes Surg [Internet]. 2024 [cited 2024 Feb 24]. https://doi.org/10.1007/s11695-023-07040-0.

16. Giannopoulos S, Pokala B, Stefanidis D. Management of gastrointestinal bleeding following bariatric surgery. Mini-Invasive Surg. 2022;6(4):22.
17. Gagner M, Deitel M, Kalberer TL, Erickson AL, Crosby RD. The second international consensus summit for sleeve gastrectomy, March 19-21, 2009. Surg Obes Relat Dis. 2009;5(4):476–85.
18. Park JY. Diagnosis and management of postoperative complications after sleeve gastrectomy. J Metab Bariatr Surg. 2022;11(1):1–12.
19. Janik MR, Walędziak M, Brągoszewski J, Kwiatkowski A, Paśnik K. Prediction model for hemorrhagic complications after laparoscopic sleeve gastrectomy: development of SLEEVE BLEED calculator. Obes Surg. 2017;27(4):968–72.
20. Yong S, Poh B, Eng A, Pasupathy S, Chan WH, Lee PC, et al. Post-operative bleeding complications in laparoscopic sleeve gastrectomy: sources, solutions and lessons learnt from a single cohort of patients. Dig Med Res [Internet]. 2019 [cited 2024 Feb 24];2. https://dmr.amegroups.org/article/view/5144.
21. Redmann JG, Lavin TE, French MS, Broussard TD, Lapointe-Gagner M. Improving hemostasis in sleeve gastrectomy with alternative stapler. JSLS. 2020;24(4):e2020.00073.
22. Córdova H, Fernández-Esparrach G. Treatment of bleeding after bariatric surgery. Tech Gastrointest Endosc. 2010;12(3):130–5.
23. Huang R, Gagner M. A thickness calibration device is needed to determine staple height and avoid leaks in laparoscopic sleeve gastrectomy. Obes Surg. 2015;25(12):2360–7.
24. Cappell MS, Friedel D. Initial management of acute upper gastrointestinal bleeding: from initial evaluation up to gastrointestinal endoscopy. Med Clin North Am. 2008;92(3):491–509, xi.
25. Fridman A, Szomstein S, Rosenthal RJ. Postoperative bleeding in the bariatric surgery patient. In: Nguyen NT, Blackstone RP, Morton JM, Ponce J, Rosenthal RJ, editors. The ASMBS textbook of bariatric surgery [internet]. New York: Springer New York; 2015 [cited 2024 Feb 24]. p. 241–7. https://link.springer.com/10.1007/978-1-4939-1206-3_21.
26. Sabry K, Hamed A, Habib H, Helmy M, Abouzeid T. Management of acute bleeding post laparoscopic sleeve gastrectomy. J Obes Weight Loss Ther. 2017;7:7.
27. Çalıkoğlu İ, Hamzaoğlu H, Yerdel MA. Combined use of endoscopy to guide laparoscopic management of intraluminal bleeding from the staple-line after sleeve gastrectomy: a video case report. Surg Obes Relat Dis. 2020;16(8):1156–7.
28. Albanopoulos K, Alevizos L, Flessas J, Menenakos E, Stamou KM, Papailiou J, et al. Reinforcing the staple line during laparoscopic sleeve gastrectomy: prospective randomized clinical study comparing two different techniques. Preliminary results. Obes Surg. 2012;22(1):42–6.
29. Gill RS, Switzer N, Driedger M, Shi X, Vizhul A, Sharma AM, et al. Laparoscopic sleeve gastrectomy with staple line buttress reinforcement in 116 consecutive morbidly obese patients. Obes Surg. 2012;22(4):560–4.
30. Romano S, Tortora G, Scaglione M, Lassandro F, Guidi G, Grassi R, et al. MDCT imaging of post interventional liver: a pictorial essay. Eur J Radiol. 2005;53(3):425–32.
31. Tasu JP, Vesselle G, Herpe G, Ferrie JC, Chan P, Boucebci S, et al. Postoperative abdominal bleeding. Diagn Interv Imaging. 2015;96(7):823–31.
32. Ladak F, Dang JT, Switzer NJ, Mocanu V, Birch DW, Karmali S. Rates of reoperation and nonoperative intervention within 30 days of bariatric surgery. Surg Obes Relat Dis. 2019;15(3):431–40.
33. Aboueisha MA, Freeman M, Allotey JK, Evans L, Caposole MZ, Tatum D, et al. Battle of the buttress: 5-year propensity-matched analysis of staple-line reinforcement techniques from the MBSAQIP database. Surg Endosc. 2023;37(4):3090–102.
34. Tasu J. Stenting post-operative abdominal bleeding: the interventional radiologist's point of view. Imaging Med [Internet]. 2015 [cited 2024 Feb 24]. https://www.semanticscholar.org/paper/Stenting-post-operative-abdominal-bleeding%3A-the-of-Tasu/321b42051ad494a069019524be2906ca38364dc4.
35. Aminian A, Brethauer SA, Sharafkhah M, Schauer PR. Development of a sleeve gastrectomy risk calculator. Surg Obes Relat Dis. 2015;11(4):758–64.

36. Ali M, El Chaar M, Ghiassi S, Rogers AM, American Society for Metabolic and Bariatric Surgery Clinical Issues Committee. American Society for Metabolic and Bariatric Surgery updated position statement on sleeve gastrectomy as a bariatric procedure. Surg Obes Relat Dis. 2017;13(10):1652–7.
37. Zeni T, Rn ST, Roberts J. Bleeding rates are increased with preoperative Lovenox administration in patients undergoing sleeve gastrectomy. Surg Obes Relat Dis. 2015;11(6):S17.
38. Steele KE, Canner J, Prokopowicz G, Verde F, Beselman A, Wyse R, et al. The EFFORT trial: preoperative enoxaparin versus postoperative fondaparinux for thromboprophylaxis in bariatric surgical patients: a randomized double-blind pilot trial. Surg Obes Relat Dis. 2015;11(3):672–83.
39. Aminian A, Vosburg RW, Altieri MS, Hinojosa MW, Khorgami Z, American Society for Metabolic and Bariatric Surgery Clinical Issues Committee. The American Society for Metabolic and Bariatric Surgery (ASMBS) updated position statement on perioperative venous thromboembolism prophylaxis in bariatric surgery. Surg Obes Relat Dis. 2022;18(2):165–74.
40. Birkmeyer NJO, Finks JF, Carlin AM, Chengelis DL, Krause KR, Hawasli AA, et al. Comparative effectiveness of unfractionated and low-molecular-weight heparin for prevention of venous thromboembolism following bariatric surgery. Arch Surg. 2012;147(11):994–8.
41. Hany M, Abouelnasr AA, Agayby ASS, Abdelsattar A, Torensma B. Towards zero thromboembolic events after bariatric metabolic surgery. Obes Surg. 2023;33(5):1606–12.
42. Nielsen AW, Helm MC, Kindel T, Higgins R, Lak K, Helmen ZM, et al. Perioperative bleeding and blood transfusion are major risk factors for venous thromboembolism following bariatric surgery. Surg Endosc. 2018;32(5):2488–95.
43. Åstedt B. Clinical pharmacology of tranexamic acid. Scand J Gastroenterol. 1987;22(sup137):22–5.
44. Chakravartty S, Sarma DR, Chang A, Patel AG. Staple line bleeding in sleeve gastrectomy—a simple and cost-effective solution. Obes Surg. 2016;26(7):1422–8.
45. Hussain A, Al-Shoek I, El-Hasani S. The use of tranexamic acid in sleeve gastrectomy. Obes Surg. 2017;27(1):198–9.
46. Klaassen RA, Selles CA, van den Berg JW, Poelman MM, van der Harst E. Tranexamic acid therapy for postoperative bleeding after bariatric surgery. BMC Obes. 2018;5:36.
47. de Brito RM, de Oliveira CMB, Moura ECR, Campelo GP, de Lima RC, Servin ETN, et al. Comparison of tranexamic acid and stapling line reinforcement in laparoscopic sleeve gastrectomy in postoperative bleeding outcomes. Braz J Anesthesiol. 2023;73(3):361–3.
48. Jossart GH. Complications of sleeve gastrectomy: bleeding and prevention. Surg Laparosc Endosc Percutan Tech. 2010;20(3):146–7.
49. Sağlam K, Kayaalp C, Gündoğan E, Sansal M, Aktaş A, Gökler C, et al. Staple line bleeding control with monopolar cautery in laparoscopic sleeve gastrectomy. Laparosc Endosc Surg Sci. 2019;26(4):181–4.
50. Okut G, Turgut E, Kaplan K, Karahan M, Bag YM, Sumer F, et al. Management of the staple line bleeding in laparoscopic sleeve gastrectomy: monopolar cautery versus oversewing. Cir Cir. 2022;90:115–20.
51. Velotti N, Manigrasso M, Di Lauro K, Vitiello A, Berardi G, Manzolillo D, et al. Comparison between LigaSure™ and Harmonic® in laparoscopic sleeve gastrectomy: a single-center experience on 422 patients. J Obes. 2019;2019:3402137.
52. Chekan E, Whelan RL. Surgical stapling device-tissue interactions: what surgeons need to know to improve patient outcomes. Med Devices (Auckl). 2014;7:305–18.
53. Gencturk M, Dalkilic MS, Erdem H, Yılmaz M, Sisik A. Correct stapling technique in laparoscopic sleeve gastrectomy: are we increasing the bleeding? A prospective cohort study. J Laparoendosc Adv Surg Tech A. 2023;33(6):561–5.
54. Roy S, Yoo A, Yadalam S, Fegelman EJ, Kalsekar I, Johnston SS. Comparison of economic and clinical outcomes between patients undergoing laparoscopic bariatric surgery with powered versus manual endoscopic surgical staplers. J Med Econ. 2017;20(4):423–33.

55. Gagner M, Deitel M, Erickson AL, Crosby RD. Survey on laparoscopic sleeve gastrectomy (LSG) at the fourth international consensus summit on sleeve gastrectomy. Obes Surg. 2013;23(12):2013–7.
56. Aiolfi A, Gagner M, Zappa MA, Lastraioli C, Lombardo F, Panizzo V, et al. Staple line reinforcement during laparoscopic sleeve gastrectomy: systematic review and network meta-analysis of randomized controlled trials. Obes Surg. 2022;32(5):1466–78.
57. Choi YY, Bae J, Hur KY, Choi D, Kim YJ. Reinforcing the staple line during laparoscopic sleeve gastrectomy: does it have advantages? A meta-analysis. Obes Surg. 2012;22(8):1206–13.
58. Simon TE, Scott JA, Brockmeyer JR, Rice RC, Frizzi JD, Husain FA, et al. Comparison of staple-line leakage and hemorrhage in patients undergoing laparoscopic sleeve gastrectomy with or without Seamguard. Am Surg. 2011;77(12):1665–8.
59. Ali A, Morris L, Hodges J, Amirkhosravi F, Yasrebi S, Khoo A, et al. Postoperative bleeding and leaks in sleeve gastrectomy are independent of both staple height and staple line oversewing. Surg Endosc. 2022;36:1–7.
60. Musella M, Milone M, Maietta P, Bianco P, Pisapia A, Gaudioso D. Laparoscopic sleeve gastrectomy: efficacy of fibrin sealant in reducing postoperative bleeding. A randomized controlled trial. Updates Surg. 2014;66(3):197–201.
61. Chen YS, Loh EW, Shen SC, Su YH, Tam KW. Efficacy of fibrin sealant in reducing complication risk after bariatric surgery: a systematic review and meta-analysis. Obes Surg. 2021;31(3):1158–67.
62. Rebibo L, Dhahri A, Chati R, Cosse C, Huet E, Regimbeau JM. Effectiveness of fibrin sealant application on the development of staple line complications after sleeve gastrectomy: a prospective randomized trial. Ann Surg. 2018;268(5):762–8.
63. De Angelis F, Abdelgawad M, Rizzello M, Mattia C, Silecchia G. Perioperative hemorrhagic complications after laparoscopic sleeve gastrectomy: four-year experience of a bariatric center of excellence. Surg Endosc. 2017;31(9):3547–51.
64. Pavone G, Gerundo A, Pacilli M, Fersini A, Ambrosi A, Tartaglia N. Bariatric surgery: to bleed or not to bleed? This is the question. BMC Surg. 2022;22(1):331.
65. Sroka G, Milevski D, Shteinberg D, Mady H, Matter I. Minimizing hemorrhagic complications in laparoscopic sleeve gastrectomy—a randomized controlled trial. Obes Surg. 2015;25(9):1577–83.
66. Kitahama S, Smith MD, Rosencrantz DR, Patterson EJ. Is bariatric surgery safe in patients who refuse blood transfusion? Surg Obes Relat Dis. 2013;9(3):390–4.
67. Sayburn A. Jehovah's witnesses and surgery. Bull R Coll Surg Engl. 2019;101(1):16–9.
68. Hanif S, Abdulla A, Sharma O, Wiggins T, Charalampakis V, Singhal R. Safety and feasibility of bariatric surgery in Jehovah's witness patients: protocols from a single surgeon practice. Obes Surg. 2024;34(1):280–1.
69. Gerin O, Rebibo L, Dhahri A, Regimbeau JM. The safety of laparoscopic sleeve gastrectomy in patients receiving chronic anticoagulation therapy: a case-matched study. Obes Surg. 2015;25(9):1686–92.
70. Shea B, Motamedi SMK, Mustafa R, Masnyj S, Sarode A, Abbas M, et al. (S029) Managing therapeutic anticoagulation in bariatric surgery patients. Surg Endosc. 2021;35(8):4779–85.

# Staple Line and Anastomotic Leaks

# 30

Edmund W. Lee and Konstantinos Spaniolas

## Introduction

Bariatric operations involve manipulation of the alimentary tract. Any staple line or gastrointestinal leak is a significant cause of morbidity in bariatric surgery. This includes increased hospital stay, discharge to rehabilitation facilities, and mortality [1–3]. Leaks are associated with a case mortality rate of approximately 5% [3]. Rates of leaks vary in the literature depending on the time of publication. As bariatric surgery evolved from open to laparoscopic, reported leak rates have overall decreased over time. Currently, leaks occur from 0.1 to 5.3% [4–8]. Any location that requires a division or anastomosis is a potential source for leak. Specific locations are reported in Table 30.1. Sleeve gastrectomy has a reported staple line leak rate of approximately 0.2–1.5% [8–11].

In a Roux-en-Y gastric bypass (RYGB), the vast majority of leaks occur proximally at the gastrojejunostomy (49–77%) [3, 12]. Other sites occur at varying frequencies depending on the series including the remnant stomach (25%), jejunojejunostomy (2–13%), and gastric pouch (9–10%) [3, 12].

In a meta-analysis of single center comparisons, the duodenal switch had a higher proximal leak rate (sleeve, duodenal bulb, duodenoileal anastomosis) 5.0% versus the RYGB 2.2% [13].

Management is dictated based on the patient's clinical condition and hemodynamics, type of surgery, timing of the current event, and extent of the leak. Data on leaks including presentation, workup, and therapies are mostly based on retrospective series, meta-analyses of these series, and investigations of databases. Randomized controlled trials would be very challenging because leak rates overall

E. W. Lee (✉) · K. Spaniolas
Department of Surgery, Stony Brook University, Stony Brook, NY, USA
e-mail: edmund.lee@stonybrookmedicine.edu



O. M. Ghanem et al. (eds.), *The SAGES Manual of Metabolic and Bariatric Surgery*, https://doi.org/10.1007/978-3-031-72309-4_30

**Table 30.1** Possible leak sites in bariatric procedures

| Surgery | Potential sites of leakage |
|---|---|
| Sleeve gastrectomy | • Gastric staple line |
| One-anastomosis gastric bypass | • Gastric staple line<br>• Gastrojejunal anastomosis |
| Roux-en-Y gastric bypass | • Gastric pouch staple line<br>• Gastrojejunal anastomosis<br>• Candy cane<br>• Jejunojejunal anastomosis<br>• Remnant stomach |
| Single-anastomosis duodenoileal bypass | • Gastric staple line<br>• Duodenoileal anastomosis<br>• Duodenal stump |
| Biliopancreatic diversion with duodenal switch | • Gastric staple line<br>• Duodenoileal anastomosis<br>• Ileoileal anastomosis<br>• Duodenal stump |

have decreased over time. At the conclusion of this chapter, the evidence-based etiologies leading to leaks, principles of management including nonsurgical and surgical, and current evidence on leak prevention will be reviewed.

## Etiology

The pathophysiology of leaks is multifactorial. Concepts in general surgical wound healing apply to bariatric cases as well. Preoperative nutritional status, use of corticosteroids, and smoking status can impact the risk for leaks [14]. Similarly, common principles of anastomotic leaks in general surgery also apply to understanding etiologies of leaks such as: excessive tension on the anastomosis, poor perfusion, or presence of distal obstruction.

Staple-line leaks can be broadly grouped into two categories: mechanical/tissue causes and ischemic causes [15]. Early leaks occurring postoperative day (POD) 1–3 are thought to be more technical in etiology (i.e., failure in technique or stapler technology and device), when collagen levels are at their lowest and the tissue is most dependent on staples/sutures. Classic ischemic leaks generally occur around POD 5–7, when wound healing transitions from inflammation to fibrosis.

Although the classic phases of wound healing (inflammation, proliferation, remodeling) were described in skin and soft tissue wound healing, healing in the gastrointestinal tract mirrors this. During the first few postoperative days, collagenase activity is high, leading to initial collagen degradation and low anastomotic strength. Therefore, the anastomosis is dependent on suture- and staple-holding strength [16]. After 3–4 days, collagen synthesis occurs rapidly and small bowel anastomosis strength approaches unwounded tissue at approximately 4 weeks after surgery [16, 17]. Any prolongation or augmentation of the phases of wound healing (i.e., systemic steroid use, poor perfusion, infection) can conceptually affect anastomotic and staple-line healing.

Sleeve gastrectomy leaks typically occur at the proximal staple line at the angle of His. They are thought to arise from a combination of ischemia, elevated pressure within the stomach, and relative distal obstruction. The division of the blood supply to the fundus via the short gastric vessels creates a relative high-risk area at the angle of His. Using a postoperative computed tomography (CT scan), a study showed significantly decreased perfusion at the angle of His when compared to other locations [18]. A 2008 study measured intraoperative basal and saline-filled stomach pressures before and after a sleeve gastrectomy and demonstrated significantly reduced distensibility of the sleeved stomach [19]. Stenosis at the incisura or pylorus can create anatomical choke points, further elevating proximal stomach pressures. Therefore, the synergy of relative ischemia of the angle of His, elevated postoperative pressures in a less-distensible stomach, and distal choke points can set up the proximal staple-line for a leak. Given that wound healing is more dependent on the integrity of the staple line during the early postoperative days, early sleeve leaks are more attributed to technical considerations such as the narrowing of the stomach at the incisura and the mechanical integrity of the staple line.

Small intestine anastomosis leaks are currently explained with general surgical principles. Tension between the inflow and outflow when bringing the stomach inferiorly and small intestine superiorly can stress staple- or suture-lines; especially early, when anastomoses have the least collagen. The division of the small intestine mesentery could set up relative ischemia of the proximal roux limb. In contrast with sleeve staple lines, the anastomosis in any bariatric procedure is in a relatively low-pressure system. However, relative distal obstruction from either a jejunojejunostomy or ileoileostomy can also apply pressure on proximal anastomoses.

## Presentation and Evaluation

One must have a high suspicion for a leak in the perioperative setting. The first clinical sign of a leak is often tachycardia. A previous retrospective study demonstrated in stepwise logistic regression that tachycardia greater than 120 bpm and respiratory distress were independent indicators of a leak [20]. The patient may have worsening abdominal pain and/or difficulty with oral intake. Peritonitis on physical exam is not reliably present in postoperative patients [20]. This can particularly be the case for patients with significant excess weight and difficult physical exams.

Initial laboratory workup may show an increasing leukocytosis and a lactic acidosis, reflecting sepsis [21]. There is evidence for use of serum C-Reactive Protein (CRP) in the early detection of colorectal anastomotic leaks, prompting an investigation into its use in bariatric leak detection. Timepoints range between POD 1–5 and cutoffs range from 71 to 225 mg/L [22, 23]. The most cited retrospective study showed that CRP > 225 mg/L on $POD_2$ has a sensitivity of 53% and specificity of 91% for postoperative complications and a sensitivity of 100% for anastomotic leaks [22]. The authors suggested that CRP could be used to select which patients to pursue imaging studies. Based on a recent systematic review and meta-analysis, the use of CRP has the highest specificity on POD1 and highest sensitivity on POD5 [23]. However, in modern enhanced recovery protocols, patients are discharged as early as POD 0–1. In addition, early detection of leaks is paramount to avoid significant morbidity and a patient with high suspicion of a possible leak will receive an imaging study regardless of CRP levels. Therefore, the only practical utility for serum CRP would seem to be to rule-out any complication in the early postoperative period.

Imaging studies involve an oral contrast study. These include an Upper Gastrointestinal Series (UGI) and a computed tomography (CT) with oral and intravenous contrast. Figure 30.1 shows extravasation of oral contrast into the left pleural space. In a systematic review and meta-analysis, the sensitivity and specificity of an UGI was found to be 54% and 100% respectively [24]. The use of high-density barium as opposed to water-soluble gastrografin may improve leak detection rate [25]. A retrospective study found that in symptomatic patients, CT had a higher sensitivity and specificity than UGI (95% and 100% vs 79% and 95%) [26]. However, in a series of 3018 patients who underwent a Roux-en-Y gastric bypass, UGI and CT were positive in only 30% and 56% of patients who had leaks [12]. When combined, both studies were still negative in 30% of patients who had leaks. This high false-negative rate shows the value of continued vigilance and clinical evaluation of the patient as opposed to relying solely on radiologic findings.

Typically the imaging of choice is based on individual institutions and availability of each other modalities. An UGI is often more time-intensive for both the patient and radiologist, who is present at the time of imaging. A CT scan has a

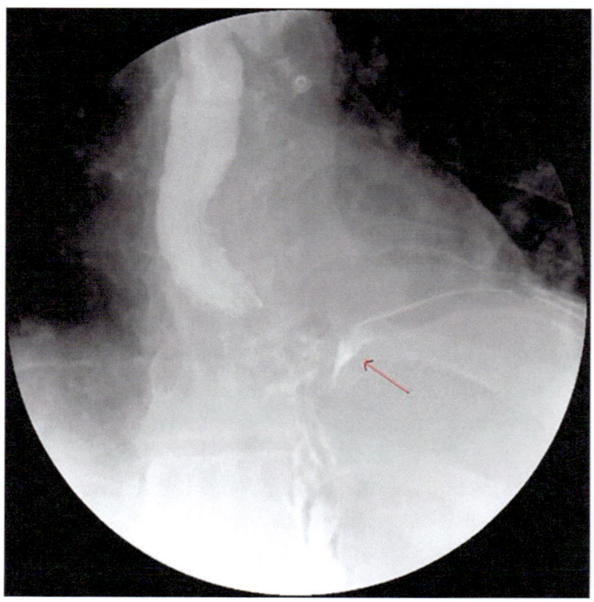

**Fig. 30.1** Upper GI Series of a sleeve gastrectomy leak into left pleural space drained with chest tube (arrow)

theoretical increased risk of aspiration, given the supine positioning. However, a CT scan can also evaluate a distal anastomosis such as a jejunojejunal or ileoileal anastomosis. Due to the proximal nature of the majority of leaks and the rapid flow of contrast through sleeves and gastrojejunal anastomoses, on-table oral contrast (where patient swallows contrast just before laying supine) should be administered to patients undergoing CT scan.

In general, routine postoperative imaging remains facility- and practitioner-dependent. There is mounting evidence that questions its routine use [27]. Given its low sensitivity in asymptomatic patients, one retrospective review demonstrated the utilization of imaging would decrease by 82%, resulting in cost-savings for the hospital [28]. In another study, routine UGI studies on POD2 were negative in two out of three gastrojejunostomy leaks [29]. Many UGIs, in this study, yielded false positives, which may prompt unnecessary prolonged hospitalizations or interventions. This data does not support routine postoperative imaging unless patients are symptomatic.

## Management

Management of leaks should consider core general surgical principles: source control, drainage, antibiotics, and nutritional support. Initially if leak is suspected, patients should be made nil per os (NPO) and broad spectrum antibiotics should be initiated. Further interventions are guided by patient factors: the patient's clinical status and stability, the size and containment of the leak, and the timing with respect to the initial surgery. For example, unstable patients in the perioperative period should be taken promptly for operative management. A combination of different strategies can be employed to manage leaks (Table 30.2).

## Nonoperative Management

Patients presenting hemodynamically stable with small abscesses or contained leaks can be managed nonoperatively. In a retrospective review, authors demonstrated that patients selectively treated nonoperatively with NPO, antibiotics, and total parenteral nutrition (TPN) were likely to resolve their leaks following gastric bypass [30]. If accessible, placement of a percutaneous drain could be considered to get source control of the infection. Figure 30.1 shows a sleeve gastrectomy leak drained with a chest tube. Resolution can be determined by assessing patient clinical status and with a negative radiologic study. In the previous study, median time to radiologic resolution was 17 days, which is a significant extension in hospital stay when compared with modern enhanced recovery pathways.

**Table 30.2** Management options for leaks

| Intervention | Management options |
|---|---|
| Nonoperative | • NPO, antibiotics, TPN<br>• Percutaneous drainage |
| Endoscopic | • Internal drainage<br>– Double-pigtail catheter<br>– Vacuum therapy<br>• Closure<br>– Over-the-scope clip<br>– Endoscopic suturing<br>• Wall defect exclusion<br>– Stent<br>• Distal feeding access<br>– Jejunostomy feeding tube |
| Operative | • Drainage<br>– Irrigation and surgical drain<br>– T-tube placement<br>• Closure<br>– Oversewing defect, omentoplasty<br>• Revision<br>– Revision of anastomosis<br>– Conversion to Gastrojejunostomy<br>• Distal feeding access<br>– Jejunostomy tube<br>– Remnant gastrostomy tube |

## Endoscopic Management

Faster resolution of a leak may be achieved with better source control. For proximal leaks (sleeve gastrectomy, gastrojejunostomy, duodenoileostomy), there have been several different tools utilized.

For **small, contained** leaks or abscesses, endoscopic internal drainage (double-pigtail catheter, transfistulary endoscopic drainage, endoscopic vacuum therapy) may be a good option [31–33]. This is advantageous for collections that cannot be accessed percutaneously. In addition, internal drainage may allow for earlier removal of surgical drains, avoiding fistulization [33]. Endoscopic vacuum therapy can be utilized for larger defects and can hasten the healing of leaks with rapid granulation [34]. However, it requires multiple reassessment and reinsertions in the endoscopy suite and a persistent nasogastric tube to supply the suction. It should not be used in patients who may not tolerate multiple anesthetic episodes or with patients who are intolerant of prolonged nasogastric tubes.

For **moderate leaks** or smaller leaks which fail to close with internal drainage, one could consider endoscopic closure methods [31, 35]. The two main types are endoscopic suturing and over-the-scope (OTS) clips. The technique employed depends on institutional availability and expertise. Smaller leaks can be closed with over-the-scope (OTS) clips. Larger leaks can be sutured closed. However, one must consider the original etiology of the leak. Anastomotic breakdown from ischemia may not heal with these closure techniques, as it may exacerbate the ischemia over the existing defect. Furthermore, for small or moderate **uncontained leaks**, a primary attempt at endoscopic closure may be preferential over internal drainage. If primary endoscopic closure is not feasible, in the setting of ill-defined containment, defect exclusion (with endoscopic stent placement) may be warranted to provide source control; this may be exchanged subsequently for internal drainage if conditions become more favorable. In such cases of endoscopic closure, infection lavage may be performed either endoscopically or via percutaneous drainage.

**Larger leaks** can be managed with wall defect exclusion via self-expandable metal stents (Fig. 30.2). The advantage to stents is that with exclusion, patients should be able to resume oral intake. Stents are replaced every 4–6 weeks until resolution. The most common complication from stents is migration. Migration rates vary in the literature, ranging from 5 to 67% [31]. Stent securement with sutures or clips may decrease the risk of migration. Currently, there are two kinds of stents: metal or polyester. Metal stents are easier to insert due to its flexibility and smaller caliber. They conceptually have a higher friction coefficient; however, migration rates between both types are similar [31]. Stenting sleeve gastrectomies are particularly challenging due to difficulties in establishing landing zones. More recently, larger stents have been adapted to accommodate sleeve anatomy.

For the successful endoscopic management of leaks, evaluation and management of distal obstructions and strictures is a key concept. This can be the case for patients with proximal sleeve leaks and distal sleeve strictures or twists. These distal irregularities may be addressed with pneumatic dilation and endoluminal stenting, in the early period.

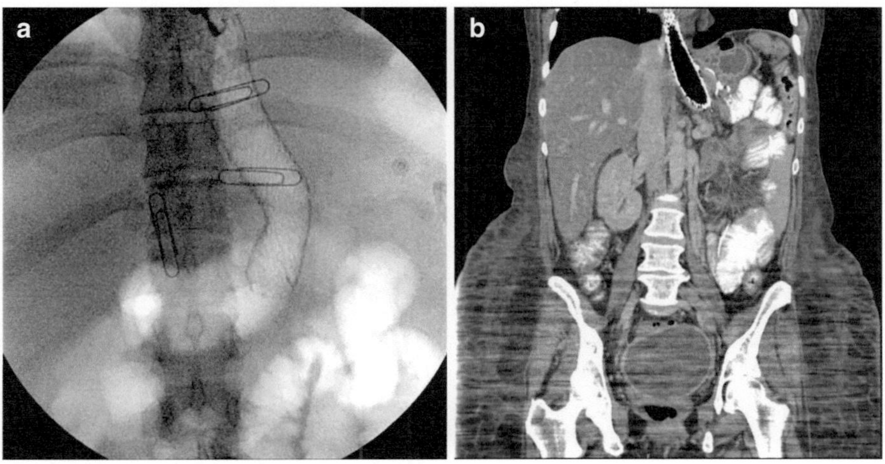


**Fig. 30.2** Endoscopic stent placement over a sleeve gastrectomy (**a**, UGI) and esophagojejunostomy (**b**, CT) leak

Depending on modalities employed and patient condition, the placement of a jejunostomy feeding tube could be considered, especially in larger defects not managed successfully with a few trials of endoscopic closure. Feeding access can be achieved transnasally or percutaneously (endoscopic or surgically placed).

## Operative Management

General surgical principles and understanding the etiologies of leaks guide the operative management of a patient. As stated above, source control, drainage, and distal feeding access guide the extent of intervention.

The minimum goal of surgical intervention is irrigation and placement of an intra-abdominal drain. Depending on the extent of adhesions, fibrinous material, and inflamed tissue integrity, it may be difficult to close the defect. Placing a T-Tube into the defect in addition to an intra-abdominal drain can control the drainage, allowing it to form a fistula [36]. If the tissue is amenable, primary closure is preferable to T-Tube insertion and fistulá formation.

The intraoperative decision to primarily close a defect or revise an anastomosis is very challenging. The operator is constantly evaluating the tissue, examining the suture- or staple-line, and possibly employing adjuncts, like indocyanine green (ICG) fluorescence. One must always consider the underlying etiology of the leak before considering definitive repair. If the core cause of the leak is ischemia, oversewing may worsen the ischemia and may only temporarily treat the leak before opening again. For example, a POD6 gastrojejunal leak found to have sutures pulled through dark tissue edges should raise suspicion for ischemic etiology and consideration of revision of the anastomosis or alternative approaches is warranted. However, a remnant stomach leak is more likely to be a technical issue such as stapler failure and may be more amenable to primary closure.

If all attempts to salvage the anatomy failed, the sleeve gastrectomy or duodenal switch can be converted to a Roux-en-Y gastric bypass anatomy. Fistulojejunostomy can also be considered to surgically address proximal staple line leak in sleeve gastrectomy. Conversion of sleeve gastrectomy to RYGB will convert a high-pressure, nondistensible stomach into a low-pressure system. Given that most sleeve leaks occur at the angle of His, an esophagojejunal anastomosis may be required. Esophagojejunal anastomoses have higher leak rates and mortality rates reported in the literature [37], likely from even more precarious blood supplies than gastrojejunal anastomoses.

## Combination Treatments

Gastrointestinal leaks following bariatric procedures can be very challenging clinical entities combining both high level technical and medical complexities. In order to optimize patient outcomes through this part of the recovery, combination approaches may be warranted. The clinician needs to remain vigilant and thinking broadly about treatment modalities and options. Combining surgical techniques for abdominal lavage and feeding access, concurrently with endoscopic procedures for source control can be a winning combination for the right patient, especially in light of severe sepsis. In other cases, staged approaches with different endoscopic modalities could provide an optimal outcome.

## Prevention

Minimizing leaks can be achieved with both patient preparation and surgical technique. A review of the Metabolic and Bariatric Surgery Accreditation and Quality Improvement Program (MBSAQIP) database found that the strongest predictors for leaks were body mass index (BMI), albumin, and age [38]. Although age is a non-modifiable risk factor, BMI and albumin could possibly be augmented through nutritional optimization and preoperative weight loss.

The learning curve of a technique plays a role in leaks. In a review of 11,800 sleeve gastrectomies, the authors found that yearly leak rates from sleeve gastrectomy decreased from 6.5 to 0.9% from 2007 to 2013 [10]. This stresses the importance of surgical technique that has been refined over the years. In a review of 750 RYGB cases, increased experience (about 100 cases) was associated with decreased operative times and technical-related complications [39].

The use of fibrin sealant as leak prophylaxis has been proposed, but the data does not support its use in this manner. Initial retrospective data showed no leaks in the areas where fibrin sealant was applied [40]. Preliminary data from a randomized control trial showed no significant difference in leak rates between the control group and fibrin sealant group and a subsequent publication from the same trial confirmed their initial findings [41, 42]. In a systematic review and meta-analysis of nine randomized control trials, fibrin sealant was shown to decrease the incidence of bleeding, but not leaks [43]. Therefore, there is no high-quality evidence for the use of fibrin sealants in bariatric surgery to prevent leaks.

Indocyanine green fluorescence imaging (ICG) has been utilized in a variety of ways in bariatric surgery. To date, there is no consensus on its use nor has there been strong evidence to support its routine use. ICG has been given intraluminally as a mechanism for leak testing [44]. A small cohort study used intravenous ICG to evaluate tissue perfusion at the gastrojejunal anastomosis [45]. Of the 30 patients, one demonstrated an ischemic area, which was confirmed with a positive methylene blue leak test, and was subsequently reinforced. Another small cohort study used intravenous ICG to evaluate gastric pouch perfusion in revisional bariatric surgery and found that none of the findings from the ICG angiography changed surgical strategy [46]. A systematic review of these small cohort studies showed the use of ICG (either intraluminally or intravenously) has changed intraoperative surgical decision making in 3.8% of patients [47]. It is impossible to form actionable conclusions from the available data.

## Sleeve Gastrectomy

It is important to size staple-load thickness appropriately. Conceptually, choosing a thinner stapler load may create a tighter staple line, but excessive compression may contribute to ischemia and introduce a weak point within the staple line. The stomach is thicker in the prepyloric region than in the fundus [48, 49]. Therefore, one should consider a thicker staple load distally, during the initial portions of the sleeve.

Larger bougie sizes were associated with significant decreases in incidence of leak without changes in weight loss [11]. In the largest study, using data from the MBSAQIP, a bougie size of 38F or greater was associated with decreased leak rates [7]. In fact, a bougie size of 40F or greater had a significantly higher percent excess BMI reduction [7]. A systemic analysis of 4888 sleeve gastrectomies found a bougie size 40F or greater was associated with a leak rate of 0.6% whereas smaller sizes were associated with a leak rate of 2.8% [50]. However, in another systematic review, bougie size had a weak linear correlation with leak rates ($r = -0.23$, $p = 0.4$) [51].

The impact of staple-line reinforcement (SLR) on leaks is mixed in the literature. In the large MBSAQIP study, leak rates were higher in the SLR cases (0.96% vs 0.65%) [7]. Another study showed no impact of buttressing materials [11]. However, in a study of cadaveric porcine stomach, ePTFE reinforcement increased the leak/bursting pressures when compared with no reinforcement [15]. A systematic review of the literature demonstrated a significantly lower leak rate with absorbable polymer membrane (APM) reinforcement when compared with bovine pericardial strips and no reinforcement [52]. In a follow-up study, the authors sought to compare the different types of reinforcement: no staple-line reinforcement (NO-SLR), suture oversewing alone (suture), bovine pericardial strips (BPS), tissue sealant (seal), and absorbable polymer membrane (APM) [53]. They found a significantly lower leak rate for the APM reinforcement (0.73%) when compared to the other modalities (suture 1.21%, NO-SLR 1.89%, seal 1.89%, and BPS 2.73%). In fact, the leak rate between the use of tissue sealant was comparable to no staple-line reinforcement at all ($p = 0.271$). The use of SLR is still up to the discretion of the surgeon.

Despite the mixed evidence, one theme is consistent in the literature: it is better to have no reinforcement at all than to both reinforce and oversew the staple line. In a single-centered study, the authors observed that both oversewing and the use of reinforcement was associated with higher leak rate [10]. This phenomenon was reproducible in the MBSAQIP study [7].

Staple-line distance from the pylorus did not impact leak rates [7, 11]. The authors categorized patients into pyloric distances of <4, 4–5, 5–6, ≥6 cm and found no differences in morbidity, leak rates, or bleed rates.

## Roux-en-Y Gastric Bypass

There is no difference in leak rates between hand-sewn versus stapled anastomoses. Initial retrospective studies showed no differences in leak rates between a hand-sewn, linear-stapled, and circular-stapled anastomosis despite an increased postoperative wound infection rate with a circular-stapled anastomosis [54–56]. A randomized trial with 119 hand-sewn and 119 circular-stapled anastomoses demonstrated no differences in leak rates, but a higher frequency of gastrointestinal bleeding (4.2% vs 0%) and wound infection (11.1% vs 3.4%) in the circular-stapled group [57]. More recently, a meta-analysis comparing the three different anastomosis types found that a hand-sewn anastomosis had a lower incidence of bleeding and wound infection when compared with a circular-stapled anastomosis. There was no differences between a hand-sewn and linear-stapled anastomosis [58].

## Conclusion

Staple line and anastomotic leaks are feared complications for a bariatric surgeon. From additional repetitions and improved operative technique, the rates of these complications have decreased over time. It remains a significant source of morbidity and sometimes mortality for patients. Constant vigilance of early signs (tachycardia, leukocytosis, and clinical symptoms for leaks) should trigger prompt imaging with PO contrast. Utilizing the foundation of wound healing principles, the etiology of leaks differs between a sleeve gastrectomy and an anastomotic surgery. This informs the different interventional options; emphasizing that one must always consider the underlying cause of the leak before committing to a specific approach. Developing operative strategies prevent leak is imperative. Because leak rates are low, prospective studies will become more difficult to conduct and the reliance on large database-based approaches will continue to drive improvements in this sector.

## References


1. Lee SW, Gregory D, Cool CL. Clinical and economic burden of colorectal and bariatric anastomotic leaks. Surg Endosc. 2020;34:4374–81. https://doi.org/10.1007/s00464-019-07210-1.
2. Nedelcu M, Manos T, Gagner M, et al. Cost analysis of leak after sleeve gastrectomy. Surg Endosc. 2017;31:4446–50. https://doi.org/10.1007/s00464-017-5495-z.
3. Carucci LR, Turner MA, Conklin RC, et al. Roux-en-Y gastric bypass surgery for morbid obesity: evaluation of postoperative extraluminal leaks with upper gastrointestinal series. Radiology. 2006;238:119–27. https://doi.org/10.1148/radiol.2381041557.
4. Hutter MM, Schirmer BD, Jones DB, et al. First report from the American College of Surgeons Bariatric Surgery Center Network: laparoscopic sleeve gastrectomy has morbidity and effectiveness positioned between the band and the bypass. Ann Surg. 2011;254:410–20; discussion 420–2. https://doi.org/10.1097/SLA.0b013e31822c9dac.
5. Gonzalez R, Nelson LG, Gallagher SF, Murr MM. Anastomotic leaks after laparoscopic gastric bypass. Obes Surg. 2004;14:1299–307. https://doi.org/10.1381/0960892042583978.
6. Marshall JS, Srivastava A, Gupta SK, et al. Roux-en-Y gastric bypass leak complications. Arch Surg. 2003;138:520–3; discussion 523–4. https://doi.org/10.1001/archsurg.138.5.520.
7. Berger ER, Clements RH, Morton JM, et al. The impact of different surgical techniques on outcomes in laparoscopic sleeve gastrectomies: the first report from the metabolic and bariatric surgery accreditation and quality improvement program (MBSAQIP). Ann Surg. 2016;264:464–73. https://doi.org/10.1097/SLA.0000000000001851.

8. Clapp B, Corbett J, Ahmad M, et al. When do leaks occur? An analysis of the metabolic and bariatric surgery accreditation and quality improvement program. Surg Obes Relat Dis. 2023;19:1128–33. https://doi.org/10.1016/j.soard.2023.04.334.
9. Rosenthal RJ, International Sleeve Gastrectomy Expert Panel, Diaz AA, et al. International sleeve gastrectomy expert panel consensus statement: best practice guidelines based on experience of >12,000 cases. Surg Obes Relat Dis. 2012;8:8–19. https://doi.org/10.1016/j.soard.2011.10.019.
10. Stroh C, Köckerling F, Volker L, et al. Results of more than 11,800 sleeve gastrectomies: data analysis of the German bariatric surgery registry. Ann Surg. 2016;263:949–55. https://doi.org/10.1097/SLA.0000000000001559.
11. Parikh M, Issa R, McCrillis A, et al. Surgical strategies that may decrease leak after laparoscopic sleeve gastrectomy: a systematic review and meta-analysis of 9991 cases. Ann Surg. 2013;257:231–7. https://doi.org/10.1097/SLA.0b013e31826cc714.
12. Gonzalez R, Sarr MG, Smith CD, et al. Diagnosis and contemporary management of anastomotic leaks after gastric bypass for obesity. J Am Coll Surg. 2007;204:47–55. https://doi.org/10.1016/j.jamcollsurg.2006.09.023.
13. Hedberg J, Sundström J, Sundbom M. Duodenal switch versus Roux-en-Y gastric bypass for morbid obesity: systematic review and meta-analysis of weight results, diabetes resolution and early complications in single-centre comparisons. Obes Rev. 2014;15:555–63. https://doi.org/10.1111/obr.12169.
14. Janik MR, Aryaie AH. The effect of smoking on bariatric surgical 30-day outcomes: propensity-score-matched analysis of the MBSAQIP. Surg Endosc. 2021;35:3905–14. https://doi.org/10.1007/s00464-020-07838-4.
15. Baker RS, Foote J, Kemmeter P, et al. The science of stapling and leaks. Obes Surg. 2004;14:1290–8. https://doi.org/10.1381/0960892042583888.
16. Thompson SK, Chang EY, Jobe BA. Clinical review: healing in gastrointestinal anastomoses, part I. Microsurgery. 2006;26:131–6. https://doi.org/10.1002/micr.20197.
17. Martens MF, Hendriks T. Postoperative changes in collagen synthesis in intestinal anastomoses of the rat: differences between small and large bowel. Gut. 1991;32:1482–7. https://doi.org/10.1136/gut.32.12.1482.
18. Saber AA, Azar N, Dekal M, Abdelbaki TN. Computed tomographic scan mapping of gastric wall perfusion and clinical implications. Am J Surg. 2015;209:999–1006. https://doi.org/10.1016/j.amjsurg.2014.05.023.
19. Yehoshua RT, Eidelman LA, Stein M, et al. Laparoscopic sleeve gastrectomy—volume and pressure assessment. Obes Surg. 2008;18:1083–8. https://doi.org/10.1007/s11695-008-9576-x.
20. Hamilton EC, Sims TL, Hamilton TT, et al. Clinical predictors of leak after laparoscopic Roux-en-Y gastric bypass for morbid obesity. Surg Endosc. 2003;17:679–84. https://doi.org/10.1007/s00464-002-8819-5.
21. Evans L, Rhodes A, Alhazzani W, et al. Surviving sepsis campaign: international guidelines for management of sepsis and septic shock 2021. Crit Care Med. 2021;49:e1063–143. https://doi.org/10.1097/CCM.0000000000005337.
22. Warschkow R, Tarantino I, Folie P, et al. C-reactive protein 2 days after laparoscopic gastric bypass surgery reliably indicates leaks and moderately predicts morbidity. J Gastrointest Surg. 2012;16:1128–35. https://doi.org/10.1007/s11605-012-1882-x.
23. Lee Y, McKechnie T, Doumouras AG, et al. Diagnostic value of C-reactive protein levels in postoperative infectious complications after bariatric surgery: a systematic review and meta-analysis. Obes Surg. 2019;29:2022–9. https://doi.org/10.1007/s11695-019-03832-5.
24. Mbadiwe T, Prevatt E, Duerinckx A, et al. Assessing the value of routine upper gastrointestinal contrast studies following bariatric surgery: a systematic review and meta-analysis. Am J Surg. 2015;209:616–22. https://doi.org/10.1016/j.amjsurg.2014.11.007.
25. Swanson JO, Levine MS, Redfern RO, Rubesin SE. Usefulness of high-density barium for detection of leaks after esophagogastrectomy, total gastrectomy, and total laryngectomy. AJR Am J Roentgenol. 2003;181:415–20. https://doi.org/10.2214/ajr.181.2.1810415.

26. Bingham J, Shawhan R, Parker R, et al. Computed tomography scan versus upper gastrointestinal fluoroscopy for diagnosis of staple line leak following bariatric surgery. Am J Surg. 2015;209:810–4; discussion 814. https://doi.org/10.1016/j.amjsurg.2015.01.004.
27. White S, Han SH, Lewis C, et al. Selective approach to use of upper gastroesophageal imaging study after laparoscopic Roux-en-Y gastric bypass. Surg Obes Relat Dis. 2008;4:122–5. https://doi.org/10.1016/j.soard.2007.10.007.
28. Singh R, Fisher BL. Sensitivity and specificity of postoperative upper GI series following gastric bypass. Obes Surg. 2003;13:73–5. https://doi.org/10.1381/096089203321136629.
29. Doraiswamy A, Rasmussen JJ, Pierce J, et al. The utility of routine postoperative upper GI series following laparoscopic gastric bypass. Surg Endosc. 2007;21:2159–62. https://doi.org/10.1007/s00464-007-9314-9.
30. Thodiyil PA, Yenumula P, Rogula T, et al. Selective nonoperative management of leaks after gastric bypass: lessons learned from 2675 consecutive patients. Ann Surg. 2008;248:782–92. https://doi.org/10.1097/SLA.0b013e31818584aa.
31. Souto-Rodríguez R, Alvarez-Sánchez M-V. Endoluminal solutions to bariatric surgery complications: a review with a focus on technical aspects and results. World J Gastrointest Endosc. 2017;9:105–26. https://doi.org/10.4253/wjge.v9.i3.105.
32. Bouchard S, Eisendrath P, Toussaint E, et al. Trans-fistulary endoscopic drainage for post-bariatric abdominal collections communicating with the upper gastrointestinal tract. Endoscopy. 2016;48:809–16. https://doi.org/10.1055/s-0042-108726.
33. Donatelli G, Dumont J-L, Cereatti F, et al. Treatment of leaks following sleeve gastrectomy by endoscopic internal drainage (EID). Obes Surg. 2015;25:1293–301. https://doi.org/10.1007/s11695-015-1675-x.
34. Markus A, Henrik BJ, Benedikt R, et al. Endoscopic vacuum therapy in salvage and standalone treatment of gastric leaks after bariatric surgery. Langenbecks Arch Surg. 2022;407:1039–46. https://doi.org/10.1007/s00423-021-02365-9.
35. Valli PV, Gubler C. Review article including treatment algorithm: endoscopic treatment of luminal complications after bariatric surgery. Clin Obes. 2017;7:115–22. https://doi.org/10.1111/cob.12182.
36. Tan JT, Kariyawasam S, Wijeratne T, Chandraratna HS. Diagnosis and management of gastric leaks after laparoscopic sleeve gastrectomy for morbid obesity. Obes Surg. 2010;20:403–9. https://doi.org/10.1007/s11695-009-0020-7.
37. Trapani R, Rausei S, Reddavid R, et al. Risk factors for esophago-jejunal anastomosis leakage after total gastrectomy for cancer. A multicenter retrospective study of the Italian research group for gastric cancer. Eur J Surg Oncol. 2020;46:2243–7. https://doi.org/10.1016/j.ejso.2020.06.035.
38. Kumar SB, Hamilton BC, Wood SG, et al. Is laparoscopic sleeve gastrectomy safer than laparoscopic gastric bypass? A comparison of 30-day complications using the MBSAQIP data registry. Surg Obes Relat Dis. 2018;14:264–9. https://doi.org/10.1016/j.soard.2017.12.011.
39. Schauer P, Ikramuddin S, Hamad G, Gourash W. The learning curve for laparoscopic Roux-en-Y gastric bypass is 100 cases. Surg Endosc. 2003;17:212–5. https://doi.org/10.1007/s00464-002-8857-z.
40. Sapala JA, Wood MH, Schuhknecht MP. Anastomotic leak prophylaxis using a vapor-heated fibrin sealant: report on 738 gastric bypass patients. Obes Surg. 2004;14:35–42. https://doi.org/10.1381/096089204772787266.
41. Silecchia G, Boru CE, Mouiel J, et al. Clinical evaluation of fibrin glue in the prevention of anastomotic leak and internal hernia after laparoscopic gastric bypass: preliminary results of a prospective, randomized multicenter trial. Obes Surg. 2006;16:125–31. https://doi.org/10.1381/096089206775565249.
42. Silecchia G, Boru CE, Mouiel J, et al. The use of fibrin sealant to prevent major complications following laparoscopic gastric bypass: results of a multicenter, randomized trial. Surg Endosc. 2008;22:2492–7. https://doi.org/10.1007/s00464-008-9885-0.

43. Chen Y-S, Loh E-W, Shen S-C, et al. Efficacy of fibrin sealant in reducing complication risk after bariatric surgery: a systematic review and meta-analysis. Obes Surg. 2021;31:1158–67. https://doi.org/10.1007/s11695-020-05098-8.
44. Pavone G, Fersini A, Pacilli M, et al. Can indocyanine green during laparoscopic sleeve gastrectomy be considered a new intraoperative modality for leak testing? BMC Surg. 2022;22:341. https://doi.org/10.1186/s12893-022-01796-5.
45. Pavone G, Fersini A, Pacilli M, et al. Anastomotic leak test using indocyanine green during laparoscopic Roux-en-Y gastric bypass: a cohort study. Ann Med Surg (Lond). 2022;84:104939. https://doi.org/10.1016/j.amsu.2022.104939.
46. Mongelli F, Garofalo F, Giacopelli P, et al. Assessment of gastric pouch blood supply with indocyanine green fluorescence in conversional and revisional bariatric surgery: a prospective comparative study. Sci Rep. 2023;13:9152. https://doi.org/10.1038/s41598-023-36442-4.
47. Hsu A, Mu SZ, James A, et al. Indocyanine green in bariatric surgery: a systematic review. Obes Surg. 2023;33:3539–44. https://doi.org/10.1007/s11695-023-06801-1.
48. Elariny H, González H, Wang B. Tissue thickness of human stomach measured on excised gastric specimens from obese patients. Surg Technol Int. 2005;14:119–24.
49. Rawlins L, Rawlins MP, Teel D 2nd. Human tissue thickness measurements from excised sleeve gastrectomy specimens. Surg Endosc. 2014;28:811–4. https://doi.org/10.1007/s00464-013-3264-1.
50. Aurora AR, Khaitan L, Saber AA. Sleeve gastrectomy and the risk of leak: a systematic analysis of 4,888 patients. Surg Endosc. 2012;26:1509–15. https://doi.org/10.1007/s00464-011-2085-3.
51. Yuval JB, Mintz Y, Cohen MJ, et al. The effects of bougie caliber on leaks and excess weight loss following laparoscopic sleeve gastrectomy. Is there an ideal bougie size? Obes Surg. 2013;23:1685–91. https://doi.org/10.1007/s11695-013-1047-3.
52. Gagner M, Buchwald JN. Comparison of laparoscopic sleeve gastrectomy leak rates in four staple-line reinforcement options: a systematic review. Surg Obes Relat Dis. 2014;10:713–23. https://doi.org/10.1016/j.soard.2014.01.016.
53. Gagner M, Kemmeter P. Comparison of laparoscopic sleeve gastrectomy leak rates in five staple-line reinforcement options: a systematic review. Surg Endosc. 2020;34:396–407. https://doi.org/10.1007/s00464-019-06782-2.
54. Kravetz AJ, Reddy S, Murtaza G, Yenumula P. A comparative study of handsewn versus stapled gastrojejunal anastomosis in laparoscopic Roux-en-Y gastric bypass. Surg Endosc. 2011;25:1287–92. https://doi.org/10.1007/s00464-010-1362-x.
55. Bendewald FP, Choi JN, Blythe LS, et al. Comparison of hand-sewn, linear-stapled, and circular-stapled gastrojejunostomy in laparoscopic Roux-en-Y gastric bypass. Obes Surg. 2011;21:1671–5. https://doi.org/10.1007/s11695-011-0470-6.
56. Awad S, Aguilo R, Agrawal S, Ahmed J. Outcomes of linear-stapled versus hand-sewn gastrojejunal anastomosis in laparoscopic Roux en-Y gastric bypass. Surg Endosc. 2015;29:2278–83. https://doi.org/10.1007/s00464-014-3942-7.
57. Abellán I, López V, Lujan J, et al. Stapling versus hand suture for gastroenteric anastomosis in Roux-en-Y gastric bypass: a randomized clinical trial. Obes Surg. 2015;25:1796–801. https://doi.org/10.1007/s11695-015-1638-2.
58. Jiang H-P, Lin L-L, Jiang X, Qiao H-Q. Meta-analysis of hand-sewn versus mechanical gastrojejunal anastomosis during laparoscopic Roux-en-Y gastric bypass for morbid obesity. Int J Surg. 2016;32:150–7. https://doi.org/10.1016/j.ijsu.2016.04.024.

# Sleeve Stenosis, Torsion, and Delayed Emptying

31

Yung Lee and Jerry T. Dang

## Introduction

Over the last decade, laparoscopic and robotic sleeve gastrectomy (SG) has become the most-performed bariatric procedure in the world. A trend analysis demonstrated consistent annual percentage increases of SG since 2013, with the most recent data showing that SG encompassed 55.4% of all bariatric procedures performed worldwide in 2018 [1]. SG is safe and efficacious, with an early postoperative mortality rate of less than 0.1% and a morbidity rate of less than 7% [2, 3]. However, despite the low risk of complications associated with SG, patients can experience significant complications such as staple line leak (0.9–2.2%), hemorrhage (<2%), as well as long-term complications such as gastroesophageal reflux disease, all of which are well described in the literature with established management strategies [4–7]. With an increasing proportion of patients undergoing SG, it is important for clinicians to be familiar with the unique postoperative challenges, as well as its range of postoperative complications.

This chapter aims to specifically explore three uncommon complications of SG: sleeve stenosis, sleeve torsion, and delayed gastric emptying. These infrequent, but critical postoperative complications require a multifaceted approach to management. This chapter will review clinical presentation, diagnosis and management strategies.

Y. Lee (✉)
Department of Surgery, McMaster University, Hamilton, ON, Canada

J. T. Dang
Digestive Disease Institute, Cleveland Clinic, Cleveland, OH, USA



O. M. Ghanem et al. (eds.), *The SAGES Manual of Metabolic and Bariatric Surgery*, https://doi.org/10.1007/978-3-031-72309-4_31

## Sleeve Stenosis and Torsion

### Presentation and Diagnosis

Sleeve stenosis, also known as gastric stenosis or stricture, requires endoscopic or surgical management in about 0.2–4% of patients after sleeve gastrectomy [8, 9]. Patients with stenosis present with symptoms such as nausea and vomiting, regurgitation, chest pain, fullness, and intolerance of oral intake. The median time from index SG to the diagnosis of sleeve stenosis was found to be approximately 47 days (range 1–114 days) [7].

Sleeve stenosis is classified into two types: anatomical and functional (i.e. sleeve torsion). Anatomical stenosis commonly occurs at the level of incisura angularis or the gastroesophageal junction of the sleeve. It results from a misplaced sleeve calibration tube (i.e. using a small bougie or endoscope) or firing staples without a calibration tube, leading to the development of a stenosed area [5]. It can also occur during the process of applying reinforcing running sutures or clips along the staple line. Anatomical stenosis can be diagnosed by use of an upper gastrointestinal (UGI) series. This often demonstrates an area of narrowing, kinking, or thinned-out segment with delayed progression of contrast depending on the degree of stenosis. Esophagogastroduodenoscopy (EGD) is useful to establish a diagnosis with direct visualisation of the narrowed incisura angularis or gastroesophageal junction.

Functional stenosis of the sleeve is commonly known as "sleeve torsion" or "gastric twist." It is hypothesized that after SG, the process of releasing the stomach from the gastrocolic ligament, gastrosplenic ligament, gastrophrenic ligament, and posterior gastric attachments can make the sleeve more prone to twisting. Moreover, the remnant stomach during the early postoperative period can develop adhesions leading to fixation of the stomach in a twisted state. It is also postulated that twisting can be caused by the progressive firing of staples in an anterior-to-posterior plane instead of a straight line when performing SG [7, 10, 11].

Despite the rare occurrence of this complication, there have been various efforts to classify different types of functional stenosis in the literature. Iannelli et al. subclassified functional stenosis into two types: Type 1: localized twisting of the gastric tube and Type 2: a spiral-shaped staple line that winds around the stomach [12]. Siqueira et al. proposed a different classification system based on the endoscopic view of the torsional stomach which includes: Degree I: mild rotation of the staple line of the stomach without shrinkage of the gastric lumen; Degree II: moderate rotation of the staple line, leading to focal area of fixed narrowing that requires additional endoscopic maneuvers for its transposition; Degree III: severe rotation of the staple line leading to stenosis, with increased difficulty for transposition or complete blockage [13]. In cases of severe stenosis, an upper GI series or CT scan may be needed if the functionally stenosed stomach does not allow for passage of an endoscope.

## Management

Initial management of anatomical sleeve stenosis consists of endoscopic balloon dilation with or without stent placement. The success rate in the resolution of stenosis and clinical improvement of symptoms ranges from 69 to 88% [14, 15]. Agnihotri et al. developed an algorithmic approach to the management of stenosis, which includes serial dilation of the stenosed segment of the sleeve with balloon sizes ranging from 30 to 35 mm. Dilation failed if there were no significant clinical improvements after three to four attempts of dilation [14]. In that case, a subsequent endoscopic stent could be placed in the stenosed segment with a self-expanding metallic stent or lumen-apposing metal stent, with repeat endoscopic evaluation every 6 months as needed. If the area of anatomical stenosis does not resolve with endoscopic management due to its severity (e.g. long or multiple segments of stenosis), surgical intervention may require revision of sleeve gastrectomy, conversion to Roux-en-Y gastric bypass, or seromyotomy [16, 17].

Patients with symptomatic functional sleeve stenosis, or sleeve torsion rarely benefit from endoscopic dilation due to the altered angulation of the sleeved stomach. Diagnostic laparoscopy is required to evaluate the orientation of the stomach once its torsional nature is confirmed via endoscopy or imaging [13, 18]. In patients with functional stenosis, a degree of organoaxial torsion secondary to adhesions is visible on diagnostic laparoscopy. Laparoscopic lysis of adhesions should be performed to return the stomach to a normal anatomic position. It is suggested in the literature to consider performing a gastropexy to the abdominal wall or surrounding anatomic structures (e.g., gastrocolic ligament, greater omentum, pancreatic fascia, left crus of the diaphragm) to prevent recurrent coiling or twisting of the stomach [19]. Conversion to Roux-en-Y gastric bypass should be considered in recurrent cases of torsion or during initial laparoscopy.

## Delayed Emptying After Sleeve Gastrectomy

### Presentation and Diagnosis

Delayed gastric emptying, also known as gastroparesis, is a gastrointestinal disorder characterized by the slow transit of food from stomach to the small intestine [20]. Impaired gastric motility can be multifactorial. In the context of previous SG, it can be idiopathic or secondary to other conditions such as diabetic neuropathy, structural complications (e.g., scarring, stenosis, malignancy), or iatrogenic postsurgical impairment of vagal gastric nerves [21, 22]. Furthermore, in the setting of SG, it is also postulated that abolishing neural innervation of the antrum or the angle of His through gastric resection can contribute to slower emptying [23]. Considering the various causes of delayed gastric emptying after SG, it is essential to conduct a thorough diagnostic assessment to identify the specific cause and tailor treatment accordingly.

Patients with delayed gastric emptying can present with long-term nausea, vomiting, regurgitation, and early satiety [24]. In the setting of the previous SG, it is important to first exclude a mechanical cause of obstruction with EGD, UGI series and/or CT scan to rule out obstruction distal to the second portion of the duodenum. In patients with no obvious cause of obstruction (e.g., sleeve stenosis or torsion, malignancy), gastric emptying scintigraphy can be conducted to establish the diagnosis of gastroparesis. Delayed gastric emptying is defined as gastric retention of greater than 10% of contents at 4 h after the test or greater than 60% at 2 h when using the standardized low-fat, scrambled egg protein meal [25]. There are currently no adjusted gastric retention percentage thresholds or other special tests for gastric emptying specific to patients with previous SG or other forms of gastric resection. As such, interpretation of test results should be completed with the help of gastrointestinal motility specialists.

## Management

Once a mechanical cause has been excluded, dietary modification and counseling should be attempted as first-line management for delayed gastric emptying after SG. Diets involving small frequent meals and based on foods that are low fat, low acidity, and low non-digestible fiber can facilitate gastric emptying and digestion [21]. It is also important to note that patients with chronic symptoms of reduced oral intake or vomiting can develop vitamin and micronutrient deficiencies. Patients with previous SG and delayed gastric emptying who can tolerate oral intake should be given enteral formula or supplements such as iron, B12, and other vitamins [26]. For patients with persistent symptoms despite dietary modifications, referral to gastroenterology and motility specialists for further investigation and medical treatment is warranted patients may also benefit from a trial of prokinetic agents (e.g., metoclopramide, domperidone) or pro-motility macrolide antibiotics (e.g., erythromycin) [21].

The overall data surrounding surgical interventions for gastroparesis in the setting of previous SG are very limited. In patients with medically refractory gastroparesis without previous SG, insertion of a gastric electrical stimulation device, intrapyloric injection of botulinum toxin, and endoscopic or laparoscopic pyloromyotomy or pyloroplasty have shown varying degrees of effectiveness [21]. For patients with delayed gastric emptying due to gastric sleeve stenosis, gastric peroral endoscopic myotomy (G-POEM) has also demonstrated some success in various case reports and case series studies [27–29]. Furthermore, conversion from SG to gastric bypass can be considered an effective surgical treatment option [30, 31].

## Conclusion

SG has emerged as the most common bariatric procedure performed worldwide due to its safety, relative technical ease, and efficacy in promoting weight loss, but is not without complications. As such, recognition and management of complications such as sleeve stenosis, torsion, and delayed gastric emptying are crucial for any provider. These complications emphasize the need for surgeons to be adept not only at performing SG, but also at managing its rare, but significant complications. These complications also demand a collaborative effort between various specialties, including gastroenterology and dieticians, to ensure optimal patient outcomes. As the field of bariatric surgery progresses, so too must our understanding and management of these complex postoperative scenarios evolve to ensure the continued success and safety of procedures like SG (Table 31.1).

**Table 31.1** Summary of the complications of sleeve gastrectomy

| Complication | Description | Diagnosis | Treatment |
|---|---|---|---|
| Sleeve stenosis | Narrowing of the sleeve causing gastric outlet obstruction | UGI series to evaluate the area of stenosis (i.e., tortuosity, angulation, narrowing)<br>EGD reveals rotation/twisting of the staple line and narrowing of the gastric lumen at the level of incisura<br>UGI series or CT scan if stenosis or torsion does not allow for the passage of the endoscope | Endoscopic dilation, possible conversion to gastric bypass or revision of sleeve gastrectomy |
| Sleeve torsion (Functional stenosis) | Axial rotation of the sleeve caused by the disruption of stomach from natural anatomic points of fixation | | Diagnostic laparoscopy, lysis of adhesions to return the sleeve to normal anatomic position ± gastropexy<br>Conversion to Roux-en-Y gastric bypass |
| Delayed gastric emptying | Marked delay in gastric motility in the absence of mechanical obstruction after sleeve gastrectomy | EGD to rule out grossly visible pathology (e.g. malignancy, stenosis) or stasis of gastric contents<br>Scintigraphy gastric emptying study<br>Investigate other potential causes of gastric motility disorders (e.g. viral, autoimmune, diabetic) | Treating the underlying cause of gastroparesis. Dietary modification, hydration, prokinetic agents, possible conversion to gastric bypass |

*UGI* upper gastrointestinal, *EGD* esophagogastroduodenoscopy, *CT* computed tomography

## References


1. Angrisani L, Santonicola A, Iovino P, Ramos A, Shikora S, Kow L. Bariatric surgery survey 2018: similarities and disparities among the 5 IFSO chapters. Obes Surg. 2021;31:1937–48. https://doi.org/10.1007/S11695-020-05207-7/TABLES/7.
2. Carlin AM, Zeni TM, English WJ, Hawasli AA, Genaw JA, Krause KR, Schram JL, Kole KL, Finks JF, Birkmeyer JD, Share D, Birkmeyer NJO. The comparative effectiveness of sleeve gastrectomy, gastric bypass, and adjustable gastric banding procedures for the treatment of morbid obesity. Ann Surg. 2013;257:791–7. https://doi.org/10.1097/SLA.0B013E3182879DED.
3. Stroh C, Köckerling F, Volker L, Frank B, Stefanie W, Christian K, Christiane B, Thomas M. Results of more than 11,800 sleeve gastrectomies: data analysis of the German bariatric surgery registry. Ann Surg. 2016;263:949–55. https://doi.org/10.1097/SLA.0000000000001559.
4. Chiu S, Birch DW, Shi X, Sharma AM, Karmali S. Effect of sleeve gastrectomy on gastroesophageal reflux disease: a systematic review. Surg Obes Relat Dis. 2011;7:510–5. https://doi.org/10.1016/J.SOARD.2010.09.011.
5. Iannelli A, Treacy P, Sebastianelli L, Schiavo L, Martini F. Perioperative complications of sleeve gastrectomy: review of the literature. J Minim Access Surg. 2019;15:1. https://doi.org/10.4103/JMAS.JMAS_271_17.
6. Kim J, Azagury D, Eisenberg D, Demaria E, Campos GM. ASMBS position statement on prevention, detection, and treatment of gastrointestinal leak after gastric bypass and sleeve gastrectomy, including the roles of imaging, surgical exploration, and nonoperative management. Surg Obes Relat Dis. 2015;11:739–48. https://doi.org/10.1016/J.SOARD.2015.05.001.
7. Rebibo L, Hakim S, Dhahri A, Yzet T, Delcenserie R, Regimbeau JM. Gastric stenosis after laparoscopic sleeve gastrectomy: diagnosis and management. Obes Surg. 2016;26:995–1001. https://doi.org/10.1007/S11695-015-1883-4.
8. Parikh A, Alley JB, Peterson RM, Harnisch MC, Pfluke JM, Tapper DM, Fenton SJ. Management options for symptomatic stenosis after laparoscopic vertical sleeve gastrectomy in the morbidly obese. Surg Endosc. 2012;26:738–46. https://doi.org/10.1007/S00464-011-1945-1/FIGURES/3.
9. Sillén L, Andersson E, Olbers T, Edholm D. Obstruction after sleeve gastrectomy, prevalence, and interventions: a cohort study of 9,726 patients with data from the Scandinavian obesity surgery registry (SOReg). Obes Surg. 2021;31:4701–7. https://doi.org/10.1007/S11695-021-05574-9.
10. Manos T, Nedelcu M, Cotirlet A, Eddbali I, Gagner M, Noel P. How to treat stenosis after sleeve gastrectomy? Surg Obes Relat Dis. 2017;13:150–4. https://doi.org/10.1016/J.SOARD.2016.08.491.
11. Subhas G, Gupta A, Sabir M, Mittal VK. Gastric remnant twist in the immediate post-operative period following laparoscopic sleeve gastrectomy. World J Gastrointest Surg. 2015;7:345. https://doi.org/10.4240/WJGS.V7.I11.345.
12. Iannelli A, Martini F, Schneck AS, Gugenheim J. Twisted gastric sleeve. Surgery. 2015;157:163–5. https://doi.org/10.1016/j.surg.2014.01.018.
13. Siqueira LT, Santa-Cruz F, Pontual JP, Aquino MAR, Dompieri LT, Kreimer F, Ferraz ÁAB. Gastric twist after sleeve gastrectomy: a proposal for endoscopic classification. Arq Bras Cir Dig. 2022;35:e1665. https://doi.org/10.1590/0102-672020210002E1665.
14. Agnihotri A, Barola S, Hill C, Neto MG, Campos J, Singh VK, Schweitzer M, Khashab MA, Kumbhari V. An algorithmic approach to the management of gastric stenosis following laparoscopic sleeve gastrectomy. Obes Surg. 2017;27:2628–36. https://doi.org/10.1007/S11695-017-2689-3/TABLES/3.
15. D'Alessandro A, Dumont JL, Dagher I, Zito F, Galasso G, Tranchart H, Cereatti F, Catheline JM, Pourcher G, Rebibo L, Calabrese D, Msika S, Rotkopf H, Tuszynski T, Pacini F, Arienzo R, D'Alessandro A, Torcivia A, Genser L, Arapis K, Chiche R, De Palma GD, Musella M,

Chevallier JM, Donatelli G. Endoscopy management of sleeve gastrectomy stenosis: what we learned from 202 consecutive patients. Surg Obes Relat Dis. 2023;19:231–7. https://doi.org/10.1016/j.soard.2022.09.015.
16. Bellorin O, Lieb J, Szomstein S, Rosenthal RJ. Laparoscopic conversion of sleeve gastrectomy to Roux-en-Y gastric bypass for acute gastric outlet obstruction after laparoscopic sleeve gastrectomy for morbid obesity. Surg Obes Relat Dis. 2010;6:566–8. https://doi.org/10.1016/j.soard.2010.05.019.
17. Dapri G, Cadière GB, Himpens J. Laparoscopic seromyotomy for long stenosis after sleeve gastrectomy with or without duodenal switch. Obes Surg. 2009;19:495–9. https://doi.org/10.1007/S11695-009-9803-0/FIGURES/3.
18. Hernandez Murcia C, Quintero PG, Rabaza J, Gonzalez A. Laparoscopic management of gastric torsion after sleeve gastrectomy. 2015. https://doi.org/10.4293/CRSLS.2014.00143.
19. Ramos AC, de Souza Bastos EL, Ramos MG, Bertin NTS, Galvão TD, de Lucena RTF, Campos JM. Technical aspects of laparoscopic sleeve gastrectomy. Arq Bras Cir Dig. 2015;28:65. https://doi.org/10.1590/S0102-6720201500S100018.
20. Horowitz M, Su YC, Rayner CK, Jones KL. Gastroparesis: prevalence, clinical significance and treatment. Can J Gastroenterol Hepatol. 2001;15:805–13. https://doi.org/10.1155/2001/628102.
21. Camilleri M, Parkman HP, Shafi MA, Abell TL, Gerson L. Clinical guideline: management of gastroparesis. Am J Gastroenterol. 2013;108:18–37. https://doi.org/10.1038/AJG.2012.373.
22. Jung HK, Choung RS, Locke GR, Schleck CD, Zinsmeister AR, Szarka LA, Mullan B, Talley NJ. The incidence, prevalence, and outcomes of patients with gastroparesis in Olmsted County, Minnesota, from 1996 to 2006. Gastroenterology. 2009;136:1225–33. https://doi.org/10.1053/j.gastro.2008.12.047.
23. Sioka E, Tzovaras G, Perivoliotis K, Bakalis V, Zachari E, Magouliotis D, Tassiopoulou V, Potamianos S, Kapsoritakis A, Poultsidi A, Tepetes K, Chatzitheofilou C, Zacharoulis D. Impact of laparoscopic sleeve gastrectomy on gastrointestinal motility. Gastroenterol Res Pract. 2018;2018:4135813. https://doi.org/10.1155/2018/4135813.
24. Lee AM, Fuchs KH, Varga G, Breithaupt W, Neki K, Broderick R, Horgan S. Sleeve gastrectomy for treatment of delayed gastric emptying—indications, technique, and results. Langenbecks Arch Surg. 2020;405:107–16. https://doi.org/10.1007/S00423-020-01856-5/TABLES/3.
25. Abell TL, Camilleri M, Donohoe K, Hasler WL, Lin HC, Maurer AH, McCallum RW, Nowak T, Nusynowitz ML, Parkman HP, Shreve P, Szarka LA, Snape WJ, Ziessman HA. Consensus recommendations for gastric emptying scintigraphy: a joint report of the American Neurogastroenterology and Motility Society and the Society of Nuclear Medicine. J Nucl Med Technol. 2008;36:44–54. https://doi.org/10.2967/JNMT.107.048116.
26. Parkman HP, Yates KP, Hasler WL, Nguyan L, Pasricha PJ, Snape WJ, Farrugia G, Calles J, Koch KL, Abell TL, McCallum RW, Petito D, Parrish CR, Duffy F, Lee L, Unalparida A, Tonascia J, Hamilton F. Dietary intake and nutritional deficiencies in patients with diabetic or idiopathic gastroparesis. Gastroenterology. 2011;141:486–498.e7. https://doi.org/10.1053/j.gastro.2011.04.045.
27. Farha J, Fayad L, Kadhim A, Şimşek C, Badurdeen DS, Ichkhanian Y, Itani MI, Kalloo AN, Khashab MA, Kumbhari V. Gastric Per-Oral endoscopic Myotomy (G-POEM) for the treatment of gastric stenosis post-laparoscopic sleeve gastrectomy (LSG). Obes Surg. 2019;29:2350–4. https://doi.org/10.1007/S11695-019-03893-6/FIGURES/2.
28. Gonzalez JM, Barthet M, Vitton V. Gastric Peroral Endoscopic Myotomy (GPOEM): a helpful tool for post laparoscopic sleeve gastrectomy gastroparesis. Obes Surg. 2021;31:403–4. https://doi.org/10.1007/S11695-020-04752-5/FIGURES/2.
29. Zhang LY, Canto MI, Schweitzer MA, Khashab MA, Kumbhari V. Gastric Per-Oral Endoscopic Myotomy (G-POEM) for the treatment of gastric sleeve stenosis: a feasibility and safety study. Endoscopy. 2022;54:376–81. https://doi.org/10.1055/A-1544-4923/ID/JR20663-3/BIB.

30. Bardaro SJ, Guerron AD, Romanelli J, Soriano I, King K, Gibbs KE, Petrick A, Menzo L, Rosenthal R, Kennedy C, Gershuni V, Daly S, Leyva-Alvizo A, Tran M, Stalin V, Kothari S, Sudan R. ASMBS guidelines/statements gastroparesis: an evidence-based review for the bariatric and foregut surgeon. Surg Obes Relat Dis. 2023;19:403. https://doi.org/10.1016/j.soard.2023.02.018.
31. Masclee GMC, Keszthelyi D, Conchillo JM, Kruimel JW, Bouvy ND, Masclee AAM. Systematic review on sleeve gastrectomy or Roux-en-Y gastric bypass surgery for refractory gastroparesis. Surg Obes Relat Dis. 2023;19:253–64. https://doi.org/10.1016/J.SOARD.2022.09.009.

# Anastomotic Stenosis and Ulcers

# 32

L. Renee Hilton-Rowe

## Abbreviations

| | |
|---|---|
| DS | Duodenal switch |
| GJ | Gastrojejunostomy |
| JJ | Jejunojejunostomy |
| MBS | Metabolic and bariatric surgery |
| MU | Marginal ulcer |
| OAGB | One anastomosis gastric bypass |
| RYGB | Roux-en-Y gastric bypass |
| SADI | Single anastomosis duodenal-ileal bypass |
| SADI-S | Single anastomosis duodenoileal bypass with sleeve gastrectomy |

## Anastomotic/Marginal Ulcers

### Epidemiology

The incidence of anastomotic ulcers also known as marginal ulcers (MU) following bariatric surgery varies widely depending on the procedure. After Roux-en-Y gastric bypass (RYGB), the incidence is 4.6% according to a systematic review of 41 studies [1]. However, it is important to note that this incidence of MU after RYGB varies widely in studies from as low as 6% to as high as 25% [2]. The gastrojejunal anastomosis site and the jejunal roux limb adjacent to the anastomosis are the most common sites for MU formation after RYGB. While MUs are most commonly

L. R. Hilton-Rowe (✉)
Center for Obesity and Metabolism, Medical College of Georgia, Augusta, GA, USA
e-mail: lhilton@augusta.edu



O. M. Ghanem et al. (eds.), *The SAGES Manual of Metabolic and Bariatric Surgery*, https://doi.org/10.1007/978-3-031-72309-4_32

associated with RYGB, ulcers can be seen after one anastomosis gastric bypass (OAGB) and duodenal switch (DS), single anastomosis duodenoileal bypass (SADI) or single anastomosis duodenoileal bypass with sleeve gastrectomy (SADI-S). The incidence of marginal ulcer after each of these procedures is 2.5% after OAGB [2–4] and 0.9% after *DS*/SADI/ SADI-S [5]. Again, these rates vary widely depending on the source; however, it is clear that MU occurs less frequently after DS/SADI/SADI-S than OAGB or RYGB.

## Etiology

There are many proposed etiologies for MUs including poor perfusion, foreign body nidus, excess acid exposure, *Helicobacter pylori* infection, medications, smoking and/or substance abuse. A meta-analysis by Beran et al. demonstrated that *Helicobacter pylori* infection, smoking, and diabetes mellitus were significant predictors of MU [6]. They also showed that there was a trend of an increased risk of MU associated with nonsteroidal anti-inflammatory drugs and a lower risk of MU with proton pump inhibitors use [6]. Knowing this list of potential causes of ulcer disease is very important for anyone evaluating and caring for postoperative patients since identifying and stopping the causal factor can lead to the resolution of the ulcer in many patients [7]. Anastomotic or surgical technique is a known etiology for increasing the risk of MU. The use of sound operative techniques and avoiding technical pitfalls are imperative to minimize MU formation. The creation of a large gastric pouch can lead to excess acid exposure. A larger gastric pouch contains more parietal cells, which results in excessive gastric acid [8]. Poor perfusion is a well-known surgical etiology for leak, ulcer, and stricture of any anastomosis including those in metabolic surgery. The gastric pouch relies on blood supplied by its pedicle, the left gastric artery. Injuring or ligating this pedicle or too many of its branches can result in poor perfusion of the gastrojejunostomy. Foreign body nidus such as retained staples, sutures, or even bezoars can cause chronic irritation and inflammation. Failure to completely divide the gastric pouch from the remnant can result in gastro-gastric fistula and result in increased acid exposure resulting in MU. Studies have shown that decreasing pouch size, using absorbable sutures, and using a linear staple fire technique can significantly decrease the rate of MU [9, 10]. *Helicobacter pylori* infection is another well-known cause of ulcers in both the stomach, duodenum and anastomoses. Preoperative screening and eradication of *H. pylori* may aid in minimizing MU formation. In the event of MU formation, testing for *H. pylori* should be done in all cases since failure to eradicate the bacteria can result in prolonged ulcers or complications of ulcer disease [11]. Nonsteroidal anti-inflammatory drugs (NSAIDs) are another suspected cause of MU after MBS. There is some ambiguity in the literature. Some studies demonstrate increased MU with NSAID use [2] and others have found no correlation [12]. While there is some ambiguity likely related to dosages and patient reporting, there is a clear correlation between high-dose NSAID use or chronic NSAID use and ulcer formation [7]. Given the numerous studies correlating NSAID use with MU formation, it is recommended that gastric bypass patients avoid NSAIDs due to the increased risk of MU in this specific population. Diabetes, especially when poorly optimized, is an independent risk factor for developing MU. In one study the authors found that for each unit rise in HbA1c above 6.0%, there was a 23% increase in the risk of developing MU [12].

Smoking is the risk factor that can be most strongly correlated to MU formation with a 4.6-fold higher risk. Numerous studies have shown that smoking leads to poor outcomes after bariatric surgery. Smoking can cause mucosal cell death, inhibit cell renewal, decrease blood flow in the GI mucosa, and interfere with the mucosal immune system [6]. Even light smoking, <10 cigarettes per day, is associated with an extraordinary risk of MU formation after RYGB [13]. Cessation is recommended in all patients undergoing MBS for at least 6 weeks preoperatively [14].

Immunosuppression is a less commonly discussed but proven independent risk factor for MU. Corticosteroid use was specifically shown to be a risk factor for MU formation after RYGB in a study by Coblijn et al. [2] In patients with ulcers that failed medical therapy compared to patients with medically responsive ulcers (both recurrent and single episodes), immunosuppression was a factor that led to recalcitrant disease and the need for surgical revision. Oral corticosteroids and inhaled corticosteroids have been linked to MU [15].

## Symptoms

Marginal ulcers can present in a variety of ways depending on the severity of the disease. Common presentation includes epigastric and/or upper left quadrant abdominal pain with nausea and/or vomiting. Pain may be worse after a meal or oral intake. Symptoms and presentation can change as disease severity progresses. Marginal ulcers, when left untreated, can progress to cause gastrointestinal bleeding, gastrojejunostomy anastomotic stenosis/stricture, and in the worse case scenario lead to perforation. Presenting symptoms of a bleeding ulcer include dark red blood in stools or black tarry stools, low hemoglobin and hematocrit, hematemesis, hypotension, vasovagal response, tachycardia and hemorrhagic shock. MU can lead to chronic anemia and death if unmanaged. A perforated marginal ulcer can present as a surgical emergency. These patients typically present with acute abdomen or severe abdominal pain. This must be managed promptly to avoid sepsis and death [2].

## Diagnosis Evaluation

Multiple imaging modalities can demonstrate signs of marginal ulcers; however, the gold standard for diagnosis is endoscopy with direct visualization of the ulcer. Most of these ulcers will be on the jejunal side of the anastomosis and are described as white or pale areas on the mucosa (Fig. 32.1).

During endoscopy, it is important to describe the location and size as well as concerning features such as eschar, bleeding, or mass. Permanent sutures,

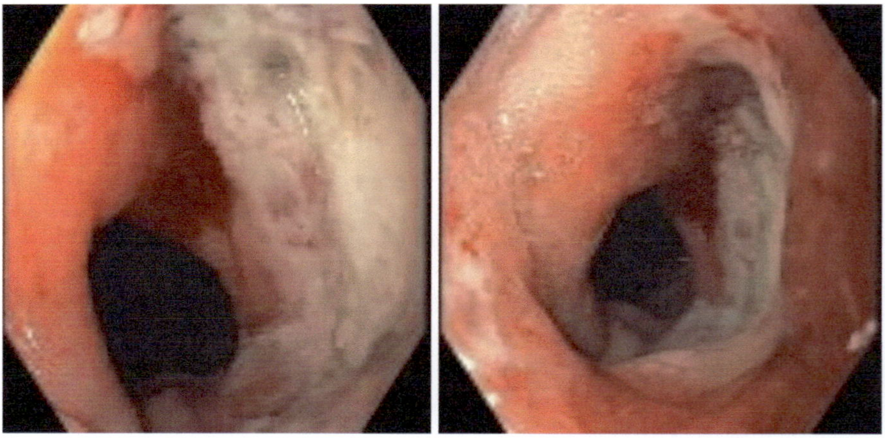

**Fig. 32.1** Large marginal ulcer comprising at least 50% of the circumference of the anastomosis

buttressing material, clips or staples at the anastomosis can serve as a nidus for ulcer formation. Any visible foreign body should be removed when possible. Endoscopic shears can be used to cut sutures flush with the mucosa and other items can be removed with snare or graspers. Food bezoars can result in chronic irritation and serve as a nidus for ulcer formation. Food can be flushed forward or removed with a basket. The reason for food or medications becoming lodged in an area should also be investigated, as this might lead to an anatomical issue contributing to ulcer formation. Foreign bodies such as mesh, gastric bands, or silastic bands can result in erosion or ischemia leading to ulcers forming at the anastomosis. If band or silastic ring erosion is leading to ulceration, operative versus endoscopic removal is advised. At the time of endoscopy, biopsy to evaluate for the presence of *H. pylori* infection is indicated when an ulcer is present. Treatment of *H. pylori* is necessary to aid with ulcer eradication. In cases when a biopsy cannot be done, a urea breath test or stool antigen testing can be obtained.While EGD is the gold standard for diagnosis, adding diagnostic imaging studies such as upper GI (UGI) or CT with contrast can rule out gastro-gastric (GG) fistula. GG fistula formation will lead to excess acid exposure and if found, should be addressed to prevent worsening of ulcer disease. In an emergency presentation with severe pain, abdominal guarding, or other symptoms concerning ulcer perforation CT scan with oral contrast is the preferred diagnostic study. CT scan will demonstrate active extravasation of contrast, inflammation, free fluid, or free air.

## Treatment of MU

Medical Management: The first step in medical management is to remove the causative agent. Smoking cessation is imperative in patients with ulcer disease. Consider referral to a formal counseling program when available. Along with immediate

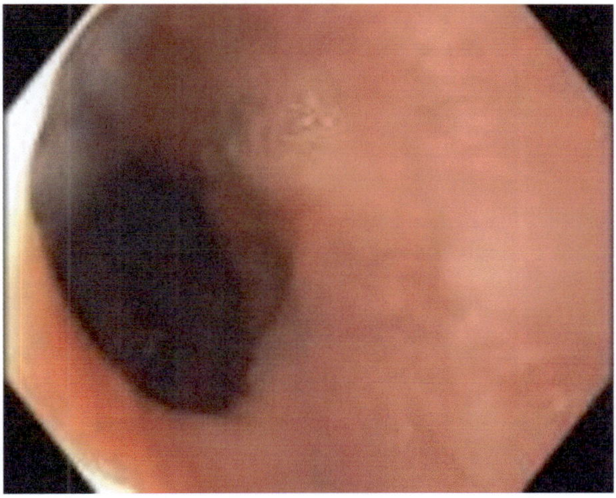

**Fig. 32.2** The same anastomosis shown in Fig. 32.1 after treatment with PPI and eradication of *H. pylori* infection. All ulcers were healed

cessation of the noxious stimuli, 6–8 weeks of oral proton pump inhibitors with sucralfate are recommended for optimal medical management (Fig. 32.2). When *H. pylori* is present, treatment with triple therapy is recommended as first-line care. After treatment, stool antigen testing or urea breath test can be used to monitor for resolution. Cases of refractory *H. pylori* infections are most commonly attributed to antibiotic resistance. American Gastroenterology Association clinical practice guidelines for escalation of treatment are recommended in these cases.

Systematic review and meta-analysis on MU for OAGB found an overall incidence rate of MU at 2.59% after OAGB. The median presentation time of MU following OAGB is within 12 months. Postoperative PPI prophylaxis was prescribed to 14.1% of patients, with variable total duration of therapy reported. Of patients with MU, 89.7% were managed conservatively with PPIs [16].

Surveillance: Repeat endoscopy is needed to ensure healing after starting medical management. Endoscopy should be repeated at 8–12 week intervals to ensure resolution of ulcers [1]. Once the ulcer has resolved, the patient can resume routine surveillance and screening as indicated with endoscopy if symptoms return. The recurrence rate of marginal ulcers varies widely in the literature from 0 to 57% of patients even with compliance with medical therapy [15]. If symptoms have returned and/or the patient has resumed smoking or NSAIDS, repeat endoscopy is warranted since the likelihood of recurrent ulcer formation is high.

## Complicated/Recalcitrant MU

In cases of persistent or nonhealing ulcers, after the removal of causative factors, and optimal medical management, endoscopic or surgical management should be discussed. Di Palma et al. suggest that patients with a history of smoking, NSAID use, and those on immunosuppressive medications are at significantly greater risk of developing a medically refractory MU following RYGB [13, 15]. Endoscopic management includes oversewing or stenting to cover the ulcer bed. This may be the only option for patients who are poor surgical candidates. Surgical management of the ulcer disease should be tailored to the individual patient. Revision of the gastrojejunostomy can treat recalcitrant MU. However, pouch revision/reduction is recommended if a large gastric pouch is present causing possible excessive acid production. In cases where modifiable risk factors such as smoking and NSAID use cannot or will not be stopped, bypass reversal is recommended. Regardless of operative intervention, surgical optimization is important prior to any revision. Revising the bypass without treating/removing the stimuli will likely result in continued ulcer disease in a new anastomosis. The patient should stop any risk factors for MU, if possible, and nutritional status should be optimized. In cases of severe chronic MU affecting oral intake, total parental nutrition (TPN) or enteral feeds may be necessary to improve nutritional status for a revision operation. Thoracoscopic truncal vagotomy is another option for patients with recalcitrant ulcers. Small studies demonstrate that thoracoscopic vagotomy may be an alternative to the revision of anastomosis with decreased operative times and similar effectiveness [17]. Despite multiple proposed operative procedures discussed in the literature for recalcitrant ulcer disease including revision of gastrojejunostomy, thoracoscopic or abdominal truncal vagotomy, subtotal or total gastrectomy, bypass reversal, conversion of bypass into sleeve gastrectomy, there is no clear consensus statement or algorithm detailing an operative treatment plan. Future randomized controlled trials are needed to determine which operation is most effective [18].

## MU Perforation

In a large survey-based paper published including 21 institutions in Italy, the marginal ulcer perforation rate was found to be very low (0.11%). In a separate systematic review of perforation of MU after RYGB and OAGB, most of the patients had undergone a Roux-en-Y gastric bypass (98%). Regardless of whether the anatomy is an RYGB or OAGB, the patient typically presents with severe abdominal pain. CT scan was the most commonly used diagnostic modality. Perforation requires prompt treatment to avoid serious complications such as sepsis and death. In hemodynamically stable patients with minimal free fluid, nonoperative surveillance with nothing per os, IV fluids, TPN, and broad-spectrum antibiotics can be used to allow time for autosealing of the perforation. In hemodynamically stable patients with localized pain and fluid collection, percutaneous drainage by interventional radiology and broad-spectrum antibiotics are appropriate management. In patients with a large perforation or hemodynamic instability, prompt diagnostic laparoscopy with drainage and closure of the perforation either primarily or with a Graham patch is the recommended management. Antibiotics should be given. Traditionally, revision of the anastomosis at the time of perforation was not advised; the tissue is friable and the leak rate is high. The patient may ultimately require a revision, but this can be delayed until all modifiable risk factors of ulcers have been stopped, the tissue is not acutely inflamed, and the patient is hemodynamically stable. In one systematic review, only 5% of patients had recurrent MU after perforation [19]. One recent publication suggested that revision at the time of exploration for perforation may be safely done. While this may be true in select cases, this is not recommended for all perforated MUs [20].

## Anastomotic Stenosis

### Epidemiology

The incidence of anastomotic stricture after bariatric surgery varies widely in the literature depending on the operation and anastomosis site. Stricture or stenosis can occur at the gastrojejunostomy or the jejunojejunostomy after RYGB although gastrojejunostomy stricture is more commonly reported. The stricture rates of gastrojejunal anastomosis vary from 3 to 7%. In a large cohort study using the Scandinavian Obesity Surgery Registry (SOReg), the incidence of stricture one year after surgery was only 0.3% [21]. After OAGB, the incidence of stricture is very low with one study reporting 0.5% [22]. In DS/SADI/SADI-S, these rates remain low. The rate of stricture after SADI-S is less predictable given the sample size in studies. The literature reports overall incidence of complications associated with loop DI was even lower than the reported incidence of anastomotic complications after Roux-en-Y gastric bypass and biliopancreatic diversion with duodenal switch [23]. Another study reported a0.09% rate of duodenoileostomy stenosis after SADI [24].

Given the lack of publications and data available, clear recommendations cannot be made for OAGB and DS/SADI/SADI-S. Future studies on risk factors, clinical presentation, investigation, and treatment of stenosis in these patient populations are recommended. The remaining portion of the chapter primarily focuses on RYGB.

Etiology: Early anastomotic strictures are generally attributed to surgical technique. This can include ischemia, tension and technical error. Stenosis can also be the result of marginal ulcers or complications of ulcer disease such as bleeding and perforation. In the SOReg study, risk factors identified for stricture formation include patient age above 60 years, circular stapled gastrojejunostomy, postoperative anastomotic leak, and marginal ulcer. The etiology of the late strictures varies, with the most common causes being very similar to chronic MU: excessive acid, nonsteroidal anti-inflammatory drug use, postoperative anastomotic leak, or continued smoking [25].

Surgical technique: There are numerous techniques described to perform both the gastrojejunostomy as well as the jejunojejunostomy. Circular stapled gastrojejunostomy has the highest rates of stricture and has been cited as an independent risk factor for stenosis [26–28]. The rate of anastomotic stricture was significantly lower using the 25-mm versus the 21-mm circular stapler [29]. The jejunojejunostomy has aptly been described as the Achilles heel of the RYGB by some authors [30]. The jejunojejunostomy creation technique varies and has been described as completely handsewn or more commonly by linear stapling. When using a linear staple, options include single-staple with suture closure of the common enterotomy, double-stapled

(stapled anastomosis and stapled closure of common enterotomy), or triple-stapled with either unidirectional or bidirectional stapling. Each of these techniques has benefits and drawbacks with the bidirectional technique having less stenosis, however, intussusception rate is higher [31]. Another technical cause of stenosis, better described as "kinking" results from omega loop creation or mesenteric defect closure. The sharp angulation from either of these techniques can lead to obstruction from mechanical twisting which can be very difficult to discern from an anastomotic stenosis on imaging.

Anastomotic leaks: Leaks result in chronic inflammation and risk of ulcer disease, which can result in stenosis. Management of leaks by both endoscopic and operative means can increase the risk of stenosis as oversewing the area of the leak will decrease the size of the anastomosis.

Ulcer complications: Chronic marginal ulcers may result in stricture due to chronic inflammation. Perforation of ulcer disease can result in stricture with or without surgical repair. Oversewing a perforation, while necessary for life-saving purposes, can result in inadvertent narrowing of the anastomosis.

Symptoms: Common symptoms of anastomotic stricture include nausea, regurgitation, vomiting, dysphagia, odynophagia, and abdominal pain. The degree of symptoms may vary based on the severity of stenosis. Solid or thick food consistency may trigger increased symptoms. Timing of the stenosis results in varied symptoms. Early stenosis is less than 90 days post-RYGB. Late stenosis occurs after the 90-day mark. The most common symptoms of the early stricture patients were dysphagia (67%), nausea (53%), and vomiting (49%), while late stenosis has a significantly greater incidence of abdominal pain and features of malnutrition at presentation [28]. Any complaints of these symptoms from a postoperative bariatric patient should raise suspicion in the surgeon and lead to a workup of stricture.

Diagnosis: Diagnosis is made based on clinical suspicion given the patient's symptoms and surgical history. The presence of stricture is confirmed by EGD, the gold standard for diagnosing stenosis is with direct visualization and measurement of stoma. Stricture can be demonstrated on radiological imaging such as upper GI or CT scan with oral contrast. The definition of a stricture varies among bariatric surgeons, but consensus was reached that a clinically significant will not allow passage of an endoscope or where the anastomosis diameter is <10 mm [28]. Diagnosis of a jejunojejunostomy stenosis is most commonly made by CT imaging with oral contrast. Upper GI with small bowel follow-through may be helpful if the diagnosis is unclear.

## Management

Medical management: Lifestyle changes such as eating smaller meals or avoiding trigger foods may alleviate symptoms. However, medical management is primarily aimed at symptom control and will not resolve the stenosis. In cases of active ulcer disease, it is recommended to treat the cause of ulcer formation since resolution of ulcer and improvement of inflammation may result in stricture resolution.

Endoscopic management: Endoscopic treatment with balloon dilation is the gold standard for stricture treatment and should be the first-line treatment in most cases. The majority of strictures can be treated with endoscopic dilation with up to 84.7% of symptom improvement [28, 32]. Early strictures have a superior response to balloon dilation versus late strictures. Stricture dilation is to be performed by a trained endoscopist or surgical endoscopist. Carrodeguas et al. have published one of the largest series of post-RYGB gastrojejunal stricture management using endoscopic balloon dilation, reporting the outcomes of 94 patients. Balloon dilation was relatively safe and effective in this series with a 2.1% risk of perforation using a through-the-scope balloon technique [17, 28]. When dilation results in perforation it can be life threatening and may result in the need for emergent surgery.

Surgical management: In cases where endoscopic dilation has failed or in cases where stenosis is so severe that dilation is not possible, surgical management is necessary. Revision of the anastomosis is usually necessary. En bloc resection of the entire gastrojejunal anastomosis and creation of a new anastomosis can be performed. Management of the jejunojejunostomy stenosis is almost always surgical. Revision of the anastomosis may be necessary for resolution of symptoms. Early or acute strictures may be managed with a Braun enteroenterostomy from the roux limb proximal to the jejunojejunostomy to the common channel. If the biliopancreatic limb is also obstructed, a similar enteroenterostomy is an option [33].

## Conclusion

Both marginal ulcers and anastomotic strictures are complications that can result in pain and life-threatening complications for the MBS patient. In most cases, prompt recognition and treatment can resolve both prior to needing revisional surgery. It is important for any surgeon managing MBS patients to recognize the signs and symptoms of both of these complications, order the appropriate diagnostic testing, and optimize medical management. Endoscopic and surgical interventions can be utilized to manage complications of ulcer disease as well as recalcitrant ulcers or strictures. The best way to avoid MU or stricture is with a sound operative technique. Before and after surgery, complications can be minimized with good pre-operative patient education, medical optimization, nutrition optimization, and ongoing follow-up.

## References

1. Salame M, Jawhar N, Belluzzi A, Al-Kordi M, Storm AC, Abu Dayyeh BK, Ghanem OM. Marginal ulcers after Roux-en-Y gastric bypass: etiology, diagnosis, and management. J Clin Med. 2023;12(13):4336. https://doi.org/10.3390/jcm12134336. PMID: 37445371; PMCID: PMC10342478.
2. Coblijn UK, Goucham AB, Lagarde SM, Kuiken SD, van Wagensveld BA. Development of ulcer disease after Roux-en-Y gastric bypass, incidence, risk factors, and patient pre-

sentation: a systematic review. Obes Surg. 2014;24(2):299–309. https://doi.org/10.1007/s11695-013-1118-5. PMID: 24234733.

3. Musella M, Vitiello A, Susa A, Greco F, De Luca M, Manno E, Olmi S, Raffaelli M, Lucchese M, Carandina S, Foletto M, Pizza F, Bardi U, Navarra G, Schettino AM, Gentileschi P, Sarro G, Chiappetta S, Tirone A, Berardi G, Velotti N, Foschi D, Zappa M, Piazza L, SICOB Collaborative group for the study of OAGB/MGB, Bagaglini G, Benavoli D, Belluzzi A, Callari C, Giusti M, Facchiano E, Licari L, Iovino G, Piatto G, Stanzione F, Uccelli M, Veroux G, Voglino C. Revisional surgery after one anastomosis/minigastric bypass: an Italian multi-institutional survey. Obes Surg. 2022;32(2):256–65. https://doi.org/10.1007/s11695-021-05779-y. Epub 2022 Jan 1. PMID: 34973123; PMCID: PMC8795019.
4. Kermansaravi M, Shahmiri SS, DavarpanahJazi AH, Valizadeh R, Berardi G, Vitiello A, Musella M, Carbajo M. One anastomosis/mini-gastric bypass (OAGB/MGB) as revisional surgery following primary restrictive bariatric procedures: a systematic review and meta-analysis. Obes Surg. 2021;31(1):370–83. https://doi.org/10.1007/s11695-020-05079-x. Epub 2020 Oct 28. PMID: 33118133; PMCID: PMC7809003.
5. Salame M, Teixeira AF, Lind R, Ungson G, Ghanem M, Abi Mosleh K, Jawad MA, Abu Dayyeh BK, Kendrick ML, Ghanem OM. Marginal ulcer and dumping syndrome in patients after duodenal switch: a multi-centered study. J Clin Med. 2023;12(17):5600. https://doi.org/10.3390/jcm12175600. PMID: 37685666; PMCID: PMC10488365.
6. Beran A, Shaear M, Al-Mudares S, Sharma I, Matar R, Al-Haddad M, Salame M, Portela R, Clapp B, Dayyeh BKA, Ghanem OM. Predictors of marginal ulcer after gastric bypass: a systematic review and meta-analysis. J Gastrointest Surg. 2023;27(6):1066–77. https://doi.org/10.1007/s11605-023-05619-7. Epub 2023 Feb 16. PMID: 36795250.
7. Sverdén E, Mattsson F, Sondén A, Leinsköld T, Tao W, Lu Y, Lagergren J. Risk factors for marginal ulcer after gastric bypass surgery for obesity: a population-based cohort study. Ann Surg. 2016;263:733–7. https://doi.org/10.1097/SLA.0000000000001300.
8. Gao X, Dai S, Wang G, Li W, Song Z, Su Z, Zhu S, Zhu L, Li P. Large versus small gastric pouch for Roux-en-Y gastric bypass in individuals with type 2 diabetes and a body mass index < 35 kg/m$^2$: six-year outcomes. Front Endocrinol. 2022;13:913062. https://doi.org/10.3389/fendo.2022.913062.
9. Sundaresan N, Sullivan M, Hiticas BA, Hui BY, Poliakin L, Thompson KJ, McKillop IH, Barbat S, Kuwada TS, Gersin KS, et al. Impacts of gastrojejunal anastomotic technique on rates of marginal ulcer formation and anastomotic bleeding following Roux-en-Y gastric bypass. Obes Surg. 2021;31:2921–6. https://doi.org/10.1007/s11695-021-05292-2.
10. Fakas S, Elias M, Lim D, Meytes V. Comparison of gastrojejunostomy techniques and anastomotic complications: a systematic literature review. Surg Endosc. 2021;35:6489–96. https://doi.org/10.1007/s00464-020-08142-x.
11. Shah SC, Iyer PG, Moss SF. AGA clinical practice update on the management of refractory Helicobacter pylori infection: expert review. Gastroenterology. 2021;160(5):1831–41. issn:0016-5085. https://doi.org/10.1053/j.gastro.2020.11.059.
12. Süsstrunk J, Wartmann L, Mattiello D, Köstler T, Zingg U. Incidence and prognostic factors for the development of symptomatic and asymptomatic marginal ulcers after Roux-en-Y gastric bypass procedures. Obes Surg. 2021;31:3005–14. https://doi.org/10.1007/s11695-021-05363-4.
13. Dittrich L, Schwenninger M-V, Dittrich K, Pratschke J, Aigner F, Raakow J. Marginal ulcers after laparoscopic Roux-en-Y gastric bypass: analysis of the amount of daily and lifetime smoking on postoperative risk. Surg Obes Relat Dis. 2020;16:389–96.
14. Carter J, Chang J, Birriel TJ, Moustarah F, Sogg S, Goodpaster K, Benson-Davies S, Chapmon K, Eisenberg D. ASMBS position statement on preoperative patient optimization before metabolic and bariatric surgery. Surg Obes Relat Dis. 2021;17:1956–76. https://doi.org/10.1016/j.soard.2021.08.024.

15. Di Palma A, Liu B, Maeda A, et al. Marginal ulceration following Roux-en-Y gastric bypass: risk factors for ulcer development, recurrence and need for revisional surgery. Surg Endosc. 2021;35:2347–53. https://doi.org/10.1007/s00464-020-07650-0.
16. Lee S, Supparamaniam S, Varghese C, et al. Marginal ulcers following one-anastomosis gastric bypass: a systematic review and meta-analysis. Obes Surg. 2023;33:2884–97. https://doi.org/10.1007/s11695-023-06762-5.
17. Bonanno A, Tieu B, Dewey E, Husain F. Thoracoscopic truncal vagotomy versus surgical revision of the gastrojejunal anastomosis for recalcitrant marginal ulcers. Surg Endosc. 2019;33(2):607–11. https://doi.org/10.1007/s00464-018-6386-7. Epub 2018 Aug 21. PMID: 30132208.
18. Fecso AB, Di Palma A, Maeda A, Englesakis M, Jackson T, Okrainec A. Operative management of recalcitrant marginal ulcers following laparoscopic Roux-en-Y gastric bypass for morbid obesity: a systematic review. Surg Obes Relat Dis. 2021;17(12):2082–90. https://doi.org/10.1016/j.soard.2021.07.017. Epub 2021 Aug 3. PMID: 34433513.
19. Martinino A, Bhandari M, Abouelazayem M, Abdellatif A, Koshy RM, Mahawar K. Perforated marginal ulcer after gastric bypass for obesity: a systematic review. Surg Obes Relat Dis. 2022;18(9):1168–75. https://doi.org/10.1016/j.soard.2022.05.024. Epub 2022 May 27. PMID: 35810084.
20. Crawford CB, Schuh LM, Inman MM. Revision gastrojejunostomy versus suturing with and without omental patch for perforated marginal ulcer treatment after Roux-en-Y gastric bypass. J Gastrointest Surg. 2023;27:1–6. https://doi.org/10.1007/s11605-022-05461-3.
21. Almby K, Edholm D. Anastomotic strictures after Roux-en-Y gastric bypass: a cohort study from the Scandinavian obesity surgery registry. Obes Surg. 2019;29(1):172–7. https://doi.org/10.1007/s11695-018-3500-9. PMID: 30206785.
22. Carbajo MA, Luque-de-León E, Jiménez JM, Ortiz-de-Solórzano J, Pérez-Miranda M, Castro-Alija MJ. Laparoscopic one-anastomosis gastric bypass: technique, results, and long-term follow-up in 1200 patients. Obes Surg. 2017;27(5):1153–67. https://doi.org/10.1007/s11695-016-2428-1. PMID: 27783366; PMCID: PMC5403902.
23. Surve A, Cottam D, Sanchez-Pernaute A, Torres A, Roller J, Kwon Y, Mourot J, Schniederjan B, Neichoy B, Enochs P, Tyner M, Bruce J, Bovard S, Roslin M, Jawad M, Teixeira A, Srikanth M, Free J, Zaveri H, Pilati D, Bull J, Belnap L, Richards C, Medlin W, Moon R, Cottam A, Sabrudin S, Cottam S, Dhorepatil A. The incidence of complications associated with loop duodeno-ileostomy after single-anastomosis duodenal switch procedures among 1328 patients: a multicenter experience. Surg Obes Relat Dis. 2018;14(5):594–601. https://doi.org/10.1016/j.soard.2018.01.020. Epub 2018 Feb 2. PMID: 29530597.
24. Liagre A, Martini F, Anduze Y, Boudrie H, Van Haverbeke O, Valabrega S, Kassir R, Debs T, Petrucciani N. Efficacy and drawbacks of single-anastomosis duodeno-ileal bypass after sleeve gastrectomy in a tertiary referral bariatric center. Obes Surg. 2021;31(6):2691–700. https://doi.org/10.1007/s11695-021-05323-y. Epub 2021 Apr 9. PMID: 33834374; PMCID: PMC8113294.
25. Cusati D, Sarr M, Kendrick M, Que F, Swain JM. Refractory strictures after Roux-en-Y gastric bypass: operative management. Surg Obes Relat Dis. 2011;7(2):165–9. https://doi.org/10.1016/j.soard.2010.11.003. Epub 2010 Nov 18. PMID: 21195672.
26. Sundaresan N, Hiticas BA, Sullivan M, Hui BY, Poliakin L, Thompson KJ, McKillop IH, Barbat S, Kuwada TS, Gersin KS, Nimeri A. Gastrojejunal anastomotic stricture following Roux-en-Y gastric bypass: an analysis of anastomotic technique at a single institution. Obes Surg. 2021;31(11):4947–52. https://doi.org/10.1007/s11695-021-05678-2. Epub 2021 Sep 13. Erratum in: Obes Surg. 2021 Sep 23. PMID: 34518993.
27. Mueller CL, Jackson TD, Swanson T, Pitzul K, Daigle C, Penner T, Urbach DR, Okrainec A. Linear-stapled gastrojejunostomy with transverse hand-sewn enterotomy closure significantly reduces strictures for laparoscopic Roux-en-Y gastric bypass. Obes Surg. 2013;23(8):1302–8. https://doi.org/10.1007/s11695-013-0920-4. PMID: 23526084.

28. Yimcharoen P, Heneghan H, Chand B, Talarico JA, Tariq N, Kroh M, Brethauer SA. Successful management of gastrojejunal strictures after gastric bypass: is timing important? Surg Obes Relat Dis. 2012;8(2):151–7. https://doi.org/10.1016/j.soard.2011.01.043. Epub 2011 Mar 11. PMID: 21441074.
29. Suggs WJ, Kouli W, Lupovici M, Chau WY, Brolin RE. Complications at gastrojejunostomy after laparoscopic Roux-en-Y gastric bypass: comparison between 21- and 25-mm circular staplers. Surg Obes Relat Dis. 2007;3(5):508–14. https://doi.org/10.1016/j.soard.2007.05.003. Epub 2007 Aug 8. PMID: 17686661.
30. Hedberg S, Xiao Y, Klasson A, Maleckas A, Wirén M, Thorell A, Laurenius A, Engström M, Olbers T. The jejunojejunostomy: an Achilles heel of the Roux-en-Y gastric bypass construction. Obes Surg. 2021;31(12):5141–7. https://doi.org/10.1007/s11695-021-05686-2. Epub 2021 Sep 3. PMID: 34480331; PMCID: PMC8595153.
31. Hedberg S, Thorell A, Engström M, Stenberg E, Olbers T. Surgical technique in constructing the jejunojejunostomy and the risk of small bowel obstruction after Roux-en-Y gastric bypass. Surg Obes Relat Dis. 2022;18(9):1151–9. https://doi.org/10.1016/j.soard.2022.05.020. Epub 2022 May 21. PMID: 35752592.
32. Goitein D, Papasavas PK, Gagné D, Ahmad S, Caushaj PF. Gastrojejunal strictures following laparoscopic Roux-en-Y gastric bypass for morbid obesity. Surg Endosc. 2005;19(5):628–32.
33. Nguyen NT, Huerta S, Gelfand D, et al. Bowel obstruction after laparoscopic roux-en-y gastric bypass. Obes Surg. 2004;14:190–6. https://doi.org/10.1381/096089204322857546.

# 33 Gastrointestinal Obstruction After Bariatric Surgery

Matthew R. Byler and Peter T. Hallowell

## Introduction

Bowel obstruction is one of the most prevalent and important complications following bariatric surgery. Although it is most common after procedures involving intestinal anastomosis, obstruction can follow any kind of bariatric operation. The severity of this complication ranges from minor self-limiting issues to critical life-threatening emergencies. Almost 380,000 bariatric operations were performed from 2020 to 2021, so all bariatric surgeons require a comprehensive understanding of all forms of bowel obstructions in this postoperative setting [1]. This knowledge is crucial for ensuring prompt assessment and appropriate treatment of the bariatric patient. This section will explore the evaluation and management of the most frequent causes of partial and complete obstruction following Roux-en-Y gastric bypass (RYGB), sleeve gastrectomy (SG), biliopancreatic diversion (BPD) with duodenal switch (DS) and single anastomosis duodeno-ileostomy (SADI).

## Obstruction After Roux-en-Y Gastric Bypass

Studies have demonstrated rates of early (within 30 days of surgery) bowel obstruction following RYGB between 0.5 and 5.2% [2–7]. A recently published retrospective analysis of 148,944 patients who underwent RYGB between 2020 and 2021 demonstrated an early bowel obstruction rate of 0.74% (406 patients) [1]. Over half (58.4%) of these patients required reoperation; therefore, it is critical that both the

M. R. Byler (✉) · P. T. Hallowell
Department of Surgery, University of Virginia, Charlottesville, VA, USA


O. M. Ghanem et al. (eds.), *The SAGES Manual of Metabolic and Bariatric Surgery*, https://doi.org/10.1007/978-3-031-72309-4_33

bariatric surgeon and general surgeon understand the nuances and unique challenges that exist in this patient population.

Understanding the clinical presentation of obstruction in gastric bypass patients is contingent upon identifying the site of the obstruction. This underscores the significance of a thorough understanding of RYGB anatomy (Fig. 33.1). In RYGB, the gastric pouch typically measures around 30 mL in volume and 5 cm in length. Ingested food passes from the esophagus into the pouch and progresses into the Roux limb. The Roux limb (also known as the alimentary limb) is a segment of the jejunum spanning 75–150 cm that extends from the gastric pouch to the jejunojejunostomy (distal anastomosis). Subsequently, food traverses the "common channel," the remaining portion of the small intestine between the jejunojejunostomy and the ileocecal valve. While the bypassed segment of stomach, known as the "gastric remnant," is no longer part of the alimentary path, it continues to secrete mucus and gastric acid. These secretions combine with bile and pancreatic fluid in the duodenum before passing into the biliopancreatic limb and meeting the alimentary limb at the jejunojejunostomy.

Obstruction of either the Roux limb or common channel typically presents with classic obstructive symptoms familiar to all general surgeons. This can include nausea, vomiting, food intolerance, abdominal pain, and distention. Obstruction of the biliopancreatic limb may differ thus posing a challenging diagnosis. Patients with an obstructed biliopancreatic limb may not exhibit classic obstructive symptoms familiar to general surgeons, given that the alimentary path may remain unblocked. In cases of biliopancreatic limb obstruction, the gastric remnant may significantly

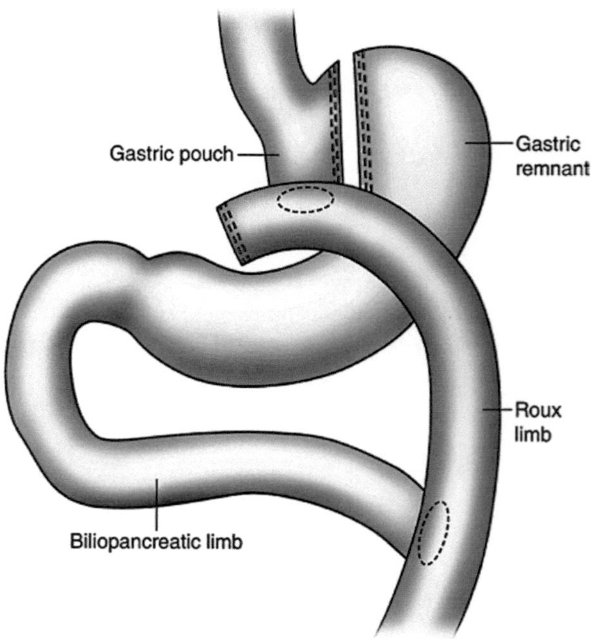


**Fig. 33.1** Anatomy of the Roux-en-Y gastric bypass

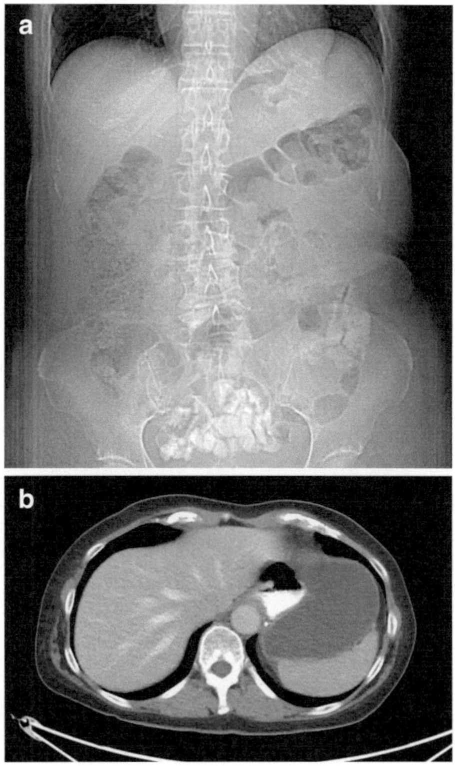


**Fig. 33.2** (**a**) Scout supine film of a patient with biliopancreatic limb obstruction that does not demonstrate a dilated remnant stomach. (**b**) CT scan of the same patient demonstrates a large fluid-filled remnant stomach due to obstruction

distend with fluid, remaining elusive on plain film (Fig. 33.2). This results in abdominal distention, hiccups, and pain, without the presence of nausea or vomiting. Biliopancreatic limb obstruction can lead to severe distension of the gastric remnant, necessitating emergent intervention.

## General Approach to the Bypass Patient with Obstruction

When evaluating intestinal obstruction in patients after RYGB, it is crucial to recognize that the clinical presentation is primarily determined by which segment of bowel is obstructed. The manifestations of Roux limb obstruction significantly differ from those of biliopancreatic limb obstruction.

Early utilization of cross-sectional imaging can delineate obstructions in the Roux limb, biliopancreatic limb, and common channel. This is commonly performed with a CT scan of the abdomen and pelvis with oral and IV contrast. However, select populations may require the use of magnetic resonance imaging (MRI) to limit radiation exposure. Plain films and upper gastrointestinal (UGI) series are of limited diagnostic value and should not be relied upon in evaluating the etiology of obstruction in the RYGB patient.

Patients experiencing abdominal pain without evident bowel distention on CT imaging may also have an internal hernia. Internal hernias induce pain through compression and eventual obstruction of intestinal vasculature, manifesting symptoms more indicative of intermittent bowel ischemia rather than straightforward obstruction. It is important to maintain a high index of suspicion for internal hernias in gastric bypass patients presenting with abdominal pain. In a bypass patient with abdominal pain, where no abnormalities are seen on CT scan, surgical exploration may still be indicated to rule out the presence of an internal hernia.

While nasogastric tube (NGT) decompression is a standard strategy for managing many general surgical patients with small bowel obstruction, its utility in obstructed gastric bypass patients is limited. The small subset of patients with a proximal alimentary tract obstruction, or common channel obstruction, causing nausea and vomiting may benefit from NGT placement. NGT decompression will be of no utility in the patient with an obstructed biliopancreatic limb. Reliance on NGT decompression for the management of patients with an internal hernia or biliopancreatic limb obstruction may result in bowel ischemia or perforation. Additionally, if NGT decompression is utilized, care must be taken during placement to avoid potential harm to a recently created gastrojejunostomy or inadvertently perforating the blind end of the Roux limb ("candy-cane end") under force.

## Obstruction from Internal Hernia

Internal hernias are the most common cause of obstruction following gastric bypass. A 2007 series from the Cleveland Clinic identified internal hernia as the leading cause of bowel obstruction in their gastric bypass patients, constituting 41% of all obstructions [8]. Recent studies, such as a survey of 594 patients, indicate internal hernia rates as high as 6.2% post-Roux-en-Y gastric bypass [9]. In gastric bypass patients with an antecolic Roux limb, two potential types of internal hernias may arise: jejunojejunal mesenteric hernia and Peterson's hernia. In gastric bypass patients with a retrocolic Roux limb, an additional hernia space is created through the transverse mesocolon.

1. **Petersen's Hernia**: This occurs in the space between the mesentery of the Roux limb and the transverse colon/mesocolon (Fig. 33.3, arrow 1).
2. **Jejunojejunal Anastomosis Mesenteric Hernia**: This involves the space between the divided mesentery of the biliopancreatic limb and the mesentery of the Roux limb at the jejunojejunal anastomosis (Fig. 33.3, arrow 2).
3. **Transverse Mesocolic Hernia**: This occurs at the created mesocolic defect through which the retrocolic Roux limb is brought up to reach the gastric pouch (Fig. 33.3, arrow 3).

Retrocolic gastric bypasses are associated with a higher rate of internal hernia, with a 2003 Mount Sinai study revealing nearly double the risk compared to antecolic placement (3.3% vs. 6.0%) [10].

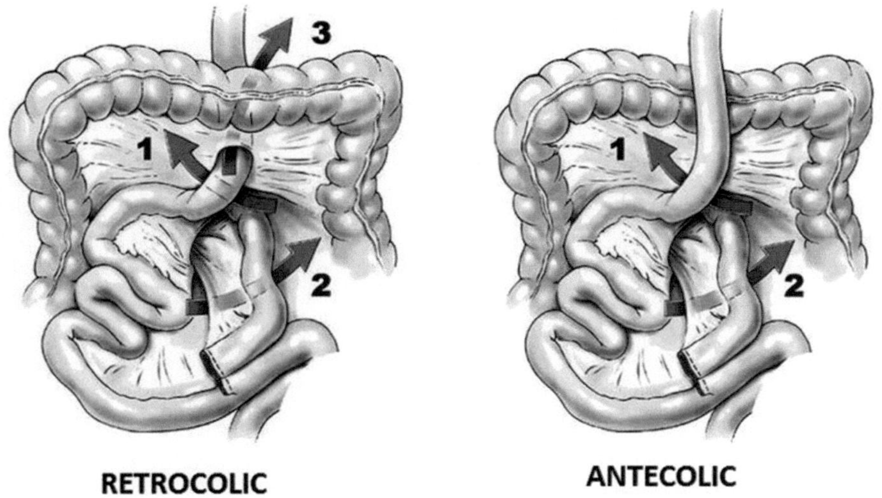


**Fig. 33.3** Arrows indicating potential spaces for internal herniation: (1) Petersen's hernia, between the Roux limb mesentery and the transverse mesocolon. (2) Jejunojejunal mesenteric hernia, at the anastomotic site between the Roux limb and biliopancreatic. (3) The opening through the transverse mesocolon when the Roux limb is retrocolic. (Image from Kim Y, Crookes PF. Complications of bariatric surgery. In: Huang, C-K, ed. Essentials and Controversies in Bariatric Surgery. https://www.intechopen.com/books/essentials-and-controversies-in-bariatric-surgery/complications-of-bariatric-surgery. © 2014 Kim Y, Crookes PF. Published under CC BY 3.0 license. https://doi.org/10.5772/58920. Accessed February 06, 2024)

Closure of internal hernia spaces with permanent suture is common amongst bariatric surgeons, although practices vary. A study in 2017 found a 2.5% internal hernia rate when mesenteric defects were closed, contrasting with almost 12% in cases without closure [11]. It is crucial to note that even with hernia defect closure, hernia defects may open over time as patients lose weight.

Internal hernias range in presentation from mild abdominal pain or food intolerance to severe peritonitis and hemodynamic instability. This broad range of presentations is due to the nature of Roux-en-Y anatomy. Herniation through internal defects may occur along the alimentary tract and present with classic symptoms of oral intolerance. However, obstruction may occur along the biliopancreatic limb and present in an insidious fashion, ranging from abdominal pain due to distention of the gastric remnant, to severe peritonitis and hemodynamic instability from intestinal ischemia.

When bowel incarceration occurs within an internal hernia, there is potential for venous outflow occlusion, leading to bowel ischemia and intense abdominal pain. Incarcerated bowel may also spontaneously reduce, bringing swift symptom resolution, or may remain incarcerated, necessitating emergent surgical intervention.

Physical examination and laboratory studies typically provide limited insight into internal hernias. For this reason, cross-sectional imaging with CT scan is preferred to evaluate the entire intestinal tract for obstruction and ischemia. These studies may show indicators such as the "swirl sign" or other mesenteric abnormalities that may be a clue about the presence of an internal hernia. It is worth noting that these studies do lack sensitivity and specificity, thus a normal CT scan does not rule out an internal hernia. Severe abdominal pain in a gastric bypass patient with a normal CT scan remains a surgical emergency.

Definitive diagnosis may require surgical exploration, either via a minimally invasive or open approach. It is important to identify the orientation of the bowel to determine if an internal hernia is present, as well as which portions of bowel are incarcerated. This may be facilitated by starting at the ileocecal junction of the terminal ileum and running the bowel retrograde until the jejunojejunostomy is identified. The Roux limb and BP limb can then be identified by continuing along each limb in a retrograde fashion. Once the intestinal orientation is noted, the incarcerated bowel should be reduced, and the hernia defect closed with a nonabsorbable suture. If the bowel is ischemic and nonviable, it should be resected and appropriate reconstruction performed. Questionably viable bowel may warrant investigation of blood supply patency during the operation and/or a "second look" within 24–48 h.

## Gastrojejunal Stricture

Gastrojejunostomy stricture is a relatively common complication post-gastric bypass, with reported incidence rates varying from 0.5 to 5% [12]. Techniques for performing the gastrojejunal anastomosis are described elsewhere in this book. A 2015 study, encompassing 1500 patients, reported a 3.4% rate of gastrojejunal stricture necessitating endoscopic intervention [13]. While the majority of cases manifest within the first 90 days post-surgery, delayed presentations, even a year or more later, are not uncommon [14]. The typical presentation occurs 4–6 weeks post-surgery, with patients progressing from solid food intolerance to liquid intolerance as the stricture narrows. Severe cases may render patients unable to swallow their oral secretions.

The etiology of gastrojejunal stricture formation remains unclear, with some attributing it to ischemia and others implicating suture material or staples. Stricture development appears to be associated with the initial size of the anastomosis, as evidenced by a 2012 study revealing a nearly four-fold incidence of intraluminal stenosis with a 21-mm circular stapler compared to a 25-mm circular stapler [15]. Staple line reinforcement materials and certain stapler characteristics, such as height, have been identified as possible influencers in the reduction of stricture rates [16, 17]. While opinions amongst surgeons differ on the likelihood of stricture formation following handsewn, linear stapled, or circular anastomoses, a meta-analysis of over 13,000 patients found no significant difference in stricture rates between handsewn and stapled anastomoses [18].

It is worth noting that obstructions labeled as "distal strictures" at the 45- to 120-mm stapled jejunojejunostomy anastomosis most likely develop as a result of a technical error causing kinking or narrowing of the common enterotomy closure. True stricture formation at the jejunojejunostomy anastomosis is exceedingly rare.

Diagnosis is primarily based on patient history and confirmed via upper endoscopy. Radiographic upper GI contrast studies may assist in diagnosis; however, this does carry the risk of contrast aspiration. Upper endoscopy proves to be the diagnostic modality of choice, enabling both diagnosis and therapeutic balloon dilation [19]. There is not currently a widely accepted, precise measurement of a gastrojejunal stricture, however, most bariatric surgeons and endoscopists consider an anastomotic stricture when it is too narrow for the passage of a standard upper endoscope (approximately 9.5 mm in diameter). Endoscopic diagnosis allows for immediate dilation via a through-the-scope dilating balloon, with diameters reaching 18–20 mm. While most patients respond to a single dilation, some may require additional treatments, and up to 13% may need four to five treatments [20].

Historically, bougie dilators were used before the widespread adoption of dilating balloons [21, 22]. Although balloon dilation is generally safe and effective, rare instances of perforation may occur. A 2012 review of 760 patients undergoing endoscopic dilation reported perforation as the most common complication, occurring in 1.8% of cases [23]. Surgical revision for recurrent stenosis was necessary in 2% of cases.

## Intussusception

Small bowel intussusception is a relatively infrequent cause of bowel obstruction following Roux-en-Y gastric bypass. The jejunojejunostomy is a frequent site of small bowel-small bowel intussusception. CT scan of the abdomen and pelvis with oral and IV contrast is frequently used to aid in diagnosing the etiology of obstruction in gastric bypass patients. The pathognomonic "target sign" is the classic finding of this condition (Fig. 33.4).

Intussusception may spontaneously resolve on serial imaging studies. However, if the intussusception is identified as the cause of bowel obstruction, or if the finding remains on serial imaging, this warrants surgical exploration. The goal of surgery is

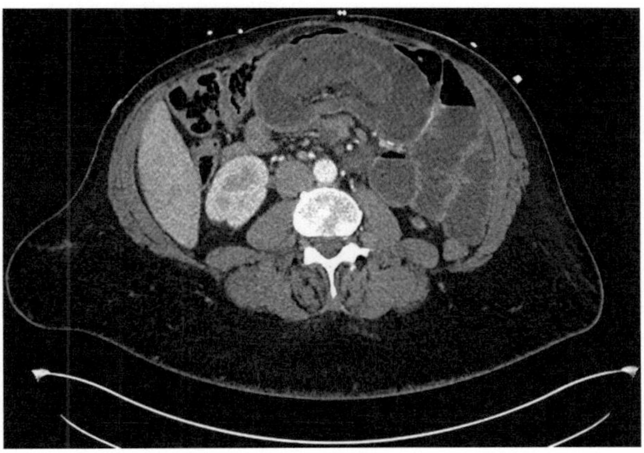

**Fig. 33.4** CT scan image showing the "target sign" consistent with intussusception

to attempt reduction of the intussusception, identify any pathologic lead points, and perform a revision of the jejunojejunostomy or resection of injured small bowel as necessary.

## Kinking at Jejunojejunostomy

Closure of the mesenteric defect created at the jejunojejunostomy site may cause an additional site for early obstruction. As the mesenteric defect is approximated, this can place tension on the intestines at the jejunojejunostomy which causes the bowel to kink forming an obstruction [24]. This has been shown to be the most common cause of early (within 30 days from surgery) bowel obstruction in patients after RYGB [1]. As previously discussed, presentation from obstruction at the jejunojejunostomy ranges from traditional symptoms from blockage of the alimentary tract causing nausea and vomiting, to vague, nonspecific abdominal symptoms as a result of biliopancreatic limb obstruction.

Several techniques to avoid kinking of the jejunojejunostomy have been discussed in the literature. These range from a bidirectional stapling technique to the placement of an anti-obstruction stitch [25, 26]. The surgeon should be aware of this potential site for obstruction during the creation of the jejunojejunostomy and closure of the mesentery, and employ the appropriate measures to mitigate the risk.

## Obstruction from Intraluminal Blood Clot or Bezoar

Obstructions due to intraluminal blood clots or food products are uncommon following gastric bypass. However, all bariatric surgeons must be keenly aware of these potential causes of bowel obstruction given the potential risks in the setting of Roux-en-Y anatomy.

Intraluminal blood clots, or hemobezoars, most commonly occur at sites of bowel anastomoses or staple lines. Obstruction from a postoperative intraluminal bleed presents early in the postoperative course, generally within the first few days. Intervention is dictated by the site of obstruction and patient presentation. Endoscopic evaluation and intervention remain an option for any intraluminal bleed if the site is endoscopically accessible. Additional options for obstruction at the jejunojejunostomy include return to the OR for remnant stomach enteral access for decompression, and/or revision of the jejunojejunostomy with clot evacuation, as dictated by the clinical scenario.

Obstruction due to phytobezoar is an extremely rare but known complication following Roux-en-Y gastric bypass. In 2016, Ben-Porat et al. reviewed 19 case reports of phytobezoar causing obstruction after gastric bypass [27]. This review demonstrated that obstruction could occur in the early postoperative period to years later. A proposed mechanism is reduced gastric motility, loss of pyloric function, and hypoacidity. Interventions include chemical enzyme therapy, endoscopic dissolution and removal, or surgical exploration. Interestingly, overconsumption of milk products to meet daily protein requirements (protein shakes) has been reported to cause lactobezoars [28]. Pre- and postoperative nutritional counseling to emphasize healthy eating habits, diverse protein source consumption, proper chewing, and avoiding the overindulgence of high-fiber foods may help prevent this complication.

## Obstruction After Sleeve Gastrectomy

Sleeve gastrectomy has become the predominant bariatric procedure in the United States since 2014 [29]. According to the ASMBS, over 150,000 sleeve gastrectomies were performed in 2021 [30]. This surgical approach entails a stapled resection of a large portion of the gastric body along the greater curve while preserving a banana-shaped stomach along the lesser curvature (Fig. 33.5). Stomach calibration is achieved by utilizing a bougie, typically 12–14 mm in diameter, along the lesser curvature during stapling.

It is essential to recognize that a considerable number of gastric sleeve patients may experience obstructive-like symptoms of nausea and vomiting within the initial postoperative period, typically occurring 1–3 days after surgery. Antiemetic medications (ondansetron, scopolamine, etc.) can be effective in alleviating these symptoms. In patients with ongoing symptoms, or in those for whom obstruction is a high concern, a fluoroscopic upper GI study is valuable in dynamically assessing for obstruction and the motility of the foregut.

**Fig. 33.5** Illustration of a stapled sleeve gastrectomy

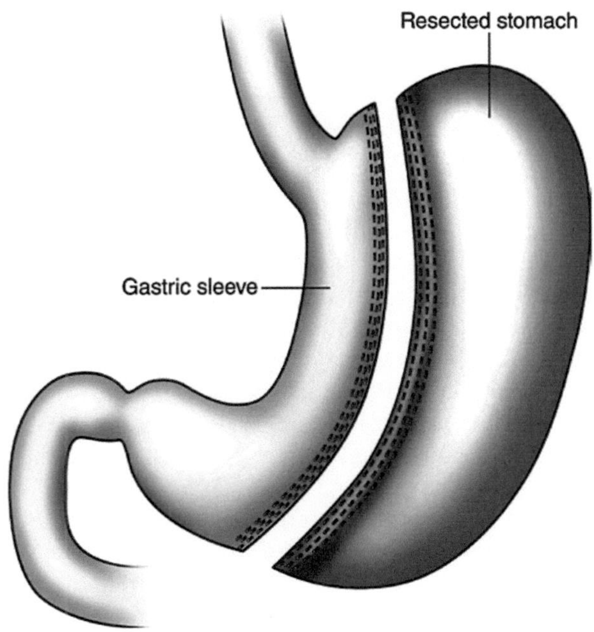

Small bowel intestinal obstructions after sleeve gastrectomy are rare, which is likely due to the minimal lower abdominal manipulation, and lack of intestinal anastomosis or mesenteric defects. A retrospective study in 2023 of 205,533 patients who underwent bariatric surgery between 2020 and 2021 found the lowest rates of early bowel obstruction in those undergoing sleeve gastrectomy with only 41 reported cases (0.03%) [1]. The most common cause of obstructive symptoms in the sleeve gastrectomy patient is due to stenosis, kinking, or twisting of the gastric sleeve. The incisura is the site at highest risk due to stapling or suturing too close to the sizing bougie. Techniques to avoid this complication are discussed elsewhere in this book.

Management of a symptomatic gastric stricture begins with endoscopic balloon dilation, which is successful in 60–80% of patients [31, 32]. Patients with symptomatic stenosis refractory to the first endoscopic dilation may require multiple dilations. Patient with ongoing stenosis refractory to dilation should be considered for conversion to RYGB. In 2013 Burgos et al. published a review of 717 patients who underwent sleeve gastrectomy and found symptomatic gastric stenosis in five patients (0.63%). Four of these patients were successfully managed endoscopically, while the fifth patient underwent conversion to RYGB [32]. A more recent study by Shnell et al. in 2021 reviewed 67 patients who required endoscopic dilation for symptomatic sleeve stenosis. Of these patients, 76.1% ($n$ = 51) were successfully managed endoscopically, while the remaining ($n$ = 16) required conversion to RYGB [31].

## Obstruction After Biliopancreatic Diversion with Duodenal Switch

Biliopancreatic diversion with duodenal switch (BPD-DS) or single anastomosis duodeno-ileostomy with sleeve gastrectomy (SADI-S) are less commonly performed surgeries, compared to RYGB. According to the ASMBS, in 2021 there were 5525 BPD-DS operations and 1025 SADI operations performed [30]. These numbers have increased over the last 2 years, as more surgeons become familiarized with the techniques.

Duodeno-ileal procedures integrate a sleeve gastrectomy followed by a division of the first portion of the duodenum, just distal to the pylorus. In the BPD-DS, a segment of small intestine is brought up to the duodenum in a Roux limb configuration (Fig. 33.6), thus establishing the alimentary, biliopancreatic, and common channel. As in the RYGB, this requires two intestinal anastomoses. In the SADI-S configuration, after performing a sleeve gastrectomy, a loop of ileum is brought up to the duodenum and an anastomosis is directly performed, hence a singular anastomosis (Fig. 33.6).

As with gastric bypass, obstructions following BPD-DS and SADI-S can be the result of internal hernias and anastomotic strictures, thus patients should be managed similarly. One notable difference is that the biliopancreatic limb ends in a duodenal stump, instead of a gastric remnant. The surgeon must be aware of this if

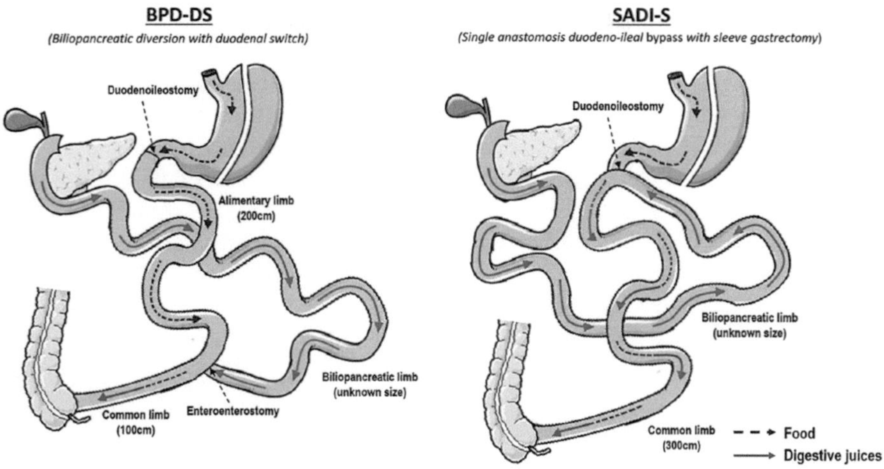


**Fig. 33.6** Illustration of the anatomy in the biliopancreatic diversion with duodenal switch (BPD_DS) and in the single anastomosis duodeno-ileal bypass with sleeve gastrectomy (SADI-S)

afferent limb dilation is demonstrated, and consider the risk of duodenal stump disruption. Despite the anatomic similarities to RYGB, as it relates to the presence of internal hernias and Roux limb anatomy, a recent study demonstrated lower rates of early bowel obstruction in BPD-DS compared to RYGB (0.4% in BPD-DS vs. 0.74% in RYGB) [1]. Similarly, there seem to be lower rates of proximal anastomotic stricture at the duodeno-ileostomy in biliopancreatic diversion than gastrojejunostomy stricture in RYGB [33]. When addressing a BPD-DS or SADI patient presenting with abdominal pain or symptoms suggestive of obstruction, the evaluation should involve the early use of cross-sectional imaging and management protocols should largely mirror those established for bypass patients.

## Small Bowel Obstruction from Adhesions Incisional Hernia

Bariatric patients can develop common complications seen in all general surgery populations, notably intraabdominal adhesions and incisional hernias causing obstructions. Published data on RYGB patients undergoing surgery for bowel obstruction found the etiology due to adhesions ranging between 8 and 47% [34, 35]. These adhesions can obstruct different parts of the gastrointestinal tract, such as the Roux limb, biliopancreatic limb, or common channel.

As previously discussed, patients can present with typical obstructive symptoms of nausea and vomiting, or vague nonspecific abdominal pain, so the surgeon must remain vigilant. Plain films and upper GI series might miss obstructions outside the alimentary path, thus CT scan with oral contrast is preferable given the efficacy in diagnosing obstruction and the ability to determine a transition zone.

Another common complication following bypass surgery, specific to a retrocolic Roux limb, is mesocolic stricture formation. Over time, this area may develop inflammatory scarring that leads to stricture formation of the Roux limb. A 2007 study of 2215 patients who underwent laparoscopic RYGB with a retrocolic Roux limb showed 20 patients (0.9%) developed symptomatic stricture of the Roux limb seen on upper GI series, secondary to compression at the transverse mesocolon. If seen, surgical exploration may be required to free the obstruction, which the authors performed laparoscopically in this series [36]. One method to mitigate this risk is to use interrupted stitches to close the mesocolic defect instead of a continuous stitch to avoid a purse-string effect. Alternatively, consideration of an antecolic Roux limb placement would eliminate the risk.

## Incisional Hernia

The prevalence of incisional hernias may be underestimated. A 2014 study using ultrasound after RYGB in 150 patients revealed a 39% incidence of trocar site hernias [37]. Although most patients were asymptomatic, it is advisable to close trocar sites 10 mm and larger to mitigate the risk of incisional herniation, although this may not entirely prevent herniation. A 2016 study reviewed 1524 patients who underwent bariatric surgery and found eight patients developed symptomatic port site hernias. One required emergency surgery [38].

The management of preexisting ventral hernias during laparoscopic Roux-en-Y gastric bypass is a debated topic. The reluctance to use prosthetic mesh during clean-contaminated operations is common among surgeons. Some prefer to delay hernia repair until significant weight loss is achieved post-surgery. Currently, bariatric surgery combined with mesh repair of ventral hernias remains controversial. In 2017, Khorgami et al. highlighted increased complications, such as higher rates of return to the operating room and longer hospital stays in patients undergoing simultaneous ventral hernia repair and bariatric surgery [39]. In a 2023 publication, Ghanem et al. similarly recommended a delayed approach to repairing abdominal wall hernias. If an abdominal wall hernia contains omentum and its location does not interfere with the bariatric operation, then its contents should be left in place and the hernia repair delayed until after completion of the bariatric operation with improvement of modifiable risk factors [40]. However, the anatomic location of the hernia, presence of intestinal contents, or a history of bowel obstruction may necessitate a temporizing concomitant hernia repair during bariatric surgery. Overall, a tailored approach analyzing the risks and benefits of concomitant bariatric surgery and hernia repair to the individual patient's condition should be considered to achieve optimal outcomes.

## Conclusion

The post-bariatric surgery population represents a unique subset of patients, with regards to the evaluation and management of postoperative bowel obstruction. The unique anatomy of these patients poses additional clinical challenges that must be taken into consideration by the surgeon. It is essential to recognize that these patients are still general surgery patients and remain susceptible to traditional causes of bowel obstruction including adhesions, and incarcerated ventral and inguinal hernias. It is crucial to explore all possible bariatric-specific causes of obstruction, while remaining vigilant about the more conventional obstruction sources.

Bowel obstruction in post-bariatric surgery patients can lead to significant morbidity and even mortality. The importance of a thorough understanding of the evaluation and management of obstruction in these patients cannot be overstated. Surgeons' increasing awareness of how best to evaluate and treat these unique complications will significantly diminish the adverse outcomes associated with gastrointestinal obstruction in bariatric patients.

## References


1. Clapp B, Abi Mosleh K, Corbett J, Salame M, Hage K, Kurian M, et al. Early bowel obstruction after bariatric surgery: an analysis of the 2020-2021 MBSAQIP database. Surg Laparosc Endosc Percutan Tech. 2023;33(5):499–504.
2. Khoraki J, Mazzini GS, Shah AS, Del Prado PAR, Wolfe LG, Campos GM. Early small bowel obstruction after laparoscopic gastric bypass: a surgical emergency. Surg Obes Relat Dis. 2018;14(8):1118–25.
3. Hwang RF, Swartz DE, Felix EL. Causes of small bowel obstruction after laparoscopic gastric bypass. Surg Endosc. 2004;18(11):1631–5.
4. Nguyen NT, Huerta S, Gelfand D, Stevens CM, Jim J. Bowel obstruction after laparoscopic Roux-en-Y gastric bypass. Obes Surg. 2004;14(2):190–6.
5. Lewis CE, Jensen C, Tejirian T, Dutson E, Mehran A. Early jejunojejunostomy obstruction after laparoscopic gastric bypass: case series and treatment algorithm. Surg Obes Relat Dis. 2009;5(2):203–7.
6. Shimizu H, Maia M, Kroh M, Schauer PR, Brethauer SA. Surgical management of early small bowel obstruction after laparoscopic Roux-en-Y gastric bypass. Surg Obes Relat Dis. 2013;9(5):718–24.
7. Nelson LG, Gonzalez R, Haines K, Gallagher SF, Murr MM. Spectrum and treatment of small bowel obstruction after Roux-en-Y gastric bypass. Surg Obes Relat Dis. 2006;2(3):377–83; discussion 83.
8. Rogula T, Yenumula PR, Schauer PR. A complication of Roux-en-Y gastric bypass: intestinal obstruction. Surg Endosc. 2007;21(11):1914–8.
9. Al-Mansour MR, Mundy R, Canoy JM, Dulaimy K, Kuhn JN, Romanelli J. Internal hernia after laparoscopic antecolic Roux-en-Y gastric bypass. Obes Surg. 2015;25(11):2106–11.
10. Comeau E, Gagner M, Inabnet WB, Herron DM, Quinn TM, Pomp A. Symptomatic internal hernias after laparoscopic bariatric surgery. Surg Endosc. 2005;19(1):34–9.
11. Aghajani E, Nergaard BJ, Leifson BG, Hedenbro J, Gislason H. The mesenteric defects in laparoscopic Roux-en-Y gastric bypass: 5 years follow-up of non-closure versus closure using the stapler technique. Surg Endosc. 2017;31(9):3743–8.
12. Sundaresan N, Hiticas BA, Sullivan M, Hui BY, Poliakin L, Thompson KJ, et al. Gastrojejunal anastomotic stricture following roux-en-Y gastric bypass: an analysis of anastomotic technique at a single institution. Obes Surg. 2021;31(11):4947–52.
13. Ribeiro-Parenti L, Arapis K, Chosidow D, Dumont JL, Demetriou M, Marmuse JP. Gastrojejunostomy stricture rate: comparison between antecolic and retrocolic laparoscopic Roux-en-Y gastric bypass. Surg Obes Relat Dis. 2015;11(5):1076–84.

14. Yimcharoen P, Heneghan H, Chand B, Talarico JA, Tariq N, Kroh M, et al. Successful management of gastrojejunal strictures after gastric bypass: is timing important? Surg Obes Relat Dis. 2012;8(2):151–7.
15. Markar SR, Penna M, Venkat-Ramen V, Karthikesalingam A, Hashemi M. Influence of circular stapler diameter on postoperative stenosis after laparoscopic gastrojejunal anastomosis in morbid obesity. Surg Obes Relat Dis. 2012;8(2):230–5.
16. Horkoff M, Purich K, Switzer N, Prasad S, Church N, Shi X, et al. A shorter circular stapler height at the gastrojejunostomy during a Roux-En-Y gastric bypass results in less strictures and bleeding complications. J Obes. 2018;2018:6959786.
17. Scott JD, Cobb WS, Carbonell AM, Traxler B, Bour ES. Reduction in anastomotic strictures using bioabsorbable circular staple line reinforcement in laparoscopic gastric bypass. Surg Obes Relat Dis. 2011;7(5):637–42.
18. Jiang HP, Lin LL, Jiang X, Qiao HQ. Meta-analysis of hand-sewn versus mechanical gastrojejunal anastomosis during laparoscopic Roux-en-Y gastric bypass for morbid obesity. Int J Surg. 2016;32:150–7.
19. Boules M, Chang J, Haskins IN, Sharma G, Froylich D, El-Hayek K, et al. Endoscopic management of post-bariatric surgery complications. World J Gastrointest Endosc. 2016;8(17):591–9.
20. Ukleja A, Afonso BB, Pimentel R, Szomstein S, Rosenthal R. Outcome of endoscopic balloon dilation of strictures after laparoscopic gastric bypass. Surg Endosc. 2008;22(8):1746–50.
21. Fernández-Esparrach G, Bordas JM, Llach J, Lacy A, Delgado S, Vidal J, et al. Endoscopic dilation with Savary-Gilliard bougies of stomal strictures after laparoscopic gastric bypass in morbidly obese patients. Obes Surg. 2008;18(2):155–61.
22. Escalona A, Devaud N, Boza C, Pérez G, Fernández J, Ibáñez L, et al. Gastrojejunal anastomotic stricture after Roux-en-Y gastric bypass: ambulatory management with the Savary-Gilliard dilator. Surg Endosc. 2007;21(5):765–8.
23. Campos JM, de Mello FST, Ferraz AAB, de Brito JN, Nassif PA, dos Passos Galvão-Neto M. Endoscopic dilation of gastrojejunal anastomosis after gastric bypass. Arq Bras Cir Dig. 2012;25(4):283–9.
24. Stenberg E, Szabo E, Ågren G, Ottosson J, Marsk R, Lönroth H, et al. Closure of mesenteric defects in laparoscopic gastric bypass: a multicentre, randomised, parallel, open-label trial. Lancet. 2016;387(10026):1397–404.
25. Munier P, Alratrout H, Siciliano I, Keller P. Bidirectional jejunojejunal anastomosis prevents early small bowel obstruction due to the kinking after closure of the mesenteric defect in the laparoscopic Roux-en-Y gastric bypass. Obes Surg. 2018;28(7):1838–44.
26. Brolin RE. The antiobstruction stitch in stapled Roux-en-Y enteroenterostomy. Am J Surg. 1995;169(3):355–7.
27. Ben-Porat T, Sherf Dagan S, Goldenshluger A, Yuval JB, Elazary R. Gastrointestinal phytobezoar following bariatric surgery: systematic review. Surg Obes Relat Dis. 2016;12(9):1747–54.
28. Kravitz SA, Song KH, Cioffi JH, Vega Colon KM, Lu MA. A bariatric curveball: a rare case of recurrent lactobezoars after Roux-en-Y gastric bypass surgery. Mil Med. 2020;185(7–8):e1294–e7.
29. Angrisani L, Santonicola A, Iovino P, Ramos A, Shikora S, Kow L. Bariatric surgery survey 2018: similarities and disparities among the 5 IFSO chapters. Obes Surg. 2021;31(5):1937–48.
30. Estimate of bariatric surgery numbers, 2011–2021: ASMBS. https://asmbs.org/resources/estimate-of-bariatric-surgery-numbers/.
31. Shnell M, Nevo N, Lahat G, Abu-Abeid S, Goldstein AL, Fishman S, et al. Endoscopic management of sleeve stenosis. Obes Surg. 2021;31(11):4749–53.
32. Burgos AM, Csendes A, Braghetto I. Gastric stenosis after laparoscopic sleeve gastrectomy in morbidly obese patients. Obes Surg. 2013;23(9):1481–6.
33. Surve A, Cottam D, Sanchez-Pernaute A, Torres A, Roller J, Kwon Y, et al. The incidence of complications associated with loop duodeno-ileostomy after single-anastomosis duodenal switch procedures among 1328 patients: a multicenter experience. Surg Obes Relat Dis. 2018;14(5):594–601.

34. Gabrielli M, Jarry C, Hurtado S, Achurra P, Muñoz R, Quezada N, et al. Small bowel obstruction following laparoscopic Roux-en-Y gastric bypass: is it always necessary to operate? A 5-year, high volume center experience. Langenbecks Arch Surg. 2021;406(6):1839–46.
35. Elms L, Moon RC, Varnadore S, Teixeira AF, Jawad MA. Causes of small bowel obstruction after Roux-en-Y gastric bypass: a review of 2,395 cases at a single institution. Surg Endosc. 2014;28(5):1624–8.
36. Ahmed AR, Rickards G, Messing S, Husain S, Johnson J, Boss T, et al. Roux limb obstruction secondary to constriction at transverse mesocolon rent after laparoscopic Roux-en-Y gastric bypass. Surg Obes Relat Dis. 2009;5(2):194–8.
37. Scozzari G, Zanini M, Cravero F, Passera R, Rebecchi F, Morino M. High incidence of trocar site hernia after laparoscopic or robotic Roux-en-Y gastric bypass. Surg Endosc. 2014;28(10):2890–8.
38. Coblijn UK, de Raaff CA, van Wagensveld BA, van Tets WF, de Castro SM. Trocar port hernias after bariatric surgery. Obes Surg. 2016;26(3):546–51.
39. Khorgami Z, Haskins IN, Aminian A, Andalib A, Rosen MJ, Brethauer SA, et al. Concurrent ventral hernia repair in patients undergoing laparoscopic bariatric surgery: a case-matched study using the National Surgical Quality Improvement Program Database. Surg Obes Relat Dis. 2017;13(6):997–1002.
40. Ghanem OM, Orenstein S, Lloyd SJ, Andalib A, Race A, Burt HA, et al. Management of abdominal wall hernias in patients with severe obesity. Surg Endosc. 2023;37(9):6619–26.

# Post-Bariatric Hypoglycemia

# 34

Lei Pei and Mary Elizabeth Patti

## Background

### Prevalence

The true prevalence of post-bariatric hypoglycemia (PBH) is uncertain, as there are differences in diagnostic methods and criteria between studies. Population-based data indicate that severe hypoglycemia that led to hospitalization occurs in 0.1–1% of bariatric patients [1, 2]. This is likely a severe underestimation, given that hypoglycemia does not usually require hospitalization. One study indicated a 25-fold increase in the prevalence of OGTT-induced hypoglycemia (defined as glucose <60 mg/dL) after Roux-en-Y gastric bypass (RYGB) compared to pre-surgery [3]. While continuous glucose monitoring can over-estimate hypoglycemia, one study of 40 post-RYGB participants detected episodes of sensor glucose <55 mg/dL in 75%; in contrast, hypoglycemia was triggered by mixed meal test in only 29% of the same participants [4]. Finally, several studies have assessed the prevalence of self-reported hypoglycemia symptoms in post-bariatric patients, ranging from 34.2% [5] to 38.5% [6]. Given that symptoms of hypoglycemia are nonspecific and instead may be linked to other aspects of post-surgical physiology, such as dumping syndrome [7], self-reported prevalence is likely to be higher than the true prevalence.

Based on the latest data as of 2021 from the American Society of Metabolic and Bariatric Surgery, sleeve gastrectomy (SG) is the predominant type of bariatric surgery (58.1%), with RYGB following closely at 21.5%. Post-bariatric hypoglycemia most commonly occurs after either RYGB or sleeve gastrectomy, but also after

L. Pei · M. E. Patti (✉)
Research Division, Joslin Diabetes Center, Boston, MA, USA

Harvard Medical School, Boston, MA, USA
e-mail: Mary.elizabeth.patti@joslin.harvard.edu


O. M. Ghanem et al. (eds.), *The SAGES Manual of Metabolic and Bariatric Surgery*, https://doi.org/10.1007/978-3-031-72309-4_34

other types of upper glycemic index (GI) surgery such as omega-loop gastric bypass [8] and fundoplication which is typically performed for reflux esophagitis [9]. While hypoglycemia prevalence is similar between RYGB and SG, hypoglycemia is typically more severe after RYGB [10]. Thus, the emergence of sleeve gastrectomy as the most performed bariatric procedure in the United States is not a safer alternative to RYGB from a hypoglycemia perspective.

## Pathophysiology of PBH

The precise mechanisms responsible for PBH remain incompletely understood. However, several mechanisms appear to dominate. First, surgical alteration of the upper gastrointestinal tract results in accelerated gastric emptying [11, 12], leading to the rapid delivery of nutrients to the absorptive intestinal mucosa. Increases in plasma glucose and amino acids are likely contributors to increased plasma insulin levels, resulting in a rapid drop in glucose levels to overt hypoglycemia 1–3 h after meals. Additionally, the rapid transit of ingested nutrients stimulates the release of GLP-1 by enteroendocrine L-cells. In the presence of hyperglycemia, these high levels of GLP-1 can further enhance insulin secretion [3, 13]. The magnitude of post-surgical increases in GLP-1 and insulin secretion are further magnified in individuals with PBH [3]. Increases in GLP1 appear to contribute significantly to meal insulin secretion; one study showed that blockade of the GLP1 receptor with the peptide antagonist exendin 9–39 resulted in ≈50% reduction in postprandial insulin secretion in patients with PBH [14]. This same compound administered to nine patients with PBH reduced OGTT-induced peak insulin levels by 57%, increased the postprandial glucose nadir by 66%, and reduced neuroglycopenic symptoms by 88% [15].

Additional mechanisms may contribute to exaggerated improvements in glucose metabolism and hypoglycemia. Studies in both humans [16] and rodents [17] have demonstrated increased glucose uptake by the intestine after surgery, potentially related to intestinal hypertrophy. One case-control cohort study evaluated glucose uptake, measured by $^{18}$F-FDG-PET-CT, in 19 patients with prior gastric surgery (mainly RYGB), in comparison to 43 age and gender-matched controls without gastric surgery. Glucose uptake was increased by 98% in the jejunum, 41% in the ascending colon, and 56% in the transverse colon of patients who had prior gastric surgery [18]. Likewise, rodent studies have demonstrated a ≈ twofold increase in glucose uptake within the Roux limb after RYGB [17].

Additional mechanisms that may contribute to hypoglycemia include reduced counterregulatory hormonal response to hypoglycemia. Abrahamsson and colleagues observed a reduction of glucagon, cortisol, and catecholamine response to hypoglycemia during a hyperinsulinemic-hypoglycemic clamp as early as 6 months post-RYGB, even in those without hypoglycemia [19]. Similarly, Salehi et al. showed that participants with a history of gastric bypass, regardless of whether they have PBH or not, have reduced glucagon levels in response to falling glucose, as compared to weight-matched nonsurgical controls [20].

Bile acids (BA) are now recognized as important signaling molecules regulating systemic metabolism via the cell surface G protein-coupled receptor TGR5 and the nuclear hormone receptor farnesoid X receptor (FXR) [21]. Following bariatric surgery in both humans and rodents, plasma levels of both total bile acids and specific bile acid species are elevated [22, 23], and levels of fibroblast growth factor 19 (FGF19), an intestinal hormone and target of BA-FXR signaling, are increased postoperatively. Moreover, experimental bile diversion to the distal intestine modulates glucose metabolism in rodents [24]. Patients with PBH may have further dysregulation of BA signaling, as postprandial plasma FGF19 levels are threefold higher in patients with PBH when compared with asymptomatic post-RYGB individuals [25].

Increased pro-inflammatory signaling may also contribute to excessive insulin response in patients with hypoglycemia after gastric bypass [26].

Autonomic dysfunction has been observed in post-bariatric patients, particularly those who have undergone gastric bypass. In a single-institution analysis, 16.3% of 4547 post-bariatric patients reported new onset of orthostatic intolerance symptoms including dizziness, orthostatic hypotension, tachycardia, bradycardia, or syncope; 4.2% remained symptomatic at 5 years [27]. A systematic review identified 87 patients diagnosed with dysautonomia; these were predominantly women post-RYGB [28]. Since the autonomic nervous system can directly influence insulin secretion and hepatic glucose production, it is possible that autonomic dysfunction could contribute to perturbations in glucose levels after meals and activity [29]. However, whether autonomic dysfunction is an underlying contributor to PBH or merely a coexisting factor remains unclear.

## Risk Factors

Identification of risk factors for hypoglycemia as a complication of surgery would be important to reduce this complication via improved preoperative screening. Studies to date have revealed that female sex, history of cholecystectomy, and lower preoperative BMI and HbA1C levels are associated with a higher risk of PBH [30, 31]. Likewise, analysis of a longitudinal cohort study of 957 RYGB patients showed that higher preoperative beta cell function and insulin sensitivity, assessed during oral glucose tolerance testing, was associated with a higher incidence of low post-load glucose levels postoperatively[31, 32]. Additional risk factors identified in 1738 patients who underwent RYGB in the LABS cohort included preoperative history of hypoglycemia symptoms (odds ratio of ten-fold for developing postoperative hypoglycemia symptoms) and use of SSRI/SNRI antidepressants (odds ratio of 1.5) [6]. Additional studies will be required to identify genetic, historical, and metabolic features indicating high risk for PBH, and to implement screening for these risk factors during preoperative evaluation in order to guide risk assessment and consider alternative obesity therapeutic approaches.

# Diagnosis of PBH

## Diagnosis of Hypoglycemia

Having postprandial symptoms alone does not make the diagnosis of PBH, given the nonspecific nature of hypoglycemia symptoms which can overlap with anxiety, arrhythmias, orthostatic hypotension, dumping syndrome, and vasomotor symptoms of menopause. Thus, it is essential to document low blood glucose at the time of symptoms to diagnose PBH. A recent study of 30 patients with a prior diagnosis of PBH analyzed CGM data collected for 50 days concurrently with autonomic, neuroglycopenic, and gastrointestinal symptoms. Interestingly, 30.6% of the postprandial periods with symptoms had normal sensor glucose levels at the time [7], suggesting non-glucose signals were contributors to symptoms after meals. Conversely, when sensor glucose was below 54 mg/dL, the frequency of symptoms in the postprandial period was only 18.9%. This study highlighted the importance of correlating the timing of symptoms with concurrent glucose levels, considering the nonspecific nature of hypoglycemia symptoms and the overlap with dumping syndrome in the post-surgical population.

Given these caveats, it is essential to first confirm the diagnosis of hypoglycemia with Whipple's triad, which includes: (1) symptoms of hypoglycemia, (2) venous glucose levels below 3.0 mmol/L (<54 mg/dL) at the time of symptoms, and (3) rapid improvement of symptoms upon normalization of glucose. A venous glucose level < 54 mg/dL is typically not seen under normal physiological conditions in individuals without diabetes and generally indicates clinically important hypoglycemia [33, 34]. Venous blood glucose is most accurate in confirming hypoglycemia, but it is often challenging to safely obtain a venous sample at the time of symptoms in the outpatient setting. Capillary glucose is an alternative, but readings can be falsely low in the setting of altered capillary flow such as Raynaud's phenomenon [35], cold temperatures, instrument error, or improper use of glucose meter [36]. CGM, especially when masked and when combined with a detailed food/activity diary, can be helpful in defining patterns of glucose excursions and provide valuable insights into the impact of meals, activity, and other factors. If masked CGM reveals no low sensor glucose levels at the time of recorded symptoms (e.g., all sensor values over 70), this may suggest that alternative factors are contributing to the patient's symptoms. However, given the inaccuracy of CGM at low glucose values, and the inherent "lag time" between blood and sensor glucose levels, we do not recommend the use of CGM for the diagnosis of hypoglycemia as low sensor glucose levels may not truly reflect capillary or venous levels, and may be falsely low due to sensor compression, altered blood flow, calibration errors or technical errors [37].

Severity of hypoglycemia has been defined by an international consensus group [33]. Level 1 hypoglycemia is defined as a blood glucose between 54 and 70 mg/dL; level 2 is a blood glucose less than 54 mg/dL; and level 3 refers to severe hypoglycemic events characterized by altered mental status and/or requiring the assistance of others.

## Glucose Patterns in PBH

Patients who have had upper gastrointestinal surgery, including those with typical PBH often exhibit a distinct glucose pattern after meals. Typically, there is a rapid initial increase in blood glucose levels within the first 30 min after eating, followed by a rapid decrease in glucose to baseline in those without hypoglycemia. Individuals with PBH have similar post-meal spikes, but rapid declines to frankly hypoglycemic levels by 1–3 h after the meal [38]. Fasting hypoglycemia is usually not observed. Low glucose levels can also be observed in response to exercise or activity.

## History and Physical Exam

A thorough medical history and examination are crucial for assessing the differential diagnosis and to rule out other causes of hypoglycemia, even in a post-surgical patient (Fig. 34.1). Information gleaned from medical history can help to define whether patterns are consistent with PBH or suggest other causes. PBH typically becomes clinically noticeable at least 1 year after bariatric surgery [38]. If hypoglycemia is observed shortly after surgery (<6 to 12 months), this suggests that an alternative diagnosis is likely and should be searched for aggressively.

Assessment of the timing of hypoglycemia episodes is helpful in differentiating between PBH and early dumping syndrome. With PBH, hypoglycemia typically occurs 1–3 h after food ingestion and is rarely observed during fasting or activity [38]. By contrast, early dumping usually occurs within an hour after consuming

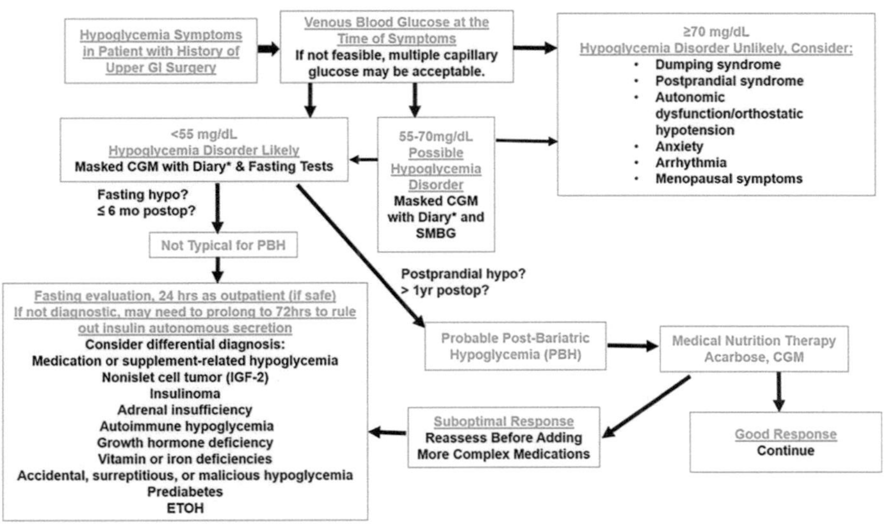


**Fig. 34.1** Suggested diagnostic evaluation of PBH. *Diary including symptoms, meals, activity. Abbreviations: *SMBG* self-monitoring blood glucose, *CGM* continuous glucose monitor, *ETOH* ethanol, *IGF-2* insulin-like growth factor 2, *GI* gastrointestinal

food. Early dumping syndrome includes a combination of gastrointestinal and vasomotor symptoms including nausea, dizziness, tachycardia, and drop in blood pressure; this syndrome is thought to be triggered by the rapid delivery of undigested nutrients to the intestine, resulting in the movement of fluid from the intravascular space to the intestinal lumen. Increases in a variety of hormones, including preproglucagon-derived peptides including glucagon like peptide 1, peptide YY, pancreatic polypeptide, vasoactive intestinal polypeptide, and neurotensin, may contribute to this syndrome [39, 40].

Detailed surgical history is important, including type of surgery, postoperative complications, and magnitude and time course of weight loss. A review of the operative report may be helpful.

For all patients, it is essential to rule out the presence of additional diagnoses that could exacerbate the severity or frequency of hypoglycemia, even in individuals with a history of upper GI surgery. These could include medication-related hypoglycemia (Table 34.1), malnutrition, adverse effects from drugs or supplements, severe systemic illness, liver or kidney disease, adrenal insufficiency [59], growth hormone insufficiency [60], autoimmune hypoglycemia [61], islet tumors (e.g., insulinoma), or non-islet cell tumors [62]. If hypoglycemia mostly occurs during fasting or is severe and refractory to initial therapy, it is important to exclude the possibility of insulinoma, which can occur in patients who have had upper gastrointestinal surgery [63]. It is important to note that insulinoma can manifest with hypoglycemia in the fasting state as well as in postprandial periods; one series reports that 6% of insulinomas only manifest hypoglycemia in the postprandial state [64].

A pertinent physical exam to assist with the above differential diagnosis includes BMI, vital signs (including orthostatic pulse and BP), skin examination for acanthosis or vitiligo, abdominal examination to detect hepatomegaly or abdominal masses,

**Table 34.1** Medications that can exacerbate hypoglycemia

| | |
|---|---|
| Antihyperglycemic medications | Insulin, sulfonylureas, meglitinide, repaglinide, metformin |
| Antimicrobials | Cibenzoline, clinafloxacin, gatifloxacin, pentamidine, artesunate/artemisinin/artemether, quinine [41] |
| Cardiovascular medications | ACE-I [42, 43], beta blockers [44] |
| Antineoplastic drugs | Imatinib [45], checkpoint inhibitors [46] |
| Analgesics | Indomethacin [47], gabapentin [48], tramadol [49], propoxyphene [50], dextropropoxyphene [51] |
| Antidepressants/mood stabilizers | SSRIs [52–54], SNRIs [55, 56], MAOIs [57], lithium [58] |
| Others | Alcohol, marijuana, herbal supplements |

*ACE-I* Angiotensin-converting enzyme (ACE) inhibitors, *SSRIs* selective serotonin reuptake inhibitors, *SNRIs* serotonin and norepinephrine reuptake inhibitors, *MAOIs* monoamine oxidase inhibitors

evaluating for galactorrhea and signs of peripheral neuropathy.

## Laboratory and Imaging Studies

After confirming hypoglycemia, lab tests are focused on ruling out other systemic disorders, which may contribute to the patient's symptoms and/or provide a clue to the etiology of hypoglycemia. We recommend a complete blood count to rule out anemia, a comprehensive chemistry panel to assess kidney and liver function, and HbA1C to screen for prediabetes as hypoglycemic phases have been reported to occur prior to the development of diabetes, but strong evidence is lacking. TSH and morning cortisol levels (8 AM or upon arising if different timing) should be conducted to rule out hypothyroidism or adrenal insufficiency. Prealbumin levels can help assess nutritional status when malnutrition is suspected. Autoimmune hypoglycemia can be evaluated by checking for insulin receptor autoantibodies. A sulfonylurea screen is highly recommended at the time of acute hypoglycemia unless there is a clearly identified alternative explanation for the hypoglycemic condition in the patient. Measurement of IGF1 can help to assess growth hormone sufficiency, while IGF2 levels and the ratio of IGF2/IGF1 can be informative for detecting non-islet cell tumor-induced hypoglycemia. Additionally, consider testing for iron and/or ferritin levels, vitamins D, B12, B1, B2, and B6, in post-bariatric patients who are at high risk for deficiencies of these factors.

While most clinicians associate insulinoma with fasting hypoglycemia, insulinoma can cause postprandial hypoglycemia [64] and multiple reports indicate that post-bariatric patients can have insulinoma [63]. Given this complexity, one needs to determine the risk. For someone deemed at low risk, measurement of glucose, insulin, C-peptide, and proinsulin levels after a 16-h overnight fast may be sufficient. Including blood glucose levels alongside insulin, measurements is crucial for accurate interpretation of the results. However, in cases of inconclusive results, or in the presence of coexisting disease making fasting more dangerous (e.g., severe CAD, seizure disorder, long QT syndrome, or other cardiac arrhythmia) extended fasting tests for 24 h or even 72 h may be necessary, with close supervision by clinicians, in a hospital setting. Likewise, even if the initial assessment suggests that insulinoma is unlikely, continued severe hypoglycemia unresponsive to medical nutrition therapy or acarbose should prompt the clinician to carefully consider whether additional testing to rule out autonomous insulin secretion is needed.

Imaging studies to rule out insulinoma are not routinely recommended unless biochemical testing supports autonomous insulin secretion. If so, accurate preoperative localization of an insulinoma is important for surgical planning and patient counseling. Noninvasive imaging procedures may include spiral computed tomography (CT), magnetic resonance imaging (MRI), and endoscopic ultrasound [65]. If these conventional imaging methods are unable to detect abnormal pancreatic lesions, Ga-68 DOTATATE PET/CT, a somatostatin-receptor-based imaging modality, may be considered [66]. If DOTATATE scan results are inconclusive, arteriography and selective arterial calcium stimulation with hepatic venous sampling can also be considered [67].

## Provocative Testing

Research studies employ provocative testing, but the similar patterns in post-bariatric patients with and without hypoglycemia make results of both glucose and meal tolerance testing inconclusive in most patients. Moreover, the stimulus type and amount are not standardized. Oral glucose tolerance testing was widely used in the past. Most studies administered 75 g glucose (ranging from 25–100 g), with insulin and C-peptide assessed at baseline and then every hour up to 4 h thereafter. However, OGTT is not recommended as it provokes postprandial hypoglycemia (2-h glucose <60 mg/dL) in 5.5% of people without diabetes, even in nonsurgical patients [68]; in post-bariatric patients, oral glucose can induce severe dumping syndrome and severe hypoglycemia, raising safety concerns for office visits.

Mixed meal testing has also been employed in research studies, typically using a liquid meal containing 40–75 g of carbohydrates as well as protein and fat. However, several studies have shown that mixed meal testing can trigger hypoglycemia in asymptomatic post-bariatric patients as well. One study showed 3 out of 9 asymptomatic RYGB individuals had glucose levels below 60 mg/dL after a liquid meal [3]. In another study, 13% of 109 individuals who were 12 months post-RYGB, had venous glucose less than 55 mg/dL after a solid mixed meal [69]. The lack of standardized meal composition definitions and glycemic cut-offs, along with high false positive rates, continue to make meal testing largely unsuitable for clinical diagnosis.

To summarize, both oral glucose and mixed meal tolerance tests are employed in research settings but are not routinely recommended for the clinical diagnosis of PBH. Rather, clinicians should focus on obtaining a comprehensive patient history, evaluating glucose patterns, and ruling out alternative causes of hypoglycemia to establish a diagnosis of PBH.

## Treatment Options for PBH

### Dietary Modification

The goal of medical nutrition therapy in PBH is to reduce the rapid and excessive rise in glucose after meals, which can contribute to increased insulin secretion and subsequent low blood glucose levels. This is often highly challenging, as gastric emptying is rapid due to altered anatomy. We highly recommend consultation with an experienced registered dietitian to review dietary habits, identify potential trigger foods, and provide customized recommendations for healthy eating after bariatric surgery. Because individual glycemic responses to foods vary greatly, a comprehensive personalized nutrition assessment is essential to elucidate each patient's postprandial blood glucose patterns in response to different foods and food combinations. Having the patient keep a detailed food diary, recording every episode of hypoglycemia and all foods eaten several hours prior, including the type and texture of food, portion size, liquids ingested with the meal, and the timing of eating, can be helpful, particularly when paired with a continuous glucose monitor.

## Modification of the Quantity and Type of Carbohydrate Based on Glycemic Index

To mitigate the rapid rise in glucose after meals related to rapid delivery and absorption of carbohydrates in the post-surgical state, it is often helpful to reduce the total quantity of carbohydrates and to completely avoid high glycemic index (GI) carbohydrates. Research conducted on individuals consuming test meals in a monitored or inpatient setting has indicated that reducing carbohydrate intake to 20–30 g per meal and 10–15 g per snack can substantially decrease or even prevent postprandial hypoglycemia [70]. One study by Marques et al. reviewed CGM tracings of nine post-RYGB patients with symptomatic hypoglycemia vs eight post-RYGB patients who remained asymptomatic. Interestingly, evaluation of the macronutrient composition of meals preceding symptomatic events identified that the symptomatic group tended to have a lower intake of protein in morning snacks (3.2 g vs 7.7 g) and a higher intake of refined carbohydrate at lunch (11.6 g vs 4.3 g) when compared with asymptomatic individuals [71].

The efficacy of a reduction in carbohydrate intake strategy may be attenuated in a home environment. In one study [72], 34 post-RYGB individuals were instructed to eat three main meals with a maximum of 30 g carbs each and three smaller meals with a maximum of 15–30 g carbs at home. Self-reported hypoglycemic events were significantly reduced, with 15% reporting complete resolution and 61% experiencing partial improvement in hypoglycemia episode frequency (to less than once a week). However, 22% of patients reported no improvement at all [72]. Reduced efficacy of carbohydrate reduction in managing PBH in the home setting may stem from several factors: (1) physical activity, which varies between individuals, could contribute to hypoglycemia in the outpatient setting and inter-individual variability, (2) maintenance of dietary adherence can be particularly challenging in the outpatient setting, especially for individuals with a history of disordered eating.

We typically recommend a reduction in carbohydrate intake to less than 30 grams per meal and complete avoidance of high glycemic index carbohydrates. However, carbohydrate intake goals should be personalized for each patient based on a thorough review of their food diary and analysis of their individual postprandial glucose patterns in response to initial changes. Some patients may require more significant carbohydrate reduction to prevent hypoglycemia (e.g., 20–25 g/meal) if the initial 30 g/meal target is not effective. Ongoing assessment is needed to make sure that greater degrees of carbohydrate restriction do not worsen hypoglycemia or induce activity-induced or nocturnal hypoglycemia, potentially via reduced glycogen stores.

Low glycemic carbohydrates are preferred as they are digested slowly, and have slower postprandial glucose rise resulting in lower-magnitude and fewer glucose spikes and therefore less postprandial insulin secretion and hypoglycemia. In contrast, high glycemic carbohydrates should be avoided as they are digested and absorbed faster, triggering more hyperglycemic "spikes" and therefore more subsequent hypoglycemia. Glycemic index information for a variety of foods can be found at www.glycemicindex.com. An additional approach to prevent hypoglycemia between meals, before exercise, and during nocturnal hours consists of uncooked cornstarch (which is a very complex, slowly metabolized carbohydrate).

Uncooked cornstarch was shown to be effective in preventing hypoglycemia events caused by a variety of disorders [73]. Two case reports demonstrated that oral intake of uncooked cornstarch (1.25–1.8 g/kg body weight per day) together with a high fiber diet led to more stable glucose levels and lower frequency of low sensor glucose on CGM [74].

Frequent dietary consultation is essential as the responses to specific foods vary considerably. Therefore, initial advice should be adjusted for each patient during subsequent follow-up visits.

## Importance of Adequate Intake of Protein and Heart-Healthy Fats

Since the dietary strategies for post-bariatric hypoglycemia focus on reducing carbohydrate intake to reduce postprandial spikes in blood glucose, the remaining calorie intake to meet nutritional goals should be met with adequate protein and heart-healthy fats.

Protein adequacy is important post-bariatric surgery as protein malnutrition is a serious complication. The American Society of Metabolic and Bariatric Surgery recommends a daily protein intake of 60–80 grams, while other guidelines suggest 1.5–2.1 grams per kilogram of ideal weight or 0.91 grams per kilogram of actual weight [75]. In a study of ten patients with PBH, a carbohydrate-reduced, high-protein (CRHP) diet (30% carbohydrate, 30% protein, 40% fat) was compared to the conventional recommended diet (55% carbohydrate, 15% protein, 30% fat). The CRHP diet reduced peak postprandial glucose by 11% and 31% at breakfast and lunch, respectively, while increasing nadir glucose by 13% and 9% compared to a conventional diet [76]. Recommended protein sources are those containing high biological value, including meat, chicken, egg whites, fish, dairy, and high-quality plant-based options such as soy protein. Liquid protein can be rapidly absorbed, and stimulate insulin secretion, so protein in solid form is strongly preferred.

Fats provide a good source of calories that typically do not stimulate insulin secretion or independently cause hypoglycemia. Therefore, increasing healthy fats can help meet calorie needs without exacerbating postprandial hypoglycemia in PBH. In addition, the order of food ingested can be important. In one study of 20 individuals with well-controlled type 2 diabetes, eating high-carbohydrate portion of the meal only after high-protein and high-fat foods resulted in reduced glycemic excursion by 18–32 mg/dL [77]. We similarly recommend that intake of protein and fats should occur prior to ingestion of carbohydrates.

## Meal Composition, Size, and Liquids

Liquid meals have more rapid transit out of the stomach or pouch and have been shown to induce higher peak GLP1 levels and higher frequency of hypoglycemia. Interestingly in one study of 32 post-RYGB individuals [78], insulin release was not different between solid and liquid meals despite the significant difference in GLP1 spikes. However, higher GLP1 levels after liquid meals may also trigger symptoms associated with dumping syndrome, including tachycardia, fatigue, nausea, and lightheadedness.

In addition, the size of the meal is a determinant of insulin secretion. Larger meals compared to smaller meals lead to more insulin secretion [78].

Since liquids can promote distention of the gastric pouch and accelerated emptying, patients should try to avoid drinking liquids during meals and for 30–60 min after each meal.

### Alcohol and Caffeine

Several studies indicate an increased risk of alcohol use disorder after bariatric surgery [79, 80]. Acutely, alcohol can reduce hepatic gluconeogenesis and therefore can increase the risk for hypoglycemia in a post-bariatric patient [81, 82]. In addition, many alcoholic drinks contain high glycemic index carbohydrates that can trigger hypoglycemia. We recommend avoidance of alcohol intake to minimize the additive risk of hypoglycemia.

Anecdotally, some patients report that caffeine increases the risk of hypoglycemia, but studies are lacking. Patients should avoid caffeine-containing beverages containing sugar.

## Acute Treatment of Hypoglycemia

Treatment of hypoglycemia in post-bariatric patients should follow similar general principles used for hypoglycemia in diabetes management. This involves consuming a small amount (5–15 g) of fast-acting carbohydrates such as glucose tablets, glucose gel, or glucose liquid, and subsequently monitoring blood glucose every 15 min to determine if additional dosing is needed. However, patients with PBH often observe that even 15 g of fast-acting carbohydrates can cause rebound hyperglycemia and subsequent hypoglycemia. Schönenberger et al. recently found that 3 of 8 patients treated with 15 g glucose experienced rebound hypoglycemia (<60 mg/dL), whereas no rebound hypoglycemia occurred when patients were given 5 g glucose plus 10 g protein. In this study, the authors suggested that 5 g of glucose appears sufficient to raise glucose out of the critical range in most patients with PBH, while also avoiding potential rebound hypoglycemia occurring with the higher 15 g doses. Additionally, complementary nutrients such as protein may provide extra glycemia-stabilizing effects. [83].

Glucagon is an essential tool for rapid treatment of hypoglycemia when patients are not able to consume glucose by mouth due to severe changes in mental status or loss of consciousness. In such cases, often a family member, partner, or roommate administers glucagon, so providing them with guidance on how to administer glucagon is necessary. Fortunately, glucagon is now available in several forms, including intranasal spray, autoinjectors, and traditional emergency kits.

## Pharmacological Therapy

### Glucosidase Inhibitors

Acarbose is a complex oligosaccharide that acts as a competitive, reversible inhibitor of pancreatic alpha-amylase and membrane-bound intestinal alpha-glucoside hydrolase. As a result, it slows carbohydrate breakdown and absorption, helping to attenuate the rise in blood glucose after meals. Acarbose is approved for the management of T2D via its effect to decrease postprandial hyperglycemia. For the same reasons, acarbose is also effective in treating PBH. One study showed that a single dose of acarbose 100 mg administered 15 min prior to a mixed meal blunted the postprandial hyperglycemic spike and decreased early postprandial secretion of GLP1 and insulin [84]. In another study of eight individuals post-RYGB, treatment with 50–100 mg acarbose three times daily before meals along with dietary counseling for 6 weeks resulted in reduction in time of CGM-derived sensor glucose over 140 mg/dL (from 13.4% to 5.2%) and a reduction in time of sensor glucose below 60 mg/dL (from 2.5% to 0.18%) [85].

In a recent retrospective study, out of 107 patients with PBH were treated with acarbose at a median dose of 150 mg daily, of whom 21% were reported to have complete resolution of all hypoglycemic events, 35% had 50–100% resolution, 20% had 20–50% resolution and 24% had 0–20% resolution [86].

The most common adverse effects of acarbose are GI intolerance, including flatulence, diarrhea, and abdominal pain [87]. A high-carbohydrate diet can worsen the gastrointestinal side effects of acarbose. Nevertheless, these symptoms typically are less severe with gradual increase in dosage and abate over time with ongoing treatment. The recommendation is to start with 25 mg three times daily at the start of the meal and then titrate up the dose as tolerated to a maximum of total daily dose of 300 mg per day.

### Somatostatin Analogues

Somatostatin analogues are approved for management of certain pituitary or gastroenteropancreatic neuroendocrine tumors. Somatostatin analogues activate specific somatostatin receptor subtypes, particularly subtypes 2 and 5 (SSTR2, SSTR5), blocking the release of several gastrointestinal hormones, such as GLP-1, gastrin [88], pancreatic polypeptide, and neurotensin [89] and changing abdominal blood flow [90]. Thus, somatostatin analogues can helpful in managing dumping syndrome, as documented in multiple studies [91, 92].

Somatostatin analogues also inhibit the secretion of glucagon (mediated by SSTR2 receptor subtypes) and insulin (SSTR2 and SSTR5). Differential activation of SSTR2/5 receptors by somatostatin analogues may contribute to differential glucose responses. Octreotide and lanreotide are more active at SSTR2 compared to SSTR5, while pasireotide activates SSTR2 and SSTR5 equally [93]. Thus, both pasireotide and octreotide can inhibit insulin release, but pasireotide is less effective at suppressing glucagon secretion, and may be less likely to cause acute hypoglycemia. Octreotide reduces antral contractility and thereby delays gastric emptying, although variable dose-dependent effects on the emptying rate have been reported [94, 95].

SSAs have been found to be effective for treatment of PBH. Administration of octreotide before an oral glucose tolerance test reduced GLP-1 and insulin responses and prevented hypoglycemia [96]. Unfortunately, a consequence of SSA therapy to prevent hypoglycemia is often induction of substantial postprandial hyperglycemia, lasting for several hours. This may be attenuated by reduction in carbohydrate intake, SSA dose reduction, or use of long-acting SSA [97]. In a multicenter, retrospective systematic review of 13 patients with recurrent severe postprandial hypoglycemia diagnosed by provocative tests, octreotide 50–100 μg administered subcutaneously every 12 h led to 3/13 (23%) patients with complete response, 5/13 (38.4%) with partial response, and 3/13 (23%) with no response [98].

In a study of 11 participants with PBH, a single dose of pasireotide 300 μg given 30 min prior to mixed meal led to significantly decreased postprandial GLP1, insulin and C-peptide as well as sustained hyperglycemia and prevention of hypoglycemia [99]. One case report demonstrated that 300 μg of pasireotide premeal was more effective in inhibiting insulin and GLP1 release, as compared with 100 μg of octreotide [100].

Long-acting preparations of somatostatin analogues are also available. Lanreotide, at a dose of 90 mg monthly, was shown to improve early postoperative dumping symptoms but not late dumping symptoms [101]. No data are available regarding its efficacy in patients with PBH.

SSAs are generally well tolerated. Side effects include injection site discomfort and erythema, gastrointestinal symptoms such as diarrhea, abdominal pain, nausea and vomiting, and biliary sludge or gallstones [102]. One report indicated that pasireotide can cause adrenal insufficiency, presumably secondary to excessive suppression of adrenocorticotropic hormone (ACTH) secretion [103]. Given that SSA can also inhibit glucagon secretion, hypoglycemia can occasionally be noted as a complication of both acute and chronic LAR dosing. Patients should be aware of this and be instructed to monitor glucose more frequently after medication initiation; if hypoglycemia occurs, a trial of pasireotide could be considered given its more balanced SSTR2/5 activity.

## Calcium Channel Blockers

Evidence of the efficacy of calcium channel blockers in PBH is limited. One case report indicated a significant reduction in frequency of hypoglycemia and amelioration of symptoms [104]. In a randomized crossover study in 11 participants with PBH, verapamil 120 mg three times a day for one week did not have any effect on hypoglycemia occurring during a mixed meal test. In the same study, CGM-derived metrics time (sensor glucose <70 mg/dL, or the rate of hypoglycemic events) did not improve vs. baseline [99].

## GLP-1 Analogues

In patients with T2D, GLP1 analogues have well-documented effects to reduce appetite, promote satiety, reduce body weight, decrease gastric emptying, and stabilize glucose levels without causing hypoglycemia [105]. Given these effects, GLP1 analogues have been used for treatment of PBH, but current data are limited to uncontrolled case series. One case series described four patients with PBH treated with liraglutide 1.2–1.8 mg daily. The patients had no symptomatic hypoglycemia during follow-up. However, hypoglycemia returned when liraglutide was temporarily stopped, demonstrating its effectiveness in preventing hypoglycemia in these patients [106]. Anecdotally, some patients have an increase in hypoglycemia when GLP1 analogues are initiated, so careful discussion of risks vs. benefits for each patient and careful monitoring upon initiation and dose escalation is recommended. In a randomized crossover study in 11 participants with PBH, liraglutide 1.2 mg for 3 weeks significantly reduced hyperglycemic events (sensor glucose >200 mg/dL), glucose variability, and modestly increased nadir glucose (from 48 to 54 mg/dL) using CGM. However, there was no significant change in percentage time of sensor glucose <70 mg/dL or rate of hypoglycemic events [99].

Studies in rodents have shown that glucagon-like peptide-1 (GLP-1) can increase beta cell mass through promoting neogenesis and proliferation and reducing apoptosis of beta cells [107, 108]. While direct data on the impact of GLP1 on the proliferation and apoptosis of beta cells in human studies is lacking, it is important to note that GLP1 receptors are expressed on the surface of insulinoma cells as well as some neuroendocrine tumors [109, 110]. Thus, it is advisable to consider ruling out insulinoma or other neuroendocrine tumors before starting GLP1 analogues given the theoretical risk of promoting proliferation of an existing but undiagnosed insulinoma in this population.

## SGLT2/1 Inhibitors

SGLT2 receptors are predominantly found in segments S1 and S2 of the proximal tubule and mediate renal tubular glucose reabsorption. SGLT1 is primarily expressed in the apical membrane of enterocytes in the small intestine where it facilitates glucose absorption in the GI tract. SGLT2/1 inhibitors have been suggested as a potential treatment option for postprandial hypoglycemia (PBH) owing to their ability to mitigate spikes in postprandial hyperglycemia by inhibiting absorption of glucose in GI tract and kidney.

One randomized, placebo-controlled study in 20 healthy participants found that canagliflozin (SGLT2 > 1 inhibitor), dosed at 300 mg treatment prior to mixed meal, reduced postprandial plasma glucose and insulin excursions [111]. Likewise, in post-RYGB individuals, a single 600 mg dose of canagliflozin resulted in reduced postprandial hyperglycemia, along with decreased postprandial secretion of insulin, C-peptide, and GLP-1 [112].

More recently, this concept has been tested in larger studies. In a pilot prospective, open-label study, without placebo control, 21 patients with PBH after RYGB were given 300 mg of canagliflozin daily for 2 weeks. Participants had reduced postprandial hyperglycemia and lower postprandial plasma insulin levels. In addition, canagliflozin reduced the frequency of hypoglycemia (glucose < 50 mg/dL) by 86% at 3 h after an oral glucose tolerance test compared to pretreatment [113]. This suggests canagliflozin may be effective for reducing hypoglycemia in patients with PBH following RYGB [113].

By contrast, Carpentieri et al. administered empagliflozin (much greater specificity for SGLT2 vs. SGLT1) 25 mg daily for 3 days to 14 post-bariatric patients (11 post-RYGB, three post-sleeve gastrectomy) [114], 7 of whom were previously diagnosed with PBH. There was a statistically significant increase in fasting glucose and mixed meal glucose area under the curve after empagliflozin treatment, but no significant impact on nadir glucose, in the PBH subgroup. Additionally, fasting insulin levels were higher after empagliflozin, possibly in response to the elevated fasting glucose. In another crossover study of 12 post-RYGB individuals, pretreatment with empagliflozin 2 h prior to mixed meal test increased nadir glucose and resulted in fewer events requiring rescue glucose administration compared to baseline (2/12 vs 7/12) [26].

In conclusion, the effectiveness of SGLT2/1 inhibitors in treating PBH remains uncertain. While some studies suggest potential effectiveness, larger randomized controlled trials are necessary to decisively determine efficacy of this approach.

## Diazoxide

Diazoxide, an agonist of the adenosine triphosphate-dependent potassium channel [115], inhibits insulin secretion and stimulates glucose release from the liver. Given that increased insulin secretion and impaired glucose production both contribute to hypoglycemia in PBH, diazoxide has been used clinically for management. However, data for its efficacy in PBH management is limited. One case report showed that diazoxide 200 mg daily in a 36-year-old patient with PBH improved hypoglycemia from severe to mild [116], while one retrospective case series review of six patients with PBH who were treated with a mean of 170 mg/day of diazoxide suggested 3/6 (50%) of the patients had partial response [98]. Common side effects of diazoxide include hypotension, palpitations, hair growth, and edema, which may lead to non-adherence to the medication [99]. Mild edema can be managed by concomitant low-dose diuretics if needed.

## Therapies in Development

### GLP-1 Receptor Antagonism

As discussed previously, a leading hypothesis for the underlying cause of PBH is overproduction of GLP-1 by L-cells in response to food intake and nutrient absorption. This leads to excessive hyperinsulinemia and subsequent post-meal hypoglycemia. Thus, blockade of the GLP1 receptor has been a target for PBH pharmacological treatment.

One such approach in development is use of the selective GLP1 receptor antagonist exendin 9–39, also known as avexitide. Avexitide has been shown to reduce insulin levels by 50% and increase nadir glucose levels by 67% in response to mixed meal tolerance tests in nine patients with PBH [14]. In a multicenter, Phase 2, randomized, placebo-controlled crossover study, 18 female participants with PBH were given placebo for 14 days followed by avexitide at 30 mg twice daily or 60 mg once daily for 14 days. Nadir glucose was increased by 21% with the 30 mg twice-daily dose and 26% with the 60 mg daily dose. Correspondingly, the postprandial insulin peak was lowered by 23% and 21%. Notably, there were significant reductions in all three levels of hypoglycemia and a 50–75% decrease in the need for rescue carbohydrates [117]. Phase III clinical trials of avexitide therapy are still in the planning stage as of this writing.

### Glucagon and Glucagon Analogues via Pump

Glucagon injection is effective in acutely raising postprandial plasma glucose in patients with PBH. However, in a single patient study, continuous glucagon infusion resulted in increased insulin levels and was unable to prevent symptomatic hypoglycemia [118].

Another approach, which may be more physiologic, is to deliver glucagon only in response to incipient hypoglycemia. A randomized, placebo-controlled crossover study in 11 post-RYGB participants with PBH with neuroglycopenia demonstrated that that a CGM-guided closed-loop glucagon rescue system was able to identify impending hypoglycemia during mixed meal tolerance test, and administer mini-doses of glucagon, effectively mitigating severe hypoglycemia [119].

Dasiglucagon, a novel stable glucagon analog in a liquid formulation, has been studied in a crossover study; a single dose of placebo, 80 or 200 μg was administered to 10 post-RYGB patients with PBH prior to a mixed meal tolerance test. Dasiglucagon was effective in increasing nadir glucose levels and reducing time spent in hypoglycemia (glucose <70 mg/dL) up to 4 h following the mixed meal [120].

## Comparison of Different Medications

It remains uncertain which approaches are the best to manage PBH. One unblinded crossover study compared the effects of acarbose, sitagliptin, verapamil, liraglutide and pasireotide on PBH after RYGB. Acarbose lowered peak glucose levels, while pasireotide increased post-meal glucose levels, but both increased nadir glucose and reduced time in hypoglycemia (glucose <70 mg/dL) after mixed meal [99]. There was no benefit of sitagliptin, which actually lowered nadir glucose. Neither verapamil nor liraglutide (titrated to 0.6–1.2 mg once daily over a 3-week period) had any significant impact on hypoglycemia, hyperglycemia or postprandial insulin secretion during mixed meal. During the 6-day CGM study, liraglutide, acarbose and sitagliptin significantly reduced hyperglycemic events (sensor glucose >200 mg/dL), while acarbose and liraglutide significantly reduced glucose variability. However, none of the treatments led to significant change in percent time with sensor glucose <70 mg/dL or rate of hypoglycemic events. [99].

## CGM as Therapy

Unmasked CGM therapy can provide information to guide patients in food choices as well as to alert them to incipient hypoglycemia. To test whether CGM could provide an actual therapeutic benefit in patients with PBH, a sequential trial in 22 individuals with PBH compared the impact of masked vs. unmasked CGM wear on glycemic patterns [121]. Access to CGM real-time data and alarms during the unmasked phase was associated with decreased time spent in low blood glucose, decreased hypoglycemia events, decreased time in hyperglycemia, and reduced glucose variability. Surprisingly, unmasking of CGM data had a greater impact on hyperglycemic excursions, potentially indicating that awareness of meal impact can guide nutritional modifications to prevent future hypoglycemia events.

Thus, use of CGM devices may improve safety in patients with PBH, especially those with impaired awareness of hypoglycemia [121]. Unfortunately, CGM therapy is often limited by lack of insurance coverage and high cost prohibiting self-purchase.

## Surgical and Endoscopic Intervention

### Enteral Feeding via Gastrostomy or Jejunostomy

A gastrostomy tube inserted into the remnant stomach in patients with history of RYGB offers a means to deliver nutrients directly to the excluded stomach and the duodenum. Delivery of a liquid mixed meal via gastrostomy results in reduced postprandial hyperglycemic spikes and significantly lower postprandial increases in GLP-1 and insulin, as compared with oral feeding [122–124].

Gastrostomy feeding into the remnant stomach has also been used to evaluate candidacy of reversal or conversion surgeries [125]. If nutrient delivery via a gastrostomy tube or J-tube for 8–12 weeks before reversal surgery resulted in symptom improvement, patients were then considered candidates for reversal or conversion surgery. In a prospective review of four post-RYGB patients with medically refractory hyperinsulinemic hypoglycemia, after showing symptom improvement with gastrostomy tube placement in the excluded stomach, patients underwent either reversal to normal anatomy or to sleeve gastrectomy. At mean follow-up of 12 months, no neuroglycopenic symptoms were reported and hypoglycemia events were reduced from 19 to 2 per week [125]. Unfortunately, this is not a fully sensitive or specific assessment as reversal does not fully correct the pathophysiology of PBH and improvement can be temporary, even if continuous tube feeding had been successful in improving hypoglycemia.

## Reversal or Conversion Surgery

Minimally-invasive reversal of RYGB anatomy with restoration of pyloric function and duodenal continuity would be expected to improve nutrient flow. Indeed, several case reports and case series support the partial success of reversal [125–127].

One prospective review of 16 PBH patients undergoing reversal surgery to normal anatomy ± sleeve gastrectomy ($n = 15$) reported that all patients had some amelioration of PBH, while 3 of 16 continued to have mild hypoglycemia (50–70 mg/dL). Five of 16 had postoperative complications (colitis, leaks, intra-abdominal hemorrhage, and mesenteric vein thrombosis). Long-term follow-up demonstrated that 2/16 had anorexia, 4/16 had GERD, 7/16 had more than 15% weight gain, and 1/16 had functional stenosis requiring endoscopic dilatation [128]. Pyloric dysfunction can arise as a complication of division of the stomach during RYGB [129], and when reversing RYGB to its original anatomy or sleeve gastrectomy, some patients may encounter severe symptoms such as nausea, vomiting, and acid reflux related to pyloric dysfunction. For a subset of these patients, pyloroplasty may be required but is often incompletely effective in yielding symptom resolution.

In summary, reversal or conversion surgery may be helpful in ameliorating medically refractory hypoglycemia in some individuals. However, reversal does not fully restore the normal anatomy or function of the upper GI tract (e.g., neuronal continuity, vascularity, adaptations of gut to previous surgery). Moreover, it is essential to weigh benefit vs risks of postoperative complications [125, 128], and weight gain can occur. Longer-term follow-up data is necessary to fully assess the safety and success of reversal or conversion surgeries.

## Transoral Outlet Reduction (TORe)

Increased size of the gastrojejunal stoma is significantly associated with weight regain as well as greater severity of dumping syndrome after RYGB [130]. As a result, surgical or endoscopic procedures aimed at reducing the size of the gastrojejunostomy have been developed.

Z'Graggen et al. reported on surgical placement of a silastic ring ($n = 8$, first two patients with additional distal pancreatectomy) or an adjustable gastric band around the pouch ($n = 4$) in 12 patients who developed severe recurrent hypoglycemia at a median interval of 2 years after RYGB. 11/12 were asymptomatic or significantly improved with respect to postprandial hypoglycemia and dumping symptoms when evaluated at 3–12 month follow-up [131]. An alternative, endoscopic approach to reduce gastrojejunostomy is transoral outlet reduction (TORe); this involves reducing the size of the opening between the stomach pouch and the small intestine to slow stomach emptying. In prior studies, TORe improved or resolved dumping syndrome symptoms in the majority of patients [132–134].

Dunn et al. reported results for 11 patients at >5 years post-RYGB who underwent TORe for severe postprandial hypoglycemia; 11/11 reported a reduction in postprandial hypoglycemic events as well as CGM-based time with glucose below 70 mg/dL at 1 year.

Furthermore, all three patients who had previously suffered seizures related to hypoglycemia achieved remission [135]. There were no adverse events requiring hospitalization; a single patient encountered persistent nausea and vomiting, necessitating dilation of the gastrojejunal anastomosis that resolved her symptoms.

In summary, endoscopic procedures such as TORe demonstrate potential for treating PBH. These approaches may lead to some weight gain, but further studies are required to determine the durability of benefit.

### Pancreatectomy

Increased beta cell mass is observed in some but not all severely affected PBH patients [136–138]. Isolated case reports, largely from patients treated early in the course of recognition of PBH as a clinical entity, showed some improvement in patients with very severe, medically refractory hypoglycemia [139–142]. Current concepts suggest that the pancreas is largely an "innocent bystander" and thus therapy should be directed at those extra-pancreatic mechanisms promoting insulin secretion, rather than resection of the pancreas. Support for this concept also comes from long-term follow-up data from a cohort of 48 patients with noninsulinoma pancreatogenous hypoglycemia of whom 33 were post-bariatric patients. Hypoglycemia symptoms were less severe than prior to pancreatectomy. However, 87% of the patients had recurrence of symptoms in long-term follow-up and the median time to recurrent symptoms was 16 months [143].

Moreover, pancreatectomy is not a benign procedure. Pancreatectomy designed to reduce beta cell mass/function also affects alpha cell number, potentially increasing risk of hypoglycemia due to reduced glucagon response [144]. Additionally, pancreatic resection carries a mortality rate ranging from 1% to 5% even in specialized units [145, 146], with overall morbidity rate of 20–40% [146]. Finally, higher percentage of pancreatic resection increase the risk for developing diabetes mellitus [147].

In summary, pancreatectomy may offer temporary improvement in hypoglycemia, but it is not a curative option and carries a high risk of hypoglycemia recurrence alongside numerous postoperative complications. Therefore, it is not recommended as a standard treatment for typical forms of PBH.

## Summary and Conclusions

Increased awareness is crucial for consideration of hypoglycemia as a potential cause of symptoms of potential hypoglycemia in patients who have undergone upper GI surgery. Diagnosis of post-bariatric hypoglycemia requires a multidisciplinary approach involving confirmation of hypoglycemia with Whipple's triad, identification of glucose patterns, and excluding other causes of hypoglycemia utilizing detailed history, physical exam, laboratory, and imaging studies.

The primary management approach for post-bariatric hypoglycemia involves dietary intervention. While various medical, surgical, and endoscopic approaches can follow medical nutrition therapy, the available data on their efficacy is limited, and side effect profiles can be challenging for long-term use. In the future, more research is needed to understand the precise pathophysiology of PBH and develop safe and effective therapies for this challenging condition.

## References

1. Lee CJ, Wood GC, Lazo M, Brown TT, Clark JM, Still C, Benotti P. Risk of post-gastric bypass surgery hypoglycemia in nondiabetic individuals: a single center experience. Obesity (Silver Spring). 2016;24(6):1342–8.
2. Marsk R, Jonas E, Rasmussen F, Naslund E. Nationwide cohort study of post-gastric bypass hypoglycaemia including 5,040 patients undergoing surgery for obesity in 1986–2006 in Sweden. Diabetologia. 2010;53(11):2307–11.
3. Goldfine AB, Mun EC, Devine E, Bernier R, Baz-Hecht M, Jones DB, Schneider BE, Holst JJ, Patti ME. Patients with neuroglycopenia after gastric bypass surgery have exaggerated incretin and insulin secretory responses to a mixed meal. J Clin Endocrinol Metab. 2007;92(12):4678–85.
4. Kefurt R, Langer FB, Schindler K, Shakeri-Leidenmuhler S, Ludvik B, Prager G. Hypoglycemia after roux-En-Y gastric bypass: detection rates of continuous glucose monitoring (CGM) versus mixed meal test. Surg Obes Relat Dis. 2015;11(3):564–9.
5. Lee CJ, Clark JM, Schweitzer M, Magnuson T, Steele K, Koerner O, Brown TT. Prevalence of and risk factors for hypoglycemic symptoms after gastric bypass and sleeve gastrectomy. Obesity (Silver Spring). 2015;23(5):1079–84.
6. Fischer LE, Wolfe BM, Fino N, Elman MR, Flum DR, Mitchell JE, Pomp A, Pories WJ, Purnell JQ, Patti ME, Investigators L. Postbariatric hypoglycemia: symptom patterns and associated risk factors in the longitudinal assessment of bariatric surgery study. Surg Obes Relat Dis. 2021;17(10):1787–98.
7. Tripyla A, Ferreira A, Schonenberger KA, Naf NH, Inderbitzin LE, Prendin F, Cossu L, Cappon G, Facchinetti A, Herzig D, Bally L. Relationship between symptom perception and postprandial glycemic profiles in patients with Postbariatric hypoglycemia after roux-en-Y gastric bypass surgery. Diabetes Care. 2023;46(10):1792–8.
8. Lazar LO, Sapojnikov S, Pines G, Mavor E, Ostrovsky V, Schiller T, Knobler H, Zornitzki T. Symptomatic and asymptomatic hypoglycemia post three different bariatric procedures: a common and severe complication. Endocr Pract. 2019;
9. Zaloga GP, Chernow B. Postprandial hypoglycemia after Nissen fundoplication for reflux esophagitis. Gastroenterology. 1983;84(4):840–2.
10. Capristo E, Panunzi S, De Gaetano A, Spuntarelli V, Bellantone R, Giustacchini P, Birkenfeld AL, Amiel S, Bornstein SR, Raffaelli M, Mingrone G. Incidence of hypoglycemia

after gastric bypass vs sleeve gastrectomy: A randomized trial. J Clin Endocrinol Metab. 2018;103(6):2136–46.
11. Chambers AP, Smith EP, Begg DP, Grayson BE, Sisley S, Greer T, Sorrell J, Lemmen L, LaSance K, Woods SC, Seeley RJ, D'Alessio DA, Sandoval DA. Regulation of gastric emptying rate and its role in nutrient-induced GLP-1 secretion in rats after vertical sleeve gastrectomy. Am J Physiol Endocrinol Metab. 2014;306(4):E424–32.
12. Kandeel AA, Sarhan MD, Hegazy T, Mahmoud MM, Ali MH. Comparative assessment of gastric emptying in obese patients before and after laparoscopic sleeve gastrectomy using radionuclide scintigraphy. Nucl Med Commun. 2015;36(8):854–62.
13. Nguyen NQ, Debreceni TL, Bambrick JE, Bellon M, Wishart J, Standfield S, Rayner CK, Horowitz M. Rapid gastric and intestinal transit is a major determinant of changes in blood glucose, intestinal hormones, glucose absorption and postprandial symptoms after gastric bypass. Obesity (Silver Spring). 2014;22(9):2003–9.
14. Salehi M, Gastaldelli A, D'Alessio DA. Blockade of glucagon-like peptide 1 receptor corrects postprandial hypoglycemia after gastric bypass. Gastroenterology. 2014;146(3):669–80.
15. Craig CM, Liu LF, Nguyen T, Price C, Bingham J, McLaughlin TL. Efficacy and pharmacokinetics of subcutaneous exendin (9–39) in patients with post-bariatric hypoglycaemia. Diabetes Obes Metab. 2018;20(2):352–61.
16. Cavin JB, Couvelard A, Lebtahi R, Ducroc R, Arapis K, Voitellier E, Cluzeaud F, Gillard L, Hourseau M, Mikail N, Ribeiro-Parenti L, Kapel N, Marmuse JP, Bado A, Le Gall M. Differences in alimentary glucose absorption and intestinal disposal of blood glucose after roux-en-Y gastric bypass vs sleeve gastrectomy. Gastroenterology. 2016;150(2):454–64.
17. Saeidi N, Meoli L, Nestoridi E, Gupta NK, Kvas S, Kucharczyk J, Bonab AA, Fischman AJ, Yarmush ML, Stylopoulos N. Reprogramming of intestinal glucose metabolism and glycemic control in rats after gastric bypass. Science. 2013;341(6144):406–10.
18. Franquet E, Watts G, Kolodny GM, Goldfine AB, Patti ME. PET-CT reveals increased intestinal glucose uptake after gastric surgery. Surg Obes Relat Dis. 2019;15(4):643–9.
19. Abrahamsson N, Borjesson JL, Sundbom M, Wiklund U, Karlsson FA, Eriksson JW. Gastric bypass reduces symptoms and hormonal responses in hypoglycemia. Diabetes. 2016;65(9):2667–75.
20. Salehi M, Woods SC, D'Alessio DA. Gastric bypass alters both glucose-dependent and glucose-independent regulation of islet hormone secretion. Obesity (Silver Spring). 2015;23(10):2046–52.
21. Lefebvre P, Cariou B, Lien F, Kuipers F, Staels B. Role of bile acids and bile acid receptors in metabolic regulation. Physiol Rev. 2009;89(1):147–91.
22. Patti ME, Houten SM, Bianco AC, Bernier R, Larsen PR, Holst JJ, Badman MK, Maratos-Flier E, Mun EC, Pihlajamaki J, Auwerx J, Goldfine AB. Serum bile acids are higher in humans with prior gastric bypass: potential contribution to improved glucose and lipid metabolism. Obesity (Silver Spring). 2009;17(9):1671–7.
23. Ryan KK, Tremaroli V, Clemmensen C, Kovatcheva-Datchary P, Myronovych A, Karns R, Wilson-Perez HE, Sandoval DA, Kohli R, Backhed F, Seeley RJ. FXR is a molecular target for the effects of vertical sleeve gastrectomy. Nature. 2014;509(7499):183–8.
24. van den Broek M, de Heide LJM, Sips FLP, Koehorst M, van Zutphen T, Emous M, van Faassen M, Groen AK, van Riel NAW, de Boer JF, van Beek AP, Kuipers F. Altered bile acid kinetics contribute to postprandial hypoglycaemia after roux-en-Y gastric bypass surgery. Int J Obes. 2021;45(3):619–30.
25. Mulla CM, Goldfine AB, Dreyfuss JM, Houten S, Pan H, Pober DM, Wewer Albrechtsen NJ, Svane MS, Schmidt JB, Holst JJ, Craig CM, McLaughlin TL, Patti ME. Plasma FGF-19 levels are increased in patients with post-bariatric hypoglycemia. Obes Surg. 2019;29(7):2092–9.
26. Hepprich M, Wiedemann SJ, Schelker BL, Trinh B, Starkle A, Geigges M, Loliger J, Boni-Schnetzler M, Rudofsky G, Donath MY. Postprandial hypoglycemia in patients after gastric bypass surgery is mediated by glucose-induced IL-1beta. Cell Metab. 2020;31(4):699–709.

27. Zhang JB, Tamboli RA, Albaugh VL, Williams DB, Kilkelly DM, Grijalva CG, Shibao CA. The incidence of orthostatic intolerance after bariatric surgery. Obes Sci Pract. 2020;6(1):76–83.
28. Addison P, Carsky K, Patti ME, Roslin M. Hypoglycemia and dysautonomia after bariatric surgery: a systematic review and perspective. Obes Surg. 2022;32(5):1681–8.
29. Rodriguez-Diaz R, Speier S, Molano RD, Formoso A, Gans I, Abdulreda MH, Cabrera O, Molina J, Fachado A, Ricordi C, Leibiger I, Pileggi A, Berggren PO, Caicedo A. Noninvasive in vivo model demonstrating the effects of autonomic innervation on pancreatic islet function. Proc Natl Acad Sci U S A. 2012;109(52):21456–61.
30. Lee CJ, Brown TT, Schweitzer M, Magnuson T, Clark JM. The incidence and risk factors associated with developing symptoms of hypoglycemia after bariatric surgery. Surg Obes Relat Dis. 2018;14(6):797–802.
31. Raverdy V, Baud G, Pigeyre M, Verkindt H, Torres F, Preda C, Thuillier D, Gele P, Vantyghem MC, Caiazzo R, Pattou F. Incidence and predictive factors of postprandial Hyperinsulinemic hypoglycemia after roux-en-Y gastric bypass: A five year longitudinal study. Ann Surg. 2016;264(5):878–85.
32. Nannipieri M, Belligoli A, Guarino D, Busetto L, Moriconi D, Fabris R, Mari A, Baldi S, Anselmino M, Foletto M, Vettor R, Ferrannini E. Risk factors for spontaneously self-reported postprandial hypoglycemia after bariatric surgery. J Clin Endocrinol Metab. 2016;101(10):3600–7.
33. International Hypoglycaemia Study, G. Glucose concentrations of less than 3.0 mmol/L (54 mg/dL) should be reported in clinical trials: a joint position statement of the American Diabetes Association and the European Association for the Study of diabetes. Diabetes Care. 2017;40(1):155–7.
34. Shah VN, DuBose SN, Li Z, Beck RW, Peters AL, Weinstock RS, Kruger D, Tansey M, Sparling D, Woerner S, Vendrame F, Bergenstal R, Tamborlane WV, Watson SE, Sherr J. Continuous glucose monitoring profiles in healthy nondiabetic participants: a multicenter prospective study. J Clin Endocrinol Metab. 2019;104(10):4356–64.
35. El Khoury M, Yousuf F, Martin V, Cohen RM. Pseudohypoglycemia: a cause for unreliable finger-stick glucose measurements. Endocr Pract. 2008;14(3):337–9.
36. Ginsberg BH. Factors affecting blood glucose monitoring: sources of errors in measurement. J Diabetes Sci Technol. 2009;3(4):903–13.
37. McGarraugh G. Alarm characterization for a continuous glucose monitor that replaces traditional blood glucose monitoring. J Diabetes Sci Technol. 2010;4(1):49–56.
38. Salehi M, Vella A, McLaughlin T, Patti ME. Hypoglycemia after gastric bypass surgery: current concepts and controversies. J Clin Endocrinol Metab. 2018;103(8):2815–26.
39. Lawaetz O, Blackburn AM, Bloom SR, Aritas Y, Ralphs DN. Gut hormone profile and gastric emptying in the dumping syndrome. A hypothesis concerning the pathogenesis. Scand J Gastroenterol. 1983;18(1):73–80.
40. Sagor GR, Bryant MG, Ghatei MA, Kirk RM, Bloom SR. Release of vasoactive intestinal peptide in the dumping syndrome. Br Med J (Clin Res Ed). 1981;282(6263):507–10.
41. Murad MH, Coto-Yglesias F, Wang AT, Sheidaee N, Mullan RJ, Elamin MB, Erwin PJ, Montori VM. Clinical review: drug-induced hypoglycemia: a systematic review. J Clin Endocrinol Metab. 2009;94(3):741–5.
42. Herings RM, de Boer A, Stricker BH, Leufkens HG, Porsius A. Hypoglycaemia associated with use of inhibitors of angiotensin converting enzyme. Lancet. 1995;345(8959):1195–8.
43. Elshimy G, Techathaveewat P, Alsayed M, Jyothinagaram S, Correa R. Simple reason for hypoglycemia: ACE inhibitor-induced severe recurrent hypoglycemia in a nondiabetic patient. Cureus. 2019;11(8):e5449.
44. Carnovale C, Gringeri M, Battini V, Mosini G, Invernizzi E, Mazhar F, Bergamaschi F, Fumagalli M, Zuccotti G, Clementi E, Radice S, Fabiano V. Beta-blocker-associated hypoglycaemia: new insights from a real-world pharmacovigilance study. Br J Clin Pharmacol. 2021;87(8):3320–31.

45. Gomez-Samano MA, Baquerizo-Burgos JE, Coronel MFC, Wong-Campoverde BD, Villanueva-Martinez F, Molina-Botello D, Avila-Rojo JA, Palacios-Baez L, Cuevas-Ramos D, Gomez-Perez FJ, Zentella-Dehesa A, Aguayo-Gonzalez A, Gulias-Herrero A. Effect of imatinib on plasma glucose concentration in subjects with chronic myeloid leukemia and gastrointestinal stromal tumor. BMC Endocr Disord. 2018;18(1):77.
46. Kamal RS, Dean A, Dutt H, Rajeh A, Fernandes R. Hypoglycemia as first presentation of presumed immune checkpoint inhibitor-induced type 1 diabetes. Clin Case Rep. 2023;11(9):e7897.
47. Hosono S, Ohno T, Kimoto H, Nagoshi R, Shimizu M, Nozawa M. Reduction in blood glucose values following indomethacin therapy for patent ductus arteriosus. Pediatr Int. 1999;41(5):525–8.
48. Scholl JH, van Eekeren R, van Puijenbroek EP. Six cases of (severe) hypoglycaemia associated with gabapentin use in both diabetic and non-diabetic patients. Br J Clin Pharmacol. 2015;79(5):870–1.
49. Senthilkumaran S, Ananth C, Menezes RG, Thirumalaikolundusubramanian P. Tramadol-induced hypoglycemia: an unusual adverse effect. J Anaesthesiol Clin Pharmacol. 2017;33(4):554–5.
50. Almirall J, Montoliu J, Torras A, Revert L. Propoxyphene-induced hypoglycemia in a patient with chronic renal failure. Nephron. 1989;53(3):273–5.
51. Laurent M, Gallinari C, Bonnin M, Soubrie C. Hypoglycemia induced by dextropropoxyphene in very old subjects. 7 cases. Presse Med. 1991;20(33):1628.
52. Deeg MA, Lipkin EW. Hypoglycemia associated with the use of fluoxetine. West J Med. 1996;164(3):262–3.
53. Pollak PT, Mukherjee SD, Fraser AD. Sertraline-induced hypoglycemia. Ann Pharmacother. 2001;35(11):1371–4.
54. Derijks HJ, Meyboom RH, Heerdink ER, De Koning FH, Janknegt R, Lindquist M, Egberts AC. The association between antidepressant use and disturbances in glucose homeostasis: evidence from spontaneous reports. Eur J Clin Pharmacol. 2008;64(5):531–8.
55. Kobylianskii J, Wu PE. Venlafaxine-induced hypoglycemia. CMAJ. 2021;193(16):E568.
56. Ozdemir S. A case report of rare adverse events associated with venlafaxine administration: hypoglycemia and lactic acidosis. Korean J Fam Med. 2022;43(1):83–5.
57. Adnitt PI. Hypoglycemic action of monoamineoxidase inhibitors (MAOI'S). Diabetes. 1968;17(10):628–33.
58. Shah JH, DeLeon-Jones FA, Schickler R, Nasr S, Mayer M, Hurks C. Symptomatic reactive hypoglycemia during glucose tolerance test in lithium-treated patients. Metabolism. 1986;35(7):634–9.
59. Tanaka S, Abe M, Kohno G, Kushimoto M, Ikeda J, Ogawa K, Suzuki Y, Ishihara H, Fujishiro M. A single episode of hypoglycemia as a possible early warning sign of adrenal insufficiency. Ther Clin Risk Manag. 2020;16:147–53.
60. Boro H, Goyal A, Khadgawat R. Isolated growth hormone deficiency presenting with recurrent hypoglycaemia in a toddler. BMJ Case Rep. 2019;12(7)
61. Basu A, Service FJ, Yu L, Heser D, Ferries LM, Eisenbarth G. Insulin autoimmunity and hypoglycemia in seven white patients. Endocr Pract. 2005;11(2):97–103.
62. Garla V, Sonani H, Palabindala V, Gomez-Sanchez C, Subauste J, Lien LF. Non-islet cell hypoglycemia: case series and review of the literature. Front Endocrinol (Lausanne). 2019;10:316.
63. Mulla CM, Storino A, Yee EU, Lautz D, Sawnhey MS, Moser AJ, Patti ME. Insulinoma after bariatric surgery: diagnostic dilemma and therapeutic approaches. Obes Surg. 2016;26(4):874–81.
64. Placzkowski KA, Vella A, Thompson GB, Grant CS, Reading CC, Charboneau JW, Andrews JC, Lloyd RV, Service FJ. Secular trends in the presentation and management of functioning insulinoma at the Mayo Clinic, 1987–2007. J Clin Endocrinol Metab. 2009;94(4):1069–73.

65. Rosch T, Lightdale CJ, Botet JF, Boyce GA, Sivak MV Jr, Yasuda K, Heyder N, Palazzo L, Dancygier H, Schusdziarra V, et al. Localization of pancreatic endocrine tumors by endoscopic ultrasonography. N Engl J Med. 1992;326(26):1721–6.
66. Nockel P, Babic B, Millo C, Herscovitch P, Patel D, Nilubol N, Sadowski SM, Cochran C, Gorden P, Kebebew E. Localization of Insulinoma using 68Ga-DOTATATE PET/CT scan. J Clin Endocrinol Metab. 2017;102(1):195–9.
67. Doppman JL, Miller DL, Chang R, Shawker TH, Gorden P, Norton JA. Insulinomas: localization with selective intraarterial injection of calcium. Radiology. 1991;178(1):237–41.
68. Parekh S, Bodicoat DH, Brady E, Webb D, Mani H, Mostafa S, Levy MJ, Khunti K, Davies MJ. Clinical characteristics of people experiencing biochemical hypoglycaemia during an oral glucose tolerance test: cross-sectional analyses from a UK multi-ethnic population. Diabetes Res Clin Pract. 2014;104(3):427–34.
69. Gasser M, Meier C, Herren S, Aubry E, Steffen R, Stanga Z. Is testing for postprandial hyperinsulinemic hypoglycemia after gastric bypass necessary? Clin Nutr. 2019;38(1):444–9.
70. Botros N, Rijnaarts I, Brandts H, Bleumink G, Janssen I, de Boer H. (2014). Effect of carbohydrate restriction in patients with hyperinsulinemic hypoglycemia after Roux-en-Y gastric bypass. Obes Surg. 2014;24(11):1850–5.
71. Marques AR, Lobato CB, Pereira SS, Guimaraes M, Faria S, Nora M, Monteiro MP. Insights from the Impact of Meal Composition on Glucose Profile Towards Post-bariatric Hypoglycemia Management." Obes Surg. 2020;30(1):249–55.
72. van Meijeren J, Timmer I, Brandts H, Janssen I, Boer H. Evaluation of carbohydrate restriction as primary treatment for post-gastric bypass hypoglycemia. Surg Obes Relat Dis. 2017;13(3):404–10.
73. Della Pepa G, Vetrani C, Lupoli R, Massimino E, Lembo E, Riccardi G, Capaldo B. Uncooked cornstarch for the prevention of hypoglycemic events. Crit Rev Food Sci Nutr. 2022;62(12):3250–63.
74. Lembo E, Lupoli R, Ciciola P, Creanza A, Silvestri E, Saldalamacchia G, Capaldo B. Implementation of low glycemic index diet together with cornstarch in post-gastric bypass hypoglycemia: two case reports. Nutrients. 2018;10(6)
75. Faria SL, Faria OP, Buffington C, de Almeida Cardeal M, Ito MK. Dietary protein intake and bariatric surgery patients: a review. Obes Surg. 2011;21(11):1798–805.
76. Kandel D, Bojsen-Moller KN, Svane MS, Samkani A, Astrup A, Holst JJ, Madsbad S, Krarup T. Mechanisms of action of a carbohydrate-reduced, high-protein diet in reducing the risk of postprandial hypoglycemia after roux-en-Y gastric bypass surgery. Am J Clin Nutr. 2019;110(2):296–304.
77. Trico D, Filice E, Trifiro S, Natali A. Manipulating the sequence of food ingestion improves glycemic control in type 2 diabetic patients under free-living conditions. Nutr Diabetes. 2016;6(8):e226.
78. Stano S, Alam F, Wu L, Dutia R, Ng SN, Sala M, McGinty J, Laferrere B. Effect of meal size and texture on gastric pouch emptying and glucagon-like peptide 1 after gastric bypass surgery. Surg Obes Relat Dis. 2017;13(12):1975–83.
79. Azam H, Shahrestani S, Phan K. Alcohol use disorders before and after bariatric surgery: a systematic review and meta-analysis. Ann Transl Med. 2018;6(8):148.
80. Svensson PA, Anveden A, Romeo S, Peltonen M, Ahlin S, Burza MA, Carlsson B, Jacobson P, Lindroos AK, Lonroth H, Maglio C, Naslund I, Sjoholm K, Wedel H, Soderpalm B, Sjostrom L, Carlsson LM. Alcohol consumption and alcohol problems after bariatric surgery in the Swedish obese subjects study. Obesity (Silver Spring). 2013;21(12):2444–51.
81. Freinkel N, Singer DL, Arky RA, Bleicher SJ, Anderson JB, Silbert CK. Alcohol hypoglycemia. I. Carbohydrate metabolism of patients with clinical alcohol hypoglycemia and the experimental reproduction of the syndrome with pure ethanol. J Clin Invest. 1963;42(7):1112–33.
82. Siler SQ, Neese RA, Christiansen MP, Hellerstein MK. The inhibition of gluconeogenesis following alcohol in humans. Am J Phys. 1998;275(5):E897–907.
83. Schonenberger KA, Ferreira A, Stebler C, Prendin F, Gawinecka J, Nakas CT, Muhlebach S, Stanga Z, Facchinetti A, Herzig D, Bally L. Nutritional strategies for correcting low glu-

cose values in patients with postbariatric hypoglycaemia: A randomized controlled three-arm crossover trial. Diabetes Obes Metab. 2023;25(10):2853–61.
84. Valderas JP, Ahuad J, Rubio L, Escalona M, Pollak F, Maiz A. Acarbose improves hypoglycaemia following gastric bypass surgery without increasing glucagon-like peptide 1 levels. Obes Surg. 2012;22(4):582–6.
85. Ritz P, Vaurs C, Bertrand M, Anduze Y, Guillaume E, Hanaire H. Usefulness of acarbose and dietary modifications to limit glycemic variability following roux-en-Y gastric bypass as assessed by continuous glucose monitoring. Diabetes Technol Ther. 2012;14(8):736–40.
86. de Heide LJM, Wouda SHT, Peters VJT, Oosterwerff-Suiker M, Gerdes VA, Emous M, van Beek AP. Medical and surgical treatment of postbariatric hypoglycaemia: retrospective data from daily practice. Diabetes Obes Metab. 2023;25(3):735–47.
87. Holmback U, Forslund A, Gruden S, Alderborn G, Soderhall A, Hellstrom PM, Lennernas H. Effects of a novel combination of orlistat and acarbose on tolerability, appetite, and glucose metabolism in persons with obesity. Obes Sci Pract. 2020;6(3):313–23.
88. Long RG, Barnes AJ, Adrian TE, Mallinson CN, Brown MR, Vale W, Rivier JE, Christofides ND, Bloom SR. Suppression of pancreatic endocrine tumour secretion by long-acting somatostatin analogue. Lancet. 1979;2(8146):764–7.
89. Adrian TE, Barnes AJ, Long RG, O'Shaughnessy DJ, Brown MR, Rivier J, Vale W, Blackburn AM, Bloom SR. The effect of somatostatin analogs on secretion of growth, pancreatic, and gastrointestinal hormones in man. J Clin Endocrinol Metab. 1981;53(4):675–81.
90. Wiest R, Tsai MH, Groszmann RJ. Octreotide potentiates PKC-dependent vasoconstrictors in portal-hypertensive and control rats. Gastroenterology. 2001;120(4):975–83.
91. Hopman WP, Wolberink RG, Lamers CB, Van Tongeren JH. Treatment of the dumping syndrome with the somatostatin analogue SMS 201-995. Ann Surg. 1988;207(2):155–9.
92. Tack J, Aberle J, Arts J, Laville M, Oppert JM, Bender G, Bhoyrul S, McLaughlin T, Yoshikawa T, Vella A, Zhou J, Passos VQ, O'Connell P, Van Beek AP. Safety and efficacy of pasireotide in dumping syndrome-results from a phase 2, multicentre study. Aliment Pharmacol Ther. 2018;47(12):1661–72.
93. Schmid HA, Brueggen J. Effects of somatostatin analogs on glucose homeostasis in rats. J Endocrinol. 2012;212(1):49–60.
94. Edmunds MC, Chen JD, Soykan I, Lin Z, McCallum RW. Effect of octreotide on gastric and small bowel motility in patients with gastroparesis. Aliment Pharmacol Ther. 1998;12(2):167–74.
95. van Berge Henegouwen MI, van Gulik TM, Akkermans LM, Jansen JB, Gouma DJ. The effect of octreotide on gastric emptying at a dosage used to prevent complications after pancreatic surgery: a randomised, placebo controlled study in volunteers. Gut. 1997;41(6):758–62.
96. Myint KS, Greenfield JR, Farooqi IS, Henning E, Holst JJ, Finer N. Prolonged successful therapy for hyperinsulinaemic hypoglycaemia after gastric bypass: the pathophysiological role of GLP1 and its response to a somatostatin analogue. Eur J Endocrinol. 2012;166(5):951–5.
97. Arts J, Caenepeel P, Bisschops R, Dewulf D, Holvoet L, Piessevaux H, Bourgeois S, Sifrim D, Janssens J, Tack J. Efficacy of the long-acting repeatable formulation of the somatostatin analogue octreotide in postoperative dumping. Clin Gastroenterol Hepatol. 2009;7(4):432–7.
98. Vilarrasa N, Goday A, Rubio MA, Caixas A, Pellitero S, Ciudin A, Calanas A, Botella JI, Breton I, Morales MJ, Diaz-Fernandez MJ, Garcia-Luna PP, Lecube A. Hyperinsulinemic hypoglycemia after bariatric surgery: diagnosis and management experience from a Spanish multicenter registry. Obes Facts. 2016;9(1):41–51.
99. Ohrstrom CC, Worm D, Hojager A, Andersen D, Holst JJ, Kielgast UL, Hansen DL. Postprandial hypoglycaemia after roux-en-Y gastric bypass and the effects of acarbose, sitagliptin, verapamil, liraglutide and pasireotide. Diabetes Obes Metab. 2019;21(9):2142–51.
100. de Heide LJ, Laskewitz AJ, Apers JA. Treatment of severe postRYGB hyperinsulinemic hypoglycemia with pasireotide: a comparison with octreotide on insulin, glucagon, and GLP-1. Surg Obes Relat Dis. 2014;10(3):e31–3.

101. Wauters L, Arts J, Caenepeel P, Holvoet L, Tack J, Bisschops R, Vanuytsel T. Efficacy and safety of lanreotide in postoperative dumping syndrome: A phase II randomised and placebo-controlled study. United European Gastroenterol J. 2019;7(8):1064–72.
102. Gomes-Porras M, Cardenas-Salas J, Alvarez-Escola C. Somatostatin analogs in clinical practice: a review. Int J Mol Sci. 2020;21(5)
103. Weaver K, Craig C, McLaughlin T. Pasireotide induced adrenal insufficiency. Clin Endocrinol (Oxf). 2016;84(6):946–7.
104. Moreira RO, Moreira RB, Machado NA, Goncalves TB, Coutinho WF. Post-prandial hypoglycemia after bariatric surgery: pharmacological treatment with verapamil and acarbose. Obes Surg. 2008;18(12):1618–21.
105. Nauck MA, Quast DR, Wefers J, Meier JJ. GLP-1 receptor agonists in the treatment of type 2 diabetes- state-of-the-art. Mol Metab. 2021;46:101102.
106. Abrahamsson N, Engstrom BE, Sundbom M, Karlsson FA. GLP1 analogs as treatment of postprandial hypoglycemia following gastric bypass surgery: a potential new indication? Eur J Endocrinol. 2013;169(6):885–9.
107. Brubaker PL, Drucker DJ. Minireview: glucagon-like peptides regulate cell proliferation and apoptosis in the pancreas, gut, and central nervous system. Endocrinology. 2004;145(6):2653–9.
108. Tourrel C, Bailbe D, Meile MJ, Kergoat M, Portha B. Glucagon-like peptide-1 and exendin-4 stimulate beta-cell neogenesis in streptozotocin-treated newborn rats resulting in persistently improved glucose homeostasis at adult age. Diabetes. 2001;50(7):1562–70.
109. Korner M, Stockli M, Waser B, Reubi JC. GLP-1 receptor expression in human tumors and human normal tissues: potential for in vivo targeting. J Nucl Med. 2007;48(5):736–43.
110. Reubi JC, Waser B. Concomitant expression of several peptide receptors in neuroendocrine tumours: molecular basis for in vivo multireceptor tumour targeting. Eur J Nucl Med Mol Imaging. 2003;30(5):781–93.
111. Polidori D, Sha S, Mudaliar S, Ciaraldi TP, Ghosh A, Vaccaro N, Farrell K, Rothenberg P, Henry RR. Canagliflozin lowers postprandial glucose and insulin by delaying intestinal glucose absorption in addition to increasing urinary glucose excretion: results of a randomized, placebo-controlled study. Diabetes Care. 2013;36(8):2154–61.
112. Martinussen C, Veedfald S, Dirksen C, Bojsen-Moller KN, Svane MS, Wewer Albrechtsen NJ, van Hall G, Kristiansen VB, Fenger M, Holst JJ, Madsbad S. The effect of acute dual SGLT1/SGLT2 inhibition on incretin release and glucose metabolism after gastric bypass surgery. Am J Physiol Endocrinol Metab. 2020;318(6):E956–64.
113. Ciudin A, Sanchez M, Hernandez I, Cordero E, Fidilio E, Comas M, Gonzalez C, Lopez N, Vilallonga R, Giralt M, Ferrer R, Hernandez C, Simo R. Canagliflozin: a new therapeutic option in patients that present postprandial Hyperinsulinemic hypoglycemia after roux-en-Y gastric bypass: a pilot study. Obes Facts. 2021;14(3):291–7.
114. Carpentieri GB, Goncalves S, Casagrande MZ, Mourad WM, Pinto LGC, Zanella MT. SGLT2 inhibition with Empagliflozin as a possible therapeutic option for postprandial hypoglycemia after bariatric surgery. Obes Surg. 2022;32(8):2664–71.
115. Hansen JB. Towards selective Kir6.2/SUR1 potassium channel openers, medicinal chemistry and therapeutic perspectives. Curr Med Chem. 2006;13(4):361–76.
116. Gonzalez-Gonzalez A, Delgado M, Fraga-Fuentes MD. Use of diazoxide in management of severe postprandial hypoglycemia in patient after roux-en-Y gastric bypass. Surg Obes Relat Dis. 2013;9(1):e18–9.
117. Craig CM, Lawler HM, Lee CJE, Tan M, Davis DB, Tong J, Glodowski M, Rogowitz E, Karaman R, McLaughlin TL, Porter L. PREVENT: A randomized, placebo-controlled crossover trial of Avexitide for treatment of Postbariatric hypoglycemia. J Clin Endocrinol Metab. 2021;106(8):e3235–48.
118. Halperin F, Patti ME, Goldfine AB. Glucagon treatment for post-gastric bypass hypoglycemia. Obesity (Silver Spring). 2010;18(9):1858–60.
119. Mulla CM, Zavitsanou S, Laguna Sanz AJ, Pober D, Richardson L, Walcott P, Arora I, Newswanger B, Cummins MJ, Prestrelski SJ, Doyle FJ, Dassau E, Patti ME. A random-

ized, placebo-controlled double-blind trial of a closed-loop glucagon system for Postbariatric hypoglycemia. J Clin Endocrinol Metab. 2020;105(4):e1260–71.
120. Nielsen CK, Ohrstrom CC, Kielgast UL, Hansen DL, Hartmann B, Holst JJ, Lund A, Vilsboll T, Knop FK. Dasiglucagon effectively mitigates Postbariatric postprandial hypoglycemia: a randomized, double-blind, placebo-controlled, crossover trial. Diabetes Care. 2022;45(6):1476–81.
121. Cummings C, Jiang A, Sheehan A, Ferraz-Bannitz R, Puleio A, Simonson DC, Dreyfuss JM, Patti ME. Continuous glucose monitoring in patients with post-bariatric hypoglycaemia reduces hypoglycaemia and glycaemic variability. Diabetes Obes Metab. 2023;25(8):2191–202.
122. Davis DB, Khoraki J, Ziemelis M, Sirinvaravong S, Han JY, Campos GM. Roux en Y gastric bypass hypoglycemia resolves with gastric feeding or reversal: confirming a non-pancreatic etiology. Mol Metab. 2018;9:15–27.
123. McLaughlin T, Peck M, Holst J, Deacon C. Reversible hyperinsulinemic hypoglycemia after gastric bypass: a consequence of altered nutrient delivery. J Clin Endocrinol Metab. 2010;95(4):1851–5.
124. Zanley E, Shah ND, Craig C, Lau JN, Rivas H, McLaughlin T. Guidelines for gastrostomy tube placement and enteral nutrition in patients with severe, refractory hypoglycemia after gastric bypass. Surg Obes Relat Dis. 2021;17(2):456–65.
125. Campos GM, Ziemelis M, Paparodis R, Ahmed M, Davis DB. Laparoscopic reversal of roux-en-Y gastric bypass: technique and utility for treatment of endocrine complications. Surg Obes Relat Dis. 2014;10(1):36–43.
126. Kantharia N, Lakdawala M, Govil A. Laparoscopic reversal of roux-en-Y gastric bypass for intractable hypoglycaemia post-operative complications. In: IFSO 22nd world congress. London, UK; 2017.
127. Mehta K, Sarr MG, Kellogg TA, Kendrick ML, McKenzie TJ. Efficacy of conversion of roux-en-Y gastric bypass to roux Jejuno-Duodenostomy for severe medically refractory postprandial hypoglycemia. Obes Surg. 2020;30(10):4141–4.
128. Vilallonga R, Rodriguez-Luna MR, Roriz-Silva R, Caubet E, Gonzalez O, Ruiz de Gordejuela A, Ciudin A, Armengol M, Fort JM. Reversal to normal anatomy (with sleeve gastrectomy) for severe hypoglycemia. Surg Innov. 2021;28(5):536–43.
129. Painter TJ, Teixeira AF, Jawad MA. Pyloric stenosis after a roux-en-Y gastric bypass: a case report. Surg Obes Relat Dis. 2015;11(1):e9–10.
130. Abu Dayyeh BK, Lautz DB, Thompson CC. Gastrojejunal stoma diameter predicts weight regain after roux-en-Y gastric bypass. Clin Gastroenterol Hepatol. 2011;9(3):228–33.
131. Z'Graggen K, Guweidhi A, Steffen R, Potoczna N, Biral R, Walther F, Komminoth P, Horber F. Severe recurrent hypoglycemia after gastric bypass surgery. Obes Surg. 2008;18(8):981–8.
132. Relly R, Mati S, Aviv CN, Fishman S. Endoscopic trans-oral outlet reduction after bariatric surgery is safe and effective for dumping syndrome. Surg Endosc. 2021;35(12):6846–52.
133. Tsai C, Steffen R, Kessler U, Merki H, Zehetner J. Short-term outcomes of endoscopic gastro-jejunal revisions for treatment of dumping syndrome after roux-En-Y gastric bypass. Surg Endosc. 2020;34(8):3626–32.
134. Vargas EJ, Abu Dayyeh BK, Storm AC, Bazerbachi F, Matar R, Vella A, Kellogg T, Stier C. Endoscopic management of dumping syndrome after roux-en-Y gastric bypass: a large international series and proposed management strategy. Gastrointest Endosc. 2020;92(1):91–6.
135. Dunn SH, Tejani S, Almandoz JP, Messiah SE, Schellinger J, Marroquin EM, Mathew M, Horton J, Tavakkoli A. Transoral gastric outlet reduction for post-prandial hypoglycemia after roux-en-Y gastric bypass. Surg Endosc. 2023;37:8285.
136. Meier JJ, Butler AE, Galasso R, Butler PC. Hyperinsulinemic hypoglycemia after gastric bypass surgery is not accompanied by islet hyperplasia or increased beta-cell turnover. Diabetes Care. 2006;29(7):1554–9.
137. Patti ME, Goldfine AB, Hu J, Hoem D, Molven A, Goldsmith J, Schwesinger WH, La Rosa S, Folli F, Kulkarni RN. Heterogeneity of proliferative markers in pancreatic beta-cells

of patients with severe hypoglycemia following roux-en-Y gastric bypass. Acta Diabetol. 2017;54(8):737–47.
138. Reubi JC, Perren A, Rehmann R, Waser B, Christ E, Callery M, Goldfine AB, Patti ME. Glucagon-like peptide-1 (GLP-1) receptors are not overexpressed in pancreatic islets from patients with severe hyperinsulinaemic hypoglycaemia following gastric bypass. Diabetologia. 2010;53(12):2641–5.
139. Alvarez GC, Faria EN, Beck M, Girardon DT, Machado AC. Laparoscopic spleen-preserving distal pancreatectomy as treatment for nesidioblastosis after gastric bypass surgery. Obes Surg. 2007;17(4):550–2.
140. Clancy TE, Moore FD Jr, Zinner MJ. Post-gastric bypass hyperinsulinism with nesidioblastosis: subtotal or total pancreatectomy may be needed to prevent recurrent hypoglycemia. J Gastrointest Surg. 2006;10(8):1116–9.
141. Patti ME, McMahon G, Mun EC, Bitton A, Holst JJ, Goldsmith J, Hanto DW, Callery M, Arky R, Nose V, Bonner-Weir S, Goldfine AB. Severe hypoglycaemia post-gastric bypass requiring partial pancreatectomy: evidence for inappropriate insulin secretion and pancreatic islet hyperplasia. Diabetologia. 2005;48(11):2236–40.
142. Service GJ, Thompson GB, Service FJ, Andrews JC, Collazo-Clavell ML, Lloyd RV. Hyperinsulinemic hypoglycemia with nesidioblastosis after gastric-bypass surgery. N Engl J Med. 2005;353(3):249–54.
143. Vanderveen KA, Grant CS, Thompson GB, Farley DR, Richards ML, Vella A, Vollrath B, Serv FJ. Outcomes and quality of life after partial pancreatectomy for noninsulinoma pancreatogenous hypoglycemia from diffuse islet cell disease. Surgery. 2010;148(6):1237–45. discussion 1245-1236.
144. Bogachus LD, Bellin MD, Vella A, Robertson RP. Deficient glucagon response to hypoglycemia during a mixed meal in total pancreatectomy/islet autotransplantation recipients. J Clin Endocrinol Metab. 2018;103(4):1522–9.
145. Buchler MW, Wagner M, Schmied BM, Uhl W, Friess H, Z'Graggen K. Changes in morbidity after pancreatic resection: toward the end of completion pancreatectomy. Arch Surg. 2003;138(12):1310–4. discussion 1315
146. Kleeff J, Diener MK, Z'Graggen K, Hinz U, Wagner M, Bachmann J, Zehetner J, Muller MW, Friess H, Buchler MW. Distal pancreatectomy: risk factors for surgical failure in 302 consecutive cases. Ann Surg. 2007;245(4):573–82.
147. Wu L, Nahm CB, Jamieson NB, Samra J, Clifton-Bligh R, Mittal A, Tsang V. Risk factors for development of diabetes mellitus (type 3c) after partial pancreatectomy: A systematic review. Clin Endocrinol. 2020;92(5):396–406.

# Reflux After Bariatric Surgery: Incidence and Workup

# 35

Daniel Praise Mowoh, Mina A. Ibrahim, and Leena Khaitan

## Introduction

In the United States, 20% of Americans report symptoms of gastroesophageal reflux disease (GERD). The prevalence of GERD amongst patients with obesity is higher and is estimated anywhere from 39% to 61% [1]. As bariatric surgery has become a primary treatment for the management of obesity, its association with GERD and its effects on the physiology of the foregut is becoming more apparent. GERD can present with symptoms such as heartburn, dysphagia, regurgitation, and cough. Understanding the cause of the symptoms allows the surgeon to better determine management strategies. The relationship between bariatric surgery and reflux is complex and multifaceted. This chapter provides an overview of reflux after bariatric surgery, discussing the various procedures and their impact on reflux, as well as potential mechanisms and management options.

## Types of Bariatric Procedures and Incidence

The incidence of reflux after bariatric surgery can vary widely depending on the type of procedure, patient characteristics, and how reflux is defined and measured. In unaltered anatomy, the contributors to reflux include patient factors (eating

D. P. Mowoh (✉)
Department of Surgery, University Hospitals Cleveland Medical Center, Cleveland, OH, USA
e-mail: Mowoh@Uhhospitals.org

M. A. Ibrahim
University Hospitals Parma Medical Center, Parma, OH, USA

L. Khaitan
Department of Surgery, University Hospitals Cleveland Medical Center, Cleveland, OH, USA

University Hospitals Parma Medical Center, Parma, OH, USA



O. M. Ghanem et al. (eds.), *The SAGES Manual of Metabolic and Bariatric Surgery*, https://doi.org/10.1007/978-3-031-72309-4_35

habits, body habitus) and mechanical contributions of hiatal hernias and lower esophageal sphincter (LES) dysfunction. In addition to these, several mechanisms may contribute to reflux after bariatric surgery:

- *Altered Anatomy*: Surgical changes to the digestive tract may disrupt the normal antireflux mechanisms, allowing gastric contents to flow back into the esophagus.
- *Increased Intra-abdominal Pressure*: Altered gastric anatomy can increase intra-abdominal pressure, promoting the development of GERD.
- *Gastric Acid Production*: Bariatric surgery can affect gastric acid production, which plays a pivotal role in GERD development and progression.
- *Gastric Emptying* Some procedures can lead to delayed gastric emptying, increasing the risk of reflux. Others may accelerate emptying.

The most common bariatric procedures performed according to ASBMS are sleeve gastrectomy, Roux-en-Y Gastric bypass, biliopancreatic Diversion with Duodenal Switch (BPD/DS), Single anastomosis Duodenal Switch (SADI) and the Adjustable Gastric Band (AGB).

## Sleeve Gastrectomy

Sleeve gastrectomy involves the removal of a large portion of the stomach, leaving a banana-shaped sleeve. The effect on reflux is mixed, with some individuals experiencing symptom relief, while others may develop or worsen GERD. The incidence of reflux after LSG varies, but some studies have reported that around 15–30% of patients may experience new or worsened reflux symptoms. Proponents that favor performing a sleeve gastrectomy in the setting of GERD suggest that GERD may improve as a decrease of intrabdominal pressure occurs with weight loss. This is viewed as GERD being more affected by obesity than the creation of the sleeve [2]. These studies note that as patients lose weight, this decreases the intra-abdominal pressure which then reduces GERD symptoms. There have been several studies showing an association between BMI and GERD, and between abdominal girth and GERD. So presumably, as these factors decrease, reflux symptoms will as well. In f multiple systematic reviews, there are many studies showing improvement in GERD and even more that show that GERD can increase after sleeve gastrectomy.

GERD may worsen and de novo GERD is reported after sleeve gastrectomy is reported in some studies as >20% [3]. Most surgeons agree the sleeve is refluxogenic and some of the causes are identified in multiple studies. Symptoms may occur or worsen due to the vertical reduction in the stomach size leading to increased pressure within the gastric lumen. It was noted as the stomach became narrow along the lesser curve, it may affect the stomach's ability to distend thereby leading to functional issues at the LES. Reflux after sleeve was also affected by the extent of disruption to the lower esophageal sphincter and crural fibers, and the presence of hiatal hernia [4]. It is important to appreciate anatomical and dynamic effects on the LES that can lead to post-sleeve gastrectomy GERD.

The incidence of reflux after sleeve is also noted to be associated with the shape of the sleeve. Within Case Western University, a study was conducted from 2011 to 2015 looking at sleeve morphology and its effects on GERD and weight loss, using postoperative UGIs to assess sleeve morphology [5]. Four unique sleeve types were described. Sleeve shape was reported as 32.6% tubular, 20.6% Dumbbell, 39.2% lower pouch, and 7.5% upper pouch (Fig. 35.1). Of the total number of patients, 62.0% had >50% excess weight loss at 1 year. Twenty-three percent of patients remained on PPI at 1 year (of which 43.3% did not have reflux preoperatively). The lower pouch shape showed a trend toward less reflux and more weight loss. In fact, if the causes of reflux after sleeve are reviewed, many point to the technical aspect of the sleeve creation [6]. In addition, according to [7], out of almost 400 patients

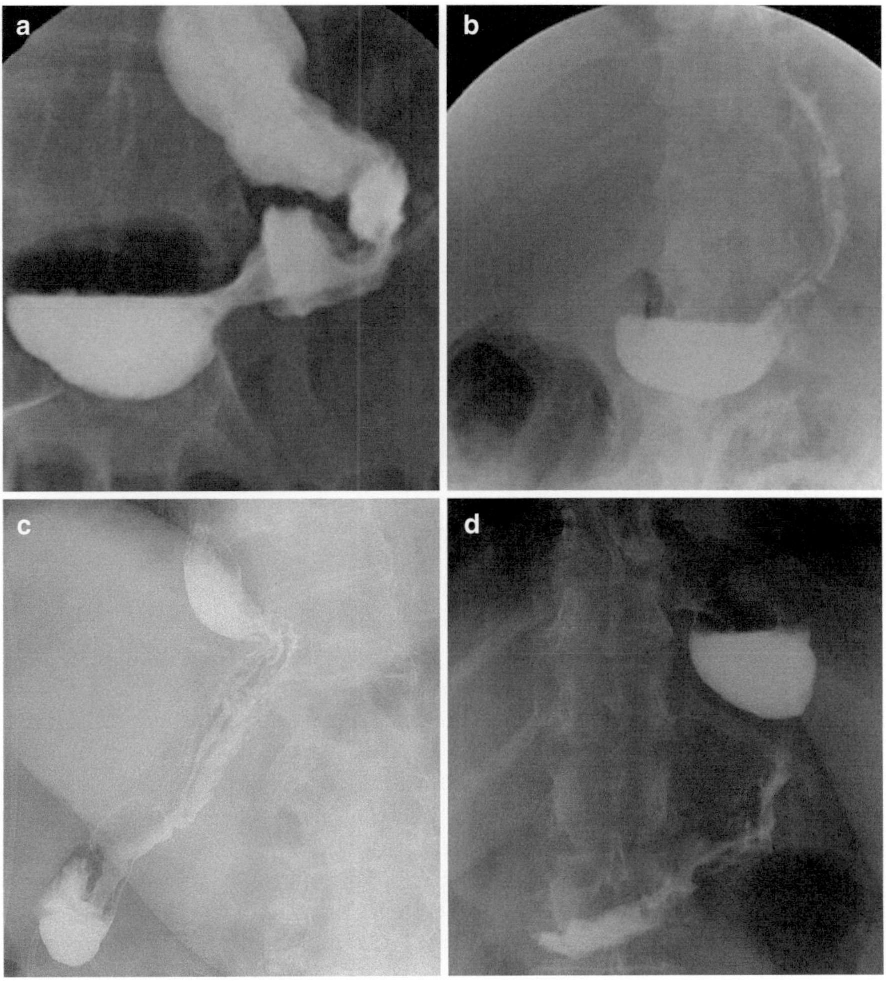


**Fig. 35.1** Sleeve gastrectomy morphology classification. Dumbbell (**a**), Lower Pouch (**b**), Tubular (**c**), and Upper Pouch (**d**) [5]

that were followed postoperatively from 6 months to 22 months, GERD can be reduced with diligent surgical technique. This study contends that surgical technique contributes to the reflux after the sleeve and not just the patient factors themselves. Careful surgical technique can decrease sleeve narrowing and angulation leading to a decrease in the development of GERD symptoms.

In many studies, hiatal hernias are noted to be one of the primary contributors to reflux symptoms. Studies suggest that with large hiatal hernias >4 cm, patients are more likely to develop postoperative GERD symptoms after sleeve. It is recommended that reduction of the hiatal hernia with restoration of the angle of His seems to be appropriate. In the presence of a concomitant hiatal hernia, there is a great debate about concomitant repair. Some suggest there is a significant improvement in GERD symptoms when a hiatal hernia is fixed, when present, at the time of sleeve gastrectomy regardless of size [3]. It has been well established that hiatal hernias are contributors to reflux in all patients, regardless of altered anatomy. There is still much debate—whether to fix all hiatal hernias at the time of sleeve. The authors believe that if the stomach is above the hiatus at all, this will affect the creation of the sleeve and those hiatal hernias should be repaired at the time of sleeve. One previous institutional studies showed that there was an association between the preoperative Hill grade seen on endoscopy and the incidence of reflux after sleeve gastrectomy [8]. In this study, patients with Hill grade 3 or 4 were noted to be more likely to have reflux after sleeve and these hiatal hernias should be fixed at the time of index surgery.

Barrett's esophagus has also been shown to increase after sleeve gastrectomy. One study suggests that the incidence of new postoperative esophagitis or BE diagnosis in patients who underwent esophagogastroduodenoscopy was higher than in the general population [9]. Although the incidence of Barrett's after sleeve varies in the literature, current guidelines suggest surveillance for Barrett's after these procedures [10].

These repeated findings lead many practitioners to suggest GERD and/or high-grade esophagitis as a relative contraindication to sleeve gastrectomy in patients with morbid obesity. The guidelines of the Society of American Gastrointestinal and Endoscopic Surgeons (SAGES) and the American Society of Metabolic and Bariatric Surgery (ASMBS) both suggest sleeve gastrectomy be avoided in patients with severe reflux [11]. In a meta-analysis looking at the incidence of GERD after sleeve, there was a 19% increase in reflux after sleeve with 23% de novo reflux [12]. The long-term prevalence of esophagitis in this study was 28% and Barrett's was 8%. Multiple factors can play a contributing role in the incidence of reflux after sleeve gastrectomy (Table 35.1). To reduce reflux after sleeve, some suggestions have been made. According to Felinska et al. [4], creating the perfect sleeve to prevent GERD, must follow six criteria. (1) Use a large bougie 40F to minimize intragastric pressure. (2) Achieve sleeve morphology in a manner that the antrum is the widest and the narrowest is the cardia to prevent functional stenosis. (3) Prevent twisting or kinking to prevent functional stenosis. (4) Preservation of the antrum to minimize intragastric pressure. (5) Repair large hiatal hernias >4 cm to restore the angle of His.

**Table 35.1** Etiologies of reflux after sleeve gastrectomy

| Causes of reflux post-sleeve |
|---|
| Patient factors such as eating habits and BMI |
| Increased intraluminal pressure due to the tubular shape |
| Sleeve morphology |
| Extent of injury to the lower esophageal sphincter |
| Concomitant presence and size of a hiatal hernia |
| Iatrogenic twisting/kinking leading to functional stenosis |

## Roux-en-Y Gastric Bypass (RYGB)

RYGB is one of the longest-standing bariatric surgeries. In addition to the weight loss effects and comorbidity resolution after RYGB, it is also known to improve [13] or resolve [14] pre-existing reflux symptoms in the majority of patients. Some studies suggest that patients with Barrett's esophagus (intestinal metaplasia of the esophagus), and even dysplasia may have complete regression 12 months after RYGB [15]. SAGES clinical practice guidelines recommend RYGB as the treatment option for patients with morbid obesity (BMI $\geq$ 35) with severe medically refractory GERD and/or patients with high-grade esophagitis [11]. These guidelines recommend RYGB as a treatment option for recurrent reflux after the initial failure of management after Nissen fundoplication [11]. The Swiss Multicenter Bypass or Sleeve Study (SM-BOSS) showed that de novo reflux is less common after gastric bypass surgery when compared to sleeve gastrectomy, with an incidence of around 10% [16]. This landmark randomized clinical trial noted patients with pre-existing GERD had significant improvement in symptoms postoperatively from bypass and fewer had new onset GERD. The mechanism by which RYGB improves GERD has been suggested to be related to a decrease in acid secretion due to a decrease in the number of parietal cells in the small gastric pouch, resultant weight loss decreasing intrabdominal pressure, and rapid emptying of the gastric pouch [17–19]. Patients presenting with reflux after RYGB can have underlying pathologies that precipitate their symptoms, such as the presence of a hiatal hernia and technical aspects of surgery with a short roux limb causing bile reflux.

Hiatal hernia is an important factor to consider for patients presenting with reflux after RYGB, as small hernias can lead to severe symptoms. Hiatal hernias cause a decrease in the lower esophageal sphincter pressure contributing to reflux. When RYGB patients develop a hiatal hernia postoperatively, even a small sliding hiatal hernia (2-3 cm) can lead to severe reflux as that equates to 40 to 80% of the gastric pouch being intrathoracic. The etiology of hiatal hernia after RYGB has been linked to several factors such as the creation of a large gastric pouch leading to higher intragastric pressure [20], disruption of normal attachments during extensive dissection of the hiatus during index RYGB [21], and small hiatal hernias missed or not repaired during index RYGB [22].

Another etiology of reflux after RYGB is secondary to the formation of a gastrogastric fistula (GGF) as gastric acid flows from the remnant stomach into the pouch.

The incidence of GGF has been estimated by some studies as ranging from 1.18% to as high as 6% [23–25]. Hence, in addition to objective and subjective evaluation of GERD, anatomical evaluations of the RYGB should be assessed for hiatal hernia and evaluation of the pouch for GGF on upper endoscopy and UGI series. GERD diagnosis is made using both subjective and objective findings. Subjective evaluations include GERD scores such as the GERD health-related quality of life scores and objective findings include a 24-h pH study with a DeMeester score ≥ 14.7.

Non-acid reflux (bile reflux) is also an important etiology that should be considered in this population of patients during the workup of reflux symptoms. This is typically related to technical aspects of the RYGB surgery with the creation of a short alimentary (roux) limb at index surgery leading to reflux of duodenal contents comprised of bile, bicarbonate, and pancreatic enzymes (Dolores Frutos [26]). The incidence of bile reflux after RYGB varies greatly, ranging from as low as 0.9% to as high as 30% [27, 28]. Objective evaluation of bile reflux can be made using impendence studies or a HIDA scan. The roux limb should be inspected for any tortuosity. Multiple studies have suggested that one of the biggest drawbacks of a one-anastomosis gastric bypass is the significant incidence of bile reflux however other studies contrast these findings with no conclusive evidence reported [27, 28]. Some studies have argued that although there may be a physiological increase in bile reflux to the stomach after one-anastomosis gastric bypass, conclusive evidence of symptomatic correlation has not been established [29, 30] and medical management is effective in controlling symptoms in all patients [31].

## Biliopancreatic Diversion with Duodenal Switch (BPD/DS)

BPD/DS is a more complex procedure to help individuals achieve significant weight loss. While this procedure has proven effective in promoting weight loss and resolving comorbidities like type 2 diabetes and hypertension, its impact on GERD has been a subject of ongoing research and debate. Some studies have reported up to 20% of patients may experience de novo reflux, while other studies suggest the resolution of GERD symptoms after weight loss similar to a sleeve gastrectomy. BPD/DS is set apart from other bariatric surgeries due to the extent of bypassing the small intestine and its efficacy in promoting weight loss. As a larger sleeve gastrectomy is part of the procedure, the debate continues on whether this procedure would benefit bariatric patients with reflux. A recent study out of the Mayo Clinic from 2009 to 2019 using a GERD-HRQL questionnaire showed that 44.7% of patients were found to be in the "GERD-resolved" subgroup, 36.8% of patients in the "No-effect" subgroup, and 18.4% patients in the "De novo GERD" subgroup suggesting satisfactory outcomes [32]. The mechanisms by which BPD/DS improves GERD are not fully understood, but several theories have been proposed: 1. Weight Loss: The significant and sustained weight loss resulting from BPD/DS may relieve pressure on the lower esophageal sphincter (LES), reducing the likelihood of acid reflux. 2. Reduced Gastric Acid Production: Since the stomach is partially removed, BPD/DS may lead to decreased acid production, thus reducing the acidity of gastric contents that could flow back into the esophagus. 3. Changes in Gut Hormones: BPD/DS can alter gut hormone levels, such as ghrelin, which plays a role in appetite and may have an impact on LES function [32, 33].

## Single Anastomosis Duodenal Switch (SADI-S)

Similar to BPD/DS, SADI-S requires a loop duodenal-ileal anastomosis with a longer common channel. This procedure has been on the rise and is used by surgeons as primary and revisional surgery after sleeve gastrectomy. While the SADI offers promising results in terms of weight loss and metabolic improvements, concerns have been raised regarding its potential association with GERD. Several studies have investigated the relationship between SADI and GERD. Some have suggested that the incidence of GERD may increase postoperatively, possibly due to the decreased transit time of food in the upper gastrointestinal tract and changes in gastric acidity. One study within a single institution and 283 patients over a several-year span showed patients to have reflux scores >8 in up to 30% of postoperative SADI patients [34]. However, these findings are not consistent across all studies, and the incidence of GERD after SADI remains a topic of ongoing research and debate.

## Adjustable Gastric Banding (AGB)

AGB used to be common but now is seldom used in bariatric surgery. One of the significant concerns associated with adjustable gastric banding is the increased risk of GERD. One study suggests that one reason the gastric band has fallen out of favor has been due to ineffective weight loss with only 11.2% of patients achieving satisfactory weight loss [35]. The mechanism of AGB aims to help individuals feel full with smaller meals and ultimately reduce calorie consumption. Factors that contribute to an association with GERD:

1. *Increased Pressure*: The constriction created by the gastric band can cause an increase in pressure within the small upper stomach pouch. This higher pressure can lead to the forced release of stomach contents into the esophagus.
2. *Reduced Sphincter Tone*: The lower esophageal sphincter (LES) is a complex mechanism that normally prevents stomach acid from refluxing into the esophagus. The pressure changes caused by the band can weaken the LES's tone, making it less effective in preventing acid reflux.
3. *Slower Gastric Emptying:* Gastric banding can delay the emptying of food from the small pouch, which increases the likelihood of GERD as food and stomach acid remain in the stomach for extended periods, allowing for more opportunities for reflux to occur.

**Table 35.2** Summary of Incidence of GERD per Bariatric Procedure

| Type of bariatric procedure | Incidence of GERD |
|---|---|
| Sleeve gastrectomy | 15–30% |
| Roux-en-Y gastric bypass (RYGB) | 2–10% |
| Biliopancreatic diversion with duodenal Switch (BPD/DS) | 20% |
| Single anastomosis duodenal switch (SADI-S) | 30% |
| Adjustable gastric banding (AGB) | 32% |

Research has shown that the incidence of GERD after gastric banding surgery can range from 10% to 40%. A previous study found that approximately 32% of patients developed GERD symptoms after gastric banding [36].

Overall, the impact of bariatric surgery on reflux is varied. The most challenging aspect of this is realizing the impact of obesity itself and how that contributes to patients' reflux symptoms. The incidence of GERD in bariatric patients is summarized in Table 35.2.

## Modalities for the Evaluation of Reflux after Bariatric Surgery

Workup for GERD after weight loss surgery should follow the principles of a traditional GERD evaluation. The findings should be put in the context of the surgical anatomy. The initial part of any GERD workup is the evaluation of patient factors. The effect of BMI on GERD has been well described. If a patient has a BMI that falls in the obese category, that should be considered a contributor to the patient's symptoms and should be optimized with nutritional counseling and lifestyle changes.

Another aspect that contributes to GERD after weight loss surgery is a patient's food choices. When patients indulge in foods such as fried foods, those with a high carbohydrate content, and sweets such as chocolate, the patients may experience more GERD symptoms. As a part of the evaluation, a careful dietary history should be reviewed to optimize the patient's food choices. Those foods that increase GERD symptoms after these procedures should be discouraged. One should offer formal dietary counseling to help the patient optimize food choices. Patients should be made aware that those foods may lead to an increase in weight and can result in adverse symptoms. It is important to note that these patient factors should be optimized even for those who have not had weight loss surgery. These lifestyle factors are even more important in those who have had weight loss surgery, as they help to contribute to the success of the weight loss operation itself.

Once a patient's lifestyle has been optimized, and symptoms persist, further evaluation is warranted. Patients who have persistent symptoms despite optimized medical/lifestyle therapy should be objectively evaluated. The workup is very similar to that used for any patient with persistent GERD. The primary difference is that the findings have to be put in the context of the altered anatomy. Furthermore, the altered anatomy affects treatment options. Evaluation can begin with endoscopy and radiologic studies such as esophagram and upper gastrointestinal series. To further document the presence of reflux and symptom correlation, objective GERD studies can be used. Esophageal motility studies can help guide therapeutic options. Sometimes a gastric emptying study can be helpful as well. Each of these studies is reviewed below and the contribution of the findings on those studies is discussed.

Finally, to quantify the symptoms of reflux, quality of life scores are very helpful in identifying the severity of symptoms. These should be tracked preoperative and postoperatively. This is important as the definitions of GERD are varied. When considering further workup in the post-bariatric patient, the need for ongoing therapy despite maximal medical management should be a part of the definition of persistent GERD. It is also important to consider objective findings of GERD on endoscopy as a part of that definition.

## Esophagogastroduodenoscopy (EGD)

EGD is a procedure used to assess reflux and anatomy in bariatric patients. During an upper endoscopy, a flexible endoscope is inserted through the mouth and down the esophagus to examine the esophagus, stomach, and the first part of the small intestine (duodenum), or the jejunum, depending on the post-surgical anatomy. An EGD can aid in reflux assessment in bariatric patients in the following ways:

1. **Visualization of the Gastroesophageal Junction** (GEJ): EGD allows direct visualization of the gastroesophageal junction to assess the integrity of the lower esophageal sphincter (LES) and the presence of any structural abnormalities such as hiatal hernias [37]. The vertical component of a hiatal hernia is one of the first aspects of evaluation. The vertical excursion can move, so it is important to evaluate the vertical excursion on initial entry as well as after the stomach has been insufflated. Assessment of the gastroesophageal flap valve is done via the Hill grade assessment. The assessment of the Hill grade is critical as it highlights the integrity and disruption of the EGJ by looking at it from a radial perspective and some authors argue is a better marker for the assessment of an antireflux barrier than assessing the axial length of hiatal hernia [38]. This requires patience and careful assessment when in the retroflex positions to truly assess this disruption. Hill Grade classification ranges from Hill Grade I–IV (Table 35.3).

   Hill Grade III and IV have been linked with esophagitis, Barrett's esophagus, symptoms of GERD, and the use of proton-pump inhibitors, while Hill Grade I & II do not have this association [37]. Many surgeons attest that Hill Grade III-IV can be surgically managed via a crural repair, helping to restore the gastroesophageal flap valve. Additionally, the authors have demonstrated greater reflux in those post sleeves if they have a Hill III or IV valve [8]. Preoperative endoscopy can help guide which patients should have hiatal hernias repaired at the time of index operation.
2. **Assessment of Esophageal Mucosa**: EGD can identify signs of esophagitis, inflammation, or mucosal damage caused by acid reflux. This is important in

**Table 35.3** Hill Grade types and description [38]

| Hill Grade classification | Description |
|---|---|
| Hill grade I | A prominent fold of tissue along the lesser curvature next to the endoscope |
| Hill grade II | The fold is less prominent and there are periods of opening and rapid closing around the endoscope |
| Hill grade III | The fold is not prominent and the endoscope is not tightly gripped by the tissue |
| Hill grade IV | There is no fold, and the lumen of the esophagus is open, often allowing the squamous epithelium to be viewed from below |

**Table 35.4** LA classification types and description [51]

| LA classification | Description |
|---|---|
| Grade A | One or more esophageal mucosal breaks $<5$ mm in length |
| Grade B | One or more mucosal breaks $>5$ mm but with continuity across mucosal folds |
| Grade C | Continuous mucosal breaks between the tops of two or more mucosal folds but involving $<75\%$ of the esophageal circumference |
| Grade D | Mucosal breaks involving more than 75% of the esophageal sphincter |

evaluating the severity of reflux and its impact on the esophagus. Once esophagitis is noted, it is important to grade the esophagitis. Esophagitis is often graded using the LA classification (Table 35.4).

Just as in those with unaltered anatomy, biopsy-proven esophagitis negates the need for objective pH studies in many cases [8]. Any mucosal abnormalities can also be biopsied at the time of procedure to examine the tissue microscopically. This helps in confirming the presence of conditions like Barrett's esophagus with or without dysplasia guiding treatment decisions. Masses in the intestinal tract can be evaluated and abnormalities in mucosa can be evaluated.

3. **Post-Bariatric Surgery Anatomic Evaluation**: All weight loss surgeries can affect the anatomy of the stomach and the risk of reflux. EGD can assess the post-surgery anatomy and any reflux-related issues. In post-sleeve gastrectomy patients, it is important to note sleeve morphology. The sleeve can be viewed as dilated, there may be stenosis or significant angulation at the incisura. Stenosis elsewhere in the stomach, particularly proximal to the incisura, can also be seen and may contribute to patient symptoms. In the post-sleeve patient, a retroflection should be performed distal to the incisura to ensure that it is not too tight or angulated. If the stomach hugs the scope, then the incisura may be too tight. It should sit loose around the scope (Fig. 35.2a, b).

   In gastric bypass patients, an EGD can aid in the detection of altered anatomy that can help to identify causes of reflux. When doing endoscopy for a bypass patient, the length of the pouch and noting the location of the diaphragmatic hiatus are important. If the pouch is too long, then excess acid burden may lead to reflux and ulcers. Hiatal hernias after bypass can lead to significant symptoms including reflux and dysphagia. It is important to note that small hiatal hernias in

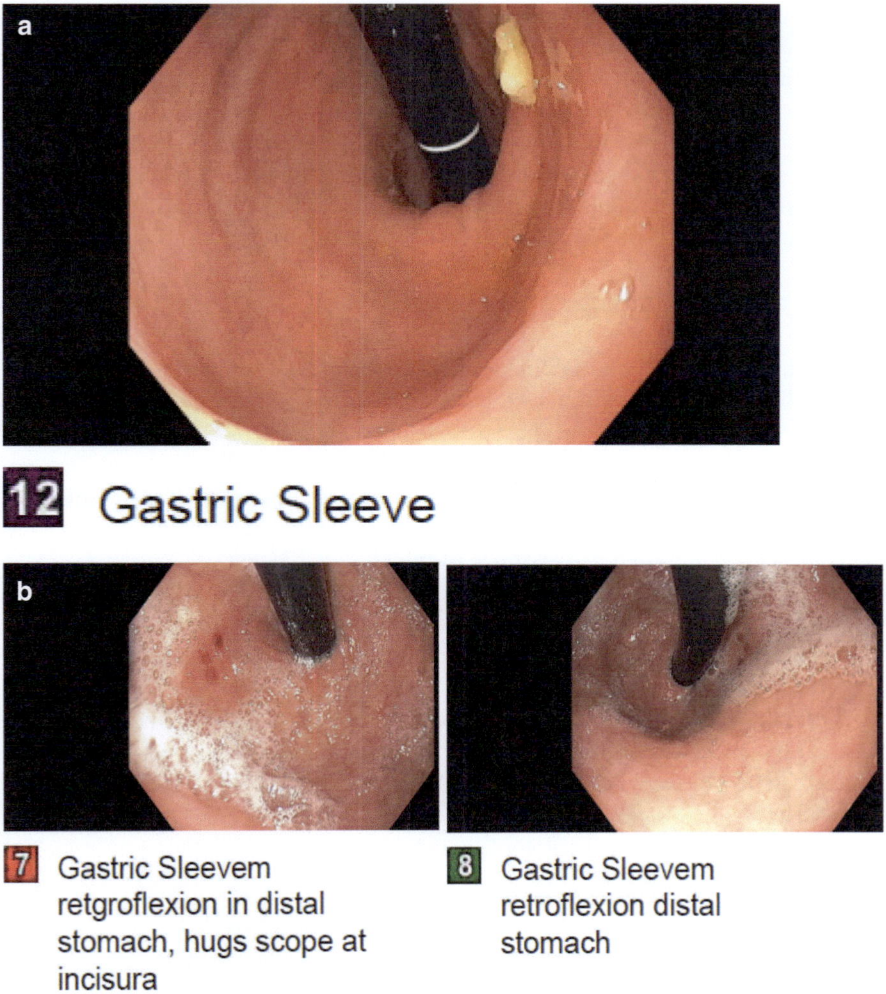


**Fig. 35.2** EGD images showing the anatomy of the incisura after a sleeve gastrectomy. (**a**) Open Incisura. (**b**) Tight incisura

gastric bypass patients may lead to increased severity of symptoms in comparison to non-surgically altered anatomy. A small intrathoracic sliding hernia of the pouch can contain a significant portion of the pouch due to its small size. A 2 cm hiatal hernia may be about 50% of the pouch and akin to a paraesophageal hernia in a normal stomach. One can also look for bile in the pouch and roux limb. This can be indicative of a gastrogastric fistula or a distal obstruction leading to bile reflux. Bile reflux can also be reflective of a short roux limb length. A less common cause of reflux after bypass is LES dysfunction. This cannot be objectively measured on endoscopy, but one can look for a patulous LES. Objectively, manometry would be used to assess this.

Following BPD/DS similar endoscopic findings mentioned post-sleeve should be noted. Bile reflux is an important thing to look for in these patients.

EGD and its ability to provide endoluminal evaluation can aid significantly in the etiology of reflux in post-bariatric patients. EGD is a valuable tool in the assessment of reflux in bariatric patients, helping clinicians diagnose, stage, and manage reflux-related issues in this patient population. This is usually the first test done in those with persistent GERD symptoms after weight loss surgery.

## The Upper Gastrointestinal Series (UGI)

The UGI, also known as a barium swallow, involves the patient swallowing a contrast medium, typically barium, which is visualized using fluoroscopic radiography. This diagnostic test allows for the assessment of the anatomy and function of the esophagus and stomach. A UGI is valuable in identifying reflux by capturing real-time images of barium flow through the esophagus and gastroesophageal junction. Reflux episodes can be observed when barium is seen flowing back into the esophagus during the exam. In the assessment of reflux, the UGI can:

1. **Quantify Reflux**: The frequency and severity of reflux episodes can be quantified using an upper GI series. Radiologists assess the degree of reflux, which can help guide treatment decisions.
2. **Evaluate Anatomic Changes**: The presence of a hiatal hernia, whether fixed or moving, can be seen radiographically. The anatomy of the GI tract and its function can be assessed. For example, a herniated gastric pouch after bypass may be easiest to see radiographically (Fig. 35.3). In addition, stenosis in the sleeve can be assessed with this technology (Fig. 35.4).

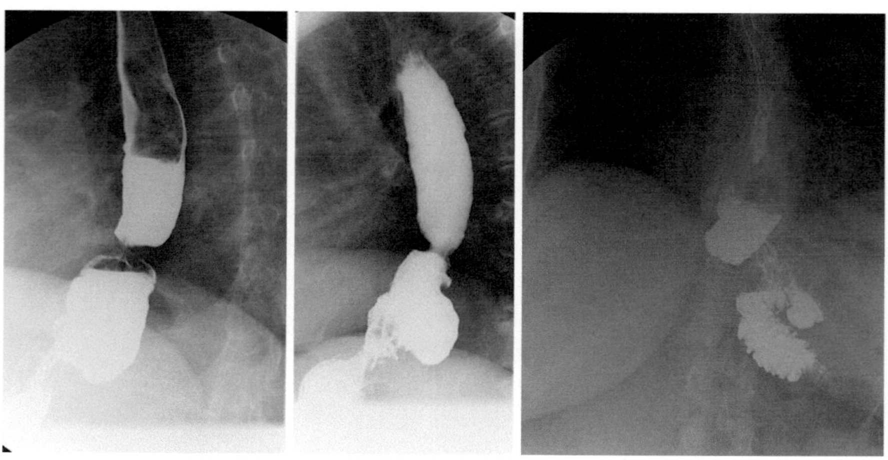

**Fig. 35.3** An UGI demonstrating a herniated gastric pouch

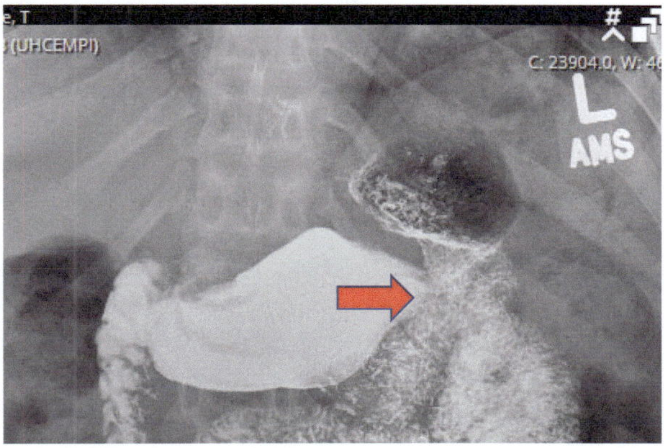


**Fig. 35.4** UGI series showing narrowing at the incisura leading to reflux

After sleeve gastrectomy, multiple studies have shown that sleeve morphology is an important contributor to reflux. The shape of the sleeve can be assessed radiographically. There are four major subtypes of sleeve morphology: Dumbbell, Lower Pouch, Tubular, or Upper Pouch (see Fig. 35.1). This information is crucial in understanding how surgical anatomy may influence GERD. In one study Dumbbell morphology has been linked with increased GERD symptoms [5]. Hiatal hernia and stenosis in the sleeve have also been associated with increased reflux. While the upper GI series is a valuable tool in assessing GERD in post-bariatric surgery patients, it has its limitations. This study is subjectively read by the radiologist in real time. This can give one general information regarding structure and function, such as the extent of the reflux. However, it cannot quantify the severity or quantity of reflux. Additionally, it is less sensitive than pH monitoring, which is considered the gold standard for diagnosing acid reflux.

Overall, this fluoroscopic study is beneficial in assessing GERD. It gives an idea of the anatomy as well as the function of the altered anatomy. Some hiatal hernias can be seen radiologically that may not have been evident endoscopically.

## Bravo PH

Bravo pH Monitoring, involves placing a small wireless pH sensor (the Bravo capsule) in the lower esophagus during an endoscopy. The capsule measures the acidity in the esophagus over a 48–96 h period and is transmitted to a recorder that the patient wears. The capsule usually falls off within 5–7 days after placement. This test can help determine the frequency and severity of acid reflux episodes. It's especially useful because it allows for monitoring over an extended period, providing a comprehensive view of reflux patterns. Patients hold their PPIs approximately 7 days before the placement of the pH sensor to accurately determine the presence of GERD during this assessment. Typical symptoms are divided in three categories (heartburn, chest pain, and regurgitation) [39]. Patients are instructed to activate the recorder while eating meals, lying down, and most importantly, when they experience typical GERD symptoms. This symptom assessment helps with correlating patients' symptoms with actual acid reflux events. This helps determine whether GERD is the primary cause of their complaints. Objective data, including acid exposure time, longest reflux episodes, supine and upright reflux help to determine a DeMeester score. This is a statistical model that helps quantify the severity of the reflux overall. Johnson-DeMeester score over 22.1, Jamieson-DeMeester scores greater than 14.7, and acid exposure time > 4.2% of the time are all considered abnormal and consistent with pathologic reflux [40]. When a patient has both objective and subjective data consistent with GERD, that is deemed an abnormal reflux burden linking the patient's symptoms to persistent GERD. If a patient has normal objective data but has a positive symptom association, that leads to a diagnosis of reflux hypersensitivity. If a patient has a normal reflux burden and negative symptom association, this is an indication that the symptoms are not due to reflux. Functional symptoms need to be explored along with an alternative diagnosis. This provides critical data to guide treatment decisions, such as medication adjustments or the need for additional surgical interventions to manage reflux in bariatric patients.

One may argue that the same definitions for pathologic reflux should be different after weight loss surgery due to the decreased parietal cell burden. In general, following sleeve gastrectomy, conventional definitions of reflux are used. After a bypass, one may consider lower acid exposure times as pathologic, however, studies have shown that conventional measures can even be used in these patients [41, 42]. The authors look to high symptom correlation as a big indicator of pathologic reflux after gastric bypass procedures.

Interestingly, although gastric bypass is considered an antireflux procedure, some patients can have reflux even after this procedure. In a recent study, [43] posits that there has been an overestimation of the resolution of reflux after gastric bypass. In this study, a review of postoperative GERD in 2454 patients from a nationwide database after RYGB showed that up to 48.8% of patients had persistent GERD within 2 years and could be persistent for up to 10 years. Postoperative GERD was defined in this study as residual or recurring symptoms of GERD with the use of acid suppression medications for beyond 6 months postoperatively. Notwithstanding this discovery of GERD prevalence in this study, the authors still report that there is a place for RYGB to be a mainstay procedure in GERD management, if not first line in select groups of patients. In addition, the SM-BOSS study still had a significant incidence of GERD in the post-bypass group.

## Esophageal Manometry

Manometry is a diagnostic technique that aids in this assessment by providing valuable information about esophageal motility and the functionality of the lower esophageal sphincter (LES). High resolution manometry provides the added benefit of seeing the motility in a graphic form and impedance adds the ability to assess esophageal clearance. In the context of bariatric surgery, manometry serves several key purposes:

1. Preoperative Assessment: Manometry is sometimes used as part of the preoperative evaluation for bariatric surgery. It helps identify pre-existing motility issues or LES dysfunction that may influence the choice of surgical procedure. This proactive approach can lead to better patient selection and personalized surgical planning. One study suggests up to 54% of obese patients have some degree of LES dysfunction [44]. We also know that obesity itself affects LES and esophageal function. Increased abdominal girth can increase reflux. Additionally, in one study, a greater BMI was associated with higher LES pressure and increased contraction amplitude [45]. That being said, the sleeve is considered refluxogenic. If the patient complains of severe reflux symptoms preoperatively and the pressure in the lower esophageal sphincter is low, the authors avoid doing a sleeve gastrectomy and choose a different weight loss procedure. The reasoning is that the pressure in the sleeve may overcome the pressure of the LES and cause more GERD.
2. Postoperative Assessment after Bariatric Surgery: Manometry has become an essential tool for evaluating patients, especially when reflux symptoms arise. The purpose of the motility study is to assess esophageal function, LES function and it is one more way evaluate hiatal hernias. Often manometrically, hiatal hernias can be seen better than on other studies such as endoscopy and esophagram (Figs. 35.5 and 35.6).

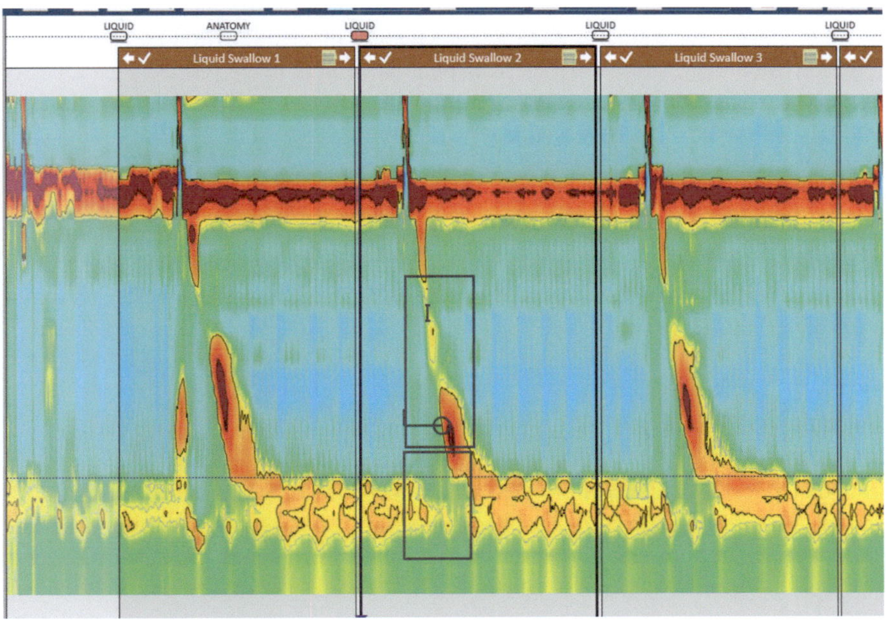


**Fig. 35.5** Manometry study showing a hypotensive LES and a small hiatal hernia after sleeve gastrectomy

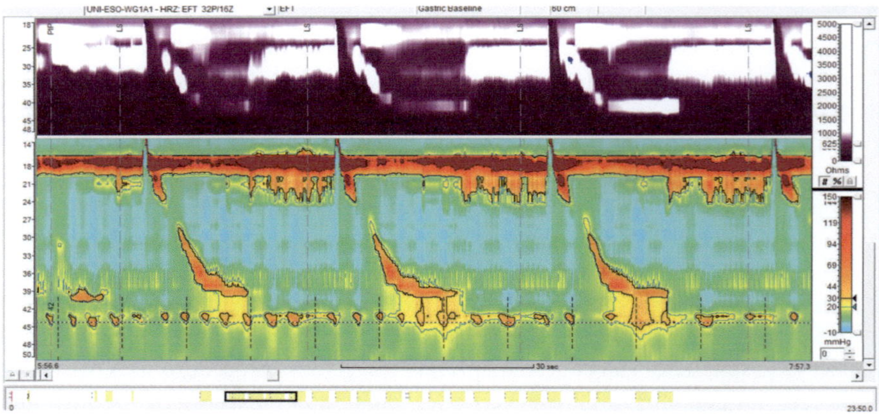

**Fig. 35.6** Manometry study showing high pressure between the LES and the hiatus in addition to a hypotensive LES and a hiatal hernia. This can lead to a choking sensation

Manometry helps to better understand esophageal function. By noting these abnormalities, the physician can have a more educated discussion about the cause of their symptoms and how to manage them. It is becoming increasingly evident that weight loss surgery can affect esophageal function. Since motility studies are not done routinely before bariatric surgery, it is not always clear if the weight loss procedure made a subclinical condition symptomatic, or is creating new problems. Changes in esophageal motility were first noted after gastric banding procedures. Since that time, more studies have shown changes in LES function and esophageal function after weight loss surgery. This phenomenon is being termed Post Obesity Surgery Esophageal Dysfunction (POSED). This is not well defined thus far and findings are mixed. This may be due to variations in surgical techniques for the various procedures. Regardless, based on manometry results, healthcare providers can develop tailored treatment plans. For example, if manometry reveals poor LES function, surgical revision, sphincter augmentation or endoscopic interventions may be recommended to address the issue and alleviate reflux symptoms [46]. Manometry can be a key diagnostic test after weight loss surgery to guide management of symptoms of GERD.

## Impedance Testing

Impedance testing measures the electrical impedance between multiple electrodes placed along the esophagus. This technology can distinguish between acid and non-acidic reflux episodes, offering a more accurate assessment of GERD compared to traditional pH monitoring alone. Through this, the movement of fluids and gases in the esophagus can be assessed allowing the detection of acidic and non-acidic reflux events, making it particularly valuable for bariatric patients who may experience different types of reflux due to altered anatomy after surgery. Much like the bravo pH study, the impedance test relies on objective and subjective data to determine if the symptoms are related to GERD [47]. Unlike the bravo pH probe, the impedance test is not wireless. The catheter probe is inserted transnasally and is left in place in the esophagus 5 cm above LES for 24 h until removal the following day. This can be somewhat uncomfortable for patients but does provide another element of information in the form of non-acidic reflux events. Acid events are noted when the pH is $<4$ and non-acid events occur when the pH is $>4$ [48]. Drops in impedance signify liquid, while increase in impedance signifies gas presence [48]. This test can identify both liquid and gas reflux, providing a more complete picture of the patient's condition. This is useful in the assessment of patients with bile reflux specifically following RYBG. Symptom correlation establishing the presence of pathologic reflux disease is the result that is the most helpful with impedance testing.

## Endoflip

The most modern technology to assess reflux after weight loss surgery is the use of impedance planimetry. This technology is another way to assess esophageal and LES function. The balloon-tipped catheter can assess the distensibility of a lumen, and this can be transduced to assess pressure within a lumen. Studies are still in their infantile stages in this space. One of the most recent studies evaluated patients with obesity using planimetry and compared them to those who had weight loss surgery [49]. In this study, the majority of patients with unaltered anatomy had preserved motility. However, after weight loss surgery, less than half had normal motility. Sleeve patients were more affected than gastric bypass patients, but those who had some sort of revision were affected the most. More data is expected to come out with this technology and will be adjunctive to our understanding of esophageal function. This will allow better management in the future.

## Gastric Emptying Studies

Gastric emptying studies (GES) have varied utility following bariatric surgery. The procedure in which they can be the most helpful is the sleeve gastrectomy. This is the only pylorus preserving procedure. Poor gastric emptying can be due to dysfunction at the pylorus and contribute to GERD. Botox injections at the pylorus have not shown significant effects in large studies in patients who are post-sleeve with GERD. Anecdotally, some have found this intervention helpful. Most of the other weight loss procedures are low pressure systems and do not have a valve at the outlet, and therefore gastric emptying is less of a concern.

## Workup Algorithm for GERD Post-Bariatric Surgery

To comprehensively assess GERD-related symptoms in post-bariatric surgery patients, it is crucial to compile a thorough medical history, emphasizing details of the patient's dietary choices. Given that poor food selections can exacerbate GERD symptoms, lifestyle adjustments may contribute to symptom resolution. After addressing modifiable factors, persistent and substantial GERD symptoms necessitate a more in-depth assessment through traditional modalities for reflux evaluation post-bariatric surgery. The subsequent algorithm provides a concise overview of diagnosing the underlying causes of GERD symptoms within this specific patient population. Figure 35.7 Algorithm outlines significant findings that should be gleaned from each of the studies. Currently, Endoflip is not included as this technology is not in our current practice. The algorithms in Fig. 35.8 incorporates the use of that technology.

Other preoperative evaluation algorithms have been proposed. All of these should be reviewed so that physicians can make an informed decision as to how to intervene for the patients' reflux. Gastric emptying studies can occasionally be helpful as well. These algorithms are specific to sleeve gastrectomy (Fig. 35.8) and gastric bypass procedures (Fig. 35.9).

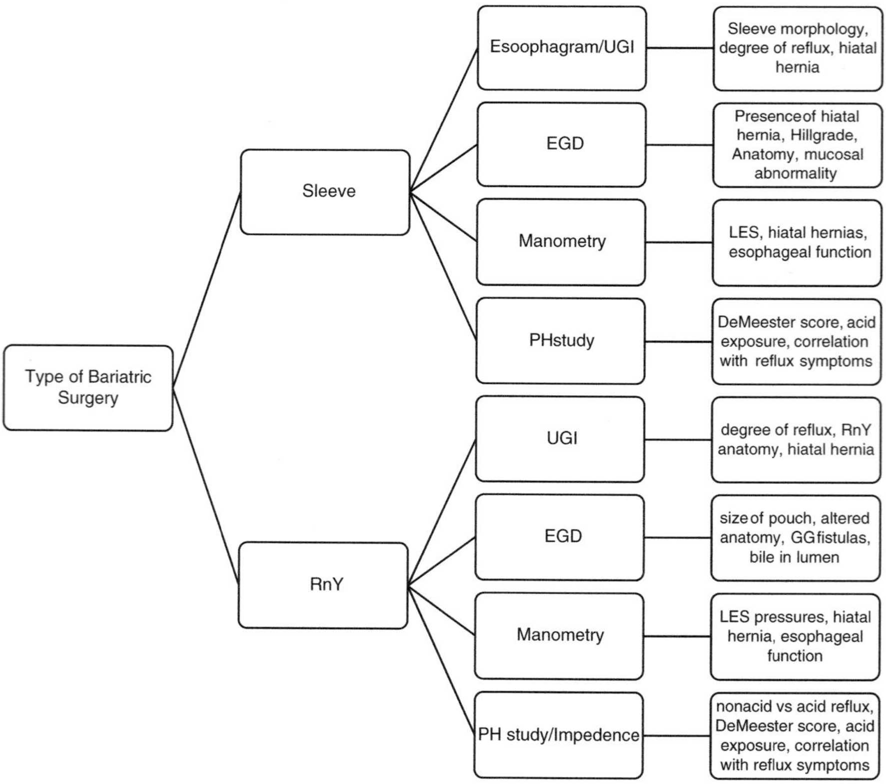


**Fig. 35.7** Most common bariatric procedures and modalities used to assess GERD causes

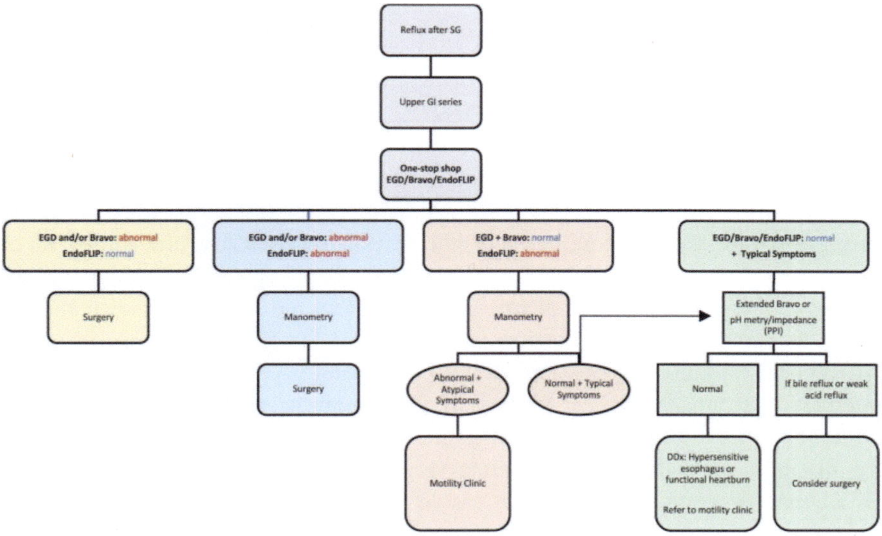


**Fig. 35.8** Algorithmic approach for the evaluation and management of GERD after SG. *GERD* gastroesophageal reflux disease, *SG* sleeve gastrectomy, *GI* gastrointestinal, *EGD* esophagogastroduodenoscopy, *PPI* proton-pump inhibitor, *DDx* differential diagnosis [50]

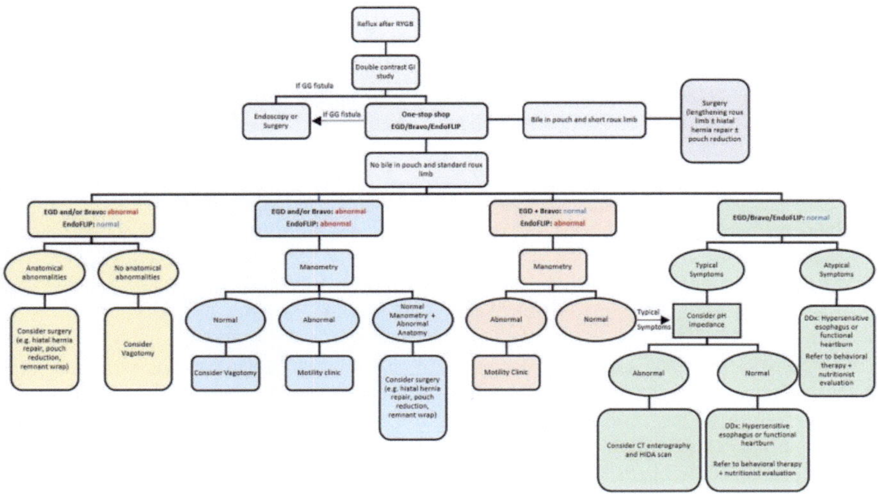


**Fig. 35.9** Algorithmic approach for the evaluation and management of GERD after RYGB. *GERD*, gastroesophageal reflux disease, *RYGB* Roux-en-Y gastric bypass, *GI* gastrointestinal, *GG* gastro-gastric, *EGD* esophagogastroduodenoscopy, *CT* computed tomography, *HIDA* hepatobiliary iminodiacetic acid, *DDx* differential diagnosis [50]

## Conclusion

This chapter has provided a comprehensive overview of reflux after bariatric surgery, encompassing the incidence of GERD after various procedures, their impact on reflux, and how to evaluate the reflux disease. The purpose of a thorough workup is to tailor management to the underlying cause of the reflux. In those with unaltered anatomy, the contributing factors to GERD include patient factors, lifestyle, hiatal hernia, and LES dysfunction. In those who have had weight loss procedures, all of these need to be considered in the context of the altered anatomy. The type of bariatric procedure plays a pivotal role in determining the incidence and nature of reflux. A comprehensive evaluation of controllable factors is essential to treating GERD after bariatric surgery. Patient lifestyle, eating habits, and weight should be optimized before any further workup. If the symptoms persist, a comprehensive evaluation utilizing all of the modalities are warranted. The physician can put all of the findings together in context of the surgical anatomy to tailor treatment and GERD management. This approach can lead to the best outcomes. Management strategies are discussed in another chapter and therefore were not reviewed here.

## References


1. Chang P, Friedenberg F. Obesity and GERD. Gastroenterol Clin N Am. 2014;43:161–73. https://doi.org/10.1016/j.gtc.2013.11.009.
2. Davrieux CF, Palermo M, Nedelcu M, Nocca D. Reflux after sleeve gastrectomy: an update. J Laparoendosc Adv Surg Tech. 2021;31:978–82. https://doi.org/10.1089/lap.2021.0478.
3. Castagneto-Gissey, L., Russo, M.F., D'Andrea, V., Genco, A., Casella, G., 2023b. Efficacy of Sleeve Gastrectomy with Concomitant Hiatal Hernia Repair versus Sleeve–Fundoplication on Gastroesophageal Reflux Disease Resolution: Systematic Review and Meta-Analysis. J Clin Med 12, 3323. doi: https://doi.org/10.3390/jcm12093323.
4. Felinska E, Billeter A, Nickel F, Contin P, Berlth F, Chand B, Grimminger P, Mikami D, Schoppmann SF, Müller-Stich B. Do we understand the pathophysiology of GERD after sleeve gastrectomy? Ann N Y Acad Sci. 2020;1482:26–35. https://doi.org/10.1111/nyas.14467.
5. Alvarez R, Youssef J, Zadeh J, Sarode A, Barger R, Abbas M, Khaitan L. Sleeve gastrectomy morphology and long-term weight-loss and gastroesophageal reflux disease outcomes. Surg Endosc. 2023b;37:5652–64. https://doi.org/10.1007/s00464-022-09555-6.
6. Altieri MS, Pryor AD. Gastroesophageal reflux disease after bariatric procedures. Surg Clin North Am. 2015;95:579–91. https://doi.org/10.1016/j.suc.2015.02.010.
7. Daes J, Jimenez ME, Said N, Dennis R. Improvement of gastroesophageal reflux symptoms after standardized laparoscopic sleeve gastrectomy. Obes Surg. 2014;24:536–40. https://doi.org/10.1007/s11695-013-1117-6.
8. Alvarez R, Ward BL, Xiao T, Zadeh J, Sarode A, Khaitan L, Abbas M. Independent association of preoperative hill grade with gastroesophageal reflux disease 2 years after sleeve gastrectomy. Surg Obes Relat Dis Off J Am Soc Bariatr Surg. 2023a;19:563–75. https://doi.org/10.1016/j.soard.2022.12.013.
9. Swei E, Helmkamp L, Samuels J, Schoen J, Scott FI, Wani S, Sullivan S. Reflux and Barrett's esophagus after sleeve gastrectomy: analysis of a statewide database. Surg Obes Relat Dis. 2023;19:1023–9. https://doi.org/10.1016/j.soard.2023.02.008.
10. Campos GM, Mazzini GS, Altieri MS, Docimo S, DeMaria EJ, Rogers AM. ASMBS position statement on the rationale for performance of upper gastrointestinal endoscopy before

and after metabolic and bariatric surgery. Surg Obes Relat Dis. 2021;17:837–47. https://doi.org/10.1016/j.soard.2021.03.007.
11. Slater BJ, Collings A, Dirks R, Gould JC, Qureshi AP, Juza R, Rodríguez-Luna MR, Wunker C, Kohn GP, Kothari S, Carslon E, Worrell S, Abou-Setta AM, Ansari MT, Athanasiadis DI, Daly S, Dimou F, Haskins IN, Hong J, Krishnan K, Lidor A, Litle V, Low D, Petrick A, Soriano IS, Thosani N, Tyberg A, Velanovich V, Vilallonga R, Marks JM. Multi-society consensus conference and guideline on the treatment of gastroesophageal reflux disease (GERD). Surg Endosc. 2023;37:781–806. https://doi.org/10.1007/s00464-022-09817-3.
12. Yeung KTD, Penney N, Ashrafian L, Darzi A, Ashrafian H. Does sleeve gastrectomy expose the distal esophagus to severe reflux? A systematic review and meta-analysis. Ann Surg. 2020;271:257–65. https://doi.org/10.1097/SLA.0000000000003275.
13. Rrezza EE, Ikramuddin S, Gourash W, Rakitt T, Kingston A, Luketich J, Schauer PR. Symptomatic improvement in gastroesophageal reflux disease (GERD) following laparoscopic roux-en-Y gastric bypass. Surg Endosc. 2002;16:1027–31. https://doi.org/10.1007/s00464-001-8313-5.
14. Perry Y, Courcoulas AP, Fernando HC, Buenaventura PO, McCaughan JS, Luketich JD. Laparoscopic roux-en-Y gastric bypass for recalcitrant gastroesophageal reflux disease in morbidly obese patients. JSLS. 2004;8:19–23.
15. Castagneto-Gissey L, Gualtieri L, Diddoro A, Lauro A, Genco A, Casella G. Y not roux-en-Y?: resolution of Barrett's esophagus after surgical conversion of gastric sleeve in two patients. Dig Dis Sci. 2023a;68:1698–704. https://doi.org/10.1007/s10620-023-07874-9.
16. Peterli R, Wölnerhanssen BK, Peters T, Vetter D, Kröll D, Borbély Y, Schultes B, Beglinger C, Drewe J, Schiesser M, Nett P, Bueter M. Effect of laparoscopic sleeve gastrectomy vs laparoscopic roux-en-Y gastric bypass on weight loss in patients with morbid obesity: the SM-BOSS randomized clinical trial. JAMA. 2018;319:255. https://doi.org/10.1001/jama.2017.20897.
17. Kim M, Navarro F, Eruchalu CN, Augenstein VA, Heniford BT, Stefanidis D. Minimally invasive roux-en-Y gastric bypass for fundoplication failure offers excellent gastroesophageal reflux control. Am Surg. 2014;80:696–703.
18. Pallati PK, Shaligram A, Shostrom VK, Oleynikov D, McBride CL, Goede MR. Improvement in gastroesophageal reflux disease symptoms after various bariatric procedures: review of the bariatric outcomes longitudinal database. Surg Obes Relat Dis. 2014;10:502–7. https://doi.org/10.1016/j.soard.2013.07.018.
19. Petersen WV, Meile T, Küper MA, Zdichavsky M, Königsrainer A, Schneider JH. Functional importance of laparoscopic sleeve gastrectomy for the lower esophageal sphincter in patients with morbid obesity. Obes Surg. 2012;22:360–6. https://doi.org/10.1007/s11695-011-0536-5.
20. Pandolfino JE, El-Serag HB, Zhang Q, Shah N, Ghosh SK, Kahrilas PJ. Obesity: a challenge to esophagogastric junction integrity. Gastroenterology. 2006;130:639–49. https://doi.org/10.1053/j.gastro.2005.12.016.
21. Santonicola A, Angrisani L, Cutolo P, Formisano G, Iovino P. The effect of laparoscopic sleeve gastrectomy with or without hiatal hernia repair on gastroesophageal reflux disease in obese patients. Surg Obes Relat Dis. 2014;10:250–5. https://doi.org/10.1016/j.soard.2013.09.006.
22. Docimo S, Rahmana U, Bates A, Talamini M, Pryor A, Spaniolas K. Concomitant hiatal hernia repair is more common in laparoscopic sleeve gastrectomy than during laparoscopic roux-en-Y gastric bypass: an analysis of 130,772 cases. Obes Surg. 2019;29:744–6. https://doi.org/10.1007/s11695-018-3594-0.
23. Capella JF, Capella RF. Gastro-gastric fistulas and marginal ulcers in gastric bypass procedures for weight reduction. Obes Surg. 1999;9:22–7. https://doi.org/10.1381/096089299765553674.
24. Chahine E, Kassir R, Dirani M, Joumaa S, Debs T, Chouillard E. Surgical Management of Gastrogastric Fistula after Roux-en-Y Gastric Bypass: 10-year experience. Obes Surg. 2018;28:939–44. https://doi.org/10.1007/s11695-017-2949-2.
25. Yao DC, Stellato TA, Schuster MM, Graf KN, Hallowell PT. Gastrogastric fistula following roux-en-Y bypass is attributed to both surgical technique and experience. Am J Surg. 2010;199:382–385; discussion 385-386. https://doi.org/10.1016/j.amjsurg.2009.09.017.

26. Bernal MD. Bile reflux after bariatric surgery. Cir Esp Engl Ed. 2023;101:S63–8. https://doi.org/10.1016/j.cireng.2023.02.014.
27. Carbajo MA, Luque-de-León E, Jiménez JM, Ortiz-de-Solórzano J, Pérez-Miranda M, Castro-Alija MJ. Laparoscopic one-anastomosis gastric bypass: technique, results, and long-term follow-up in 1200 patients. Obes Surg. 2017;27:1153–67. https://doi.org/10.1007/s11695-016-2428-1.
28. Ghiassi S, Nimeri A, Aleassa EM, Grover BT, Eisenberg D, Carter J. American Society for Metabolic and Bariatric Surgery position statement on one-anastomosis gastric bypass. Surg Obes Relat Dis. 2023;S1550728923007931:319. https://doi.org/10.1016/j.soard.2023.11.003.
29. Fuchs K-H, Maroske J, Fein M, Tigges H, Ritter MP, Heimbucher J, Thiede A. Variability in the composition of physiologic duodenogastric reflux. J Gastrointest Surg. 1999;3:389–96. https://doi.org/10.1016/S1091-255X(99)80055-9.
30. Schindlbeck NE, Heinrich C, Stellaard F, Paumgartner G, Muller-Lissner SA. Healthy controls have as much bile reflux as gastric ulcer patients. Gut. 1987;28:1577–83. https://doi.org/10.1136/gut.28.12.1577.
31. Carbajo M, García-Caballero M, Toledano M, Osorio D, García-Lanza C, Carmona JA. One-anastomosis gastric bypass by laparoscopy: results of the first 209 patients. Obes Surg. 2005;15:398–404. https://doi.org/10.1381/0960892053576677.
32. Badaoui JN, Kellogg TA, Abu Dayyeh BK, Maroun JW, McKenzie TJ, Harmsen WS, Kendrick ML, Ghanem OM. The outcomes of laparoscopic biliopancreatic diversion with duodenal switch on gastro-esophageal reflux disease: the Mayo Clinic experience. Obes Surg. 2021;31:4363–70. https://doi.org/10.1007/s11695-021-05581-w.
33. Anderson B, Gill RS, De Gara CJ, Karmali S, Gagner M. Biliopancreatic diversion: the effectiveness of duodenal switch and its limitations. Gastroenterol Res Pract. 2013;2013:1–8. https://doi.org/10.1155/2013/974762.
34. Admella V, Lazzara C, Sobrino L, Acrich E, Biondo S, Pujol-Gebellí J, Osorio J. Patient-reported outcomes and quality of life after single-anastomosis Duodeno-ileal bypass with sleeve gastrectomy (SADI-S): a cross-sectional study with 283 patients from a single institution. Obes Surg. 2023;33:1754–63. https://doi.org/10.1007/s11695-023-06554-x.
35. Kowalewski PK, Olszewski R, Kwiatkowski A, Gałązka-Świderek N, Cichoń K, Paśnik K. Life with a gastric band. Long-term outcomes of laparoscopic adjustable gastric banding—a retrospective study. Obes Surg. 2017;27:1250–3. https://doi.org/10.1007/s11695-016-2435-2.
36. Angrisani L, Cutolo PP, Formisano G, Nosso G, Vitolo G. Laparoscopic adjustable gastric banding versus roux-en-Y gastric bypass: 10-year results of a prospective, randomized trial. Surg Obes Relat Dis Off J Am Soc Bariatr Surg. 2013;9:405–13. https://doi.org/10.1016/j.soard.2012.11.011.
37. Brännström L, Werner M, Wallner B, Franklin KA, Karling P. What is the significance of the hill classification? Dis Esophagus. 2023;36:doad004. https://doi.org/10.1093/dote/doad004.
38. Hansdotter I, Björ O, Andreasson A, Agreus L, Hellström P, Forsberg A, Talley N, Vieth M, Wallner B. Hill classification is superior to the axial length of a hiatal hernia for assessment of the mechanical anti-reflux barrier at the gastroesophageal junction. Endosc Int Open. 2016;04:E311–7. https://doi.org/10.1055/s-0042-101021.
39. Pandolfino JE, Kwiatek MA. Use and utility of the bravo™ pH capsule. J Clin Gastroenterol. 2008;42:571–8. https://doi.org/10.1097/MCG.0b013e31815bb602.
40. Boström M, Thorsson O, Toth E, Agardh D. Clinical value of wireless pH-monitoring of gastro-esophageal reflux in children before and after proton pump inhibitors. BMC Gastroenterol. 2014;14:3. https://doi.org/10.1186/s12876-014-0225-7.
41. King K, Sudan R, Bardaro S, Soriano I, Petrick AT, Daly SC, Lo Menzo E, Davis D, Leyva-Alvizo A, Gonzalez-Urquijo M, Eisenberg D, El Chaar M. Assessment and management of gastroesophageal reflux disease following bariatric surgery. Surg Obes Relat Dis. 2021;17:1919–25. https://doi.org/10.1016/j.soard.2021.07.023.
42. Raj PP, Bhattacharya S, Misra S, Kumar SS, Khan Mohd J, Gunasekaran SC, Palanivelu C. Gastroesophageal reflux–related physiologic changes after sleeve gastrectomy and roux-

en-Y gastric bypass: a prospective comparative study. Surg Obes Relat Dis. 2019;15:1261–9. https://doi.org/10.1016/j.soard.2019.05.017.
43. Holmberg D, Santoni G, Xie S, Lagergren J. Gastric bypass surgery in the treatment of gastro-oesophageal reflux symptoms. Aliment Pharmacol Ther. 2019;50:159–66. https://doi.org/10.1111/apt.15274.
44. Hong D, Khajanchee YS, Pereira N, Lockhart B, Patterson EJ, Swanstrom LL. Manometric abnormalities and gastroesophageal reflux disease in the morbidly obese. Obes Surg. 2004;14:744–9. https://doi.org/10.1381/0960892041590854.
45. Herbella FAM, Sweet MP, Tedesco P, Nipomnick I, Patti MG. Gastroesophageal reflux disease and obesity. Pathophysiology and implications for treatment. J Gastrointest Surg. 2007;11:286–90. https://doi.org/10.1007/s11605-007-0097-z.
46. Grover K, Khaitan L. Magnetic sphincter augmentation as treatment of gastroesophageal reflux disease after sleeve gastrectomy. Dis Esophagus. 2023;36:doad030. https://doi.org/10.1093/dote/doad030.
47. Hobbs P, Gyawali CP. The role of esophageal pH-impedance testing in clinical practice. Curr Opin Gastroenterol. 2018;34:249–57. https://doi.org/10.1097/MOG.0000000000000441.
48. Villa N, Vela MF. Impedance-pH testing. Gastroenterol Clin North Am. 2013;42:17–26. https://doi.org/10.1016/j.gtc.2012.11.003.
49. Brunaldi VO, Abboud DM, Abusaleh RR, Al Annan K, Razzak FA, Ravi K, Valls EJV, Storm AC, Ghanem OM, Abu Dayyeh BK. Post-bariatric surgery changes in secondary esophageal motility and Distensibility parameters. Obes Surg. 2024;34:347–54. https://doi.org/10.1007/s11695-023-06959-8.
50. Ghanem OM, Ghazi R, Abdul Razzak F, Bazerbachi F, Ravi K, Khaitan L, Kothari SN, Abu Dayyeh BK. Turnkey algorithmic approach for the evaluation of gastroesophageal reflux disease after bariatric surgery. Gastroenterol Rep. 2023;11:goad028. https://doi.org/10.1093/gastro/goad028.
51. Azer SA, Reddivari AKR. Reflux esophagitis. In: In: StatPearls. StatPearls: Publishing, Treasure Island (FL); 2024.

# Reflux After Bariatric Surgery: Management Options

# 36

Jorge Cornejo, Lorna A. Evans, and Enrique F. Elli

## Introduction

The management of gastroesophageal reflux (GERD) following bariatric surgery can range from medical therapy to endoscopic options to surgical options [1, 2]. First-line treatment of this condition is similar to that of the general population and involves dietary and lifestyle modifications, followed by acid-reducing medications [3]. When medical treatment fails, other therapies are considered [4]. This chapter focuses on a detailed review of the surgical options for post-bariatric surgery reflux and a proposed algorithm summarizing the decision-making is presented in Fig. 36.1. The chapter will discuss management following the most popular bariatric procedures performed today: Sleeve Gastrectomy (SG), Roux-en-Y gastric bypass (RYGB), and Duodenal Switch (DS). The initial evaluation in patients with reflux after bariatric surgery consists of an upper gastrointestinal (UGI) series, esophagogastroduodenoscopy (EGD) with Bravo-pH study, and manometry.

J. Cornejo · L. A. Evans · E. F. Elli (✉)
Department of General Surgery, Mayo Clinic, Jacksonville, FL, USA
e-mail: elli.enrique@mayo.edu


O. M. Ghanem et al. (eds.), *The SAGES Manual of Metabolic and Bariatric Surgery*, https://doi.org/10.1007/978-3-031-72309-4_36

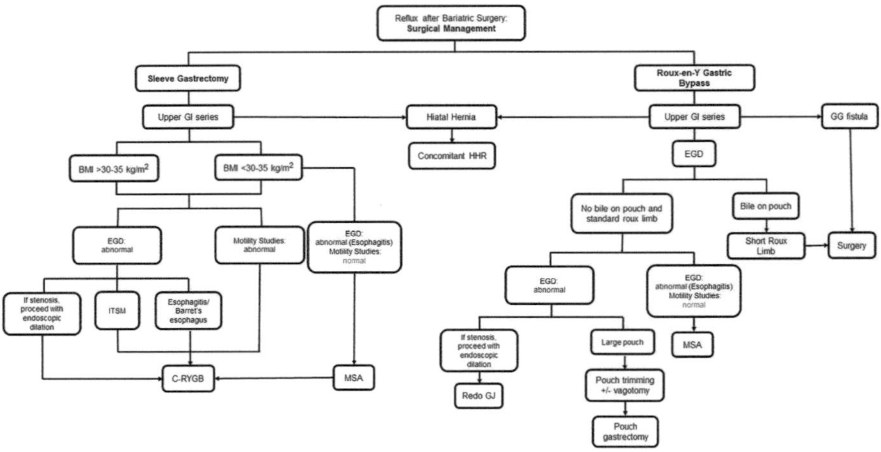


**Fig. 36.1** Algorithm management for post bariatric surgery gastroesophageal reflux disease patients. *BMI* body mass index, *EGD* esophagogastroduodenoscopy, *ITSM* intrathoracic sleeve migration, *MSA* magnetic sphincter augmentation, *C-RYGB* conversion to RYGB, *GG* gastro-gastric, *GJ* gastrojejunostomy

## Management of Reflux After Sleeve Gastrectomy

The anatomical structures of the gastroesophageal junction that comprised the anti-reflux barrier are the lower esophageal sphincter (LES), the sling fibers at the cardia, the diaphragmatic crura, and the gastroesophageal flap valve (GEFV) [5]. Impairment in any of these mechanisms may contribute to the development of de novo GERD or worsening of pre-existing GERD in patients after SG [6].

If a large hiatal hernia (HH) is found in the contrast study, this should be repaired during the reoperation because the presence of a simultaneous hiatal defect contributes to an incompetent gastroesophageal junction (GEJ) and decreased lower esophageal sphincter (LES) pressure leading to an impaired esophageal acid clearance [5, 7, 8]. In addition, Golas et al. reported that post-bariatric hiatal hernia repair resulted in the marked improvement of bloating, abdominal pain, regurgitation, and food intolerance or dysphagia (BARF) in most patients [9]. Body mass index (BMI) range of 30–35 kg/m$^2$ is helpful to determine the type of surgical management the patient will undergo.

### Conversion from Sleeve Gastrectomy to Roux-en-Y Gastric Bypass

Several studies reported that patients who underwent conversion to RYGB showed an improvement in reflux symptoms of 70–100% [10–12]. The mechanisms behind the successful reduction in GERD symptoms include the diversion of bile from the Roux limb, weight loss, lower acid production in the gastric pouch, rapid pouch emptying, and decreased abdominal pressure over the LES [13]. Huynh et al. found an objective reduction in the GERD-HRQL score at 15 months after the conversion to RYGB and reported that an interval of 3 months or greater between SG and the onset of symptoms was associated with a limited response after surgery [14]. While conversion of SG to RYGB is effective for GERD symptoms, it doesn't confer an optimal long-term weight loss, regardless of the indication [15]. Important technical details during this procedure are the hiatal hernia repair, transection of the stomach above potential strictures, and the creation of a small pouch. Studies reported that a small pouch in RYGB is associated with faster gastric emptying, greater weight loss maintenance, better diabetes mellitus resolution, and lower rates of marginal ulcer [16, 17].

This procedure is considered in two scenarios: *abnormal EGD (sleeve stenosis, intrathoracic sleeve migration, or esophagitis/Barret's esophagus) or abnormal motility studies*, regardless of the BMI before the reoperation. Gastric stenosis occurs in 0.7–4% of patients that undergo SG as a result of progressive rotation of the staple line and scarring of the sleeve in a kinked fashion, or due to imbrications of the staple line and over-retraction of the greater curvature during stapling [18]. The stenosis site is most often located in the middle portion of the sleeve and some radiological patterns of gastric sleeves are described to be correlated with GERD symptoms [5]. RYGB is the revisional procedure of choice for post-sleeve strictures due to the high success rate [19]. However, endoscopic techniques such as stents or achalasia balloon dilations are preferred as the initial management of this complication [20]. The complexity of gastric sleeve stenosis leads to a relatively high percentage of conversion to RYGB, as described in two small case series with surgical conversion rates of 11.8% and 14.28% [18, 19]. Intrathoracic sleeve migration (ITSM) is a sliding HH that occurs after SG and represents an important pathogenic factor in the development of GERD [21, 22]. The incidence of ITSM range between 5% and 45% and is considered as evidence of migration of the gastric tube ≥2 cm above the hiatal area [22]. Conversion to RYGB in case of complicated ITSM is shown to be safe and effective in terms of GERD and endoscopic lesion resolution [21, 22].

Furthermore, RYGB is associated with the regression of erosive esophagitis and Barrett's [23]. A recent meta-analysis performed by the International Federation for the Surgery of Obesity and Metabolic Disorders (IFSO) Barrett's Esophagus task force, described a 62.9% remission of Barrett's esophagus after RYGB [24]. It is encouraged to perform a conversion to RYGB in the case of a preoperative finding of Barrett's esophagus after SG. Sleeve gastrectomy's (SG) effect on esophageal function can present as a worsening of GERD. This was described in a study of 37 patients with preoperative esophageal dysmotility disorder who underwent SG which resulted in the persistence of achalasia and GERD symptoms after surgery [25]. Current data shows that conversion to RYGB is the gold standard procedure for patients with known esophageal dysmotility, as it not only prevents but can improve esophageal disorders [26].

## Magnetic Sphincter Augmentation (MSA)

Following SG, refractory GERD has traditionally been treated with conversion to gastric bypass. One suggested alternative is the use of magnetic lower esophageal sphincter augmentation (MSA) to treat reflux in this subset of patients [27]. This procedure is considered in patients with a BMI range of <30–35 kg/m$^2$ with *abnormal EGD (esophagitis) and normal motility studies*. Reddy et al. proposed an algorithm for MSA in patients with reflux after bariatric surgery and recommended that device implantation should be done when sleeve-related anatomic defects and esophageal dysmotility have been ruled out [28]. Studies showed the effectiveness of this surgical alternative through the postoperative reduction of GERD score questionnaires and medication usage [29, 30]. Important technical details during this procedure are hiatal hernia repair, identification of the posterior vagus nerve, and placement of an appropriately sized MSA device. If GERD persists after MSA placement, a conversion to RYGB is offered.

## Management of Reflux after Roux-en-Y Gastric Bypass

Some studies report that patients who underwent RYGB can experience persisting or worsening pre-existing GERD, or might develop de novo GERD [31–33]. The Swiss Multicenter Bypass or Sleeve Study (SM-BOSS) of 217 patients reported de novo GERD in 10.7% of patients who underwent RYGB [32]. Proposed etiologies include a dilated gastric pouch, G-cell inhibition, gastric outlet obstruction, gastric pouch herniation into the mediastinum, esophageal dysmotility, development of a gastro-gastric (GG) fistula, and bile reflux due to a short Roux limb [13, 34].

If a large HH is found in the contrast study, this should be repaired during the reoperation. An upper GI series is useful to diagnose a gastro-gastric fistula (GGF), which occurs in 1–2.6% and is evidenced by the passage of contrast into the gastric remnant on imaging [35, 36]. A GGF < 1 cm can be successfully treated endoscopically with a reported high success rate of 76% with endoscopic stenting [37, 38]. However, a fistula size greater than 1 cm is less likely to heal endoscopically [38], and surgical revision may be necessary [34]. Likewise, EGD is especially relevant because it allows the identification of bile in the pouch that could be indicative of a GGF or a short Roux limb. To date, studies have reported a bile reflux incidence of 3.4–5% after RYGB [39, 40]. These patients may benefit from Roux-limb lengthening [41].

On the other hand, if no evidence of bile is seen through EGD, the following surgical options are proposed:

### Redo-Gastrojejunostomy

This procedure is considered in patients with the following scenario: *abnormal EGD (gastrojejunal [GJ] stenosis)*. Anatomical defects such as stenosis commonly occur post RYGB at the gastrojejunal (GJ) anastomosis. This narrowing in a range of 3–28% after RYGB and the contributing factors include anastomotic tension, tissue ischemia, foreign body reaction, and chronic GJ ulcers [42, 43]. Typically, patients have symptoms of nausea, vomiting, reflux, and progressive dysphagia, and may experience higher weight loss than expected. GJ stenosis often becomes symptomatic when the luminal diameter is < 1 cm [35]. Endoscopic management is considered the most effective tool in the diagnosis and initial management of the stenosis in the GJ anastomosis, with balloon dilation used first and stent representing a salvage for failed endoscopic dilation. Failure of endoscopic management, reported in 5–6.5% of cases, may be adequately treated with reconstruction of the GJ anastomosis [44, 45].

## Pouch Trimming and Vagotomy

This procedure is considered in patients with the following scenario: *abnormal EGD (large pouch)*. The restriction in the RYGB is determined by the size of the pouch and the diameter of the gastrojejunal anastomosis [46]. Generally, the gastric pouch in RYGB measures between 3 and 4 cm or less, and when enlarged may result in increased acid production from retained parietal cells [47]. Long gastric pouches can produce GERD and suboptimal weight loss [35]. Surgical revision has been described in cases of weight regain or insufficient weight loss [35]. Some studies reported improvement in reflux symptoms after either endoscopic or surgical resizing of the gastric pouch [48, 49]. Vagotomy may be performed in conjunction with pouch trimming to reduce symptoms of GERD [50, 51]. If reflux persists after pouch trimming and vagotomy, a pouch gastrectomy can be offered.

## Magnetic Sphincter Augmentation (MSA)

A similar algorithm of MSA after SG is used for post-gastric bypass reflux [28]. Thus, this procedure is considered in patients with the following scenario: *abnormal EGD (esophagitis) and normal motility studies*. Small case series compared GERD-related outcomes in patients who underwent MSA with previous bariatric surgery versus those without it. Both groups showed a comparable improvement in GERD-related questionnaires (70% vs 84%), medication cessation (90% vs 94%), and rates of postoperative dysphagia [52]. Similar results were reported by Broderick et al., and also showed 100% overall patient satisfaction post-procedure [27]. Therefore, MSA combined with crural repair appears to be an encouraging therapeutic option in patients with refractory GERD following bariatric surgery [53].

## Management of Reflux after Duodenal Switch

Patients with Single Anastomosis Duodenoileal Bypass with Sleeve Gastrectomy (SADI-S) can be managed with MSA in the same way as those who have received SG. In addition, more technically complex options can be performed such as conversion of SADI-S to conventional Duodenal Switch (DS) when bile reflux is found in a 24-h pH-impedance study or to RYGB when acid reflux is obtained on the Bravo-pH study. If a pathologic hiatal hernia is found, this should be repaired.

## References

1. El Chaar M, Stoltzfus J, Claros L, Miletics M. Indications for revisions following 630 consecutive laparoscopic sleeve gastrectomy cases: experience in a single accredited center. J Gastrointest Surg. 2017;21:12–6.
2. Langer FB, Bohdjalian A, Shakeri-Leidenmühler S, Schoppmann SF, Zacherl J, Prager G. Conversion from sleeve gastrectomy to Roux-en-Y gastric bypass—indications and outcome. Obes Surg. 2010;20:835–40.
3. King K, Sudan R, Bardaro S, Soriano I, Petrick AT, Daly SC, et al. Assessment and management of gastroesophageal reflux disease following bariatric surgery. Surg Obes Relat Dis. 2021;17(11):1919–25.
4. Treitl D, Nieber D, Ben-David K. Operative treatments for reflux after bariatric surgery: current and emerging management options. J Gastrointest Surg. 2017;21:577–82.
5. Felinska E, Billeter A, Nickel F, Contin P, Berlth F, Chand B, et al. Do we understand the pathophysiology of GERD after sleeve gastrectomy? Ann N Y Acad Sci. 2020;1482(1):26–35.
6. Lipan MJ, Reidenberg JS, Laitman JT. Anatomy of reflux: a growing health problem affecting structures of the head and neck. Anat Rec Part B: New Anatomist. 2006;289(6):261–70.
7. Hyun JJ, Bak Y-T. Clinical significance of hiatal hernia. Gut Liver. 2011;5(3):267.
8. Patti MG, Goldberg HI, Arcerito M, Bortolasi L, Tong J, Way LW. Hiatal hernia size affects lower esophageal sphincter function, esophageal acid exposure, and the degree of mucosal injury. Am J Surg. 1996;171(1):182–6.
9. Golas A, El-Attrache B-FM, Jorge J, Dietrick J, Gonzalvo JP, Murr MM. Repair of post–bariatric surgery, recurrent, and de novo hiatal hernias improves bloating, abdominal pain, regurgitation, and food intolerance. Surg Obes Relat Dis. 2021;17(4):683–91.
10. Boru CE, Greco F, Giustacchini P, Raffaelli M, Silecchia G. Short-term outcomes of sleeve gastrectomy conversion to RY gastric bypass: multi-center retrospective study. Langenbeck's Arch Surg. 2018;403:473–9.
11. D'Urso A, Vix M, Perretta S, Ignat M, Scheer L, Mutter D. Indications and long-term outcomes of conversion of sleeve gastrectomy to Roux-en-Y gastric bypass. Obes Surg. 2021;31(8):3410–8.
12. Carandina S, Soprani A, Montana L, Murcia S, Valenti A, Danan M, et al. Conversion of sleeve gastrectomy to Roux-en-Y gastric bypass in patients with gastroesophageal reflux disease: results of a multicenter study. Surg Obes Relat Dis. 2020;16(6):732–7.
13. Altieri MS, Pryor AD. Gastroesophageal reflux disease after bariatric procedures. Surg Clin. 2015;95(3):579–91.
14. Huynh D, Mazer L, Tung R, Cunneen S, Shouhed D, Burch M. Conversion of laparoscopic sleeve gastrectomy to Roux-en-Y gastric bypass: patterns predicting persistent symptoms after revision. Surg Obes Relat Dis. 2021;17(10):1681–8.
15. Parmar CD, Mahawar KK, Boyle M, Schroeder N, Balupuri S, Small PK. Conversion of sleeve gastrectomy to Roux-en-Y gastric bypass is effective for gastro-oesophageal reflux disease but not for further weight loss. Obes Surg. 2017;27:1651–8.

16. Gao X, Dai S, Wang G, Li W, Song Z, Su Z, et al. Large versus small gastric pouch for Roux-en-Y gastric bypass in individuals with type 2 diabetes and a body mass index < 35 kg/m$^2$: six-year outcomes. Front Endocrinol. 2022;13:913062.
17. Riccioppo D, Santo MA, Rocha M, Buchpiguel CA, Diniz MA, Pajecki D, et al. Small-volume, fast-emptying gastric pouch leads to better long-term weight loss and food tolerance after Roux-en-Y gastric bypass. Obes Surg. 2018;28:693–701.
18. Agnihotri A, Barola S, Hill C, Neto MG, Campos J, Singh VK, et al. An algorithmic approach to the management of gastric stenosis following laparoscopic sleeve gastrectomy. Obes Surg. 2017;27:2628–36.
19. Hamed H, Elghadban H, Ezzat H, Attia M, Sanad A, El Sorogy M. Gastric stenosis after sleeve gastrectomy: an algorithm for management. Obes Surg. 2020;30:4785–93.
20. Manos T, Nedelcu M, Cotirlet A, Eddbali I, Gagner M, Noel P. How to treat stenosis after sleeve gastrectomy? Surg Obes Relat Dis. 2017;13(2):150–4.
21. Saber AA, Shoar S, Khoursheed M. Intra-thoracic sleeve migration (ITSM): an underreported phenomenon after laparoscopic sleeve gastrectomy. Obes Surg. 2017;27:1917–23.
22. Termine P, Boru CE, Iossa A, Ciccioriccio MC, Campanelli M, Bianciardi E, et al. Transhiatal migration after laparoscopic sleeve gastrectomy: myth or reality? A multicenter, retrospective study on the incidence and clinical impact. Obes Surg. 2021;31:3419–26.
23. Rebecchi F, Ugliono E, Morino M. Reflux following bariatric surgery. Mini-Invasive Surg. 2022;6:30.
24. Fisher OM, Chan DL, Talbot ML, Ramos A, Bashir A, Herrera MF, et al. Barrett's oesophagus and bariatric/metabolic surgery—IFSO 2020 position statement. Obes Surg. 2021;31(3):915–34.
25. Sans A, Frey S, De Montrichard M, Takoudju C, Coron E, Blanchard C. Impact on sleeve gastrectomy in patients with esophageal motor disorder. Surg Obes Relat Dis. 2021;17(11):1890–6.
26. Naik RD, Choksi YA, Vaezi MF. Impact of weight loss surgery on esophageal physiology. Gastroenterol Hepatol. 2015;11(12):801.
27. Broderick RC, Smith CD, Cheverie JN, Omelanczuk P, Lee AM, Dominguez-Profeta R, et al. Magnetic sphincter augmentation: a viable rescue therapy for symptomatic reflux following bariatric surgery. Surg Endosc. 2020;34:3211–5.
28. Reddy NC, Sujka J, DuCoin C. Magnetic sphincter augmentation algorithm for post-bariatric surgery gastroesophageal reflux disease patients. Obes Surg. 2022;32(9):3185–7.
29. Hawasli A, Sadoun M, Meguid A, Dean M, Sahly M, Hawasli B. Laparoscopic placement of the LINX® system in management of severe reflux after sleeve gastrectomy. Am J Surg. 2019;217(3):496–9.
30. Desart K, Rossidis G, Michel M, Lux T, Ben-David K. Gastroesophageal reflux management with the LINX® system for gastroesophageal reflux disease following laparoscopic sleeve gastrectomy. J Gastrointest Surg. 2015;19:1782–6.
31. Rrezza E, Ikramuddin S, Gourash W, Rakitt T, Kingston A, Luketich J, et al. Symptomatic improvement in gastroesophageal reflux disease (GERD) following laparoscopic Roux-en-Y gastric bypass. Surg Endosc. 2002;16:1027–31.
32. Peterli R, Wölnerhanssen BK, Peters T, Vetter D, Kröll D, Borbély Y, et al. Effect of laparoscopic sleeve gastrectomy vs laparoscopic Roux-en-Y gastric bypass on weight loss in patients with morbid obesity: the SM-BOSS randomized clinical trial. JAMA. 2018;319(3):255–65.
33. Ehlers AP, Thumma JR, Finks JF, Carlin AM, Ghaferi AA, Varban OA. Evaluation of patient reported gastroesophageal reflux severity at baseline and at 1-year after bariatric surgery. Ann Surg. 2022;275(6):1143–8.
34. Ghanem OM, Ghazi R, Abdul Razzak F, Bazerbachi F, Ravi K, Khaitan L, et al. Turnkey algorithmic approach for the evaluation of gastroesophageal reflux disease after bariatric surgery. Gastroenterology. Report. 2023;11:goad028.
35. Del Gobbo GD, Kroh M. Reflux after gastric bypass: Roux en-Y and one-anastomosis gastric bypass. In: The SAGES manual of physiologic evaluation of foregut diseases; 2023. p. 573–90. https://doi.org/10.1007/978-3-031-39199-6_42.

36. Sweigert PJ, Bakhos F, Marcotte E, Chand B. Revisional bariatric surgery for management of late complications. In: The ASMBS textbook of bariatric surgery; 2020. p. 309–20.
37. Okazaki O, Bernardo WM, Brunaldi VO, Junior CCDC, Minata MK, de Moura DT, et al. Efficacy and safety of stents in the treatment of fistula after bariatric surgery: a systematic review and meta-analysis. Obes Surg. 2018;28:1788–96.
38. Pauli EM, Beshir H, Mathew A. Gastrogastric fistulae following gastric bypass surgery—clinical recognition and treatment. Curr Gastroenterol Rep. 2014;16:1–8.
39. Keleidari B, Mahmoudieh M, Davarpanah Jazi AH, Melali H, Nasr Esfahani F, Minakari M, et al. Comparison of the bile reflux frequency in one anastomosis gastric bypass and Roux-en-Y gastric bypass: a cohort study. Obes Surg. 2019;29:1721–5.
40. Eldredge TA, Bills M, Ting YY, Dimitri M, Watson MM, Harris MC, et al. Once in a bile—the incidence of bile reflux post-bariatric surgery. Obes Surg. 2022;32(5):1428–38.
41. Swartz DE, Mobley E, Felix EL. Bile reflux after Roux-en-Y gastric bypass: an unrecognized cause of postoperative pain. Surg Obes Relat Dis. 2009;5(1):27–30.
42. Boules M, Chang J, Haskins IN, Sharma G, Froylich D, El-Hayek K, et al. Endoscopic management of post-bariatric surgery complications. World J Gastrointest Endosc. 2016;8(17):591.
43. Brethauer SA, Kothari S, Sudan R, Williams B, English WJ, Brengman M, et al. Systematic review on reoperative bariatric surgery: American society for metabolic and bariatric surgery revision task force. Surg Obes Relat Dis. 2014;10(5):952–72.
44. de Moura EG, Orso IR, Aurélio EF, de Moura ET, de Moura DT, Santo MA. Factors associated with complications or failure of endoscopic balloon dilation of anastomotic stricture secondary to Roux-en-Y gastric bypass surgery. Surg Obes Relat Dis. 2016;12(3):582–6.
45. Rosenthal RJ. Dilating the stenotic gastrojejunostomy after laparoscopic Roux-en-Y gastric bypass for morbid obesity: when things go wrong. J Gastrointest Surg. 2009;13:1561–3.
46. Iannelli A, Schneck A-S, Hébuterne X, Gugenheim J. Gastric pouch resizing for Roux-en-Y gastric bypass failure in patients with a dilated pouch. Surg Obes Relat Dis. 2013;9(2):260–7.
47. Suter M. Gastroesophageal reflux disease, obesity, and Roux-en-Y gastric bypass: complex relationship—a narrative review. Obes Surg. 2020;30(8):3178–87.
48. Mikami D, Needleman B, Narula V, Durant J, Melvin WS. Natural orifice surgery: initial US experience utilizing the StomaphyX TM device to reduce gastric pouches after Roux-en-Y gastric bypass. Surg Endosc. 2010;24:223–8.
49. Al-Bader I, Khoursheed M, Al Sharaf K, Mouzannar DA, Ashraf A, Fingerhut A. Revisional laparoscopic gastric pouch resizing for inadequate weight loss after Roux-en-Y gastric bypass. Obes Surg. 2015;25:1103–8.
50. Okafor PN, Lien C, Bairdain S, Simonson DC, Halperin F, Vernon AH, et al. Effect of vagotomy during Roux-en-Y gastric bypass surgery on weight loss outcomes. Obes Res Clin Pract. 2015;9(3):274–80.
51. Salame M, Jawhar N, Belluzzi A, Al-Kordi M, Storm AC, Abu Dayyeh BK, et al. Marginal ulcers after Roux-en-Y gastric bypass: etiology, diagnosis, and management. J Clin Med. 2023;12(13):4336.
52. Kuckelman JP, Phillips CJ, Derickson MJ, Faler BJ, Martin MJ. Esophageal magnetic sphincter augmentation as a novel approach to post-bariatric surgery gastroesophageal reflux disease. Obes Surg. 2018;28:3080–6.
53. Riva CG, Asti E, Lazzari V, Aquilino K, Siboni S, Bonavina L. Magnetic sphincter augmentation after gastric surgery. J Soc Laparoendosc Surg. 2019;23(4)

# Malnutrition: Incidence, Diagnosis, and Management

# 37

Joel Brockmeyer and Thomas O'Hara

Malnutrition is a relatively common complication following any metabolic or bariatric surgery, especially for patients who are not following appropriate postoperative supplementation and laboratory evaluation guidelines. The American Society of Metabolic and Bariatric Surgeons (ASMBS), Obesity Society, American Association of Clinical Endocrinologists, Obesity Medicine Association, and American Society of Anesthesiologists publish clinical practice guidelines for perioperative nutritional support for patients undergoing bariatric procedures [1]. At a minimum, all patients undergoing metabolic or bariatric procedures should undergo nutritional testing before surgery and have their nutritional status optimized by supplementation. The need for long-term nutritional monitoring is required for all procedures and support can be greater with a more extensive bypass of the small intestine. In this chapter, operative intraabdominal procedures will be reviewed along with individual deficiencies and their treatment.

## Preoperative Risk of Malnutrition

Patients with obesity are at risk for malnutrition prior to any metabolic or bariatric surgery interventions. Multiple studies have shown lower-than-normal levels of vitamin B12, folate, vitamin D, hemoglobin, and iron, but the severity and rate of deficiencies vary across these studies [2]. One study of 100 preoperative patients found six patients with iron deficiency, one with ferritin deficiency, one with folate

J. Brockmeyer (✉)
Department of Surgery, D.D. Eisenhower Army Medical Center, Ft. Eisenhower, GA, USA
e-mail: joel.r.brockmeyer.mil@health.mil

T. O'Hara
Department of General Surgery, D.D. Eisenhower Army Medical Center,
Ft. Eisenhower, GA, USA



O. M. Ghanem et al. (eds.), *The SAGES Manual of Metabolic and Bariatric Surgery*, https://doi.org/10.1007/978-3-031-72309-4_37

deficiency, six with thiamine deficiency, 22 patients with vitamin D deficiency, six patients with anemia, and no patients with vitamin B12 deficiency. Large portions of the patient population were found to have lower than recommended dietary intake of iron, calcium, folate, vitamin B1, and vitamin B12 preoperatively [3]. Another study of 169 patients found anemia in 4% of patients, iron deficiency in 5%, vitamin D deficiency in 74%, and vitamin B12 deficiency in 12%. Twenty two percentage of patients also had hyperparathyroidism [4]. While the rates of individual nutritional deficiencies can be low in preoperative bariatric surgery patients, it is important to evaluate for the presence of any malnutrition with preoperative laboratory analysis. Oral supplementation for any deficiencies should be started immediately upon diagnosis.

## Metabolic Surgeries

Surgeries such as sleeve gastrectomy (SG) and gastric banding (LAGB), have less risk of the development of malnutrition compared to those that incorporate intestinal bypass (Roux-en-Y gastric bypass (RYGB), one-anastomosis gastric bypass (OAGB), biliopancreatic diversion/duodenal switch (BPD/DS)) which can be considered hypoabsorptive. Several studies have been completed showing that SG patients have less risk of developing nutritional deficiencies when compared to RYGB patients [5]. However, with decreased oral intake, these patients are still at risk for the development of nutritional deficiencies. SG patients are predominantly at risk for the development of vitamin B12 deficiency, decreased ferritin, and decreased transferrin. These deficiencies may be present prior to surgery or can develop in patients postoperatively [6].

Following SG, nutritional supplementation is recommended and likely necessary to prevent vitamin deficiencies. The minimum recommendation from the ASMBS Clinical Practice Guidelines is a twice-daily adult multivitamin that contains iron, folic acid, and thiamine, calcium citrate with 1200–1500 mg of elemental calcium per day, 2000–3000 international units (IU) of vitamin D, and vitamin B12 supplementation. These recommendations are the same for patients with gastric banding, except only on a single daily adult multivitamin instead of two [1].

While LAGB and SG carry a lower overall risk of malnutrition and nutritional deficiencies, long-term follow-up with yearly nutritional labs should be completed. Minimum recommendations include yearly testing for a chemistry panel (SMA-21), complete blood counts (CBC), vitamin B12, and thiamine, especially if any signs of deficiency are present [1]. Table 36.1 shows many of the common nutritional deficiencies and commonly accepted normal levels. While LAGB and SG may have some risk of developing nutritional deficiencies, the risk can increase significantly with procedures with a hypoabsorptive component. The most performed hypoabsorptive procedure is the Roux-en-Y gastric bypass (RYGB). About 25% of all the bariatric procedures in 2021 were primary hypoabsorptive procedures, such as the RYGB or BPD-DS. The RYGB made up 88% of these primary procedures [7].

**Table 36.1** Vitamins and minerals commonly deficient after bariatric surgery [44]

| | Major site of absorption | Deficiency symptoms | Normal levels |
|---|---|---|---|
| Iron | Duodenum | Microcytic anemia, fatigue, pallor, glossitis, koilonychias | Serum Iron: 60–170 μg/dL<br>Ferritin: 20–335 μg/L |
| Vitamin B12 | Ileum | Megaloblastic anemia, fatigue, glossitis, paresthesias, ataxia | 200–900 ng/mL |
| Thiamine | Jejunum | Wet beriberi (cardiac insufficiency)<br>Dry beriberi (neuritis and neuropathy)<br>Wernicke-Korsakoff Syndrome (nystagmus, ataxia, mental status changes) | 2.5–7.5 μg/dL |
| Zinc | Duodenum | Rash, acne, hair loss, change in taste, immune deficiency | 60–130 μg/dL |
| Selenium | Duodenum | Anemia, fatigue, bone disease, mood disorders cardiomyopathy | 70–150 ng/mL |
| Copper | Duodenum | Hypochromic anemia, neutropenia, pancytopenia, hypopigmentation (skin, hair, nails) | 85–180 μg/dL |
| Calcium | Duodenum | Muscle cramps, tetany, neuromuscular hyperexcitability, osteomalacia, osteoporosis | 9.0–10.5 mg/dL |
| Vitamin D | Ileum | Osteomalacia, secondary hyperparathyroidism | 25-OH Vitamin D: 25–40 ng/mL |
| Vitamin K | Ileum | Increased bleeding | 0.2–3.2 ng/mL |
| Vitamin A | Ileum | Vision changes, endophthalmitis, poor wound healing | Plasma retinol: 20–80 μg/dL |
| Vitamin E | Ileum | Dry fragile hair, hair loss, hyporeflexia, gait disturbances, muscle weakness, decreased proprioception | Plasma alpha-tocopherol: 5.5–17 μg/mL |
| Protein | Ileum | Organ dysfunction (particularly liver and pancreas), edema. | Albumin: 3.5–5.0 g/dL |
| Vitamin B9 (folate) | Throughout small intestine, mostly jejunum | Megaloblastic anemia, glossitis, changes in skin pigmentation | 2–20 ng/mL |

RYGB increases the risk of nutritional deficiencies compared to SG. A meta-analysis evaluating anemia risk following either RYGB or SG found that RYGB patients had a higher risk of vitamin B12 deficiency but found no difference in iron or folate deficiencies [8]. However, another meta-analysis looking specifically for individual deficiencies found that RYGB patients had higher rates of decreased hemoglobin, iron, and vitamin B12. The study found no difference in folate deficiency or vitamin D deficiency, but RYGB patients had higher parathyroid hormone (PTH) levels [5].

When considering hypoabsorptive procedures, the risk for malnutrition increases as alimentary or Roux limb lengths increase. In a study evaluating Roux limb lengths of RYGB, one study found that Roux limb lengths of >250 cm were associated with an increased risk of deficiencies of vitamin D, vitamin A, vitamin B12, iron, and calcium. There was also a risk of zinc and selenium deficiency with lengthening Roux limbs [9]. Biliopancreatic diversion with duodenal switch (BPD/DS) further demonstrates the increased risk of malnutrition when the alimentary limb length is increased at the expense of the common channel length. Patients who underwent BPD/DS compared to RYGB are at increased risk of requiring inpatient care for nutritional deficiencies even though the risk of deficiencies between the two surgeries may not be statistically different. One study found equal amounts of iron deficiency and vitamin B12/folate deficiency in several thousand patients who underwent BPD/DS or RYGB [10]. In a study of 116 BPD/DS patients, nearly every patient was found to have vitamin D deficiency and osteoporosis was present in 41.4% of the patients despite patients reporting compliance with the recommended supplementation. These patients were also found to have a high rate of zinc, vitamin A, calcium, and vitamin B12 deficiency. While many of the patients had iron deficiency, only 13% had anemia. 34/116 required reoperation and 29.3% of those reoperations were for malnutrition [11]. This reinforces that nutritional deficiencies may require reoperations for revision of anatomy, usually lengthening common channels or in the case of the RYGB, reversal.

Oral supplementation of individual vitamins and minerals can resolve deficiencies. Vitamin D and B12 both improve significantly with oral supplementation. One study found that 74% of 169 preoperative patients had vitamin D deficiency. After RYGB, the percentage decreased to 56% with a daily multivitamin and no additional vitamin D or calcium [4]. Oral supplementation, in one study of 427 RYGB patients, was found to resolve vitamin D and B12 deficiencies in more than 80% of patients. Anemia also resolved in over 60% of the patients with additional oral iron supplementation [12]. In BPD/DS patients, another study found that very large amounts of nutritional supplementation could prevent most nutritional deficiencies in 65 patients followed for 5 years postoperatively. This supplementation regimen included an over-the-counter multivitamin twice daily, an additional daily proprietary multivitamin, a daily capsule of vitamin A, a daily ferrous fumarate, and a weekly capsule of vitamin D 50,000 international units (IU) [13]. In a long-term study of 490 RYGB patients for 12 years postoperatively, patients routinely taking their supplementation were compared to those not taking their supplementation. Seventy four percent of the patients were adherent. The supplementation in the study included an over-the-counter multivitamin twice daily, calcium with vitamin D daily, and vitamin B12 injections. Supplementation decreased the rate of vitamin D deficiency from 78% to 52%. Folate, vitamin B12, and vitamin B6 deficiencies without supplementation were 34%, 52%, and 52%, respectively, but the deficiencies decreased to 11%, 29%, and 17%, respectively, with supplementation [14]. While oral supplementation will not completely mitigate the risk of nutritional deficiencies after all surgeries, it is imperative that patients follow the current clinical practice guidelines as there is a significant risk of deficiencies without any supplementation.

The recently internationally accepted (OAGB) and single anastomosis duodenal interposition-sleeve (SADI-S) also carry the risk of nutritional deficiencies. The length of the common channel has been found to matter in determining the risk of these deficiencies. One study evaluating the evolution of the OAGB at a single institution found significant rates of iron and calcium deficiency over a 20-year period [15]. With the OAGB, as with the BPD/DS and RYGB, the length of the common channel was found to influence rates of nutritional deficiencies. In a meta-analysis comparing OAGB with biliopancreatic limb lengths of 150 vs 200 centimeters, longer biliopancreatic limb length was found to correlate with a significantly increased risk of ferritin and folate deficiency [16]. It is reasonable to assume that the OAGB and SADI-S will carry the risk of malnutrition and nutritional deficiency similar to RYGB and BPD/DS.

## Protein Malnutrition

Following bariatric surgeries, patients are at risk for protein malnutrition, particularly if they undergo a hypoabsorptive procedure [17]. This is secondary to poor protein digestion and absorption due to bypassed anatomy, with pancreatic and biliary function significantly altered postoperatively [17]. However, patients with procedures such as SG may also develop protein malnutrition, as a result of postoperative eating habits, such as avoidance of protein-rich food sources, failure to take protein supplements, or protracted vomiting [17, 18]. Aging, the amount of weight lost after surgery, and dumping syndrome can contribute to protein malnutrition [18]. Overall, protein deficiency is reported to be 13% in the postoperative bariatric population [18, 19]. The rates of malnutrition after LAGB or SG are low, ranging from 0 to 2% [20]. Conversely, the incidence is as high as 18–25% in patients who underwent RYGB or BPD/DS [18, 19]. The degree of malnutrition can be correlated to the length of the bypassed intestine [19]. Notably, there is a higher incidence in patients who undergo BPD/DS and in patients who undergo distalization procedures due to weight loss failure after index surgery [21, 22]. Patients with greater weight loss following surgery are also more likely to develop hypoalbuminemia [23]. Protein malnutrition is the most severe macronutrient complication seen after bariatric surgery and is associated with an annual hospitalization rate of 1% per year in the postoperative population, significant morbidity, and overall poor outcomes [17, 20].

The clinical signs of protein malnutrition are significant edema of the bilateral lower extremities, such that the patient may have notable weight regain, and hearing loss [17, 21]. Additionally, protein deficiency influences immune function, resulting in an insufficient barrier response leading to increased bacterial translocation into the bloodstream and reducing adaptive immunity. Protein malnutrition does not influence phagocytic activity, however [18].

Protein malnutrition is characterized by an albumin level of <3.5 g/dL that is not otherwise explained by hepatic failure, renal loss, or gastrointestinal loss [20]. Deficiency is stratified as mild (albumin between 3.0 and 3.5 g/dL), moderate (between 2.5 and 3/0 g/dL), and severe (<2.5 g/dL) [20]. Patients may demonstrate hypoalbuminemia immediately postoperatively during their initial weight loss, but this often normalizes within 3 months of surgery [23]. Prealbumin is another marker that can be used to evaluate protein malnutrition. It is particularly useful to assess acute malnutrition, as it has a half-life of 24–48 h [18]. However, prealbumin is an acute-phase reactant and may be misleading in the presence of inflammation or infection.

Prevention of protein malnutrition following bariatric surgery requires a daily protein intake of 60 to 120 grams of protein daily, or between 1.1 and 1.5 g/kg ideal body weight [17–19]. Between 10% and 35% of the patient's total energy intake should be provided by protein intake [19]. Patients who underwent BPD/DS require an additional 30% protein to meet their daily needs [17, 20]. An emphasis should be placed on regular weight training and aerobic exercise, for the purpose of preserving lean muscle mass [17]. Patients with mild hypoalbuminemia benefit from oral protein supplementation [20]. Collagen is gaining popularity as an oral protein source due to its rapid absorption in the intestinal tract and bioavailability [18]. Patients with severe disease, or without improvement with oral supplementation alone should be managed with modular protein supplements that are rich in branch-chain amino acids, with possible progression to 24-hour enteral feeding or parental nutrition, if they do not improve with oral supplementation [17, 20, 22].

## Vitamin B1 (Thiamine)

Thiamine is a water-soluble vitamin that plays an essential role as a cofactor in the metabolism of carbohydrates and branched-chain fatty acids [24]. Thiamine is absorbed throughout the intestine, primarily in the duodenum and the first portion of the jejunum, via carried-mediated active transport [17, 24]. Notably, thiamine plays a key role in glucose oxidation, which becomes pertinent in patients with acute thiamine deficiency [24]. Administration of intravenous glucose in a patient with an acute thiamine deficiency, without concomitant administration of parenteral thiamine, can further deplete thiamine stores and lead to lysis of neuronal cells [21, 24]. Given this concern, bariatric patients should never receive intravenous glucose without accompanying thiamine [25].

Thiamine deficiency is reported to be as high as 29% in patients preoperatively [26]. Incidence ranges from <1% to 49% postoperatively in the bariatric population, varying by type of surgery performed [17, 26]. Deficiency in the bariatric population occurs because of bypassing the primary sites of absorption, again the duodenum and proximal jejunum, or due to limited intake from persistent emesis [17, 21]. Risk of thiamine deficiency is increased in female patients, patients with postoperative protein malnutrition, noncompliance with postoperative multivitamins, patients with excessive and/or rapid weight loss, patients with excessive alcohol consumption, and patients with heart failure, particularly those treated with furosemide [25, 26]. Deficiency may occur secondary to small bowel bacterial overgrowth, as well [26].

Early symptoms of thiamine deficiency are nausea and constipation [17]. Patients may develop dry beriberi with brisk tendon reflexes, peripheral neuropathy, polyneuritis, paresthesia, muscle weakness, pain of extremities, gait ataxia, and convulsions, or wet beriberi with heart failure with high cardiac output, edema in the lower extremities, changes in heart rate, lactic acidosis, dyspnea, cardiac hypertrophy, dilation of the right ventricle, respiratory distress, systemic venous hypertension, and bounding arterial pulsations [26]. Gastroenterological symptoms are common, with nausea, emesis, slow gastric emptying, jejunal dilation, constipation, or megacolon possible [26]. Patients may progress to more advanced deficiency, which leads to neurologic complications and occurs in up to 4% of postoperative patients [21]. Advanced acute thiamine deficiency is known as Wernicke's encephalopathy, characterized by polyneuropathy, ataxia, ocular changes such as nystagmus or ophthalmoplegia, and short-term memory loss [21, 26]. The classic triad for Wernicke's includes confusion, ataxia and ophthalmoplegia, but this presentation is infrequent [21, 25]. Chronic severe thiamine deficiency, known as Korsakoff syndrome, includes psychosis and hallucinations [26].

The normal laboratory range of plasma thiamine is 4–15 nmol/L, and the whole blood or erythrocyte thiamine range is 2.5–7.5 μg/dL (74–222 nmol/L). Erythrocytes contain 80–90% of total thiamine, in the form of thiamine diphosphate (TDP). TDP, the biologically active form of thiamine, is not found in measurable concentrations in plasma and is best determined with whole blood specimens. The normal range for TDP is 70–180 nmol/L [26]. Additional laboratory values then can be used for diagnosing thiamine deficiency include transketolase (normal is >150 nmol/L), erythrocyte transketolase activity (ETKA)/activity coefficient (normal is <1.15), and urinary thiamine. Values indicative of thiamine deficiency include TDP <70 nmol/L, transketolase <120 nmol/L, ETKA/activity coefficient >12.5, or urinary thiamine <40 μg [26]. In patients with evidence of encephalopathy, MRI findings are inconsistent and, therefore, unreliable for diagnosis [25].

Given the high incidence of preoperative thiamine deficiency in patients seeking bariatric surgery, routine preoperative thiamine screening is recommended for all patients [26]. Postoperatively, routine screening is recommended for all patients with risk factors for thiamine deficiency, such as female sex, not attending postoperative nutritional clinics, cardiac failure, or persistent gastrointestinal symptoms. If symptoms of, or risk factors for, thiamine deficiency are present, thiamine status should be assessed within the first six months postoperatively, then every three to six months until symptoms resolve [26].

Routine thiamine supplementation above the recommended daily amount is recommended postoperatively for bariatric patients to prevent deficiency. All patients should take at least 12 mg of thiamine daily, and preferably a B-complex vitamin once or twice daily that includes 50 mg of thiamine [26].

In patients with suspected thiamine deficiency, the recommended dose and route of therapy are based on the severity of patient symptoms [26]. Given the difficulty with confirmatory testing for thiamine deficiency, all patients with suspected deficiency should be empirically treated based on their symptoms [25, 26]. For mild deficiency, oral thiamine 100mg two or three times per day is recommended, until symptoms resolve. For more advanced diseases, doses of intravenous thiamine from 200mg three times daily up to 500mg once or twice daily, are given for 3–5 days, followed by 250 mg per day for three to five days or until symptoms resolve [26]. Intravenous therapy is followed by 100 mg oral thiamine indefinitely, or until risk factors for deficiency have resolved. Intramuscular thiamine may be considered, dosed as 250 mg daily for 3–5 days, or 100–250 mg monthly. Simultaneous administration of magnesium, potassium and phosphorus should be considered for patients at risk for refeeding syndrome [26].

## Vitamin B9 (Folic Acid)

Folate is a water-soluble vitamin that plays a key role in cellular division and replication of DNA. It is primarily obtained via dietary intake, mostly from leafy green vegetables such as kale or spinach, as well as the liver. Folate may also be produced by colonic microbiota [18]. Folate is primarily absorbed throughout the small intestine [17].

Folate deficiency is reported to be as high as 54% in all patients with obesity [26]. The incidence of folate deficiency after bariatric surgery ranges from 9% to 65% [17, 26]. Patients with a preoperative deficiency are particularly at risk for a deficiency postoperatively [12]. Deficiency is primarily driven by poor dietary intake and non-adherence to postoperative multivitamins, rather than malabsorption [17, 26]. Folate deficiency may be exacerbated by vitamin B12 deficiency, as B12 is necessary for the conversion of inactive methyltetrahydrofolic acid to active tetrahydrofolic acid [17].

Folate deficiency primarily affects fast-replicating tissues, such as the skin and bone marrow [18, 26]. Common findings of folate deficiency include changes in skin pigmentation, skin ulceration, glossitis, and megaloblastic anemia [17, 18, 26]. Symptoms of anemia include fatigue, pallor, and dyspnea on exertion, though mild anemia may be asymptomatic [17]. Anemia may lead to impaired circulation, ultimately leading to delayed tissue healing. [18] Deficiency in pregnant patients may cause fetal neural tube defects [17, 18].

The normal red blood cell folate range is 340–1020 nmol/mL for patients 18 years or older. Values <305 nmol/mL are consistent with folate deficiency, and values below 227 nmol/mL are consistent with anemia. Serum values will range from 2 to 20 ng/mL [26]. Laboratory evaluation may demonstrate increased serum homocysteine and normal methylmalonic acid (MMA) levels [26].

Given the high incidence of preoperative folate deficiency in patients seeking bariatric surgery, routine preoperative folate screening is recommended for all patients. Routine screening is also recommended for all patients postoperatively, with particular attention given to females of childbearing age, given the risk of fetal neural tube defects [26].

Folate supplementation is recommended for all bariatric patients. Patients should receive 400–800 μg daily from their multivitamin [26]. Women of childbearing age should take a greater amount, 800–1000 μg daily [26]. Folate deficiency can generally be addressed with oral repletion alone [17, 18]. The recommended repletion dose is 1000 μg daily until folate levels have normalized, followed by resumption of the standard supplementation dose [26]. Folate supplementation above one mg daily is not recommended in bariatric patients due to the potential masking of vitamin B12 deficiency [26].

## Vitamin B12

Cobalamin or vitamin B12 is a water-soluble vitamin that serves as a cofactor for the enzymatic conversion of MMA to succinyl-CoA and for the conversion of homocysteine to methionine [18]. Its primary role is in cellular DNA synthesis [27]. It is found in different chemical forms in foods derived from animal sources such as eggs and dairy products [18]. The typical Western diet contributes 3–30 μg cobalamin daily [28].

Cobalamin is ingested in a protein-bound form [27]. Gastric acid and pepsin break down the bond between cobalamin and the animal carrier protein, releasing free cobalamin. Cobalamin binds to R-binder (also known as haptocorrin or transcobalamin I), a product of the salivary cells and the gastric parietal cells. The R-binder-cobalamin complex advances to the duodenum, where it is joined by additional R-binder-cobalamin complexes secreted in the bile. Both dietary and biliary complexes are broken down by pancreatic proteases, releasing free cobalamin [27, 28]. Free cobalamin binds to the intrinsic factor (IF) that has been produced by gastric parietal cells [27]. Though produced in the stomach, IF can only weakly bind to cobalamin in the presence of R-binder, until R-binder is broken down by the pancreatic proteases [28]. The cobalamin-IF complexes transit to the distal ileum undisturbed, where they attach to ileal enterocyte receptors and cobalamin is bound to transport proteins transcobalamin I, II, and III [27, 28]. 1–5% of cobalamin is absorbed in the small intestine independent of IF transport [19]. Cobalamin is subsequently transported systemically via the portal system, where the circulating R-binder attaches to 80% of available cobalamin, rendering it unavailable, while the remaining active fraction of cobalamin is bound to transcobalamin II [27, 28].

Prior to bariatric surgery, the incidence of vitamin B12 deficiency is noted to be between 2–18% of patients with obesity and 6–30% of patients on proton-pump inhibitors [26]. Deficiency is also associated with several drugs used to treat obesity-related comorbidities, including metformin, proton-pump inhibitors, angiotensin-converting enzyme inhibitors, and colchicine [29]. The use of acid-reducing medications decreases the ability for cobalamin to be released from its initial animal protein-cobalamin bond, preventing the formation of R-binder-cobalamin complexes [27]. Other causes of deficiency include congenital deficiencies of transcobalamin II or previous ileal resections [28]. The prevalence of B12 deficiency one year following bariatric surgery is 11%, but some studies demonstrate long-term rates as high as 70% [17, 27, 29]. Deficiency after bariatric surgery is typically associated with hypoabsorptive procedures, through multiple mechanisms. These include decreased secretion of intrinsic factors, limited gastric acidity, and bypassing of the duodenum [17, 27]. Inadequate dietary intake is a leading cause in postoperative bariatric patients. Notably, patients who develop postoperative intolerances to meat have notably lower B12 levels compared to those who do not [27].

B12 deficiency is classically associated with megaloblastic anemia [17, 26–28]. Other clinical manifestations include glossitis, numbness or paresthesia of the extremities, ataxia, changes in reflexes, lightheadedness or vertigo, tinnitus, and palpitations [26]. Patients may develop subacute degeneration of the spinal cord, and if not treated promptly, may develop spastic paresis and loss of proprioception and fine touch [27]. Advanced signs and symptoms of B12 deficiency include angina, symptoms of congestive heart failure, and altered mental status, ranging from mild forgetfulness to frank psychosis [26].

The normal range of serum B12 is 200–900 pg/mL, with a serum B12 of <200 pg/mL indicating deficiency. However, serum vitamin B12 levels alone may not be adequate to identify a B12 deficiency [26]. Serum MMA is recommended for any patient with suspected B12 deficiency, as an elevated MMA level may be a reliable indicator of B12 deficiency because it indicates a metabolic change that is highly specific to this deficiency. A serum MMA >0.376 μmol/L is indicative of B12 deficiency. Increased serum homocysteine may also be used, with levels >13.2 μmol/L indicative of B12 deficiency [26].

Preoperative screening for vitamin B12 deficiency is recommended for all patients planning to undergo bariatric surgery. Postoperatively, screening for B12 deficiency is recommended every three months for the first year, and then at least annually or as clinically indicated [26].

All postoperative bariatric patients should take B12 supplementation, and dosing varies based on the route of administration [26]. Oral dosing (whether disintegrating tablet, sublingual, or liquid) is 350–500 μg daily [19, 26]. Vitamin B12 nasal sprays are available and should be taken as directed by the manufacturer. Parenteral formulations are available for either subcutaneous or intramuscular administration, and these are administered in monthly doses of 1000 μg [26]. For patients with B12 deficiency, the traditional dosing for repletion was intramuscular B12 dosed at 1000 μg daily for 1 week, followed by 1000 μg weekly for 1 month [28]. Alternatively, patients can take 1000 μg of oral B12 until their B12 levels have normalized, which has been noted to be successful in up to 85% of patients [12, 26].

## Iron

Iron is a trace element that is essential for multiple cellular and enzymatic processes. Mostly notably, iron plays a key structural role in myocytes and erythrocytes, via the proteins myoglobin and hemoglobin, respectively. Ferritin serves as an iron storage protein, while transferrin acts as an iron transporter in plasma [30].

Iron is mainly absorbed in the duodenum and proximal jejunum. Iron can only be absorbed by the gastrointestinal tract in its ferrous form, $Fe^{2+}$, and transformation to this form occurs within the acidic environment of the stomach [18].

Iron deficiency is noted to be present in up to 45% of all patients with obesity [26]. This is attributed to the significant chronic inflammation associated with obesity [31]. The proinflammatory adipokine hepcidin is elevated in obesity due to chronic low-grade inflammation, which leads to decreased expression of ferroportin, an iron transporter that promotes iron absorption in the small bowel. This process leads to decreased iron absorption. Additionally, high levels of hepcidin inhibit the release of recycled iron from macrophages after phagocytosis, as well as prevent the mobilization of stored iron from hepatocytes [29]. Bariatric surgery improves this chronic inflammation, but iron deficiency remains prevalent postoperatively, albeit due to different mechanisms [31]. Iron deficiency is reported in up to 50% of patients postoperatively but varies by type of procedure [28]. Patients who undergo RYGB have reported rates of iron deficiency from 13% to 62% postoperatively [26]. Mechanisms for deficiency following bariatric surgery include decreased gastric acid secretion leading to less luminal $Fe^{2+}$, exclusion of the duodenum and proximal jejunum, and decreased dietary iron intake from iron-rich foods, such as red meat [17–19, 29, 30]. Proton-pump inhibitors have also been linked to iron deficiency in non-bariatric patients, secondary to suppression of gastric acid, which leads to decreased absorption of iron. This may also occur with $H_2$ blockers but has been noted to occur less frequently [31]. Patients with preoperative iron deficiency are significantly more likely to develop deficiency postoperatively, as well [12]. Additional risk factors are female sex, younger age, and greater degree of postoperative weight loss [19, 32].

The primary clinical manifestation associated with iron deficiency is microcytic anemia [26]. Symptoms include fatigue, dysphagia, palpitations, dyspnea on exertion, impaired learning ability, decreased work performance and gastrointestinal upset. Clinical signs include pallor, glossitis, koilonychias (spoon-shaped nails), vertical ridges on nails, and decreased immune function [17, 26].

Testing for iron status should include a panel of tests, to include a serum iron, transferrin, total iron binding capacity (TIBC) and ferritin. Ferritin levels alone should not be used to diagnose iron deficiency, because ferritin is an acute-phase reactant and may fluctuate with age, inflammation, and infection [26]. A complete blood count should be obtained to evaluate for microcytic anemia. Given the high incidence of iron deficiency in the population with obesity, preoperative screening is recommended for all patients. Postoperative screening is recommended within three months of surgery, every three to six months for the first postoperative year, and then annually. Postoperatively, patients should be closely monitored for signs or symptoms of iron deficiency [26].

Iron deficiency is broken down into five stages based on clinical and laboratory findings. The normal range of serum iron is 60–170 μg/dL, and levels below 50 μg/dL are consistent with iron deficiency [26]. Normal transferrin levels range from 200 to 360 μg/dL, and transferrin saturation ranges from 20% to 50%. The critical threshold for TIBC is <450 μg/dL [26]. Stage I deficiency is characterized as a serum ferritin decreased to 20 ng/mL. Stage II deficiency is defined as serum iron decreased to 50 μg/dL with an associated transferrin saturation <16%. Stage III has the presence of a normocytic anemia with normal appearing red blood cells, and microcytosis marks the progression to Stage IV deficiency. Stage V deficiency occurs when the deficiency reaches the end organs and slows clinical signs of deficiency [26].

All postoperative patients should receive iron supplementation, although deficiency may occur despite this precaution [26, 28]. Patients at low risk for iron deficiency, such as male patients without history of anemia, should receive at least 18 mg of iron from their multivitamin [26]. Menstruating female patients and those who have had a RYGB or a BPD/DS should take at least 45 to 60 mg of elemental iron daily cumulatively, between their multivitamin and additional iron supplements [26]. In patients with iron deficiency, oral supplementation should be increased to provide 150–200 mg elemental iron daily and can be increased up to 300 mg three times daily, if needed. Oral supplementation should be taken in divided doses, separate from calcium supplements, acid-reducing medications, and foods rich in phytates or polyphenols [26]. Notably, adherence to oral iron supplements is often low secondary to digestive intolerance. [28]. If the deficiency does not respond to oral therapy, intravenous iron infusions should be considered [26].

## Vitamin D and Calcium

Vitamin D is a fat-soluble vitamin that plays a key role in bone mineral homeostasis, as well as within the immunoregulatory response, where it can induce macrophages to synthesize antimicrobial peptides [18, 33]. Vitamin D levels are closely related to calcium levels, based on the mechanism of parathyroid hormone (PTH).

Vitamin D is primarily synthesized by the skin, through a process which requires ultraviolet rays [34]. A small amount of vitamin D is obtained from the diet, supplied by fortified dairy products and eggs [18, 34].

Calcium is absorbed through both active and passive mechanisms throughout the small intestine [35]. Active, transcellular transport occurs primarily in the duodenum and proximal jejunum, and is stimulated by 1,25-dihydroxyvitamin D, whereas passive paracellular absorption occurs through the length of the small bowel independently of vitamin D [35]. In RYGB patients, where the duodenum and proximal jejunum are bypassed, adaptation takes place via increased PTH secretion, leading to increased 1,25-dihydroxyvitamin D and more efficient calcium absorption [36]. However, this effect is lost in patients who have post-surgical hypoparathyroidism secondary to parathyroidectomy. Passive calcium absorption alone is typically insufficient to maintain appropriate calcium homeostasis [36].

Vitamin D deficiency is reported to be as high as 90% in patients with obesity [26]. Remarkably, the incidence is reported to be up to 100% postoperatively for bariatric patients in some literature [26]. Elevated PTH levels have been reported in up to 49% of patients preoperatively [37]. Causes of postoperative vitamin D deficiency include low sun exposure due to a sedentary lifestyle, pre-existing altered vitamin D metabolism, fat malabsorption due to bypass of duodenum and proximal jejunum, and bacterial overgrowth [34]. Calcium deficiency, on the other hand, has a much lower incidence, occurring in only 10% of patients. Calcium absorption is significantly affected by bypassing the duodenum and proximal jejunum and may be exacerbated if patients cannot tolerate dairy products after surgery [17].

Patients with vitamin D deficiency are often asymptomatic. When patients become symptomatic, it is often as a result of hypocalcemia, which leads to muscle cramps, tetany, and neuromuscular hyperexcitability [26]. Long-term effects include osteoporosis and osteomalacia, which can present with muscle weakness and bone pain. Patients may even develop immunosuppression [26, 38]. Patients with vitamin D deficiency are noted to have a higher percentage of respiratory tract infections, and bariatric patients with deficiency are noted to have a three times higher risk of nosocomial infections [18, 38]. Vitamin D deficiency has been demonstrated to have a negative effect on weight loss at two years postoperatively [38].

Given the high incidence of deficiency, all patients should be screened preoperatively for vitamin D and calcium deficiencies, as well as hyperparathyroidism, with special attention paid to peri- and post-menopausal women [26, 33]. Screening should include serum vitamin D, 25-hydroxylase vitamin D, alkaline phosphatase, PTH, and 24-hour urine calcium [26]. Serum calcium alone is not a reliable marker for deficiency, nor does it correlate to adequate calcium intake or absorption, because calcium balance is a complex relationship between gut absorption, bone resorption, and renal reabsorption [33]. 25-hydroxylase vitamin D is the preferred biochemical assay of vitamin D. In peri- and post-menopausal women, increase bone resorption can be evaluated via urinary and/or serum type I collagen N-telopeptide levels, which are high in patients with decreasing estrogen production. Postoperatively, all patients should be routinely screened for deficiency as well [26].

The normal range for serum calcium, in patients without renal disease, is 9.0–10.5 mg/dL. Calcium may be falsely decreased in patients with hypoalbuminemia; and in those instances, ionized calcium is a more reliable test. Vitamin D insufficiency is defined as vitamin D levels 20–30 ng/mL, and deficiency occurs when levels decrease below 20 ng/mL. Deficiency may be accompanied by decreased serum phosphorus, increased serum alkaline phosphatase, and decreased urinary calcium. Serum PTH >65 pg/mL is also indicative of hypocalcemia [26].

After bariatric surgery, all patients are recommended to take calcium and vitamin D supplements. For calcium, the recommended dose varies by procedure, with patients who undergo SG or RYGB taking 1200 –1500 mg per day, while patients who undergo BPD/DS receive 1800–2400 mg per day [26]. To enhance calcium absorption in bariatric patients, it is recommended that calcium be given in divided doses, with preference for calcium citrate. Calcium carbonate supplements must be taken with meals. Calcium citrate doses can be taken with or without meals [26]. The recommended supplemental dose of vitamin D depends on the patient's preoperative vitamin D status and the formulation used. The recommended vitamin D3 dose is 3000 IU daily, or until blood levels of 25-hydroxylase vitamin D levels are >30 ng/mL. Vitamin D3 is more frequently used, as the dosage of vitamin D3 needed, when compared to vitamin D2, is 70–90% lower to achieve a similar effect. However, both forms of vitamin D can be efficacious, despite differences in frequency and dosage [26].

Bariatric patients with hypocalcemia first need correction of any vitamin D deficiency, to achieve normalization of their calcium. All patients with vitamin D deficiency following weight loss surgery should be repleted with at least 3000 IU daily, but up to 6000 IU daily of oral vitamin D3 [26]. Alternatively, vitamin D deficiency can be treated with 50,000 IU vitamin D2, one to three times weekly. Calcium deficiency should be treated with similar doses as recommended for supplementation: taking 1200–1500 mg daily for SG and RYGB patients, and 1800–2400 mg daily for BPD/DS patients [26].

## Other Fat-Soluble Vitamins (Vitamins A, E, K)

Vitamins A, E, and K are essential, fat-soluble vitamins. Vitamin A promotes neoangiogenesis, enhances fibroblast activity and replication, increases production and deposition of collagen and expansion of the extracellular matrix, and controls neutrophil maturation [18]. Vitamin E plays an important role in gene expression and cell signaling and contributes to wound healing [18]. Vitamin K is a critical agent for the coagulation cascade, particularly for prothrombin, factors VII, IX, and X, and proteins C and S. Vitamin K contributes to bone mineralization and inhibition of vascular calcification [39].

Vitamin A cannot be synthesized in the human body and must be obtained through diet. It can be obtained through animal products such as eggs, dairy products, and fish liver oil, as well as fruits and vegetables [18]. Vitamin A is absorbed through the small intestine as either retinol (if from an animal-derived product) or carotene (if from a plant-based source). Once absorbed, it is converted to retinyl palmitate and hydrolyzed, bound to retinyl-binding protein and transported to peripheral tissues [40].

Vitamin E is also not produced by the human body and obtained through the diet. Vitamin E is found in plant-based products such as fresh vegetables, cereals, and nuts [18].

Vitamin K occurs in two natural forms, known as K1 and K2, and one synthetic form, known as K3 [39]. Vitamin K1, also known as phylloquinone, is the primary source of vitamin K in Western diets, and occurs in dark green leafy vegetables, such as kale, spinach, and broccoli. Vitamin K2, also known as menaquinone, is typically of microbial origin, and found in animal-based foods, such as dairy products and meats. The majority of vitamin K2 is synthesized by specific gut flora, with *Bacteroides* the most common bacteria implicated [39]. Dietary vitamin K is primarily absorbed in the jejunum and ileum, with very poor absorption occurring in the colon. This vitamin is dependent on bile and pancreatic enzymes for digestion prior to absorption. Once absorbed, vitamin K travels via chylomicrons to the liver and other target tissues [39].

The incidence of deficiency varies between the fat-soluble vitamins. Prior to surgery, 14% of patients may be deficient in vitamin A but only 2.2% are found to be deficient in vitamin E [26]. There is no data evaluating the rates of vitamin K deficiency in preoperative bariatric patients; however, vitamin K deficiency is extremely rare in general [26]. Vitamin A deficiency increases in prevalence postoperatively, with up to 70% of bariatric patients developing a deficiency [18, 26]. Vitamin E and vitamin K deficiency are very uncommon after bariatric surgery [26]. Deficiency of these vitamins after bariatric surgery is primarily caused by fat malabsorption, particularly in RYGB and BPD/DS, though bacterial overgrowth may contribute [39, 41]. Additional patients who may be at risk for vitamin K deficiency include those with liver disease and those on medications that may affect vitamin K metabolism, such as long-term antibiotics, bile acid sequestrants, and warfarin [39].

Vitamin A deficiency typically manifests with ophthalmologic symptoms [26]. Early symptoms include night blindness, Bitot's spots (foamy white spots on the sclera), endophthalmitis, and poor wound healing [17, 26]. Patients may additionally develop hyperkeratinized skin or loss of taste [26]. Advanced deficiency leads to corneal damage, xerosis, keratomalacia, corneal perforation and, ultimately, blindness [26, 42]. Vitamin A deficiency is associated with an increased infection rate, impaired metabolism in the bone, thyroid and pancreas, and increased rates of skin cancer [18]. Increased infection may be linked to impaired neutrophil maturation, as patients may have an increased neutrophil count but with diminished phagocytic activity. Natural killer cell function is also impaired with vitamin A deficiency [18].

Vitamin E deficiency is characterized by dry, fragile hair and hair loss [18]. Patients may also develop paresthesias in their extremities, hyporeflexia, gait disturbances, muscle weakness, and diminished proprioception and sense of vibration. In advanced deficiency, patients may develop hemolytic anemia, ophthalmoplegia, nystagmus or night blindness [26].

Vitamin K deficiency most commonly presents with bleeding complications. Typical signs are mucosal bleeding, easy bruising, delayed blood clotting, heavy menstruation, nose bleeds, and spontaneous internal bleeding [26, 39].

All patients are recommended to be screened for fat-soluble vitamin deficiency prior to bariatric surgery [26]. Vitamin A should be measured in all patients within the first postoperative year, and then routinely in patients who underwent a hypoabsorptive procedure. Given the rarity of postoperative vitamin E or vitamin K deficiency, only symptomatic patients should be screened for deficiency following surgery [26].

Vitamin A levels are best tested via plasma retinol, with a normal range of 20 to 80 μg/dL. Retinol <10 μg/dL is considered deficiency [26]. Retinol binding protein may also provide insight into vitamin A levels. Vitamin E levels are assessed via plasma alpha-tocopherol. Ranges may vary, but an alpha-tocopherol levels <5 μg/mL is generally considered criteria for vitamin E deficiency [26]. Plasma lipid levels may also be considered during workup for vitamin E deficiency. Vitamin K deficiency is typically assessed using prothrombin; however, it is not a very specific marker for vitamin K and may be altered for a variety of other reasons [26].

Postoperative supplementation of the fat-soluble vitamins is typically dosed based on the procedure the patient underwent. LAGB patients are recommended to take 5,000 IU daily of vitamin A and 90–120 μg daily of vitamin K [26]. SG and RYGB patients are recommended to take 5,000–10,000 IU daily of vitamin A and

90 to 120 µg daily of vitamin K [26]. BPD/DS patients are recommended to take 10,000 IU daily of vitamin A and 300 µg daily of vitamin K [26]. Notably, a dose of 15 mg daily of vitamin E is recommended for all patients, regardless of procedure. Higher maintenance doses of any of these vitamins may be necessary in patients who had preoperative deficiencies, and special attention should be paid to vitamin A and vitamin K in pregnant females [26].

Recommended doses for repletion of fat-soluble vitamin deficiencies in bariatric patients vary by clinical presentation. For vitamin A deficiency, patients must be evaluated for corneal changes. Patients without corneal changes are treated with 10,000–25,000 IU daily of oral vitamin A until clinical improvement, which typically occurs in 1–2 weeks [26]. Patients who have corneal changes receive a higher dose of 50,000–100,000 IU daily as an intramuscular injection for three days, followed by 50,000 IU daily for one week. Patients with vitamin A deficiency should also be evaluated for concurrent iron and copper deficiencies, as these mineral deficiencies may impair resolution of vitamin A deficiency [26]. For vitamin E deficiency, there is not a clearly defined therapeutic dosage for bariatric patients. However, there is a potential antioxidant effect when taking vitamin E supplements of 100–400 IU daily, and this is a dose that is higher than a standard multivitamin contains [26]. Patients with vitamin K deficiency are treated based on the chronicity of their malabsorption. With acute malabsorption, patients are treated with a parental dose of 10mg vitamin K. For chronic malabsorption, the recommended regimen is one to two mg daily of oral vitamin K or one to two mg per week parenterally [26].

## Zinc

Zinc is a trace mineral that has multiple functions for the immune system and wound healing. It is important for collagen production, fibroblast proliferation and proliferation of lymphocytes [18]. Zinc has antioxidant and antiatherogenic properties, related to its stimulation of apoptosis resistance and production of acute response proteins and metalloproteases. Zinc is abundant in seafood and red meats [18]. It is primarily absorbed in the duodenum and proximal jejunum [26].

Up to 24% and 50% of all patients seeking bariatric surgery have preoperative zinc deficiencies, and that increases to 74% of patients seeking BPD/DS [18, 26]. Postoperatively, 35% of patients are noted to have zinc deficiency, but again, BPD/DS patients have a significantly higher incidence of 70% [18, 26].

Early zinc deficiency presents with rashes, acne, changes in or absence of taste, immune deficiency with increased infections, infertility, growth retardation and delayed sexual maturation. Signs of advanced disease include hypogonadism, alopecia, bullous pustular dermatitis, acrodermatitis enteropathica, diarrhea, anorexia, and night blindness [26]. The increased risk of infection is linked to decreased cellular and humoral immunity. Specifically, zinc deficiency is associated with decreased natural killer cell activity, decreased lymphocyte proliferation, and decreased IL-2 production [18]. Patients may have impaired wound healing due to reduction in fibroblast proliferation and collagen production.

Preoperative screening for zinc deficiency is recommended for all patients undergoing RYGB or BPD/DS, as these procedures have the greatest risk of postoperative deficiency. These same patients should also be screened for deficiency yearly following surgery [26]. Serum and plasma zinc are the most appropriate biomarkers to obtain. Zinc assays should be interpreted with the knowledge that patients with obesity have lower zinc levels and lower plasma concentrations of zinc compared to leaner patients. Normal plasma zinc ranges from 60 to 130 μg/dL. Deficiency is associated with zinc levels <70 μg/dL [26].

All post-bariatric patients should have zinc supplementation. For patients who received SG, LAGB, or RYGB, the recommendation is 8–22 mg daily, which increases to 16–22 mg for BPD/DS patients [26]. There is not a standard zinc repletion dose for postoperative bariatric patients. However, copper and zinc deficiencies may coexist, copper should be supplemented with 1 mg copper per eight to 15 mg of elemental zinc [26].

## Copper

Copper is a trace element that plays multiple keys roles within the body. Some of these roles include melanin synthesis, ATP synthesis, electron transport, conversion of dopamine to norepinephrine, iron oxidation, free radical scavenging and many more. In the body, it is found primarily in the liver [43].

Most dietary copper is absorbed throughout the small intestine, though some is absorbed in the stomach. The acidic environment of the stomach causes copper to release from food complexes, allowing for absorption of copper in the duodenum. As intestinal pH increases, the proportion of available copper that is absorbed decreases, which leads to decreased rates of copper absorption in the distal small bowel. Copper crosses the intestinal apical membrane via copper transporter Ctr1, which is an active process. Passive diffusion does also occur, particularly with high amounts of copper ingestion. Copper is then stored inside the enterocyte by combining with metallothionein, an intracellular cytoplasmic protein, until it interacts with copper-transporting ATPase and is placed into systemic circulation via the portal system and eventually undergoes enterohepatic recycling [43].

The preoperative incidence of copper deficiency is as high as 70% in female patients desiring BPD/DS. Postoperatively, that figure increases up to as much as 90% of patients who undergo BPD/DS [26]. RYGB patients can develop copper deficiency at a rate of 10–20% [26]. Deficiency associated with bariatric surgery is typically because of decreased intestinal absorption, which is caused by bypassing of the proximal small bowel, decreased acidic environment, and reduced dietary copper intake [43].

Early signs of copper deficiency include hypochromic anemia, neutropenia, and pancytopenia [26, 43]. Additional signs include hypopigmentation of the hair, skin and nails, hypercholesterolemia, and impaired bone metabolism [26]. Advanced deficiency presents with neurologic dysfunction, with peripheral neuropathy, encephalopathy, and central nervous system demyelination. Neurological symptoms typically do not present until many years of deficiency. Slow and subclinical deficiency likely occurs well before symptoms become apparent [43].

Patients planning to undergo BPD/DS should be evaluated for copper deficiency in the preoperative period, given the high incidence of deficiency both preoperatively and postoperatively in this population [26]. Postoperatively, patients with intestinal bypass procedures should be screened at least annually. Both serum or plasma copper and ceruloplasmin, a copper transport protein, can be used to evaluate for copper deficiency. It should be noted that both copper and ceruloplasmin are acute-phase reactants and may be affected by age, anemia, inflammation, and infection [26]. The normal serum range for copper is 11.8–22.8 mmol/L, and the normal range for ceruloplasmin is 75–145 μg/dL. Deficiency is noted as serum copper <10 mmol/L or ceruloplasmin <75 μg/dL [26].

All bariatric patients should receive copper supplementation postoperatively. Patients with adjustable gastric band or sleeve gastrectomy should receive at least one mg daily of copper, and patients with intestinal bypass procedures should receive at least two mg daily. Patients with mild deficiency should be treated with three to eight mg daily of oral copper gluconate or copper sulfate until their serum levels return to normal. Severe deficiency should be addressed with two to four mg daily of intravenous copper for six days, or until serum levels return to normal and neurologic symptoms are resolved. Once serum copper levels have normalized, levels should be checked every three months to monitor for recurrent deficiency [26].

## Selenium

Selenium is a trace element that plays an important role in immune regulation. It contributes to muscle metabolism, thyroid function, protein synthesis and serves as an antioxidant. Selenium is a cofactor in multiple enzymatic processes, most notably antioxidant reactions such as glutathione peroxidase. Serving in this capacity, selenium blocks immunosuppression secondary to oxidative stress [18]. It is found in meat, fish, and cereals. Deficiency is uncommon but is reported to occur in approximately 3% of patients after bariatric surgery [18]. Selenium supplementation has been shown to improve both the adaptive and innate response, even in patients with optimal selenium levels. Supplementation with 100 mg daily has also been shown to lead to a lower wound infection rate [18].

## References

1. Mechanick J, Apoviam C, Brethauer S, et al. Clinical Practice Guidelines for the perioperative nutrition, metabolic, and nonsurgical support of patients undergoing bariatric procedures—2019 update. Surg Obes Rel Dis. 2020;16:175–247.

2. Argyrakopoulou G, Konstantinidou S, Dalamaga M, et al. Nutritional deficiencies before and after bariatric surgery: prevention and treatment. Curr Nutr Rep. 2022;11:95–101.
3. Dagan S, Zelber-Sagi S, Webb M, et al. Nutritional status prior to laparoscopic sleeve gastrectomy surgery. Obes Surg. 2016;26:2119–26.
4. Arias P, Domeniconi E, Garcia M, et al. Micronutrient deficiencies after Roux-en-Y gastric bypass: long-term results. Obes Surg. 2020;30:169–73. https://doi.org/10.1007/s11695-019-04167-x.
5. Gu L, Fu R, Chen P, et al. In terms of nutrition, the most suitable method for bariatric surgery: laparoscopic sleeve gastrectomy or Roux-en-Y gastric bypass? A systematic review and meta-analysis. Obes Surg. 2020;30:2003–14.
6. Antoniewicz A, Kalinowski P, Kotulecka K, et al. Nutritional deficiencies in patients after Roux-en-Y gastric bypass and sleeve gastrectomy during 12-month follow-up. Obes Surg. 2019;29:3277–84.
7. Estimate of Bariatric Surgery Numbers, 2011–2021. 2022. The ASMBS Website. https://asmbs.org/resources/estimate-of-bariatric-surgery-numbers. Accessed 01 Oct 2023.
8. Kwon Y, Ha J, et al. Comparative risk of anemia and related micronutrient deficiencies after Roux-en-Y gastric bypass and sleeve gastrectomy in patients with obesity: an updated meta-analysis of randomized controlled trials. Obes Rev. 2022;23:e13419. https://doi.org/10.1111/obr.13419.
9. van der Burg Y, Boerboom A, et al. Weight loss and malnutrition after conversion of the primary Roux-en-Y gastric bypass to distal gastric bypass in patients with morbid obesity. Surg Obes Relat Dis. 2020;16:381–8. https://doi.org/10.1016/j.soard.2019.12.009.
10. Skogar M, Sundbom M. Early complications, long-term adverse events, and quality of life after duodenal switch and gastric bypass in a matched national cohort. Surg Obes Relat Dis. 2020;16:614–9. https://doi.org/10.1016/j.soard.2020.02.001.
11. Süsstrunk J, Schneider R, et al. Long-term outcome after biliopancreatic diversion with duodenal switch: a single-center experience with up to 20 years follow-up. Surg Obes Relat Dis. 2023;19:83–90. https://doi.org/10.1016/j.soard.2022.10.020.
12. van der Beek E, Monpellier V, et al. Nutritional deficiencies in gastric bypass patients: incidence, time of occurrence, and implications for post-operative surveillance. Obes Surg. 2015;25:818–23. https://doi.org/10.1007/s11695-014-1456-y.
13. Joret M, Nanayakkara A, et al. Duodenal switch combined with systematic post-operative supplementation and regular patient follow-up results in good nutritional outcomes. Obes Surg. 2022;32:2226–36. https://doi.org/10.1007/s11695-022-06063-3.
14. Bjerkan K, Sandvik J, et al. Vitamin and mineral deficiency 12 years after Roux-en-Y gastric bypass, a cross-sectional multicenter study. Obes Surg. 2023;33:3178–85. https://doi.org/10.1007/s11695-023-06787-w.
15. Almuhanna M, Soong T, et al. Twenty years' experience of laparoscopic 1-anastomosis gastric bypass: surgical risk and long-term results. Surg Obes Relat Dis. 2021;17:968–75. https://doi.org/10.1016/j.soard.2021.01.010.
16. Salman M, Salman A, et al. One Anastomosis Gastric Bypass (OAGB) with a 150-cm Biliopancreatic Limb (BPL) versus a 200-cm BPL, a systematic review and meta-analysis. Obes Surg. 2023;33:1846–56. https://doi.org/10.1007/s11695-023-06556-9.
17. Lupoli R, Lembo E, et al. Bariatric surgery and long-term nutritional issues. World J Diabetes. 2017;8:464–74. https://doi.org/10.4239/wjd.v8.i11.464.
18. Toninello P, Montanari A, et al. Nutritional support for bariatric surgery patients: the skin beyond the fat. Nutrients. 2021;13:1565. https://doi.org/10.3390/nu13051565.
19. Handzlik-Orlik G, Holecki M, et al. Nutrition management of the post-bariatric surgery patient. Nutr Clin Pract. 2015;30:383–92. https://doi.org/10.1177/0884533614564995.
20. Kuin C, den Ouden F, et al. Treatment of severe protein malnutrition after bariatric surgery. Obes Surg. 2019;29:3095–102. https://doi.org/10.1007/s11695-019-04035-8.
21. Kassir R, Debs T, et al. Complications of bariatric surgery: presentation and emergency management. Int J Surg. 2016;27:77–81. https://doi.org/10.1016/j.ijsu.2016.01.067.

22. Ghiassi S, Higa K, et al. Conversion of standard Roux-en-Y gastric bypass to distal bypass for weight loss failure and metabolic syndrome: 3-year follow-up and evolution of technique to reduce nutritional complications. Surg Obes Relat Dis. 2018;14:554–61. https://doi.org/10.1016/j.soard.2018.01.004.
23. Shah M, Sharma A, et al. Hypocalcemia after bariatric surgery: prevalence and associated risk factors. Obes Surg. 2017;27:2905–11. https://doi.org/10.1007/s11695-017-2705-7.
24. Iannelli A, Addeo P, et al. Wernicke's encephalopathy after laparoscopic Roux-en-Y gastric bypass: a misdiagnosed complication. Obes Surg. 2010;20:1594–6. https://doi.org/10.1007/s11695-010-0116-0.
25. Nuzzo A, Czernichow S, et al. Prevention and treatment of nutritional complications after bariatric surgery. Lancet Gastroenterol Hepatol. 2021;6:238–51. https://doi.org/10.1016/S2468-1253(20)30331-9.
26. Parrott J, Frank L, et al. American Society for metabolic and bariatric surgery integrated health nutritional guidelines for the surgical weight loss patient 2016 update: micronutrients. Surg Obes Relat Dis. 2017;13:727–41. https://doi.org/10.1016/j.soard.2016.12.018.
27. Majumder S, Soriano J, et al. Vitamin B12 deficiency in patients undergoing bariatric surgery: preventive strategies and key recommendations. Surg Obes Relat Dis. 2013;9:1013–9. https://doi.org/10.1016/j.soard.2013.04.017.
28. Fernández-Bañares F, Monzón H, Forné M. A short review of malabsorption and anemia. World J Gastroenterol. 2009;15:4644–52. https://doi.org/10.3748/wjg.15.4644.
29. Deledda A, Pintus S, et al. Nutritional management in bariatric surgery patients. Int J Environ Res Public Health. 2021;18:12049. https://doi.org/10.3390/ijerph182212049.
30. Bjørklund G, Peana M, et al. Iron deficiency in obesity and after bariatric surgery. Biomol Ther. 2021;11:613. https://doi.org/10.3390/biom11050613.
31. Sharma N, Chau WY, Dobruskin L. Effect of long-term proton pump inhibitor therapy on hemoglobin and serum iron levels after sleeve gastrectomy. Surg Obes Relat Dis. 2019;15:1682–9. https://doi.org/10.1016/j.soard.2019.06.019.
32. Enani G, Bilgic E, et al. The incidence of iron deficiency anemia post-Roux-en-Y gastric bypass and sleeve gastrectomy: a systematic review. Surg Endosc. 2020;34:3002–10. https://doi.org/10.1007/s00464-019-07092-3.
33. Kim J, Brethauer S, et al. ASMBS Clinical Issues Committee: American Society for Metabolic and Bariatric Surgery Clinical Issues Committee, Position Statement. Metabolic bone changes after bariatric surgery. Surg Obes Relat Dis. 2015;11:406–11. https://doi.org/10.1016/j.soard.2014.03.010.
34. Chakhtoura M, Rahme M, El-Hajj Fuleihan G. Vitamin D metabolism in bariatric surgery. Endocrinol Metab Clin N Am. 2017;46:947–82. https://doi.org/10.1016/j.ecl.2017.07.006.
35. Balsa JA, Botella-Carretero JI, et al. Role of calcium malabsorption in the development of secondary hyperparathyroidism after biliopancreatic diversion. J Endocrinol Investig. 2008;31:845–50. https://doi.org/10.1007/BF03346429.
36. Zaarour M, Zaharia R, et al. Laparoscopic revision of bariatric surgeries in two patients with severe resistant hypocalcemia after endocrine cervical surgery. Obes Surg. 2020;30:1616–20. https://doi.org/10.1007/s11695-019-04132-8.
37. Kim J, Nimeri A, et al. American Society for Metabolic and Bariatric Surgery (ASMBS) Clinical Issues Committee. Metabolic bone changes after bariatric surgery: 2020 update, American Society for Metabolic and Bariatric Surgery Clinical Issues Committee position statement. Surg Obes Relat Dis. 2021;17:1–8. https://doi.org/10.1016/j.soard.2020.09.031.
38. Schaaf C, Gugenheim J. Impact of preoperative serum vitamin D level on postoperative complications and excess weight loss after gastric bypass. Obes Surg. 2017;27:1982–5. https://doi.org/10.1007/s11695-017-2600-2.
39. Sherf-Dagan S, Goldenshluger A, et al. Vitamin K-what is known regarding bariatric surgery patients: a systematic review. Surg Obes Relat Dis. 2019;15:1402–13. https://doi.org/10.1016/j.soard.2019.05.031.

40. Zalesin KC, Miller WM, et al. Vitamin A deficiency after gastric bypass surgery: an underreported postoperative complication. J Obes. 2011;2011:760695. https://doi.org/10.1155/2011/760695.
41. Machado JD, Campos CS, et al. Intestinal bacterial overgrowth after Roux-en-Y gastric bypass. Obes Surg. 2008;18:139–43. https://doi.org/10.1007/s11695-007-9365-y.
42. Silva ACF, Kazmarek LM, et al. Dermatological manifestations relating to nutritional deficiencies after bariatric surgery: case report and integrative literature review. Sao Paulo Med J. 2022;140:723–33. https://doi.org/10.1590/1516-3180.2021.0616.R1.17022022.
43. Btaiche IF, Yeh AY, et al. Neurologic dysfunction and pancytopenia secondary to acquired copper deficiency following duodenal switch: case report and review of the literature. Nutr Clin Pract. 2011;26:583–92. https://doi.org/10.1177/0884533611416127.
44. Brockmeyer J. Malnutrition. In: Lim R, Jones D, editors. Metabolic and bariatric surgery exam and board review. New York: McGraw Hill; 2023. p. 222–34.

# Part IV

# Weight Recurrence

# Weight Recurrence and Metabolic and Bariatric Surgery: Definition, Evaluation, and Implications

# 38

Karimatu Jalloh and Maria S. Altieri

## Introduction

Obesity persists as one of the most daunting health challenges of the twenty-first century, an enduring pandemic both in the United States and worldwide. The prevalence of obesity in the United States surged from 30.5% in 2000 to a staggering 42.4% in 2018 [1], mirroring a global trend [2–4]. The surge in obesity is not unique to one generation but spans across generations, marking a rapid escalation of the problem [4]. Projections based on National Health and Education Examination data estimated that by 2030, 86% of Americans would be overweight or obese, while the National Center for Health Statistics, in 2015, estimated that 72% of Americans were already overweight or obese [1].

In the quest to address this health crisis, bariatric surgery has emerged as the most effective method for weight loss and maintaining weight loss among overweight and obese individuals. The popularity of bariatric surgery is evidenced by the fact that over 600,000 surgeries are performed worldwide annually, with more than 256,000 performed in the United States in 2019 [5]. While this surgical approach has produced significant weight reduction in patients, especially by ameliorating weight-related comorbid conditions, some patients subsequently experience weight regain [1]. We define recurrence as gaining weight after initially achieving an expected weight loss through surgery. This phenomenon can develop gradually over time, leading to a return of obesity or a substantial increase in body weight, with or without the resurgence of health-related comorbidities that were initially alleviated or improved by surgical intervention [6].

Despite extensive efforts to address obesity, healthcare providers continue to witness the recurrence of the condition. The absence of a universally accepted standard

K. Jalloh · M. S. Altieri (✉)
Department of Surgery, University of Pennsylvania, Philadelphia, PA, USA
e-mail: Maria.Altieri@pennmedicine.upenn.edu



O. M. Ghanem et al. (eds.), *The SAGES Manual of Metabolic and Bariatric Surgery*, https://doi.org/10.1007/978-3-031-72309-4_38

definition for weight recurrence and a consensus on treatment guidelines exacerbates the issue. Establishing a standardized definition for weight recurrence (WR) is of paramount importance for understanding the phenomenon and devising effective treatment plans [1, 6, 7].

While a standard definition is lacking, there are several definitions for weight recurrence outlined in the literature. Examples of these definitions encompass criteria such as an increase of 10 kg from the nadir weight, an increase of 25% excess weight loss (EWL) from the nadir weight, an increase in body mass index (BMI) exceeding 5 $kg/m^2$ from the nadir weight, a return to a BMI of 35 $kg/m^2$, any weight gain after the remission of type 2 diabetes, any degree of weight recurrence, changes in weight from the nadir to 5 years postoperatively expressed as alterations in BMI or percent of total weight loss (%TWL), variations in percent excess BMI lost or %EWL, patients regaining over 10% of their lowest postoperative weight 2 years after a Roux-en-Y gastric bypass (RYGB), and, at 2 years following a sleeve gastrectomy (SG), and an increase in weight of 5 kg from the nadir weight [8–16]. These definitions vary in terms of when they assess weight recurrence, and the lack of a consensus definition remains a fundamental challenge in the development of treatment plans and research protocols.

## Risk Factors

Weight regain is multifactorial including patient-related factors, such as disordered eating habits and reduced physical activity; psychiatric-related factors; procedure-related factors; and hormonal adaptations. A systematic review published in 2021 showed that at least one in six patients had ≥10% weight regain following metabolic and bariatric surgery. The authors further identified several risk factors, which they placed into five categories: anatomical, genetic, dietary, psychiatric, and temporal. Other specific factors like gastrojejunal stoma diameter, gastric volume following sleeve, anxiety, time after surgery, emotional eating and increased sweet consumption, portion size, food urges, binge eating, loss of control/disinhibition when eating, and genetics have been positively associated with weight regain. On the contrary, postprandial GLP-1, eagerness to change physical activity habits, self-esteem, social support, fruit and zinc consumption, HDL, and quality of life have been negatively associated [17].

Abnormal eating behaviors are frequently reported by individuals who have undergone bariatric surgery. These behaviors include uncontrolled eating and repetitively consuming small amounts of food between regular mealtimes. Notably, research indicates that more than half of the patients who have received bariatric surgery had a history of binge eating before the procedure, and some transition to grazing or uncontrolled eating patterns after surgery [5, 18]. The prevalence of grazing behavior in post-bariatric surgery patients varies, with estimates ranging from 17% to 47%, depending on the assessment methods utilized [5, 19, 20]. Loss of control eating refers to situations where individuals find it challenging to resist or halt their eating, leading to unplanned eating episodes and difficulties in stopping. This behavior is often accompanied by subjective distress [20] and has been linked to unfavorable outcomes for individuals post-bariatric surgery, including the recurrence of weight gain [5]. These findings underscore the significance of addressing these abnormal eating behaviors in the post-bariatric surgery population to support better long-term success and weight maintenance. Other common risk factors contributing to weight recurrence include eating disorders, such as binge eating disorder, night eating syndrome, postsurgical eating avoidance disorder, and soft food syndrome. Non-compliance with dietary recommendations, a return to previous unhealthy eating habits, and a sedentary lifestyle also play significant roles [21, 22]. Additionally, psychiatric disorders such as depression, alcohol misuse, and the use of certain psychotropic and antidepressant medications have all been identified as factors influencing weight recurrence following bariatric surgery [5, 8, 15, 16, 22–27].

Procedure-related weight regain can be due to complications following metabolic and bariatric surgery, such as gastric band slippage, gastrogastric fistula formation, dilation of the gastric fundus, and enlargement of the gastric pouch [8, 23–30].

Furthermore, hormonal and metabolic imbalances are also known to influence weight recurrence. While decreased food intake due to upregulation of satiety hormones like pancreatic peptide YY, GLP, and GIP, and the downregulation of hunger-inducing ghrelin after anatomical exclusion of the foregut in bariatric surgery help in weight loss, these hormonal alterations diminish over time, causing WR [23, 27, 31–35]. Hypoglycemia due to the altered carbohydrate metabolism after bariatric surgery triggers inappropriate insulin surges to downregulate blood glucose levels. These irregularities heighten the hunger response a few hours after meals, resulting in weight recurrence in most patients [27, 36].

## Evaluation of Weight Recurrence

Since WR after MBS can be multifactorial, regular long-term follow-up and timely treatment by a multidisciplinary team is of the essence. As soon as WR is noticed, an office visit with the team is important in order to identify risk factors for WR. A multidisciplinary discussion between the surgeon, the registered dietitian, the psychologist, and the patient can provide clues on the causes of WR. This will help address any maladaptive lifestyle behaviors. In addition, contrast-based imaging studies such as an Upper Gastrointestinal series (UGI) and upper gastrointestinal endoscopy are necessary [37]. Depending on the causes of weight regain, an individualized plan can be created.

## Treatment Plans for Weight Recurrence

The issue of weight recurrence following bariatric surgery is multifaceted and influenced by various factors. To manage and address weight recurrence post-bariatric surgery, healthcare providers have established guidelines to emphasize the importance of follow-up appointments with a team of healthcare professionals, including surgeons, obesity medicine specialists, dietitians, and psychologists. Lifestyle modifications, dietary adjustments, and physical activity play a central role in weight management for post-bariatric surgery patients. In cases of moderate to rapid weight regain, interventions such as pharmacotherapy and surgical revisions may be considered [16, 35].

Following surgery, maladaptive lifestyle behaviors can be a contributing factor to weight recurrence, and it is of great importance that patients preparing for bariatric surgery understand the dietary behaviors that are paramount in achieving and maintaining an optimal weight. Patients need appropriate nutritional education, dietary behavior coaching, and lifelong follow-up with the bariatric multidisciplinary team to provide them with the knowledge, skill, and support they need to optimize their weight loss process [27, 38, 39].

Due to the alteration of the GI anatomy post-bariatric surgery, the reduced stomach capacity imposes limitations on the food choices and eating behaviors of the patients. Patients are advised to practice eating slowly, chewing thoroughly, avoiding larger volumes of food, and following specific food restrictions post-bariatric surgery. In order to avoid post-bariatric surgery dumping syndrome and hypoglycemia, patients are advised to refrain from consuming simple sugars. The established general dietary guidelines for patient's post-bariatric surgery include limiting portion size to one-half cup (125 g) per 30 min, selecting protein-rich and high-fiber-containing foods such as fish, poultry, eggs, lean meat, low-fat dairy, legumes, fruits, vegetables, and whole grains. Also, proper spacing of meals ranging from about 4 to 6 meals daily is necessary to help develop satiety and enhance food tolerance in patients post-bariatric surgery [21, 38–45]. Certain complications, such as reflux or vomiting can contribute to maladaptive behaviors and improper food choices, further contributing to weight recurrence.

Pharmacotherapeutic intervention post-bariatric surgery can be considered as an adjunct while correcting dietary and lifestyle behaviors. Studies have shown that pharmacotherapy can be effective in decreasing the progression of rapid weight recurrence. However, this intervention post-bariatric surgery is still limited, the reason being that there are no standard guidelines and recommendations on the use of anti-obesity medications (AOM) after bariatric surgery. Additionally, some bariatric surgery centers do not have obesity medicine specialists which limits the utilization of obesity medication as some bariatric surgeons may not be familiar with them [16, 39, 46].

## Anti-Obesity Medications

Currently, the United States Food and Drug Administration (FDA) has several approved anti-obesity medications (AOMs): phentermine/topiramate, naltrexone/bupropion, orlistat, and liraglutide. Phentermine is a sympathomimetic amine that increases the secretion of catecholamine in the hypothalamus and causes appetite suppression. It was approved in 1959 and has been utilized for the prevention of weight recurrence since as a single-agent treatment for obesity. Topiramate is a migraine and anti-epileptic medication that has been used with phentermine for the treatment of weight recurrence as studies have shown that the combination of these two drugs improved weight loss after bariatric surgery when the desired result was not achieved. This combination was FDA-approved in 2012 [46–51].

Liraglutide is an injectable GLP-1 agonist that was approved by the FDA as an anti-obesity medication. Prescribed at a dosage of 3.0 mg, Liraglutide can target appetite regulation between the peripheral and central nervous system (CNS) pathways. It is utilized post-bariatric surgery for patients who experience inadequate weight loss and weight recurrence as one of the effective interventions to prevent weight recurrence, although there is limited data suggesting that GLP-1 agonists can aid in preventing hypoglycemia post-bariatric surgery [52–56].

Orlistat is an FDA-approved lipase inhibitor that promotes the malabsorption of 25–30% of fat ingested from the GI tract. There is no data supporting evidence of orlistat being an effective treatment for weight recurrence. Orlistat is known to increase the risk of vitamin deficiencies after bariatric surgery, and hence cannot be considered for first-line management of weight recurrence [57].

Naltrexone SR/Bupropion SR is another FDA-approved medication combination of anti-obesity medication. Each medication is approved independently for the treatment of different disorders and each medication affects the CNS. Naltrexone as a single agent is FDA-approved for treating alcohol use disorder (AUD) and opioid use disorder while Bupropion is approved for smoking cessation and unipolar major depression. Due to its independent properties and its effect on the CNS, a synergistic effect has been hypothesized in humans based on animal studies conducted on the pro-opiomelanocorth receptor it shows that the effect induces satiety and blocks feedback inhibition. However, there is no data supporting evidence of the significance and impact of the combination of these two drugs in the treatment of weight recurrence post-bariatric surgery [51–53].

## Revisional Surgery

Another intervention utilized to treat and manage weight recurrence post-bariatric surgery is revisional surgery. Revisional surgery is used to repair anatomic abnormalities such as gastrogastric (GG) fistula when identified in endoscopy or upper GI tract, enlarged gastric pouch, and dilated stoma [58]. These abnormalities can be treated using either a minimally invasive or endoscopic approach resulting in improved short-term weight loss but inconsistent results in long-term weight loss. In laparoscopic procedures, gastrojejunal anastomosis is mostly taken down which results in the resizing of the gastric pouch. While this may help with WR in a short period, the long-term durability is yet to be confirmed. The complication rate of laparoscopic revisional surgical procedures in bariatric surgery has declined significantly. As a result, revisional surgery poses a lesser risk of improving weight loss than before [59, 60].

Even without the occurrence of anatomic abnormalities in primary bariatric surgery, procedures such as distalization of the jejunojejunostomy for a gastric bypass, vertical sleeve gastrectomy (VSG) conversion to a gastric bypass, and single anastomosis duodeno-ileal (SADI), bypass is done to increase the hypoabsorptive component of the initial procedure. In distal gastric bypass, the jejunojejunostomy is altered to either increase the length of the biliopancreatic limb or the alimentary limb with a shorter common channel. Even though weight loss has been achieved in revisional surgery using these procedures, there are still issues experienced by patients such as protein-calorie malnutrition and micronutrient deficiencies by 20% [61, 62].

In consideration of revisional surgery as a treatment option for weight recurrence, it is essential to identify whether the patient has acid reflux disease or is undergoing surgery due to weight recurrence alone. For patients who experience acid reflux disease following SG, gastric bypass is the most recommended intervention. The RYGB is a well-established option in bariatric surgery, known for its safety and effectiveness in both primary and revisional procedures [63, 64]. Importantly, it offers significant benefits for patients with gastroesophageal reflux disease (GERD) by bypassing much of the parietal cell mass of the stomach, making it the preferred choice to alleviate GERD symptoms.

Another option for patients with weight recurrence following LSG is conversion to a SADI bypass. The surgical complications and malnutrition rates associated with SADI-S are similar to those associated with gastric bypass, hence single SADI is another option for treating inadequate weight loss after VSG [62, 65].

## Outcomes

Revisional bariatric surgery is a complex procedure associated with a higher risk of postoperative complications compared to primary surgeries, with perioperative morbidity rates ranging from 19% to 50% [66–69]. However, recent advancements in laparoscopic surgical techniques and the expertise of well-trained bariatric surgeons have made laparoscopic revisions a safer option. Complication rates for laparoscopic revisions range from 14.3% to 46.3%, with conversions to laparotomy occurring at a rate of 3.0–27.8% [70–75].

As the number of bariatric procedures performed continues to rise, there's an increasing demand for revisional procedures. These revisions are necessary not only to address early surgical complications but also for reasons such as insufficient weight loss, weight recurrence, delayed implant-related issues, or intolerable side effects, often occurring months or years after the initial surgery. Revisional bariatric surgery constitutes 5–15% of all bariatric cases currently [66, 76, 77]. The revision rates vary among procedures, with 20–60% after laparoscopic adjustable gastric banding (LAGB) [78–83], 9–17% after RYGB [71, 78, 82, 84], and 9–11% after sleeve gastrectomy (SG) [85, 86]. Despite numerous studies on initial bariatric procedures for morbid obesity, research on the best choices for revisional surgery after a previous primary procedure remains limited. It is crucial to establish a tailored revision strategy for various indications to assist bariatric surgeons in making informed decisions following primary surgeries.

## Limb Distalization Following RYGB

In studies exploring the challenges of insufficient weight loss after RYGB, recent findings suggest that performing distalization of limbs following RYGB, offers promising outcomes for renewed weight loss compared to other revisional procedures [87, 88]. However, it's essential to cautiously assess the long-term consequences, including potential malabsorption and patient safety [87]. A retrospective analysis of RYGB distalization with biliopancreatic limb (BP limb) lengthening and common limb (CL) shortening revealed that 13.6% of patients developed nutritional deficiencies, necessitating corrective surgery [89]. This underscores the risks associated with solely extending the biliopancreatic limb (Type I DRYGB revision). Additionally, the Type II DRYGB revision showed suboptimal weight loss outcomes [62, 90–92].

In the Type II DRYGB revision category, elongating the alimentary limb (AL) alone did not significantly impact weight loss, emphasizing the limited effectiveness of this approach [90–92]. On the other hand, Type III DRYGB revision, involving lengthening both the AL and biliopancreatic limb (BPL), was deemed crucial for reducing the risk of nutritional deficiencies and enhancing weight loss [87, 88]. In Category I of DRYGB revision, the malabsorptive distal gastric bypass, with an extended AL and unmeasured BP limb, led to common nutritional deficiencies in 18% of patients, necessitating reintervention [93]. Long-term outcomes reported a 32% incidence of postoperative nutritional deficiencies requiring revision and limb lengthening [94]. The studies highlight the complexities of DRYGB revisions, emphasizing the importance of careful consideration of factors such as limb lengthening and patient safety to achieve optimal outcomes in terms of weight loss and nutritional well-being.

## Pouch Revision Following RYGB

Gastric pouch and anastomotic revision involve the laparoscopic reduction of an enlarged pouch and dilated gastrojejunal anastomosis, limiting its size to 1.5 cm or less. A study conducted by Morales et al. indicated that laparoscopic pouch revision is comparable in both safety and effectiveness to open revisional procedures [60]. Another study by Iannelli et al. suggested that laparoscopic pouch revision is a short-term option for addressing weight regain after Roux-en-Y gastric bypass, with both studies reporting %EWL >72% at the 12-month follow-up. However, complications, such as intra-abdominal abscess and pulmonary embolism, were observed in 30% of patients, with no perioperative mortalities [95]. In contrast, a study by Parikh et al. reported that gastric pouch revision procedures were ineffective for failed RYGB, achieving only a %EWL of <26% after 12 months [96].

Another study, covering a 1-year follow-up period with 25 patients, initially showed promising results with a mean drop of 8 BMI points. However, at the 2-year follow-up, there were no statistically significant differences from the pre-revision weights. Instead, patients had a higher BMI than at the initial time of the revision

[59]. Initially, the %EBMIL was 43.3% at 1 year but dropped drastically to 14% at 3 years, emphasizing that gastric pouch revision is promising for the short term but may not be an effective method for the long term [97].

## Sleeve to RYGB

Laparoscopic SG is the most common bariatric procedure, mainly due to its surgical simplicity [98]. However, in long-term follow-up, challenges such as GERD and weight recurrence have become notable concerns associated with the procedure [61, 99–103]. Randomized controlled trials have indicated that there may not be a discernible difference in weight loss between SG and RYGB when treating obesity [104–106].

While the conversion of SG to RYGB effectively tackles GERD, research suggests that there might be no additional weight loss achieved after the revision. Additionally, there is a scarcity of reported data regarding the outcomes following the conversion of SG to RYGB [107]. Recent studies, however, propose that a gastric bypass with an extended biliopancreatic (BP) limb surpasses standard or short BP limb gastric bypasses in terms of weight loss and glycemic control [108–110]. The prolonged BP limb is believed to amplify weight loss by increasing bile acid circulation, leading to the deactivation of digestive enzymes [109, 110]. Despite the potential efficacy of a longer BP limb in weight loss and diabetes control, it comes with an elevated risk of diarrhea and nutritional deficiencies [111, 112]. However, the utilization of a modified RYGB with an extended BP limb may aid in weight reduction and glycemic control, particularly in patients concurrently managing obesity and diabetes [98, 113].

In a recent study, a complete resolution of GERD was observed in 60% of patients after converting from SG to RYGB, while the remaining 40% experienced residual symptoms and occasionally required proton pump inhibitor (PPI) medication. These findings align with other studies indicating that 30–50% of patients undergoing RYGB for GERD after SG may still need medication for residual symptoms [105, 114, 115].

## Sleeve to BPD/DS

BPD/DS involves a partial SG with pylorus preservation, establishing a roux limb, a long biliopancreatic (BP) limb, and a short common channel [116]. In a 14-year study from 2006 to 2019, 549 SGs were performed, with 84 patients (15.3%) opting for conservation. During the study, 19 patients (26.8%) underwent a conversion from SG to BPD/DS, resulting in a significant increase in both %TWL and %EWL [117]. However, complications emerged, with two patients experiencing chronic diarrhea and malnutrition post-SG to BPD/DS conversion, necessitating small intestine interposition [118].

The study identified a 15.3% conversion rate after an average of 5.2 years post-SG, mainly for GERD (33.8%) and IWL (32.4%) or a combination of both (31.0%). Significant weight loss was observed after conversion, especially with the addition of a hypoabsorptive component like BPD/DS. Studies by Andalib et al. and Shimon et al. reported higher total weight loss (TWL) after BPD/DS compared to RYGB [119, 120]. Some cases in other studies reported severe malnutrition and steatorrhea after BPD/DS [117, 119, 120]. BPD/DS showed promising results in addressing medical problems, with remission rates of up to 94.0% for T2D and up to 87.5% for HTN [121, 122]. Another study reported a remission rate of 83.3% for T2D and 25.0% for HTN in patients undergoing BPD/DS [117].

Parikh et al. and Keshishian et al. shared their experiences with this revision in 12 and 47 patients, respectively [116, 123]. The reported %EWL was excellent at 62.7% at 1 year and 71% at up to 3 years, corresponding to %EBMIL of 63.7% and 76%, respectively. Major complications were relatively low at 4.0%. Despite offering the best long-term weight loss with an acceptable complication profile, revision using BPD/DS has not gained wide acceptance due to the procedure's complexity and concerns about long-term severe malnutrition [62].

## Sleeve to SADI-S

SADI-S (single anastomosis duodenal-ileal bypass with sleeve), introduced by Sánchez-Pernaute and Torres et al. in 2007, is a relatively new surgical technique aiming to achieve results comparable to BPD/DS in excess weight loss but with lower complication rates [124]. Hypoabsorptive bariatric operations like SADI-S are linked to a high prevalence of nutritional deficiencies due to altered gastrointestinal anatomy and reduced absorptive capacity. Post-surgery, patients experience reduced food intake and dyspepsia, potentially leading to severe malnutrition from decreased caloric intake or nutrient deficiency [29, 125].

Outcomes related to nutritional deficiencies are variable and conflicting in studies. Balibrea et al. presented midterm results of 30 SADI procedures in patients with high BMI, revealing a correlation between common channel length and nutritional deficiencies. Deficiencies reported included total protein (58.33%), folate (18.18%), Vitamin B12 (33.33%), Vitamin D (55.56%), and calcium (45.45%) [126]. Moon et al. reported 2-year outcomes in 140 primary laparoscopic and robot-assisted SADI, showing lower levels of albumin (20.0%), total protein (12.0%), and calcium (16%) [127]. Sánchez-Pernaute reported midterm results of 97 patients with T2DM following SADI, indicating deficiencies of 34% in total protein, 13.7% in albumin, and 50% in vitamin D [124]. In a cohort of 286 patients, Zaveri et al. demonstrated lower levels of calcium (4.89%), total protein (5.59%), albumin (3.46%), vitamin B12 (0%), and vitamin D (15.03%) after a 2-year follow-up [128].

Results may vary due to differences in patient selection and management protocols [129]. A study at 24 months post-surgery showed BMI ranging from 28.6 to 32.7 kg/m$^2$, %EWL from 73.91% to 85.96%, and %TWL from 25.8% to 46.3% [128, 130, 131]. Another study found that SADI procedure demonstrates a more substantial reduction in weight loss. Patients undergoing SADI exhibited %TWL of 30.0 ± 18.4, %EWL of 66.2 ± 21.7, and a BMI of 12.2 ± 8.9 [132]. This result supports previous research suggesting the effectiveness of SADI in achieving significant weight loss, as reported by Dijkhorst et al. [65], who successfully used SADI-S as a revisional bariatric procedure [65, 128]. This study aligns with previous research, with two prior studies also reporting an EWL% of 66.2 ± 21.7 following the SADI-S procedure over a 5-year period [132].

In patients undergoing the SADI procedure, a study by Sánchez-Pernaute found a higher resolution for comorbidities such as T2D, with a 52% remission after a 5-year follow-up. Zaveri et al. reported an 81% remission rate of T2D over a 4-year follow-up period after SADI [133, 134]. However, complications emerged as six patients in the cohort (14%) experienced diarrhea/steatorrhea [134].

## Implications of Weight Recurrence

Weight recurrence following metabolic and bariatric surgery can have significant implications for patients' health, well-being, and healthcare costs. It often leads to the return of obesity-related comorbidities, such as type 2 diabetes (T2D), hypertension, and dyslipidemia, resulting in increased healthcare expenses. These expenses include follow-up appointments, diagnostic tests, and potential revisional surgeries, which can significantly impact a patient's financial situation and negatively affect their quality of life and emotional well-being [133, 135–141].

It is essential for both patients and healthcare providers to be aware of these implications and collaborate on strategies to prevent or effectively address weight recurrence. Some studies have identified various complications that can lead to hospital readmissions following bariatric surgery. These complications may include abdominal pain, high fever, or persistent nausea. In one study, during the first year of post-bariatric surgery, 16.7% of complications occurred after SADI-S, and 17.6% were reported after RYGB. In some cases, patients who underwent SADI required reoperation in the form of a re-sleeve procedure due to insufficient weight loss. Another patient who underwent SADI developed severe chronic diarrhea and subsequently underwent duodenojejunostomy to facilitate enteral feeding [65].

## Limitations and Challenges

Much like any scientific inquiry, research on weight recurrence post-bariatric surgery is not without its set of challenges and limitations. This emerging field faces several constraints. Weight recurrence has had several definitions, which makes it difficult to compare studies. Many studies grapple with limited sample sizes and the absence of control groups for comparative analysis, which restricts the applicability of their findings to a broader population of bariatric surgery patients. Moreover, weight recurrence can be a protracted issue, and numerous studies have relatively short follow-up periods, rendering it challenging to gauge the full scope of weight recurrence and its enduring consequences.

Another noteworthy limitation is the retrospective nature of some research, relying on retrospective data, which can introduce biases and compromise data quality and availability. Some studies may also exhibit selection bias by including only patients who continued attending follow-up appointments. Published systematic review studies often grapple with incomplete datasets, with data gaps regarding factors contributing to weight recurrence, such as mortality rates, the proportion of patients lost to follow-up, and reoperation rates [142].

Furthermore, bariatric surgery encompasses a variety of procedures, each with its unique mechanisms and outcomes. Pooling data from different procedures can complicate the ability to draw precise conclusions about the effectiveness of interventions for managing weight recurrence and identifying the most suitable approaches. The inconsistency in the definition of weight recurrence across various studies further complicates accurate comparisons [105]. Acknowledging these limitations is crucial, as the field of bariatric surgery and weight management continues to evolve. Future research endeavors hold the potential to offer a more comprehensive understanding of weight recurrence and its management, building on these insights.

## Future Directions

The field of addressing weight recurrence after bariatric surgery is relatively new, and both healthcare providers and researchers are actively working to better comprehend the multifaceted factors contributing to this issue. While current research underscores the effectiveness of bariatric surgery in managing obesity, significant strides are being made to refine patient care and enhance long-term outcomes. Future directions in this realm include personalized treatment plans, tailoring both surgical procedures and postoperative care to the unique physiological and psychological needs of each individual. This entails using tools like genetic profiling, metabolic testing, and psychological assessments to create highly individualized treatment regimens.

Pharmacological interventions, particularly the use of anti-obesity medications following bariatric surgery, are emerging as a promising approach to combat weight recurrence and help patients maintain their weight loss. However, rigorous research and testing are necessary to evaluate the effectiveness of these medications and assess potential health consequences. Developing and fine-tuning medications that can regulate appetite and metabolism is a dynamic field of research. Such medications may make it easier for patients to sustain their weight loss post-surgery. Simultaneously, nutritional education and support play a crucial role. Innovative strategies are being explored to assist patients in making healthier dietary choices and adapting to new dietary requirements. This may also involve incorporating exercise programs to enhance the long-term success of weight management.

Long-term follow-up care is another promising direction. Establishing interdisciplinary collaborations among various healthcare providers and researchers can help create comprehensive, long-term follow-up care plans for bariatric surgery patients. This continuous monitoring and support can help identify potential issues and provide guidance on maintaining weight loss. Exploring the role of the gut microbiome in weight recurrence after bariatric surgery holds potential. This avenue of research may lead to targeted interventions, such as the use of probiotics or dietary modifications, to support long-term weight loss.

Furthermore, ensuring equal access to bariatric surgery and postoperative care for all individuals is of paramount importance in addressing weight recurrence. Collaborative efforts between researchers and providers are necessary to reduce healthcare disparities and broaden the accessibility of bariatric surgery for diverse populations. Research in these areas will contribute to a deeper understanding of the factors contributing to weight recurrence after bariatric surgery and the development of more effective strategies to prevent and manage this challenge.

## Conclusion

Weight recurrence is a critical and complex phenomenon within the context of obesity as a chronic disease and bariatric surgery. Bariatric surgery remains a highly effective treatment for obesity, leading to sustained weight loss and the amelioration of weight-related comorbidities. However, a substantial proportion of patients experience significant weight recurrence post-bariatric surgery during long-term follow-up. The lack of a standardized definition for weight recurrence has posed a challenge, both for researchers and healthcare providers, in understanding and addressing this issue comprehensively. The prevalence of weight recurrence varies widely depending on the definition and the time since surgery, making it crucial to establish a common understanding of this concept.

While there may be cases of weight recurrence attributed to anatomical and surgical causes, the primary contributors to weight recurrence appear to be postoperative factors, including increased caloric intake due to heightened appetite, maladaptive or dysregulated eating habits, inadequate physical activity, and psychosocial stresses. The development of a universally accepted standard definition for weight recurrence is essential. This common framework will enable researchers and healthcare providers to identify the stages at which weight recurrence can lead to comorbidities and which comorbidities are more likely to return. With a standardized definition in place, a personalized care plan and interdisciplinary collaboration can be established, facilitating more effective management and support for postoperative bariatric surgery patients.

In light of these considerations, there is a clear need for further exploration and research into weight recurrence to enhance our understanding of this phenomenon, improve patient care, and ultimately contribute to the long-term success of bariatric surgery as a treatment for obesity.

## References


1. Majid SF, et al. Current state of the definition and terminology related to weight recurrence after metabolic surgery: review by the POWER Task Force of the American Society for Metabolic and Bariatric Surgery. Surg Obes Relat Dis. 2022;18(7):957–63.
2. Brebal KMM, et al. Weight gain and changes in nutritional status of Brazilian adults after 20 years of age: a time-trend analysis (2006–2012). Rev Bras Epidemiol. 2020;23:e200045.
3. Chen Y, et al. The prevalence and increasing trends of overweight, general obesity, and abdominal obesity among Chinese adults: a repeated cross-sectional study. BMC Public Health. 2019;19(1):1293.
4. Kranjac AW, Wagmiller RL. Decomposing trends in adult body mass index, obesity, and morbid obesity, 1971–2012. Soc Sci Med. 2016;167:37–44.
5. Noria SF, et al. Weight regain after bariatric surgery: scope of the problem, causes, prevention, and treatment. Curr Diab Rep. 2023;23(3):31–42.
6. Sugerman HJ. Bariatric surgery for severe obesity. J Assoc Acad Minor Phys. 2001;12(3):129–36.
7. Monaco-Ferreira DV, Leandro-Merhi VA. Weight regain 10 years after Roux-en-Y gastric bypass. Obes Surg. 2017;27(5):1137–44.
8. Lauti M, et al. Weight regain following sleeve gastrectomy-a systematic review. Obes Surg. 2016;26(6):1326–34.
9. Shantavasinkul PC, et al. Predictors of weight regain in patients who underwent Roux-en-Y gastric bypass surgery. Surg Obes Relat Dis. 2016;12(9):1640–5.
10. da Silva FB, Gomes DL, de Carvalho KM. Poor diet quality and postoperative time are independent risk factors for weight regain after Roux-en-Y gastric bypass. Nutrition. 2016;32(11–12):1250–3.
11. Thomas DD, et al. Weight recidivism after Roux-en-Y gastric bypass surgery: an 11-year experience in a multiethnic medical center. Obesity (Silver Spring). 2019;27(2):217–25.
12. Christian NJ, et al. Validity of self-reported weights following bariatric surgery. JAMA. 2013;310(22):2454–6.
13. Voorwinde V, et al. Definitions of long-term weight regain and their associations with clinical outcomes. Obes Surg. 2020;30(2):527–36.
14. Monpellier VM, et al. Weight change after Roux-en Y gastric bypass, physical activity and eating style: is there a relationship? Obes Surg. 2019;29(2):526–33.
15. King WC, Hinerman AS, Courcoulas AP. Weight regain after bariatric surgery: a systematic literature review and comparison across studies using a large reference sample. Surg Obes Relat Dis. 2020;16(8):1133–44.
16. Istfan NW, et al. Approach to the patient: management of the post-bariatric surgery patient with weight regain. J Clin Endocrinol Metab. 2021;106(1):251–63.
17. Athanasiadis DI, et al. Factors associated with weight regain post-bariatric surgery: a systematic review. Surg Endosc. 2021;35(8):4069–84.
18. Colles SL, Dixon JB, O'Brien PE. Grazing and loss of control related to eating: two high-risk factors following bariatric surgery. Obesity (Silver Spring). 2008;16(3):615–22.
19. Pizato N, et al. Effect of grazing behavior on weight regain post-bariatric surgery: a systematic review. Nutrients. 2017;9(12)
20. Conceição EM, et al. What is "grazing"? Reviewing its definition, frequency, clinical characteristics, and impact on bariatric surgery outcomes, and proposing a standardized definition. Surg Obes Relat Dis. 2014;10(5):973–82.
21. Freire RH, et al. Food quality, physical activity, and nutritional follow-up as determinant of weight regain after Roux-en-Y gastric bypass. Nutrition. 2012;28(1):53–8.
22. Sarwer DB, et al. Psychopathology, disordered eating, and impulsivity as predictors of outcomes of bariatric surgery. Surg Obes Relat Dis. 2019;15(4):650–5.
23. Karmali S, et al. Weight recidivism post-bariatric surgery: a systematic review. Obes Surg. 2013;23(11):1922–33.

24. Suter M. Laparoscopic band repositioning for pouch dilatation/slippage after gastric banding: disappointing results. Obes Surg. 2001;11(4):507–12.
25. Yimcharoen P, et al. Endoscopic findings and outcomes of revisional procedures for patients with weight recidivism after gastric bypass. Surg Endosc. 2011;25(10):3345–52.
26. Heneghan HM, et al. Influence of pouch and stoma size on weight loss after gastric bypass. Surg Obes Relat Dis. 2012;8(4):408–15.
27. El Ansari W, Elhag W. Weight regain and insufficient weight loss after bariatric surgery: definitions, prevalence, mechanisms, predictors, prevention and management strategies, and knowledge gaps-a scoping review. Obes Surg. 2021;31(4):1755–66.
28. Weiner RA, et al. Laparoscopic sleeve gastrectomy—influence of sleeve size and resected gastric volume. Obes Surg. 2007;17(10):1297–305.
29. Braghetto I, et al. Evaluation of the radiological gastric capacity and evolution of the BMI 2–3 years after sleeve gastrectomy. Obes Surg. 2009;19(9):1262–9.
30. Braghetto I, et al. Is laparoscopic sleeve gastrectomy an acceptable primary bariatric procedure in obese patients? Early and 5-year postoperative results. Surg Laparosc Endosc Percutan Tech. 2012;22(6):479–86.
31. Tsouristakis AI, et al. Long-term modulation of appetitive hormones and sweet cravings after adjustable gastric banding and Roux-en-Y gastric bypass. Obes Surg. 2019;29(11):3698–705.
32. Jirapinyo P, et al. A meta-analysis of GLP-1 after Roux-En-Y gastric bypass: impact of surgical technique and measurement strategy. Obes Surg. 2018;28(3):615–26.
33. Bohdjalian A, et al. Sleeve gastrectomy as sole and definitive bariatric procedure: 5-year results for weight loss and ghrelin. Obes Surg. 2010;20(5):535–40.
34. Santo MA, et al. Weight regain after gastric bypass: influence of gut hormones. Obes Surg. 2016;26(5):919–25.
35. Lombardo M, Bellia A, Mattiuzzo F, et al. Frequent follow-up visits reduce weight regain in long-term management after bariatric surgery. Bariatr Surg Pract Patient Care. 2015;10(3):119–25.
36. Roslin M, et al. Abnormal glucose tolerance testing following gastric bypass demonstrates reactive hypoglycemia. Surg Endosc. 2011;25(6):1926–32.
37. Díaz R, et al. Endoscopy after bariatric surgery: what the endoscopist must know. Rev Med Chile. 2020;148(1):83–92.
38. Aills L, et al. ASMBS Allied Health Nutritional guidelines for the surgical weight loss patient. Surg Obes Relat Dis. 2008;4(Suppl. 5):S73–108.
39. Mechanick JI, et al. Clinical practice guidelines for the perioperative nutrition, metabolic, and nonsurgical support of patients undergoing bariatric procedures—2019 update: cosponsored by American Association of Clinical Endocrinologists/American College of Endocrinology, The Obesity Society, American Society for Metabolic & Bariatric Surgery, Obesity Medicine Association, and American Society of Anesthesiologists. Surg Obes Relat Dis. 2020;16(2):175–247.
40. Bosnic G. Nutritional requirements after bariatric surgery. Crit Care Nurs Clin North Am. 2014;26(2):255–62.
41. Mechanick JI, et al. Clinical practice guidelines for the perioperative nutritional, metabolic, and nonsurgical support of the bariatric surgery patient—2013 update: cosponsored by American Association of Clinical Endocrinologists, The Obesity Society, and American Society for Metabolic & Bariatric Surgery. Obesity (Silver Spring). 2013;21(01):S1–27.
42. Magallares A, Schomerus G. Mental and physical health-related quality of life in obese patients before and after bariatric surgery: a meta-analysis. Psychol Health Med. 2015;20(2):165–76.
43. Parkes E. Nutritional management of patients after bariatric surgery. Am J Med Sci. 2006;331(4):207–13.
44. Zalesin KC, Franklin BA, Miller WM, et al. Preventing weight regain after bariatric surgery: an overview of lifestyle and psychosocial modulators. Am J Lifestyle Med. 2010;4(2):113–20.
45. Leahy CR, Luning A. Review of nutritional guidelines for patients undergoing bariatric surgery. AORN J. 2015;102(2):153–60.

46. Istfan NW, et al. The mitigating effect of phentermine and topiramate on weight regain after Roux-en-Y gastric bypass surgery. Obesity (Silver Spring). 2020;28(6):1023–30.
47. Srivastava G, Apovian CM. Current pharmacotherapy for obesity. Nat Rev Endocrinol. 2018;14(1):12–24.
48. Toth AT, et al. Weight loss medications in young adults after bariatric surgery for weight regain or inadequate weight loss: a multi-center study. Children (Basel). 2018;5(9)
49. Schwartz J, et al. Pharmacotherapy in conjunction with a diet and exercise program for the treatment of weight recidivism or weight loss plateau post-bariatric surgery: a retrospective review. Obes Surg. 2016;26(2):452–8.
50. Grilo CM, Reas DL, Mitchell JE. Combining pharmacological and psychological treatments for binge eating disorder: current status, limitations, and future directions. Curr Psychiatry Rep. 2016;18(6):55.
51. Stanford FC, et al. The utility of weight loss medications after bariatric surgery for weight regain or inadequate weight loss: a multi-center study. Surg Obes Relat Dis. 2017;13(3):491–500.
52. Miras AD, et al. Adjunctive liraglutide treatment in patients with persistent or recurrent type 2 diabetes after metabolic surgery (GRAVITAS): a randomised, double-blind, placebo-controlled trial. Lancet Diabetes Endocrinol. 2019;7(7):549–59.
53. Wharton S, et al. Liraglutide 3.0 mg for the management of insufficient weight loss or excessive weight regain post-bariatric surgery. Clin Obes. 2019;9(4):e12323.
54. Abrahamsson N, et al. GLP1 analogs as treatment of postprandial hypoglycemia following gastric bypass surgery: a potential new indication? Eur J Endocrinol. 2013;169(6):885–9.
55. Ahrén B, et al. Semaglutide induces weight loss in subjects with type 2 diabetes regardless of baseline BMI or gastrointestinal adverse events in the SUSTAIN 1 to 5 trials. Diabetes Obes Metab. 2018;20(9):2210–9.
56. O'Neil PM, et al. Efficacy and safety of semaglutide compared with liraglutide and placebo for weight loss in patients with obesity: a randomised, double-blind, placebo and active controlled, dose-ranging, phase 2 trial. Lancet. 2018;392(10148):637–49.
57. Avenell A, et al. Bariatric surgery, lifestyle interventions and orlistat for severe obesity: the REBALANCE mixed-methods systematic review and economic evaluation. Health Technol Assess. 2018;22(68):1–246.
58. Ribeiro-Parenti L, et al. Classification, surgical management and outcomes of patients with gastrogastric fistula after Roux-En-Y gastric bypass. Surg Obes Relat Dis. 2017;13(2):243–8.
59. Hamdi A, et al. Midterm outcomes of revisional surgery for gastric pouch and gastrojejunal anastomotic enlargement in patients with weight regain after gastric bypass for morbid obesity. Obes Surg. 2014;24(8):1386–90.
60. Morales MP, et al. Laparoscopic revisional surgery after Roux-en-Y gastric bypass and sleeve gastrectomy. Surg Obes Relat Dis. 2010;6(5):485–90.
61. Himpens J, et al. Outcomes of revisional procedures for insufficient weight loss or weight regain after Roux-en-Y gastric bypass. Obes Surg. 2012;22(11):1746–54.
62. Tran DD, et al. Revision of Roux-En-Y gastric bypass for weight regain: a systematic review of techniques and outcomes. Obes Surg. 2016;26(7):1627–34.
63. Still CD, et al. Clinical factors associated with weight loss outcomes after Roux-en-Y gastric bypass surgery. Obesity (Silver Spring). 2014;22(3):888–94.
64. Puzziferri N, et al. Long-term follow-up after bariatric surgery: a systematic review. JAMA. 2014;312(9):934–42.
65. Dijkhorst PJ, et al. Failed sleeve gastrectomy: single anastomosis duodenoileal bypass or Roux-en-Y gastric bypass? A multicenter cohort study. Obes Surg. 2018;28(12):3834–42.
66. Spyropoulos C, et al. Revisional bariatric surgery: 13-year experience from a tertiary institution. Arch Surg. 2010;145(2):173–7.
67. Schwartz RW, et al. Gastric bypass revision: lessons learned from 920 cases. Surgery. 1988;104(4):806–12.
68. Owens BM, Owens ML, Hill CW. Effect of revisional bariatric surgery on weight loss and frequency of complications. Obes Surg. 1996;6(6):479–84.

69. Sugerman HJ, et al. Conversion of failed or complicated vertical banded gastroplasty to gastric bypass in morbid obesity. Am J Surg. 1996;171(2):263–9.
70. Victorzon M. Revisional bariatric surgery by conversion to gastric bypass or sleeve—good short-term outcomes at higher risks. Obes Surg. 2012;22(1):29–33.
71. Gagner M, et al. Laparoscopic reoperative bariatric surgery: experience from 27 consecutive patients. Obes Surg. 2002;12(2):254–60.
72. Mognol P, Chosidow D, Marmuse JP. Laparoscopic conversion of laparoscopic gastric banding to Roux-en-Y gastric bypass: a review of 70 patients. Obes Surg. 2004;14(10):1349–53.
73. Van Dessel E, et al. Roux-en-Y gastric bypass as a re-do procedure for failed restricive gastric surgery. Surg Endosc. 2008;22(4):1014–8.
74. Hii MW, et al. Laparoscopic conversion of failed gastric banding to Roux-en-Y gastric bypass: short-term follow-up and technical considerations. Obes Surg. 2012;22(7):1022–8.
75. Tran TT, et al. Revisional weight loss surgery after failed laparoscopic gastric banding: an institutional experience. Surg Endosc. 2013;27(11):4087–93.
76. Behrns KE, et al. Reoperative bariatric surgery. Lessons learned to improve patient selection and results. Ann Surg. 1993;218(5):646–53.
77. Radtka JF, et al. Revisional bariatric surgery: who, what, where, and when? Surg Obes Relat Dis. 2010;6(6):635–42.
78. Sjöström L, et al. Effects of bariatric surgery on mortality in Swedish obese subjects. N Engl J Med. 2007;357(8):741–52.
79. Boza C, et al. Laparoscopic adjustable gastric banding (LAGB): surgical results and 5-year follow-up. Surg Endosc. 2011;25(1):292–7.
80. Van Nieuwenhove Y, et al. Long-term results of a prospective study on laparoscopic adjustable gastric banding for morbid obesity. Obes Surg. 2011;21(5):582–7.
81. Himpens J, et al. Long-term outcomes of laparoscopic adjustable gastric banding. Arch Surg. 2011;146(7):802–7.
82. Romy S, et al. Roux-en-Y gastric bypass vs gastric banding for morbid obesity: a case-matched study of 442 patients. Arch Surg. 2012;147(5):460–6.
83. O'Brien PE, et al. Long-term outcomes after bariatric surgery: fifteen-year follow-up of adjustable gastric banding and a systematic review of the bariatric surgical literature. Ann Surg. 2013;257(1):87–94.
84. Higa K, et al. Laparoscopic Roux-en-Y gastric bypass: 10-year follow-up. Surg Obes Relat Dis. 2011;7(4):516–25.
85. Weiner RA, Theodoridou S, Weiner S. Failure of laparoscopic sleeve gastrectomy—further procedure? Obes Facts. 2011;4(Suppl. 1):42–6.
86. van Rutte PW, et al. Indications and short-term outcomes of revisional surgery after failed or complicated sleeve gastrectomy. Obes Surg. 2012;22(12):1903–8.
87. Ngomba Muakana JA, et al. Distalization of standard Roux-en-Y gastric bypass: indications, technique, and long-term results. Obes Surg. 2023;33(5):1373–81.
88. Hamed H, Ali M, Elmahdy Y. Types, safety, and efficacy of limb distalization for inadequate weight loss after Roux-en-Y gastric bypass: a systematic review and meta-analysis with a call for standardized terminology. Ann Surg. 2021;274(2):271–80.
89. Shin RD, et al. Revision of Roux-en-Y gastric bypass with limb distalization for inadequate weight loss or weight regain. Obes Surg. 2019;29(3):811–8.
90. Brolin RE. Comment on: Long-term results of malabsorptive distal Roux-en-Y gastric bypass in superobese patients. Surg Obes Relat Dis. 2011;7(2):193–4.
91. Svanevik M, et al. Patient-reported outcome measures 2 years after standard and distal gastric bypass-a double-blind randomized controlled trial. Obes Surg. 2018;28(3):606–14.
92. Gadiot RPM, et al. Does the length of the common channel as part of the total alimentary tract matter? One year results from the multicenter Dutch Common Channel Trial (DUCATI) comparing standard versus distal Roux-en-Y gastric bypass with similar biliopancreatic bowel limb lengths. Obes Surg. 2020;30(12):4732–40.
93. Sugerman HJ, Kellum JM, DeMaria. Conversion of proximal to distal gastric bypass for failed gastric bypass for superobesity. J Gastrointest Surg. 1997;1(6):517–24. discussion 524–6

94. Kellum JM, et al. Long-term results of malabsorptive distal Roux-en-Y gastric bypass in superobese patients. Surg Obes Relat Dis. 2011;7(2):189–93.
95. Iannelli A, et al. Gastric pouch resizing for Roux-en-Y gastric bypass failure in patients with a dilated pouch. Surg Obes Relat Dis. 2013;9(2):260–7.
96. Parikh M, Heacock L, Gagner M. Laparoscopic "gastrojejunal sleeve reduction" as a revision procedure for weight loss failure after roux-en-y gastric bypass. Obes Surg. 2011;21(5):650–4.
97. Amor IB, et al. Midterm outcomes of gastric pouch resizing for weight regain after Roux-en-Y gastric bypass. Obes Surg. 2020;30(7):2723–8.
98. Lee MH, Almalki OM, Lee WJ, Soong TC, Chen SC. Outcomes of laparoscopic revisional conversion of sleeve gastrectomy to Roux-en-Y gastric bypass: different strategies for obese and non-obese Asian patients. Asian J Surg. 2023;46(2):761–6.
99. Mahawar KK, et al. Sleeve gastrectomy and gastro-oesophageal reflux disease: a complex relationship. Obes Surg. 2013;23(7):987–91.
100. Arman GA, et al. Long-term (11+years) outcomes in weight, patient satisfaction, comorbidities, and gastroesophageal reflux treatment after laparoscopic sleeve gastrectomy. Surg Obes Relat Dis. 2016;12(10):1778–86.
101. Felsenreich DM, et al. Outcome of sleeve gastrectomy converted to Roux-en-Y gastric bypass and one-anastomosis gastric bypass. Obes Surg. 2022;32(3):643–51.
102. Genco A, et al. Gastroesophageal reflux disease and Barrett's esophagus after laparoscopic sleeve gastrectomy: a possible, underestimated long-term complication. Surg Obes Relat Dis. 2017;13(4):568–74.
103. Chang DM, et al. Thirteen-year experience of laparoscopic sleeve gastrectomy: surgical risk, weight loss, and revision procedures. Obes Surg. 2018;28(10):2991–7.
104. Ignat M, et al. Randomized trial of Roux-en-Y gastric bypass versus sleeve gastrectomy in achieving excess weight loss. Br J Surg. 2017;104(3):248–56.
105. Salminen P, et al. Effect of laparoscopic sleeve gastrectomy vs laparoscopic Roux-en-Y gastric bypass on weight loss at 5 years among patients with morbid obesity: The SLEEVEPASS randomized clinical trial. JAMA. 2018;319(3):241–54.
106. Peterli R, et al. Effect of laparoscopic sleeve gastrectomy vs laparoscopic Roux-en-Y gastric bypass on weight loss in patients with morbid obesity: the SM-BOSS randomized clinical trial. JAMA. 2018;319(3):255–65.
107. Parmar CD, et al. Conversion of sleeve gastrectomy to Roux-en-Y gastric bypass is effective for gastro-oesophageal reflux disease but not for further weight loss. Obes Surg. 2017;27(7):1651–8.
108. Caruana JA, et al. Distal small bowel bypass for weight regain after gastric bypass: safety and efficacy threshold occurs at <70% bypass. Surg Obes Relat Dis. 2015;11(6):1248–55.
109. Ise I, et al. Changes in enterohepatic circulation after duodenal-jejunal bypass and reabsorption of bile acids in the bilio-pancreatic limb. Obes Surg. 2019;29(6):1901–10.
110. Ueno T, et al. Mechanism of bile acid reabsorption in the biliopancreatic limb after duodenal-jejunal bypass in rats. Obes Surg. 2020;30(7):2528–37.
111. Miyachi T, et al. Biliopancreatic limb plays an important role in metabolic improvement after duodenal-jejunal bypass in a rat model of diabetes. Surgery. 2016;159(5):1360–71.
112. Ahuja A, et al. MGB-OAGB: effect of biliopancreatic limb length on nutritional deficiency, weight loss, and comorbidity resolution. Obes Surg. 2018;28(11):3439–45.
113. Fehervari M, et al. Weight loss specific to indication, remission of diabetes, and short-term complications after sleeve gastrectomy conversion to Roux-en-Y gastric bypass: a systematic review and meta-analysis. Surg Obes Relat Dis. 2023;19(4):384–95.
114. Carandina S, et al. Conversion of sleeve gastrectomy to Roux-en-Y gastric bypass in patients with gastroesophageal reflux disease: results of a multicenter study. Surg Obes Relat Dis. 2020;16(6):732–7.
115. Lim CH, et al. Resolution of erosive esophagitis after conversion from vertical sleeve gastrectomy to Roux-en-Y gastric bypass. Obes Surg. 2020;30(12):4751–9.
116. Keshishian A, et al. Duodenal switch is a safe operation for patients who have failed other bariatric operations. Obes Surg. 2004;14(9):1187–92.

117. Dirnberger AS, et al. Mid-term outcomes after conversion procedures following laparoscopic sleeve gastrectomy. Obes Surg. 2023;33(9):2679–86.
118. Dindo D, Demartines N, Clavien PA. Classification of surgical complications: a new proposal with evaluation in a cohort of 6336 patients and results of a survey. Ann Surg. 2004;240(2):205–13.
119. Andalib A, et al. Short-term outcomes of revisional surgery after sleeve gastrectomy: a comparative analysis of re-sleeve, Roux en-Y gastric bypass, duodenal switch (Roux en-Y and single-anastomosis). Surg Endosc. 2021;35(8):4644–52.
120. Shimon O, et al. Long-term effectiveness of laparoscopic conversion of sleeve gastrectomy to a biliopancreatic diversion with a duodenal switch or a Roux-en-Y gastric bypass due to weight loss failure. Obes Surg. 2018;28(6):1724–30.
121. Biertho L, et al. Second-stage duodenal switch for sleeve gastrectomy failure: a matched controlled trial. Surg Obes Relat Dis. 2018;14(10):1570–9.
122. Osorio J, et al. Revisional laparoscopic SADI-S vs. duodenal switch following failed primary sleeve gastrectomy: a single-center comparison of 101 consecutive cases. Obes Surg. 2021;31(8):3667–74.
123. Parikh M, Pomp A, Gagner M. Laparoscopic conversion of failed gastric bypass to duodenal switch: technical considerations and preliminary outcomes. Surg Obes Relat Dis. 2007;3(6):611–8.
124. Sánchez-Pernaute A, et al. Proximal duodenal-ileal end-to-side bypass with sleeve gastrectomy: proposed technique. Obes Surg. 2007;17(12):1614–8.
125. Schweiger C, et al. Nutritional deficiencies in bariatric surgery candidates. Obes Surg. 2010;20(2):193–7.
126. Balibrea JM, et al. Mid-term results and responsiveness predictors after two-step single-anastomosis duodeno-ileal bypass with sleeve gastrectomy. Obes Surg. 2017;27(5):1302–8.
127. Moon RC, et al. Safety and effectiveness of single-anastomosis duodenal switch procedure: 2-year result from a single US Institution. Obes Surg. 2018;28(6):1571–7.
128. Zaveri H, et al. Mid-term 4-year outcomes with single anastomosis duodenal-ileal bypass with sleeve gastrectomy surgery at a single US center. Obes Surg. 2018;28(10):3062–72.
129. Marincola G, et al. Medium-term nutritional and metabolic outcome of single anastomosis duodeno-ileal bypass with sleeve gastrectomy (SADI-S). Nutrients. 2023;15(3):742.
130. Spinos D, et al. The effectiveness of single-anastomosis duodenoileal bypass with sleeve gastrectomy/one anastomosis duodenal switch (SADI-S/OADS): an updated systematic review. Obes Surg. 2021;31(4):1790–800.
131. Kasalický M, Koblihová E, Pažin J. SADIS Single anastomosis duodeno-ileal bypass with sleeve gastrectomy as a second step after sleeve gastrectomy. Rozhl Chir. 2019;98(2):52–7.
132. Salama AF, et al. Comparative analysis of 5-year efficacy and outcomes of single anastomosis procedures as revisional surgery for weight regain following sleeve gastrectomy. Surg Endosc. 2023;37(10):7548–55.
133. Sánchez-Pernaute A, et al. Single-anastomosis duodenoileal bypass as a second step after sleeve gastrectomy. Surg Obes Relat Dis. 2015;11(2):351–5.
134. Shoar S, et al. Single anastomosis duodeno-ileal switch (SADIS): a systematic review of efficacy and safety. Obes Surg. 2018;28(1):104–13.
135. Shah M, Simha V, Garg A. Review: long-term impact of bariatric surgery on body weight, comorbidities, and nutritional status. J Clin Endocrinol Metab. 2006;91(11):4223–31.
136. DiGiorgi M, et al. Re-emergence of diabetes after gastric bypass in patients with mid- to long-term follow-up. Surg Obes Relat Dis. 2010;6(3):249–53.
137. Jiménez A, et al. Long-term effects of sleeve gastrectomy and Roux-en-Y gastric bypass surgery on type 2 diabetes mellitus in morbidly obese subjects. Ann Surg. 2012;256(6):1023–9.
138. Sheppard CE, et al. The economic impact of weight regain. Gastroenterol Res Pract. 2013;2013:379564.
139. Karlsson J, et al. Ten-year trends in health-related quality of life after surgical and conventional treatment for severe obesity: the SOS intervention study. Int J Obes. 2007;31(8):1248–61.

140. Jirapinyo P, Abu Dayyeh BK, Thompson CC. Weight regain after Roux-en-Y gastric bypass has a large negative impact on the Bariatric Quality of Life Index. BMJ Open Gastroenterol. 2017;4(1):e000153.
141. Alexandrou A, et al. What is the actual fate of super-morbid-obese patients who undergo laparoscopic sleeve gastrectomy as the first step of a two-stage weight-reduction operative strategy? Obes Surg. 2012;22(10):1623–8.
142. Angrisani L, et al. Laparoscopic adjustable gastric banding versus Roux-en-Y gastric bypass: 10-year results of a prospective, randomized trial. Surg Obes Relat Dis. 2013;9(3):405–13.

# 39 Endoscopic Management of Weight Regain Post-Bariatric Surgery

Margaret G. Keane and Barham K. Abu Dayyeh

As rates of obesity grow, more patients are undergoing bariatric surgery [1, 2]. Although a very effective treatment for severe obesity and its associated co-morbidities [3–6], weight recurrence and failure to achieve sustained weight loss occur is common [7, 8] and becomes more likely with increased time from surgery [9]. Weight recurrence and return of obesity-related co-morbidities has important health consequences for patients and is expensive and burdensome on healthcare systems [10].

The cause of weight recurrence following bariatric surgery is often multifactorial. Nutritional and lifestyle noncompliance, hormonal and metabolic factors, psychological factors as well as anatomic factors can contribute. A multidisciplinary approach to management is recommended to address all relevant factors in each case, to halt weight recurrence and achieve sustained weight loss long-term. Several novel endoscopic approaches to manage anatomical factors leading to treat weight recurrence have been developed over the last two decades. This chapter will describe these minimally invasive endoscopic revisional therapies that can be used to treat post-surgical weight recurrence.

## Roux-en-Y Gastric Bypass

Roux-en-Y gastric bypass (RYGB) is a successful procedure for weight loss, but patients may regain 20–30% of the maximal weight they initially lost, and in some studies, a third of patients regained almost all of the weight they lost [11, 12].

M. G. Keane
Johns Hopkins Hospital, Baltimore, MD, USA

B. K. Abu Dayyeh (✉)
Mayo Clinic, Rochester, MN, USA

Interventional Gastroenterology, Cedars Sinai Medical Center, Los Angeles, USA
e-mail: barham.abudayyeh@cshs.org


O. M. Ghanem et al. (eds.), *The SAGES Manual of Metabolic and Bariatric Surgery*, https://doi.org/10.1007/978-3-031-72309-4_39

Anatomically, a dilated gastrojejunal anastomosis (GJA) and elongated pouch have been associated with weight regain [13, 14]. A cohort study of 205 who underwent RYGB patients found stomal dilation in 59%, an enlarged pouch in 29% and enlarged pouch and stoma in 12% at a mean follow-up of 6.9 ± 3.7 years post-surgery. Multivariate analysis showed pre-RYGB BMI, longer duration from RYGB and stomal dilation predicted weight regain post-RYGB, but stomal dilation was the most important factor [15]. To treat stomal dilation associated with weight regain, revisional bariatric surgery can be pursued and the rate of revisional surgeries has increase three fold in the past decade [16]. Surgical revision involves suturing or stapling the gastric pouch or GJ anastomosis to reduce it in size. Although weight loss outcomes can be promising, these procedures have higher rates of complications, in comparison to primary bariatric surgery [15, 17]. Also by its nature, revisional surgery often limits future obesity interventions due to alterations of the GI tract and abdominal cavity, which is important in a chronic relapsing condition like obesity [17]. There has therefore been a growing interest in the development of minimally invasive, and anatomy-preserving alternative revisional therapies. As in primary obesity, endoscopic revisional therapies become a useful tool to address weight regain after bariatric surgery and offer an intermediate option between medical and surgical interventions.

## Transoral Outlet Reduction (TORe)

The transoral outlet reduction (TORe) procedure is a minimally invasive endoscopic technique that can reduce the diameter of the GJ anastomosis. It can be combined with a gastric pouch size reduction during the same procedure. The technique aims to delay emptying of the gastric pouch to enhancing the sensation of satiety [18–20], leading to improvements in cognitive restraint [21]. Its superior safety profile compared with conventional surgical revision (Table 39.1), has led to it becoming the preferred approach for stoma and pouch reduction in many centers [22].

As the procedure has evolved, the technique and devices used to perform the intervention have steadily improved, leading to greater weight loss and improved durability of the procedure. Currently, the most performed TORe techniques are the full-thickness TORe (FT TORe) and the argon plasma coagulation TORe (APC-TORe), which omits endoscopic suturing.

In the FT- TORe, firstly APC is applied circumferentially to the gastric side of the GJA at 35–80 W to induce a 1 cm tissue char. This injury leads to the de-epithelization of the gastric mucosa, which on healing induces tissue fibrosis and circumferential scaring of the outlet, hence reducing it in diameter. In the second part of the procedure, the stoma is oversewn with a full-thickness suturing device (Overstitch™; Boston Scientific, Marlborough, MA, USA) using one or more sutures. Using argon plasma coagulation (APC) in combination with suturing, rather than suturing alone is preferable as it leads to greater weight loss [20]. The sutures are then tightened or "cinched" over a through the scope balloon, reducing the outlet to 8–12 mm to size (Fig. 39.1). The final reduction in size of the GJ

**Table 39.1** Outcomes for Full Thickness TORe

| | Year | Study design | No. | Age (years) | Female (%) | Baseline BMI (kg/m$^2$) | Weight regain | Baseline GJA (mm) | Treatment protocol | No. of sessions | Suture pattern | APC | Severe AEs | AEs |
|---|---|---|---|---|---|---|---|---|---|---|---|---|---|---|
| Goyal et al. [50] | 2016 | RC | 25 | 53.0 | 80.0 | 40.8 | – | – | Single session | | Interrupted and running | Yes | None | None |
| Watson et al. [51] | 2017 | RC | 15 | 46.3 | 93.3 | 43.7 | 36.6 kg | 26.3 | Single session | | Pursestring | Yes | None | None |
| Staudenmann et al. [52] | 2017 | RC | 22 | 43.6 | 90.9 | 34.9 | 18.7 kg | 24.3 | Single session | | Interrupted | Yes | None | Perforation (1) |
| Vargas et al. [53] | 2017 | RC | 130 | 47.1 | 88.0 | 36.8 | 38.8% | 28.0 | Single session | | Interrupted or figure of eight | 50 W, 1 L | None | Nausea/vomiting (13), pain (23), stricture (5), superficial esophageal tear (1) |
| Espinet Col El et al. [54] | 2018 | RC | 13 | 50.5 | 61.5 | 37.1 | 21.6 kg | 36.0 | Single session | | Interrupted | 60 W, 1.6 L | None | None |
| Fayad et al. [55] | 2019 | RC | 44 | 48.5 | 90.9 | 41.5 | 51.1% | 28.9 | Every 8 weeks until GJA ≤12 mm with APC | 2.1 | 2-fold running | 50 W, 1 L | None | Stricture (3), ulcer (3), gastrogastric fistula (1) |
| Hollenbach et al. [33] | 2019 | RC | 26 | 50.8 | 76.9 | NA | – | 39.6 | In 12 weeks with APC if dilated GJA | 1.3 | Interrupted | 30 W, 0-8-1 L | None | None |
| Jirapinyo et al. [30] | 2020 | RC | 443 | 49.0 | - | 41.8 | 43.9% | 25.0 | Single session | | Pursestring (83.9%), interrupted (16.1%) | Yes | None | None |
| Brunaldi et al. [56] | 2020 | RCT | 19 | 42.5 | 89.7 | 44.8 | 56.4 kg | 21.7 | Single session | | Figure of eight | 50 W, 1.5 L | None | Stricture (1) |
| Maselli et al. [57] | 2023 | RC | 284 | 51.3 | 91.9 | 39.3 | - | 33.4 | Single session | | Pursestring | 80W, 1.2L | Persistent vomiting requiring overnight admission (1) | Stricture (11) |

[a]*RC* retrospective cohort, *RCT* randomized controlled trial, *APC* argon plasma coagulation, *Kg* kilograms, *AE* adverse events

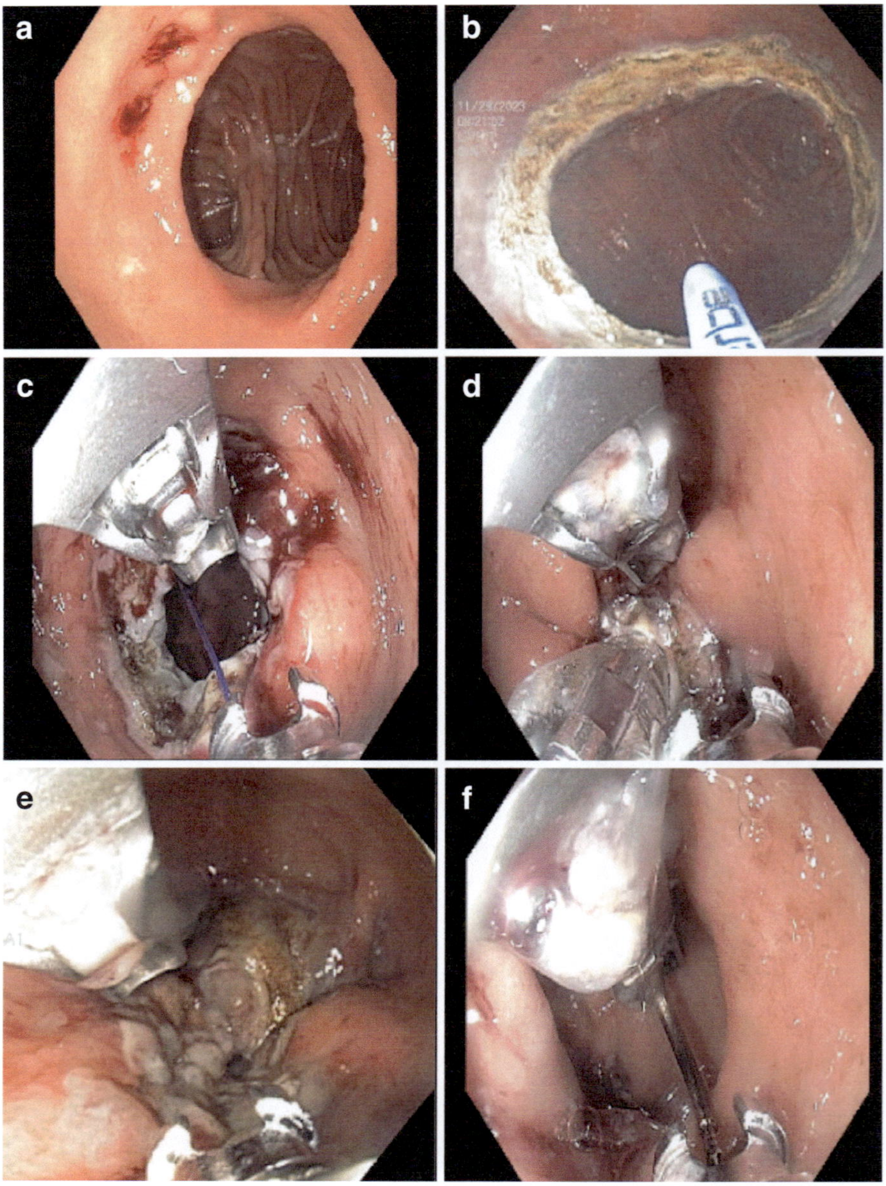

**Fig. 39.1** Full-thickness transoral outlet reduction (TORe) procedure: (**a**) Dilated GJA; (**b**) ablation of the gastric rim via APC; (**c**) suturing the anastomosis with the Overstitch™ system (Boston Scientific, Marlborough, MA, USA); (**d**) sizing of the gastrojejunal anastomosis using an CRE balloon; (**e**) narrowed GJA following TORe (**f**) gastric pouch following gastric pouch reduction

*anastomosis* size on multivariate analysis is an important predictor of weight loss following TORe, and can be useful treatment target [21, 23]. Use of a controlled radial expansion (CRE) balloon allows for accurate sizing of the outlet reduction, while reducing the potential for overtightening which can lead to complications such as a stomal stenosis (Fig. 39.1).

In 2013, a prospective, multicenter, randomized, blinded, sham-controlled trial (RESTORe trial) provided level I evidence for the efficacy of TORe for managing weight regain post-RYGB. This trial included 50 patients. Those undergoing TORe achieved significantly more weight loss (3.5%; 95% CI, 1.8–5.3%) compared to the sham control group (0.4%; 95% CI, 2.3% weight gain to 3.0% weight loss) ($P = 0.021$). 83% of TORe subjects also said they would undergo the procedure again, and 78% said they would recommend the procedure to a friend. The groups had similar rates of adverse events [24]. This trial defined the TORe procedure as a safe and effective alternative procedure to surgical revision.

One limitation of this study was it used a first-generation endoscopic suturing device which obtained only partial-thickness sutures. This device has been superseded by a full-thickness suturing device, which has demonstrated better weight loss outcomes [25], that have steadily improved with time and improvements in technique (Table 39.1).

A subsequent large multicentre international experience and meta-analysis included 130 consecutive patients who underwent FT TORe. Average weight lost at 6, 12, and 18 months after TORe was 9.31 ± 6.7 kg ($N = 84$), 7.75 ± 8.4 kg ($N = 70$), 8 ± 8.8 kg ($N = 46$) ($P < 0.01$ for all three-time points), respectively. The meta-analysis component of the study included 330 patients and the pooled weight lost at 12 months was 8.4 kg (95% CI 6.5–10.3). No serious adverse events occurred [26]. A recent meta-analysis of TORe using the FT TORe technique described above included thirteen studies and 850 patients undergoing 877 TORe procedures. The pooled rate of technical success was 99.89%. The absolute weight loss (kg) at 3, 6, and 12 months was 6.14, 10.15, and 7.14, respectively. Total body weight loss at 3, 6, and 12 months was 6.69%, 11.34%, and 8.55%, respectively. The pooled rate of adverse events was 11.4% with abdominal pain being the most common adverse event [27]. When TORe is implemented as part of a multidisciplinary intervention, it is a safe, reproducible, and effective approach to managing weight recidivism after RYGB and likely should be utilized early in the management algorithm for weight regain.

The durability of the TORe procedure has been questioned and several studies have reported evidence of weight recurrence even at the 12-month mark [20, 28, 29]. While other studies have demonstrated more durable weight loss including one longitudinal 5-year study of 331 patients, that reported 8.5 ± 8.5%, 6.9 ± 10.1%, and 8.8 ± 12.5% total body weight loss at 1, 3, and 5 years, respectively [30]. Weight regain post-TORe, like post-RYGB, is likely multifactorial and driven by a lack of dietary compliance, and genetic and psychological factors. However, technique and suture breakage/migration is likely an important factor, leading to redilation of the GJA and weight regain [28, 31–33]. In a subgroup analysis of a longitudinal study of TORe patients, improved durability was observed with a purse string suture pattern compared to an interrupted suture pattern [29]. In the study described above with 5-year durability, most patients underwent purse string suturing. In addition, to maintain weight loss long-term post TORe 39.3% underwent adjunctive pharmacotherapy and 3.6% ultimately required a repeat full-thickness TORe to address a weight plateaus [30].

Argon plasma coagulation can be applied to the outlet alone to facilitate gastric outlet reduction (APC-TORe). A retrospective cohort study also showed that high-dose APC (70–80 W) compared to low-dose APC (45–55 W) induced higher total body weight loss (10% vs. 5%) [34]. A recent RCT compared the APC TORe to a standard multidisciplinary diet for weight regain and found significantly more weight loss [9.73 kg vs. 1.38 kg], a reduction in the anastomosis diameter ($P < 0.001$), improved early satiation [0.77 vs. −0.59, $P < 0.001$], and improvement of quality of life with APC TORe [35] (Table 39.2).

To address the lack of comparative data between FT TORe and APC TORe, a metanalysis was undertaken comparing the two techniques. It included nine studies of FT TORe ($n = 737$) and 7 of APC-TORe ($n = 888$) studies. APC TORe required a mean of 1.2–3 sessions whereas FT TORe was mostly undertaken in a single session. Percentage total body weight loss was 8.0% (95% CI, 6.3–9.7%), 9.5% (95% CI, 8.1–11.0%), and 5.8% (95% CI, 4.3–7.1%) after FT TORe and 9.0% (95% CI, 4.1–13.9%), 10.2% (95% CI, 8.4–12.1%), and 9.5% (95% CI, 5.7–13.2%) after APC TORe at 3, 6, and 12 months, respectively. There was no difference in weight loss at 3 and 6 months between the two techniques ($P > 0.05$). Stricture formation was the most common AE occurring in 3.3% of patients after FT TORe and 4.8% after APC-TORe ($P = 0.38$). All were successfully treated by endoscopic dilation or conservative *treatment*. Only one severe adverse event occurred (GI bleeding 14 days after the procedure, which was successfully treated endoscopically with epinephrine injection, followed by *intensive care unit* admission for supportive care.) after an APC-TORe. No severe AEs occurred after FT TORe. FT TORe and APC TORe have comparable weight-loss outcomes with an excellent and comparable safety profile, but APC TORe typically requires multiple endoscopic sessions to achieve the same outcome [23].

To enhance weight loss and improve technique durability, several modifications to the TORe technique have been explored. Replacing APC with sclerotic agents such as sodium morrhuate circumferentially around the stoma, to induce fibrosis and decrease stoma size has been proposed [21, 36]. In one study of 28 patients the procedure, the outlet was successfully reduced to <12 mm in 18 of 28 patients (64%). The procedure was repeated up to three times, as required. Only one adverse event occurred, a case of symptomatic stomal stenosis, which was successfully managed with two sessions of balloon dilation [36]. In a further study of 43 patients, 9 underwent a TORe using endoscopic suturing and 34 a TORe with sclerotherapy. Patients had 10.4 ± 2.2% of their total body weight loss following suturing compared to 2.7 ± 5.5% TBW ($P < 0.01$) following sclerotherapy TORe. The diameter of the gastric outlet was also significantly reduced with suturing compared to sclerotherapy [15.0 ± 6.7 mm vs. 2.6 ± 5.7 mm ($P < 0.01$)] [21]. As endoscopic suturing provided greater weight loss, sclerotherapy TORe has not been widely adopted.

In some instances, APC has also been replaced with cryoablation, a technique more commonly used for the eradication of Barrett's or adenomas. The cryoablation balloon is placed at the level of GJA and the outlet is treated circumferentially like

**Table 39.2** APC-TORe outcome

| | Year | Study design | No. | Age (years) | Female (%) | Baseline BMI (kg/m$^2$) | Weight regain | Baseline GJA (mm) | Treatment protocol | No. of sessions | APC | Severe AEs | AEs |
|---|---|---|---|---|---|---|---|---|---|---|---|---|---|
| Fittipaldi-Fernandez et al. [58] | 2015 | RC | 40 | 42.4 | 87.5 | 36.3 | 46.6% | 36.2 | Every 8 weeks until GJA 8-12 mm | 2.4 | 80 W, 2 L then 70 W, 2 L | None | Stricture (1) |
| Moon et al. [59] | 2018 | RC | 558 | 40.9 | 81.5 | 34 | NA | 24.4 | NA | 2 | 70 W, 2 L | None | Of 333 patients: stricture (9), ulcer (3), leakage (2), vomiting (3), bleeding (1) |
| Fittipaldi-Fernandez et al. [58] | 2019 | RCT | 20 | 46.7 | 80.0 | 36.1 | 24.9 kg | 34.3 | Every 8 weeks for 3 sessions | 3 | 90 W, 2.5 L | None | Stricture (1) |
| Fayad et al. [55] | 2019 | RC | 11 | 46.7 | 90.9 | 38.5 | 51.5% | 28.1 | Every 8 week until GJA ≤12 mm | 2.4 | 50 W, 1 L | None | Stricture (1) |
| de Quadros et al. [60] | 2020 | RCT | 22 | 41.0 | 68.2 | 36.4 | 19.5 kg | 21.7 | Every 8 weeks until GJA 10-14 mm or early satiety | 2.4 | 80 W, 1 L | None | None |

| | Year | Study design | No. | Age (years) | Female (%) | Baseline BMI (kg/m$^2$) | Weight regain | Baseline GJA (mm) | Treatment protocol | No. of sessions | APC | Severe AEs | AEs |
|---|---|---|---|---|---|---|---|---|---|---|---|---|---|
| Jirapinyo et al. [30] | 2020 | RC | 217 (116 low APC, 101 high APC) | 48.0 | 89.0 | 36.5 | 41.4% | 17.0 (low APC), 20.8 (high APC) | Every 10-12 weeks until target weight or GJA ≤10 mm | 1.9 | 45-55 W, 0.8 L (low APMC); 70-80 W, 0.8 L (high APC) | None | Stricture (19), bleeding (11), mucosal coagulation (1), esophagitis (1) |
| Brunaldi et al. [56] | 2020 | RCT | 20 | 45.9 | 89.7 | 40.9 | 45.1 kg | 20.3 | Every 6 weeks until GJA ≤12 mm, up to 3 sessions | 1.2 | 50 W, 1.5 L | Bleeding (1) | Stricture (1), prolonged drowsiness after procedure (1), bleeding (1) |

[a] *RC* retrospective cohort, *RCT* randomized controlled trial, *APC* argon plasma coagulation, *Kg* kilograms, *AE* adverse events

with APC. The treatment can also be extended into the gastric pouch, as required. The freeze and thaw treatment is thought to induce a submucosal injury and fibrosis resulting in a significant reduction of both sizes of GJA diameter (24–17 mm, $P < 0.001$) and pouch length (5–4 cm, $P < 0.05$). In an initial cohort study of 22 patients, short-term total body weight loss was 8.1% at two months. However, three severe AEs (13.6%) occurred, one was GJA stenosis requiring endoscopic dilation, and two with bleeding from the treated area requiring transfusion and endoscopic evaluation, although no intervention was performed and patients were discharged on high-dose proton pump inhibitors [32].

Barola et al. described a modification of the TORe technique using a two-fold running suture TORe to improve durability. Although the technique resulted in a significant reduction in BMI (5.5 + 5.0%, $P < 0.001$ at a mean follow-up of 113.2 ± 75.7 days), 15.4% of the patients developed gastric stenosis, although all were managed with balloon dilation [37].

To enhance weight loss and address concerns about the durability of the TORe procedure, recently, some groups have evaluated a modification of the technique to replace APC with endoscopic submucosal dissection (ESD) before applying endoscopic sutures (the ESD-TORe) [33, 38]. A retrospective study compared patients who underwent modified ESD-TORe vs. APC -TORe. At 12 months, the ESD-TORe group experienced greater weight loss compared with the traditional TORe group (12.1 ± 9.3% vs. 7.5 ± 3.3% TBWL). However, this technique resulted in a higher rate of major complications (21.1% for ESD-TORe vs. 8.77% for APC-TORe) [38]. Further studies are needed on this promising technique to evaluate possible concerns with safety and efficacy before widespread adoption. Adoption may also be limited due to local skills and the technical difficulty of ESD.

The majority of TORe studies to date have performed the suturing component with the Overstitch™ endoscopic suturing device (Boston Scientific, Marlborough, MA, USA). Recently two further endoscopic full-thickness tissue approximation devices have been cleared by the U.S. Food and Drug Administration for use; the Incisionless Operating Platform™ (IOP) endoscopic plication device (USGI Medical, San Clemente, Calif, USA) and the endomina™ platform (EndoTools Therapeutics, Belgium). Compared with suturing, which opposes tissue in a mucosa-to-mucosa fashion, plication opposes tissue and is approximated in a serosa-to-serosa fashion. The IOP device has been used to perform a Plication TORe (P-TORe), also known as restorative obesity surgery endoluminal. The IOP consists of four parts: the transport-R (a 54F endoscope with four working channels that can be steered in four directions), the 16-mm g-Prox (for grasping and approximating tissue), the g-Lix (for grasping tissue and pulling it into the jaws of the g-Prox), and the g-Cath (for deploying suture anchors). In 2010, a 9-center observational study of 116 patients who underwent P-TORe for the treatment of weight regain after RYGB. In this registry series, the amount of weight loss was 18% excess weight loss (EWL) in 1 year [39]. Since then, the newer generation of IOP has been introduced, which allows for easier device usage, larger tissue anchor surface areas, and integrated suture cutting. This device was evaluated in a cohort study of 111 RYGB patients who underwent P-TORe. Patients achieved 9.5 ± 8.5% TBWL at 12 months.

Adverse events occurred in 12.6%. These included GJA stenosis (9.9%), melena because of marginal ulceration (1.8%), and deep vein thrombosis (0.9%). P-TORe appears to be technically feasible, safe, and effective at treating weight regain after RYGB, but larger comparative studies and long-term studies are required to fully evaluate this novel technique.

## Combination Therapy

In a study of 145 RYGB patients who underwent combination therapy with TORe and pharmacotherapy (topiramate, phentermine/topiramate, phentermine, or liraglutide), at 12 months, patients experienced 15.2 ± 7.4% total body weight loss. Ninety percent of patients achieved ≥5% TWL at 12 months. Combination therapy was associated with greater weight loss than pharmacotherapy alone (15.2% vs. 6.8%; $P < 0.0001$) or TORe alone (15.2% vs. 8.7%; $P < 0.0001$). Rates of serious adverse events were similar for combination therapy vs. AOM alone vs. TORe alone being 2.1% vs. 4.7% vs. 0.6% ($P > 0.05$). Combination therapy also yielded similar weight loss outcomes to surgical revision (15.2% vs. 16.4% TBWL; $P = 0.34$), with a lower serious adverse event rate (2.1% vs. 14.3%; $P = 0.0004$) [40]. Therefore, in patients with a higher BMI (>50 kg/m$^2$) where enhanced weight loss is needed, or in patients post TORe who encounter a weight loss plateaus combination therapy should be considered.

Type 1 surgical distalization of the Roux limb with biliopancreatic limb elongation offers the best weight loss and nutritional profile option, if surgical revision is being considered post-RYGB [41]. Combining TORe with distalization of the Roux limb has been explored in a case report of a morbidly obese patient. They achieved 17.3% of total body weight loss 6 months post-TORe and 4 months after distalization. They encountered no adverse events. Further studies are needed to evaluate this technique for weight regain post-RYGB in higher BMI patients [42].

## Sleeve Gastrectomy

Weight regain after laparoscopic sleeve gastrectomy affects up to 2/3 of patients over time. The gastric sleeve may dilate, and the size of the gastric sleeve is linearly correlated with post-operative BMI [43, 44]. Over time, the natural history of the sleeve is that it will dilate. It is hypothesized that the increase in the size of the sleeve will reduce the restrictive effect of the procedure allowing patients to consume a larger volume of calories and regain weight. Health practitioners typically assess for sleeve dilation with an upper gastrointestinal endoscopy and radiographic upper gastrointestinal series. The most common surgical solution for this problem is conversion to RYGB or a repeat sleeve gastrectomy, so-called "re-sleeving" to reduce the gastric reservoir using surgical staplers. Conversion to an RYGB does lead to a satisfactory return to weight loss [45]. However, revisional surgery post laparoscopic sleeve is associated with a higher rate of adverse events, seen in 15%

of patients [46]. Minimally invasive endoscopic approaches have therefore been explored as an alternative.

## Endoscopic Revision Post Gastric Sleeve

Endoscopic revision of the sleeve is an alternative to a surgical "resleeve" or conversion to RYGB. In 2017 the first series of five patients was published, showing the efficacy of Endoscopic Sleeve Gastrectomy (ESG) after Sleeve Gastrectomy [47]. The procedure is analogous to the one performed for primary weight loss. The ESG is typically performed with the Overstitch™ endoscopic suturing device (Boston Scientific, Marlborough, MA, USA). Lines of full-thickness endoscopic sutures begin at the incisura on the anterior wall of the sleeve, with subsequent bites progressing along the greater curvature and over the staple line to the posterior wall and potentially returning to the anterior wall in a "U shaped" pattern. Approximately 6–10 bites per suture are performed (Fig. 39.2). In a retrospective study of 34 patients who successfully underwent ESG following sleeve gastrectomy, technical success was 100% with a TBWL of greater than 10% at 1 year in 82.4% of patients [48]. A larger prospective multicenter study of 82 patients with weight regain after sleeve gastrectomy reported a TBWL of 15.7% at 12 months. Only one moderate AE occurred, a stricture at the level of the gastroesophageal junction, managed with a single session of endoscopic dilation [49]. Revision ESG is a safe and effective means of managing weight recidivism after sleeve gastrectomy, with sustained weight loss for up to 1 year. This is a good option for patients who do not want to consider more invasive surgical revisional options.

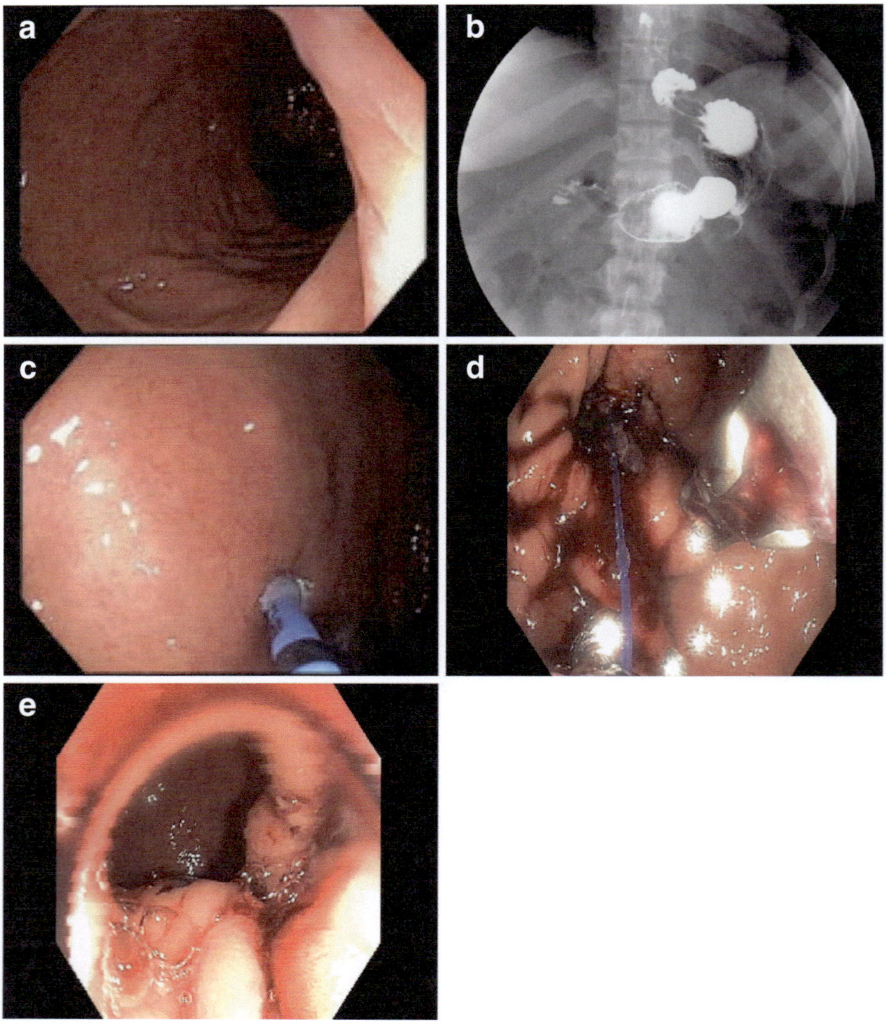


**Fig. 39.2** Endoscopic sleeve gastroplasty post laparoscopic sleeve gastrectomy (**a**) Dilated sleeve during endoscopy; (**b**) Dilated sleeve on UGIS (**c**) Marking of the sleeve with APC (**d**) suturing the anastomosis with the Overstitch™ system (Boston Scientific, Marlborough, MA, USA); (**e**) endoscopic view post revision sleeve

## Conclusion

Weight recurrence may occur in up to one-third of patients after bariatric surgery and etiology is multifactorial. Revisional surgery is associated with higher rates of morbidity than primary procedures. Minimally invasive endoscopic approaches are effective for weight loss, are reproducible, and are associated with lower rates of adverse events.

## References


1. Chooi YC, Ding C, Magkos F. The epidemiology of obesity. Metabolism. 2019;92:6–10.
2. Finucane MM, et al. National, regional, and global trends in body-mass index since 1980: systematic analysis of health examination surveys and epidemiological studies with 960 country-years and 9.1 million participants. Lancet. 2011;377(9765):557–67.
3. Sjostrom L, et al. Lifestyle, diabetes, and cardiovascular risk factors 10 years after bariatric surgery. N Engl J Med. 2004;351(26):2683–93.
4. Pope GD, et al. Life expectancy benefits of gastric bypass surgery. Surg Innov. 2006;13(4):265–73.
5. Adams TD, et al. Long-term mortality after gastric bypass surgery. N Engl J Med. 2007;357(8):753–61.
6. Buchwald H, et al. Bariatric surgery: a systematic review and meta-analysis. JAMA. 2004;292(14):1724–37.
7. Tran DD, et al. Revision of Roux-En-Y gastric bypass for weight regain: a systematic review of techniques and outcomes. Obes Surg. 2016;26(7):1627–34.
8. King WC, et al. Comparison of the performance of common measures of weight regain after bariatric surgery for association with clinical outcomes. JAMA. 2018;320(15):1560–9.
9. Monaco-Ferreira DV, Leandro-Merhi VA. Weight regain 10 years after Roux-en-Y gastric bypass. Obes Surg. 2017;27(5):1137–44.
10. Karmali S, et al. Weight recidivism post-bariatric surgery: a systematic review. Obes Surg. 2013;23(11):1922–33.
11. Adams TD, Davidson LE, Hunt SC. Weight and metabolic outcomes 12 years after gastric bypass. N Engl J Med. 2018;378(1):93–6.
12. Sjostrom CD, et al. Reduction in incidence of diabetes, hypertension and lipid disturbances after intentional weight loss induced by bariatric surgery: the SOS Intervention Study. Obes Res. 1999;7(5):477–84.
13. Abu Dayyeh BK, Lautz DB, Thompson CC. Gastrojejunal stoma diameter predicts weight regain after Roux-en-Y gastric bypass. Clin Gastroenterol Hepatol. 2011;9(3):228–33.
14. Heneghan HM, et al. Influence of pouch and stoma size on weight loss after gastric bypass. Surg Obes Relat Dis. 2012;8(4):408–15.
15. Yimcharoen P, et al. Endoscopic findings and outcomes of revisional procedures for patients with weight recidivism after gastric bypass. Surg Endosc. 2011;25(10):3345–52.
16. Surgery, A.S.f.M.a.B., Estimate of Bariatric Surgery Numbers, 2011–2021.
17. Brethauer SA, et al. Systematic review on reoperative bariatric surgery: American Society for Metabolic and Bariatric Surgery Revision Task Force. Surg Obes Relat Dis. 2014;10(5):952–72.
18. Abu Dayyeh BK, Jirapinyo P, Thompson CC. Plasma Ghrelin levels and weight regain after Roux-en-Y gastric bypass surgery. Obes Surg. 2017;27(4):1031–6.
19. Barrichello S, et al. Increased gastric retention capacity, assessed by scintigraphy, after APC treatment of dilated gastrojejunal anastomosis. GE Port J Gastroenterol. 2018;25(6):327–30.
20. Brunaldi VO, et al. Endoscopic treatment of weight regain following Roux-en-Y gastric bypass: a systematic review and meta-analysis. Obes Surg. 2018;28(1):266–76.
21. Jirapinyo P, Dayyeh BK, Thompson CC. Gastrojejunal anastomotic reduction for weight regain in Roux-en-y gastric bypass patients: physiological, behavioral, and anatomical effects of endoscopic suturing and sclerotherapy. Surg Obes Relat Dis. 2016;12(10):1810–6.
22. Jirapinyo P, et al. Evaluation of an endoscopic suturing device for transoral outlet reduction in patients with weight regain following Roux-en-Y gastric bypass. Endoscopy. 2013;45(7):532–6.
23. Jaruvongvanich V, et al. Endoscopic full-thickness suturing plus argon plasma mucosal coagulation versus argon plasma mucosal coagulation alone for weight regain after gastric bypass: a systematic review and meta-analysis. Gastrointest Endosc. 2020;92(6):1164–75.
24. Thompson CC, et al. Endoscopic suturing for transoral outlet reduction increases weight loss after Roux-en-Y gastric bypass surgery. Gastroenterology. 2013;145(1):129–137 e3.

25. Kumar N, Thompson CC. Comparison of a superficial suturing device with a full-thickness suturing device for transoral outlet reduction (with videos). Gastrointest Endosc. 2014;79(6):984–9.
26. Vargas EJ, et al. Transoral outlet reduction with full thickness endoscopic suturing for weight regain after gastric bypass: a large multicenter international experience and meta-analysis. Surg Endosc. 2018;32(1):252–9.
27. Dhindsa BS, et al. Efficacy of transoral outlet reduction in Roux-en-Y gastric bypass patients to promote weight loss: a systematic review and meta-analysis. Endosc Int Open. 2020;8(10):E1332–40.
28. Tsai C, et al. Endoscopic Gastrojejunal Revisions Following Gastric Bypass: Lessons Learned in More Than 100 Consecutive Patients. J Gastrointest Surg. 2019;23(1):58–66.
29. Callahan ZM, et al. Five-year results of endoscopic gastrojejunostomy revision (transoral outlet reduction) for weight gain after gastric bypass. Surg Endosc. 2020;34(5):2164–71.
30. Jirapinyo P, et al. Five-year outcomes of transoral outlet reduction for the treatment of weight regain after Roux-en-Y gastric bypass. Gastrointest Endosc. 2020;91(5):1067–73.
31. Espinet Coll E, et al. Efficacy and safety of transoral outlet reduction via endoscopic suturing in patients with weight regain after a surgical Roux-en-Y gastric bypass. Rev Esp Enferm Dig. 2018;110(9):551–6.
32. Fayad L, et al. Cryoballoon ablation for gastric pouch and/or outlet reduction in patients with weight regain post Roux-en-Y gastric bypass. Endoscopy. 2020;52(3):227–30.
33. Hollenbach M, et al. Endoscopic full-thickness transoral outlet reduction with semicircumferential endoscopic submucosal dissection. Endoscopy. 2019;51(7):684–8.
34. Jirapinyo P, et al. Dose response for argon plasma coagulation in the treatment of weight regain after Roux-en-Y gastric bypass. Gastrointest Endosc. 2020;91(5):1078–84.
35. de Quadros LG, et al. Endoscopic Argon Plasma Coagulation vs. Multidisciplinary Evaluation in the Management of Weight Regain After Gastric Bypass Surgery: a Randomized Controlled Trial with SHAM Group. Obes Surg. 2020;30(5):1904–16.
36. Catalano MF, et al. Weight gain after bariatric surgery as a result of a large gastric stoma: endotherapy with sodium morrhuate may prevent the need for surgical revision. Gastrointest Endosc. 2007;66(2):240–5.
37. Barola S, et al. Demonstration of transoral gastric outlet reduction: 2-fold running suture technique. VideoGIE. 2017;2(1):2–3.
38. Jirapinyo P, de Moura DTH, Thompson CC. Endoscopic submucosal dissection with suturing for the treatment of weight regain after gastric bypass: outcomes and comparison with traditional transoral outlet reduction (with video). Gastrointest Endosc. 2020;91(6):1282–8.
39. Horgan S, et al. Incisionless revision of post-Roux-en-Y bypass stomal and pouch dilation: multicenter registry results. Surg Obes Relat Dis. 2010;6(3):290–5.
40. Jirapinyo P, Thompson CC. Combining transoral outlet reduction with pharmacotherapy yields similar 1-year efficacy with improved safety compared with surgical revision for weight regain after Roux-en-Y gastric bypass (with videos). Gastrointest Endosc. 2023;98(4):552–8.
41. Hamed H, Ali M, Elmahdy Y. Types, safety, and efficacy of limb distalization for inadequate weight loss after Roux-en-Y Gastric bypass: a systematic review and meta-analysis with a call for standardized terminology. Ann Surg. 2021;274(2):271–80.
42. Abu Dayyeh B, et al. A novel approach for weight regain after Roux-en-Y gastric bypass: Staged transoral outlet reduction (TORe) followed by surgical type 1 distalization. VideoGIE. 2022;7(4):135–7.
43. Weiner RA, et al. Laparoscopic sleeve gastrectomy—influence of sleeve size and resected gastric volume. Obes Surg. 2007;17(10):1297–305.
44. Braghetto I, et al. Evaluation of the radiological gastric capacity and evolution of the BMI 2-3 years after sleeve gastrectomy. Obes Surg. 2009;19(9):1262–9.
45. Langer FB, et al. Conversion from sleeve gastrectomy to Roux-en-Y gastric bypass—indications and outcome. Obes Surg. 2010;20(7):835–40.

46. Lee Y, et al. Single- or double-anastomosis duodenal switch versus Roux-en-Y gastric bypass as a revisional procedure for sleeve gastrectomy: a systematic review and meta-analysis. Surg Obes Relat Dis. 2019;15(4):556–66.
47. Eid G. Sleeve gastrectomy revision by endoluminal sleeve plication gastroplasty: a small pilot case series. Surg Endosc. 2017;31(10):4252–5.
48. de Moura DTH, et al. Endoscopic sleeve gastroplasty in the management of weight regain after sleeve gastrectomy. Endoscopy. 2020;52(3):202–10.
49. Maselli DB, et al. Revisional endoscopic sleeve gastroplasty of laparoscopic sleeve gastrectomy: an international, multicenter study. Gastrointest Endosc. 2021;93(1):122–30.
50. Goyal D, et al. Mo1950 combined endoscopic Trans-Oral Outlet Reduction With Gastroplasty (TORe-G) produces robust weight loss in patients with Roux-en-Y Gastric Bypass (RYGB) failure. Gastroenterology. 2016;150(4 Suppl. 1):S825.
51. Watson RR, et al. Sa2003 Comparison of Transoral Outlet Reduction (TORE) Alone Versus Tore With Gastroplasty (Tore-G): a matched cohort analysis. Gastrointest Endosc. 2017;85(Suppl. 5):AB271-AB272.
52. Staudenmann D, et al. Transoral outlet reduction (TORe) partially reverses weight regain after bariatric Roux-en-Y gastric bypass (RYGB). First clinical experience from a tertiary referral center. In: Swiss medical weekly. Muttenz, Switzerland: Emh Swiss Medical Publishers Ltd; 2017.
53. Vargas EJ, et al. Su2039—transoral oulet reduction with full thickness endoscopic suturing for weight regain after gastric bypass: a large multicenter international experience and meta-analysis. Gastroenterology. 2017;152(5 Suppl. 1):S637.
54. Espinet-Coll E, et al. Efficacy and safety of transoral outlet reduction via endoscopic suturing in patients with weight regain after a surgical Roux-en-Y gastric bypass. Rev Espanola Enferm Digest (REED). 2018;110(9):551–7.
55. Fayad L, et al. A real-world, insurance-based algorithm using the two-fold running suture technique for transoral outlet reduction for weight regain and dumping syndrome after Roux-En-Y gastric bypass. Obesity Surg. 2019;29:2225–32.
56. Brunaldi V, et al. Argon plasma coagulation alone versus endoscopic suturing plus argon plasma coagulation to treat weight regain after Roux-en-Y gastric bypass: a prospective randomized trial (with videos). Gastrointest Endosc. 2020;92:97–107.
57. Maselli DB, et al. Transoral outlet reduction: outcomes of endoscopic Roux-en-Y gastric bypass revision in 284 patients at a community practice. World J Gastrointest Endosc. 2023;15(10):602–13.
58. Fittipaldi-Fernandez RJ, Diestel CF. Tu1471 a new approach in the treatment of weight regain after bariatric surgery: the argon plasma coagulation of the anastomosis. Gastroenterology. 2015;148(4):S-901.
59. Moon RC, et al. Efficacy of utilizing argon plasma coagulation for weight regain in Roux-en-Y gastric bypass patients: a multi-center study. Obesity Surg. 2018;28:2737–44.
60. de Quadros LG, et al. Endoscopic argon plasma coagulation vs. multidisciplinary evaluation in the management of weight regain after gastric bypass surgery: a randomized controlled trial with SHAM group. Obesity Surg. 2020;30:1904–16.

# Revisions and Conversions After Adjustable Gastric Band

**40**

Tanyaradzwa M. Kajese, Luke S. Crawford, Erik B. Wilson, and Shinil K. Shah

## Introduction

Once a very popular surgery for the treatment of obesity, the laparoscopic adjustable gastric band (LAGB) has declined in popularity in recent years. In 2021, the LAGB made up only 0.43% of all bariatric surgical procedures performed in the United States [1]. While it was regarded as a safe and technically straight-forward procedure, LAGB placement is associated with several complications. These include gastric band slippage, pouch dilation, port or tubing malfunction, band erosion, stomal obstruction, and/or port infection [2]. Furthermore, the LAGB has shown to have inferior results in regards to overall weight loss and subsequent weight recurrence when compared to other bariatric surgical procedures [3]. Revisions or conversions are often required because of these outcomes. The focus of this chapter is to review the types of revisions and conversions that are typically employed to treat complications of LAGB placement as well as weight recidivism.

T. M. Kajese · L. S. Crawford · E. B. Wilson
Division of Minimally Invasive and Elective General Surgery, Department of Surgery, McGovern Medical School at UT Health, Houston, TX, USA

S. K. Shah (✉)
Division of Minimally Invasive and Elective General Surgery, Department of Surgery, McGovern Medical School at UT Health, Houston, TX, USA

Michael E. DeBakey Institute for Comparative Cardiovascular Science and Biomedical Devices, Texas A&M University, College Station, TX, USA
e-mail: shinil.k.shah@uth.tmc.edu


O. M. Ghanem et al. (eds.), *The SAGES Manual of Metabolic and Bariatric Surgery*, https://doi.org/10.1007/978-3-031-72309-4_40

## Revisions

Reoperations in bariatric surgery are not uncommon. The type of re-operative surgery is categorized based on the anatomic modifications that are performed at the time of the re-operation. In the case of revisions, the basic anatomy of the primary surgery is maintained. These are usually employed in the case of chronic complications of an initially effective primary procedure [4]. For the LAGB, revisions include band repositioning and band replacement. These revisional approaches should only be considered in patients with adequate primary weight loss who are now experiencing a band complication. Conversely, for LAGB patients who experience inadequate initial weight loss, the optimal treatment option is conversion to another bariatric/metabolic procedure.

Revisions of the LAGB may be considered straightforward reoperations. However, a high incidence of morbidity has been reported in this particular patient population. Up to two-thirds of the patients undergoing revision will experience additional complications, such as recurrent prolapse, erosion, or failure of weight loss. Eventually, the majority of patients who undergo revision of their LAGB will require conversion [5].

## Band Repositioning

When a LAGB has been in position for an extended period, certain conditions may occur that ultimately require repositioning in order to help a patient resume or maintain successful weight loss. Each component of the LAGB can potentially require revision. The band encircling the proximal stomach may slip, and this can result in gastric prolapse. The intraabdominal tubing can develop adhesions, resulting in potential bowel obstruction. Furthermore, when significant weight loss occurs, the subcutaneous port can flip or turn on its axis. This makes port access difficult or no longer possible for band adjustments. The port can also protrude more, thus resulting in pain.

When a slip occurs, it can result in gastric prolapse which may cause symptoms of gastric outlet obstruction (nausea, vomiting, dysphagia, odynophagia or gastroesophageal reflux). Band repositioning at the proximal stomach can be performed laparoscopically. With this minimally invasive approach, the previously placed gastro-gastric plication stitches are removed. The band can then be unbuckled and opened. This will allow for a reduction of the gastric prolapse and confirmation of the viability of the stomach. The band is repositioned in its proper anatomical position approximately 2 cm distal to the gastroesophageal junction. The gastro-gastric plication stitches can then be replaced with the use of 2-0 permanent sutures to approximate the distal fundus of the stomach to the superiorly located gastric pouch. These plication stitches will create a protective tunnel for the anterior, left-lateral aspect of the band, and should be placed without tension. It is important to ensure that the buckle is not covered by these imbrication sutures [6].

On rare occasions, the LAGB tubing can result in intraabdominal adhesions that cause a small bowel obstruction [7]. Abdominal imaging will assist with this diagnosis. A laparoscopic approach is recommended to perform the exploration. However, if there is significant bowel dilation, an open approach may need to be employed to avoid bowel injury with laparoscopic entry. As in the case of any surgery for adhesive small bowel obstruction, the small intestine should be examined initially from the distal ileocecum, with the surgeon running the bowel proximally until the transition zone is identified. This is recognized by the site where the small intestine changes caliber (normal/decompressed to dilated). The adhesions are released from the involved LAGB tubing. The tubing is then repositioned in a new location, free from previous scar tissue.

The final component of the LAGB that may require repositioning is the port. Traditionally, the LAGB port is sutured to the anterior fascia of the abdominal wall using non-absorbable sutures [8]. On occasion, this subcutaneous port can flip or migrate under the skin, making needle access for band adjustment difficult or impossible. Furthermore, as patients lose significant weight, the overlying subcutaneous adipose tissue shrinks. This may cause the previously buried port to protrude and cause pain. These two scenarios may require repositioning of the port. This intervention generally does not require intraabdominal access. A superficial skin incision is created over the prior port incision. The port is identified and the overlying scar capsule is removed. The port is then repositioned appropriately on the anterior abdominal wall in a nearby site and secured in position to the rectus sheath fascia with interrupted non-absorbable stitches.

## Band Replacement

Certain scenarios can occur with a LAGB which may require band replacement to help a patient resume successful weight loss/maintenance of weight loss. These include band infection and/or erosion, or a leak in any component of the device. Infection is identified by overlying skin changes such as erythema, port dehiscence, or purulent drainage. Any presumed infection should be considered a band erosion until proven otherwise. Band erosion is generally diagnosed with endoscopic evaluation or cross-sectional imaging of the abdomen. In addition to infection at the subcutaneous port site, patients with band erosion may present with symptoms of gastric outlet obstruction. A leak is identified when serial band fills do not result in any restriction, or when the amount of saline infused into the port cannot be aspirated back out.

LAGB replacement includes both an intraabdominal approach and a superficial approach to ensure that all components of the previously placed LAGB are removed prior to placing the new device. The underlying subcutaneous port must be removed and the tubing is cut at the level of the anterior abdominal wall. Laparoscopically, the intraabdominal tubing and band encircling the stomach are then removed. The previously placed gastro-gastric plication stitches must be released, and the underlying scar tissue (cicatrix) should be transected and released as well. If the cicatrix is left in place, patients may continue to experience symptoms of gastric outlet obstruction. When placing the new LAGB, the pars flaccida technique is generally employed. The new LAGB is placed superior to the left gastric artery and caudal to the gastroesophageal junction. The buckle is locked anteriorly. Gastro-gastric plication stitches are placed between the distal fundus of the stomach and the superiorly located gastric pouch. The free end of the tubing is then externalized and connected to the port without tension. The port is then sutured to the anterior fascia with non-absorbable sutures [6]. The LAGB is then tested with a fill using a non-coring needle to rule out any sites of leak or device malfunction.

It should be noted that in the cases of band erosion and/or infection, replacement with a new band should be conducted in a staged procedure after the removal of and band and all components. Band replacement typically should be delayed until 6 weeks after the band removal. This allows time for gastric healing from the erosion and/or clearance of the infectious process prior to placing a new LAGB device. Depending on the patient's symptoms and or duration of symptoms, the surgeon should consider testing for esophageal dysfunction and or gastric emptying delay prior to replacing a LAGB.

## Conversions

When discussing re-operative bariatric surgery, conversions refer to procedures where the structural anatomy of the primary operation is changed to a different type of operation. Conversions are typically required when there has been inadequate weight loss or weight recidivism. They are also utilized in scenarios where a post-operative complication arises that is directly associated with the underlying anatomy of the primary surgery [4]. In the case of LAGB, conversions refer to removal of the LAGB device with subsequent vertical sleeve gastrectomy (SG), Roux-en-Y gastric bypass (RYGB), duodenal switch (DS), or single anastomosis duodenoileal bypass with sleeve gastrectomy (SADI-S). Conversion to one anastomosis gastric bypass can also be performed. The details of this operation are covered in Chap. 24.

Several factors to consider when choosing the type of LAGB conversion for a potential patient include weight loss associated with the LAGB, patient body mass index and weight loss goals, potential complications, comorbidities, anatomy and patient preference. For those patients who are undergoing conversion for weight recurrence, an operation that includes a hypoabsorptive mechanism such as the RYGB, DS or SADI-S will likely have superior weight loss results as compared to SG. A systematic review compared the conversion of LAGB to SG, RYGB and DS in terms of excess weight loss with results of 35.5%, 48.2%, and 78.4% respectively [9]. Potential complications should be considered and vary between the three procedures. All three have a risk of staple line or anastomotic leak; however, the RYGB and DS/SADI-S have a higher risk of nutritional deficiencies and internal hernias, while the RYGB has an additional higher risk of marginal ulcers. Patients with severe gastroesophageal reflux, pseudo-achalasia or other motility disorders of the esophagus may be poor candidates for conversion to an SG. Conversions due to a prior eroded LAGB should not be converted to an SG. Conversion to RYGB should be avoided in patients who chronically take NSAIDS, are current smokers or are likely to relapse due to the risk of marginal ulcers and subsequent bleeding, obstruction, and/or perforation. Finally, patients may favor one conversion to others based on history of complications from prior surgery, anecdotal evidence from family members or friends, and/or personal research. All of these factors play a significant role and should be considered when counseling patients on their conversion/revision options.

There is continued debate if a one-stage or two-stage LAGB conversion should be performed. A recent meta-analysis of LAGB conversions did not show a statistically significant difference in leak rate between one or two-staged conversions and reported an overall leak rate of 1.95% [10]. Advocates of a one-stage procedure argue that it is more advantageous for the patient as only one surgery is required and interval weight regain between procedures is avoided [10]. Variability in insurance coverage is another important factor to consider. Most insurance providers cover a second weight-loss procedure due to a complication from the index operation, but a smaller number cover an additional procedure to due weight recurrence [11]. Additionally, gastro-gastric plication may not be as easily identified in an operative field that has already been operated on twice before [12]. Those supporting a two-stage conversion note that inflammation of the gastric tissue will have time to decrease, resulting in a decreased risk of staple line leak, especially in patients being converted to SG. Additionally, it is theorized that improved vascularization of previously fibrotic areas of stomach may result in a more robust perfusion of the anastomosis in the setting of an RYGB [10]. In situations where the band has significantly slipped or is associated with gastric ischemia, a two-stage procedure may allow the stomach to convert back to a more anatomically correct and/or perfused state.

Upper endoscopy should be considered prior to proceeding to LAGB conversion to assess for band erosion, esophagitis and the presence of a hiatal hernia. Esophageal manometry may be obtained when considering converting to SG, DS, or SADI-S, especially when patient history suggests an esophageal motility disorder or if there are concerns for pseudo-achalasia. This is to assess for possible esophageal motility disorders, which may dissuade the surgeon from SG.

## Conversion to Sleeve Gastrectomy

After laparoscopic or robotic ports are placed, an internal or external liver retractor can be utilized to help facilitate exposure. Once visualization is optimized, the LAGB is removed in the same fashion as noted previously in this chapter. It is essential to restore normal anatomy by releasing the gastro-gastric plication and performing an excision of the cicatrix of the greater curvature of the stomach and the angle of His. At this point, if a hiatal hernia was noted on preoperative endoscopy or seen intra-operatively, it is repaired. The greater omentum is taken down off the greater curvature of the stomach beginning four to six centimeters proximal to the pylorus and carried cranially to the left crus. Once completed, a sizing tube (bougie) of the surgeon's choice is inserted and used to stent the lesser curve of the stomach. Stapled division of the stomach is performed using the surgeon's preferred stapler with or without staple line reinforcement. It is important to note that the staple line will invariably cross the site of the prior gastric band. Thus, proper excision of the cicatrix will decrease the risk of having inappropriate staple height and decrease the risk of bleeding and leak [13]. Upper endoscopy with a leak test can subsequently be performed to evaluate the new sleeve anatomy.

## Conversion to Roux-en-Y Gastric Bypass

After ports are placed, an internal or external liver retractor can be utilized to help facilitate exposure. Once the visualization is optimized, the LAGB is removed. Similar to conversion to SG, hiatal hernias can then be repaired if indicated, and normal anatomy is restored by taking down the gastric plication sutures and excising the cicatrix. The pars flaccida is then incised and the vessels adjacent to the lesser curve are divided using a vascular staple load/energy device. Alternatively, a peri-gastric approach may be utilized based on the surgeon's preference. The dissection is continued posteriorly until the posterior attachments to the stomach are all divided to the angle of His. The gastric pouch is then created using multiple staple cartridges with or without staple line reinforcement. The size of the gastric pouch is determined by surgeon preference and is often created with the use of a bougie or sizing tube. Depending on the surgeon's technique and minimally invasive approach, the jejunojejunostomy and gastrojejunostomy are constructed. An upper endoscopy with a leak test can then be performed to evaluate the gastric pouch and gastrojejunostomy.

## Conversion to Duodenal Switch or Single Anastomosis Duodenoileal Bypass with Sleeve Gastrectomy

Both the traditional DS and SADI-S have the same initial steps (sleeve gastrectomy). As mentioned in the prior section, after port placement and internal/external liver retraction, the LAGB device is removed (including the takedown of the gastric plication and dissection and excision of the cicatrix), hiatal hernia is identified and repaired if indicated, and an SG is then performed, utilizing the same operative technique as aforementioned in this chapter. The distal stomach is then further mobilized to the first portion of the duodenum. The duodenum is then circumferentially mobilized at this location. The duodenum is then transected 2 cm distal to the pylorus. Either a traditional DS or SADI-S is then performed, techniques of which are discussed in Chaps. 22 and 23, respectively. Upper endoscopy with a leak test can then be performed to assess the anatomy and anastomosis.

## Conclusion

The LAGB is a weight-loss procedure that has declined in popularity, largely secondary to long-term weight loss/weight recidivism as well as complications such as slip and erosion. Patients with an LAGB require an individualized surgical approach based on complications, anatomy, associated medical comorbidities, body mass index, weight-loss goals, and personal preferences. Surgeons who take care of patients with LAGBs should be aware of the variety of options and techniques when approaching revisions, replacement and conversions in patients who have undergone prior LAGB.

## References


1. ASMBS. Estimate of Bariatric Surgery Numbers, 2011–2021. https://asmbs.org/resources/estimate-of-bariatric-surgery-numbers. Published 2022. Accessed November 5, 2023.
2. Kodner C, Hartman DR. Complications of adjustable gastric banding surgery for obesity. Am Fam Physician. 2014;89(10):813–8.
3. O'Brien PE, Hindle A, Brennan L, et al. Long-term outcomes after bariatric surgery: a systematic review and meta-analysis of weight loss at 10 or more years for all bariatric procedures and a single-centre review of 20-year outcomes after adjustable gastric banding. Obes Surg. 2019;29(1):3–14.
4. Aleman R, Menzo EL, Szomstein S, Rosenthal RJ. Reoperative bariatric surgery. In: Nguyen NT, Brethauer SA, Morton JM, Ponce J, Rosenthal RJ, editors. The ASMBS textbook of bariatric surgery. Cham: Springer International Publishing; 2020. p. 265–80.
5. Patel S, Eckstein J, Acholonu E, Abu-Jaish W, Szomstein S, Rosenthal RJ. Reasons and outcomes of laparoscopic revisional surgery after laparoscopic adjustable gastric banding for morbid obesity. Surg Obes Relat Dis. 2010;6(4):391–8.
6. Seeras K, Acho RJ, Prakash S. Laparoscopic gastric band placement. StatPearls Publishing; 2023. StatPearls Web site. https://www.ncbi.nlm.nih.gov/books/NBK526062/. Published 2023. Updated 2023 Jan 19. Accessed November 5, 2023
7. Suter KJ, Rajasagaram N, Nottle P. Gastric band connection tube results in small bowel obstruction: an acute emergency. J Surg Case Rep. 2016;2016(5)
8. Akkary E, Olgers F. Subcutaneous placement of lap band port without fascial fixation provides safe and durable access. Obes Surg. 2014;24(11):1987–91.
9. Elnahas A, Graybiel K, Farrokhyar F, Gmora S, Anvari M, Hong D. Revisional surgery after failed laparoscopic adjustable gastric banding: a systematic review. Surg Endosc. 2013;27(3):740–5.
10. Zadeh J, Le C, Ben-David K. Safety of adjustable gastric band conversion surgery: a systematic review and meta-analysis of the leak rate in 1- and 2-stage procedures. Surg Obes Relat Dis. 2020;16(3):437–44.
11. Gebran SG, Knighton B, Ngaage LM, et al. Insurance coverage criteria for bariatric surgery: a survey of policies. Obes Surg. 2020;30(2):707–13.
12. Spaniolas K, Yang J, Zhu C, et al. Conversion of adjustable gastric banding to stapling bariatric procedures: single- or two-stage approach. Ann Surg. 2021;273(3):542–7.
13. Gangemi A, Russel S, Patel K, Khalaf H, Masrur M, Hassan C. Conversion to laparoscopic sleeve gastrectomy after failure of laparoscopic gastric band: a systematic review of the literature and cost considerations. Obes Res Clin Pract. 2018;12(5):416–20.

# 41 Weight Recurrence After Sleeve Gastrectomy

Abdulaziz Karam Ali and Amin Andalib

## Introduction

In the realm of revisional bariatric surgery, insufficient weight loss (IWL) has emerged as a significant factor for revision after primary procedures [1–4]. A recent national data analysis conducted by Ghanem and colleagues revealed that IWL and weight recurrence (WR) were the primary reasons for revisional surgeries after sleeve gastrectomy (SG) followed by gastroesophageal reflux disease (GERD) [5]. IWL not only diminishes a patient's quality of life but can also lead to the recurrence of associated comorbidities, subsequently driving up medical costs [6, 7].

Revisional surgery following SG can be challenging and complex at times and requires advanced skills and expertise from surgeons. Moreover, these challenges have also sparked an increased exploration of non-surgical interventions as viable alternatives. Despite these options, the demand for surgical expertise remains paramount [8]. Therefore, a comprehensive understanding of both surgical and non-surgical approaches is essential to navigate the intricate landscape of revisional bariatric procedures.

It is important to clarify that until now, there have been no universally agreed-upon definitions for IWL or a clinically important WR. Furthermore, there is no established standard timeframe for assessing such weight outcomes after surgery, mainly because comprehensive large-scale studies in this field are scarce. The prevalence of poor weight outcomes varies considerably in existing literature, primarily due to the diverse definitions employed [9, 10].

A. K. Ali
Bariatric/MIS Fellow, Department of Surgery, McGill University, Montreal, QC, Canada

A. Andalib (✉)
Centre for Bariatric Surgery, Department of Surgery, McGill University, Montreal, QC, Canada
e-mail: amin.andalib@mcgill.ca



O. M. Ghanem et al. (eds.), *The SAGES Manual of Metabolic and Bariatric Surgery*, https://doi.org/10.1007/978-3-031-72309-4_41

## Nomenclature for Poor Weight Outcomes after Bariatric Surgery [11]

As previously mentioned, there are no universally agreed-upon definitions for IWL or clinically important WR. In addition, there is no clear standard timeframe for assessing such weight outcomes after surgery. It is more convenient to begin by defining successful weight loss after bariatric surgery. In most studies, achieving greater than 50% excess weight loss (EWL) in the first 2 years after surgery is considered a successful surgical outcome [12, 13]. After SG, successful weight loss can also be measured using the bariatric Analysis and Reporting Outcome System (BAROS) score higher than three points. The BAROS score is a comprehensive measure that considers factors such as resolution of comorbidities, percentage EWL, Moorehead-Ardelt quality of life score, and the presence of any postoperative complications or repeat surgeries [14].

It is crucial to identify the two types of poor weight outcomes after bariatric surgery along with the most commonly recognized definitions [11]:

- *Insufficient weight loss*: defined as EWL < 50% 18–24 months after bariatric surgery.
- *Weight recurrence*: defined as progressive weight regain (≥20%) that occurs after the achievement of an initially successful weight loss (defined as EWL > 50%).

## Nomenclature for Revisional Bariatric Surgery [15]

- Conversion surgery: Procedures that change from an index procedure to a different type of procedure.
- Corrective surgery: Procedures addressing complications or incomplete treatment effects of a previous bariatric operation.
- Reversal surgery: Procedures that restore original anatomy. This is not applicable to SG.

## Prevalence of Poor Weight Outcomes After SG

In a recent nationwide study conducted in France, Lazzati and colleagues examined all patients who had undergone SG over a 10-year period (2008–2018). The focus of the study was to analyze the rate of revisions performed after the index surgery. The observed rates for revisional surgery were 4.7%, 7.5%, and 12.2%, at 5, 7, and 10 years after initial SG respectively. Notably, these rates were higher among patients with a previous gastric banding history prior to their SGs, with revisional rates reaching 9.9%, 14.5%, and 20.7% at the same time intervals. In their analysis, Lezzati and colleagues highlighted the primary reasons for revisions, which mainly included WR, GERD, and anatomical complications such as stenosis and fistulas [16].

However, the prevalence of the need for revisional surgery after SG may not be consistent across various studies. For instance, Felsenreich and colleagues observed a high revision rate in their 15-year follow-up cohort, totaling 49%. The primary indications for revisions were WR (26.4%) followed by symptomatic GERD (18.9%), and early leak necessitating acute conversion surgery (3.8%). However, it's important to note that their sample size was relatively small [17].

Clapp and colleagues, along with Matar et al., have both conducted a meta-analysis which included their own data. The former meta-analysis revealed a revision rate of 20%, from which 13% were attributed to WR and 3% were due to GERD symptoms [4]. According to Matar et al., the most common complications related to SG necessitating revisional surgery were GERD and IWL/WR, accounting for 30.4% and 52% of the conversions, respectively [18]. Hence, poor weight outcomes constitute a significant challenge often necessitating salvage revisional procedures after SG.

Furthermore, only a limited number of studies have investigated the preoperative predictive factors for WR following bariatric procedures, specifically SG. However, among those that have, there are certain common factors that include older age, male sex, higher preoperative Body Mass Index (BMI) especially BMI > 50kg/m$^2$, mental health issues, and the presence of certain comorbidities (diabetes mellitus, hypertension, and obstructive sleep apnea [19–24].

## Causes for Poor Weight Outcomes After SG

Understanding the factors behind WR after bariatric procedures is crucial for improving long-term patient outcomes. Various elements can influence weight management after surgery. Exploring these factors carefully provides essential insight into tailoring effective strategies to mitigate WR and enhance the overall success of bariatric interventions.

### Surgical/Anatomic Factors

#### Gastric Sleeve Dilatation

Gradual enlargement of the remaining gastric sleeve following the initial SG is a prominent concern, often necessitating revisional surgery for approximately 4.5% of individuals [25, 26]. The continued expansion of the gastric pouch is considered a significant factor contributing to the IWL after surgery [27]. However, the link between gastric sleeve dilation and WR remains uncertain [28].

#### High Residual Gastric Volume and Retained Fundus

Existing literature has consistently explored the residual stomach volume as a predictive factor for WR following SG. Studies by Obeidat et al. & Abdullah et al. investigated the impact of a large gastric sleeve on weight loss outcomes and the likelihood of WR over time [29, 30]. Their findings indicated that radical antral resection, when combined with SG, enhances the restrictive effect, potentially leading to more significant and sustained weight loss [29]. Additionally, Abdullah et al. conducted a randomized control trial involving two groups of SG patients, highlighting that increasing the size of the resected antrum improved weight loss without significantly raising the complication rate [30]. This aligns with the recommendations from the 2012 sleeve gastrectomy summit, which suggested using a 36 Fr bougie and leaving a pyloric antral segment of less than 5 cm, a practice endorsed by 59.5% of surgeons. [31]

Also, the role of the retained fundus in bariatric surgery, particularly in procedures that include SG, has garnered significant attention in understanding weight loss outcomes. Fundus is responsible for the production the hunger-stimulating hormones, such as ghrelin. Ghrelin plays a pivotal role in regulating appetite and influencing weight loss after surgery. In a poorly performed SG where the fundus is retained, the levels of ghrelin might not be adequately suppressed. This hormonal imbalance can affect weight loss efforts [32]. Moreover, the higher residual gastric volume can also negatively impact the weight outcomes.

### Bougie Size

The size of the bougie is often considered a potential factor affecting the weight outcomes after SG. Numerous studies have analyzed the percent EWL in relation to bougie size [31, 33, 34]. In a retrospective study spanning up to 7 years, Abd Ellatif et al. investigated long-term predictors of success after SG [35]. Their findings indicated that a smaller bougie size (36Fr) and a smaller remaining antrum were both linked to a significantly higher percent EWL [35]. Nevertheless, it is crucial to interpret these data with caution due to studies indicating an association between a smaller bougie size and a higher risk of leak [36, 37].

## Hormonal/Metabolic Factors

### Ghrelin

The impact of ghrelin on weight loss and maintenance after SG remains insufficiently explored, lacking clear identification of its effects. However, Bohdjalian and colleagues undertook a study observing 26 individuals for 5 years. Within this period, 19.2% of the participants had WR. Furthermore, plasma ghrelin levels were measured in 12 patients. The researchers observed a notable decline in ghrelin levels shortly after SG, which persisted throughout the 5-year follow-up. Although there were slightly elevated ghrelin levels in those who experienced WR. However, drawing definitive conclusions is challenging due to the limited sample size [38].

### Serotonin

In a prospective cohort study led by Demerdash et al., individuals who underwent SG were divided into two categories based on their weight loss outcomes. One group included 78 patients who maintained consistent weight loss, while the other group comprised of 14 patients who experienced WR two years after surgery [39]. The study demonstrated significantly elevated levels of serotonin in the group experiencing WR compared to the group with maintained weight loss. Moreover, a positive correlation between serotonin levels and BMI was observed in both groups. These results supported the researchers' hypothesis, indicating that serotonin might play a crucial role in regulating weight loss and maintenance after SG [39].

#### Obesity-Related Immune Cell Phenotypes in Adipose Tissue

Obesity is characterized by the infiltration of immune cells, including macrophages in the adipose tissue [40]. Even after weight loss, certain aspects of the immune profile remain unchanged and studies in both mice and humans suggest the existence of an 'obesogenic memory, which contributes to the risk of WR. One potential mechanism involves enzymes secreted by macrophages that modify the extracellular matrix, some of which may belong to the cathepsin protease family. However, further experimental research is necessary to fully understand the persistent immune cell profile, especially in humans, and its role in the process of WR [40].

### Behavioral/Mood Factors

#### Eating Disorder

Different types of eating disorders and behaviors such as binge eating, loss-of-control eating, and night eating syndrome have been reported to be related to poor weight outcomes after bariatric surgery. However, most of the studies included patients who underwent Roux en-Y gastric bypass and only a few had SG [41]. Conversely, alterations in the upper gastrointestinal tract after bariatric surgery can lead to new eating patterns, notably consuming smaller quantities of food over extended periods, termed "grazing," as observed in other studies [42].

Some studies have proposed that preoperative binge eating disorder could be a risk factor for the development of grazing after surgery [43]. Additionally, grazing has been associated with suboptimal weight loss [44].

#### Energy Consumption and Expenditure

It is widely recognized that higher caloric intake is linked to inferior weight outcomes. Alvarez and colleagues revealed that individuals undergoing SG face a higher risk of WR if they tend to consume a diet rich in fat and energy, in contrast to those who successfully maintain their weight [45]. Expanding on this notion, Essayli et al. investigated the connection between behavioral weight management skills and weight loss following SG. Their study indicated that participants with WR were prone to adopting unhealthy eating habits, resulting in higher caloric intake. Moreover, these individuals were more likely to cease self-weighing and daily food intake recording in contrast to those who effectively maintained their weight loss [46]. These observations emphasize the pivotal role of behavioral strategies in managing weight after SG.

### Mood

Research has indicated that patients' mood, including feelings of depression and anxiety, can negatively influence their weight outcomes [47]. Alvarez and colleagues classified patients into normal, borderline, or clinically disturbed categories based on their depression and anxiety scores obtained from standardized questionnaires. After segregating patients into two groups according to median WR, the study discovered that the group experiencing higher WR showed elevated levels of clinical or borderline anxiety, unlike the group with less WR [45]. Interestingly, there was no notable difference in depression levels between both groups. However, after adjusting for confounding, neither anxiety nor depression exhibited a significant association with WR [45].

### Follow-Up Support

Following SG, like all other bariatric procedures, it is crucial to provide comprehensive follow-up care, encompassing both medical and if needed, psychosocial interventions, to sustain a healthy lifestyle and help maintain post-surgical weight loss. Discontinuation of regular follow-up appointments has been linked to potential WR after the surgery [48].

In conclusion, a multifaceted approach considering anatomic, hormonal, behavioral, and psychosocial factors is pivotal in addressing WR after SG. Tailoring interventions to individual patient's needs, supported by meticulous surgical planning and robust follow-up care, are essential in ensuring sustained weight loss and improved quality of life after bariatric surgery including SG.

## Treatment Options for Poor Weight Outcomes After SG

Different treatment options have been suggested to address IWL/WR after SG. For a more organized discussion in this chapter, we will categorize these treatment options into non-surgical and surgical approaches. Non-surgical interventions offer emerging and ground-breaking ways to tackle IWL/WR after bariatric surgery. Medical interventions, supervised by healthcare professionals, may involve medications that control appetite or inhibit fat absorption [49]. Additionally, endoscopic interventions are emerging as a growing field in the realm of revisional bariatric procedures [50–52]. The most common therapeutic option to address IWL/WR after SG remains the revisional surgeries. The choice and type of revisional surgery are often influenced by various factors such as co-existing refractory GERD after SG. Various non-surgical and surgical options to address IWL/WR after SG are summarized below.

## Non-surgical Therapeutic Options

### Pharmacotherapy and Gut Hormone (Co)agonists

Surgical revisions are often considered the most effective intervention to address IWL/WR after SG, although revisional procedures are associated with higher complications compared to the initial surgery itself. Consequently, pharmaceutical agents especially the emerging gut hormone (co)agonists may present potentially safer alternatives for addressing poor weight outcomes in this patient population.

While disparities in weight loss outcomes among specific surgical procedures are well-documented, there is limited research examining the effects of weight management medications in the context of different surgical techniques. Pharmacological agents assist in weight loss by targeting various physiological mechanisms related to obesity [53]. Common FDA-approved medications for obesity treatment include orlistat, phentermine/topiramate, liraglutide 3.0 mg, naltrexone/bupropion, and semaglutide 2.4 mg, with other novel agents either undergoing approval processes or being used off-label. Despite a growing body of literature, there is no consensus or standardized algorithm for selecting pharmaceutical options after bariatric procedures. The choice often depends on individual patient factors and existing comorbidities.

Most level I evidence regarding the use of gut hormone receptor agonists is primarily focused on patients with diabetes with a less severe burden of obesity including class I obesity [49]. However, in a recent comprehensive review published in Nature Metabolism with a focus on only the weight loss effect from these gut hormone receptors (co)agonists from phase 3 trials in patients without diabetes, semaglutide, and tirzepatide both have promising results at 68 and 72 weeks, respectively [54]. Semaglutide is a glucagon-like peptide-1 (GLP-1) receptor agonist and its weekly injections at 2.4 mg dosing resulted in 15kg weight loss at 68 weeks. More impressively, tirzepatide which is a glucose-dependent insulinotropic polypeptide (GIP) and GLP-1 receptor co-agonist, showed a dose-dependent response with 5, 10, or 15 mg weekly dosing up to 72 weeks resulting in 21% total weight loss (TWL) [54]. These results especially those from the tirzepatide are highly encouraging and can certainly play a part in addressing IWL/WR in patients after SG. However, literature from real-world data and outside randomized control trials and even findings from trial extensions involving semaglutide, suggest that the impact of these pharmaceutical agents is less profound outside the trials with only 3–5% TWL and there is significant WR in a short time interval of 6 months following the stoppage of such gut hormone agonists [55, 56]. These findings suggest that the beneficial impact of such pharmaceutical agents is dependent on their continuous use.

### Endoscopic Revisional Procedures

Abu Dayyeh and colleagues were the first to explore the feasibility of the endoscopic sleeve gastroplasty (ESG) procedure as an alternative to traditional SG in 2013 [50]. However, the role of revisional ESG after SG was first reported by Sharaiha et al. with a successful endoscopic sleeve plication after a prior SG, which allowed for an added weight loss of 9 kg [51]. In a recent multicenter study, 82 patients who had undergone revisional ESGs for WR after an initial SG were examined. The study revealed that 81% of patients achieved a TWL of $\geq$ 10% 1 year after the intervention. These findings underscore the safety and effectiveness of revisional ESG as a short-term management option [52].

The purpose of this section on the non-surgical interventions is not to diverge from the revisional surgeries. Instead, it aims to shed light on some alternative and complimentary tools. These tools could assist physicians in managing WR after metabolic/bariatric surgery, allowing for various available options based on the patient's characteristics and wishes. This is especially important as some patients may not be suitable candidates for another revisional surgery due to different reasons.

## Surgical Revisional Options

### Re-sleeve Gastrectomy (ReSG)

The idea of redo SG was first introduced by Ganger et al. in 2003 to address inadequate weight loss following duodenal switch (DS). This approach was specifically designed for patients presenting with a considerably enlarged gastric pouch linked to gradual WR [57]. In a similar context, Baltasar and colleagues noted the potential need for ReSG when the residual gastric sleeve dilates or the initial reduction in gastric volume proves to be insufficient [58]. Hence, laparoscopic ReSG can be a practical solution, particularly when the initial gastric sleeve becomes excessively large or dilates over time or in the case of a large, retained fundus [59].

Primary dilation refers to the inadequate removal of the fundus during the initial surgery, signifying a technical flaw in dissecting the upper posterior gastric pouch completely. It is crucial to ascertain if proximal dilation is associated with a twist or stricture in the stomach's mid-body. Opting for a ReSG procedure in these situations could elevate the risk of upstream leak due to heightened intraluminal pressure..In contrast, secondary dilation is characterized by a uniformly enlarged gastric tube, exceeding 250 ml in volume as determined by radiographic measurements. Noel and colleagues published a case series detailing the medium-term outcomes over 5 years of patients who underwent ReSG due to IWL or WR after their initial SG [60]. On average, ReSG was performed 28 months after the primary SG, and the revisional ReSG resulted in and added 9 kg/m$^2$ drop in the BMI equivalent to a mean excess body mass index loss (EBMIL) of 64% 5 years after ReSG. Notably, (72%) of the patients who underwent ReSG achieved > 50% EBMIL at five-year follow-up [60]. Similar findings were also described by other studies with an added 57–66% EWL albeit at a short-term follow-up of 1 year after ReSG [61, 62].

In 2015 Nedelcu et al. proposed an algorithm for selecting which patients should be considered for ReSG when faced with IWL or WR after the primary SG [63]. An integral part of the algorithm was an upper gastrointestinal contrast study to assess the existing gastric sleeve dimensions. ReSG was proposed as a revisional option if the barium swallow indicated dilation in the upper gastric pouch or a significant retained fundus. In cases where the barium swallow did not reveal a major dilation in the upper part of the sleeve or the results were inconclusive, a follow-up computed tomography scan volumetry was performed. ReSG was contemplated if the existing sleeve's volumetrics surpassed 250 ml. If the volume was less than 250 ml and/or based on other symptoms like GERD, the patient would then undergo an upper endoscopy and based on overall characteristics would be considered for other more appropriate bypass-type revisional procedures [63].

Various studies in the literature have compared the outcomes of ReSG versus other bypass-type revisional surgeries. These studies again recommend ReSG as an effective option in situations where the existing gastric sleeve is very dilated or a large, retained fundus exists. However, most of the studies show that bypass-type revisional procedures compared to ReSG, are more effective in addressing poor weight outcomes after a primary SG [61, 64, 65]. As a revisional surgery, ReSG offers advantages such as shorter procedure time, and further volume reduction of the remaining gastric sleeve, while lowering the chance of dumping syndrome due to the preservation of the pylorus. Additionally, there is a decreased risk of vitamin deficiencies. However, it is crucial to weigh these benefits against the heightened risk of staple-line sleeve leaks after ReSG, necessitating careful counseling of patients [14].

### Roux en-Y Gastric Bypass (RYGB)

The conversion of primary SG to RYGB is typically considered in cases of IWL, WR, or complications like refractory GERD, leaks, spiraling staple-line, or strictures that do not respond to medical treatment or endoscopic procedures [66]. While numerous studies have demonstrated the safety of conversion to RYGB as a revisional surgery after a primary SG, it is important to note that complication rates are higher compared to primary RYGB [67, 68]. In a recent study using data from The Metabolic and Bariatric Surgery Accreditation and Quality Improvement Program (MBSAQIP), Dang et al, reported that revisional RYGB after primary SG is associated with a higher rate of serious complications compared to primary RYGB [69]. The overall complication rate was low at (7.2%) and considered acceptable without a significant difference in 30-day mortality. Interestingly, they found that the main reason for a conversion of SG to RYGB was in fact GERD followed by WR or IWL [69].

While some studies have shown an added 20% TWL after using RYGB as a revisional procedure following an unsuccessful SG and up to medium-term follow-up [70], most studies have shown a wide range of added weight loss that are often not great ranging from 7–24% [66, 71, 72]. Predicting the exact extent of additional weight loss with confidence proves challenging, primarily due to the variability in documenting weight loss after revisional surgeries and some technical factors of the operation including the choice of the small bowel limb length for the alimentary or the biliopancreatic limb and the common channel. However, the literature is unequivocal in stating that the conversion to RYGB after SG due to refractory GERD is the revisional procedure of choice and is highly successful in alleviating the reflux symptoms and their sequelae [73, 74].

## One Anastomosis Gastric Bypass (OAGB)

The OAGB, sometimes known as mini-gastric bypass (MGB), was initially introduced by Mason and Ito in 1967 [75]. While the minimally invasive approach was pioneered by Rutledge in 2001 [76], it has only been endorsed and recognized by prominent international bariatric societies over the past few years. OAGB is also considered a viable revisional procedure after an unsuccessful SG. In a retrospective multicenter study by Poublon et al comparing the outcomes for OAGB versus RYGB for IWL/WR after primary restrictive procedures, they found that while both revisional procedures were equally effective at 1 year, the OAGB resulted in a significantly lower BMI by the second and third year after revision equivalent to an average of 2–3 kg/m$^2$ lower BMI units compared to conversions to RYGB [77]. However, a recent randomized controlled trial conducted by Hany and colleagues reported on 2-year outcomes of revisional RYGB compared to OAGB performed for WR after SG [78]. OAGB was found to be a shorter operation by an average of 20 min and while at the 6-month mark, it resulted in a superior weight loss compared to RYGB, these differences gradually diminished over time and were no longer significantly different between both revisions by the second year. By two years after the revisional surgery, both groups also exhibited substantial improvements in dyslipidemia, hypertension, and diabetes when compared to before the revision [78].

Despite the positive outcomes observed, concerns about bile reflux after OAGB remain a major point of concern and are reported to range between 2–56% [78, 79]. While plagued with poor documentation and a lack of proper objective testing in the literature, bile reflux remains a leading cause for reoperation after OAGB, as reported in the literature [80].

## Duodenal Switch (DS)

Classic DS is shown to be more effective than other common malabsorptive procedures such as RYGB in achieving both durable weight loss and resolving comorbidities, especially for patients suffering from extreme obesity with BMI $\geq$ 60kg/m$^2$ [72, 81, 82]. Marceau and colleagues conducted a study examining the long-term outcomes of over 1,400 patients who underwent classic DS, with a mean follow-up of 7.3 years (ranging from 2 to 15 years). The mean baseline BMI in this group was 51 kg/m$^2$. The study revealed a substantial 73% EWL% with 80% of patients achieving success and maintaining a weight loss of over > 50% EWL throughout the follow-up. Similar profound improvements in obesity-related comorbidities were also documented [83].

When primary metabolic surgery does not achieve sufficient weight loss, classic DS stands out as one of the most effective revisional procedures for weight loss. Homan and colleagues explored this topic in a retrospective single-center study, detailing their findings on secondary surgeries following SG. Three years after revision and as compared to RYGB, they reported significantly higher median EWL of 59% for DS versus 23% and 27% TWL versus 9%, respectively [84]. However, the DS group showed a higher incidence of vitamin and mineral deficiencies in comparison to the RYGB group [84]. Other comparative studies have also demonstrated that at both short and medium-term follow-ups after revisional surgeries performed for IWL/WR after SG, classic DS achieves the best added weight loss [64, 85].

However, certain reservations against the classic DS procedure such as technical complexities and potential side effects such as frequent bowel movements, fat, micronutrient, and protein-calorie malnutrition render it unpopular and its practice scattered into only a handful of high-volume centers worldwide. As a result, classic DS comprises less than 5% of the annual bariatric procedures performed globally [86, 87]. The modifications introduced via other DS derivative procedures may further increase the uptake of DS-type surgeries with similar beneficial outcomes but with fewer side effects.

### Single Anastomosis Duodenal Switch (SADS)

Certain modifications have been introduced to the classic DS procedure via SADS derivatives, which have shown promising results while addressing some of the apprehensions towards classic DS procedure such as technical issues, long-term malnutrition and gastrointestinal side effects [88–90]. The most established of these derivatives are the single anastomosis duodeno-ileal bypass with sleeve gastrectomy (SADI-S) and stomach intestinal pylorus-preserving surgery (SIPS) [91, 92].

In a separate chapter, a more detailed exploration of the efficacy of SADI-S as a primary procedure will be presented. However, a recent single-center prospective study reported on long-term outcomes of SADS versus classic DS up to 5 years after surgery and it included procedures performed as a second-stage procedure at a median of 2 years after a previous SG [89]. They found that at long-term follow-up, both SADS and DS resulted in a similar and profound overall weight loss of 20–24 kg/m$^2$ drop in BMI points and similar added TWL but, SADS was associated with fewer nutritional deficiencies (especially fat-soluble vitamins) and GI symptoms (daily bowel movements) as compared to classic DS [89].

Another multicenter prospective study by Gebelli et al., also recently reported on 5-year outcomes of SADS versus classic DS although all the procedures were primary one-stage operations [90]. Conversely, they found that while the weight outcomes were similar between both procedures up to 3 years after surgery, classic DS resulted in higher weight loss thereafter until 5 years after surgery and compared to SADS [90]. Despite the fact that classic DS may be associated with higher added weight loss for the treatment of IWL or WR after an initial SG, it is associated with an increased operative time, more frequent bowel movement and steatorrhea, more fat-soluble vitamin deficiencies, and hypoproteinemia [88, 89, 93–95]. Considering all these factors, along with the technical complexities associated with DS, many surgeons have embraced SADS as a preferred bypass-type procedure as a salvage revisional surgery after an unsuccessful SG.

## Summary

In conclusion, poor weight outcomes after SG as defined by IWL and WR are not infrequent, and their causes are multifactorial. Revisional and conversional surgery after SG due to IWL or WR can be complex, and the procedure choice should be tailored to the patient's needs after a thorough evaluation. Proper consideration of patient-specific factors and the pattern of WR is crucial. It's essential to approach the situation meticulously, utilizing all available treatment options supported by scientific evidence. By understanding the unique needs of each patient and staying informed about the latest research findings, medical professionals can navigate this challenging territory effectively, ensuring the best possible outcomes for their patients.

## References


1. Altieri MS, Yang J, Nie L, Blackstone R, Spaniolas K, Pryor A. Rate of revisions or conversion after bariatric surgery over 10 years in the state of New York. Surg Obes Relat Dis. 2018;14(4):500–7.
2. Hjorth S, Näslund I, Andersson-Assarsson JC, Svensson P-A, Jacobson P, Peltonen M, et al. Reoperations after bariatric surgery in 26 years of follow-up of the Swedish Obese Subjects Study. JAMA Surg. 2019;154(4):319–26.
3. Kapała J, Maroszczuk T, Lewandowska J, Lech P, Dowgiałło-Gornowicz N. Weight regain in the second year after sleeve gastrectomy could be a predictor of long-term outcomes? Medicina. 2023;59(4):766.
4. Clapp B, Wynn M, Martyn C, Foster C, O'Dell M, Tyroch A. Long term (7 or more years) outcomes of the sleeve gastrectomy: a meta-analysis. Surg Obes Relat Dis. 2018;14(6):741–7.
5. Clapp B, Cottam S, Salame M, Marr JD, Galvani C, Ponce J, et al. Comparative analysis of sleeve conversions of the Metabolic and Bariatric Surgery Accreditation and Quality Improvement Program 2020 database. Surg Obes Relat Dis. 2023;
6. Wang YC, McPherson K, Marsh T, Gortmaker SL, Brown M. Health and economic burden of the projected obesity trends in the USA and the UK. Lancet. 2011;378(9793):815–25.
7. Collaborators GBDD. Global, regional, and national burden of diabetes from 1990 to 2021, with projections of prevalence to 2050: a systematic analysis for the Global Burden of Disease Study 2021. Lancet. 2023;402(10397):203–34.
8. Zhang L, Tan WH, Chang R, Eagon JC. Perioperative risk and complications of revisional bariatric surgery compared to primary Roux-en-Y gastric bypass. Surg Endosc. 2015;29(6):1316–20.
9. Tolvanen L, Christenson A, Surkan PJ, Lagerros YT. Patients' experiences of weight regain after bariatric surgery. Obes Surg. 2022;32(5):1498–507.
10. El Ansari W, Elhag W. Weight regain and insufficient weight loss after bariatric surgery: definitions, prevalence, mechanisms, predictors, prevention and management strategies, and knowledge gaps—a scoping review. Obes Surg. 2021;31(4):1755–66.
11. Nedelcu M, Khwaja HA, Rogula TG. Weight regain after bariatric surgery—how should it be defined? Surg Obes Relat Dis. 2016;12(5):1129–30.
12. Voglino C, Badalucco S, Tirone A, Ciuoli C, Cantara S, Benenati N, et al. Follow-up after bariatric surgery: is it time to tailor it? Analysis of early predictive factors of 3-year weight loss predictors of unsuccess in bariatric patients. Updat Surg. 2022;74(4):1389–98.
13. van de Laar AW, van Rijswijk AS, Kakar H, Bruin SC. Sensitivity and specificity of 50% excess weight loss (50%EWL) and twelve other bariatric criteria for weight loss success. Obes Surg. 2018;28(8):2297–304.
14. Noel P, Nedelcu M, Nocca D, Schneck A-S, Gugenheim J, Iannelli A, et al. Revised sleeve gastrectomy: another option for weight loss failure after sleeve gastrectomy. Surg Endosc. 2014;28(4):1096–102.
15. Brethauer SA, Kothari S, Sudan R, Williams B, English WJ, Brengman M, et al. Systematic review on reoperative bariatric surgery: American Society for Metabolic and Bariatric Surgery Revision Task Force. Surg Obes Relat Dis. 2014;10(5):952–72.

16. Lazzati A, Bechet S, Jouma S, Paolino L, Jung C. Revision surgery after sleeve gastrectomy: a nationwide study with 10 years of follow-up. Surg Obes Relat Dis. 2020;16(10):1497–504.
17. Felsenreich DM, Artemiou E, Steinlechner K, Vock N, Jedamzik J, Eichelter J, et al. Fifteen years after sleeve gastrectomy: weight loss, remission of associated medical problems, quality of life, and conversions to Roux-en-Y gastric bypass—long-term follow-up in a multicenter study. Obes Surg. 2021;31(8):3453–61.
18. Matar R, Monzer N, Jaruvongvanich V, Abusaleh R, Vargas EJ, Maselli DB, et al. Indications and outcomes of conversion of sleeve gastrectomy to Roux-en-Y gastric bypass: a systematic review and a meta-analysis. Obes Surg. 2021;31(9):3936–46.
19. Cadena-Obando D, Ramírez-Rentería C, Ferreira-Hermosillo A, Albarrán-Sanchez A, Sosa-Eroza E, Molina-Ayala M, Espinosa-Cárdenas E, et al. Are there really any predictive factors for a successful weight loss after bariatric surgery? BMC Endocr Disord. 2020;20:1–8.
20. Ortega E, Morínigo R, Flores L, Moize V, Rios M, Lacy AM, et al. Predictive factors of excess body weight loss 1 year after laparoscopic bariatric surgery. Surg Endosc. 2012;26(6):1744–50.
21. Courcoulas AP, King WC, Belle SH, Berk P, Flum DR, Garcia L, et al. Seven-year weight trajectories and health outcomes in the longitudinal assessment of bariatric surgery (LABS) study. JAMA Surg. 2018;153(5):427–34.
22. Ochner CN, Jochner MCE, Caruso EA, Teixeira J, Xavier P-SF. Effect of preoperative body mass index on weight loss after obesity surgery. Surg Obes Relat Dis. 2013;9(3):423–7.
23. Marek RJ, Ben-Porath YS, Dulmen MHMV, Ashton K, Heinberg LJ. Using the presurgical psychological evaluation to predict 5-year weight loss outcomes in bariatric surgery patients. Surg Obes Relat Dis. 2017;13(3):514–21.
24. Odom J, Zalesin KC, Washington TL, Miller WW, Hakmeh B, Zaremba DL, et al. Behavioral predictors of weight regain after bariatric surgery. Obes Surg. 2010;20(3):349–56.
25. Braghetto I, Cortes C, Herquiñigo D, Csendes P, Rojas A, Mushle M, et al. Evaluation of the radiological gastric capacity and evolution of the BMI 2–3 years after sleeve gastrectomy. Obes Surg. 2009;19(9):1262–9.
26. Gumbs AA, Gagner M, Dakin G, Pomp A. Sleeve gastrectomy for morbid obesity. Obes Surg. 2007;17(7):962–9.
27. Tassinari D, Berta RD, Nannipieri M, Giusti P, Di Paolo L, Guarino D, et al. Sleeve gastrectomy: correlation of long-term results with remnant morphology and eating disorders. Obes Surg. 2017;27(11):2845–54.
28. Langer FB, Bohdjalian A, Felberbauer FX, Fleischmann E, Reza Hoda MA, Ludvik B, et al. Does gastric dilatation limit the success of sleeve gastrectomy as a sole operation for morbid obesity? Obes Surg. 2006;16(2):166–71.
29. Obeidat F, Shanti H, Mismar A, Albsoul N, Al-Qudah M. The magnitude of antral resection in laparoscopic sleeve gastrectomy and its relationship to excess weight loss. Obes Surg. 2015;25(10):1928–32.
30. Abdallah E, El Nakeeb A, Yousef T, Abdallah H, Ellatif MA, Lotfy A, et al. Impact of extent of antral resection on surgical outcomes of sleeve gastrectomy for morbid obesity (a prospective randomized study). Obes Surg. 2014;24(10):1587–94.
31. Gagner M, Deitel M, Erickson AL, Crosby RD. Survey on laparoscopic sleeve gastrectomy (LSG) at the Fourth International Consensus Summit on Sleeve Gastrectomy. Obes Surg. 2013;23(12):2013–7.
32. Lin E, Gletsu N, Fugate K, McClusky D, Gu LH, Zhu J-L, et al. The effects of gastric surgery on systemic Ghrelin levels in the morbidly obese. Arch Surg. 2004;139(7):780–4.
33. Rosenthal R. Laparoscopic sleeve gastrectomy: does Bougie size affect mean percentage of excess weight loss? Short-term outcomes. Surg Obes Relat Dis. 2008;4(5):687–8.
34. Al-Tai S, Axer S, Szabo E, Ottosson J, Stenberg E. The impact of the bougie size and the extent of antral resection on weight-loss and postoperative complications following sleeve gastrectomy: results from the Scandinavian Obesity Surgery Registry. Surg Obes Relat Dis. 2023;
35. Abd Ellatif ME, Abdallah E, Askar W, Thabet W, Aboushady M, Abbas AE, et al. Long term predictors of success after laparoscopic sleeve gastrectomy. Int J Surg. 2014;12(5):504–8.

36. Yuval JB, Mintz Y, Cohen MJ, Rivkind AI, Elazary R. The effects of bougie caliber on leaks and excess weight loss following laparoscopic sleeve gastrectomy. Is there an ideal Bougie size? Obes Surg. 2013;23(10):1685–91.
37. Berger ER, Clements RH, Morton JM, Huffman KM, Wolfe BM, Nguyen NT, et al. The impact of different surgical techniques on outcomes in laparoscopic sleeve gastrectomies: the first report from the metabolic and bariatric surgery accreditation and quality improvement program (MBSAQIP). Ann Surg. 2016;264(3):464–73.
38. Bohdjalian A, Langer FB, Shakeri-Leidenmühler S, Gfrerer L, Ludvik B, Zacherl J, et al. Sleeve gastrectomy as sole and definitive bariatric procedure: 5-year results for weight loss and Ghrelin. Obes Surg. 2010;20(5):535–40.
39. Demerdash HM, Sabry AA, Arida EA. Role of serotonin hormone in weight regain after sleeve gastrectomy. Scand J Clin Lab Invest. 2018;78(1–2):68–73.
40. van Baak MA, Mariman ECM. Obesity-induced and weight-loss-induced physiological factors affecting weight regain. Nat Rev Endocrinol. 2023;19(11):655–70.
41. Beck NN, Mehlsen M, Støving RK. Psychological characteristics and associations with weight outcomes two years after gastric bypass surgery: Postoperative eating disorder symptoms are associated with weight loss outcomes. Eating Behav. 2012;13(4):394–7.
42. Saunders R. "Grazing": a high-risk behavior. Obes Surg. 2004;14(1):98–102.
43. Nicolau J, Ayala L, Rivera R, Speranskaya A, Sanchís P, Julian X, et al. Postoperative grazing as a risk factor for negative outcomes after bariatric surgery. Eating Behav. 2015;18:147–50.
44. de Zwaan M, Hilbert A, Swan-Kremeier L, Simonich H, Lancaster K, Howell LM, et al. Comprehensive interview assessment of eating behavior 18–35 months after gastric bypass surgery for morbid obesity. Surg Obes Relat Dis. 2010;6(1):79–85.
45. Alvarez V, Carrasco F, Cuevas A, Valenzuela B, Muñoz G, Ghiardo D, et al. Mechanisms of long-term weight regain in patients undergoing sleeve gastrectomy. Nutrition. 2016;32(3):303–8.
46. Essayli JH, LaGrotte CA, Fink-Miller EL, Rigby A. Patients' reported usage of weight management skills following bariatric surgery. Obes Surg. 2018;28(2):584–8.
47. Alhalel N, Schueller SM, O'Brien MJ. Association of changes in mental health with weight loss during intensive lifestyle intervention: does the timing matter? Obes Sci Pract. 2018;4(2):153–8.
48. Lauti M, Stevenson S, Hill AG, MacCormick AD. Patient perspectives about follow-up care and weight regain following sleeve gastrectomy. Obes Surg. 2016;26(11):2724–31.
49. Muller TD, Bluher M, Tschop MH, DiMarchi RD. Anti-obesity drug discovery: advances and challenges. Nat Rev Drug Discov. 2022;21(3):201–23.
50. Abu Dayyeh BK, Rajan E, Gostout CJ. Endoscopic sleeve gastroplasty: a potential endoscopic alternative to surgical sleeve gastrectomy for treatment of obesity. Gastrointest Endosc. 2013;78(3):530–5.
51. Sharaiha RZ, Kedia P, Kumta N, Aronne LJ, Kahaleh M. Endoscopic sleeve plication for revision of sleeve gastrectomy. Gastrointest Endosc. 2015;81(4):1004.
52. Maselli DB, Alqahtani AR, Abu Dayyeh BK, Elahmedi M, Storm AC, Matar R, et al. Revisional endoscopic sleeve gastroplasty of laparoscopic sleeve gastrectomy: an international, multicenter study. Gastrointest Endosc. 2021;93(1):122–30.
53. Schwartz MW, Seeley RJ, Zeltser LM, Drewnowski A, Ravussin E, Redman LM, et al. Obesity pathogenesis: an endocrine society scientific statement. Endocr Rev. 2017;38(4):267–96.
54. Nogueiras R, Nauck MA, Tschop MH. Gut hormone co-agonists for the treatment of obesity: from bench to bedside. Nat Metab. 2023;5(6):933–44.
55. Powell W, Song X, Mohamed Y, Walsh D, Parks EJ, McMahon TM, et al. Medications and conditions associated with weight loss in patients prescribed semaglutide based on real-world data. Obesity. 2023;31(10):2482–92.
56. Wilding JPH, Batterham RL, Davies M, Van Gaal LF, Kandler K, Konakli K, et al. Weight regain and cardiometabolic effects after withdrawal of semaglutide: the STEP 1 trial extension. Diabetes Obes Metab. 2022;24(8):1553–64.

57. Gagner M, Rogula T. Laparoscopic reoperative sleeve gastrectomy for poor weight loss after biliopancreatic diversion with duodenal switch. Obes Surg. 2003;13(4):649–54.
58. Baltasar A, Serra C, Pérez N, Bou R, Bengochea M. Re-sleeve gastrectomy. Obes Surg. 2006;16(11):1535–8.
59. Rebibo L, Dhahri A, Robert B, Regimbeau J-M. Repeat sleeve gastrectomy: optimization of outcomes by modifying the indications and technique. Surg Obes Relat Dis. 2018;14(4):490–7.
60. Noel P, Nedelcu A, Eddbali I, Gagner M, Danan M, Nedelcu M. Five-year results after resleeve gastrectomy. Surg Obes Relat Dis. 2020;16(9):1186–91.
61. AlSabah S, Alsharqawi N, Almulla A, Akrof S, Alenezi K, Buhaimed W, et al. Approach to poor weight loss after laparoscopic sleeve gastrectomy: re-sleeve vs. gastric bypass. Obes Surg. 2016;26(10):2302–7.
62. Rebibo L, Fuks D, Verhaeghe P, Deguines J-B, Dhahri A, Regimbeau J-M. Repeat sleeve gastrectomy compared with primary sleeve gastrectomy: a single-center, matched case study. Obes Surg. 2012;22(12):1909–15.
63. Nedelcu M, Noel P, Iannelli A, Gagner M. Revised sleeve gastrectomy (re-sleeve). Surg Obes Relat Dis. 2015;11(6):1282–8.
64. Andalib A, Alamri H, Almuhanna Y, Bouchard P, Demyttenaere S, Court O. Short-term outcomes of revisional surgery after sleeve gastrectomy: a comparative analysis of re-sleeve, Roux en-Y gastric bypass, duodenal switch (Roux en-Y and single-anastomosis). Surg Endosc. 2021;35(8):4644–52.
65. Antonopulos C, Rebibo L, Calabrese D, Ribeiro-Parenti L, Arapis K, Dhahri A, et al. Comparison of repeat sleeve gastrectomy and Roux-en-Y gastric bypass in case of weight loss failure after sleeve gastrectomy. Obes Surg. 2019;29(12):3919–27.
66. Abdemur A, Han S-M, Lo Menzo E, Szomstein S, Rosenthal R. Reasons and outcomes of conversion of laparoscopic sleeve gastrectomy to Roux-en-Y gastric bypass for nonresponders. Surg Obes Relat Dis. 2016;12(1):113–8.
67. Frieder JS, Aleman R, Gomez CO, Ferri F, Okida LF, Funes DR, et al. Outcomes of reoperative surgery in severely obese patients after sleeve gastrectomy: a single-institution experience. Surg Obes Relat Dis. 2020;16(8):983–90.
68. de Raaff CAL, Coblijn UK, de Vries N, Heymans MW, van den Berg BTJ, van Tets WF, et al. Predictive factors for insufficient weight loss after bariatric surgery: does obstructive sleep apnea influence weight loss? Obes Surg. 2016;26(5):1048–56.
69. Dang JT, Vaughan T, Mocanu V, Mubashir H, Barajas-Gamboa JS, Codina RC, et al. Conversion of sleeve gastrectomy to Roux-en-Y gastric bypass: indications, prevalence, and safety. Obes Surg. 2023;33(5):1486–93.
70. Diaz Del Gobbo G, Mahmoud N, Barajas-Gamboa JS, Klingler M, Barrios P, Abril C, et al. Conversion of sleeve gastrectomy to Roux-en-Y gastric bypass to enhance weight loss: single enterprise mid-term outcomes and literature review. Bariatr Surg Pract Patient Care. 2022;17(4):197–205.
71. Parmar CD, Mahawar KK, Boyle M, Schroeder N, Balupuri S, Small PK. Conversion of sleeve gastrectomy to Roux-en-Y gastric bypass is effective for gastro-oesophageal reflux disease but not for further weight loss. Obes Surg. 2017;27(7):1651–8.
72. Dijkhorst PJ, Boerboom AB, Janssen IMC, Swank DJ, Wiezer RMJ, Hazebroek EJ, et al. Failed sleeve gastrectomy: single anastomosis duodenoileal bypass or Roux-en-Y gastric bypass? A multicenter cohort study. Obes Surg. 2018;28(12):3834–42.
73. Pallati PK, Shaligram A, Shostrom VK, Oleynikov D, McBride CL, Goede MR. Improvement in gastroesophageal reflux disease symptoms after various bariatric procedures: review of the bariatric outcomes longitudinal database. Surg Obes Relat Dis. 2014;10(3):502–7.
74. Goonawardena J, Ward S. Effect of Roux-en-Y gastric bypass on Barrett's esophagus: a systematic review. Surg Obes Relat Dis. 2021;17(1):221–30.
75. Mason EE, Ito C. Gastric bypass in obesity. Surg Clin North Am. 1967;47(6):1345–51.
76. Rutledge R. The mini-gastric bypass: experience with the first 1274 cases. Obes Surg. 2001;11(3):276–80.

77. Poublon N, Chidi I, Bethlehem M, Kuipers E, Gadiot R, Emous M, et al. One anastomosis gastric bypass vs. Roux-en-Y gastric bypass, remedy for insufficient weight loss and weight regain after failed restrictive bariatric surgery. Obes Surg. 2020;30(9):3287–94.
78. Hany M, Zidan A, Elmongui E, Torensma B. Revisional Roux-en-Y Gastric bypass versus revisional one-anastomosis gastric bypass after failed sleeve gastrectomy: a randomized controlled trial. Obes Surg. 2022;32(11):3491–503.
79. Keleidari B, Dehkordi MM, Shahraki MS, Ahmadi ZS, Heidari M, Hajian A, et al. Bile reflux after one anastomosis gastric bypass surgery: a review study. Ann Med Surg (Lond). 2021;64:102248.
80. Johnson WH, Fernanadez AZ, Farrell TM, MacDonald KG, Grant JP, McMahon RL, et al. Surgical revision of loop ("mini") gastric bypass procedure: multicenter review of complications and conversions to Roux-en-Y gastric bypass. Surg Obes Relat Dis. 2007;3(1):37–41.
81. Mingrone G, Panunzi S, De Gaetano A, Guidone C, Iaconelli A, Nanni G, et al. Bariatric-metabolic surgery versus conventional medical treatment in obese patients with type 2 diabetes: 5 year follow-up of an open-label, single-centre, randomised controlled trial. Lancet. 2015;386(9997):964–73.
82. Torres A, Rubio MA, Ramos-Levi AM, Sanchez-Pernaute A. Cardiovascular risk factors after single anastomosis duodeno-ileal bypass with sleeve gastrectomy (SADI-S): a new effective therapeutic approach? Curr Atheroscler Rep. 2017;19(12):58.
83. Marceau P, Biron S, Hould F-S, Lebel S, Marceau S, Lescelleur O, et al. Duodenal switch: long-term results. Obes Surg. 2007;17(11):1421–30.
84. Homan J, Betzel B, Aarts EO, van Laarhoven KJHM, Janssen IMC, Berends FJ. Secondary surgery after sleeve gastrectomy: Roux-en-Y gastric bypass or biliopancreatic diversion with duodenal switch. Surg Obes Relat Dis. 2015;11(4):771–7.
85. Dirnberger AS, Süsstrunk J, Schneider R, Poljo A, Klasen JM, Slawik M, et al. Mid-term outcomes after conversion procedures following laparoscopic sleeve gastrectomy. Obes Surg. 2023;33(9):2679–86.
86. Angrisani L, Santonicola A, Iovino P, Formisano G, Buchwald H, Scopinaro N. Bariatric surgery worldwide 2013. Obes Surg. 2015;25(10):1822–32.
87. Khorgami Z, Shoar S, Andalib A, Aminian A, Brethauer SA, Schauer PR. Trends in utilization of bariatric surgery, 2010–2014: sleeve gastrectomy dominates. Surg Obes Relat Dis. 2017;13(5):774–8.
88. Andalib A, Bouchard P, Alamri H, Bougie A, Demyttenaere S, Court O. Single anastomosis duodeno-ileal bypass with sleeve gastrectomy (SADI-S): short-term outcomes from a prospective cohort study. Surg Obes Relat Dis. 2021;17(2):414–24.
89. Andalib A, Safar A, Bouchard P, Demyttenaere S, Court O. Single anastomosis duodenal switch versus classic duodenal switch: long-term outcomes from a prospective comparative cohort study. Obes Surg. 2023;
90. Gebellí JP, Lazzara C, de Gordejuela AGR, Nora M, Pereira AM, Sánchez-Pernaute A, et al. Duodenal Switch vs. Single-Anastomosis Duodenal Switch (SADI-S) for the treatment of grade IV obesity: 5-year outcomes of a multicenter prospective cohort comparative study. Obes Surg. 2022;32(12):3839–46.
91. Sánchez-Pernaute A, Rubio Herrera MA, Pérez-Aguirre E, García Pérez JC, Cabrerizo L, Díez Valladares L, et al. Proximal duodenal–ileal end-to-side bypass with sleeve gastrectomy: proposed technique. Obes Surg. 2007;17(12):1614–8.
92. Mitzman B, Cottam D, Goriparthi R, Cottam S, Zaveri H, Surve A, et al. Stomach Intestinal Pylorus Sparing (SIPS) surgery for morbid obesity: retrospective analyses of our preliminary experience. Obes Surg. 2016;26(9):2098–104.
93. Baltasar A, Bou R, Bengochea M, Arlandis F, Escrivá C, Miró J, et al. Duodenal switch: an effective therapy for morbid obesity—intermediate results. Obes Surg. 2001;11(1):54–8.
94. Magee CJ, Barry J, Brocklehurst J, Javed S, Macadam R, Kerrigan DD. Outcome of laparoscopic duodenal switch for morbid obesity. Br J Surg. 2010;98(1):79–84.
95. Osorio J, Lazzara C, Admella V, Franci-León S, Pujol-Gebellí J. Revisional laparoscopic SADI-S vs. duodenal switch following failed primary sleeve gastrectomy: a single-center comparison of 101 consecutive cases. Obes Surg. 2021;31(8):3667–74.

# Revisions/Conversions from Roux-en-Y Gastric Bypass due to Weight Recurrence

# 42

Rana C. Pullatt, Karl Hage, and Amanda Belluzzi

## Introduction

The Roux-en-Y gastric bypass (RYGB) is one of the most efficient metabolic and bariatric surgeries (MBS) in terms of short-, mid-, and long-term weight-loss outcomes. It stands as the gold-standard for sustained weight loss and overall obesity-related medical conditions resolution [1]. Nevertheless, the excellent weight-loss results associated with RYGB are not without the possibility of eventual weight recurrence [2]. Indeed, multiple studies reporting the long-term outcomes of RYGB demonstrate that a proportion of patients experience either inadequate weight loss (IWL) or weight recurrence (WR). In a large prospective study following patients who underwent RYGB, less than half of the patients were able to maintain at least 30% weight loss after 12 years of surgery [3]. These results echo those demonstrated by multiple other retrospective studies showing that the rate of IWL/WR after 5 years of RYGB varies between 15–30% and can reach up to 40–50% at the 10-year mark [4, 5]. WR after RYGB represents a challenging situation both for the patient and the treating physician. Fortunately, there are multiple available options to address this issue including behavioral interventions, medications, endoscopic interventions, and surgical revision/conversion to counter some of the factors that resulted in WR.

R. C. Pullatt (✉)
Foregut & Metabolic Surgery, Department of Surgery Medical University of South Carolina, Charleston, USA

K. Hage · A. Belluzzi
Department of Surgery, Mayo Clinic, Rochester, MN, USA



O. M. Ghanem et al. (eds.), *The SAGES Manual of Metabolic and Bariatric Surgery*, https://doi.org/10.1007/978-3-031-72309-4_42

## Non-surgical Approaches to Manage WR After RYGB

### Behavioral Interventions

Emerging studies have shown that addressing psychosocial and behavioral factors implicated in WR after MBS is associated with significant and sustained benefit. In the multicentered Longitudinal Assessment of Bariatric Surgery 2 (LABS-2) study, behavioral modifications were examined to evaluate the durability of health changes after MBS [6]. Results demonstrated that patients who adhered to behavioral interventions such as self-weighing and portion control lost significantly more weight than those who did not engage in such interventions (38.8% vs. 24.6% weight loss) [6]. Others also examined the outcomes of acceptance-based strategies and different modes of intervention delivery, such as online and by phone, to optimize patient follow-up. In the current era, a multidisciplinary approach to WR after RYGB is required. Non-judgmental behavioral intervention specific to each patient is necessary to offer the optimal results for patients following MBS.

### Medications

Since the early 2010s, several new medications have been added to the options of non-surgical therapeutic options to optimize weight loss. Indeed, there exist several medications such as lorcaserin hydrochloride, phentermine-topiramate, and bupropion hydrochloride-naltrexone hydrochloride which act as appetite suppressants. Other drugs such as liraglutide also have additional peripheral actions by inhibiting gastric emptying [7]. These medications have been compared to placebo and have shown a modest additional weight loss when coupled with lifestyle modifications (between 4–10% excess weight loss) [7]. Despite small studies showing promising results, there remains a lack of large, randomized control trials that evaluate the efficacy of these medications for WR after MBS.

### Endoscopic Approach: TORe

Gastrojejunal stoma size enlargement is a common anatomical change seen after RYGB that contributes largely to WR by reducing the patient's satiety and increasing the volume of food consumed during each meal. A novel approach to reduce the diameter of the stoma and address these changes has emerged using advanced endoscopic suturing techniques. The transoral outlet reduction (TORe) endoscopy is an outpatient procedure used to plicate the gastrojejunal anastomosis and reduce the stoma surface to 1 cm. In a recent multicentered study evaluating the weight-loss outcomes 18 months after TORe, patients demonstrated satisfactory weight loss with a mean of 8 ± 8.8 kg lost along with a favorable risk profile [8, 9].

### Endoscopic Approach: Others

In addition to the TORe procedure, there are also other endoscopic options available such as sclerotherapy, Restorative Obesity Surgery Endoscopic (ROSE), and endoscopic gastric plication. Endoscopic sclerotherapy is performed by injecting sodium morrhuate into the rim of the gastrojejunal anastomosis to reduce the stoma diameter [10]. Similarly, ROSE, and endoscopic gastric plication aim to create tissue folds and reduce the pouch and stoma size. However, studies have shown that after 12 months, the stoma size typically returns to its pre-interventional size leading to a high rate of failure to maintain the weight loss [11].

## Surgical Approaches to Manage WR After RYGB

Commensurate with the increase in bariatric procedures over time, the numbers of revisional bariatric surgery have steadily climbed. In fact, revisional bariatric surgery currently constitutes 11–17% of all performed MBS procedures [12]. In a large cohort study evaluating 10-year outcomes of 22,768 patients who underwent RYGB, 4.9% of patients had a revision/conversion with the most common indication being IWL/WR [13]. Thus, revisional/conversional surgery can be offered to patients who have not experienced sufficient weight loss following their primary RYGB or to those who regained a significant amount of weight after initial weight loss.

### Preoperative Assessment

Patients who meet the criteria for revisional/conversional bariatric surgery must undergo an extensive preoperative assessment by a multidisciplinary team, including the bariatric surgeon, a registered dietician, nurse educators, and other specialized providers [14]. In addition to a thorough medical history and physical examination, certain tests must also be performed to identify and manage the patients' obesity-related medical conditions. Metabolic assessment includes a complete blood count, complete metabolic panel, fasting blood glucose, hemoglobin A1c, lipid panel, urinalysis, and coagulation studies. It is also paramount to evaluate the patient's overall nutritional status with serum vitamin B12, folic acid, vitamin D, iron studies, serum albumin and prealbumin levels [15]. Patients with a history of GERD should also undergo a preoperative esophagogastroduodenoscopy (EGD) to evaluate the presence of a concomitant hiatal hernia, *H. pylori* disease, Barett esophagus, or other upper GI diseases [16]. Indeed, some of these findings might dictate procedure choice and postoperative management. Preoperative mental and emotional assessments are also strongly recommended to address any underlying mood or eating disorders that might negatively affect surgical outcomes and attention must be paid to discuss the physical changes to the patient's skin and body after MBS [17]. Lastly, specific recommendations such as avoidance of pregnancy in the immediate preoperative period and up to 18 months after surgery as well as smoking cessation for a minimum of 6 weeks prior to the procedure should be mandated [18].

## Revisional/Conversional Procedures for Weight Recurrence After RYGB

Revisional/conversional surgical procedures for weight recurrence after initial RYGB can be categorized into four groups:

1. Laparoscopic pouch resizing and/or revision of gastrojejunal anastomosis (GJA).
2. Adjustable or non-adjustable gastric band (AGB) over pouch ± pouch/GJA resizing.
3. Distalizing RYGB (DRGB) ± Band or pouch/GJA resizing.
4. Conversion to biliopancreatic diversion with duodenal-switch (BPD-DS) or single-anastomosis duodeno-ileal bypass with sleeve gastrectomy (SADI-S).

Multiple etiologies for WR after RYGB have been reported including gastric pouch dilatation >5 cm in diameter, gastric fistula and wide GJ stoma [19]. The following surgical revisions and conversions aim to address some of the anatomic changes implicated in WR.

### Laparoscopic Pouch Resizing and/or Revision of Gastrojejunal Anastomosis (GJA)

This option was reported to be the most commonly performed revisional surgery procedure after RYGB before 2015. In most cases, gastric and candy cane resection is performed by using a linear stapler in patients with gastric pouch >5 cm or dilated GJA (>2 cm) [20, 21]. The gastric pouch is then resized to the volume of 20–40 mL after calibration with a 32–36 French bougie. The anastomosis is then resized to a diameter of 1.5 cm and the resection of the candy cane is performed when present. The outcome in terms of BMI reduction is inferior to most of the other surgical revisional procedures, especially in the long term [22]. Amor et al. reported a mean excess weight loss (EWL) at 1, 3, and 5 years follow-up of 38.6%, 52% and 43% with an 8% rate of overall complications and no mortality [20]. Laparoscopic GJA plication has also been described by some authors as an effective and safe procedure when compared to the previously described surgical technique with a median EWL at 6 months of 46.2% [23, 24]. In conclusion, despite the promising short-term results of this surgical option, the long-term efficacy of this revisional procedure is inferior when compared to other techniques [19].

### Adjustable or Non-adjustable Gastric Band Over Pouch ± Pouch/GJA Resizing

This procedure takes advantage of the well-known restrictive component of the laparoscopic gastric banding in which a prosthetic band is positioned proximal to the gastrojejunostomy. After the placement of 4 to 5 trocars, the dissection of the previous gastric bypass from liver parenchyma is started to identify the anatomical landmarks. The pouch is then freed circumferentially paying attention to spare the blood supply to the pouch. The lateral aspect of the pouch is resized after the insertion of a 35 French bougie using linear staplers. After downsizing the pouch, a Fobi-ring or similar device is placed 0.5–1 cm above the gastrojejunostomy in a perigastric technique without the need for additional sutures. The length of the ring can vary between 5.5 and 6.5 cm, taking into consideration the amount of scar tissue at the surgical site. The rationale of this procedure is based on the prevention of post-prandial dilation, thus maintaining the restrictive effect of the procedure. Moon et al. reported a mean EWL of 23.4, 39 and 18.9% at 6, 12, and 24 months after surgery respectively associated with a high rate of complications and reoperation due to stricture and perforated ulcers [25].

In a large series by Schmidt et al., weight loss was observed in 97% of patients who underwent LAGB placement after failed RYGB with a median EWL of 37.7% after 2.5 years of follow-up with 46.4% of them maintaining an EWL percentage >30% [26]. Due to the acceptable safety profile, lower surgical risks, and no change in nutrient absorption, this surgical option may represent an attractive option compared to other procedures in selected patients. However, band erosion should be monitored in the long run.

## Distalizing RYGB (DRGB)

Distalization of RYGB is defined by the shortening of the common channel, increasing the malabsorptive component of the initial surgery.

There are two main types of distalization: **type 1 distalization** was first described by Sugerman et al. in the early 1980s in which the jejunojejunostomy is taken down at the end of the alimentary limb and the limb is reanastomosed to the distal ileum, at a point 150 cm proximal to the ileocecal valve. In this type of distalization the alimentary limb maintains its original size of 100–150 cm, the common channel with a 150 cm length, and an unmeasured biliopancreatic limb [27].

**Type 2 distalization** was initially suggested by Brolin et al. as a variation in which the jejunojejunostomy is taken down at the end of the biliopancreatic limb (BP limb), then the BP limb is reanastomosed to a point of 75 cm proximal to the ileocecal valve, thus creating a shorter common channel, while maintaining the length of the BP limb and the sum of common and alimentary limbs unchanged [28].

Both techniques are commonly performed laparoscopically and have demonstrated safety. Excellent and durable results have been reported with both types even in the mid-term. Nevertheless, the curve of weight loss is suggested to be steeper with type 1 and associated with better quality of life as long as the length of the common channel is anywhere between 100–150 cm. Moreover, in type I distalization, EWL ranged from 61% to 90% and from 68% to 85% at 1 and 5 years respectively [29]. In the work by Srikanth et al., an EWL of 77% was still reported to be significant at a follow-up of more than 10 years [30].

Despite promising long-term outcomes, most reported DRYGB, either with type 1 or type 2 distalization, resulted in a high rate of severe Protein Energy Malnutrition (PEM), hypoalbuminemia, and mortality often requiring revisions. For the above reasons, some authors recommend a common channel length >200 cm or a total alimentary limb length (TALL) which is defined as the sum of roux limb and common channel length. In the work by Shin et al., the total alimentary limb (roux limb plus common channel) lengths (TALL) ranged from 200 to 300 cm with a mean of 255.8 cm, while in the cohort of patients described by van der Burgh, the TALL was of 350–400 cm [31, 32]. In a recent systematic review by Franken et. al, severe malnutrition was reported in 18% of cases after DRYGB, reoperation was needed in 21% and reversal of distalization was performed in 15% of all patients [33]. Therefore, accurate measurement of the intestinal limbs is paramount.

In conclusion, DRGYB is to be considered the most effective approach in the short and long term, with the potential risk of PEM requiring revision. Therefore, it is advisable to maintain a TALL of 350 cm and reserve this kind of revisional procedure for experienced centers which can ensure good follow-up.

### Conversion to Biliopancreatic Diversion with Duodenal-Switch (BPD-DS) or Single-Anastomosis Duodeno-ileal Bypass with Gastric Sleeve (SADI-S)

BPD-DS is categorized as one of the most effective procedures in the spectrum of bariatric surgery due to its hypoabsorptive component. Conversion of RYGB to BPD-DS can be challenging due to the complexity of the redo operations. For the surgical procedure, five trocars are usually placed: right, left lower, and left upper quadrant and two midlines, 1 immediately below the xiphoid process for liver retraction and one for the camera port midway between the latter one and the umbilicus. Initially, lysis of adhesion is performed to free the left liver lobe and identify the gastrojejunal anastomosis. The ileocecal valve is identified, and the ileum measured proximally 100 cm. This site is marked with a suture for further identification. An additional 150 cm is measured proximally along the ileum and the ileum is divided at a total of 250 cm from the ileocecal junction. Digestive continuity is restored with the take down of the GJ anastomosis, the construction of a gastro-gastric anastomosis followed by a sleeve gastrectomy, and the division of the first portion of duodenum using a tunnel dissection 3–4 cm distal to the pylorus. An end-to-side duodeno-ileal anastomosis is performed and finally, the biliopancreatic limb is taken down to the previously 100-cm mark and a side-to-side entero-enterotomy is created.

A variation of the sleeve gastrectomy can be performed by dividing the excluded stomach at the mid-body of the stomach and respecting the upper half of the stomach including all the fundus. The remnant is then reanastomosed to the gastric pouch in standard fashion either within a 2-layer sutured anastomosis or using a linear stapler and closing the common enterotomy with absorbable sutures. This accomplishes the purpose of a sleeve gastrectomy by reducing the volume of the stomach and removing the fundus without compromising the blood supply of the remnant or the GG anastomosis. The original roux limb of the gastric bypass can then be resected if short or the biliopancreatic limb can be detached from the jejunojejunostomy, and the proximal end of the roux limb can be reanastomosed to the biliopancreatic limb taking care to correctly orient the mesentery to establish full continuity and reversal of the bypass.

The SADI-S was first described and then introduced into clinical practice by the group of Sànchez-Pernaute and Torres in 2007 [34]. Their technique eliminated the Roux-en-Y reconstruction of the original BPD described by Scopinaro [35] and instead, perform a one-loop duodeno ileostomy with pylorus preservation. At the beginning of their experience, a common limb of 200 cm was used, later many surgeons preferred to move the length to 250–300 cm given that longer common channels have proved to minimize the risk of malnutrition and persistent diarrhea without significantly affecting weight loss [36].

A Roux-en-Y gastric bypass can be converted to a SADI after reversal of the bypass and conversion to a sleeve gastrectomy as described above. The duodenal transection is performed using a tunnel dissection past the pylorus. With the proper identification and preservation of the gastroduodenal artery, the duodenal transection can be safely performed. It is a surgeon's preference to take down the right gastric artery to allow a vertical position of the duodenum. Next, the ileo-cecal valve is identified and 300 cm are counted from that point proximally and a loop configuration duodeno-ileal anastomosis is performed. The selected loop is anchored to the proximal sectioned duodenum and a double-layer manual end-to-side antecolic duodeno-ileal anastomosis is performed. Experience with BPD-DS and SADI-S conversions has been described by Surve et al. and Topart et al. reporting a mean EWL as high as 56.4% and 61.5% after 2 years of follow-up [37, 38]. Keshishian et al. reported an EWL of 71% after 3 years in a cohort of 47 patients who underwent conversional BPD-DS due to weight recurrence after RYGB with a 4% rate of major complications [39]. Overall, although long-term weight-loss outcomes are excellent after revisional/conversional BPD-DS and SADI-S, their profound technical difficulties and associated early and late complications limit their widespread use [40].

## Postoperative Assessment

In the immediate postoperative course, patients who undergo revisional/conversional bariatric surgery are placed on a venous thromboembolism (VTE) prevention regimen which includes early ambulation (within the first 4–6 h), compression devices and administration of low molecular weight or unfractionated heparin [41]. Patients are typically started on a clear liquid diet for the first 24 h followed by a progression to a low-fat, full-liquid diet. After discharge, patients are required to adhere to prescribed protein supplements, a vitamin regimen, and gradual progression in food consistency over the next month. Outpatient post-op visits occur between 2 and 6 weeks after discharge with additional checkups at 3 and 6 months. Patients will also be examined bi-annually for a period of two years after MBS and then annually thereafter [42].

## Quality of Life After Revisional/Conversional Bariatric Surgery

Quality of life assessments after revisional/conversional surgery can occur using validated questionnaires such as the short-form health survey (SF-36) or Moorehead-Ardelt II (MA-II) survey. Both surveys take into account different factors such as physical appearance, social functioning, and physical and mental health. One of the goals of successful revisional surgery for our patients is the attainment of a good self-reported quality of life. Recent studies have confirmed, using these validated surveys, that the quality of life 5 years after revisional RYGB was similar to that after primary RYGB, and that it was also similar to the general population's quality of life [43, 44].

## Conclusion

Overall, it appears that many therapeutic modalities are effective for weight loss in the short term following RYGB. Endoscopic approaches show lower rates of complications, but also lower efficacy. On the other hand, surgical revisional/conversional procedures are effective in the short- and mid-term and are associated with higher rates of complications and malnutrition in the long-term.

## References

1. Noria SF, Shelby RD, Atkins KD, Nguyen NT, Gadde KM. Weight regain after bariatric surgery: scope of the problem, causes, prevention, and treatment. Curr Diab Rep. 2023;23(3):31–42.
2. Guimarães M, Osório C, Silva D, Almeida RF, Reis A, Cardoso S, et al. How sustained is Roux-en-Y Gastric bypass long-term efficacy? Roux-en-Y gastric bypass efficacy. Obes Surg. 2021;31(8):3623–9.
3. Sjöström L, Narbro K, Sjöström CD, Karason K, Larsson B, Wedel H, et al. Effects of bariatric surgery on mortality in Swedish obese subjects. N Engl J Med. 2007;357(8):741–52.
4. Maciejewski ML, Arterburn DE, Van Scoyoc L, Smith VA, Yancy WS Jr, Weidenbacher HJ, et al. Bariatric surgery and long-term durability of weight loss. JAMA Surg. 2016;151(11):1046–55.
5. Monaco-Ferreira DV, Leandro-Merhi VA. Weight regain 10 years after Roux-en-Y gastric bypass. Obes Surg. 2017;27(5):1137–44.
6. King WC, Hsu JY, Belle SH, Courcoulas AP, Eid GM, Flum DR, et al. Pre- to postoperative changes in physical activity: report from the longitudinal assessment of bariatric surgery-2 (LABS-2). Surg Obes Relat Dis. 2012;8(5):522–32.
7. Moon S, Lee J, Chung HS, Kim YJ, Yu JM, Yu SH, et al. Efficacy and safety of the new appetite suppressant, liraglutide: a meta-analysis of randomized controlled trials. Endocrinol Metab (Seoul). 2021;36(3):647–60.
8. Abboud DM, Yao R, Rapaka B, Ghazi R, Ghanem OM, Abu Dayyeh BK. Endoscopic management of weight recurrence following bariatric surgery. Front Endocrinol (Lausanne). 2022;13:946870.
9. Vargas EJ, Bazerbachi F, Rizk M, Rustagi T, Acosta A, Wilson EB, et al. Transoral outlet reduction with full thickness endoscopic suturing for weight regain after gastric bypass: a large multicenter international experience and meta-analysis. Surg Endosc. 2018;32(1):252–9.
10. Abu Dayyeh BK, Jirapinyo P, Weitzner Z, Barker C, Flicker MS, Lautz DB, et al. Endoscopic sclerotherapy for the treatment of weight regain after Roux-en-Y gastric bypass: out-

comes, complications, and predictors of response in 575 procedures. Gastrointest Endosc. 2012;76(2):275–82.
11. Gallo AS, DuCoin CG, Berducci MA, Nino DF, Almadani M, Sandler BJ, et al. Endoscopic revision of gastric bypass: Holy Grail or Epic fail? Surg Endosc. 2016;30(9):3922–7.
12. Clapp B, Ponce J, DeMaria E, Ghanem O, Hutter M, Kothari S, et al. American Society for Metabolic and Bariatric Surgery 2020 estimate of metabolic and bariatric procedures performed in the United States. Surg Obes Relat Dis. 2022;18(9):1134–40.
13. Altieri MS, Yang J, Nie L, Blackstone R, Spaniolas K, Pryor A. Rate of revisions or conversion after bariatric surgery over 10 years in the state of New York. Surg Obes Relat Dis. 2018;14(4):500–7.
14. Schlottmann F, Nayyar A, Herbella FAM, Patti MG. Preoperative evaluation in bariatric surgery. J Laparoendosc Adv Surg Tech A. 2018;28(8):925–9.
15. Mechanick JI, Youdim A, Jones DB, Garvey WT, Hurley DL, McMahon MM, et al. Clinical practice guidelines for the perioperative nutritional, metabolic, and nonsurgical support of the bariatric surgery patient—2013 update: cosponsored by American Association of Clinical Endocrinologists, The Obesity Society, and American Society for Metabolic & Bariatric Surgery. Obesity (Silver Spring). 2013;21(01):S1–27.
16. Moulla Y, Lyros O, Mehdorn M, Lange U, Hamade H, Thieme R, et al. Preoperative upper-GI endoscopy prior to bariatric surgery: essential or optional? Obes Surg. 2020;30(6):2076–84.
17. Fabricatore AN, Crerand CE, Wadden TA, Sarwer DB, Krasucki JL. How do mental health professionals evaluate candidates for bariatric surgery? Survey results. Obes Surg. 2006;16(5):567–73.
18. Mechanick JI, Youdim A, Jones DB, Timothy Garvey W, Hurley DL, Molly McMahon M, et al. Clinical practice guidelines for the perioperative nutritional, metabolic, and nonsurgical support of the bariatric surgery patient—2013 update: cosponsored by American Association of Clinical Endocrinologists, the Obesity Society, and American Society for Metabolic & Bariatric Surgery. Surg Obes Relat Dis. 2013;9(2):159–91.
19. Kermansaravi M, Davarpanah Jazi AH, Shahabi Shahmiri S, Eghbali F, Valizadeh R, Rezvani M. Revision procedures after initial Roux-en-Y gastric bypass, treatment of weight regain: a systematic review and meta-analysis. Updat Surg. 2021;73(2):663–78.
20. Amor IB, Petrucciani N, Kassir R, Malyshev E, Mazoyer C, Korkmaz C, et al. Midterm outcomes of gastric pouch resizing for weight regain after Roux-en-Y Gastric bypass. Obes Surg. 2020;30(7):2723–8.
21. Hamdi A, Julien C, Brown P, Woods I, Hamdi A, Ortega G, et al. Midterm outcomes of revisional surgery for gastric pouch and gastrojejunal anastomotic enlargement in patients with weight regain after gastric bypass for morbid obesity. Obes Surg. 2014;24(8):1386–90.
22. Al-Bader I, Khoursheed M, Al Sharaf K, Mouzannar DA, Ashraf A, Fingerhut A. Revisional laparoscopic gastric pouch resizing for inadequate weight loss after Roux-en-Y gastric bypass. Obes Surg. 2015;25(7):1103–8.
23. Ferraz AA, de Siqueira LT, Nunes Filho E, de Araújo JG Jr, Campos JM, de Barros-Correia TX, et al. Revision surgery for treatment of weight regain after Roux-en-Y gastric bypass. Obes Surg. 2014;24(1):2–8.
24. León F, Maiz C, Daroch D, Quezada N, Gabrielli M, Muñoz C, et al. Laparoscopic hand-sewn revisional gastrojejunal plication for weight loss failure after Roux-en-Y gastric bypass. Obes Surg. 2015;25(4):744–9.
25. Moon RC, Teixeira AF, Jawad MA. Treatment of weight regain following roux-en-Y gastric bypass: revision of pouch, creation of new gastrojejunostomy and placement of proximal pericardial patch ring. Obes Surg. 2014;24(6):829–34.
26. Schmidt HJ, Lee EW, Amianda EA, Nyirenda TL, Talishinskiy T, Novack RC Jr, et al. Large series examining laparoscopic adjustable gastric banding as a salvage solution for failed gastric bypass. Surg Obes Relat Dis. 2018;14(12):1869–75.
27. Sugerman HJ, Kellum JM, DeMaria EJ. Conversion of proximal to distal gastric bypass for failed gastric bypass for superobesity. J Gastrointest Surg. 1997;1(6):517–24. discussion 24–6

28. Brolin RE, Cody RP. Adding malabsorption for weight loss failure after gastric bypass. Surg Endosc. 2007;21(11):1924–6.
29. Tran DD, Nwokeabia ID, Purnell S, Zafar SN, Ortega G, Hughes K, et al. Revision of Roux-En-Y gastric bypass for weight regain: a systematic review of techniques and outcomes. Obes Surg. 2016;26(7):1627–34.
30. Srikanth MS, Oh KH, Fox SR. Revision to malabsorptive Roux-en-Y gastric bypass (MRNYGBP) provides long-term (10 years) durable weight loss in patients with failed anatomically intact gastric restrictive operations: long-term effectiveness of a malabsorptive Roux-en-Y gastric bypass in salvaging patients with poor weight loss or complications following gastroplasty and adjustable gastric bands. Obes Surg. 2011;21(7):825–31.
31. Shin RD, Goldberg MB, Shafran AS, Shikora SA, Majumdar MC, Shikora SA. Revision of Roux-en-Y gastric bypass with limb distalization for inadequate weight loss or weight regain. Obes Surg. 2019;29(3):811–8.
32. van der Burgh Y, Boerboom A, de Boer H, Witteman B, Berends F, Hazebroek E. Weight loss and malnutrition after conversion of the primary Roux-en-Y gastric bypass to distal gastric bypass in patients with morbid obesity. Surg Obes Relat Dis. 2020;16(3):381–8.
33. Franken RJ, Franken J, Sluiter NR, de Vries R, Euser S, Gerdes VEA, et al. Efficacy and safety of revisional treatments for weight regain or insufficient weight loss after Roux-en-Y gastric bypass: a systematic review and meta-analysis. Obes Rev. 2023;24(10):e13607.
34. Sánchez-Pernaute A, Rubio Herrera MA, Pérez-Aguirre E, García Pérez JC, Cabrerizo L, Díez Valladares L, et al. Proximal duodenal-ileal end-to-side bypass with sleeve gastrectomy: proposed technique. Obes Surg. 2007;17(12):1614–8.
35. Scopinaro N, Adami GF, Marinari GM, Gianetta E, Traverso E, Friedman D, et al. Biliopancreatic diversion. World J Surg. 1998;22(9):936–46.
36. Gebellí JP, Lazzara C, de Gordejuela AGR, Nora M, Pereira AM, Sánchez-Pernaute A, et al. Duodenal switch vs. single-anastomosis duodenal switch (SADI-S) for the treatment of grade IV obesity: 5-year outcomes of a multicenter prospective cohort comparative study. Obes Surg. 2022;32(12):3839–46.
37. Surve A, Zaveri H, Cottam D, Belnap L, Medlin W, Cottam A. Mid-term outcomes of gastric bypass weight loss failure to duodenal switch. Surg Obes Relat Dis. 2016;12(9):1663–70.
38. Topart P, Becouarn G. One-stage conversion of Roux-en-Y gastric bypass to a modified biliopancreatic diversion with duodenal switch using a hybrid sleeve concept. Surg Obes Relat Dis. 2016;12(9):1671–8.
39. Keshishian A, Zahriya K, Hartoonian T, Ayagian C. Duodenal switch is a safe operation for patients who have failed other bariatric operations. Obes Surg. 2004;14(9):1187–92.
40. Alexandrou A, Sakarellos P, Davakis S, Vailas M, Dimitriou N, Papalampros A, et al. Revision of Roux-en-Y gastric bypass for inadequate weight loss or weight regain. In Vivo. 2022;36(1):30–9.
41. Bartlett MA, Mauck KF, Daniels PR. Prevention of venous thromboembolism in patients undergoing bariatric surgery. Vasc Health Risk Manag. 2015;11:461–77.
42. Poitou Bernert C, Ciangura C, Coupaye M, Czernichow S, Bouillot JL, Basdevant A. Nutritional deficiency after gastric bypass: diagnosis, prevention and treatment. Diabetes Metab. 2007;33(1):13–24.
43. Mohos E, Schmaldienst E, Prager M. Quality of life parameters, weight change and improvement of co-morbidities after laparoscopic Roux Y gastric bypass and laparoscopic gastric sleeve resection—comparative study. Obes Surg. 2011;21(3):288–94.
44. Chew CAZ, Shabbir A. Revisional bariatric surgery: focus on quality of life. J Obes Metab Syndr. 2017;26(2):97–101.

# Surgical Revisions After Endoscopic Primary Procedures

43

Natan Zundel, Felipe J. Cantu Jr, and Juan D. Hernandez

## Introduction

It is clear to all stakeholders involved in the study and treatment of the obesity epidemic that it has exceeded the capacity of response of health systems around the world. Part of the response is bariatric surgery, which has already proven the most effective and durable method to produce significant and enduring weight loss.

Despite sustained efforts, bariatric surgery has only reached around 1% [1] of the population in need of such an intervention. On the other hand, there are patients who will not undergo bariatric surgery for different reasons including severe medical conditions, lack of resources, and insurance issues. There are also patients out of the traditional parameters widely accepted as indications to undergo surgery. Additionally, many candidates for surgery will not accept it [2]. Reasons found are unavailability, lack of confidence due to the risk of complications, and excessive cost, among others. The GBD Obesity Collaborators (Global Burden of Diseases, Injuries and Risk Factors Study of the University of Washington), a group that studies the burden of diseases in the world, state that any excess of BMI over 25 has a

N. Zundel (✉)
Department of Surgery, University of Buffalo, Buffalo, NY, USA

JNMC, Miami, FL, USA

F. J. Cantu Jr
Department of Surgery, Hospital Christus Muguerza, Reynosa, Mexico

Universidad Mexico Americana del Norte UMAN, Reynosa, Tamaulipas, Mexico

J. D. Hernandez
Division of General Surgery, Hospital Universitario Fundacion Santa Fe de Bogota, Bogotá, Colombia

Department of Surgery and Anatomy, Universidad de los Andes School of Medicine, Bogotá, Cundinamarca, Colombia


O. M. Ghanem et al. (eds.), *The SAGES Manual of Metabolic and Bariatric Surgery*, https://doi.org/10.1007/978-3-031-72309-4_43

progressive increase in the risk of cardiovascular disease, diabetes, and death [1]. This statement means that patients in overweight or level I obesity with no comorbidities, will benefit from a more effective treatment than just lifestyle changes including diet and exercise, that has proven insufficient [3], and they likely will not be candidates for surgery.

The void in obesity treatment caused by system insufficiency or the lack of options to offer to a population that won't be operated on, is progressively being filled by new alternatives. Still in its infancy and unlikely to replace surgery in the foreseeable future, hormonal treatments are appearing. GLP 1 analogs are being used in the treatment of diabetes and obesity with favorable results, but the effects are not sustained without continued treatment. These medications are successful if maintained for longer periods [4]. However, it is still unknown how effective these treatments will be in the long term, and if they will be safe and cost-effective.

Endoscopic procedures, initially of low complexity, have been available for several years with different levels of success and durability. Endoscopy technology progressed along with robotic surgery and natural orifice transluminal endoscopic surgery (NOTES) but developed independently and to a higher level, to produce devices that allow endoscopists to carry out actual endoscopic surgical interventions. Along with technology, endoscopists and surgeons have more practice and have gained skills in advanced procedures that allow them to practice procedures that usually require surgery, like treating achalasia with POEM (peroral endoscopic myotomy) [5] or other endoscopic extraluminal interventions.

Albeit progressing, technology has been slow in becoming available on a larger scale, so publications are scarce and with low levels of evidence. To date, these procedures are considered non-surgical, safe with lower risk, and mostly lower in cost compared to a surgical intervention. Procedures have a variable rate of success in their outcomes and therefore are still looking for a place in the armamentarium to treat obesity. Additionally, these techniques are still not as effective as surgery but seem to be finding indications of use, and their own space.

Current evidence indicates that endoscopic bariatric devices and techniques, although better than diet and change of habits, are not universally efficacious and have temporary success, with many patients with weight recurrence or experiencing pain or other symptoms. These scenarios motivate physicians, as in any other chronic disease, to seek further interventions or mixed therapeutics and escalate treatment according to the patient's individual circumstances. The next step in the therapeutics of obesity, after medications and counseling, may be endoluminal therapies with varying degrees of success. Conversion to a surgical procedure is increasingly common as endoscopic techniques proliferate. The decision and timing to take the patient to a bariatric procedure is influenced by the kind of endoscopic procedure the patient underwent before and the planned surgical conversion. This chapter will explore how to approach these patients with a focus on the unique aspects of the previous endoluminal intervention and outcomes of surgical conversion.

## Endoscopic Bariatric Procedures and Devices

The search for less invasive procedures to treat mild to moderate obesity has taken many forms, through different lines of investigation and inventions. Researchers' interests have gone from temporary methods to more durable solutions. There have been different approaches to a variety of indications. Some strategies have been difficult to accept or tolerate by patients. Indications can be temporary weight loss before a major operation, use as a first stage for a planned bariatric surgery, and for other indications, including as a weight-loss method to facilitate pregnancy in the short term, or prior to orthopedic surgery to improve outcomes, for example. Other indications include weight loss in mild obesity with more severe metabolic disease, older and fragile patients that require weight loss, or potentially as a cosmetic method of reducing weight. Endoscopic devices appeal to a broad group of patients because they are less invasive and potentially reversible, and the procedure duration and hospital stay are short compared to surgery.

### Intragastric Balloon (IGB)

The intragastric balloon is the longest available endoscopic device, first proposed as an obesity treatment in the 1980's. It has been likened to a bezoar [6] since it occupies a large space in the stomach, decreasing gastric volume and creating satiety. Balloons as devices have seen improvement and can be found in swallowable and adjustable versions. Most balloons are designed to remain in place for 4–6 months, with some designed to last for 1 year in the stomach before retrieval. In the Spanish consensus on IGB [7], over 20,000 patients were reported. In this large series, patients reached a mean percentage of TBWL of 17%, with minimum and maximum %TBWL of 0% and 52% respectively. Intragastric balloons are only effective while in place, however, balloons can be implanted sequentially, and no specific number of balloons has been defined as maximal. Regarding adverse events, early removal may occur in up to 4% of patients and often occurs early after implantation. The most common major adverse event is gastric ulceration (0.4%) which varies between brands and requires balloon removal. Intragastric balloons can also produce gastric perforation or bowel obstruction if passed distally [7], especially if the balloon is not removed in planned time intervals (Fig. 43.1a, b). An important consideration when choosing balloon treatment for obesity is that there is limited treatment duration and that weight regain is common upon removal and cessation of therapy.

### Endoscopic Sleeve Gastroplasty (ESG)

Endoscopic sleeve gastroplasty (ESG) is an endoscopic procedure first described by Abu Dayyeh in 2013 [8]. Initially, the procedure was carried out with mucosal-only stitches using a suturing device (Overstitch™; Apollo Endosurgery, Austin, TX).

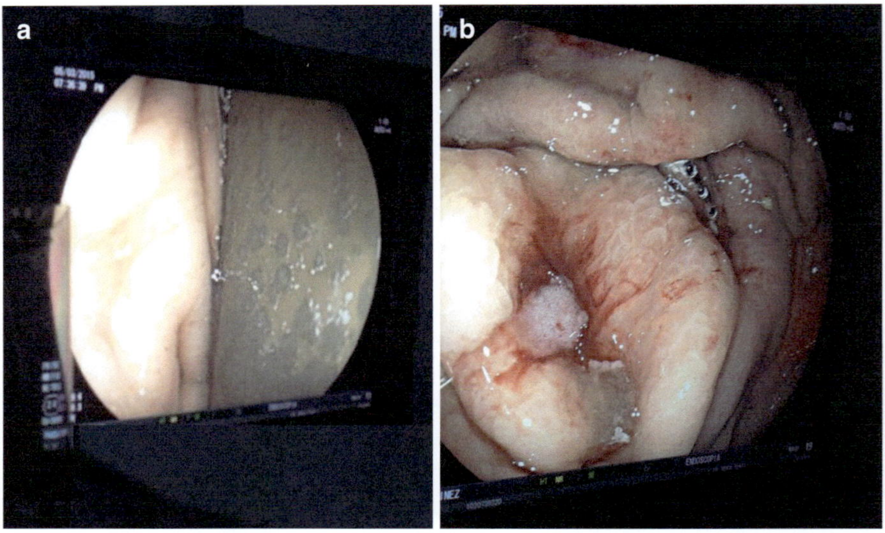

**Fig. 43.1** (**a**) Intragastric balloon showing changes of being seven months in the stomach. The long stay produced a perforated ulcer. (**b**) Endoscopy showing the perforated ulcer, with a laparoscopic suction device going through it. On the left, there is a second ulcer

After a description of the initial concept, the technique was modified to include transmural stitches, plicating the greater curve of the stomach, starting near the incisura angularis and progressing proximally to the fundus, with preservation of the angle of His. The final result is an invagination of the greater curvature of the stomach with a remaining 20% of the lumen [9]. A systematic review by Jalal and Edye´s showed a 6-month total body weight loss (TBWL) of 13.7–15.2%, which is significantly less than laparoscopic sleeve gastrectomy (LSG). They also found significantly less complications (Clavien-Dindo 2 and up) in ESG than in LSG (2.0–2.7% vs. 9.2–16.9%). As a full-thickness stitches procedure, complications include bleeding, perforation, and leaks. Alqahtani [10] and Sharaiha [11] reported good control and/or remission of diabetes, hypertension and dyslipidemia, in a post-procedure period of 3–12 months. As with other procedures, there are also non-responder patients to the procedure.

Another endoscopic procedure with similar results and complications is the primary obesity surgery endolumenal (POSE) procedure. The differences between POSE and ESG include the delivery device, the suturing mechanism and the location of stitches in the stomach. While ESG creates a tubularized "sleeve" with a curved needle, POSE uses a different endoscopic stitching device known as the g-Cath™ EZ Delivery Catheter and Snowshoe Suture Anchor™ (USGI Medical, San Clemente, CA) to reduce the size of the fundus and part of the body of the stomach [12]. In a randomized, sham-controlled study, Sullivan et al. [13] randomized 332 patients and demonstrated a significantly higher %TBWL in the treatment group than in the sham group. There are still unanswered questions on long-term results, durability, and how training will influence outcomes.

## Aspire System (AspireAssist® System—Aspire Bariatrics, Inc. King of Prussia, PA)

Aspire Assist is a modified gastrostomy placed by endoscopy similar to the classic percutaneous endoscopic gastrostomy (PEG), with a larger bore inner cannula. It is designed to extract part of the food ingested. Once installed, the PEG-like device is left to heal. Once ready for use, it is attached to an external pump after each meal (Fig. 43.2). Food content mixes stomach fluid with the addition of water. Once infused, then this is aspirated with extraction of food particles and therefore decreased caloric intake. Though the literature is limited, a one-year study with 207 patients showed that the AspireAssist™ group reached a significantly greater weight loss than the control group, treated with lifestyle counseling alone [14]. A four-year follow-up multicenter European study [15] showed that weight loss is maintained during the use of the therapy, even after 4 years of continuous use.

In 2022, Aspire Bariatrics, the company making AspireAssist™, withdrew the system, and therefore future implantations will cease and limited supplies will exist, with resultant removals of the device. However, revisions/interventions will continue to be needed.

## Small Bowel Directed Therapies for Obesity

Small bowel-directed therapies for obesity are based on the foregut theory, in which exclusion of the duodenum prevents absorption in the proximal bowel [16]. The aims of the endoscopic procedures and devices utilizing this concept are to exclude the duodenum and proximal jejunum from absorbing nutrients, and also to deliver those nutrients rapidly into the ileum [17]. Clever designs have produced devices that include:

Endobarrier™ (GI Dynamics, Lexington, MA) [18] is a duodenal-jejunal bypass liner, and the gastro-duodeno-jejunal sleeve (ValenTx™, Inc., Maple Grove, MN). Both are impermeable, tubular polymeric devices anchored to the mucosa that divert nutrients and prevent mucosal contact, with digestion by biliary and pancreatic

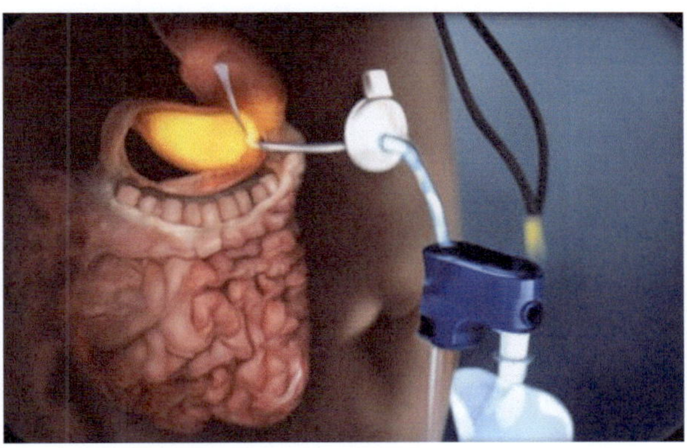

**Fig. 43.2** Aspire assist system showing the PEG installed in the stomach and connected to the aspiration device

secretion occurring at the end of the tube. Endobarrier™ is anchored distal to the pylorus in the duodenal bulb and has a length of 60 cm resulting in the exclusion of the duodenum and proximal jejunum. ValenTx™ is fixed laparoscopically with guided transmural anchors at the gastroesophageal junction, with a 120 cm tube extending to the jejunum. These devices have shown successful results in weight loss and diabetes control with reduction of glycosylated hemoglobin. A recent study with 1022 patients from 10 countries showed that the Endobarrier™ achieved a mean weight loss of 13.3 kg, with a statistically significant reduction in systolic blood pressure, HbA1C, cholesterol, and weight [19]. Complications include liner migration and obstruction, bleeding, perforation, and liver abscess from the anchoring mechanism. This last complication has limited the device expansion. The authors recommend removing the device at 9 months to reduce the risk of portal contamination.

Duodenal mucosal resurfacing is an endoscopic technique using the Revita DMR™ (Fractyl, Waltham, MA) device that results in ablation of 10 cm of duodenal mucosa distal to the ampulla of Vater [18]. A balloon catheter is advanced endoscopically and inflated, circulating hot water to produce mucosal ablation. The objective of delivering therapy to the mucosal lining is to facilitate the formation of new enterocytes and reestablish a healthy neuroendocrine axis. A systematic review composed of four studies [20] showed a significant reduction in HbA1C and fasting plasma glucose after 6 months, 3.1 kg mean weight reduction after 3 months, but no significant weight loss after 6 months. A significant decrease in hepatic steatosis was also noted after 3 months.

## Considerations When Selecting an Endoscopic Procedure for the Treatment of Obesity

The aim of endoscopic bariatric procedures to date is to improve the quality of life of patients with obesity and to slow down the deleterious effects of obesity on cardiovascular and other systems through weight reduction and control of comorbidities. The duration and impact of this effect is less with endoscopic procedures than with surgery. It should be considered that in some cases, the beneficial effects of endoscopic procedures have a limited duration. As such, repetition of the initial endoscopic procedure, conversion to or addition of an alternative endoscopic procedure, and proceeding to a surgical bariatric intervention all are safe possibilities for patient treatment [21].

As with any new procedure, there is a possibility that when these endoscopic complex and technically demanding procedures expand to a larger number of endoscopists, a higher number of complications or recurrences may be reported.

## Revision after Endoscopic Metabolic Procedures

Weight recurrence and complications are the main causes for conversion of an endoscopic to a surgical procedure. Therefore, for each endoscopic procedure there should be established goals and objectives. Once a decision to move on to a surgical procedure is made, patients need to be evaluated according to the reason for conversion. It is recommended that all patients have a preoperative endoscopy and upper GI fluoroscopy series as part of that work up. Additional studies may include CT, pH probe, manometry, and MRI as indicated.

### Intragastric Balloon

The presence of the device creates dilatation of the stomach and changing the characteristics of the muscle wall including edema and thickening of the gastric wall when the device is in place for longer periods of time. In a study to establish if there is benefit of using IGB in super-obese patients to improve risk prior to bariatric surgery, authors found more complications in the balloon group, including leaks, bleeding, and abscess during the conversion [22]. Based on such outcomes, it is suggested to wait several weeks and up to 2 months until inflammation is reduced enough to safely operate and reduce the risk of leaks or bleeding after surgery. Selecting the correct staple height on the stomach after the IGB removal is crucial to prevent failure of the staple line formation leading to fistulas and bleeding (Fig. 43.3) It is recommended to have a variety of staple loads during these procedures, especially cartridges for thick tissue, and be prepared to reinforce the staple lines with suture, reinforcement materials or in some scenarios a laparoscopic totally hand-sewn technique is required in case the stomach wall is exceedingly thick.

### Endoscopic Sleeve Gastroplasty (ESG)

Endoscopic Sleeve Gastroplasty (ESG) is increasingly commonly performed and therefore may be a more routinely performed conversion to surgery. ESG requires skill and training to create a symmetric sleeve, small enough to produce weight loss. Alqahtani has described how this is both a reversible and repeatable intervention and may require the removal of sutures and other hardware before another intervention [23].

Indications for ESG reversal or conversion include severe abdominal pain, insufficient weight loss or patient´s dissatisfaction. However, before considering a conversion when insufficient weight loss is the indication, Lopez-Nava et al. suggest a repeat ESG [24] based on a short cohort of their patients. They did a second ESG on patients who did not achieve initial weight loss and for those patients with weight recurrence. In this group of redo ESG, all patients were able to achieve some degree of weight loss.

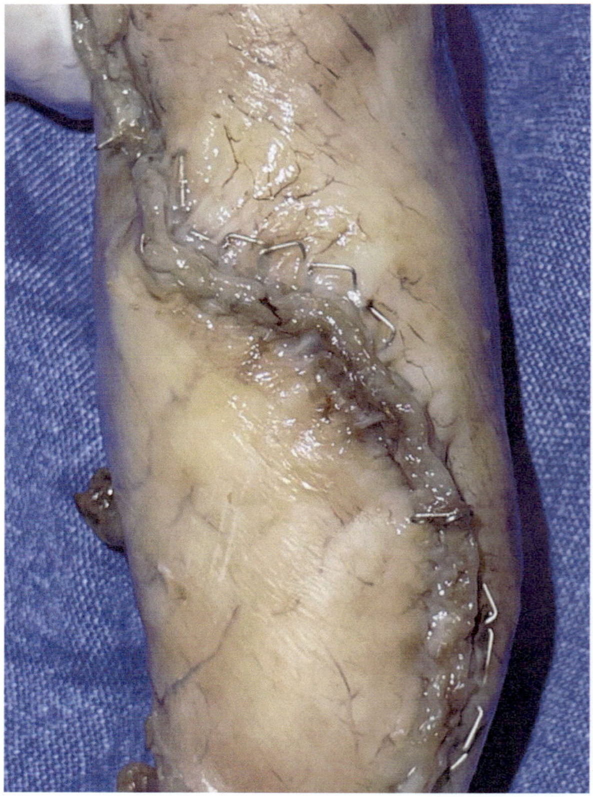

**Fig. 43.3** Specimen after vertical sleeve gastrectomy with exceedingly thick gastric wall. Incomplete formation of surgical staples in a patient who underwent an IGB removal 6 weeks before the sleeve gastrectomy

Zerrweck et al., describe the conditions, preparation, and surgical technique considerations for patients undergoing conversion after ESG [25]. It has been recommended that an endoscopy be performed prior to surgery to remove all hardware, or intraoperative as a hybrid procedure (Fig. 43.4). In our experience, we found that it is not simple to remove all hardware and that bleeding can occur. Currently, we perform a hybrid technique, with the endoscope at the time of laparoscopy to identify and avoid any anchor, cinch, T-fastener or suture material. As part of the conversion, the stomach should be released of all adhesions, especially to the posterior wall, that tends to have more and thicker attachments that may alter gastric anatomy (Fig. 43.5). Sometimes removal of sutures includes dissecting them from the stomach serosal layer, with long threads firmly adhered to it (Fig. 43.6). We also recommend using a higher staple height for gastric division as the wall is thicker. Staple line should go medially to where endoscopic suturing was done and where hardware is found. If stapler cannot be placed and deployed safely preserving an appropriate sleeve lumen, a gastric bypass should be considered instead.

A word of caution was voiced by Grille et al. [21], on a case report of a conversion of ESG. They describe how it was impossible to remove the sutures and T-fasteners endoscopically, and were not visible on laparoscopy, possibly because they were not full-thickness. They had to perform a partial gastrectomy due to this

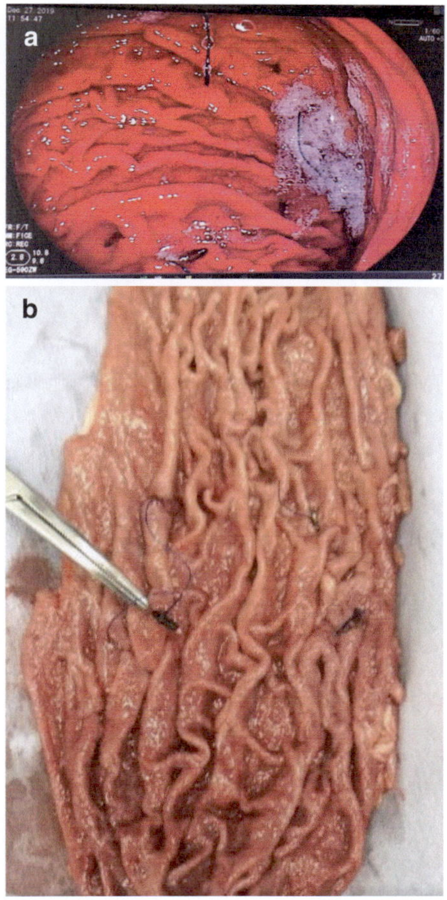


**Fig. 43.4** (**a**) Endoscopy of a failed ESG from the authors´ experience. It shows loose sutures and T- fasteners, with a completely undone gastroplasty. (**b**) Same patient after the LSG

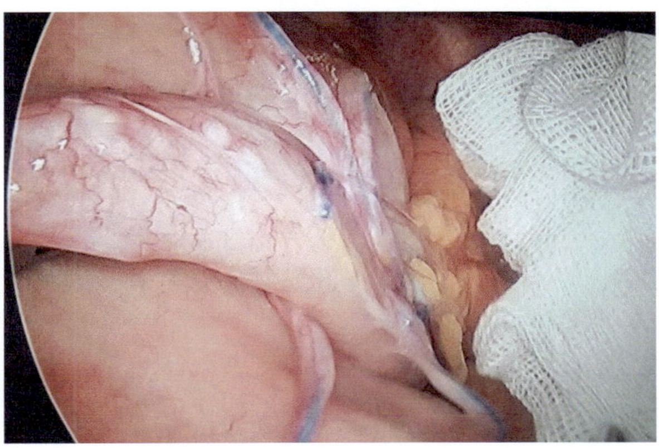

**Fig. 43.5** Same patient as Fig. 43.4, on a laparoscopic view, showing severe adhesions formed by full-thickness sutures

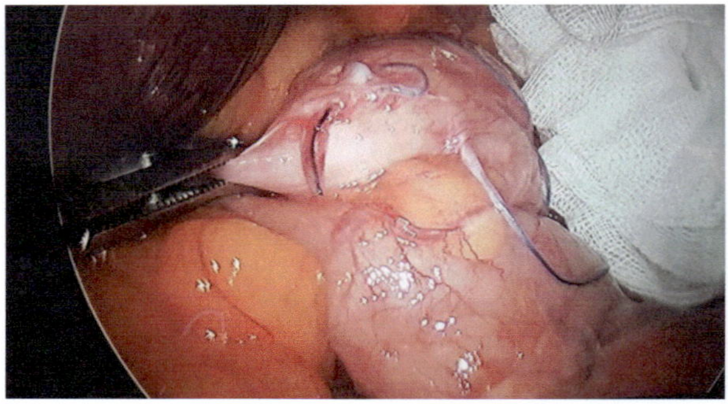

**Fig. 43.6** Long threads of ESG sutures adhered to the stomach serosal layer that could create severe adhesions

finding. In a similar report from Australia [26], conversion of ESG to LSG was successful in two patients, and authors had to remove hardware that had progressed into the abdominal wall.

## Aspire

As mentioned above, the current and future lack of supplies to the system make it compulsory to remove the PEG-like device. The removal of the gastrostomy tube (called the A-tube) is done endoscopically, and a group of authors in a case report [27] recommend the de-epithelialization of the PEG tract and closure of the stoma with a suturing device to avoid the formation of a chronic fistula. They specifically used the X-Tack Endoscopic HeliX Tacking System (Apollo Endosurgery, Austin, TX, USA).

When considering conversion to surgery, the A-tube preferably has been removed weeks before the operation to reduce the amount of scarring and inflammation. Adhesions will be found to the abdominal wall and freed to completely expose the stomach [28]. When performing a sleeve gastrectomy, the part of the stomach where the stoma was should be part of the resection, as long as its location allows for a viable gastric conduit.

## Small Bowel as Target for Endoscopic Bariatric Devices

In the techniques described above, the anchoring of the devices or the ablation of the mucosa produce inflammation, and therefore carrying out any procedure (sleeve, bypass or single anastomosis duodeno-ileal bypass with sleeve gastrectomy -SADI-S-) will have the risk to find inflammation and changes in the normal anatomy or tissue thickness. This may result in complications of the staple line, including bleeding, leaks, or fistula. There are no published reports specifically dedicated to conversion to surgical procedures, but the recommendation is to wait until the device is removed and inflammation Has subsided, before carrying out a bariatric surgical interventions.

## Conclusions

Bariatric endoscopic procedures and devices have been improving with time and new technologies. These advancements have expanded a niche for their application and are becoming available to a larger number of professionals and being used by more people around the world.

These devices must be safe and effective in the hands of appropriately trained endoscopists. Additionally, as endoscopic procedures, they should reduce time exposure to the effects of obesity in treated patients, improving quality of life and treating or delaying the appearance of comorbidities. Additionally, every endoscopic procedure should: (1) be repeatable, that is, used sequentially if adequate, (2) should permit revisions and when required, must allow to safely conduct a laparoscopic or open bariatric procedure. As with any obesity treatment, patients should be treated within a multidisciplinary program and followed to make the necessary adjustments should they be required. A number of patients will need laparoscopic bariatric surgery after endoscopic interventions. If the endoscopic bariatric procedure was properly done, the risk of complications during surgery will be less.

Endoscopic bariatric interventions are becoming part of the obesity treatment continuum. Obesity is a chronic disease and with time, many patients will need more than one therapeutic intervention. Each endoscopic procedure has and will have unique indications, contraindications, and outcomes to best fit individual patient needs. Continued studies and rigorous outcomes must be reviewed to identify the best intervention to treat obesity in an individual patient.

## References

1. GBD 2015 Obesity Collaborators. Health effects of overweight and obesity in 195 countries over 25 years. N Engl J Med. 2017;377(1):13–27.
2. Rozier MD, Ghaferi AA, Rose A, et al. Patient preferences for bariatric surgery: findings from a survey using discrete choice experiment methodology. JAMA Surg. 2019;154:e184375.
3. Langeveld M, DeVries JH. The long-term effect of energy restricted diets for treating obesity. Obesity. 2015;23:1529–38.
4. Rubino D, Abrahamsson N, Davies M, Hesse D, Greenway FL, Jensen C, Lingvay I, Mosenzon O, Rosenstock J, Rubio MA, Rudofsky G, Tadayon S, Wadden TA, Dicker D, STEP 4 Investigators. Effect of continued weekly subcutaneous semaglutide vs placebo on weight loss maintenance in adults with overweight or obesity: the STEP 4 randomized clinical trial. JAMA. 2021;325:1414–25. https://doi.org/10.1001/jama.2021.3224.
5. Crespin OM, Liu LWC, Parmar A, Jackson TD, Hamid J, Shlomovitz E, Okrainec A. Safety and efficacy of POEM for treatment of achalasia: a systematic review of the literature. Surg Endosc. 2017;31(5):2187–201. https://doi.org/10.1007/s00464-016-5217-y.
6. Silva LB, Neto MG. Intragastric balloon. Minim Invasive Ther Allied Technol. 2022;31(4):505–14. https://doi.org/10.1080/13645706.2021.1874420.
7. Espinet Coll E, Del Pozo García AJ, Turró Arau R, Nebreda Durán J, Cortés Rizo X, Serrano Jiménez A, Escartí Usó MÁ, Muñoz Tornero M, Carral Martínez D, Bernabéu López J, Sierra Bernal C, Martínez-Ares D, Espinel Díez J, Marra-López Valenciano C, Sola Vera J, Sanchis Artero L, Domínguez Jiménez JL, Carreño Macián R, Juanmartiñena Fernández JF, Fernández Zulueta A, Consiglieri Alvarado C, Grecco E, Bezerra Silva L, Neto MG. Spanish

Intragastric Balloon Consensus Statement (SIBC): practical guidelines based on experience of over 20000 cases. Rev Esp Enferm Dig. 2023;115(1):22–34. https://doi.org/10.17235/reed.2022.9322/2022.
8. Abu Dayyeh BK, Rajan E, Gostout CJ. Endoscopic sleeve gastroplasty: a potential endoscopic alternative to surgical sleeve gastrectomy for treatment of obesity. Gastrointest Endosc. 2013;78(3):530–5. https://doi.org/10.1016/j.gie.2013.04.197.
9. Jalal MA, Cheng Q, Edye MB. Systematic review and meta-analysis of endoscopic sleeve gastroplasty with comparison to laparoscopic sleeve gastrectomy. Obes Surg. 2020;30(7):2754–62. https://doi.org/10.1007/s11695-020-04591-4.
10. Alqahtani A, al-Darwish A, Mahmoud AE, et al. Short-term outcomes of endoscopic sleeve gastroplasty in 1000 consecutive patients. Gastrointest Endosc. 2019;89(6):1132–8.
11. Sharaiha RZ, Kumta NA, Saumoy M, et al. Endoscopic sleeve gastroplasty significantly reduces body mass index and metabolic complications in obese patients. Clin Gastroenterol Hepatol. 2017;15(4):504–10.
12. Lopez Nava G, Arau RT, Asokkumar R, et al. Prospective multicenter study of the Primary Obesity Surgery Endoluminal (POSE 2.0) procedure for treatment of obesity. Clin Gastroenterol Hepatol. 2023;21(1):81–9.
13. Sullivan S, Swain JM, Woodman G, Antonetti M, De La Cruz-Muñoz N, Jonnalagadda SS, Ujiki M, Ikramuddin S, Ponce J, Ryou M, Reynoso J, Chhabra R, Sorenson GB, Clarkston WK, Edmundowicz SA, Eagon JC, Mullady DK, Leslie D, Lavin TE, Thompson CC. Randomized sham-controlled trial evaluating efficacy and safety of endoscopic gastric plication for primary obesity: the ESSENTIAL trial. Obesity. 2017;25(2):294–301. https://doi.org/10.1002/oby.21702.
14. Thompson CC, Abu Dayyeh BK, Kushner R, Sullivan S, et al. Percutaneous gastrostomy device for the treatment of class II and class III obesity: results of a randomized controlled trial. Am J Gastroenterol. 2017;112(3):447–57. https://doi.org/10.1038/ajg.2016.500.
15. Nyström M, Machytka E, Norén E, Testoni PA, Janssen I, Turró Homedes J, Espinos Perez JC, Turro Arau R. Aspiration therapy as a tool to treat obesity: 1- to 4-year results in a 201-patient multi-center post-market European registry study. Obes Surg. 2018;28(7):1860–8. https://doi.org/10.1007/s11695-017-3096-5.
16. Cohen R, le Roux CW, Papamargaritis D, et al. Role of proximal gut exclusion from food on glucose homeostasis in patients with type 2 diabetes. Diabet Med. 2013;30:1482–6.
17. Forgione A, Cummings DE, et al. The mechanism of diabetes control after gastrointestinal bypass surgery reveals a role of the proximal small intestine in the pathophysiology of type 2 diabetes. Ann Surg. 2006;244:741–9.
18. Edmundowicz SA. Small bowel target devices and techniques. Gastrointest Endosc Clin N Am. 2017;27:289–97. the EndoBarrier (GI Dynamics, Lexington, MA)
19. Ryder REJ, Laubner K, Benes M, Haluzik M, Munro L, et al. Endoscopic duodenal-jejunal bypass liner treatment for type 2 diabetes and obesity: glycemic and cardiovascular disease risk factor improvements in 1022 patients treated worldwide. Diabetes Care. 2023;46(4):e89–91.
20. De Oliveira GHP, de Moura DTH, Funari MP, McCarty TR, Ribeiro IB, Bernardo WM, et al. Metabolic effects of endoscopic duodenal mucosal resurfacing: a systematic review and meta-analysis. Obes Surg. 2021;31(3):1304–12. https://doi.org/10.1007/s11695-020-05170-3.
21. Grille VJ, You D, Kipnis S. Endoscopic sleeve gastroplasty requiring conversion to partial gastrectomy with paraesophageal hernia repair. J Surg Case Rep. 2021;5:1–3.
22. Coffin B, Maunoury V, Pattou F, Hébuterne X, Schneider S, Coupaye M, Ledoux S, Iglicki F, Mion F, Robert M, Disse E, Escourrou J, Tuyeras G, Le Roux Y, Arvieux C, Pouderoux P, Huten N, Alfaiate T, Hajage D, Msika S. Impact of intragastric balloon before laparoscopic gastric bypass on patients with super obesity: a randomized multicenter study. Obes Surg. 2017;27(4):902–9. https://doi.org/10.1007/s11695-016-2383-x.
23. Alqahtani A, Elahmedi M, Alqahtani YA, et al. Laparoscopic sleeve gastrectomy after endoscopic sleeve gastroplasty: technical aspects and short-term outcomes. Obes Surg. 2019;29(11):3547–52.

24. Lopez-Nava G, Asokkumar R, Negi A, Normand E, Bautista I. Re-suturing after primary endoscopic sleeve gastroplasty (ESG) for obesity. Surg Endosc. 2021;35:2523–30. https://doi.org/10.1007/s00464-020-07666-6.
25. Zerrweck C, Galvao M, Bandari M, Zundel N. Conversion from endoscopic sleeve gastroplasty to sleeve. In: Gagner M, Ramos Cardoso A, Palermo M, Noel P, Nocca D, editors. The perfect sleeve gastrectomy; 2020. p. 453–61. https://doi.org/10.1007/978-3-030-28936-2.
26. Alhayo S, Devadas M. Laparoscopic sleeve gastrectomy following multiple failed endoscopic sleeve gastroplasties. JSCR. 2019;12:1–3.
27. Waseem A, Wawrzynski J, Maselli DB, Kucera A, Wooley C, McGowan. Endoscopic removal of a weight-loss device with stoma closure using a tack-and-suture device. Video GIE. 2023;8(11):441–2. https://doi.org/10.1016/j.vgie.2023.07.005.
28. Villalonga R, Bademci R, Roriz-Silva R, Sanchez-Cordero S, Curbelo Y, Almanza A. Conversion of aspireassist system® to sleeve gastrectomy: technical video description. Obes Surg. 2019;29(8):2715–7. https://doi.org/10.1007/s11695-019-03993-3.

# Revisions and Conversions After One Anastomosis Gastric Bypass (OAGB), Single Anastomosis Duodenal Ileostomy (SADI-S) and Biliopancreatic Diversion-Duodenal Switch (BPD-DS)

44

Diana Kantarovich, Katherine Carsky, Vikrom Dhar, Lamorna Coyle, and Mitchell Roslin

## Introduction

Bariatric surgery stands in opposition to the norms of other surgical procedures. Where other operations are performed to remove or repair a diseased portion of the body, weight loss or metabolic surgery rearranges the intestinal tract to create a controlled anatomical and physiological abnormality. Bariatric surgeries are generally divided into restrictive and hypoabsorptive operations. For restrictive procedures the stomach is reduced in size, while for hypoabsorptive procedures restriction is combined with the bypassing of a significant portion of the small intestine—resulting in food traveling a shorter path before reaching the colon. As these latter procedures change both the stomach size and reroute the small intestine, they produce the highest weight loss and lowest rates of recidivism while leading to the greatest improvement in diabetes and other metabolic parameters [1]. Unfortunately, bypassing absorption in the small intestine also leads to the highest risk of micronutrient deficiencies, anemia, and loss of lean muscle mass and bone [2–4]. Balancing these outcomes remains a challenge for bariatric surgeons.

One difficulty of bariatric surgery is the range of reasons for revisions following a procedure. This includes technical issues such as strictures and chronic obstruction, as well as the development of non-healing ulcers, gastroesophageal reflux disease (GERD), or bile reflux gastritis [5, 6]. An increasing proportion of revisions following restrictive procedures including Laparoscopic Sleeve Gastrectomy (LSG)

D. Kantarovich · K. Carsky · V. Dhar · M. Roslin (✉)
Department of General Surgery, Northwell Health, Lenox Hill Hospital, New York, NY, USA
e-mail: dkantarovich@northwell.edu

L. Coyle
Donald and Barbara Zucker School of Medicine at Hofstra/Northwell, Hempstead, NY, USA



O. M. Ghanem et al. (eds.), *The SAGES Manual of Metabolic and Bariatric Surgery*, https://doi.org/10.1007/978-3-031-72309-4_44

and Laparoscopic Adjustable Gastric Banding (LAGB) are done for inadequate weight loss and weight regain. In contrast, the majority of revisions performed following hypoabsorptive procedures are done for symptoms of short bowel including nutritional deficiencies, diarrhea, irritable bowel disease, anemia, and bone loss [7].

One Anastomosis Gastric Bypass (OAGB), Single Anastomosis Duodenal Ileal Bypass with Sleeve (SADI- S) and Biliopancreatic Diversion with Duodenal Switch (BPD-DS) are perhaps the three most robust bariatric procedures accepted by major surgical organizations. They combine a reduction in stomach capacity with a bypass of a minimum of 150 centimeters (cm) of the proximal small intestine. As a result, these procedures offer excellent weight loss results. Therefore, patients that do require surgical revision following these procedures usually do so because of nutritional issues rather than inadequate weight loss or recurrence. Careful assessment of body composition and muscle function is mandatory before considering a revision for weight recurrence after these malabsorptive procedures. In this chapter, we will detail the dominant anatomical configurations of these procedures, explain the most prevalent issues, and detail the best reconstructive and revisional techniques.

## Evaluation of the Post-Operative Patient

Although the objective of weight loss is to lose excess fat while preserving lean muscle mass and bone, it would be naïve to assume that there is no component of muscle and bone loss as weight loss occurs. The reduction in adipose tissue after surgery leads to reduction in leptin levels and an increase in adiponectin levels which may lead to increased bone resorption [8]. The Longitudinal Assessment of Bariatric Surgery (LABS) study revealed that Roux-en-y Gastric Bypass (RYGB) and LSG patients lost 20% of their muscle mass one year following surgery [9]. While the majority of patients undergoing bariatric surgery have proportionally more fat loss than muscle or bone mass loss, these complications cannot be overlooked.

Patient evaluation is crucial at regular intervals. In addition to measuring weight, a directed physical exam should be completed. This includes examination of a patient's dentition and jaw. We have found that patients with symptoms of short bowel tend to have protrusion of their lower mouth, retraction of the mandible and loss of dentition. As part of the physical exam, patients should be asked to go from a sitting to standing position without the assistance of their arms to evaluate gluteal muscle strength. To evaluate balance, they should be asked to stand on one leg. Additionally, it is imperative to ask about activity levels and to describe bowel habits. Importantly, laboratory values are not always reliable markers of nutritional status. Meaningful deficiencies must be addressed; however, normal results do not eliminate the possibility of a serious problem. Patients may be using their reserve, catabolizing normal tissues, and relying on other compensatory mechanisms. Eating disorder experts that handle anorectic patients often note that they are surprised that laboratory tests can remain normal until very late in the disease process [10, 11]. As part of a typical follow-up routine, a physician may recommend four visits in the first year with blood testing at 3 months and 12 months. Following this, they should complete a yearly evaluation which often includes dual x-ray absorptiometry (DEXA) scans for analysis of bone and body composition. Unfortunately, DEXA scans are difficult to obtain due to reimbursement issues. While it would be informative to use bioelectrical impedance analysis (BIA) to measure the changes in body composition after bariatric surgery, its accuracy remains controversial.

## One Anastomosis Gastric Bypass (OAGB)

OAGB has become an increasingly popular international procedure but has established limited penetration in the United States. The procedure was first described by the American surgeon Robert Rutledge, who in 1997 named the procedure Mini-Gastric Bypass (MGB) as the original technique was completed through a mini-laparotomy [12]. For multiple reasons this procedure has been controversial and poorly received in the United States (US). The procedure was compared to Billroth II reconstructions, utilized in early bariatric procedures, and primarily criticized for biliary reflux with concerns for malignancy in the long term. After many years of debate, the operation was finally accepted by the American Society of Metabolic and Bariatric Surgeons in 2022. Its place in clinical practice in the United States is still evolving.

The operation involves creating a long gastric sleeve that reflects the lesser curvature of the stomach (Fig. 44.1a). The pouch is long and begins 2–3 cm distal to the angularis incisura and extends to the "angle of His". The remnant stomach remains in place. By design, the pouch is longer (15–18 cm) and narrower (36–40

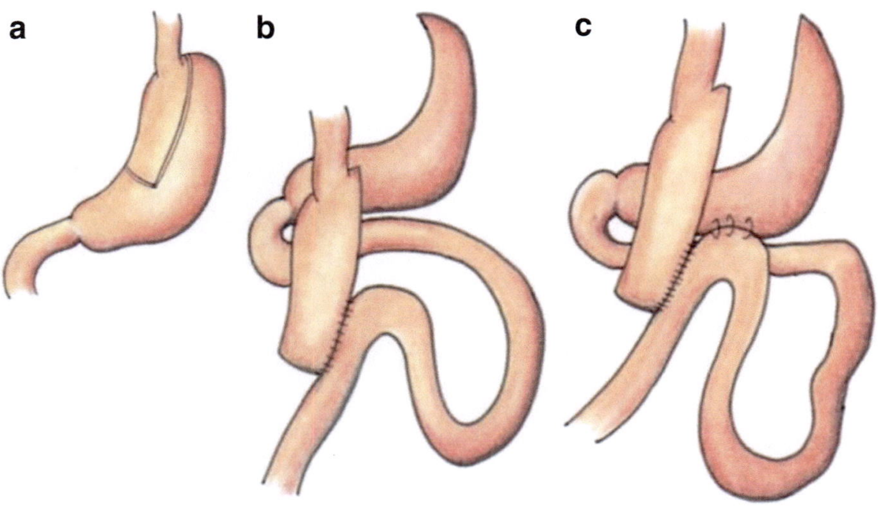


**Fig. 44.1** (**a**) Creation of the gastric pouch in OAGB. (**b**) Anastomosis is created between the distal lateral pouch and the small bowel 150–250 cm from the ligament of Treitz. (**c**) The orientation of the proximal small bowel is fixed superiorly to help reduce bile reflux

French bougie) than a classic RYGB pouch, with some labeling it a "pencil pouch". The small bowel is measured, and a single ante-colic anastomosis is created from the distal lateral corner of the gastric pouch to the jejunum, generally between 150 cm and 250 cm distal to the ligament of Treitz (Fig. 44.1b). The anastomosis is not meant to be restrictive, and measures from 3 to 5 cm wide. The orientation of the proximal small bowel to the anastomosis is fixed superiorly to help reduce bile reflux (Fig. 44.1c). Advocates for the procedure highlight these nuances to relieve fear about the consequences of bile reflux and gastroesophageal reflux. They argue that a long narrow pouch, combined with a non-restrictive anastomosis, limit the bile stream from reaching the esophagus (Fig. 44.2). Furthermore, as compared to procedures performed years ago, the biliopancreatic (BP) limb is longer. This dilutes the bile and allows for a significant portion of bile to be reabsorbed by the small bowel prior to reaching the stomach pouch.

The combination of a narrow pouch, non-restrictive anastomosis, elimination of the antrum and fundus and absence of a pylorus makes food move more rapidly following OAGB. As a result, as compared to duodenal switch (DS) type procedures, a longer common channel is required (300–350 cm). In a randomized controlled trial performed by experienced surgeons, a 200 cm OAGB was compared to an RYGB with 50 cm BP limb. The weight loss, improvement in metabolic disease, and reduction in HgBA1c was significantly greater in OAGB. However, the rate of malnutritional parameters was far greater and approached 20% in patients having

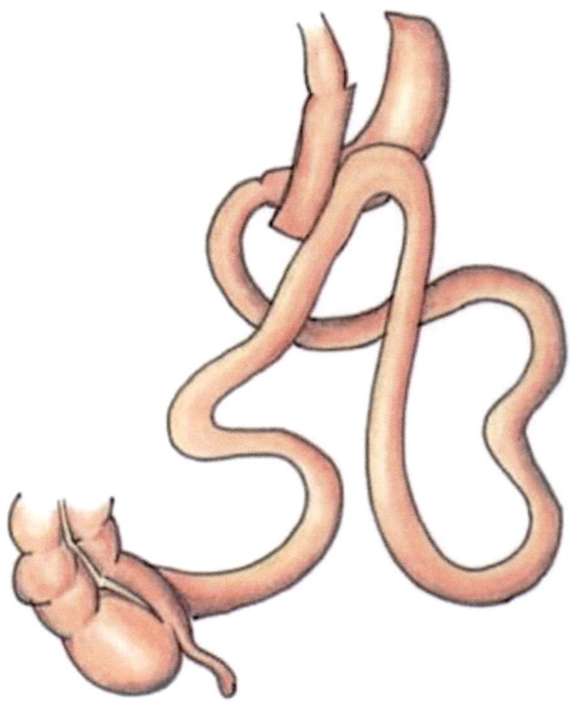

**Fig. 44.2** The completed One Anastomosis Gastric Bypass (OAGB)

complications related to OAGB surgery [13]. While longer limb length can result in better weight loss, length over 200–250 cm can also lead to greater risk of malnutrition.

## Revisions for Diarrhea, Malnutrition, Vitamin Deficiency, Irritable Bowel Syndrome, Anemia or Bone Loss

As discussed, hypoabsorptive procedures offer the best weight loss and potentially the best treatment for many patients with energy imbalance who continue to consume high calorie foods. Lifelong follow-up, however, is imperative. Without follow-up there may be increased risk for Wernicke Encephalopathy, iron deficiency anemia and hypoalbuminemia [14]. A minority of patients are subject to the risks seen with short bowel syndrome including frequent bowel movements, malnutrition, fatigue, and chronic anemia. Hypoalbuminemia with peripheral swelling should be treated with total parenteral nutrition until swelling is relieved prior to considering surgical revision. Diarrhea not amenable to nutritional alteration can also be an indication for revision.

The key feature in surgical revision is increasing the length of bowel that comes into contact with food. This can be achieved by moving the loop backwards. The site of the original anastomosis is divided and an entero-enterostomy is performed. The loop is reattached 100–150 cm more proximal along the BP limb (Fig. 44.3). This technique is appropriate for those patients whose BP limb is more than 200 cm. However, for those with BP limbs <200 cm, moving a meter back may lead to an increased risk of bile reflux. As mentioned, the length of the BP limb allows for dilution and reabsorption of bile, thus the longer length of the BP limb in OAGB is partially responsible for the low levels of reported bile reflux gastritis and esophagitis.

Another option, which in our opinion is preferable for patients with BP limbs that are <200 cm and that can be used in all circumstances, is to create what has been called "kissing cousins". To do so, the small bowel is divided just proximal to the loop anastomosis (Fig. 44.4a). That end of bowel is taken and attached 75 cm distal to the anastomosis. From this point, measure back on the BP limb 100–150 cm and attach it about 30 cm distal to the anastomosis with a side-to-side anastomosis. The gastrojejunostomy is left intact, but two small bowel attachments are created (Fig. 44.4b). This approach has also been used for malnutrition and diarrhea following BPD-DS [15].

## Management of Bile Reflux Gastritis and GERD

Overall incidence of bile reflux after OAGB is 1–4%, and has been shown to be associated with pouches shorter than 9 cm and presence of pre-operative GERD [16]. The initial treatment consists of dietary changes and the use of proton pump inhibitors (PPIs). If medical management fails, a reversal or revision to RYGB may be considered. This is done by dividing the small bowel proximal to the anastomosis

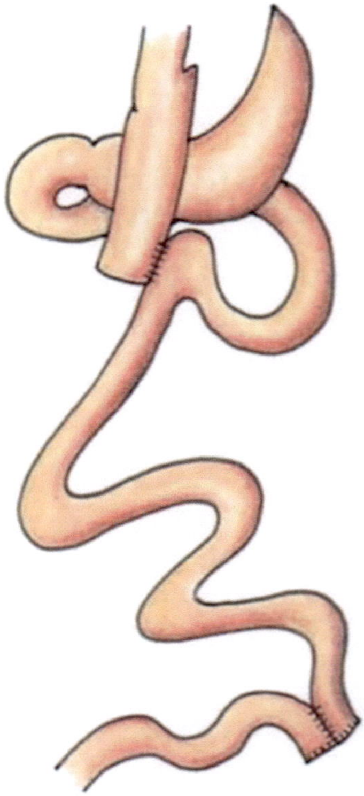

**Fig. 44.3** Revision of OAGB involving moving the loop backwards to create a new anastomosis, shorter BP limb, and longer common channel

and then performing an entero-enterostomy, preferably 75 cm distal to the anastomosis to limit any retrograde flow.

Reports of revision for GERD following OAGB are not frequent. If this occurs, a repair of the hiatal hernia can be performed. A plication with the remnant stomach can be done. Another method is placing a LINX device around the esophagus, which is a magnetic sphincter augmentation system intended to increase sphincter tone, thereby preventing reflux. Additionally, a recent experimental approach used the round ligament to provide a pseudoplication [17]. Without a traditional fundoplication, however, the surgical repair of the hiatus can be unsuccessful long term. If there is evidence of severe esophagitis we would suggest converting to a RYGB with repair of the hiatal hernia. During the repair, the hernia is reduced with mobilization of the intra-thoracic esophagus to obtain at least a 3 cm segment of intra-abdominal esophagus before the crura is then reapproximated. In addition, we suggest placing a suture at the gastroesophageal (GE) junction to the base of the crura to further prevent esophageal migration.

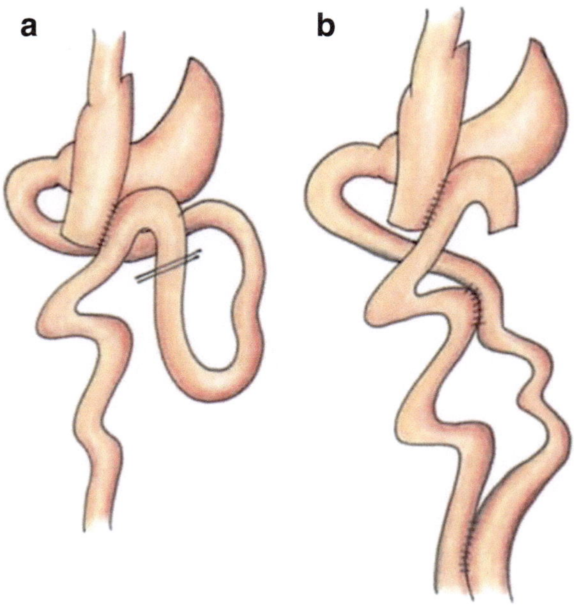


**Fig. 44.4** (**a**) Division of small bowel just proximal to the anastomosis, leaving the gastrojejunostomy intact. (**b**) Creation of a second anastomosis 100–150 cm proximal on BP limb and 30 cm distal to the prior GJ anastomosis, leaving two anastomoses and two common channels

## Management of Marginal Ulcers

Marginal ulcers (MU) can be a significant complication following OAGB with rates reported as high as 3–10%. Many marginal ulcers can be managed conservatively with diet modification, PPIs and H2 blockers [18]. Additionally, patients must be tested for H. pylori to help guide medical therapy. If the ulcer persists, surgical management is more complex and the portion of the bowel with the ulcer may require formal resection and re-anastomosis. To adequately treat, both the pouch and the small bowel require resection. Thus, as the pouch will be shorter and smaller, we suggest converting to a RYGB. Some also suggest vagotomy or remnant gastrectomy to reduce the risk of recurrent ulcers. For emergency perforation, patching can be done, but stricture is a risk.

## Management of Weight Regain or Inadequate Weight Loss

OAGB is a very effective weight loss operation. However, as with any procedure, there can be inadequate weight loss or weight regain. Prior to consideration of revision, it is imperative to re-evaluate these patients and determine the causes of their inadequate results. Patients may require dietary consultation as they often may be consuming high levels of refined carbohydrates and processed foods. Additionally, these patients can optimize their weight loss with glucagon-like peptide (GLP) analogues that appear to have reasonable efficacy following bariatric procedures. Revision may be considered as a final resort.

The optimal strategy to increase weight loss is lengthening the BP limb. This comprises of separating the small bowel from the pouch, closing the small bowel with an entero-enterostomy, and creating a loop attachment 100–150 cm more distally. However, this increases the risk of malnutrition and short bowel symptoms, as previously described. The therapeutic range where fat loss occurs, minimal lean tissue is lost, and there are no symptoms of short bowel may be very small. As a result, it is our suggestion that these patients should be followed carefully and that having body composition measurements may also be insightful to their progress.

## Biliopancreatic Diversion with Duodenal Switch (BPD-DS) and Single Anastomosis Duodenal Ileal Bypass with Sleeve (SADI-S)

Biliopancreatic diversion was first described by Scopinaro in 1979. This procedure combined a horizontal gastric resection with the closure of a duodenal stump, gastroileal anastomosis, and an ileoileal anastomosis to create a 50 cm common channel and a 250 cm alimentary channel. The duodenal switch procedure was first described by DeMeester in 1987 as a treatment for bile gastritis. Hess later adapted this procedure for bariatric surgery [19]. The BPD-DS procedure includes a sleeve gastrectomy (40–54 French bougie), the transection of the duodenum distal to the pylorus, and the creation of an alimentary limb, enzymatic or BP limb and a common channel (Fig. 44.5). Hess measured the entire small bowel, finding that the added length of the alimentary and common channel was 40% of the total bowel. Ten percent of the total was then used to create the common channel. This was adapted by Marceau and several others to have a common channel that ranged from 75 to 100 cm. More recently, with the understanding that fat consumption is not necessarily responsible for obesity, the common channel has been lengthened.

The Single Anastomosis Duodenal Ileal Bypass with Sleeve (SADI-S) was first described in 2007 [20]. It was developed with the hope that it would offer weight loss similar to BPD-DS and that lengthening the common channel might lead to a reduction of nutritional disorders. In lieu of a Roux construction such as in BPD-DS, in SADI-S a loop of bowel that is 250–300 cm from the ileocecal valve is attached to the divided duodenum (Fig. 44.6). Although there is promising data, both procedures can still have patients that develop critical nutritional deficiencies [21].

Both procedures combine a longitudinal gastrectomy that is generally less restrictive than primary Laparoscopic Sleeve Gastrectomy (LSG) with a post-pyloric intestinal bypass. The smallest guiding diameter should be a 40 French (Fr) bougie. Larger sizes up to 54 Fr are also acceptable. The more accommodating sleeve offers several potential benefits; leak rates decrease with increasing bougie size and the potential for GERD is reduced [22]. Additionally, adequate intake is required to optimize nutrition, as a narrow sleeve can increase gastric emptying [23]. Thus, even with the pylorus intact, a small diameter sleeve that does not have a fundus or any antrum can promote rapid passage, increasing the potential for malabsorption when combined with a shortened intestinal pathway.

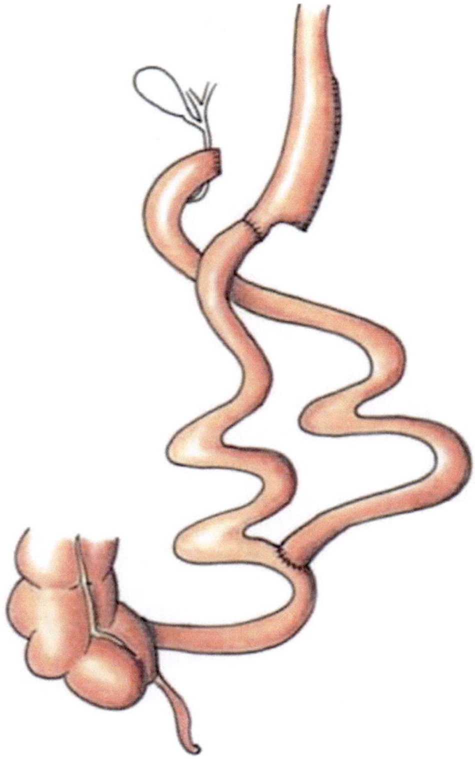

**Fig. 44.5** BPD-DS

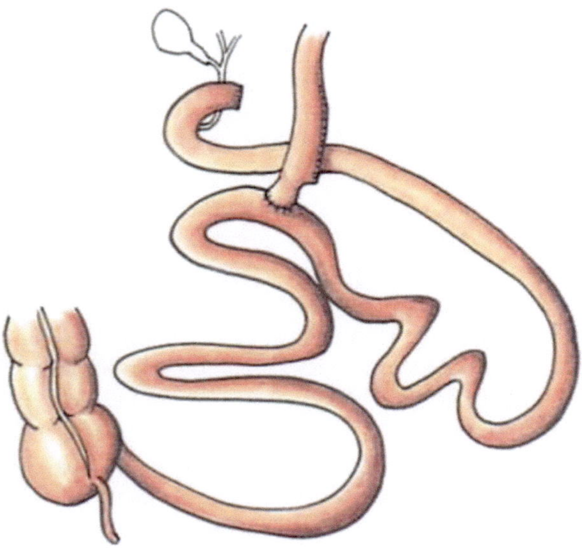

**Fig. 44.6** SADI-S

The second aspect of the procedure is the intestinal bypass. Food should encounter at least 250–300 cm of small bowel in its journey through the body. On occasion, this number is increased in low BMI patients with a metabolic syndrome. For BPD-DS, the shortest acceptable limb lengths are an alimentary or Roux limb of 150 cm and a common channel of 100 cm. Lengthening the common channel in BPD-DS is increasingly common. A recent randomized study demonstrated reduced vitamin deficiencies and similar weight loss when the common channel is increased to 200 cm [24].

In SADI-S, a loop that is a minimum of 250 cm from the start of the terminal ileum is attached to the post-pyloric duodenum. Many suggest using a 300 cm loop. This results in a BP limb that can be considered the afferent limb, and a digestive limb or common channel which is also the efferent limb. The duodenum is anastomosed to the proximal aspect of the ileum. In this configuration, a majority of the duodenum and the jejunum are bypassed.

Many substances are preferentially absorbed in the bypassed segments in both procedures. These include divalent cations and the majority of vitamins with the exception of B12 [25]. Fat-soluble vitamins, such as vitamins A, D, E and K, are best absorbed with the assistance of bile and fat. However, most of the bile is absorbed in the afferent limb in SADI-S or the BP limb in BPD-DS, making supplementation of fat-soluble vitamins mandatory. Advantages of these procedures include approximately 30% greater weight loss than LSG, as well as greater lasting resolution of metabolic conditions such as Type II diabetes [21, 26].

## Revisions for Diarrhea, Malnutrition, Vitamin Deficiency, Irritable Bowel Syndrome, Anemia or Bone Loss

While adding an intestinal bypass to a sleeve gastrectomy results in greater weight loss and resolution of certain comorbid conditions, the risk of complications of short bowel syndrome increases, similar to OAGB. These complications include frequent bowel movements, flatulence, and anal rectal pathology as well as deficiency of micronutrients, divalent cations, and hypoproteinemia [15].

It is key to assess the relationship between food intake and bowel movements. Fat malabsorption and steatorrhea are characterized by abundant dense stool that floats after eating. Lactose deficiency presents with frequent watery diarrhea 40 min following eating. However, watery diarrhea following a bariatric procedure is more often associated with malabsorption of carbohydrates leading to an osmotic gradient promoting fluid entry into the gastrointestinal tract (GI), also known as early dumping syndrome. This results in diarrhea about 10–30 min after eating.

Additionally, increased gut bacteria in the small bowel and the colon cause fermentation of carbohydrates, releasing methane. Small intestinal bacterial overgrowth (SIBO) can be diagnosed by a breath test for lactulose which, if positive, should lead to an antibiotic treatment. Treatment also includes alteration of diet and the use of motility agents such as Imodium and Lomotil. A histamine two-blocker and proton-pump inhibitor should be prescribed. Physicians should emphasize a low-fat diet that limits the fermentation-causing carbohydrate intake, a so-called FODMAP diet [27]. If diarrhea persists, other medications including clonidine, octreotide and GLP agonists can be utilized. The GLP-1 agonists delay gastric emptying and reduce motility. The GLP-2 analog (teduglutide) is rarely used following bariatric surgery [28]. Although its usage does lead to short-term gut hypertrophy and increased absorption, it is expensive and must be used indefinitely or the effect will dissipate. Therefore, if surgical revision is practical, it is preferred, and the use of the GLP-2 analog is reserved for patients who do not have a surgical alternative. Prior to surgery these patients often require several weeks of parenteral nutrition to stabilize and provide an optimal surgical environment.

The earliest laboratory signs of poor nutrition following bariatric surgery are low BUN and hypokalemia. These are typically noted before there is a decrease seen in total protein or albumin levels. Chronic patients can usually compensate but may present with low bicarbonate and potassium from diarrhea. Iron, magnesium, and calcium can also be abnormal. Iron is predominately absorbed in the duodenum and proximal intestine, which are bypassed during these cases. Hence, anemia, stemming from iron deficiency, is common. Calcium is also preferentially absorbed in the proximal intestine and can be further lowered by abnormal vitamin D absorption. Additionally, calcium binds to the increased levels of fatty acids that are present in the GI tract from fat malabsorption. Magnesium, which is preferentially absorbed in a lower portion of the GI tract, also can be abnormal because of its binding to fatty acids and increased excretion. As discussed with OAGB, hypoproteinemia following these hypoabsorptive procedures can lead to peripheral edema. When this occurs, treatment is mandatory. This is the leading indication for revision following BPD-DS and can also occur following SADI-S [15].

The absence of bile salts to form micelles and reduced absorptive capacity can lead to a deficiency of fat-soluble vitamins A, D, E, and K even with high-dose supplementation. Vitamin D deficiency complicates calcium deficiency and increases bone turnover and the risk of metabolic bone disease. Vitamin K deficiency can lead to alteration in blood clotting that can be further exacerbated if there is increasing steatosis or cholestasis in the liver from malnutrition. It is essential that supplements should be water soluble versions to maximize the probability of absorption [29].

As opposed to the majority of water-soluble vitamins that are absorbed in the proximal small bowel, B12 is preferentially absorbed in the ileum [30]. However, it requires the presence of an intrinsic factor, which is decreased after the creation of the sleeve, to be absorbed. Additionally, if there is a bacterial overgrowth, the bacteria may compete for B12 and can further compromise the levels. Deficiency can potentiate anemia and cause neurologic symptoms. Supplementation is best done through the nose, sublingual, or by injection.

Critical deficiencies of the trace elements zinc, copper, and selenium can certainly occur. In general, they are rarely isolated and are representative of a lengthy period of inadequate nutrition. Zinc deficiency is the most common. Copper deficiency can be a cause of peripheral neuropathy and weakness many years after bariatric surgery. Similarly, selenium deficiency can lead to heart failure.

Administration of trace elements is usually given with parenteral nutrition. Clinically significant deficiencies are rarely encountered in patients who do not have multiple problems [31].

All bariatric procedures that bypass the duodenum and proximal intestine can increase the incidence of osteomalacia, osteoporosis, osteopenia, and secondary hyperparathyroidism. As discussed above, calcium absorption is compromised, and vitamin D absorption is hindered by bile diversion. In general, supplements are effective in mitigating damage. To minimize the risk of hungry bones it is essential to optimize calcium and vitamin D. Routine monitoring and serial bone density measurements are suggested.

Malabsorption can also lead to nephrolithiasis. This can be exacerbated by the promotion of foods that are high in oxalate. If there is fat malabsorption, calcium will bind to free fatty acids—creating a soap-like consistency. That leaves oxalate free which can then be absorbed by the colon. Oxalate enters the bloodstream, is filtered by the kidney, and then binds to calcium inside the urinary tract, potentially resulting in stones or calcinosis of the kidney [32]. The treatment for this is a low oxalate diet and increased calcium intake in order to increase the binding of oxalate. Finally, brisk hydration to prevent hypovolemia is essential. Early detection is necessary as this can progress to renal failure. Surgical restoration of bowel length may be required.

Malabsorption treatment can start with nutritional supplements such as total parenteral nutrition (TPN). These must begin gradually to prevent refeeding syndrome. Thiamine must be given prior to administering any high-dextrose solution or concentrated feeding. Placing an enteral feeding tube should be delayed until edema resolves, and nutrition improves. With severe hypoalbuminemia, leaky gut is common [33]. Thus, the best approach is the slow initiation of TPN which has 100 g of amino acids, 40 g of fat, and limits dextrose to 140 g or less. Simultaneously, diuretics can be given with albumin to improve peripheral edema. These patients should be hospitalized and daily laboratory studies must be obtained. They should be kept on a regular diet that is low in fat and fermentable carbohydrates while high in protein, with calorie counts and the number and consistency of bowel movements recorded.

The cause of these symptoms is not always malabsorption, however. Patients may actually be experiencing poor intake quantity and quality. Once repleted, following rescue therapy, they may not require surgical revision. In addition, it is important to screen for substance abuse in these cases. Generally speaking, malnutrition this severe will occur within 2 years of surgery. If delayed, there is likely a secondary cause.

Often, endoscopy and CT scans are performed to rule out a mechanical cause for malnutrition. Colonoscopy can be considered to make sure there is no other cause such as inflammatory bowel disease. TPN should be maintained until laboratory values are normalized and oral intake improves or there is a plan for surgical revision.

For patients that require surgical revision for malabsorption for BPD-DS, the distal anastomosis is located and the Roux and BP limbs are identified. A minimum of 150 cm is measured moving from the anastomosis to the proximal portion of the BP limb. This point is now closer to the ligament of Treitz and is attached using a side-to-side anastomosis to the Roux limb approximately 30 cm distal from the duodenal anastomosis (similar to the revision displayed in Fig. 44.4b). There is no need to divide the Roux limb [15].

For patients that have a SADI-S, revisions include several potential options for lengthening the BP limb. The first is to take down the duodenal enteral anastomosis. We advise a staple line here, fired transversely, rather than simple suture closure to avoid distal obstruction, before then performing another single anastomosis 100–150 cm proximally (Fig. 44.7).

Alternatively, two small bowel anastomoses can be performed. The small bowel can be transected immediately proximal to the anastomosis and then attached approximately 50 cm downstream, converting to a Roux configuration (Fig. 44.8a). Then, similarly to the revision of a standard DS, 150 cm is measured proximally on the BP limb. This point is then attached to the now proximal Roux limb (Fig. 44.8b). Again, a feeding jejunostomy can be placed to supplement feedings. There is no need to transect the Roux limb and food can go down either conduit (Fig. 44.8c). This is usually extremely effective for frequent bowel movements and malnutrition.

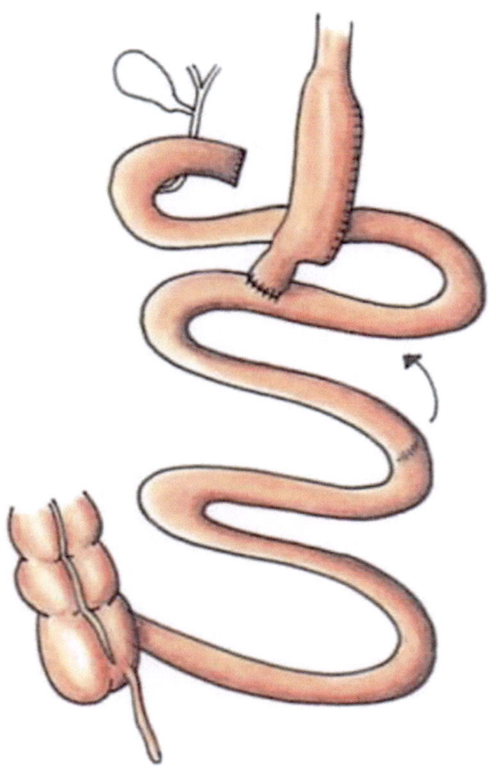

**Fig. 44.7** SADI-S modification involving taking down the anastomosis and creating a new anastomosis proximally

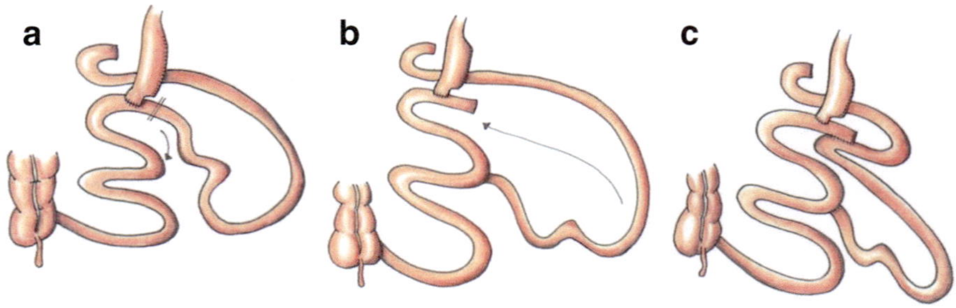


**Fig. 44.8** (**a**) Alternative SADI-S modification starts by dividing the small bowel proximal to the anastomosis to reattach it 50 cm downstream on the common channel. (**b**) Next, 150 cm upstream on the BP limb is measured and attached to the proximal Roux limb. (**c**) Final configuration of the alternative SADI-S modification

Another option, which we have not utilized but could be appropriate in a compromised individual, is to take a proximal loop of small bowel and attach it to the gastric pouch. We would suggest that this method only has short term benefits, and that other complications may be observed such as bile reflux gastritis and marginal ulcers. However, this is a simple approach that may be used in rare circumstances.

## Management of Bile Reflux and Gastroesophageal Reflux Disease (GERD)

Both procedures have very low risk of developing bile reflux. Bile reabsorption is hindered when it binds to lipids [34]. The long afferent limb in SADI-S or BP limb in BPD-DS does not contain food or lipid, hence a large fraction of secreted bile is absorbed prior to reaching the ileum. Additionally, the loop attachment is placed to the duodenum, past the pylorus, making the incidence of clinically significant bile reflux extremely low. Should this occur there should be a prompt investigation for an obstructive focus or kink in the anastomosis that is preferentially favoring emptying of the afferent limb into the gastric pouch.

Given both procedures require a sleeve as part of the procedure, patients can present with symptoms of GERD. Most patients will respond to medical therapy. However, for severe GERD that is refractory to medical treatment, there are numerous proposals for treating reflux following sleeve gastrectomy which include endoscopic procedures such as Stretta™. This is an endoscopic radiofrequency procedure used to increase thickening of the lower esophageal sphincter (LES) and decrease transient lower esophageal sphincter relaxation rate, therefore reducing esophageal acid exposure. A meta-analysis of controlled and cohort studies of patients with GERD showed a significant reduction in erosive esophagitis, reduced esophageal acid exposure, increased LES as well as subjective improvements in heartburn symptoms and reduced proton-pump inhibitor use [35]. Another approach is placing a LINX device around the esophagus. A retrospective review of seven patients showed subjective improvement in GERD-related symptoms [36]. Finally, a surgical approach can be used which involves a hiatal hernia repair. A recent experimental approach is to use the round ligament to provide a pseudoplication [17]. However, without true fundoplication, the surgical repair of the hiatus can be unsuccessful long term.

For patients with severe esophagitis after SADI-S, refractory to medications, conversion to RYGB can be offered. In this procedure the vertical sleeve gastrectomy (VSG) is divided to create a pouch, and the Roux limb is constructed from the previous BP limb. The distal sleeve is resected and an entero-enterostomy is completed where the loop was to prevent distal obstruction (Fig. 44.9a, b). This is a procedure that is also indicated if there is a chronic stricture or asymmetry of the sleeve causing the GERD. Higher complication rates are reported with this procedure.

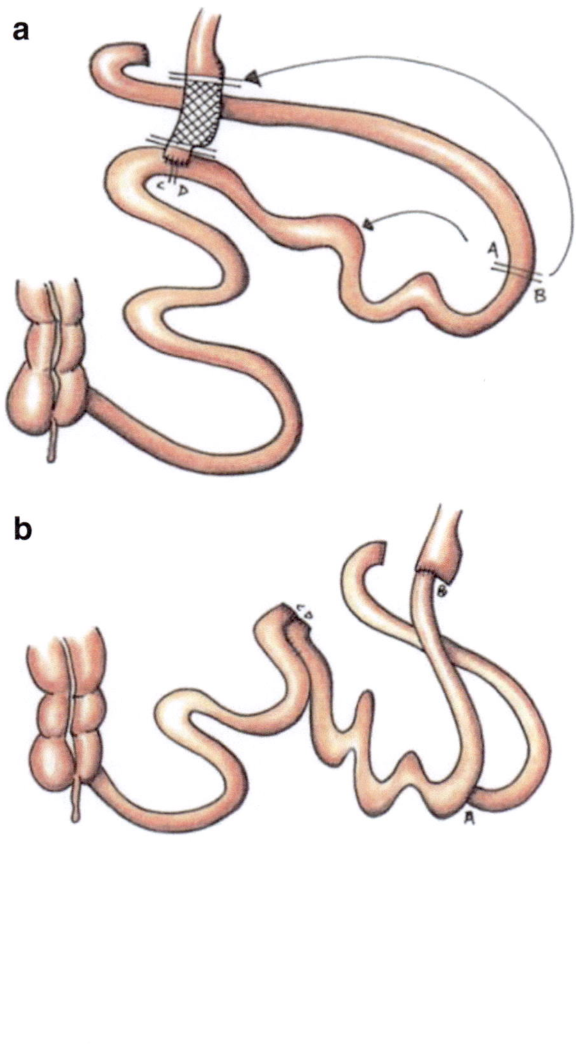


**Fig. 44.9** (**a**) SADI-S conversion to RYGB by dividing VSG to create a pouch and constructing a Roux limb from the previous BP with an entero-enterostomy created at prior loop site to prevent distal obstruction. (**b**) Final configuration of SADI-S conversion to RYGB

## Management of Marginal Ulcers

Marginal ulcer formation should be a very rare event when there is a proper duodenal cuff. The proximal duodenum secretes a bicarbonate rich fluid while the longitudinal gastrectomy further reduces acid production, contributing to decreased risk of ulcers. Similarly, anastomotic strictures are very unusual in both procedures [37]. If an ulcer does occur medical management should be initiated as described for cases with OAGB.

## Management of Weight Recurrence

Many have suggested for weight recurrence following SADI-S to convert to BPD-DS with a 100 cm common channel. Although we do believe this will result in nominal weight loss, we question whether this would result in quality weight loss or just loss of functional reserve. In the future, it is our contention that patients being considered for these procedures be followed with a DEXA body composition study and functional testing. The devastating impact of severe obesity has been well documented. However, in a study in press we report that while most of our 90-year-olds are obese or overweight, none are morbidly obese. Additionally, gaining one pound per year after the age of 80 has been shown to be related to improved longevity [38]. Effectively this reminds us that less is not always more and that having a certain adipose reserve is important.

For weight regain following BPD-DS many of these same factors must be considered. For patients many years out, especially those that had sleeves done over very large bougies, we have seen near normal stomach capacity. When nutritionally repleted, and with good body composition, we have had reasonable results with reducing gastric capacity and re-sleeving the gastric pouch. This is mostly effective in patients that have documentation that the fundus has reformed or has become grossly dilated.

## Management of Small Bowel Obstruction

A major long-term issue with bariatric procedures that involve the intestine is the risk of small bowel obstruction resulting in mesenteric volvulus and small bowel ischemia. A commonly mentioned advantage of SADI-S, as compared to BPD-DS, is that it does not require division of the mesentery. As a result, there is no mesenteric defect, lowering the potential spaces for internal herniation. However, this does not eliminate the possibility of small bowel obstruction. Many patients have had previous procedures which may act as a source for adhesions. Torsion of the afferent limb herniating under the anastomosis has also been reported [39]. This potential space can be considered a Peterson's defect. This has been handled with laparoscopy with no reports of bowel ischemia to date. In fact, several proponents of the procedure have advocated closing this potential space. Another technique advocates for fixation of the afferent limb by placing an additional stich between the gastric pouch antrum and the afferent limb, making torsion less likely.

In BPD-DS many have hypothesized that the obstruction rate is higher than RYGB [40]. The significant weight loss and disappearance of internal fat possibly allow for greater movement of intestinal loops. However, such data is hard to accumulate, as this can occur years after the primary procedure. As compared to SADI-S, the mesenteric defect and area under the Roux represent two potential spaces for migration. Closure of the spaces at the time of surgery is suggested, but massive weight loss and loss of fat may make permanent fixation difficult.

## Conclusions

The above procedures alter both the stomach and small bowel anatomy resulting in robust weight loss. However, nutritional issues and symptoms consistent with short bowel syndrome can occur and surgical revisions may become necessary. OAGB more so than SADI-S and BPD-DS can require revision for bile reflux and marginal ulcer. Revisions for GERD are not common for any of these procedures. Revisions for weight regain are also uncommon and practitioners should be careful to measure muscle function, nutritional reserve, and bone composition before considering increasing the degree of the intestinal bypass.

## References

1. Wolfe BM, Kvach E, Eckel RH. Treatment of obesity: weight loss and bariatric surgery. Circ Res. 2016;118(11):1844–55. https://doi.org/10.1161/CIRCRESAHA.116.307591.
2. Lupoli R, Lembo E, Saldalamacchia G, Avola CK, Angrisani L, Capaldo B. Bariatric surgery and long-term nutritional issues. World J Diabetes. 2017;8(11):464–74. https://doi.org/10.4239/wjd.v8.i11.464.
3. Paccou J, Martignène N, Lespessailles E, et al. Gastric bypass but not sleeve gastrectomy increases risk of major osteoporotic fracture: French population-based cohort study. J Bone Miner Res Off J Am Soc Bone Miner Res. 2020;35(8):1415–23. https://doi.org/10.1002/jbmr.4012.
4. Jammah AA. Endocrine and metabolic complications after bariatric surgery. Saudi J Gastroenterol Off J Saudi Gastroenterol Assoc. 2015;21(5):269–77. https://doi.org/10.4103/1319-3767.164183.
5. Palermo M, Acquafresca PA, Rogula T, Duza GE, Serra E. Late surgical complications after gastric by-pass: a literature review. Arq Bras Cir Dig ABCD Braz Arch Dig Surg. 2015;28(2):139–43. https://doi.org/10.1590/S0102-67202015000200014.
6. Eldredge TA, Bills M, Ting YY, et al. Once in a bile—the incidence of bile reflux post-bariatric surgery. Obes Surg. 2022;32(5):1428–38. https://doi.org/10.1007/s11695-022-05977-2.
7. Blom-Høgestøl IK, Aasbrenn M, Chahal-Kummen M, et al. Irritable bowel syndrome-like symptoms and health related quality of life two years after Roux-en-Y gastric bypass—a prospective cohort study. BMC Gastroenterol. 2019;19(1):204. https://doi.org/10.1186/s12876-019-1103-0.
8. Holanda N, Crispim N, Carlos I, Moura T, Nóbrega E, Bandeira F. Musculoskeletal effects of obesity and bariatric surgery—a narrative review. Arch Endocrinol Metab. 2022;66(5):621–32. https://doi.org/10.20945/2359-3997000000551.

9. Belle S. Longitudinal assessment of bariatric surgery. NIDDK Central Repository. https://doi.org/10.58020/VV2F-YM41. Published online January 13, 2023:367907462 MB
10. Gentile MG, Manna GM, Pastorelli P, Oltolini A. Laboratory evaluation in patients with anorexia nervosa: usefulness and limits. Clin Ter. 2011;162(5):401–7.
11. Miller KK, Grinspoon SK, Ciampa J, Hier J, Herzog D, Klibanski A. Medical findings in outpatients with anorexia nervosa. Arch Intern Med. 2005;165(5):561–6. https://doi.org/10.1001/archinte.165.5.561.
12. Rutledge R. The mini-gastric bypass: experience with the first 1274 cases. Obes Surg. 2001;11(3):276–80. https://doi.org/10.1381/096089201321336584.
13. Efficacy and safety of one anastomosis gastric bypass versus Roux-en-Y gastric bypass for obesity (YOMEGA): a multicentre, randomised, open-label, non-inferiority trial. Accessed November 15, 2023. https://pubmed.ncbi.nlm.nih.gov/30851879/
14. Salgaonkar H, Sharples A, Marimuthu K, Rao V, Balaji N. One anastomosis gastric bypass (OAGB). In: Lomanto D, Chen WTL, Fuentes MB, editors. Mastering endo-laparoscopic and thoracoscopic surgery: ELSA manual. Springer Nature; 2023. p. 297–304. https://doi.org/10.1007/978-981-19-3755-2_43.
15. Topart PA, Becouarn G. Revision and reversal after biliopancreatic diversion for excessive side effects or ineffective weight loss: a review of the current literature on indications and procedures. Surg Obes Relat Dis Off J Am Soc Bariatr Surg. 2015;11(4):965–72. https://doi.org/10.1016/j.soard.2015.01.015.
16. Musella M, Susa A, Manno E, et al. Complications following the mini/one anastomosis gastric bypass (MGB/OAGB): a multi-institutional survey on 2678 patients with a mid-term (5 years) follow-up. Obes Surg. 2017;27(11):2956–67. https://doi.org/10.1007/s11695-017-2726-2.
17. Gálvez-Valdovinos R, Cruz-Vigo JL, Marín-Santillán E, Funes-Rodríguez JF, López-Ambriz G, Domínguez-Carrillo LG. Cardiopexy with ligamentum teres in patients with hiatal hernia and previous sleeve gastrectomy: an alternative treatment for gastroesophageal reflux disease. Obes Surg. 2015;25(8):1539–43. https://doi.org/10.1007/s11695-015-1740-5.
18. Lee S, Supparamaniam S, Varghese C, Mahawar K. Marginal ulcers following one-anastomosis gastric bypass: a systematic review and meta-analysis. Obes Surg. 2023;33(9):2884–97. https://doi.org/10.1007/s11695-023-06762-5.
19. Hess DS, Hess DW. Biliopancreatic diversion with a duodenal switch. Obes Surg. 1998;8(3):267–82. https://doi.org/10.1381/096089298765554476.
20. Sánchez-Pernaute A, Rubio Herrera MA, Pérez-Aguirre E, et al. Proximal duodenal-ileal end-to-side bypass with sleeve gastrectomy: proposed technique. Obes Surg. 2007;17(12):1614–8. https://doi.org/10.1007/s11695-007-9287-8.
21. Cottam D, Roslin M, Enochs P, Metz M, Portenier D, Smith D. Single anastomosis duodenal switch: 1-year outcomes. Obes Surg. 2020;30(4):1506–14. https://doi.org/10.1007/s11695-019-04352-y.
22. Yuval JB, Mintz Y, Cohen MJ, Rivkind AI, Elazary R. The effects of bougie caliber on leaks and excess weight loss following laparoscopic sleeve gastrectomy. Is there an ideal bougie size? Obes Surg. 2013;23(10):1685–91. https://doi.org/10.1007/s11695-013-1047-3.
23. Sioka E, Tzovaras G, Perivoliotis K, et al. Impact of laparoscopic sleeve gastrectomy on gastrointestinal motility. Gastroenterol Res Pract. 2018;2018:4135813. https://doi.org/10.1155/2018/4135813.
24. Lebel S, Dion G, Marceau S, Biron S, Robert M, Biertho L. Clinical outcomes of duodenal switch with a 200-cm common channel: a matched, controlled trial. Surg Obes Relat Dis Off J Am Soc Bariatr Surg. 2016;12(5):1014–20. https://doi.org/10.1016/j.soard.2016.01.014.
25. Hjelt K, Krasilnikoff PA. Vitamin B12 absorption capacity in healthy children. J Pediatr Gastroenterol Nutr. 1986;5(2):274–7.
26. Dorman RB, Rasmus NF, al-Haddad BJS, et al. Benefits and complications of the duodenal switch/biliopancreatic diversion compared to the Roux-en-Y gastric bypass. Surgery. 2012;152(4):758–65.; discussion 765–767. https://doi.org/10.1016/j.surg.2012.07.023.
27. Barrett JS. How to institute the low-FODMAP diet. J Gastroenterol Hepatol. 2017;32(Suppl. 1):8–10. https://doi.org/10.1111/jgh.13686.

28. Drucker DJ. The discovery of GLP-2 and development of teduglutide for short bowel syndrome. ACS Pharmacol Transl Sci. 2019;2(2):134–42. https://doi.org/10.1021/acsptsci.9b00016.
29. Homan J, Betzel B, Aarts EO, et al. Vitamin and mineral deficiencies after biliopancreatic diversion and biliopancreatic diversion with duodenal switch—the rule rather than the exception. Obes Surg. 2015;25(9):1626–32. https://doi.org/10.1007/s11695-015-1570-5.
30. Hardlei TF, Mørkbak AL, Bor MV, Bailey LB, Hvas AM, Nexo E. Assessment of vitamin B(12) absorption based on the accumulation of orally administered cyanocobalamin on transcobalamin. Clin Chem. 2010;56(3):432–6. https://doi.org/10.1373/clinchem.2009.131524.
31. Kumar N. Nutrients and neurology. Contin Minneap Minn. 2017;23(3):822–61. https://doi.org/10.1212/01.CON.0000520630.69195.90.
32. Lieske JC, Mehta RA, Milliner DS, Rule AD, Bergstralh EJ, Sarr MG. Kidney stones are common after bariatric surgery. Kidney Int. 2015;87(4):839–45. https://doi.org/10.1038/ki.2014.352.
33. Prendergast AJ, Kelly P. Interactions between intestinal pathogens, enteropathy and malnutrition in developing countries. Curr Opin Infect Dis. 2016;29(3):229–36. https://doi.org/10.1097/QCO.0000000000000261.
34. Ferrannini E, Camastra S, Astiarraga B, et al. Increased bile acid synthesis and deconjugation after biliopancreatic diversion. Diabetes. 2015;64(10):3377–85. https://doi.org/10.2337/db15-0214.
35. Perry KA, Banerjee A, Melvin WS. Radiofrequency energy delivery to the lower esophageal sphincter reduces esophageal acid exposure and improves GERD symptoms: a systematic review and meta-analysis. Surg Laparosc Endosc Percutan Tech. 2012;22(4):283–8. https://doi.org/10.1097/SLE.0b013e3182582e92.
36. Warren HF, Brown LM, Mihura M, Farivar AS, Aye RW, Louie BE. Factors influencing the outcome of magnetic sphincter augmentation for chronic gastroesophageal reflux disease. Surg Endosc. 2018;32(1):405–12. https://doi.org/10.1007/s00464-017-5696-5.
37. Surve A, Zaveri H, Cottam D, Belnap L, Cottam A, Cottam S. A retrospective comparison of biliopancreatic diversion with duodenal switch with single anastomosis duodenal switch (SIPS-stomach intestinal pylorus sparing surgery) at a single institution with two year follow-up. Surg Obes Relat Dis Off J Am Soc Bariatr Surg. 2017;13(3):415–22. https://doi.org/10.1016/j.soard.2016.11.020.
38. Crow RS, Petersen CL, Cook SB, et al. Weight change in older adults and risk of frailty. J Frailty Aging. 2020;9(2):74–81. https://doi.org/10.14283/jfa.2019.44.
39. Surve A, Cottam D, Horsley B. Internal hernia following primary laparoscopic SADI-S: the first reported case. Obes Surg. 2020;30(5):2066–8. https://doi.org/10.1007/s11695-020-04444-0.
40. Strain GW, Torghabeh MH, Gagner M, Ebel F, Dakin GF, Abelson JS, Connolly D, Pomp A. The impact of biliopancreatic diversion with duodenal switch (BPD/DS) over 9 years. Obes Surg. 2017;27(3) https://doi.org/10.1007/s11695-016-2371-1.

# Part V

# Special Considerations

# 45 Concomitant Treatment of the Hiatus

K. Paige Mihalsky and Laura E. Fischer

## Background

Hiatal hernias are very common in patients with obesity. A hiatal hernia is characterized by a protrusion of any abdominal structure other than the esophagus into the thoracic cavity through a widening of the hiatus of the diaphragm, most commonly the upper stomach. A wide range of patients with obesity (up to 50%) are found to have a hiatal hernia at the time of bariatric surgery [1–6]. While many of these patients report symptoms of gastroesophageal reflux disease (GERD), a large number of these hernias are incidentally found, either during pre-bariatric surgery evaluation or during a weight-loss procedure.

Obesity is an independent risk factor for the development of hiatal hernias and GERD, with 60% of patients with a hiatal hernia reporting symptoms of GERD. These symptoms include a burning sensation in the chest, regurgitation, chronic cough, and wheezing. This is due to acidic gastric contents refluxing into the esophagus with higher frequency and volume than baseline physiologic reflux. Several factors contribute to the development of hiatal hernias in obesity, including increased intra-abdominal pressure, esophageal shortening secondary to chronic GERD, obstructive sleep apnea, and congenital or acquired abnormalities in the function of the lower esophageal sphincter (LES).

K. P. Mihalsky
Department of Surgery, University of Oklahoma Health Science Center, Oklahoma City, OK, USA

L. E. Fischer (✉)
Department of Surgery, University of Oklahoma Health Science Center, Oklahoma City, OK, USA

Mercy Hospital Oklahoma City, Oklahoma City, USA


O. M. Ghanem et al. (eds.), *The SAGES Manual of Metabolic and Bariatric Surgery*, https://doi.org/10.1007/978-3-031-72309-4_45

Hiatal hernias vary significantly in their anatomic presentation, with a sliding hiatal hernia, or type I, being the most common. Widening of the hiatal opening in the diaphragm allows the upper stomach to intermittently slide into the mediastinum, with the gastroesophageal junction migrating above the diaphragm during breath inhalation [7]. The negative pressure environment of the thoracic cavity combined with the positive pressure of the abdominal cavity exacerbates this axial movement over time. Intrathoracic location and the loss of the anatomic attachments of the angle of His render the LES functionally incompetent. Hiatal hernia types II through IV, also known as paraesophageal hernias (PEH), occur when any portion of the gastrointestinal (GI) tract or any intra-abdominal organ migrates through the hiatus to reside next to the esophagus; this can be stomach, omentum, colon, and small bowel or more rarely, pancreas, liver, adrenal glands or other organs. Types II through IV PEH can be more concerning than a type I sliding hernia, as the normal anatomic blood supply to the herniated organ(s) may be compromised. Normal function of the incarcerated organ(s) may also be altered due to obstruction or compression.

Evaluation and management of hiatal hernias is a topic of great importance for bariatric surgeons as the surgical options for weight loss have a direct impact on the anatomy and physiology of the esophagus and stomach. Of particular concern is the risk of developing esophagitis and Barrett's esophagus after vertical sleeve gastrectomy (SG) potentially placing patients at risk for later development of esophageal cancer. Initial reports on the worsening and new development of erosive esophagitis and Barrett's esophagus (BE) after SG were published in 2017. Genco *et al* reported an increase in GERD symptoms from 34% to 68%, increase in PPI use from 19% to 57%, increases in esophagitis in all classes (A: 13–46%, B: 8–33%, C: 4–12%, and D: 0-9.1%), as well as an unexpected 17% incidence of new BE seen at a mean of 58 months after surgery [8]. A 5-year multicenter study showed similar results with 18.8% incidence of new BE (no difference among five centers) and an increase in GERD symptoms, erosive esophagitis, and PPI use (22–76%, 10–41%, 22–52%, respectively) [9]. Subsequent prospective studies have reported that SG has similar rates of de novo BE compared with RYGB, however, SG patients do have significantly higher rates of GERD, esophagitis, PPI use, and bile reflux that may also be associated with post-operative weight regain [10, 11]. Additionally, the risk of esophageal cancer with non-dysplastic BE is unknown as compared with the known increased risk of BE with dysplasia; currently, the AGA does not recommend endoscopic treatment for non-dysplastic BE [12]. Overall, the long-term risk of GERD, erosive esophagitis, and BE should not be discounted by bariatric surgeons and consideration for life-long health factors should be a part of the surgical decision-making process.

## Preoperative Evaluation

Despite hiatal hernias being closely linked to GERD, many patients who present for the consideration of bariatric surgery are asymptomatic with regard to reflux disease even in the presence of a hiatal hernia, esophagitis, or Barrett's esophagus [13]. Therefore, it can be valuable to evaluate the presence of a hiatal hernia as part of pre-surgical planning.

EGD allows a visual assessment of the mucosa of the esophagus, stomach, and duodenum. A hiatal hernia is diagnosed on EGD when evaluating the distance between the esophagogastric junction (EGJ) and the diaphragmatic pinch, which is the extrinsic compression of the diaphragmatic hiatus on the gastric wall. Additional information about the hiatus can be obtained by retroflexing the endoscope and visualizing the gastroesophageal flap valve (GEFV). The GEFV is a flat musculo-mucosal fold wrapping 180° around the EGJ and extending 3–4 cm superiorly on the lesser curve [14]. Hill classification is utilized as a reproducible endoscopic grading system for EGJ morphology and competence. The Hill valve grade can also be a better predictor of GERD than LES pressure. Hill classification specifies whether the GEFV is normal (grade I/II) or abnormal (grade III/IV) by evaluating the GEFV in relation to the endoscope and movement of the GEFV with respirations [14]:

- *Grade I* defines the GEFV as being a prominent fold oriented tightly around the endoscope and extending 3–4 cm along the lesser curvature with a competent valve that does not open with respiration.
- *Grade II* defines the GEFV as being a visible fold oriented loosely around the endoscope that opens and closes periodically with respiration.
- *Grade III* has a loss of the GEFV with an absence of any visible tissue fold and without tight closure of the EGJ tissues around the endoscope.
- *Grade IV* has a large diaphragmatic hiatus and the tissue in this area is widely open around the endoscope; the squamous mucosa of the esophagus can be visualized through this opening. The gastric folds can often be seen to migrate into the thoracic cavity with inspiration during the retroflexed view.

Despite these definitions, some pathologic conditions can complicate the endoscopic diagnosis of a hiatal hernia. Patients with severe GERD-causing BE may have a blurred or elevated EGJ which is difficult to precisely define [15]. A wide separation of the crura can make the diaphragmatic pinch difficult to recognize [16]. Additionally, endoscopic insufflation can reduce hiatal hernias back into the abdominal cavity for the duration of the procedure, masking its presence. For these reasons, EGD alone is insufficient for the diagnosis of a hiatal hernia.

While EGD is an important aspect of hiatal hernia diagnosis prior to bariatric surgical planning, it can also assist in the definitive diagnosis of GERD and/or BE which may further affect surgical decision-making. In the updated Lyon Consensus Guidelines (2023), the modern definition of 'actionable GERD' requires "conclusive evidence of reflux-related pathology on endoscopy and/or abnormal reflux monitoring (using Lyon consensus thresholds) in the presence of troublesome symptoms" [17]. Common GERD symptoms include heartburn, chest pain, and regurgitation and potential, but less common symptoms, include belching, chronic cough, and wheezing. The symptoms of globus sensation, voice hoarseness, nausea, abdominal pain, and indigestion are noted to be unlikely to be related to the pathology of GERD. On endoscopy, Los Angeles (LA) grade B, C, and D esophagitis, BE, and benign peptic stricture are all conclusive evidence of GERD and do not require additional confirmation with reflux monitoring. Additionally, a hiatal hernia noted on endoscopy is considered supportive evidence for GERD. With the ability to definitively diagnose GERD on endoscopy, preoperative evaluation with EGD is a valuable tool.

Contrast studies, including the UGI series, are helpful to gauge the size and reducibility of hiatal hernias and precisely localizing the EGJ in relation to the esophageal hiatus [18]. Contrast studies are reported to be more sensitive than endoscopy in detecting type I sliding hiatal hernias in the bariatric population [2]. UGI can be used in conjunction with routine preoperative EGD when there is concern for a large hiatal hernia that will require surgical intervention.

The necessity of routine preoperative esophagogastroduodenoscopy (EGD) and upper gastrointestinal series (UGI) in the evaluation of hiatal hernia among bariatric surgery candidates is debated as most are detected during surgery and the sensitivity of both studies is limited (47–64% for EGD and 14–32% for UGI) [4–6]. However, the specificity of these tests is relatively high (74–94% for EGD and 94–98% for UGI) [2, 4–6], so when used together, they can assist in preoperative planning, especially for high-risk patients. The arguments against routine EGD and UGI include added cost, low sensitivity, potential morbidity, and an absence of improvement in operative times or post-operative complications [4–6].

The role of additional diagnostic techniques including computed tomography (CT), high-resolution esophageal manometry (HRM), and pH testing vary widely and depend heavily on the clinical presentation of the patient. If additional information is needed for clinical decision-making, CT imaging can aid with diagnosis of a paraesophageal hernia with volvulus or other emergent presentations beyond the scope of this discussion.

Care should be taken by the bariatric surgeon to align their surgical goals of care to the individual needs of each patient and the preoperative evaluation should allow for appropriate surgical decision-making. The decision to perform a RYGB vs SG, single-anastomosis duodenoileal bypass with sleeve gastrectomy (SADI-S), duodenal switch (DS), one-anastomosis gastric bypass (OAGB), or adjustable gastric banding (AGB) in patients with self-reported symptoms of GERD and presence of a hiatal hernia remains complex. Identifying the presence of a hiatal hernia prior to surgery may help guide operative decision-making with regard to bariatric procedure selection – generally, SG, SADI-S, DS, OAGB, and AGB procedures can exacerbate reflux symptoms while Roux-en-Y gastric bypass (RYGB) can alleviate symptoms [19–21].

SG is an effective weight-loss procedure; however, it has been associated with increased incidence of GERD post-operatively, with up to 41% of patients reporting new symptoms and 19–30% reporting worsened symptoms [22–28]. Hill grade III and IV and the presence of a hiatal hernia are associated with post-SG GERD [28]. In fact, post-SG GERD symptoms correlate with hiatal hernia recurrence as well as a high rate of erosive esophagitis and BE [29]. RYGB may offer better GERD resolution with equivalent or improved weight loss benefit [3, 22, 30, 31].

Traditionally, RYGB remains the operation of choice for patients with a known type III or IV paraesophageal hernia, as the anatomic changes of an RYGB markedly reduce the risk of significant GERD. Additionally, the Los Angeles (LA) Classification of esophagitis is determined preoperatively on EGD to aid with surgical planning. If LA grade C (one or more mucosal breaks < 75% circumference) or grade D (one or more mucosal breaks ≥ 75% circumference) esophagitis is observed, a diagnosis of severe esophagitis is made, and RYGB is the preferred operation [32]. GERD is the most common complication following SG and is often not considered the procedure of choice for patients with a documented type III or IV paraesophageal hernia, medication-refractory GERD symptoms, erosive esophagitis, or BE.

Relief of GERD-related symptoms after RYGB is thought to be related to the anatomy of the gastric pouch—there are significantly fewer parietal cells in the cardia as compared with the gastric antrum. Separation of the cardia from the gastric remnant eliminates access to the majority of acid-producing gastric cells from the esophagus. Additionally, replacement of the distal esophagus and LES within the positive-pressure abdominal cavity, re-approximation of the bilateral crural pillars, and reduction in intra-abdominal pressure with weight loss all contribute to a reduction or cessation of pathologic reflux. RYGB alone is an established surgical treatment for GERD and can even improve symptoms in the absence of a hiatal hernia repair.

## Principles of Repair

For small type I hiatal hernias, a primary, posterior, sutured crural repair at the time of bariatric surgery is indicated. This typically includes mobilization of the esophagus circumferentially into the mediastinum and posterior re-approximation of the hiatus with permanent suture. Type of suture, type of repair (running vs. interrupted), and use of materials such as pledgets or mesh are per surgeon preference. Previous studies have shown that posterior re-approximation has improved GERD outcomes 1 year after concomitant HHR and SG [33]. Anterior repair alone has no clear benefit and additionally has resulted in increased complications including hemorrhage and readmission [27, 33].

For large, type II-IV PEHs, a high mediastinal dissection of the esophagus should be performed to achieve adequate intra-abdominal length without upward tension. Additionally, the hernia sac should be dissected from the mediastinal structures and excised when possible. Hernia sac dissection as a first operative step greatly facilitates intra-operative reduction of the hernia as well as decreases the risk of early recurrence. Prior to addressing the sac and the crural pillar on the right side of the esophagus, the left gastric vasculature should be identified and reduced into the abdomen to prevent injury. At times, sac excision can be difficult, and excision is not feasible. It is imperative, however, that the peritoneal lining of the sac is disconnected from the crura to reduce recurrence risk.

The use of mesh for reinforcement of large hiatal hernia repairs leads to decreased short-term recurrence rates; however, there is inadequate long-term data to support the use of mesh for all hiatal hernia repairs [34]. Recurrence rates of primary repair may be as high as 42% [35, 36]. Reinforcement of the crural repair may be indicated for large crural defects or recurrent hiatal hernias. On-lay resorbable mesh is the traditional reinforced repair, however, the use of pledget buttress sutures in the primary repair may be an alternative reinforcement with a lower complication rate. For hernia defects under tension, posterior on-lay application of a 'U'-shaped resorbable biologic mesh is indicated and leads to fewer recurrences than suture cruroplasty alone (2% vs. 14%, respectively) [37]. For giant type IV paraesophageal hernias where tension-free crural repair is unattainable, reconstruction of the hiatus with the ligamentum teres as a vascularized autologous flap is also a potential option [38, 39]. With this, the risks and increased cost associated with mesh are no longer a factor [40]. With this technique, a vascularized autologous on-lay flap is safe and effective for the closure of the crural defect. Mobilization of the falciform ligament from the anterior abdominal wall is performed to prevent lateral tension on the flap, with caution taken to avoid devascularization. Then, interrupted vertical mattress sutures are used to fix the falciform ligament to the left and right crural pillars. An alternative method is to create a relaxing incision in the diaphragm lateral to the crural pillar to allow for a tension-free midline closure. The relaxing incision can then be closed with a bridging mesh. This technique is safe and effective in long-term follow-up studies [41].

For all hiatal hernia repairs, an EGD can be performed upon completion of the procedure to confirm appropriate tightening of the diaphragm around the esophagus, evaluate for esophageal angulation over a posterior cruroplasty, as well as evaluate suture line integrity related to the concomitant bariatric procedure. A size 36 French endoscope should traverse the EJG easily but without excess space. This ensures an appropriate re-approximation of the crural pillars without causing obstruction.

Early postoperative dysphagia is the most common complication following hiatal hernia repair, with dehydration being the most common cause of readmission following bariatric surgery. To ensure adequate nutritional intake to maintain hydration, all patients should be monitored overnight to ensure appropriate *per os* fluid intake prior to discharge. Early postoperative dysphagia following hiatal hernia repair is reported in up to 50% of patients, and therefore the general recommendation is to slowly advance a diet from liquids to soft solids over the first 2 weeks postoperatively.

Following hiatal hernia repair, there are no long-term imaging requirements for asymptomatic patients to evaluate recurrence. Contrast studies or endoscopy can be considered for patients reporting recurrence or new-onset symptoms including burning chest pain, dysphagia, or signs and symptoms of a leak or perforation.

## Concomitant Operative Treatment

In addition to selecting the most appropriate weight loss procedure for each patient, the bariatric surgeon must also consider whether to repair hiatal hernias concomitantly. Hiatal hernias and GERD are correlated to obesity, BMI, and each other, with increased intra-abdominal pressure noted as a leading cause of both hiatal hernias and GERD [31, 42]. Some studies have shown that hiatal hernia-related symptoms improve after weight-loss surgery alone, deeming repair of the hiatus unnecessary at the time of operation. This theory avoids the potential increase in morbidity and mortality during hiatal hernia repair in a high-risk patient with obesity. However, because untreated hiatal hernias often progress to symptomatic GERD, there is an increased risk of reoperation following bariatric surgery [43, 44]. For this reason, many surgeons choose to concomitantly repair hiatal hernias with bariatric surgery when the risk profile of the patient is acceptable [34].

Repair of a hiatal hernia is an important factor in an effort to prevent the effects of GERD on the esophagus. Erosive esophagitis following bariatric surgery is an objective measure of the anti-reflux mechanism of the EGJ. One study showed that severe esophagitis (LA Grade C or D) was three times more prevalent after SG compared with RYGB (10.7% vs. 3.1%, $p = 0.0007$) [45]. Additionally, the prevalence of erosive esophagitis among patients with a hiatal hernia diagnosed postoperatively was 51% following SG and 37% following RYGB, as compared to 34% and 16% respectively for those without a hiatal hernia.

A stand-alone bariatric procedure without concomitant hiatal hernia repair can be considered if there is a high risk of increased morbidity and mortality, however, in patients with acceptable risk, identification and dissection of the hiatus with a primary posterior crural reconstruction is preferred. The safety and effectiveness of a concomitant hiatal hernia repair has been demonstrated [46]. Multiple studies have evaluated outcomes of RYGB with hiatal hernia repair, and there is no significant difference with regard to morbidity, mortality, 30-day readmission rates, duration of stay, and cost of the concomitant technique when performed at the time of initial bariatric procedure [46, 47]. Another study showed acceptable morbidity (17%) and mortality (2.5%) when combining RYGB with HHR in patients over age 65 [48].

Concomitant SG and hiatal hernia repair is also feasible and safe [49, 50]. One large registry analysis showed a small increase in 30-day readmission (4% vs. 3%), reoperation (1.1% vs. 0.7%), and morbidity (1.9% vs. 1.5%), but no increased risk of death with the combined repair [51]. Previous studies have shown that concomitant hiatal hernia repair is more common with SG (21% repair), despite a higher rate of GERD diagnosis preoperatively in patients who underwent RYGB (10.8% repair) [52]. Due to the perception that SG may worsen or induce GERD symptoms, the higher rate of hiatal hernia repair may reflect an effort to mitigate the risk of post-SG GERD. However, while it is associated with improved GERD symptoms (70% vs. 64%) and statistically lower rates of *de novo* GERD (28% vs. 30%), concomitant hiatal repair cannot be guaranteed to remediate or prevent new-onset GERD. Additionally, multiple studies have shown little or no difference in post-SG GERD symptoms with or without HHR [25–28].

Overall, recent studies have suggested that concomitant repair of hiatal hernia with RYGB has the lowest rate of complication or reoperation when compared to SG [53] and concomitant repair is becoming more common as surgeons become comfortable with the techniques [54]. However, a recent global, multi-institutional study showed an overall increase in 30-day complications when bariatric surgery is combined with another procedure, including hiatal hernia repair (12.7% vs. 4.7%)

[55]. There is high variability in bariatric surgeon choice to perform concomitant surgery, with higher rates of preoperative endoscopy associated with a higher rate of concomitant hiatal hernia repair (33% vs. 17%) [56] .Overall, the surgeon's hiatal hernia repair rate ranged from 8% to 57% and remained broad even when the patient had a documented hiatal hernia (20–91%). Decision-making should be undertaken with full understanding regarding risks and outcomes and care should be taken to carefully consider each patient's risk profile prior to undertaking a combination procedure.

## Post-Bariatric Hiatal Hernia Management

Due to the high prevalence of hiatal hernias in this patient population, the lack of concomitant repair in some patients, and the high rate of hiatal hernia recurrence, many patients will be diagnosed with a new or recurrent hiatal hernia after their bariatric procedure. Diagnosis is often performed using endoscopy, UGI, and CT imaging when patients present with GERD symptoms. Primary repair, consisting of reduction of the neo-stomach into the abdomen and posterior cruroplasty (with or without mesh), has been shown to be safe and effective in resolving symptoms [57, 58], and post-bariatric hiatal hernias seem to develop more commonly in SG patients compared with RYGB [58].

In most cases, there is not sufficient fundus to perform an anti-reflux procedure in these patients, so alternative methods to augment the lower esophageal sphincter have been devised. Augmentation with the ligamentum teres has been described in multiple publications with acceptable long-term results. This procedure involves wrapping the ligamentum teres around the distal esophagus in a semi-circle and fixing it with a permanent suture to the diaphragmatic crura bilaterally, either anteriorly or posteriorly. Results include an improvement or resolution of GERD symptoms in 50–80% with no change in symptoms in only 12–20% of patients [59–61]. There are also reports of using a magnetic sphincter device to treat reflux in SG patients [62], however, comprehensive long-term studies on this technique are limited. Early studies show a decrease in PPI use (88–25%) at 3 years and resolution of GERD symptoms with no adverse events [63]. Another study reported PPI use decreased from 100% to 20% and quality of life improved [64]. Additional studies should be performed to maximize symptom improvement and reduce the rate of recurrence for post-bariatric hiatal hernia repairs.

## Conclusion

Overall, concomitant posterior repair of all hiatal hernias present at the time of bariatric surgery is recommended when the patient has an acceptable risk profile. Indications for mesh are complex and the decision to use resorbable biologic or synthetic mesh during a hiatal hernia repair varies. For hiatal hernias diagnosed preoperatively, patients should be counseled about the potential benefit of RYGB as compared with alternative weight-loss procedures as it has the potential to improve or cure GERD in addition to its other metabolic and weight-loss benefits. However, for hiatal hernias noted incidentally at the time of bariatric operation, RYGB and SG are both safe and effective procedures to perform in combination with a hiatal hernia repair [53]. Alternatives to fundoplication, such as magnetic sphincter and ligamentum teres augmentation, for the treatment or prevention of GERD, require additional long-term studies to confirm efficacy.

## References

1. Che F, Nguyen B, Cohen A, Nguyen NT. Prevalence of hiatal hernia in the morbidly obese. Surg Obes Relat Dis. 2013;9(6):920–4.
2. Fornari F, Gurski RR, Navarini D, Thiesen V, Mestriner LH, Madalosso CA. Clinical utility of endoscopy and barium swallow X-ray in the diagnosis of sliding hiatal hernia in morbidly obese patients: a study before and after gastric bypass. Obes Surg. 2010;20(6):702–8.
3. Bakhos CT, Patel SP, Petrov RV, Abbas AE. Management of paraesophageal hernia in the morbidly obese patient. Thorac Surg Clin. 2019;29(4):379–86.
4. Imam A, Asfour G, Imam R, Bilitzky-Kopit A, Pines G, Sapojnikov S, et al. Hiatal hernia evaluation before bariatric surgery: should it be routinely done? Obes Surg. 2021;31(3):1013–20.
5. Mizrahi I, Abubeih A, Rachmuth J, Plotkin Y, Beglaibter N, Grinbaum R, et al. Routine upper gastrointestinal fluoroscopy before laparoscopic sleeve gastrectomy: is it necessary? Obes Surg. 2019;29(6):1704–8.
6. Mani VR, Kalabin A, Nwakanama C, Suman P, Ahmed L. Preoperative versus intraoperative diagnosis of hiatal hernia in bariatric population. Surg Obes Relat Dis. 2019;15(11):1949–55.
7. Kavic SM, Segan RD, George IM, Turner PL, Roth JS, Park A. Classification of hiatal hernias using dynamic three-dimensional reconstruction. Surg Innov. 2006;13(1):49–52.
8. Genco A, Soricelli E, Casella G, Maselli R, Castagneto-Gissey L, Di Lorenzo N, et al. Gastroesophageal reflux disease and Barrett's esophagus after laparoscopic sleeve gastrectomy: a possible, underestimated long-term complication. Surg Obes Relat Dis. 2017;13(4):568–74.
9. Sebastianelli L, Benois M, Vanbiervliet G, Bailly L, Robert M, Turrin N, et al. Systematic endoscopy 5 years after sleeve gastrectomy results in a high rate of Barrett's esophagus: results of a multicenter study. Obes Surg. 2019;29(5):1462–9.
10. Wolnerhanssen BK, Meyer-Gerspach AC, Nussbaumer R, Sauter M, Thumshirn M, Bueter M, et al. Prospective clinical cohort study: low incidence of Barrett esophagus but high rate of reflux disease at 5-year follow-up after sleeve gastrectomy versus Roux-en-Y gastric bypass. Surg Obes Relat Dis. 2023;19(7):707–15.
11. Ferrer JV, Acosta A, Garcia-Alementa EM, Garcia AT, Del Castillo D, Espelta MV, et al. High rate of de novo esophagitis 5 years after sleeve gastrectomy: a prospective multicenter study in Spain. Surg Obes Relat Dis. 2022;18(4):546–54.
12. Rubenstein JH, Sawas T, Wani S, Eluri S, Singh S, Chandar AK, et al. AGA clinical practice guideline on endoscopic eradication therapy of Barrett's esophagus and related neoplasia. Gastroenterology. 2024;166(6):1020–55.
13. Chandar AK, Keerthy K, Gupta R, Grady WM, Canto MI, Shaheen NJ, et al. Patients with esophageal adenocarcinoma with prior gastroesophageal reflux disease symptoms are similar to those without gastroesophageal reflux disease: a cross-sectional study. Am J Gastroenterol. 2024;119(5):823–9.
14. Hill LD, Kozarek RA, Kraemer SJ, Aye RW, Mercer CD, Low DE, et al. The gastroesophageal flap valve: in vitro and in vivo observations. Gastrointest Endosc. 1996;44(5):541–7.

15. Wallner B, Sylvan A, Janunger KG. Endoscopic assessment of the "Z-line" (squamocolumnar junction) appearance: reproducibility of the ZAP classification among endoscopists. Gastrointest Endosc. 2002;55(1):65–9.
16. Kahrilas PJ, Kim HC, Pandolfino JE. Approaches to the diagnosis and grading of hiatal hernia. Best Pract Res Clin Gastroenterol. 2008;22(4):601–16.
17. Gyawali CP, Yadlapati R, Fass R, Katzka D, Pandolfino J, Savarino E, et al. Updates to the modern diagnosis of GERD: Lyon consensus 2.0. Gut. 2024;73(2):361–71.
18. Mittal SK, Awad ZT, Tasset M, Filipi CJ, Dickason TJ, Shinno Y, et al. The preoperative predictability of the short esophagus in patients with stricture or paraesophageal hernia. Surg Endosc. 2000;14(5):464–8.
19. Admella V, Lazzara C, Sobrino L, Acrich E, Biondo S, Pujol-Gebelli J, et al. Patient-reported outcomes and quality of life after single-anastomosis duodeno-ileal bypass with sleeve gastrectomy (SADI-S): a cross-sectional study with 283 patients from a single institution. Obes Surg. 2023;33(6):1754–63.
20. Genco A, Castagneto-Gissey L, Gualtieri L, Lucchese M, Leuratti L, Soricelli E, et al. GORD and Barrett's oesophagus after bariatric procedures: multicentre prospective study. Br J Surg. 2021;108(12):1498–505.
21. Madalosso CA, Gurski RR, Callegari-Jacques SM, Navarini D, Thiesen V, Fornari F. The impact of gastric bypass on gastroesophageal reflux disease in patients with morbid obesity: a prospective study based on the Montreal Consensus. Ann Surg. 2010;251(2):244–8.
22. Aili A, Maimaitiming M, Maimaitiyusufu P, Tusuntuoheti Y, Li X, Cui J, et al. Gastroesophageal reflux related changes after sleeve gastrectomy and sleeve gastrectomy with fundoplication: a retrospective single center study. Front Endocrinol (Lausanne). 2022;13:1041889.
23. Peterli R, Wolnerhanssen BK, Peters T, Vetter D, Kroll D, Borbely Y, et al. Effect of laparoscopic sleeve gastrectomy vs laparoscopic Roux-en-Y gastric bypass on weight loss in patients with morbid obesity: the SM-BOSS randomized clinical trial. JAMA. 2018;319(3):255–65.
24. Salminen P, Gronroos S, Helmio M, Hurme S, Juuti A, Juusela R, et al. Effect of laparoscopic sleeve gastrectomy vs Roux-en-Y gastric bypass on weight loss, comorbidities, and reflux at 10 years in adult patients with obesity: the SLEEVEPASS randomized clinical trial. JAMA Surg. 2022;157(8):656–66.
25. Snyder B, Wilson E, Wilson T, Mehta S, Bajwa K, Klein C. A randomized trial comparing reflux symptoms in sleeve gastrectomy patients with or without hiatal hernia repair. Surg Obes Relat Dis. 2016;12(9):1681–8.
26. Samakar K, McKenzie TJ, Tavakkoli A, Vernon AH, Robinson MK, Shikora SA. The effect of laparoscopic sleeve gastrectomy with concomitant hiatal hernia repair on gastroesophageal reflux disease in the morbidly obese. Obes Surg. 2016;26(1):61–6.
27. Hider AM, Bonham AJ, Carlin AM, Finks JF, Ghaferi AA, Varban OA, et al. Impact of concurrent hiatal hernia repair during laparoscopic sleeve gastrectomy on patient-reported gastroesophageal reflux symptoms: a state-wide analysis. Surg Obes Relat Dis. 2023;19(6):619–25.
28. Alvarez R, Ward BL, Xiao T, Zadeh J, Sarode A, Khaitan L, et al. Independent association of preoperative Hill grade with gastroesophageal reflux disease 2 years after sleeve gastrectomy. Surg Obes Relat Dis. 2023;19(6):563–75.
29. Angrisani L, Santonicola A, Borrelli V, Iovino P. Sleeve gastrectomy with concomitant hiatal hernia repair in obese patients: long-term results on gastroesophageal reflux disease. Surg Obes Relat Dis. 2020;16(9):1171–7.
30. Nadaleto BF, Herbella FA, Patti MG. Gastroesophageal reflux disease in the obese: Pathophysiology and treatment. Surgery. 2016;159(2):475–86.
31. El-Hadi M, Birch DW, Gill RS, Karmali S. The effect of bariatric surgery on gastroesophageal reflux disease. Can J Surg. 2014;57(2):139–44.
32. Sami SS, Ragunath K. The Los Angeles classification of gastroesophageal reflux disease. Video J Encycl GI Endosc. 2013;1(1):103–4.

33. Ehlers AP, Bonham AJ, Ghaferi AA, Finks JF, Carlin AM, Varban OA. Impact of hiatal hernia repair technique on patient-reported gastroesophageal reflux symptoms following laparoscopic sleeve gastrectomy. Surg Endosc. 2022;36(9):6815–21.
34. Kohn GP, Price RR, DeMeester SR, Zehetner J, Muensterer OJ, Awad Z, et al. Guidelines for the management of hiatal hernia. Surg Endosc. 2013;27(12):4409–28.
35. Hashemi M, Peters JH, DeMeester TR, Huprich JE, Quek M, Hagen JA, et al. Laparoscopic repair of large type III hiatal hernia: objective followup reveals high recurrence rate. J Am Coll Surg 2000;190(5):553–60; discussion 60–1.
36. Wiechmann RJ, Ferguson MK, Naunheim KS, McKesey P, Hazelrigg SJ, Santucci TS, et al. Laparoscopic management of giant paraesophageal herniation. Ann Thorac Surg 2001;71(4):1080–6; discussion 6–7.
37. Clapp B, Kara AM, Nguyen-Lee PJ, Alvarado L, Marr JD, Annabi HM, et al. Does the use of bioabsorbable mesh for hiatal hernia repair at the time of bariatric surgery reduce recurrence rates? A meta-analysis Surg Obes Relat Dis. 2022;18(12):1407–15.
38. Varga G, Cseke L, Kalmar K, Horvath OP. Prevention of recurrence by reinforcement of hiatal closure using ligamentum teres in laparoscopic repair of large hiatal hernias. Surg Endosc. 2004;18(7):1051–3.
39. Varga G, Cseke L, Kalmar K, Horvath OP. Laparoscopic repair of large hiatal hernia with teres ligament: midterm follow-up: a new surgical procedure. Surg Endosc. 2008;22(4):881–4.
40. Park AE, Hoogerboord CM, Sutton E. Use of the falciform ligament flap for closure of the esophageal hiatus in giant paraesophageal hernia. J Gastrointest Surg. 2012;16(7):1417–21.
41. McKay SC, DeMeester SR, Sharata A, DeSouza ML, Bradley DD, Reavis KM, et al. Diaphragmatic relaxing incisions for complex hiatal reconstruction: longer-term follow-up confirms safety, efficacy and rare complications. Surg Endosc. 2023;37(11):8636–43.
42. Gagner M, Deitel M, Erickson AL, Crosby RD. Survey on laparoscopic sleeve gastrectomy (LSG) at the Fourth International Consensus Summit on Sleeve Gastrectomy. Obes Surg. 2013;23(12):2013–7.
43. DuPree CE, Blair K, Steele SR, Martin MJ. Laparoscopic sleeve gastrectomy in patients with preexisting gastroesophageal reflux disease : a national analysis. JAMA Surg. 2014;149(4):328–34.
44. Obeid T, Krishnan A, Abdalla G, Schweitzer M, Magnuson T, Steele KE. GERD is associated with higher long-term reoperation rates after bariatric surgery. J Gastrointest Surg 2016;20(1):119–24; discussion 24.
45. Matar R, Maselli D, Vargas E, Veeravich J, Bazerbachi F, Beran A, et al. Esophagitis after bariatric surgery: large cross-sectional assessment of an endoscopic database. Obes Surg. 2020;30(1):161–8.
46. Kothari V, Shaligram A, Reynoso J, Schmidt E, McBride CL, Oleynikov D. Impact on perioperative outcomes of concomitant hiatal hernia repair with laparoscopic gastric bypass. Obes Surg. 2012;22(10):1607–10.
47. Boules M, Corcelles R, Guerron AD, Dong M, Daigle CR, El-Hayek K, et al. The incidence of hiatal hernia and technical feasibility of repair during bariatric surgery. Surgery 2015;158(4):911–6; discussion 6–8.
48. Hage K, Cornejo J, Allotey JK, Castillo-Larios R, Caposole MZ, Iskandar M, et al. Feasibility and outcomes of simultaneous gastric bypass with paraesophageal hernia repair in elderly patients. Obes Surg. 2023;33(9):2734–41.
49. Pham DV, Protyniak B, Binenbaum SJ, Squillaro A, Borao FJ. Simultaneous laparoscopic paraesophageal hernia repair and sleeve gastrectomy in the morbidly obese. Surg Obes Relat Dis. 2014;10(2):257–61.
50. Dakour Aridi HN, Tamim H, Mailhac A, Safadi BY. Concomitant hiatal hernia repair with laparoscopic sleeve gastrectomy is safe: analysis of the ACS-NSQIP database. Surg Obes Relat Dis. 2017;13(3):379–84.
51. Janik MR, Ibikunle C, Aryaie AH. Safety of concurrent sleeve gastrectomy and hiatal hernia repair: a propensity score-matched analysis of the MBSAQIP registry. Surg Obes Relat Dis. 2020;16(3):365–71.

52. Docimo S Jr, Rahmana U, Bates A, Talamini M, Pryor A, Spaniolas K. Concomitant hiatal hernia repair is more common in laparoscopic sleeve gastrectomy than during laparoscopic Roux-en-Y gastric bypass: an analysis of 130,772 cases. Obes Surg. 2019;29(2):744–6.
53. Lewis KH, Callaway K, Argetsinger S, Wallace J, Arterburn DE, Zhang F, et al. Concurrent hiatal hernia repair and bariatric surgery: outcomes after sleeve gastrectomy and Roux-en-Y gastric bypass. Surg Obes Relat Dis. 2021;17(1):72–80.
54. Clapp B, Liggett E, Barrientes A, Aguirre K, Marwaha V, Tyroch A. Concomitant hiatal hernia repair with sleeve gastrectomy: a 5-year analysis. JSLS. 2020;24(4)
55. Martinino A, Nanayakkara KDL, Madhok B, Wong GYM, Abouelazayem M, Pereira JPS, et al. Global 30-day morbidity and mortality of primary bariatric surgery combined with another procedure: the BLEND study. Obes Surg. 2024;
56. Valukas CS, Vitello D, Sanchez J, Soetikno A, Prinz J, Hungness ES, et al. Surgeon variability in repair of hiatal hernia at the time of bariatric surgery. Surg Endosc. 2024;
57. Clapp B, Vo LU, Lodeiro C, Harper B, Montelongo S, Lee I, et al. Late-term hiatal hernia after gastric bypass: an emerging problem. Surg Obes Relat Dis. 2020;16(4):471–5.
58. Golas A, El-Attrache BM, Jorge J, Dietrick J, Gonzalvo JP, Murr MM. Repair of post-bariatric surgery, recurrent, and de novo hiatal hernias improves bloating, abdominal pain, regurgitation, and food intolerance. Surg Obes Relat Dis. 2021;17(4):683–91.
59. Chaudhry S, Farsi S, Nakanishi H, Parmar C, Ghanem OM, Clapp B. Ligamentum teres augmentation for hiatus hernia repair after bariatric surgery: a systematic review and meta-analysis. Surg Laparosc Endosc Percutan Tech. 2024;
60. Hawasli A, Foster R, Lew D, Peck L. Laparoscopic Ligamentum Teres cardiopexy to the rescue; an old procedure with a new use in managing reflux after sleeve gastrectomy. Am J Surg. 2021;221(3):602–5.
61. Mackey EE, Dore FJ, Kelly JF, Crawford AS, Cohen P, Czerniach D, et al. Ligamentum teres cardiopexy for post vertical sleeve gastrectomy gastroesophageal reflux. Surg Endosc. 2023;37(9):7247–53.
62. Ndubizu GU, Petrick AT, Horsley R. Concurrent magnetic sphincter augmentation and hiatal hernia repair for refractory GERD after laparoscopic sleeve gastrectomy. Surg Obes Relat Dis. 2020;16(1):168–70.
63. Ibrahim MA, Mowoh DP, Al Khadem M, Abbas M, Khaitan L. Long-term outcomes of magnetic sphincter augmentation in sleeve gastrectomy and Roux-en-Y gastric bypass patients: a comprehensive analysis. Surg Endosc. 2024;
64. Peine BS, Denning MT, Brea F, Wolf SE, Bethea JP, Speicher JE, et al. Esophageal magnetic sphincter augmentation following bariatric surgery improves quality of life and reduces proton pump inhibitor usage. J Gastrointest Surg. 2024;28(1):72–4.

# 46 Robotic-Assisted Metabolic and Bariatric Surgery

Michelle Nessen, Valeria Noguera, Abdallah Attia, and Carlos Galvani

## Introduction

Worldwide obesity has tripled since 1975, and in 2020, the prevalence of obesity in the United States was 41.9% [1, 2]. Rates of obesity have escalated globally, posing a public health challenge of immense proportions [3]. Obesity predisposes patients to obesity-related comorbidities, such as diabetes mellitus, hypertension, obstructive sleep apnea, and dyslipidemia. Bariatric surgery is a safe and effective weight loss and obesity management modality. Laparoscopic techniques allowed the field bariatric surgery field to rapidly grow since the mid-1990s, and minimally invasive bariatric surgery has since served as the cornerstone of obesity management. The subsequent introduction of robotic surgery has allowed surgeons to overcome some of the technical limitations associated with laparoscopic surgery, and potentially flattening the learning curve.

The history of robotics in the United States dates back to the early 2000s, with the FDA's approval of the da Vinci Surgical System for general laparoscopic surgery. Prior to that, Drs. Cadiere et al. described robotic-assisted laparoscopic gastric banding Belgium in 1998 [4]. Horgan first introduced the use of the da Vinci system in the United States for bariatrics and other advanced laparoscopic procedures such as Heller myotomy, nephrectomy and adrenalectomy in 2001 [5]. This marked the beginning of a new chapter in minimally invasive surgery, offering enhanced precision, control, and visualization. Since then, the field of robotic surgery has expanded rapidly, with continual upgrades in robotic technology and increasing adoption by

M. Nessen · V. Noguera · A. Attia
Division of Minimally Invasive Surgery, Tulane University, New Orleans, LA, USA
e-mail: Mnessen@tulane.edu; Vnoguera@tulane.edu; Aattia@tulane.edu

C. Galvani (✉)
Division of General Surgery, LSU Health, Department of Surgery, New Orleans, LA, USA
e-mail: cgalva@lsuhsc.edu


O. M. Ghanem et al. (eds.), *The SAGES Manual of Metabolic and Bariatric Surgery*, https://doi.org/10.1007/978-3-031-72309-4_46

bariatric surgeons worldwide. A review of the utilization rate of robotic bariatric surgery based on MBSAQIP data between 2015 and 2020 demonstrated an increase in the use of robotics for sleeve gastrectomy (SG) from 6.0 to 17.2% and Roux-en-Y gastric bypass (RYGB) from 6.8 to 16.7%. The greatest annual increase in procedures over this time was seen in revisional surgery, which can be more variable in complexity, which was noted to rise by 3.7-fold, from 4.7% of procedures to 17.4% [6].

## Technical Advantages of Robotic-Assisted Surgery

Robotic technology, at its core, offers several advantages over traditional laparoscopic approaches. While laparoscopic instruments are limited in their degrees of motion, robotic platforms offer up to 7 degrees of freedom, comparable to the human arm. Other benefits include three-dimensional view and magnification of the operative field, improved dexterity and precision of instrument movements, and ergonomic comfort for the surgeon, potentially reducing operative fatigue [7, 8]. In the bariatric population, robotics can mitigate work-related injuries by decreasing the stress caused by torque against thick abdominal walls. Moreover, the robotic platform's ability to scale movements and filter tremors translates into more delicate and precise surgical maneuvers [8].

The advent of robotic staplers in bariatric surgery has additionally improved the autonomy for the operating surgeon, reducing the need for stapling done by a bedside assistant. Recent updates to the stapler technology include monitoring tissue compression prior to and during staple firing to optimize staple lines [8]. Surgeons can use real time feedback from the staplers to guide staple heights based on tissue compression. Suturing on the robotic platform is more easily facilitated compared to laparoscopy, regardless of surgeon experience level [9]. The surgeon is also able to control the three working arms and camera without need for an experienced assistant. The integration of table motion with robotic arms has also increased efficiency in robotic bariatrics. Taken together, these advantages have increased surgeons' autonomy, potentially decreasing the number of cases needed to overcome learning curves. When considered altogether, these advantages have the potential to offer clinical value by decreasing operative times, hospital stay and the morbidity of bariatric procedures.

Multiple robotic platforms exist, with Intuitive's da Vinci system as the most commonly utilized in the United States. Most notably for bariatrics, the fourth generation Xi system has allowed for multi-quadrant single set up procedures, advanced energy devices, and fluorescence imaging that can be utilized for assessment of tissue perfusion or intraluminal leak tests [10].

## Robotic Bariatric Program Setup

Implementation of robotic bariatric surgery requires new competencies related to technical skills, knowledge, teamwork, distinct approach to communication, training, and problem resolution. Understanding the distinct processes related to robotic surgery enables the development of standard practices that can increase patient safety, improve efficiency, and reduce costs. Of course, this will require a multidisciplinary approach where surgeons, anesthesiologists, and the operating room staff (nurses, scrub technicians) are focused in collaborating to foster growth through innovation, and efficiencies (e.g. efficient well-run rooms, experienced and highly trained staff, safe and organized patient care, predictable and familiar operating environment, core robotics OR team). To integrate robotics into a bariatric surgical practice, it is paramount for surgeons to acquire sound technical skills, along appropriate patient selection and regularity of cases. Most experts recommend starting with simple cases and believe it is not logical to only use the robot for complex cases such as revisions or large BMI patients since these cases are likely to lengthen the learning curve.

## Surgeon Feedback

The robotic platform and its associated technology give providers more feedback into their practices and progress compared open or traditional laparoscopic procedures. Some systems allow case details to be synced with online and mobile device-based applications. Reports for each surgery can include console time, active time, number of instruments utilized, and number of times exchanged (Fig. 46.1). Operative times are tracked over time and compared to national averages (Fig. 46.2). Number and types of staplers used per case can also be tracked. This data can be used to determine areas of improvement for individual surgeons, such as ways to improve efficiency of procedures with more thoughtful use of instruments. Trainees should be provided with accounts and can similarly track progress with different procedures over time.

Additional feedback tools include surgical video recording, review and collaboration between providers in real time by sharing live cases. The technological additions of integrated intelligence reflect the incorporation of this technology in various medical and non-medical fields in recent years.

## Procedures Overview

The surgical techniques in RABS are diverse and continually evolving. As mentioned, the newer robotic systems have allowed single docking for both restrictive and anastomotic procedures. Like open or laparoscopic bariatric surgery, modification in specific instruments and steps, including anastomotic technique and order in which portions of the procedure are carried out, can vary by institution and surgeon.

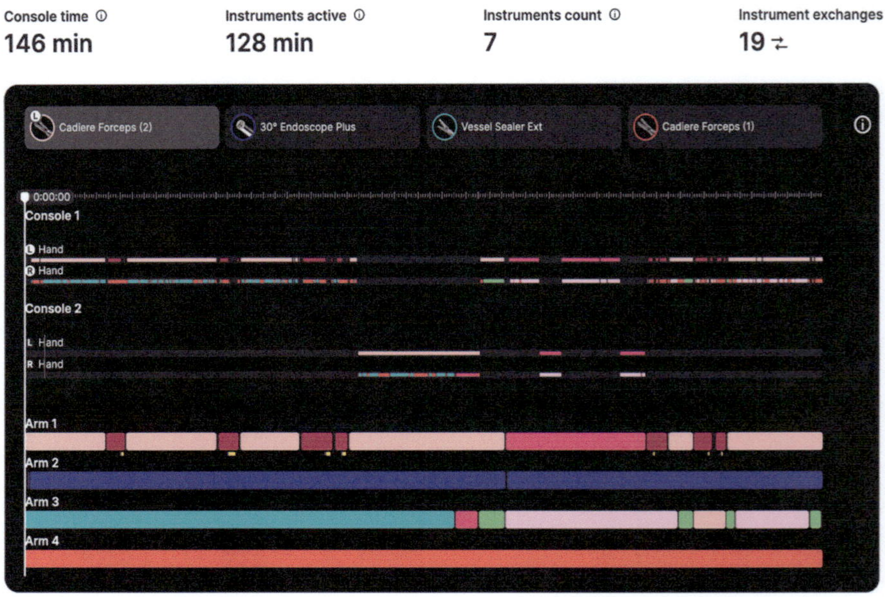


**Fig. 46.1** My Intuitive App Case Tracking Function. Both primary surgeon and trainee can see different instruments used over time per case

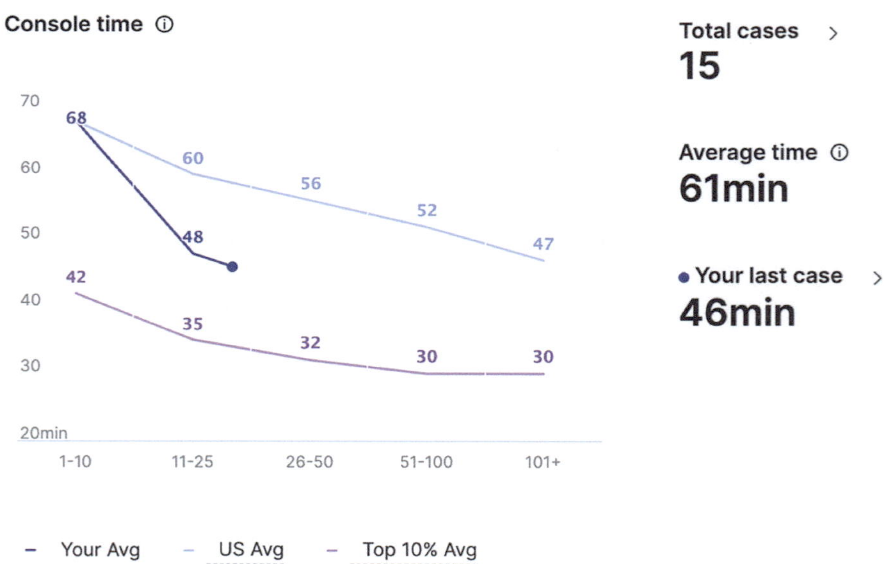


**Fig. 46.2** My Intuitive App Total Console Time Per Case. Surgeon's console time is tracked over operative experience and volume and compared to national averages

The primary goal is to streamline robotic patient positioning, port placement and instrumentation as much as possible to increase efficiency in the operating room.

## Operating Room Setup

A larger operating room is preferable when performing robotic surgery. More space allows the various robotic components to be stored effectively and personnel to move freely around the room. Preferably, there will be ceiling-mounted flat panel monitors and equipment booms to house insufflators, electrosurgical units, laparoscopic camera equipment and light sources. Anesthesia equipment is located at the head of the operating table (Fig. 46.3).

An operating room table that can accommodate patients with severe obesity is mandatory. The table must also be able to provide steep reverse Trendelenburg and have the capability to attach a foot board. When available, integrated table motion available allows for patient positioning throughout the case and feedback on table angles for the teams. In addition, a transfer matt should be used for repositioning and lateral transfer of the patient. Prior to induction of anesthesia, the patient should be secured to the table, pneumatic compression devices placed on the lower legs, and systemic anticoagulation administered.

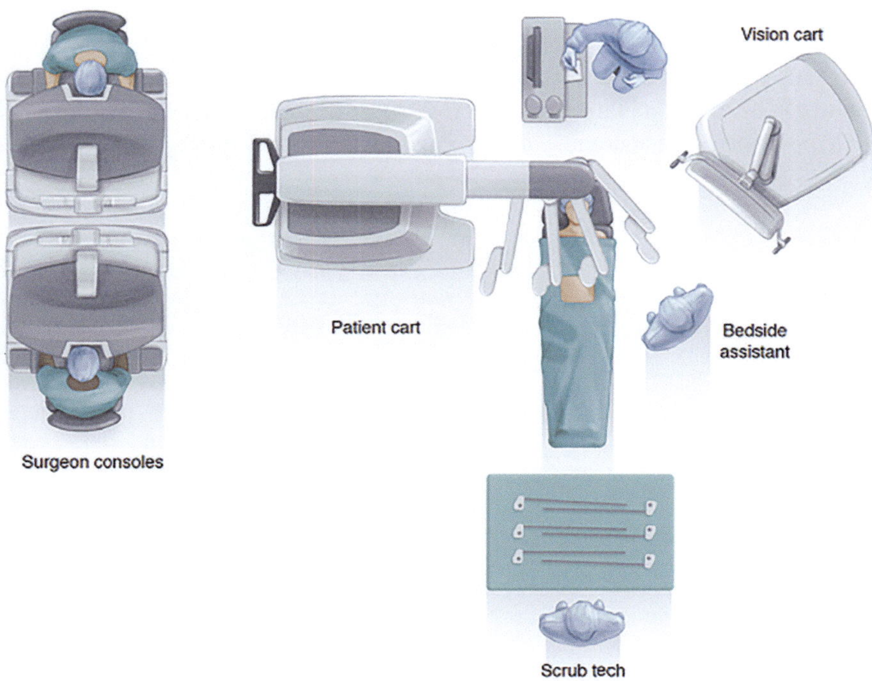


**Fig. 46.3** Operating Room Components and Set Up

Once intubated, the patient is positioned with arms out, with padding to pressure points added as necessary, and secured at the thighs. Some providers choose to additionally secure patients at the chest and right above the ankles. While universally employed in laparoscopic bariatric procedures given higher degrees of reverse Trendelenburg, a footboard may not be necessary in robotic bariatric surgery. An upper body warming device should be placed above the nipples with adequate exposure to the xiphoid. An 36 French suction and calibration tube is placed to decompress the stomach. This tube is also used for sizing of the stomach and stenting of anastomoses. If unavailable, the stomach may initially be decompressed with a standard orogastric sump tube and switched out to a bougie later in the procedure. The abdomen is prepped widely with chlorhexidine-based solution before sterile drapes applied.

## Access and Port Placement

Access to the abdomen can be gained via closed or open techniques, depending on provider preference. Insufflating using a Veress needle at Palmer's prior to optical or blind entry is feasible. In patients with suspected adhesive disease from prior open surgery or intraperitoneal mesh, the first entry port is placed left subcostal.

Our preferred method of entry involves direct optical entry with an 8 mm robotic trocar using a 5 mm 30-degree handheld laparoscope. This first port (Arm #2) is placed in the left mid-abdomen, two fingerbreadths lateral to the umbilicus and one palm-width (~15 to 18 cm) inferior to the left costal margin (Fig. 46.4). This port is ultimately used for the robotic camera. During optical entry at this location, insufflation can be turned on through the robotic trocar to allow for separation of planes while inserting in the abdominal cavity. Pressure is set to 15 mmHg.

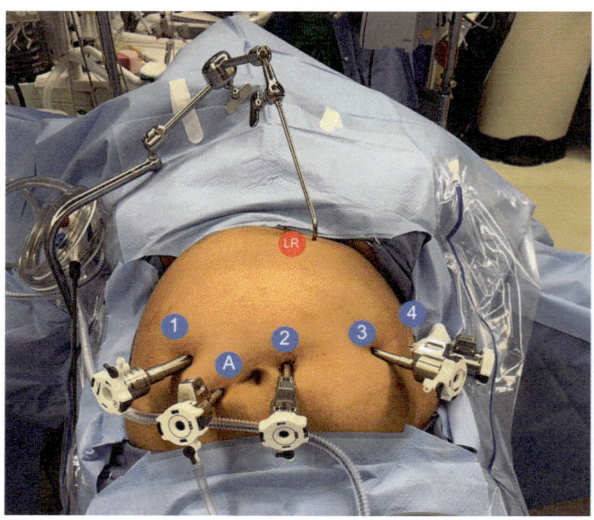


**Fig. 46.4** Standard Robotic Port Placement and Liver Retractor Set Up. Arm #1 12 mm trochar (accommodates SureForm stapler); Arm #2 (Camera) 8 mm trochar; Arm #3 8 mm trochar (working port); Arm #4 8 mm trochar (retracting arm); 8 mm bedside assist sits caudal to Arm #1 and #2; Subxiphoid self-retaining liver retractor

**Table 46.1** General instrumentation

| |
|---|
| 5 mm 30-degree handheld laparoscope |
| 30° robotic camera (Arm #2) |
| 3–4 8-mm trocars |
| 1–2 12-mm trocars |
| Nathanson liver retractor |
| Force bipolar (Arm #1) |
| Vessel sealer or SynchroSeal (Arm #3) |
| Monopolar scissors (Arm #3) |
| 2 needle drivers (Arm #3, ±Arm #1), |
| Mega Suturecut |
| Large needle driver |
| Cadiere or Prograsp or Tip-Up fenestrated gasper (Arm #4) |
| 60 mm stapler with reloads (Arm #1) |

Two 8-mm trocars and one 12-mm trocar are then placed at the same level of the camera port as follows: 12-mm port on the right midclavicular line (Arm #1), one on the left midclavicular line (Arm #3), and one in the left anterior axillary line (Arm #4). A 5-mm subxiphoid incision is used for the placement of the Nathanson liver retractor with the patient in 15–20° of reverse Trendelburg position. A self-retaining liver stitch may also be utilized and is generally easier to place robotically compared to traditional laparoscopy.

For certain procedures (RYGB, Single Anastomosis duodenal switch, Revisions), an 8-mm trocar assist port is placed caudally either between Arms #1 and #2 or #2 and #3 for the bedside assistant. Using the robotic 8-mm trocar allows for easy passing of needles and suction/irrigation, without the need to close the fascia or use disposables.

The da Vinci Xi Surgical system can be docked from the patient's right or left side. All described techniques here utilize a two right-hands approach, with the camera maintained in Arm #2 (Table 46.1).

Upper endoscopy may be utilized at any point during the procedure if anatomy is unclear. Intraoperative endoscopic images may be projected onto the robotic console and the screens in the room offering picture-in-picture at any point during the case.

## Operative Techniques

### Concomitant Hiatal Hernia Repair

When hiatal hernias are encountered, it is recommended to fully mobilize the proximal stomach and esophagus and perform crural approximation with permanent suture. For large hernias, a mesh may be utilized. Visualization of and in the mediastinum and suturing are both enhanced using the robotic platform.

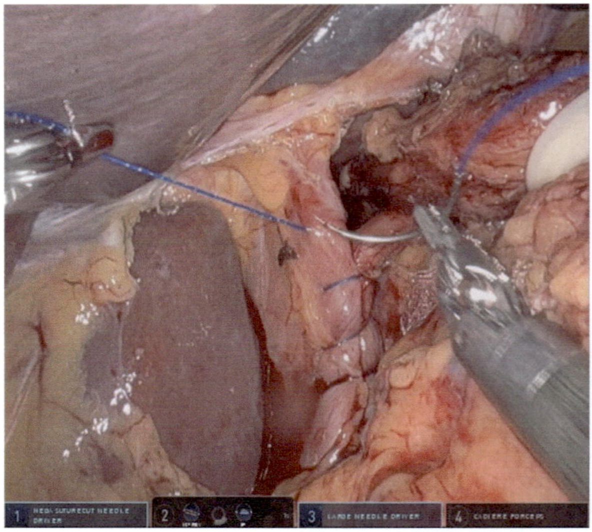


**Fig. 46.5** Posterior Crural Repair. Running barbed suture is used to reapproximate the posterior crura in a running fashion

## Technique

After opening pars flaccida identifying the right crus, it is dissected carefully off the esophagus. This dissection is typically carried out from anterior to posterior along the right crus starting at the right side of the phrenoesophageal membrane until fully exposing the right crus. After complete exposure of the right crus, a retroesophageal window is created and extended exposing the confluence of the crura. At this point the Penrose drain is passed behind the esophagus and used to encircle the esophagus and vagus nerves. Then attention is focused on the left crura, typically the dissection starts from posterior to anterior, and is continued in a circular manner around the rim of the hiatus with complete takedown of the phrenoesophageal membrane. The dissection is continued with a combination of blunt dissection and the vessel sealer until complete exposure of the left crus is achieved. Transhiatal dissection of the esophagus is started and continued in a cephalad direction. The articulated vessel sealer device and the fenestrated bipolar grasper are used for the circumferential dissection of the esophagus. Mobilization of the esophagus can typically be accomplished using blunt dissection of relatively thin alveolar tissue by exercising traction and countertraction maneuvers always dissecting away from the esophagus. The esophageal mobilization is completed only after 2–3 cm of intraabdominal esophagus is observed without tension. The esophagus is retracted anteriorly and to the left by Arm #4, and the vessel sealer is replaced with a suture cut needle driver. Closure of the diaphragmatic defect is started at the junction of the right and left crus to decrease tension on every stitch and is carried out anteriorly. The closure is performed using running non-absorbable barbed suture. A "shoe lacing technique" is used to decrease tension of the repair (Fig. 46.5).

## Sleeve Gastrectomy

Sleeve gastrectomy (SG) is currently the most commonly performed bariatric procedure worldwide, and in the United States 160,609 procedures were performed in 2022 as reported by the ASMBS. [11] The robotic approach to SG has been found to be safe and feasible, including in patients with higher BMI (>50 kg/m$^2$) [3]. Between 2015 and 2020, there was a 2.87 fold increase in SG being performed robotically [6]. Some of the advantages include a relatively fast learning curve, improved visualization for complete fundal dissection and ease of oversewing the staple line [12]. Staple line reinforcement can utilize, including commercially available bioabsorbable buttress or oversewing of parts or all of the staple line. For surgeons new to robotic bariatric surgery, SG may be a good steppingstone to the robotic RYGB or other procedures.

### Setup

Four robotic trocars and a liver retractor are placed as described above. Initial instruments include:

- Arm #1: Fenestrated bipolar; stapler
- Arm #2: Camera
- Arm #3: Vessel sealer (or SynchroSeal)
- Arm #4: Cadiere (or Tip-Up)

### Technique

Robotic SG is carried out in similar steps to laparoscopic procedures. The anterior stomach is grasped by Arm #1 and retracted to enter the lesser sac with energy on Arm #3. The omentum is freed proximally to the left crural pillar and distally to approximately 4 cm from the pylorus. A 36F calibration tube is used to size the sleeve, which is passed down to the antrum. Arm #1 is then used to fire sequential 60 mm staple loads. If utilizing buttress material, a black load with buttress is the first load, followed by additional black and then green or blue loads depending on the thickness of the tissue. Built in technology monitors tissue compression before and during firing, adjusting to optimize staple height in real time. Force fire may be employed with black reloads if tissue is found to be too thick to continue, or a switch to a larger reload should be employed (Fig. 46.6a). If no buttress material is utilized, current trends recommend downsizing of the staple line to prevent bleeding complications. A green/blue/white load algorithm may first be utilized depending on tissue thickness and stapler pauses for compression.

Regardless of the specific technique, it is critical to exclude the fundus and avoid close proximity to the GE-junction as the proximal stomach is approached.

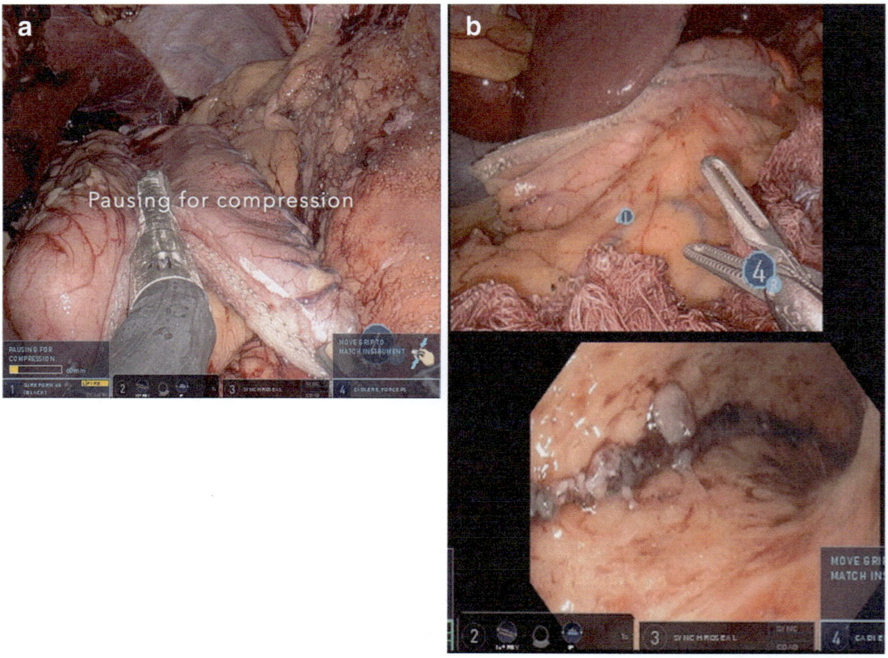


**Fig. 46.6** (**a**) Sleeve Gastrectomy Utilizing Buttress Material for Staple Line Reinforcement. It is critical as the GE junction is approached to exclude the posterior fundus. (**b**) Completed Sleeve Gastrectomy with Intraoperative EGD. The TilePro™ function allows for simultaneous viewing of surgical field and endoscopic images. Angulation and width of sleeve as well as staple line bleeding is evaluated after completion of sleeve

Staple line reinforcement via the oversewing technique may be utilized if no buttress material is employed. Options include proximal imbrication of the staple line, suturing around parts or all the staple line, or oversewing with concurrent omentopexy to the cut edge of the omentum.

Endoscopy can be used to visualize the staple line for intraluminal bleeding and evaluate the angulation at the incisura (Fig. 46.6b). Leak tests after sleeve may be employed based on provider discretion. If a leak test is performed with endoscopy, the upper abdomen is submerged, distal stomach clamped, and insufflation applied while looking for bubbles. Intraluminal administration of indocyanine green while looking for evidence of immunofluorescence extravasation can also be used as a leak test. Reports of 100% sensitivity and 98.28% specificity using this method have been described [13].

## Outcomes

Overall, robotic SG is a safe and effective procedure for the treatment of obesity. The learning curve associated with SG is passed by about 20 cases [12]. Overall, use of staple line reinforcement is associated with reduced risk of some adverse outcomes, including organ-space infection and 30-day reoperation [14]. In a review of the ASMBS database comparing patients undergoing laparoscopic versus robotic SG with BMI >50 kg/m$^2$, robotic cases were found to have longer operative times and length of stay with no difference between overall morbidity and mortality. After adjustment, the robotic approach was found to be an independent risk factor for organ-space surgical site infection. Large scale retrospective reviews have yielded mixed results on other outcomes. Some studies have suggested that on top of longer operative times, robotic sleeves are associated with increased risk of reoperation and readmission at 30 days compared to laparoscopy. [15]

Different techniques utilize robotic SG via three incisions to improve efficiency, costs, and pain without sacrificing safety outcomes. As with any new technology, advances over time have helped improved outcomes in robotic bariatric surgery [12].

## Roux-en-Y Gastric Bypass

### Intro

Robotic-assisted RYGB was first introduced in 2001, but it was slow to initially to be incorporated into widespread use by bariatric surgeons. In the last decade, however, there has been greater utilization with a 2.46-fold increase in the proportion of procedures performed robotically between 2015 and 2020 [6]. One of the main advantages of the robot for RYGB is the shorter learning curve to perform advanced maneuvers such fully hand-sewn anastomoses. The robotic platform also improves surgeon autonomy in these procedures, decreases variability and improves surgeon ergonomics [16]. Visualization and retraction particularly during pouch creation may also be facilitated by the robotic approach. The procedure here describes a completely hand-sewn gastrojejunal approach and fully stapled jejuno-jejunostomy, but variations in technique can vary widely.

### Setup

The described technique utilizes four 8 mm trocars, including one to serve as the assist port, a liver retractor and one 12 mm trocar.

- Arm #1: Fenestrated bipolar; stapler
- Arm #2: Camera
- Arm #3: Vessel sealer (or SynchroSeal); monopolar scissors
- Arm #4: Cadiere (or Tip-Up)

The assist port is used for both passing sponges/sutures and suction and, specifically for the RYGB, may be used to aid in exposure during closure of Petersen's space.

## Technique

- *Pouch Creation*
- If no hiatal hernia is present, the procedure proceeds with dissection of the peritoneum off the diaphragm at the angle of His to expose the left crus. This will facilitate the division of the most cephalad part of the gastric pouch. To create a 20- to 30-mL gastric pouch, the stomach is transected about 4–5 cm distal to gastroesophageal junction. A perigastric dissection is performed along the lesser curvature by creating a window behind the stomach just below the first hepatic branch using vessel sealer or SynchroSeal and blunt dissection. Care should be taken to stay caudal to the left gastric artery. The stomach then is divided transversely at about 40 mm widgth via Arm #1 and 1–1/2 fires of 60 mm staplers (with buttressing if desired) towards the angle of His. A 36F calibration tube is used to avoid narrowing the pouch and avoid injury to the esophagus. Staple line reinforcement material is used to prevent bleeding from the staple line between the pouch and remnant stomach (Fig. 46.7). The articulation afforded by robotic staplers requires using only one 12 mm trocar.
- *Creation of omega loop and blind loop (candy cane)*
- Robotic RYGB is created via an omega loop confirmation. The greater omentum and the transverse colon are retracted cephalad. The greater omentum is divided as needed. Arm #4 retracts the transverse mesocolon and the greater omentum while Arm #1 and #3 identify the ligament of Treitz. The jejunum is then run distally, and a loop is chosen that will be able to reach to the upper abdomen (70–125 cm from the ligament) without tension. This jejunal segment is sutured in a running fashion to the gastric pouch with an absorbable 9 inch 3-0 barbed suture. This will become the outer posterior layer of the gastrojejunal anastomosis. Then the small bowel is divided with robotic linear stapler white load just to

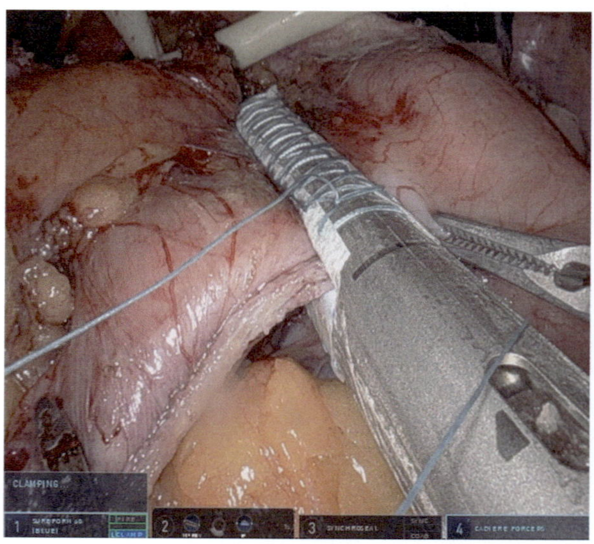


**Fig. 46.7** Creation of Gastric Pouch. SureForm stapler with buttress material firing towards angle of His to create pouch. 36F bougie is positioned within pouch to size and guide stapler

the left of the gastric pouch to separate the bilio-pancreatic limb from the alimentary limb and to create the blind loop. The mesentery of the small bowel is generally not divided.

- *Creation of the jejuno-jejunostomy and closure of the mesenteric defects*
- Once the omega loop is divided, the alimentary (Roux) limb is constructed. About 120–150 cm is measured starting at the gastrojejunostomy towards the distal jejunum. This is performed using two graspers in Arms #1 and #4, while monopolar scissors are introduced in Arm #3. Enterotomies are created the scissors and a stapled side-to-side jejuno-jejunostomy is created with a 60-white load. Following creation of the jejuno-jejunostomy, the common enterostomy is closed with another 60-white load. The jejuno-jejunal mesenteric defect and Petersen's space are closed with non-absorbable 6-inches 3-0 barbed suture (Fig. 46.8).
- Depending on provider practice, the gastrojejunostomy may be completed in totality before the jejuno-jejunostomy as described above.
- *Creation of the gastrojejunostomy*
- The next step is the completion of the gastrojejunostomy. A gastrotomy and jejunotomy are created with monopolar scissors (Fig. 46.9). The gastrotomy is created against traction with the calibration tube. A 1.5–2 cm gastrojejunostomy is "hand-sewn" in two layers using two needle drivers (Arms #1 and #3) and absorbable 6-inch barbed sutures (×2). Starting from lateral to medial, an inner posterior layer of running 3-0 absorbable barbed suture is created with full thickness bites between stomach and jejunum (Fig. 46.10). Once the inner posterior layer is completed the bougie is advanced into the jejunum to stent the anastomosis. Finally, two anterior layers (inner/outer) of running seromuscular (Lembert sutures) are created. The outer anterior row is fashioned as a continuation of the outer posterior row 9-inch suture.

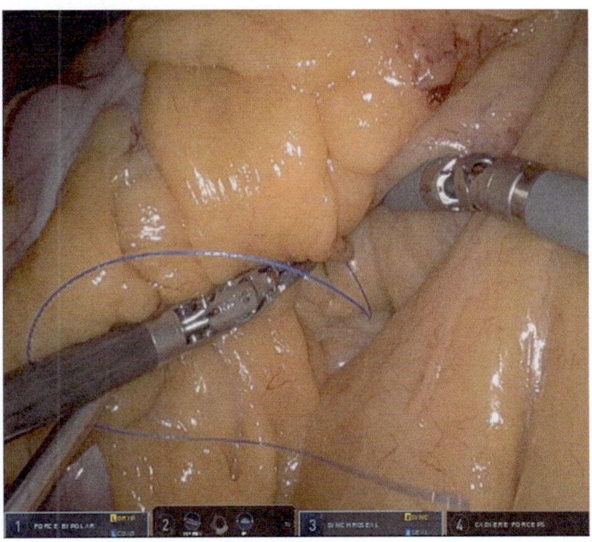

**Fig. 46.8** Closure of Petersen's Defect. Running permanent barbed suture is used to close the defect between the mesentery of the alimentary limb and transverse mesocolon. The assist port may be utilized to help visualize this potential space

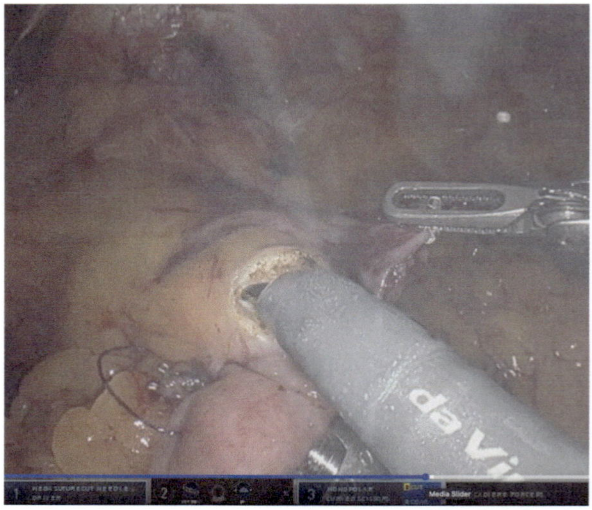

**Fig. 46.9** Gastrotomy Creation. Monopolar cautery is used with the scissors to create the gastrotomy with counterforce from the intraluminal bougie

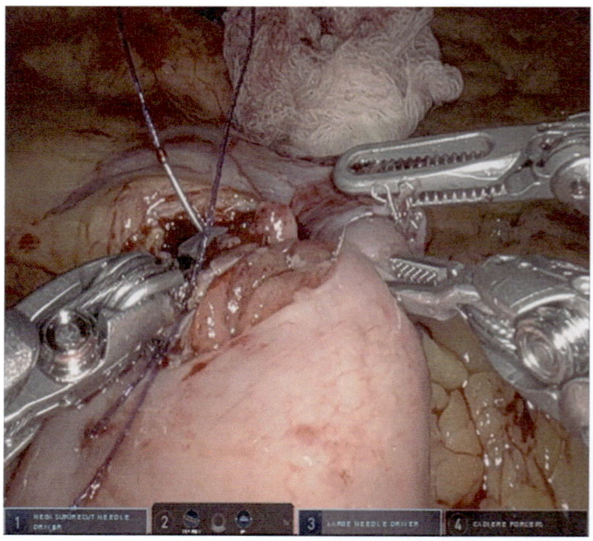

**Fig. 46.10** Creation of Fully Hand Sewn Gastrojejunostomy. Running absorbable 3-0 barbed suture is used to fashion the gastrojejunostomy. Two needle drivers (in Arm #1 and Arm #3) are employed for suturing for safe and effective turning around corners

The alimentary limb is clamped just distal to the gastrojejunal anastomosis, and the upper abdomen filled with water to perform an air leak test. The gastroscope is inserted into the patient's esophagus insufflating along the way. The gastric pouch is entered, and the anastomosis is traversed while evaluating for intraluminal bleeding and leak (Fig. 46.11).

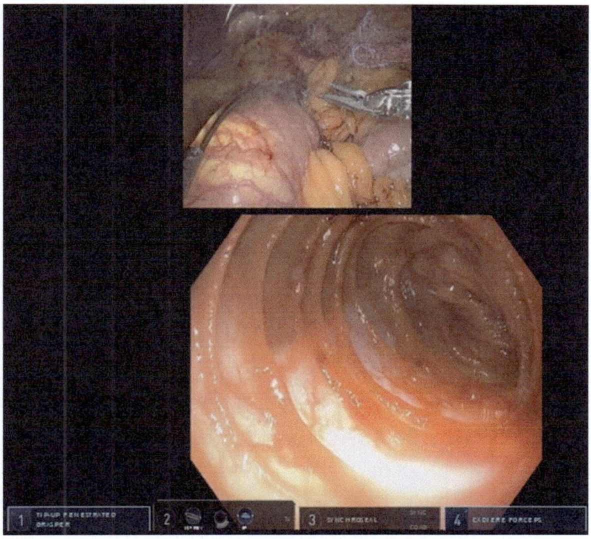

**Fig. 46.11** Leak Test. The alimentary limb is clamped and submerged via irrigation instilled from assist port. The TilePro function allows for simultaneous viewing of endoscopic images and operative field

## Outcomes

The robotic RYGB has been found to be safe and effective for the treatment of obesity. Reported advantages of its use have been included a shorter learning curve and a lower complication rate at the gastrojejunostomy. A meta-analysis comparing RA-RYGB vs LA-RYGB showed that the learning curve for RA-RYGB is between 10 and 30 surgeries [17]. A comparative study which included 389 laparoscopic and 388 RA-RYGB also showed a significantly reduced conversion rate in the robotic arm compared with the laparoscopic arm (less than 1% versus almost 5%) although operative time was longer [18]. The hand-sewn anastomosis has the advantages of allowing for direct examination of the anastomosis, reducing the risk of bleeding, and can be used in situations where the use of a stapled anastomosis would be contraindicated, and decreased long-term rates of strictures [19].

A large retrospective review utilizing propensity-matched analysis of MBSAQIP data demonstrated mixed results when comparing laparoscopic and robotic RYGB. While rates of postoperative morbidity and mortality were similar between the groups, the robotic platform associated with increased risk of reoperation and readmission as well as organ/space surgical site infection, septic shock, anastomotic leak and bowel obstruction [20]. As technological advances continue, costs and technical challenges with the robotic RYGB continue to improve, with increased surgeon autonomy and reproducibility, with the potential to further improve outcomes.

## SADI-S/BPD-DS

The biliopancreatic diversion with duodenal switch (BPD-DS) is considered the most effective treatment modality for patients with obesity and is generally reserved for those with high BMI (>50 kg/m$^2$). The modern BPD-DS involves creating a SG, transection of the duodenum distal to the pylorus and creation of a short alimentary limb (~150 cm) and common channel (~100 cm). Early cases were performed open, and then with possible laparoscopic SG followed by open duodeno-ileal and ilio-ileal anastomoses. The single anastomosis duodenal-ileal bypass with sleeve (SADI-S) was later introduced, that involves creation of a SG followed by duodeno-ileal anastomosis in a loop configuration (common channel ~300 cm). Based on ASMBS data, the number of BPD-DS and SADI-S procedures has steadily increased over recent years, with 6100 BPD-DS procedures performed in 2022 compared to 2272 in 2019. 1600 SADI-S procedures were performed in 2022 [21]. The proportion of these procedures done robotically has also increased over time [6]. The procedures can be performed in a staged fashion, with SG performed in a separate setting or in the same operation. Careful patient selection regarding adherence to lifelong supplementation and follow-up is critical. The robot approach is well-suited for these complex procedures as it helps reduce stress from torque on the abdominal wall in high BMI patients, the use of fluorescence to trace and determine blood supply to the duodenum, and aids in visualization during the duodenal dissection and hand-sewn duodeno-ileal anastomoses.

## Setup

BPD-DS: The described technique utilizes three 8 mm trocars, including one to serve as the assist port, a liver retractor and two 12 mm trocars. The stapler in Arm #3 is specifically used for the creation of ileo-ileal anastomosis and may also be used for the sleeve or duodenal transection.

- Arm #1 (12 mm): Fenestrated bipolar; stapler
- Arm #2: Camera
- Arm #3 (12 mm): Vessel sealer (or SynchroSeal); monopolar scissors; stapler
- Arm #4: Cadiere (or Tip-Up)

SADI-S: The setup for a SADI-S is similar to an R-RYGB, utilizing four 8 mm trocars, including one to serve as the assist port, a liver retractor and one 12 mm trocar. The stapler in Arm #1 can be used to fashion the sleeve and staple across the duodenum.

## BPD-DS Technique

After port placement, the abdomen is inspected for adhesions to ensure that the distal bowel will be mobile enough to create the duodeno-ileal anastomosis without tension. In patients with prior pelvic or lower abdominal surgery, it may not be feasible to run the bowel proximally from the terminal ileum. In patients with previously performed SG, cholecystectomy or other procedures in the upper abdomen, adhesions between the liver and stomach/duodenum may need to be taken down.

The robot can be used to run the bowel from the terminal ileum proximally to measure a common channel of 100 cm, which is marked with a suture. The bowel should be rotated in a counterclockwise fashion while handling. The bowel is run an additional 150 cm for the alimentary limb, which is brought up and secured to the omentum near the pylorus. Additional suture markers can be sued to help orient the bowel as keeping it in the proper configuration for the anastomosis is critical. Table motion can be utilized to place the patient into mild Trendelburg to localize the terminal ileum. Alternatively, the bowel may be run laparoscopically, and clips used to mark distances before docking the robot and proceeding with the upper abdominal portions of the procedure. It is recommended to use standardized measuring techniques while counting the bowel to prevent malabsorption and severe nutritional deficiencies if undercounted. Pre-measured umbilical tape-marked instruments or a ruler are all options to measure with.

The order in which parts of the dissection are carried out may vary from provider to provider. Typically, the lesser sac is entered as the usual first step of the SG. The dissection is carried distally towards the pylorus using the energy device in Arm #3 along the greater curve. Arm #4 is used to grasp the antrum anterolaterally, exposing the underside of the pylorus and the first portion of the duodenum. Energy is used to divide any adhesions to the pancreas and along the outer border of the pylorus and duodenum. Perforators from the gastroduodenal artery become visible as the dissection nears the pancreaticoduodenal groove, which serves as the landmark to complete the dissection (Fig. 46.12). At least 2–3 cm of the first portion of the duodenum should be achieved for adequate length for the anastomosis. Arm #4 then retracts the antrum down to expose the lesser curve, where the peritoneum is opened along the first portion of the duodenum. The instrument in Arm #1 can then tunnel posteriorly and come out along the lesser curve to ensure the route for the stapler.

Assuming a single-stage procedure, an SG is performed as previously described prior to division of the duodenum. When performed as part of a BPD-DS, a "generous" sleeve is preferred, either by using a larger bougie (40–56F) or by keeping further distance from the lesser curve by visual inspection.

Attention is turned back to the division of the duodenum. A white staple load is deployed through Arm #1 through the previously defined tunnel, ensuring adequate duodenal length (Fig. 46.13). Buttress material may be used at this location, particularly for maintenance of the duodenal stump to help prevent bleeding or stump blowout. Care should be taken to avoid structures such as the porta hepatis. After

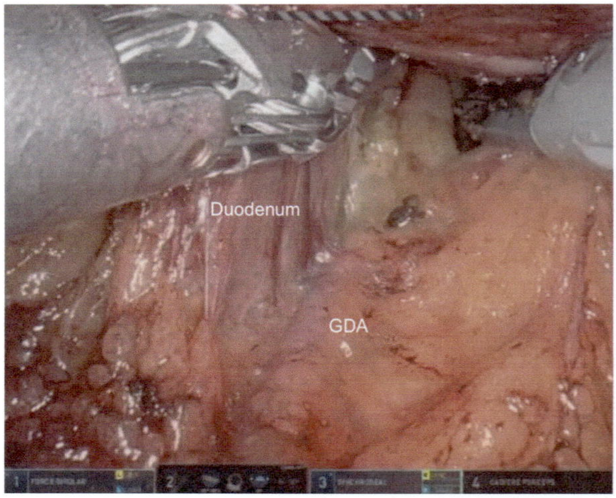


**Fig. 46.12** Gastroduodenal Artery (GDA) Visualized Along Pancreaticoduodenal Groove. The landmark for completion of the posterior dissection is the GDA, which lies perpendicular to the duodenum. Perforators can first be seen as the dissection is carried distally running parallel to the bowel

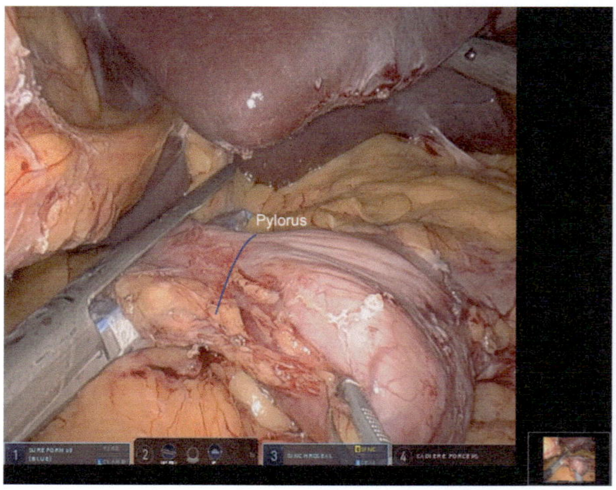


**Fig. 46.13** Extent of Duodenal Dissection and Division. 2–3 cm duodenal cuff ensured prior to division with SureForm stapler

division, the freedom of movement is evaluated for the creation of the anastomosis. The peritoneum can be divided further proximally along the lesser curve and division of the right gastric may be necessary for adequate mobilization.

The ileum is then freed either from the assist port or robotic scissors to be able to fashion the hand-sewn duodeno-ileostomy. If there is any question about the proper orientation of the bowel, it may be run proximally or distally such that the biliopancreatic limb (BP) is entering from the screen right and there is no twisting of the mesentery. A 9-inch 3-0 absorbable barbed suture is used to run the posterior outer layer of the anastomosis with a needle driver in Arm #3 by going around the staple line of the duodenum to the ileum (Fig. 46.14a). Monopolar cautery on scissors in Arm #3 is then used to create enterotomies that typically span almost the full width

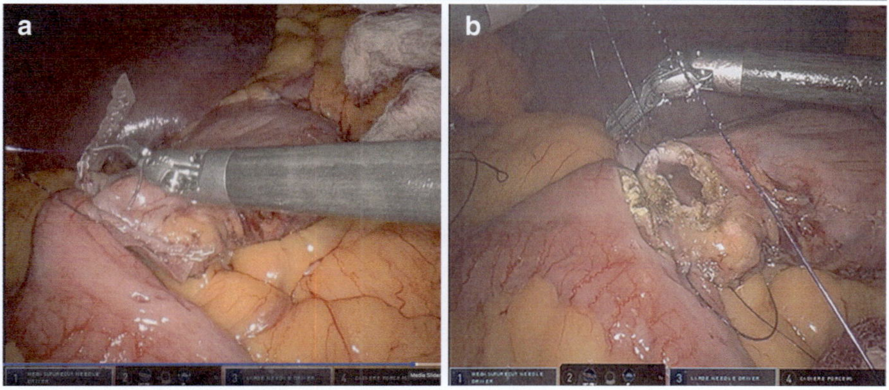


**Fig. 46.14** Hand Sewn Duodeno-Ileostomy Setup. (**a**) Posterior outer layer. (**b**) Duodenotomy and mirrored enterotomy closed with running 3-0 absorbable barbed suture

of the duodenum (Fig. 46.14b). The remainder of the anastomosis is completed similarly to the described RYGB, with two-needle drivers (Arm #1 and #3) used to sew a full-thickness posterior inner layers with 3-0 absorbable barbed suture. The initial posterior layer 9-inch 3-0 suture can be used to wrap around to complete the anterior outer layer taking seromuscular bites.

For a BPD-DS procedure, the BP limb is then divided from the alimentary limb with a 60 mm white load via Arm #1 or #3. Upper endoscopy is performed, and a leak test is completed with the anastomosis submerged in water and the alimentary limb clamped.

Attention is then turned to the creation of the ileo-ileostomy. The alimentary limb is then run distally to the previously marked division for the common channel, which is divided with an additional white staple load. Enterotomies are then made with hot scissors in Arm #3 at the antimesenteric portions of the bowel for the creation of a fully stapled ileo-ileostomy, usually fired most comfortably via Arm #3 with white loads for the anastomosis and common enterotomy. Alternatively, the common enterotomy can be hand-sewn in two layers with an absorbable suture.

The resulting mesenteric defects between the alimentary limb and the transverse mesocolon and at the ileo-ileostomy are closed with permanent suture.

## SADI-S

The operative technique for the duodenal dissection for a SADI-S procedure is the same as described for BPD-DS. The major difference is that only one anastomosis (the duodeno-ileostomy) is fashioned and in a loop configuration. The typical length for the common channel is 300 cm, again counted from the terminal ileum proximally. There will be only one resulting mesenteric defect to be closed.

## Outcomes

When compared to other bariatric procedures the BPD-DS and SADI-S result in superior weight loss and improvement of metabolic disease. Randomized control trials have demonstrated this effect up to 15 years following BPD-DS versus RYGB. Nutritional deficiencies such as fat-soluble vitamin deficiency, hypoalbuminemia and anemia are more common after these procedures [9]. The introduction of the Xi system has made these complex anastomotic procedures more accessible to bariatric surgeons who may not have previously performed BPD-DS or SADI-S. A series of 179 one-stage robotically assisted BPD-DS performed between 2007 and 2013 demonstrated the overall feasibility of the procedure, with all cases successfully completed, without major intraoperative complications. Medial length of stay was 2.7 days. In this series, there was no BBD-DS-related mortality up to 36 months following the procedure [22]. The learning curve of the BPD-DS may be longer than with other more commonly performed bariatric surgeries. In a retrospective review, out of a single institution, surgeons who had performed at least 50 cases had improved outcomes in regard to operative time, length of stay and leak rate. This 2023 review also highlighted a global complication rate of 7.9%, which is significantly less than previously reported rates of 15.3% in a 2020 cohort study. As with all newer procedures on evolving technology, outcomes improve over time [23].

## Revisional Bariatric Surgery

Due to an ever-increasing number of bariatric procedures performed and the length of follow-up, the number of patients who need revisional surgery is climbing. The first step for patients being evaluated for revisional surgery is to perform a detailed history and physical examination. It is important to obtain the operative reports from previous operations to better understand the surgical technique used in the initial surgery. One should also investigate the patient's dietary habits, percentage of initial weight loss and subsequent weight regain, and symptoms such as dysphagia, GERD, food regurgitation and postprandial abdominal pain. An upper gastrointestinal endoscopy and barium swallow are initial tests that clarify surgical anatomy and diagnosis of some of the above conditions.

Revisional bariatric surgery accounts for up to 25% of bariatric procedures in the modern era and has increased 311% since 2011 [3]. The rate of revisional surgery varies with the index bariatric procedure. It could be as high as 40% after adjustable gastric band (AGB), 10–20% after RYGB, and 5.5% after SG [24]. There are two overarching reasons for revisional bariatric surgery: (1) complications after primary bariatric surgery, not including immediate postoperative complications, and (2) patients who have insufficient weight loss or weight regain after primary bariatric surgery.

Revisional bariatric procedures can also be classified as;

- Conversion: Procedures that change from an index procedure to a different type of procedure.

- Corrective: Procedures addressing complications or incomplete treatment effects of a previous bariatric operation.
- Reversal: Procedures that restore original anatomy.

Like primary cases, the utilization of robotics for revisional cases has increased over time, a 3.7-fold increase from 2015 to 2020 [6]. Thorough pre-operative evaluation to define anatomy is crucial before any procedure and should include imaging studies such as an upper GI series and endoscopy. Understanding anatomic abnormalities, such as narrowing or dilation of a sleeve and gastro-gastric fistula or stomal stenosis in a bypass, allows for a more streamlined setup and follow-through of procedures. Of course, one must be diligent during any dissection and adapt to unexpected findings. The robotic platform again offers an advantage in these often-difficult cases given increased visual acuity, suturing ability and, particularly in the case of revisional surgery, utilization of the immunofluorescence to evaluate for perfusion of tissue.

## Patient Selection

The first step for patients being evaluated for revisional surgery is to perform a detailed history and physical examination. It is important to obtain the operative reports from previous operations to better understand the surgical technique used in the initial surgery. One should also investigate the patient's dietary habits, percentage of initial weight loss and subsequent weight regain, and symptoms such as dysphagia, GERD, food regurgitation and postprandial abdominal pain. These symptoms could be signs of anatomical issues such as stenosis at the anastomosis, hiatal hernia, marginal ulcer, pouch dilation, gastro-gastric fistula in patients with a history of gastric bypass or inadequate removal of gastric fundus in initial sleeve gastrectomy.

An upper gastrointestinal endoscopy and barium swallow are initial tests that clarify surgical anatomy and diagnosis of some of the above conditions. The endoscopy can detect sequel of GERD such as esophagitis, stricture and Barrett's esophagus, hiatal hernia, marginal ulcer or anastomotic stenosis, bleeding, and gastro-gastric fistula. A barium swallow is a complementary study to better understand the altered surgical anatomy. It can also delineate anatomical and functional stenosis, obstruction or fistula. If a patient has dysphagia without obvious mechanical reasons, esophageal manometry or gastric emptying study can be beneficial to rule out functional issues.

Reviewing the operative report(s) from previous surgeries is always valuable in understanding the surgical technique used in the primary operation. For example, in the case of RYGB, it is useful to know how the bypass was reconstructed (retrocolic vs antecolic, etc.) or whether the mesenteric defects were closed. In the case of a sleeve gastrectomy, it is important to know what size bougie was used to construct the sleeve and whether a hiatal hernia was identified and repaired. This will allow the surgeon to appropriately prepare preoperatively.

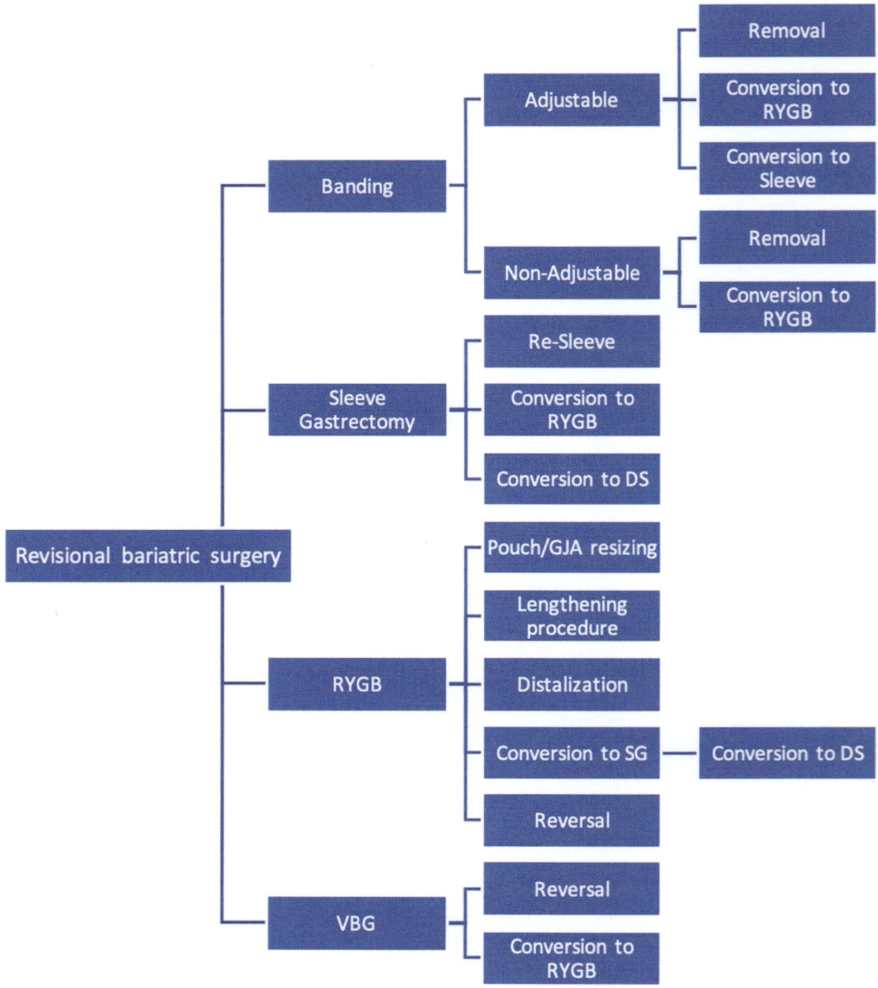


**Fig. 46.15** Revisional Surgery Decision Tree. Revisional bariatric surgery is highly dependent on primary procedure type, anatomy and symptoms

Figure 46.15 demonstrates the various options for revisions after primary bariatric surgery. Anatomy and symptoms will guide decision making and intraoperative findings may also alter the initial plans. It is important to include and discuss all possible portions of the procedure, as well as their complications, during the consent process.

## Setup

Four robotic trocars, a liver retractor and an assist port are utilized in revisional cases. Setup and port placement for revisional cases are generally similar to the setup for RYGB. It is recommended to use an assistant port for easy access to bedside suctioning and insertion and removal of sponges/sutures.

## Technique

Entry to the abdomen may depend on prior surgery. If history of open surgery, the entry to the abdominal cavity will migrate to the left upper quadrant, right upper quadrant or sometimes periumbilical using a Hassan technique.

One of the most challenging aspects of revisional bariatric surgery is adhesiolysis. Previous open surgery lends itself toward midline adhesions. Some degree of adhesions are almost always present between the liver and stomach. Other common areas for adhesions are at the angle of His and retrogastric to the pancreas. Adhesiolysis can be started laparoscopically to create space for the insertion of the robotic trocars. However, we endeavor to dock the robot as early as possible to facilitate the adhesiolysis and shorten operative time. Sometimes this can represent starting with two working arms.

Adhesiolysis then continues with monopolar scissors in Arm #3 and a fenestrated bipolar in Arm #1. The main advantages of the robotic system are self-assisting, better exposure/visualization of structures and the articulated energy device. These benefits may decrease the incidence of iatrogenic perforation and bleeding.

The procedure is highly dependent upon prior anatomy and intended revision. Intraoperative EGD can be used to further delineate anatomy, such as the location of the gastroesophageal junction. It is also important to be cognizant of previous staple lines, suture materials, clips, and silastic/mesh banding which could cause staplers to jam, misfire and damage tissue. Irrespective of the index procedure, it is critical to identify and preserve the left gastric artery. Intravenous administration of indocyanine green can facilitate the identification of the vascular supply.

Common revisional procedures include SG to RYGB, AGB to SG or RYGB, SG to BPD-DS or SADI-S and RYGB revision including pouch reduction or distalization.

Examples of specific revisional procedures:

- AGB: Excision of the peri-gastric capsule created by the band is essential to prevent staple misfiring (Fig. 46.16). Common conversion procedures post LAGB removal are SG and RYGB. Usual stapler reloads for either RYGB or sleeve conversion are blue, green or black depending on tissue thickness.
- SG: Conversion to RYGB; Adhesiolysis is performed from the antrum of the stomach progressing in a cephalad direction until the angle of His. If a neofundus is present it should be completely freed and excised during the creation of the gastric pouch. The usual stapler reloads for pouch creation are either blue or green. Care must be taken to identify clips on the staple line from the index procedure. In patients with chronic sleeve fistulas, conversion to esophagojejunostomy must be considered (Fig. 46.17).

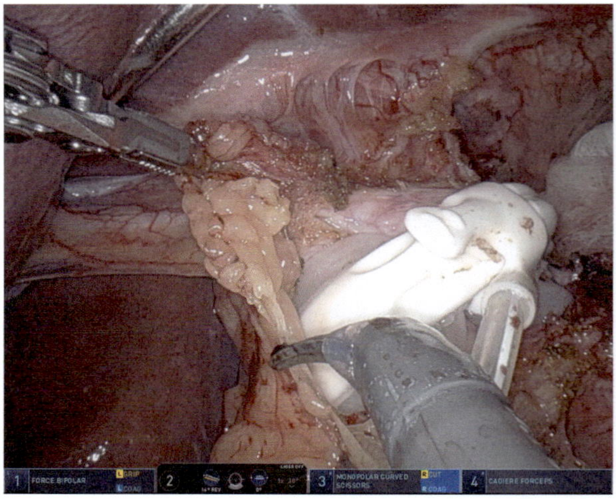


**Fig. 46.16** Removal of Adjustable Gastric Band. Takedown of plication sutures and capsulotomy important steps in removal of AGB

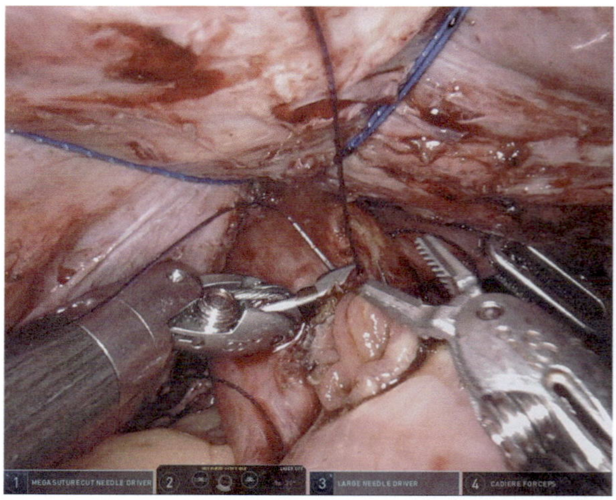


**Fig. 46.17** Hand Sewn Esophagojejunostomy. In the setting of severe sleeve complications, conversion to esophagojejunostomy is a save approach

- Vertical Banded Gastroplasty (VBG): Conversion to RYGB; the gastric pouch must be created proximal to the stoma and medial to the gastro-gastric staple line of the VBG. It is our practice to excise the fundus and most of the body of the stomach includes the previous staple line. For this purpose, the short gastric vessels are taken down with vessel sealer. Stapler reloads for the gastric resection are usually black or green.
- RYGB: It is crucial to delineate the anatomy of the RYGB at the beginning of the procedure. Revision may include pouch shortening with a re-creation of the gastrojejunal anastomosis. This often requires lysis of adhesions between the pouch and liver anteriorly and pouch and gastric remnant posteriorly. If the RYGB reconstruction was done retrocolic/retrogastric, further dissection may be necessary to be able to perform the reconstruction with no tension. Once the anasto-

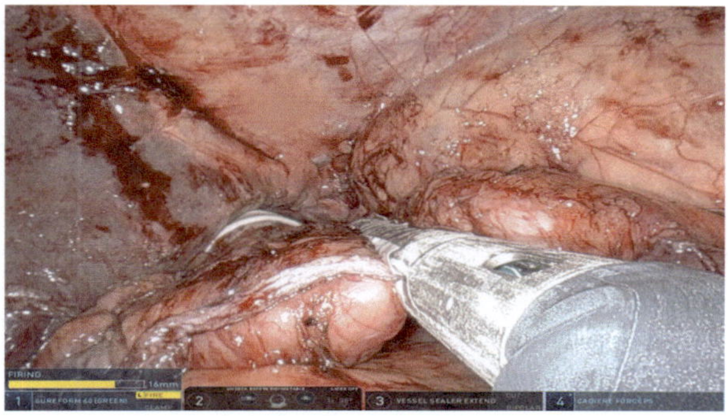

**Fig. 46.18** RYGB Pouch Revision. Recreation of gastric pouch after resection of prior anastomosis, including distal pouch and proximal alimentary limb

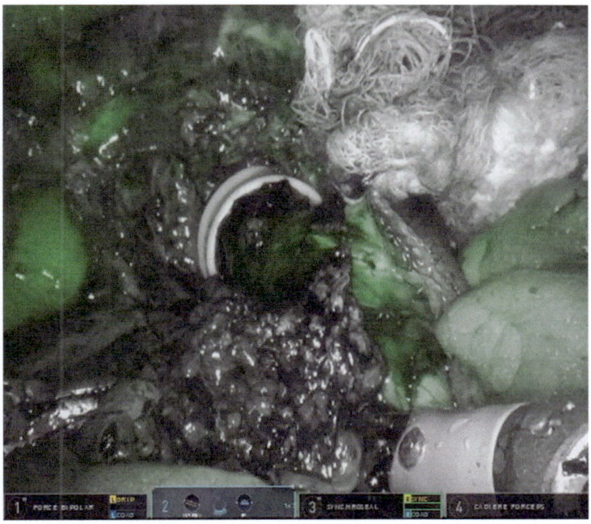

**Fig. 46.19** Indocyanine Green Evaluation of Pouch. Perfusion of the gastric pouch can be evaluated using intravenously administered indocyanine green. An esophagojejunostomy should again be considered if there is evidence of poor blood supply to avoid leaks and strictures

mosis is freed, the gastric pouch is transected proximal to the anastomosis with a linear stapler. The proximal jejunum is also transected along with its mesentery. The pouch can be revised to reduce complications of a wide pouch, such as in the setting of marginal ulcer (Fig. 46.18). If concern for vascular supply, indocyanine green can be administered intravenously and perfusion evaluated (Fig. 46.19). The anastomosis must then be refashioned. Distalization procedures may be performed in conjunction with pouch revision, and most commonly involve shortening the common channel and increasing the biliopancreatic limb length to decrease the total alimentary length.

## Outcomes

Revisional surgery may be technically challenging, and the introduction of robotics has helped make these procedures more technically feasible via minimally invasive techniques. [25] Rates of complication for revisional surgery are generally higher than for primary procedures, and the types of procedures included in individual studies should be scrutinized when trying to generalize outcomes. AGB is converted to a different procedure most often for insufficient weight loss, and reflux is the main cause of patients who have undergone SG. Early reviews demonstrated significant weight loss after revisional surgery, with mean BMI decreasing from 44.8 to 29 kg/m$^2$ after 3 years in a series of 99 robotic revisional procedures. In this group, 17% of patients experienced minor complications, but none experienced significant postoperative bleed or leak [18].

Overall, data strongly in favor of the robotic over laparoscopic approach has been mixed. In a large systematic review and met-analysis comparing robotic to laparoscopic outcomes in revisional bariatric surgery that included large numbers of patients in both groups, no difference was found between the groups when comparing length of stay. However, the robotic group was noted to have higher conversion rates to open, reoperation, and readmission [26]. In a review of outcomes from the MBSAQIP database, there was no difference in postoperative complications between robotic and laparoscopic revision cases; however, robotic cases were associated with longer operative times and slightly increased lengths of stays [27]. One argument against the use of robots for revisional cases is their increased associated operative time, however, these cases have higher proportions of technically complex procedures which can account for increased times.

## Challenges to Robotic Bariatric Surgery

### Accessibility

Access to any developing technology may have multiple barriers preventing its more widespread application. Some of the barriers that have been described pertaining to robotic-assisted surgery include the upfront cost of equipment and long-term economic viability, variable outcomes-based evidence, relationships between clinicians and managerial staff, and personal views on the usefulness of the platform in the future [28]. Building a successful robotic program goes far beyond the surgeon to involve all aspects of perioperative care such as instrument management, industry representatives, operating room nurses and techs and trainees. Upfront and maintenance costs are heavily scrutinized by administrators. Many existing operating rooms may not be able to physically store and efficiently deploy the various components of the robot, limiting its use. Hospitals and surgery centers may also have providers "competing" for robot time if there is a mismatch between availability and providers across multiple specialties, including urologists, gynecologists, and colorectal surgeons, who utilize robotic-assisted surgery. This particular point could represent a real challenge for busy and proficient laparoscopic bariatric surgeons.

Recent technological advancements have rapidly progressed, and the global medical robotics market continues to grow annually improving access to the robot is growing both in the United States and internationally [29]. As the technology continues to be more widely accepted and implemented, early investments can help drive productivity and attract those with new skill sets to help promote growth.

## Cost

The cost-benefit ratio of robotic-assisted surgery remains one of the largest considerations in the field. While robotic surgery offers numerous benefits, it also comes with higher operational costs, including the initial investment in the robotic system, maintenance expenses, and the cost of disposable instruments. It is important to take total costs into account, such as length of stay and price of reintervention, when comparing different approaches. Differences between cost effectiveness between procedures also exist, such as studies that have demonstrated less cost benefit of the robotic approach specifically for SG when taking rare but serious complications into consideration [30]. Using technology to improve efficiency to cut down on operative time mitigates cost. In a 2024 review of costs over time for robotic bariatric surgery, the total cost for the robotic approach was 1.5 times higher compared to laparoscopy for both RYGB and SG. However, trends over time demonstrated a decrease in total and operative costs in robotic surgery at a higher rate than laparoscopic costs [31]. As with improving efficiency and outcomes over time, costs can be expected to continue to improve and allow for greater implementation of robotic-assisted surgery.

## Conclusion

Robotic-Assisted Bariatric Surgery is a dynamic and rapidly advancing field, with the potential to offer the advantages of minimally invasive surgery to a larger number of patients. As the technology continues to evolve and become more accessible, it holds the potential to become a mainstay in bariatric surgery, offering improved outcomes for patients with obesity.

## References

1. World Health Organization. Obesity and overweight. 2021 [cited 2024 02/29/2026]. https://www.who.int/news-room/fact-sheets/detail/obesity-and-overweight.
2. CDC. Adult obesity facts. 2022 [cited 2024 29-2-2024]. https://www.cdc.gov/obesity/data/adult.html.
3. English WJ, et al. American Society for Metabolic and Bariatric Surgery estimation of metabolic and bariatric procedures performed in the United States in 2016. Surg Obes Relat Dis. 2018;14(3):259–63.
4. Cadiere GB, et al. The world's first obesity surgery performed by a surgeon at a distance. Obes Surg. 1999;9(2):206–9.

5. Horgan S, Vanuno D. Robots in laparoscopic surgery. J Laparoendosc Adv Surg Tech A. 2001;11(6):415–9.
6. Bauerle WB, et al. Current trends in the utilization of a robotic approach in the field of bariatric surgery. Obes Surg. 2023;33(2):482–91.
7. Dimou FM, et al. Understanding the current role of robotic-assisted bariatric surgery. Obes Surg. 2021;31(7):3130–7.
8. Iranmanesh P, et al. Robotic primary and revisional bariatric surgery. Surg Clin North Am. 2020;100(2):417–30.
9. Moller SG, et al. Laparoscopic versus robotic-assisted suturing performance among novice surgeons: a blinded, cross-over study. Surg Laparosc Endosc Percutan Tech. 2020;30(2):117–22.
10. Niclauss N, et al. A comparison of the da Vinci Xi vs. the da Vinci Si Surgical System for Roux-En-Y gastric bypass. Langenbecks Arch Surg. 2019;404(5):615–20.
11. ASMBS. Estimate of Bariatric Surgery Numbers, 2011–2022. 2022 [cited 2024. https://asmbs.org/resources/estimate-of-bariatric-surgery-numbers/.
12. Giudicelli G, et al. Global benchmarks in primary robotic bariatric surgery redefine quality standards for Roux-en-Y gastric bypass and sleeve gastrectomy. Br J Surg. 2024;111(1):znad374.
13. Kalmar CL, et al. Intraluminal indocyanine green for intraoperative staple line leak testing in bariatric surgery. Surg Endosc. 2020;34(9):4194–9.
14. Bennett WC, et al. Comparison of robot-assisted sleeve gastrectomy outcomes in multiple staple line treatment modalities from 2015 to 2019: a 5-year propensity score-adjusted MBSAQIP® analysis. Surg Endosc. 2023;37(2):1401–11.
15. Nasser H, et al. Comparative analysis of robotic versus laparoscopic revisional bariatric surgery: perioperative outcomes from the MBSAQIP database. Surg Obes Relat Dis. 2020;16(3):397–405.
16. Doumouras AG, et al. Mastery in bariatric surgery: the long-term surgeon learning curve of Roux-en-Y gastric bypass. Ann Surg. 2018;267(3):489–94.
17. Wang L, et al. Robotic versus laparoscopic Roux-en-Y gastric bypass for morbid obesity: a systematic review and meta-analysis. Obes Surg. 2018;28(11):3691–700.
18. Snyder B, et al. Robotically assisted revision of bariatric surgeries is safe and effective to achieve further weight loss. World J Surg. 2013;37(11):2569–73.
19. Tieu K, et al. Robotic-assisted Roux-en-Y gastric bypass: update from 2 high-volume centers. Surg Obes Relat Dis. 2013;9(2):284–8.
20. Aeschbacher P, et al. Laparoscopic versus robotic-assisted primary bariatric-metabolic surgery. are we still expecting to overcome the learning curve? A propensity score-matched analysis of the MBSAQIP database. Surg Obes Relat Dis. 2024;20(9):831–9.
21. Clapp B, et al. American Society for Metabolic and Bariatric Surgery 2022 estimate of metabolic and bariatric procedures performed in the United States. Surg Obes Relat Dis. 2024;20(5):425–31.
22. Antanavicius G, Rezvani M, Sucandy I. One-stage robotically assisted laparoscopic biliopancreatic diversion with duodenal switch: analysis of 179 patients. Surg Obes Relat Dis. 2015;11(2):367–71.
23. Teixeira A, et al. Analysis of the impact of the learning curve on the safety outcome of the totally robotic-assisted biliopancreatic diversion with duodenal switch: a single-institution observational study. Obes Surg. 2023;33(9):2742–8.
24. Park JY, Song D, Kim YJ. Causes and outcomes of revisional bariatric surgery: initial experience at a single center. Ann Surg Treat Res. 2014;86(6):295–301.
25. Vanetta C, et al. Current status of robot-assisted revisional bariatric surgery. J Clin Med. 2022;11(7):1820.
26. Ataya K, et al. Robotic versus laparoscopic revisional bariatric surgeries: a systematic review and meta-analysis. J Minim Invasive Surg. 2023;26(4):198–207.
27. Clapp B, et al. Comparison of robotic revisional weight loss surgery and laparoscopic revisional weight loss surgery using the MBSAQIP database. Surg Obes Relat Dis. 2019;15(6):909–19.
28. Lawrie L, et al. Barriers and enablers to the effective implementation of robotic assisted surgery. PLoS One. 2022;17(8):e0273696.

29. Surgical Robotics Market By Component (Systems, Accessories, Services); By surgery type: gynecology surgery, urology surgery, neurosurgery, orthopedic surgery, general surgery, other surgeries. Surgical Robotics Market. 2023 [cited 2024. https://www.precedenceresearch.com/surgical-robotics-market#:~:text=The%20global%20surgical%20robotics%20market,forecast%20period%202023%20to%202032.
30. Acevedo E, et al. Outcomes in conventional laparoscopic versus robotic-assisted revisional bariatric surgery: a retrospective, case-controlled study of the MBSAQIP database. Surg Endosc. 2020;34(4):1573–84.
31. Read MD, et al. The downtrending cost of robotic bariatric surgery: a cost analysis of 47,788 bariatric patients. J Robot Surg. 2024;18(1):63.

# Bariatric Emergencies for the General Surgeon

# 47

Oliver Knoell and Pearl Ma

## Introduction to Bariatric Surgery

Obesity is a widespread global disease. According to the World Health Organization, over 1 billion people worldwide suffer from obesity [1]. Bariatric and metabolic surgeries provide the most effective treatment for significant and sustained weight loss as well as significant reduction or even resolution of obesity-related diseases [2].

According to the International Federation for the Surgery of Obesity and Metabolic Disorders (IFSO) eighth global registry report for 2023, 480,970 bariatric operations were performed worldwide [3]. In 2022, the American Society for Metabolic and Bariatric Surgery (ASMBS) reported that over 280,000 bariatric and metabolic operations were performed in the United States [4]. The most commonly performed primary metabolic and bariatric surgery (MBS) operations are the sleeve gastrectomy (SG) (57.4%), Roux-en-Y gastric bypass (RYGB) (22.2%) and biliopancreatico-duodenal switch (BPD/DS) (2.2%) with significant decline in adjustable band placement (AGB) at 0.9%. Recently, the ASMBS has endorsed newer operations such as the one anastomosis gastric bypass (OAGB) and the intragastric balloon with a rise in revisional MBS operations for weight recurrence or complications of the primary operation. Overall complication rates of bariatric surgery remain low, estimated at 4% across all operations with 0.1% mortality [5]. Complication rates compare similarly to other common operations such as appendectomy, cholecystectomy, and knee arthroplasty [4, 6].

With the wide variety of operations and particular anatomical modifications of each operation, healthcare professionals caring for a post-MBS patient may need to be more familiar with the potential short- and long-term complications that may

O. Knoell · P. Ma (✉)
Fresno Heart and Surgical Hospital/Community Health Partners, Fresno, CA, USA

University of California-San Francisco-Fresno Medical Education Program, Fresno, CA, USA



O. M. Ghanem et al. (eds.), *The SAGES Manual of Metabolic and Bariatric Surgery*, https://doi.org/10.1007/978-3-031-72309-4_47

arise. These complications may not necessarily be a direct complication of the operation itself. However, the anatomical changes may challenge general surgeons for intraoperative and postoperative management for non-bariatric-related surgeries. For example, an endoscopic retrograde cholangiopancreatography (ERCP) for choledocholithiasis may require transgastric access to the remnant stomach in an RYGB patient. Ideally, MBS patients with bariatric emergencies are managed by their primary operating surgeon or an experienced bariatric surgeon. However, in reality, patients often present to their local hospital and require management by the general surgeon, who may be unable to transfer the patient to a bariatric center due to limited bed capacities or acuity of the patient's clinical status. A recent survey of Canadian general surgeons taking acute care surgery call found that 25% of the polled surgeons were uncomfortable managing post-MBS complications despite most stating that management of MBS complications should be within the general surgeons' scope of practice [7].

With the growing number and types of MBS operations, including increased medical tourism operations, the general surgeon will most likely be called upon to deal with a bariatric surgery emergency at some time in their career. This chapter will highlight common early and late postoperative complications after most frequently performed MBS operations and serve as a reference for the general surgeon. Other parts of this textbook find more detailed descriptions of the individual MBS complications.

## Postoperative Complications

### Roux-en-Y Gastric Bypass (RYGB): Bleeding

Rates of bleeding in patients undergoing RYGB in a review of a prospectively maintained database of 4466 patients over ten years were reported at 0.94%. The sources of bleeding in RYGB can commonly occur at either the gastrojejunostomy or jejunojejunostomy, either within the bowel lumen or extraluminal at the staple line. Additionally, bleeding may originate from adjacent organs, including the liver or spleen and the mesentery of the small bowel or transverse colon [8]. Patients would present with signs of gastrointestinal bleeding, including melena or hematochezia. Depending on the patient's clinical stability, most patients can be managed conservatively with or without blood transfusions, cessation of anticoagulation medications, and intravenous fluid resuscitation. Early postoperative bleeding was clinically diagnosed at one center from 19 to 38 hours postoperatively, and 93% of the cases were managed conservatively [9].

Endoscopic control of intraluminal bleeds is an option for gastrojejunostomy anastomotic bleeds. However, endoscopic evaluation of the jejunojejunostomy or remnant stomach may be complex, given that the roux limb length is generally around 100 cm or more and a biliopancreatic limb 50 cm or more. Blood clot bezoars can obstruct the jejunojejunostomy and may require decompression, surgically or endoscopically. Endoscopic evaluation of the jejunojejunostomy may be performed intraoperatively by an experienced endoscopist if surgical exploration is warranted. Care should be taken to avoid disruption of the healing gastrojejunal anastomosis. Remnant stomach bleeding is most likely due to staple line bleeding and, therefore, requires oversewing the staple line with absorbable sutures.

## Bleeding After Sleeve Gastrectomy

Bleeding in the postoperative bariatric patient, while relatively rare, can incur significant morbidity or even mortality if not recognized and treated promptly. Bleeding is the most common major complication after SG. A recent survey of the MBSAQIP data analyzed over 175,000 SG procedures, in which the reported rate of bleeding after SG was 0.6%, though rates vary in the literature. Bleeding after SG can commonly occur from the staple line either intraluminally or intraabdominally. The most feared source of bleeding in a patient who has recently undergone SG is unrecognized bleeding from the short gastric pedicle or spleen, which can result in significant and life-threatening hemorrhage. Treatment options include laparoscopic oversewing of the staple line, intraabdominal hematoma evacuation, and drain placement with endoscopic evaluation. If bleeding cannot be controlled laparoscopically, then an open approach should be taken to rescue the patient with life-threatening hemorrhage.

## RYGB Gastrointestinal Leaks

Gastrointestinal leaks after bariatric surgery can challenge the surgical provider in diagnosis and management. The care of these patients often benefits from a multidisciplinary team with subspecialty training and familiarity with managing these complications. Early bariatric surgery consultation or transfer to tertiary bariatric centers should be pursued when the patient's physiologic parameters allow. However, surgical intervention should not be delayed in hemodynamically unstable patients.

The incidence of leaks after RYGB is reported at about 1% [10]. Leaks may occur within the first week of surgery. However, most leaks will be detected after hospital discharge [11]. Sustained tachycardia >120 bpm, shortness of breath, left-sided pleural effusion, abdominal pain, oral intolerance, and fevers may be presenting symptoms. A high degree of suspicion in any patient displaying these symptoms within 30 days of bariatric surgery is warranted. Evaluation of a patient with a suspected leak should begin with a thorough diagnostic evaluation with labs and a clinical exam of the patient. Radiographic investigation is best evaluated with a computed tomography (CT) scan of the abdomen and pelvis with and without contrast. Oral water-soluble contrast, not barium sulfate, should be administered when suspecting a gastrointestinal leak, as chemical peritonitis can occur [12].

Upper gastrointestinal (UGI) series may also be considered; however, a recent meta-analysis indicated that CT may be more sensitive and specific in detecting gastrointestinal leaks in patients with high clinical suspicion [13]. The gastrointestinal and jejunostomy anastomosis should be evaluated in any series. Leaks at the remnant stomach are difficult to radiologically assess. Therefore, supportive care with IV fluid resuscitation, early initiation of broad-spectrum antibiotics, and source control of sepsis/shock should be initiated promptly. The surgeon should have a low threshold for operative exploration in a patient suspected of gastrointestinal leak after bariatric surgery. Laparoscopic exploration is safe in experienced hands, and negative exploration should be commended as a safe surgical practice rather than punitive quality measures [14]. In an infected postoperative field, we recommend adherence to principles of infection control with drain placement followed by prompt transfer to a tertiary center. Consideration should also be given to placement of a remnant feeding gastrostomy if feasible in the event that prolonged bowel rest is anticipated.

## SG Leak

SG leak rates are around 1.5% [15]. Leaks after SG compared to RYGB can be more severe and are treated with different considerations. Due to the presence of both the pylorus and the lower esophageal sphincter, the sleeve leak is a high-pressure system. Further, many sleeve leaks result from functional gastric outlet obstruction due to narrowing at the incisura angularis, twisting, or kinking. While gastrojejunostomy leak after RYGB might be adequately managed with Graham patch and drainage, this is unlikely to be successful in a leak after SG. Timing of leak after SG will dictate management steps. Source control with drainage is the first line of management. Parenteral nutrition will likely be necessary as well. Additional treatment modalities may be considered in the tertiary center setting. Endoscopic stenting with either laparoscopically or radiographically placed external drainage has been described as an option for the treatment of these patients. In some cases, prolonged leaks from SG may require subtotal or total gastrectomy with conversion to Roux-en-Y with either gastrojejunostomy or esophagojejunostomy. Consultation with an advanced gastroenterologist and bariatric surgeon is advised.

## Wound Infections

Wound infection is the second most common 30-day complication after bariatric surgery, according to a review of MBSAQIP data, with a rate of 0.5% [16]. Laparoscopic techniques have significantly reduced wound infections compared to the open era of bariatric surgery [17]. Signs of wound infection are similar to those of any other abdominal surgery, including erythema, warmth, drainage, fever, and fluctuance. Treatment includes drainage and initiation of antibiotics when cellulitis or immunocompromised state are present. Intraabdominal infection or abscess should raise the concern for staple line or anastomotic leak and be investigated further.

## Gastrointestinal Obstruction

The presentation of gastrointestinal obstruction in a patient who has had prior metabolic and bariatric surgery can be highly variable depending on the type of operation as well as the surgical techniques used. Operations such as the adjustable gastric band and sleeve gastrectomy do not alter the anatomy of the small bowel or its mesentery. However, gastric obstruction can still occur with these operations and should be considered. If the fluid reservoir of the gastric band is filled excessively, the stomach can become obstructed. Over time, dense scar tissue can form surrounding the band near the hiatus and develop a stricture of the proximal stomach. The first step in managing these patients should involve emptying the fluid via the subcutaneous port using a Huber needle, often relieving symptoms. Eventually, band removal may be indicated if recurrent gastric obstruction occurs or symptoms persist despite complete emptying of the band of fluid. Sleeve gastrectomy can also be susceptible to gastric obstruction. Although this is a rare event, it will usually occur at the incisura angularis when the stomach is divided too close to the lesser curve of the stomach. Functional obstruction can also occur with twisting or kinking of the stomach due to staple line creation. Management of gastric stricture after sleeve gastrectomy has multiple options depending on the time of surgery and available resources. Endoscopic dilation can be an option [18]. Seromyotomy is also a technique described to manage this challenging problem [19]. Conversion to a Roux-en-Y gastric bypass may be necessary if the sleeve cannot be salvaged [18, 20]. If nasogastric decompression is warranted, we recommend that this is never placed blindly in the recent postoperative setting, to avoid iatrogenic gastric perforation at the staple line. Endoscopic nasogastric decompression may be considered.

Anastomotic bariatric operations are susceptible to internal hernia, closed-loop obstruction, and intussusception. Although the mesenteric spaces are now routinely closed with permanent sutures, this was not always standard practice. In RYGB and DS, the enteroenterostomy mesenteric spaces can serve as a source of internal hernia. In the RYGB, an additional mesenteric defect is created when the roux limb is brought to the pouch to create the gastrojejunostomy. In the antecolic technique, the roux limb mesentery and the transverse colon create a significant potential space (Petersen's space) that can turn into an internal hernia if it is not closed (Fig. 47.1).

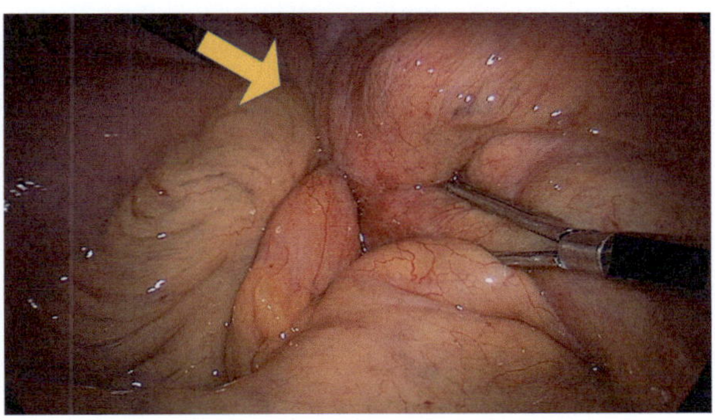

**Fig. 47.1** Demonstrated above is an internal hernia at the Petersen's space in a patient who had undergone antecolic antegastric laparoscopic Roux-en-Y gastric bypass 7 days prior. The arrow indicates common channel herniation through an incompletely closed Petersen's space

The retrocolic RYGB delivers the roux limb into the lesser sac via an opening created in the thin part of the transverse mesocolon. This space can serve as a source of potential internal hernia if not effectively closed. During the reduction of an internal hernia, running the bowel retrograde from the ileocecal valve will assist in reducing the hernia. Permanent sutures are used to close the open mesenteric defects. If there is a concern for prolonged postoperative ileus, a gastrostomy tube is placed in the remnant stomach for decompression.

As with all operations, adhesive bowel disease can occur in any patient with prior bariatric surgery. Though minimally invasive techniques decrease the burden of adhesive disease, this does not eliminate the possibility of adhesive small bowel obstruction. The approach to bowel obstruction in the bariatric patient may differ significantly from that of the non-bariatric patient. In patients who have undergone an RYGB, the small gastric pouch is approximately 10–30 ml in volume, and therefore, nasogastric decompression of the pouch and roux limb may not provide significant symptom relief or decompression. Additionally, it does not address the biliopancreatic limb. In the event of complete obstruction of the biliopancreatic limb managed with nasogastric decompression, perforation of the gastric remnant due to overdistension is a dreaded complication that can occur [21]. The surgeon's approach to managing bowel obstruction in bariatric patients should err on the side of surgical exploration rather than non-operative management.

Intussusception after RYGB may occur most commonly at the jejunojejunostomy, with telescoping of the bowel immediately involving the anastomosis. Diagnosis can be challenging, as symptoms mimic many other gastrointestinal complications after gastric bypass. Non-specific symptoms such as nausea, abdominal pain, vomiting, and diarrhea may be the only clinical signs. Imaging is frequently non-diagnostic, although a "target sign" may be captured on cross-sectional imaging. A high degree of suspicion and a low threshold for diagnostic laparoscopy may be necessary to confirm intussusception [22]. Even in the event of radiographic confirmation, intussusception is frequently transient and may not be present during surgical exploration. If there is concern for bowel compromise or ischemia, then prompt surgical exploration is warranted. As with all exploratory or diagnostic operations in bariatric patients, a complete survey of the relevant anatomy should be conducted, including inspection of all mesenteric defects and anastomoses. If the jejunojejunostomy is confirmed to be the source of obstruction, then reduction of the intussusception should be performed and small bowel examined. In the event of irreversible ischemia, complete resection of the jejunojejunostomy is necessary with complete revision of the anastomosis and anastomosis of the roux limb to prior common channel, then a second anastomosis of the biliopancreatic limb at least 10 cm distal to the prior anastomosis to create a new common channel, by either a hand-sewn or stapled technique [23]. Mesenteric defects should be closed with non-absorbable sutures.

## Nutritional and Metabolic Emergencies

Gastrointestinal anatomical restriction and alterations in enterohormonal signaling after surgery can lead to drastic reductions in calorie intake. Malabsorption contributes to the weight loss mechanism in operations with the added factor of intestinal bypass. Although these effects are the mechanism of action that makes bariatric operations the most effective treatment of obesity and related metabolic diseases, it is a double-edged sword. Gastrointestinal intolerance is common after bariatric surgery. Vomiting, loss of appetite, changes in bowel habits, and maladaptive eating habits can lead to malnutrition and vitamin deficiencies. In some cases, these can be severe and life-threatening.

Malnutrition has the potential to be most pronounced in patients who have undergone gastrointestinal bypass operations, particularly the biliopancreatic diversion with duodenal switch (BPD/DS) or distal gastric bypass. The modern BPD/DS involves a generously sized sleeve gastrectomy with a 250 cm roux limb anastomosed to the first portion of the duodenum and a 75–100 cm common channel with a long biliopancreatic limb. Scopinaro's original biliopancreatic diversion involved an even shorter common channel of 50 cm but created a gastrojejunostomy to a 300–500 cc proximal gastric pouch instead of a sleeved stomach with duodenoileostomy. Severe protein malnutrition may be a potential consequence of any bariatric operation but should be of particular concern in patients with gastrointestinal bypass. Patients may present with hair loss, fatigue, weakness, and temporal wasting. Significant hypoalbuminemia may be present. In severe cases in which oral protein-calorie supplementation is ineffective, treatment with nasoenteric or parenteral nutrition may be required. Gastrostomy placement and feeding are other considerations for patients with a remnant stomach. These patients should be monitored carefully in an inpatient setting for refeeding syndrome. Some patients may ultimately require reversing their bariatric operation or conversion to a less malabsorptive procedure once malnutrition is corrected.

Micronutrient deficiencies are numerous and can be related to deficiencies of fat-soluble vitamins A, D, E, and K, as well as water-soluble vitamins and trace elements such as calcium, copper, folate, magnesium, phosphorus, thiamin, vitamin B12, and Vitamin B6. Of these, deficiencies in thiamin, B12, and copper are of particular concern due to the potential for severe or even life-threatening neurological complications [24].

Vitamin B1, or thiamin deficiency, can present with peripheral motor and sensory deficits, cardiomyopathy, and heart failure. Wernicke encephalopathy may also be a clinical presentation of thiamin deficiency with symptoms of gait ataxia, nystagmus, ophthalmoplegia, and confusion. B1 deficiency can result in permanent neurologic impairment or even death and requires emergency treatment with thiamin supplementation. Importantly, avoid dextrose-containing fluids until thiamin is administered in a patient suspected of being deficient in thiamin to avoid precipitating Wernicke encephalopathy.

Vitamin B12 deficiency may result in post-gastrectomy or gastric bypass patients due to the inability of B12 to be freed from its protein-bound state due to low hydrochloric acid levels. Symptoms of B12 deficiency can include glossitis, leukopenia, macrocytic anemia, thrombocytopenia, paresthesia, and irreversible neuropathy. If unrecognized, B12 deficiency can result in progressive ascending polyneuropathy that can end with respiratory failure and death.

Copper deficiency is rare but can present with myelopathy. Replacement can be achieved with oral elemental copper supplementation. Zinc and iron may interfere with copper absorption [25].

## Marginal Ulcer

Marginal ulceration is an inflammatory ulcer on the jejunal side of a gastrojejunal anastomosis (Fig. 47.2a). The rate of marginal ulceration in RYGB patients varies widely in the literature; however, in a systematic review of 41 studies, the average rate of marginal ulcer was 4.6% [26]. Marginal ulcer typically presents several months to years after RYGB. Presenting symptoms may include upper abdominal pain, upper GI bleeding, nausea, early satiety/stenosis, or sepsis with perforation. Early marginal ulcers can occur, usually attributable to technical factors such as tension on the gastrojejunal anastomosis, compromised blood supply, or foreign body (such as permanent suture material, staples) involving the anastomosis. Most marginal ulcers present several months to years after RYGB. Risk factors typically include non-steroidal anti-inflammatory medication use, tobacco consumption/smoking, steroids, and *H. pylori* infection [27]. Larger gastric pouch volume has also been demonstrated to correlate to higher ulcer rates [26]. Surgical exploration should not be delayed in patients presenting with perforation, peritonitis, and sepsis. Ideal surgical management is still debated, but the principles of source control and limiting contamination apply. Broad-spectrum antibiotics and antifungals are the initial treatments. Laparoscopic omental patch repair and drain placement are the most commonly performed operations to treat perforated ulcers in the emergency setting (Fig. 47.2b) If there is a concern for the sturdiness of the patch or repair, a

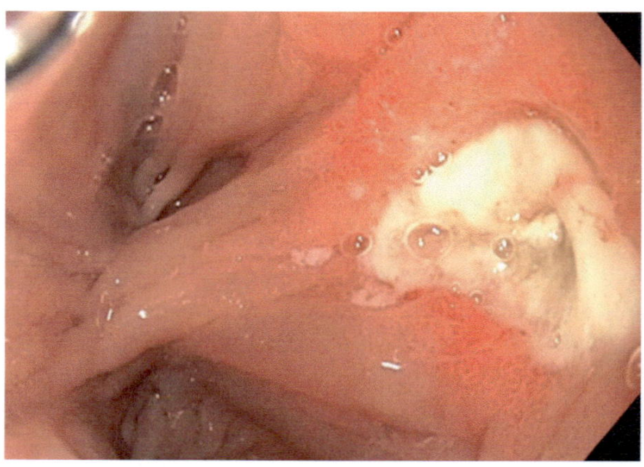

**Fig. 47.2a** Endoscopic image of a perforated marginal ulcer

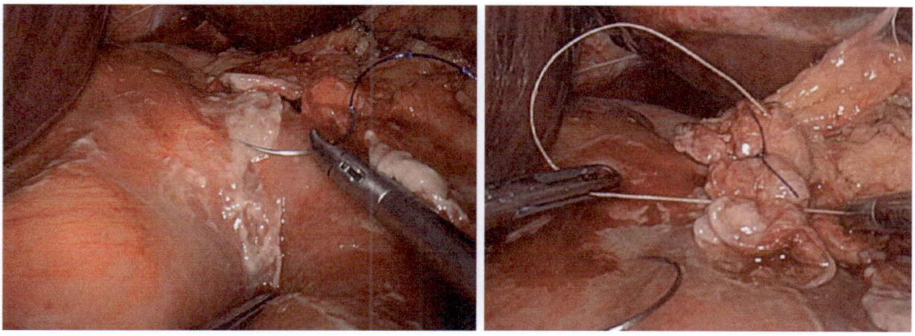

**Fig. 47.2b** Intraoperative image of a small perforated marginal ulcer before and after repair with graham patch

remnant gastrostomy tube may be placed for feeding. Endoscopy is often a helpful adjunct to delineate anatomy and test any repairs during surgical exploration. UGI series can be performed 3–5 days after repair to reassure the surgeon of a negative leak before starting clear liquids. Recent retrospective evidence has suggested that laparoscopic revision of gastrojejunostomy may result in a lower likelihood of ulcer recurrence compared to omental patch [28]. The surgeon should aim first and foremost to control sepsis, recognizing their own particular skillset and hospital resources.

## Pulmonary Embolism and Deep Venous Thrombosis (DVT)

Risk factors for venous thromboembolism include BMI > 50, venous stasis, pulmonary hypertension, prior venous thromboembolism (VTE), poor functional status, and prolonged operative times. The bariatric surgery patient frequently has at least one, if not several, risk factors. The rate of VTE has been estimated at around 1.1% in the postoperative bariatric patient population [29]. VTE is frequently diagnosed after hospital discharge, averaging 21 to 28 days from the time of presentation [30]. Multiple predictive scoring systems have been investigated in the bariatric patient population to attempt to select patients who may benefit from extended chemical DVT prophylaxis after bariatric surgery [31–33]. Deep vein thrombosis and pulmonary embolism should be considered in any patient within a month of bariatric surgery who presents with symptoms of dyspnea, tachycardia, hypoxia, or pleuritic chest pain. Prompt diagnosis and treatment with therapeutic anticoagulation are critical, as the risk of untreated thromboembolism is a higher cause of mortality than the risk of postoperative surgical bleeding [34].

## Portomesenteric Thrombosis

Portal or mesenteric vein thrombosis (PMVT) may occur after bariatric surgery, however, with a higher incidence after SG. Although overall incidence is rare, this can be a highly morbid or potentially fatal condition. The rate of PVT in the post-sleeve gastrectomy patient has varied in the literature from 0.3 to 0.4% [35, 36]. Acute portal vein thrombosis may be partial or complete. The presenting symptom is frequently epigastric pain. If the superior mesenteric vein is occluded, there may be additional symptoms of sharp, intermittent abdominal pain or loose stool [37]. In severe cases, bowel ischemia can occur due to venous outflow obstruction. Presentation generally occurs 10–20 days after surgery and diagnosis with IV contrasted cross-sectional imaging (Fig. 47.3). Treatment with anticoagulation is required. Anticoagulation in patients without complete occlusion for at minimum 3–6 months. When complete occlusion and bowel compromise are present, intervention with thrombectomy and thrombolysis are recommended [38]. Long-term effects of PVT include a cavernous transformation of the portal vein [39].

## Gallstone Disease After Bariatric Surgery

Rapid weight loss following bariatric surgery causes cholesterol concentration within the biliary tree, decreased gallbladder contraction due to decreased cholecystokinin secretion, and altered enterohepatic bile salt recycling [40]. Further, patients with obesity are at higher risk for gallstone formation. Concomitant

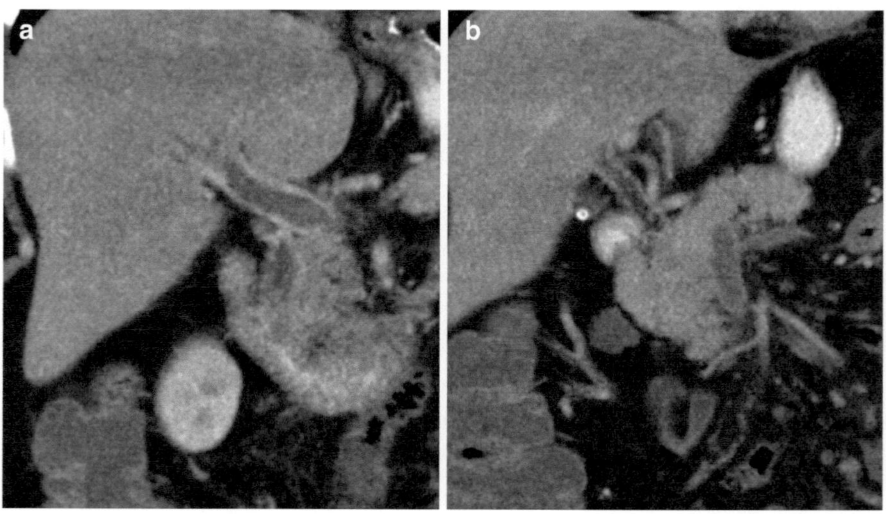


**Fig. 47.3** (**a**) Nearly-occlusive portal vein thrombus. (**b**) Nearly-occlusive mesenteric vein thrombus. These images were obtained from the same patient 30 days after they underwent laparoscopic sleeve gastrectomy. Presenting symptoms were generalized abdominal pain and poor oral intake. The patient was treated with apixaban and recovered well

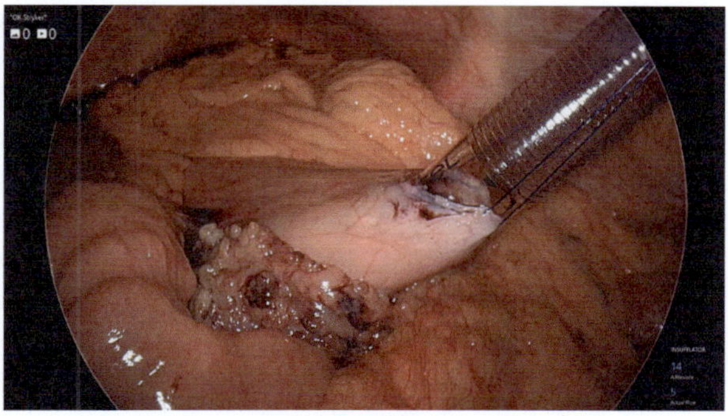

**Fig. 47.4** Laparoscopic placement of a 15-mm port into the remnant stomach allows endoscopic access to the duodenum for cholangiopancreatography and treatment of choledocholithiasis

cholecystectomy at the time of bariatric surgery has been a topic of debate among the bariatric surgery community. While concomitant cholecystectomy was previously standard, more recent trends suggest that a conservative approach is becoming more common [41]. Gallstone disease in patients with previous SG can be treated similarly to most other patients with gallstone disease. In the event of choledocholithiasis, the biliary tree is still easily accessed with standard ERCP if needed. In the RYGB patient with long roux and biliopancreatic limb lengths, oral endoscopic access to the biliary tree is not straightforward or always feasible. Simple cholelithiasis or acute cholecystitis in the RYGB patient may be managed similarly to non-bariatric cases. It is our practice to perform an intraoperative cholagiogram during cholecystectomy for any patient with intestinal bypass anatomy. The common bile duct stone management in a patient with RYGB anatomy requires coordination between the advanced endoscopy and surgical teams. In the event of common bile duct stones, laparoscopic-assisted transgastric ERCP may be necessary with laparoscopic placement of a 15 mm port into the remnant stomach (Fig. 47.4). The surgeon should attempt to provide the endoscopist enough distance from the pylorus and a suitable trajectory to allow easy navigation into the duodenum (see picture below). Advanced endoscopic techniques such as single or double balloon enteroscope-assisted ERCP and endoscopic ultrasound-directed transgastric ERCP (EDGE) have been described with advanced GI capabilities [42, 43].

In some cases, transhepatic access with the interventional radiologist may also be viable. Care of these patients requires knowledge of the resources and abilities of the multidisciplinary team within the healthcare system. Early referral to a tertiary center may be indicated when the necessary resources are unavailable at the presenting facility.

## Psychosocial and Behavioral Emergencies

Patients with obesity have a higher risk for depression, anxiety, eating disorders, and other mental health diseases compared to the general population [44]. While pre-operative screening and mental health evaluation are standard practice in most metabolic and bariatric surgery centers, these are chronic conditions that may persist after bariatric surgery. Some studies have even demonstrated an increased incidence of self-injurious behavior or suicide after bariatric surgery [45, 46]. Additionally, the incidence of alcohol use disorder (AUD) is increased in patients undergoing RYGB. Rates of AUD are similar in RYGB and SG patients [47].

Interestingly, a higher incidence of AUD in RYGB patients has been demonstrated compared to adjustable gastric band patients [48]. The mechanism of increased AUD incidence after bariatric surgery is likely multifactorial; however, part of the mechanism may be due to changes in alcohol pharmacokinetics related to decreased gastric alcohol dehydrogenase in the post-gastrectomy patient [49]. It is important to recognize mental health crises or substance abuse concerns promptly. Awareness of the increased prevalence of these diseases in the bariatric population is essential in order to recognize and treat them early with the consultation of licensed mental health professionals.

## Patient Education and Follow-Up

Obesity is a chronic disease; subsequently, the bariatric surgery patient should have access to lifelong multidisciplinary care from providers with specialized knowledge and training. Any patient interested in bariatric surgery should be extensively counseled about the chronicity of obesity, the multiple factors contributing to obesity, and the potential risks and benefits of all therapies (surgical, medical, and otherwise). For patients who elect to undergo a bariatric/metabolic operation, the surgeon should educate them about the specific complications of the operation that the patient and surgeon agree are most suited to their needs. Immediate postoperative complications must be disclosed, but so should the more delayed or subacute complications discussed above and elsewhere throughout this text. These patients require lifelong surveillance. We advocate for frequent follow-up in the early postoperative period, which is gradually extended to annual follow-up. Post-surgical patients should have lifelong surveillance for vitamin deficiencies, bone mineral density deficiency, dietary counseling, mental health screening, and periodic endoscopic surveillance to evaluate post-surgical anatomy. Bariatric surgery centers should be equipped to provide easy access to multidisciplinary care to facilitate and encourage lifelong follow-up.

## Conclusion

The complications of patients who have undergone bariatric and metabolic surgery can pose significant challenges in diagnosis and treatment. Complications can occur in the immediate postoperative setting or many years/decades after surgery. Whether early or late complications, patients may present to the emergency room with anything from bowel perforation or obstruction to Wernicke encephalopathy, dumping syndrome, or mental health crisis. The general surgeon should be aware of the many potential complications related to bariatric surgery to promptly diagnose and treat these conditions and, in effect, limit the morbidity and mortality these complications can incur. Endoscopic and radiologic interventions may also assist in treatment management. When the patient's condition allows, consultation or referral to a bariatric surgery referral center should be considered if the complexity of the patient's condition exceeds the capabilities of the hospital resources. In unstable patients, damage control, drain placement, and temporary abdominal closure followed by prompt transfer to a tertiary facility may be the safest option.

## References


1. World Health Organization. (2022). World Obesity Day 2022—accelerating action to stop obesity. https://www.who.int/news/item/04-03-2022-world-obesity-day-2022-accelerating-action-to-stop-obesity.
2. Arterburn DE, Olsen MK, Smith VA, Livingston EH, Van Scoyoc L, Yancy WS Jr, Eid G, Weidenbacher H, Maciejewski ML. Association between bariatric surgery and long-term survival. JAMA. 2015;313(1):62–70. https://doi.org/10.1001/jama.2014.16968.
3. International Federation for Surgery for Obesity and Metabolic Disorders. IFSO—8th Global Registry Report; 2023. https://www.ifso.com/pdf/8th-ifso-registry-report-2023.pdf.
4. Clapp B, Ponce J, Corbett J, Ghanem OM, Kurian M, Rogers AM, Peterson RM, LaMasters T, English WJ. American Society for Metabolic and Bariatric Surgery 2022 estimate of metabolic and bariatric procedures performed in the United States. Surg Obes Relat Dis. 2024:S1550-7289(24)00036-4. Advance online publication. https://doi.org/10.1016/j.soard.2024.01.012.
5. American Society for Bariatric and Metabolic Surgery. Obesity in America; 2021. https://asmbs.org/resources/obesity-in-america/.
6. Aminian A, Brethauer SA, Kirwan JP, Kashyap SR, Burguera B, Schauer PR. How safe is metabolic/diabetes surgery? Diabetes Obes Metab. 2015;17:198–201. https://doi.org/10.1111/dom.12405.
7. Poole M, Fasola L, Zevin B. Management of complications after bariatric surgery: a survey of comfort and educational needs of general surgeons in Ontario, Canada. Obes Surg. 2022;32(7):2407–16. https://doi.org/10.1007/s11695-022-06095-9.
8. Heneghan HM, Meron-Eldar S, Yenumula P, Rogula T, Brethauer SA, Schauer PR. Incidence and management of bleeding complications after gastric bypass surgery in the morbidly obese. Surg Obes Relat Dis. 2012;8(6):729–35. https://doi.org/10.1016/j.soard.2011.05.011.
9. Pereira A, Santos RF, Costa-Pinho A, Silva A, Nogueiro J, Carneiro S, Lima-da-Costa E, Santos-Sousa H, Preto J. Early postoperative bleeding after laparoscopic Roux-En-Y gastric bypass: a single Center Analysis. Obes Surg. 2022;32(6):1902–8. https://doi.org/10.1007/s11695-022-05973-6.
10. Smith MD, Adeniji A, Wahed AS, Patterson E, Chapman W, Courcoulas AP, Dakin G, Flum D, McCloskey C, Mitchell JE, Pomp A, Staten M, Wolfe B. Technical factors associated with anastomotic leak after Roux-en-Y gastric bypass. Surg Obes Relat Dis. 2015;11(2):313–20. https://doi.org/10.1016/j.soard.2014.05.036.
11. Aurora AR, Khaitan L, Saber AA. Sleeve gastrectomy and the risk of leak: a systematic analysis of 4,888 patients. Surg Endosc. 2012;26(6):1509–15. https://doi.org/10.1007/s00464-011-2085-3.
12. Kalff MC, de Raaff CAL, de Vries CEE, Coblijn UK, Willink MT, Fauquenot-Nollen JMB, Jensch S, de Castro SMM, van Veen RN. Diagnostic value of computed tomography for detecting anastomotic or staple line leakage after bariatric surgery. Surg Obes Relat Dis. 2018;14(9):1310–6. https://doi.org/10.1016/j.soard.2018.05.007.

13. Musella M, Cantoni V, Green R, Acampa W, Velotti N, Maietta P, Cuocolo A. Efficacy of postoperative Upper Gastrointestinal Series (UGI) and Computed Tomography (CT) scan in bariatric surgery: a meta-analysis on 7516 patients. Obes Surg. 2018;28(8):2396–405. https://doi.org/10.1007/s11695-018-3172-5.
14. Gonzalez R, Sarr MG, Smith CD, Baghai M, Kendrick M, Szomstein S, Rosenthal R, Murr MM. Diagnosis and contemporary management of anastomotic leaks after gastric bypass for obesity. J Am Coll Surg. 2007;204(1):47–55. https://doi.org/10.1016/j.jamcollsurg.2006.09.023.
15. Gagner M, Kemmeter P. Comparison of laparoscopic sleeve gastrectomy leak rates in five staple-line reinforcement options: a systematic review. Surg Endosc. 2020;34(1):396–407. https://doi.org/10.1007/s00464-019-06782-2.
16. Daigle CR, Brethauer SA, Tu C, Petrick AT, Morton JM, Schauer PR, Aminian A. Which postoperative complications matter most after bariatric surgery? Prioritizing quality improvement efforts to improve national outcomes. Surg Obes Relat Dis. 2018;14(5):652–7. https://doi.org/10.1016/j.soard.2018.01.008.
17. Nguyen NT, Goldman C, Rosenquist CJ, Arango A, Cole CJ, Lee SJ, Wolfe BM. Laparoscopic versus open gastric bypass: a randomized study of outcomes, quality of life, and costs. Ann Surg. 2001;234(3):279–91. https://doi.org/10.1097/00000658-200109000-00002.
18. Parikh A, Alley JB, Peterson RM, Harnisch MC, Pfluke JM, Tapper DM, Fenton SJ. Management options for symptomatic stenosis after laparoscopic vertical sleeve gastrectomy in the morbidly obese. Surg Endosc. 2012;26(3):738–46. https://doi.org/10.1007/s00464-011-1945-1.
19. Dapri G, Cadière GB, Himpens J. Laparoscopic seromyotomy for long stenosis after sleeve gastrectomy with or without duodenal switch. Obes Surg. 2009;19(4):495–9. https://doi.org/10.1007/s11695-009-9803-0.
20. Barajas-Gamboa JS, Landreneau J, Abril C, Raza J, Corcelles R, Kroh M. Conversion of sleeve gastrectomy to Roux-en-Y gastric bypass for complications: outcomes from a tertiary referral center in the Middle East. Surgery for obesity and related diseases : official journal of the American Society for Bariatric Surgery. 2019;15(10):1690–5. https://doi.org/10.1016/j.soard.2019.07.027.
21. Jones KB. Biliopancreatic limb obstruction in gastric bypass at or proximal to the jejunojejunostomy: a potentially deadly, catastrophic event. Obes Surg. 1996;6(6):485–93. https://doi.org/10.1381/096089296765556386.
22. Stephenson D, Moon RC, Teixeira AF, Jawad MA. Intussusception after Roux-en-Y gastric bypass. Surg Obes Relat Dis. 2014;10(4):666–70. https://doi.org/10.1016/j.soard.2014.01.026.
23. Facchiano E, Soricelli E, Leuratti L, Caputo V, Quartararo G, Lucchese M. Intussusception after Roux-en-Y gastric bypass: laparoscopic management. Obes Surg. 2018;28(7):2145–7. https://doi.org/10.1007/s11695-018-3265-1.
24. Tack J, Deloose E. Complications of bariatric surgery: dumping syndrome, reflux and vitamin deficiencies. Best Pract Res Clin Gastroenterol. 2014;28(4):741–9. https://doi.org/10.1016/j.bpg.2014.07.010.
25. Bemeur C, Butterworth RF. Thiamin. In: Ross AC, Caballero B, Cousins RJ, et al., editors. Modern nutrition in health and disease. 11th ed. Lippincott Williams & Wilkins. p. 317.
26. Salame M, Jawhar N, Belluzzi A, Al-Kordi M, Storm AC, Abu Dayyeh BK, Ghanem OM. Marginal ulcers after Roux-en-Y gastric bypass: etiology, diagnosis, and management. J Clin Med. 2023;12(13):4336. https://doi.org/10.3390/jcm12134336.
27. Rodrigo DC, Jill S, Daniel M, Kimberly C, Maher EC. Which factors correlate with marginal ulcer after surgery for obesity? Obes Surg. 2020;30(12):4821–7. https://doi.org/10.1007/s11695-020-04960-z.
28. Crawford CB, Schuh LM, Inman MM. Revision Gastrojejunostomy Versus Suturing With and Without Omental Patch for Perforated Marginal Ulcer Treatment After Roux-en-Y Gastric Bypass. J Gastrointest Surg. 2023;27(1):1–6. https://doi.org/10.1007/s11605-022-05461-3.

29. Froehling DA, Daniels PR, Mauck KF, Collazo-Clavell ML, Ashrani AA, Sarr MG, Petterson TM, Heit JA. Incidence of venous thromboembolism after bariatric surgery: a population-based cohort study. Obes Surg. 2013;23(11):1874–9. https://doi.org/10.1007/s11695-013-1073-1.
30. Birkmeyer NJ, Finks JF, English WJ, Carlin AM, Hawasli AA, Genaw JA, Wood MH, Share DA, Birkmeyer JD, Collaborative MBS. Risks and benefits of prophylactic inferior vena cava filters in patients undergoing bariatric surgery. J Hosp Med. 2013;8(4):173–7.
31. Caruana JA, Anain PM, Pham DT. The pulmonary embolism risk score system reduces the incidence and mortality of pulmonary embolism after gastric bypass. Surgery. 2009;146(4):678–85. https://doi.org/10.1016/j.surg.2009.07.011.
32. Aminian A, Andalib A, Khorgami Z, Cetin D, Burguera B, Bartholomew J, Brethauer SA, Schauer PR. Who should get extended thromboprophylaxis after bariatric surgery?: a risk assessment tool to guide indications for post-discharge pharmacoprophylaxis. Ann Surg. 2017;265(1):143–50. https://doi.org/10.1097/SLA.0000000000001686.
33. Finks JF, English WJ, Carlin AM, Krause KR, Share DA, Banerjee M, Birkmeyer JD, Birkmeyer NJ, Michigan Bariatric Surgery Collaborative, & Center for Healthcare Outcomes and Policy. Predicting risk for venous thromboembolism with bariatric surgery: results from the Michigan Bariatric Surgery Collaborative. Ann Surg. 2012;255(6):1100–4. https://doi.org/10.1097/SLA.0b013e31825659d4.
34. Buchwald H, Estok R, Fahrbach K, Banel D, Sledge I. Trends in mortality in bariatric surgery: a systematic review and meta-analysis. Surgery. 2007;142(4):621–35. https://doi.org/10.1016/j.surg.2007.07.018.
35. Goitein D, Matter I, Raziel A, Keidar A, Hazzan D, Rimon U, Sakran N. Portomesenteric thrombosis following laparoscopic bariatric surgery: incidence, patterns of clinical presentation, and etiology in a bariatric patient population. JAMA Surg. 2013;148(4):340–6. https://doi.org/10.1001/jamasurg.2013.1053.
36. Luo L, Li H, Wu Y, Bai Z, Xu X, Wang L, Mendez-Sanchez N, Qi X. Portal venous system thrombosis after bariatric surgery: a systematic review and meta-analysis. Surgery. 2021;170(2):363–72. https://doi.org/10.1016/j.surg.2021.03.005.
37. Primignani M. Portal vein thrombosis revisited. Dig Liver Dis. 2010;42(3):163–70. https://doi.org/10.1016/j.dld.2009.08.003.
38. Belnap L, Rodgers GM, Cottam D, Zaveri H, Drury C, Surve A. Portal vein thrombosis after laparoscopic sleeve gastrectomy: presentation and management. Surg Obes Relat Dis. 2016;12(10):1787–94. https://doi.org/10.1016/j.soard.2016.03.005.
39. Ramos R, Park Y, Shazad G, Garcia A, C., & Cohen, R. Cavernous transformation of portal vein secondary to portal vein thrombosis: a case report. J Clin Med Res. 2012;4(1):81–4. https://doi.org/10.4021/jocmr775w.
40. Guzmán HM, Sepúlveda M, Rosso N, San Martin A, Guzmán F, Guzmán HC. Incidence and risk factors for cholelithiasis after bariatric surgery. Obes Surg. 2019;29(7):2110–4. https://doi.org/10.1007/s11695-019-03760-4.
41. Worni M, Guller U, Shah A, Gandhi M, Shah J, Rajgor D, Pietrobon R, Jacobs DO, Ostbye T. Cholecystectomy concomitant with laparoscopic gastric bypass: a trend analysis of the nationwide inpatient sample from 2001 to 2008. Obes Surg. 2012;22(2):220–9. https://doi.org/10.1007/s11695-011-0575-y.
42. Inamdar S, Slattery E, Sejpal DV, Miller LS, Pleskow DK, Berzin TM, Trindade AJ. Systematic review and meta-analysis of single-balloon enteroscopy-assisted ERCP in patients with surgically altered GI anatomy. Gastrointest Endosc. 2015;82(1):9–19. https://doi.org/10.1016/j.gie.2015.02.013.
43. Lopes TL, Baron TH. Endoscopic retrograde cholangiopancreatography in patients with Roux-en-Y anatomy. J Hepatobiliary Pancreat Sci. 2011;18(3):332–8. https://doi.org/10.1007/s00534-010-0361-6.
44. Dawes AJ, Maggard-Gibbons M, Maher AR, Booth MJ, Miake-Lye I, Beroes JM, Shekelle PG. Mental health conditions among patients seeking and undergoing bariatric surgery: a meta-analysis. JAMA. 2016;315(2):150–63. https://doi.org/10.1001/jama.2015.18118.

45. Bhatti JA, Nathens AB, Thiruchelvam D, Grantcharov T, Goldstein BI, Redelmeier DA. Self-harm emergencies after bariatric surgery: a population-based cohort study. JAMA Surg. 2016;151(3):226–32. https://doi.org/10.1001/jamasurg.2015.3414.
46. Adams TD, Gress RE, Smith SC, Halverson RC, Simper SC, Rosamond WD, Lamonte MJ, Stroup AM, Hunt SC. Long-term mortality after gastric bypass surgery. N Engl J Med. 2007;357(8):753–61. https://doi.org/10.1056/NEJMoa066603.
47. Ibrahim N, Alameddine M, Brennan J, Sessine M, Holliday C, Ghaferi AA. New onset alcohol use disorder following bariatric surgery. Surg Endosc. 2019;33(8):2521–30. https://doi.org/10.1007/s00464-018-6545-x.
48. King WC, Chen JY, Courcoulas AP, Dakin GF, Engel SG, Flum DR, Hinojosa MW, Kalarchian MA, Mattar SG, Mitchell JE, Pomp A, Pories WJ, Steffen KJ, White GE, Wolfe BM, Yanovski SZ. Alcohol and other substance use after bariatric surgery: prospective evidence from a U.S. multicenter cohort study. Surg Obes Relat Dis. 2017;13(8):1392–402. https://doi.org/10.1016/j.soard.2017.03.021.
49. Ivezaj V, Benoit SC, Davis J, Engel S, Lloret-Linares C, Mitchell JE, Pepino MY, Rogers AM, Steffen K, Sogg S. Changes in alcohol use after metabolic and bariatric surgery: predictors and mechanisms. Curr Psychiatry Rep. 2019;21(9):85. https://doi.org/10.1007/s11920-019-1070-8.

# Adolescents and Bariatric Surgery: Techniques and Outcomes

# 48

Nestor de la Cruz-Munoz, Sarah Messiah, and Eli Monzon Canales

## Definition of Childhood Obesity

The Centers for Disease Control and Prevention (CDC) defines childhood obesity as a condition where a child's body mass index (BMI) exceeds the 95th percentile for their age and sex, indicating a significantly elevated weight relative to peers. BMI is calculated by dividing a person's weight in kilograms by the square of their height in meters (BMI = weight in kg / (height in meters)^2) or by dividing weight in pounds by the square of height in inches and multiplying by 703 for the imperial system (BMI = (weight in lbs. / (height in inches)^2) * 703) and serves as a key metric in identifying obesity in children and adolescents. The CDC's definition of obesity underscores the importance of BMI assessment in diagnosing childhood obesity taking sex-and age-specific growth into consideration, emphasizing the percentile cutoff to identify those at risk. Severe obesity, defined as ≥120% of the 95th percentile of body mass index (BMI) adjusted for age and sex or a BMI >35 kg/m$^2$, is the fastest growing subcategory of obesity in the United States (US) pediatric population [1]. Specifically, the American Academy of Pediatrics (AAP) divides

N. de la Cruz-Munoz (✉)
DeWitt Daughtry Family Department of Surgery, Division of Laparoendoscopic and Bariatric Surgery, University of Miami Miller School of Medicine, Miami, FL, USA
e-mail: ndelacruz@med.miami.edu

S. Messiah
School of Public Health, The University of Texas Health Science Center at Houston (UTHealth), Dallas, TX, USA

Center for Pediatric Population Health, School of Public Health, The University of Texas Health Science Center at Houston, Dallas, TX, USA

E. Monzon Canales
Center for Pediatric Population Health, School of Public Health, The University of Texas Health Science Center at Houston, Dallas, TX, USA



O. M. Ghanem et al. (eds.), *The SAGES Manual of Metabolic and Bariatric Surgery*, https://doi.org/10.1007/978-3-031-72309-4_48

obesity into two classes based on severity; Class 2 (≥120% to <140% of the 95th percentile or a BMI ≥35 to ≤39 kg/m$^2$) and Class 3 (≥140% of the 95th percentile or BMI ≥40 kg/m$^2$) [2, 3]. It should be noted that while BMI is a valuable screening tool, it does not directly measure body fat and may not account for variations in muscle mass or bone density, thus necessitating comprehensive evaluation by healthcare professionals. Severe obesity in the pediatric years is associated with many cardiometabolic comorbidities, liver and kidney disease, lower sleep quality, and mental health comorbidities, resulting in lower quality of life scores [4–6]. Moreover, severe obesity during adolescence tracks strongly into adulthood and is associated with adult asthma, arthritis, and poorer cardiometabolic and psychological risk profiles, as well as lower life expectancy [7–12].

## Epidemiology

In many countries, just a few decades ago, the age-standardized prevalence of thinness was greater than that of obesity. Furthermore, the age-standardized prevalence of obesity surpassed 10% in very few countries. Yet, from 1990–2022, obesity has doubled in most countries with increases in girls in 186 countries (93%) and in boys in 195 countries (98%) with a posterior probability of at least 0·80 [13]. The prevalence of severe obesity among United States adolescents has almost doubled from 4.7% to 9.2% over the past decade [14]. National Health and Nutrition Examination Survey (NHANES) data shows the overall severe obesity rate among US adolescents (ages 13–19) increased between 2015 (5.6%) to 2018 (6.5% which = about 4.8 million youth; *P*-trend <0.001); the largest increase was among Hispanics (4.1% in 1999–2000 to 10.7% in 2017–18, *P*-trend <0.001), followed by non-Hispanic blacks (6.7% to 10.2%, *P*-trend <0.001) and non-Hispanic whites (2.6% to 4%) [15]. Obesity disparities result from a complex interplay of genetic, social, and economic factors.

## Etiology/Predictors/Risk Factors

The etiology of childhood obesity is multifactorial, including genetic, biological, psychological, socioecological, and environmental factors. An individual exposed to one or a combination of etiological factors can result in alterations in immunologic, metabolic, and epigenetic processes that alter the body's energy regulation leading to obesity. Genetic predispositions play a significant role in determining an individual's susceptibility to obesity, influencing factors such as metabolism, fat storage, and appetite regulation. Social determinants, such as access to healthy foods, opportunities for physical activity, and cultural norms surrounding body image, also exert profound effects. Moreover, economic factors, including income level, education, and neighborhood environments, shape lifestyle choices and access to healthcare services, further exacerbating disparities in obesity rates. Finally, structural determinants such as weight bias, discrimination and stigma can also play a critical role in obesity development throughout childhood [16, 17]. This intricate interplay underscores the need for comprehensive approaches to address obesity, recognizing the intersecting influences of genetics, social and structural dynamics, and economic conditions. Such strategies should encompass not only individual behavior change but also broader systemic interventions aimed at promoting equitable access to healthy environments and resources for all communities. Starting obesity prevention early in life is important as studies show that if a child has obesity at ages 6–11-years they have a 30–50% chance of having obesity as an adult [18]. This risk significantly increases if obesity is present in adolescence, ranging from 50–80% depending on the severity of obesity playing a determining role [19, 20]. These statistics underscore the critical importance of addressing obesity prevention and intervention strategies early in life to mitigate long-term health risks.

Heritability studies have suggested that genetics may contribute 40–70% to an individual's obesity risk and that 25–40% of BMI may be heritable [21–23]. Genomic studies have been able to identify 32 loci that can predispose an individual to obesity [24]. Although various research studies have determined that genetics can play a role in the development of obesity, genetic predisposition often needs to be coupled with contributing environmental and behavioral factors to influence weight. Polygenetic causes are by far more frequent than single gene defects or monogenetic syndromes, such as Melanocortin 4 receptor (MC4R) deficiency, Leptin deficiency, proopiomelanocortin (POMC) deficiency, Prader-Willi syndrome, Bardet-Biedl syndrome, etc., that typically account for less than 5% of cases of childhood obesity [25].

Instead, the best predictor for childhood obesity is parental obesity. If children have one parent with obesity, the children tend to have future obesity, and may even be more predictive than the child's weight. Family factors such as types of foods available, mealtime structure, and sedentary family habits can contribute significantly [21, 26, 27]. Meanwhile, psychological factors, depression, anxiety, low self-esteem, or eating disorders, appear to have more of an impact in the adolescent population, however it is unclear whether obesity is a cause or a consequence of disease [28, 29].

## Health Impact of Childhood Obesity

Pediatric obesity profoundly impacts health, increasing short- and long-term risks of physical, social, and emotional well-being. The global rise in pediatric obesity is linked to numerous medical conditions, such as cardiovascular disease, dyslipidemia, insulin resistance, Type 2 Diabetes Mellitus (T2DM), non-alcoholic fatty liver disease (NAFLD), cholelithiasis, skin issues, obstructive sleep apnea, renal disease, menstrual irregularities, and orthopedic problems [30, 31].

## Cardiometabolic/Cardiovascular

Excess weight characterized as metabolically unhealthy includes increased visceral fat, adipocyte hypertrophy, inflammatory factor secretion, and ectopic fat deposition. These features increase the risk of cardiovascular and cardiometabolic diseases including dyslipidemia, hypertension (HTN), and T2DM. In children, this excess body fat can increase atherogenic lipoproteins, dysglycemia, and accelerate vascular aging. The accumulation of metabolic markers such as high LDL-cholesterol, low HDL-cholesterol, high triglycerides, and high blood pressure can lead to progressive atherosclerotic cardiovascular disease and increased morbidity [30, 32, 33].

## Endocrinological/Diabetes

It has been well established that there is a strong correlation between childhood obesity and insulin resistance and T2DM. Rapid weight gain, the physiologic decline in insulin sensitivity of puberty, and a relative decline in insulin secretion unable to compensate for the increased demand can lead to progressive glucose intolerance, microvascular injury, and eventual insulin insensitivity [30, 34, 35]. Both cross-sectional and longitudinal cohort studies have shown cumulative exposure to insulin resistance and dysglycemia leads to deterioration of vascular structure and function, which are major factors in accelerated vascular aging, cardiovascular remodeling, and diminished cardiovascular function [30, 34, 36, 37].

Obesity can influence the clinical and biochemical phenotype of endocrine and metabolic abnormalities therefore amplifying disease. Endocrinologically, childhood obesity may predispose youth to accelerated linear growth, advanced skeletal maturation, and, in girls, early onset of sexual maturation or even the development of adolescent polycystic ovarian syndrome (PCOS) [38–40].

## Pulmonary

Children with elevated BMI have a significantly higher prevalence of Obstructive Sleep Apnea (OSA) (45% among those with obesity compared to 9% among those with a healthy weight) [41]. Moreover, OSA severity increases with BMI. During sleep, reduced airway muscle tone in children with OSA leads to airway narrowing and obstruction, causing intermittent hypoxemia and arousals, disrupting sleep [42]. OSA is linked to neurocognitive impairment, reduced quality of life, and cardiovascular issues. Among children with obesity, OSA may exacerbate cardiovascular and metabolic burden by inducing systemic hypertension, altering ventricular structure, increasing arterial stiffness, and contributing to metabolic syndrome [43].

## Gastrointestinal

MAFLD, or Metabolic Associated Fatty Liver Disease, is increasingly recognized as a significant concern in the pediatric population. It refers to a spectrum of liver conditions characterized by fat accumulation in the liver along with metabolic abnormalities such as insulin resistance, dyslipidemia, and obesity. In children, MAFLD is associated with various adverse health outcomes, including liver inflammation, fibrosis, and an increased risk of developing advanced liver disease later in life. Obesity significantly increases the risk of developing MAFLD in children due to associated factors such as insulin resistance, dyslipidemia, adipokine imbalance, oxidative stress, and alterations in gut microbiota [44]. These factors create a metabolic environment conducive to fat accumulation in the liver and the progression of liver disease.

Managing MAFLD in pediatric patients requires a multifaceted approach involving lifestyle modifications, dietary interventions, and sometimes pharmacological treatments to address underlying metabolic issues and prevent disease progression. Early identification and intervention are crucial in mitigating the long-term consequences of MAFLD in pediatric patients.

## Musculoskeletal

Childhood obesity increases the risk of various musculoskeletal problems including impairments in mobility and flexibility, changes in postural balance leading to increased prevalence of fractures, lower extremity joint pain, lower extremity malalignment, and overall decrease in range of motion in comparison to children with normal BMI [45, 46]. A common hip disorder that has been attributed to excess mechanical stress caused by obesity is Slipped Capital Femoral Epiphysis (SCFE). If untreated, this condition can progress to avascular necrosis of the femur, amputation, and life-long disabilities. Childhood obesity has also been associated with decreases in bone ossification and reduction of mechanical strength of bones and joints that could lead to the tibial growth disorder, Blount Disease [47, 48]. Although the exact mechanism of the disorder is not known, the incidence of infantile Blount disease is rising in parallel to the increasing obesity in children [49].

## Socioemotional/Mental Health

Socioemotional consequences of childhood obesity vary among individuals. Children who are overweight or with obesity face numerous difficulties including, but not limited to, bullying, discrimination, negative stereotypes, or even ostracization from peers [29]. Due to the various consequences of childhood obesity, children may often be excluded from a variety of activities, which can contribute to the development of many negative features. These negative social consequences can manifest into low self-esteem, low self-confidence, a negative body image, anxiety, depression, and can also affect academic performance. A cross-sectional study of 106 children and adolescents (57 males) between the ages of 5 and 18 years concluded that overweight and children with obesity were four times more likely to report having problems at school than their normal weight peers, and are more likely to miss school more frequently, especially those with chronic health conditions such as diabetes and asthma, which also affect academic performance [50].

### Healthcare Costs/Utilization

Childhood obesity is associated with high healthcare utilization and costs. According to Finkelstein et al. [51] systematic literature search, the incremental lifetime direct medical cost from the perspective of a 10-year-old child with obesity relative to a 10-year-old normal weight child ranges from $12,660 to $19,630 when weight gain through adulthood among normal weight children is accounted for, and from $16,310 to $39,080 when such weight is not accounted for. According to these estimations, the total lifetime costs of a cohort of ten-year-olds with obesity to be in the range of $9 to $14 billion. Lightwood et al. [52] estimates that, in the United States, the cumulative attributable cost related to direct medical care and lost productivity from childhood obesity could exceed $250 billion. Obesity-associated comorbidities are typically progressive conditions that increase morbidity and the risk of premature death. The comorbidities that increase costs and utilization of healthcare resources that mainly cooccur with obesity are cardiometabolic diseases, mood disorders, asthma, pregnancy, and malignancies, such as leukemia, Hodgkin's disease, colorectal cancer, and breast cancer [2, 53].

## Medical and Behavioral Therapy

The treatment of childhood obesity necessitates a nuanced approach, tailored to individual needs and circumstances. It is imperative to consider various factors, including medical, socioeconomic, developmental, and environmental influences, when devising therapeutic strategies.

### Behavioral Therapy

Behavioral therapy, coupled with lifestyle modifications, serves as a foundational approach to achieving weight reduction in children. This method involves regular visits with family involvement to promote healthier eating habits and increased physical activity. Nutritional management focuses on minimizing cardiometabolic risk factors and comorbidities while ensuring optimal growth and development. Strategies include reducing intake of sugary beverages and processed foods, encouraging daily moderate-to-vigorous physical activity, limiting sedentary behaviors, and incorporating diverse lean protein sources. Nearly all effective treatments for childhood obesity incorporate this behavioral component [2]. Lifestyle modification or behavioral-based monotherapy have shown modest improvements in BMI status with infrequent resolution of severe obesity classification, or individuals often regain weight after therapy completion [5].

## Pharmacotherapy

According to AAP clinical practice guidelines in 2023, children ages 8 through 11 years of age with obesity can be offered pharmacotherapy for weight management and as an adjunct to health behavior and lifestyle treatment [2].

Glucagon-like peptide-1 receptor agonists (GLP-1 agonists) (e.g. liraglutide, exenatide, dulaglutide, semaglutide, and tirzepatide) enhance insulin secretion and decrease hunger by slowing gastric emptying and by acting on targets in the central nervous system (arcuate nucleus of the hypothalamus, limbic/reward system in amygdala and the cortex), and they are approved for pediatric patients aged 12 and older [2, 54]. The weight-loss potential for several GLP-1 agonist is ~ 3–5% of body weight for youth compared to adults with an associated improvement in the glycemic and cardiometabolic profile [30]. However, recent clinical trial results of Semaglutide in adolescents demonstrated a mean change in BMI of − 16.1% compared to 0.6% with placebo [55].

Other medications such as Orlistat, Phentermine, combination Phentermine/Topiramate, etc. are pharmacological options listed in the AAP clinical practice guideline for the evaluation and treatment of children and adolescents with obesity but are not as frequently used [2]. Another medication referenced off-label for weight loss in childhood obesity is Metformin. The results of Metformin have been modest (<5% weight reduction) and inconsistent, such that many reserve its use for T2DM or PCOS [2].

Behavioral and lifestyle interventions alone or with concomitant pharmacological intervention are cornerstones of treatment for childhood obesity. Yet, while pharmacological interventions are still rapidly evolving, children with more immediate and life-threatening comorbidities and affected by severe obesity may require additional therapeutic options. Furthermore, once childhood obesity is established, it is often refractory to treatment leading to only a brief period of weight loss, followed by rapid re-accumulation of the lost weight after the termination of therapy [56].

## Bariatric Surgery

While prevention remains the core of obesity therapy in children who develop severe obesity, several studies have clearly demonstrated that metabolic and bariatric surgery (MBS) is a safe and effective safe, effective, and viable treatment alternative for childhood obesity. Disappointing outcomes related to the application of nonsurgical treatment modalities alone (e.g. nutritional counseling, exercise, pharmacological, and behavioral and lifestyle modification) have highlighted MBS as more than a treatment of last resort [12]. Furthermore, several studies have demonstrated it is the only available therapy that has exhibited long-term safety and a sustained reduction in BMI for 10–18 years postoperatively [57–59]. The two most prevalent procedures performed are vertical sleeve gastrectomy (VSG) and Laparoscopic Roux-en-Y gastric bypass and have resulted in significant and sustained weight loss and improvement and/or resolution of numerous related comorbid conditions [4, 12, 60]. Laparoscopic adjustable gastric band (LAGB) procedures have declined due to worse long-term outcomes, higher complication rates, and higher reintervention rates.

## Indications

The indications for MBS in adolescents, 10-to-19 years of age (WHO), are similar to those for adults. The American Society for Metabolic and Bariatric Surgery (ASMBS) pediatric guidelines states MBS should be considered in adolescents with a BMI ≥120% of the 95th percentile with hyperlipidemia, HTN, T2D, insulin resistance, depressed Health-related quality of life (HRQOL), GERD, OSA, NAFLD, orthopedic disease, idiopathic intracranial hypertension (IIH), or a BMI ≥140% of the 95th percentile [12]. Contraindications to MBS include a medically correctable cause of obesity, an ongoing substance abuse problem (within the preceding year), a medical, psychiatric, psychosocial, or cognitive condition that prevents adherence to postoperative dietary and medication regimens, and current or planned pregnancy within 12-to-18 months of the procedure [4, 12].

## Outcomes

For the past several years, VSG has been the most common MBS procedure for severe childhood obesity. It has been viewed as a more attractive procedure due to its lower risk of perioperative and long-term complications and a relatively low reintervention rate. Studies have demonstrated mean BMI reductions between 13–20 kg/m$^2$, 30-day complication rates under 5%, and reintervention rates ranging from 1–11% [61, 62]. Although VSG has comparable weight loss to RYGB, it has a slightly lower comorbidity resolution rate and an increase in postoperative development of GERD [63]. Although VSG long-term outcome data is quickly emerging, current data demonstrates that, for the adolescent population, it is an effective therapy for the reduction or resolution of cardiometabolic diseases that heavily impact this population [12].

Roux-en-Y gastric bypass is the second most common MBS procedure currently performed for the treatment of childhood/adolescent obesity. Studies have demonstrated that RYGB has resulted in mean BMI reductions of 15–16 kg/m$^2$, 30-day complication rates ranging from 9–11%, and reintervention rates under 20%, which include endoscopic dilations [12, 61]. Long-term research has demonstrated that many of these individuals are able to maintain the BMI loss, approximately 13 kg/

$m^2$ [59, 62]. Due to higher complication rates, such as nutritional deficiencies, caution should be used in adolescents with noncompliance tendencies. Another major consideration is preexisting GERD, where RYGB is the superior treatment to other MBS therapies.

Laparoscopic adjustable gastric band is the least frequently used MBS therapy. Studies have demonstrated a mean BMI loss of 10–11.6 kg/$m^2$, 30-day complication rates of 10–11%, and intervention rates that vary from 14.7–42%, highest among the MBS procedures [4, 12, 64]. Although LAGB has been proven to be safe and effective, given the high failure rate and increased need for reintervention, it is not considered the preferred therapy [2]. Furthermore, in 2022, ASMBS estimated only 2500 individuals underwent LAGB and is not likely being performed in the adolescent population.

Among the three most common MBS, the negative adverse effects are quite similar by procedure type. Most postoperative complications are minor (15%), such postoperative dehydration, nausea, and vomiting. Approximately 8% of individuals suffer from major perioperative complications. Other negative outcomes range from gastrointestinal problems, vitamin deficits, reduction in lean body mass, and postoperative GERD [12, 60].

## Therapeutic Disparities

Childhood obesity disproportionately affects racial minority groups, especially Hispanic and Black, via numerous factors, such as genetics, pre- and perinatal factors, socioeconomic status, and other childhood factors. For example, consumption of increased processed foods and sugar-sweetened beverages is more common in Hispanic and Non-Hispanic Black children in comparison to White children. It has been demonstrated that healthier, nutritious food alternatives are far more expensive and less affordable than those that contain added sugars, trans fats, or saturated fats leading to a greater food insecurity in low-income families [2, 16]. Due to an accumulation of factors, these populations have a propensity towards severe obesity that require medical intervention.

These at-risk and already resource-limited individuals are mainly treated at the primary-care level since referral to an advanced level of care is infrequent as individuals are more likely to have limited access, or poor insurance coverage [65]. Successful behavioral and lifestyle modification intervention requires frequent in-person provider visits within an established timeframe, access to parks or open spaces for physical activity, and strong-family engagement, which may not be conducive for certain populations. Furthermore, in recent years, the use of anti-obesity medications (AOM) has been utilized in pediatric patients as an adjunct therapy. Outcome data among children and adolescents of different ethnicities is currently being investigated. Data from a recent large retrospective study performed using electronic health records demonstrated that AOM prescription rates are lower among Hispanics compared to non-Hispanic Whites, while there was no statistical significance when comparing non-Hispanic Whites to other races [66]. Yet, it is suggested that the largest barrier for pharmacological intervention is the cost of anti-obesity medications that disproportionately affect low-income populations. Currently, only a few states have Medicaid coverage for anti-obesity medications [16].

Bariatric surgery, on other the hand, is the only available therapy having demonstrated long-term weight loss with comorbidity improvement or resolution in various ethnicities [15, 67]. Although the most effective treatment for severe obesity, access to care is multifactorial, with race and socioeconomic status being principal considerations. Just under 50% of pediatric patients who qualify for surgery receive insurance coverage following initial request for authorization [16]. White females with private insurance have the highest acceptance rate, while Hispanic and Non-Hispanic Black with Medicaid are less likely to receive authorization regardless of comparable outcome results [16, 68]. Obesity disproportionately affects racial minority groups, specifically Black, Hispanic, and multiracial adolescents, and recent studies have demonstrated that these groups largely benefit from access to MBS with sustained weight loss, comorbidity reductions, and a low long-term complication rate for up to almost two decades [16, 57, 65, 67].

## Challenges

The decision-making process for MBS is rooted in a framework of thoughtful, shared decision making between the patient, parents, and medical and surgical providers [4, 12]. Yet, there are several obstacles that impede this therapeutic process, such as access being limited further by primary provider concerns and beliefs on surgical intervention. National survey information from various countries suggest that many physicians are reluctant to refer adolescent patients for MBS with concerns for altered development, a lack of awareness of MBS as a viable option, insufficient knowledge on the surgical procedures, complications, or follow-up required, or even provider weight bias that weight is a personal responsibility rather than a medical pathology [4]. Another common occurrence is the lack of progression from long-term lifestyle management to medical intervention, where no progress is achieved and carried over into adulthood. However, current research has demonstrated that MBS is safe, efficacious, has no impact on linear growth, and a small percentage of long-term complications [69].

After a referral, a comprehensive and multidisciplinary assessment that includes a physiologic and psychosocial component is performed to gauge eligibility and provide further information [4, 12]. During this phase, it is paramount to determine the patient's and family's capacity to understand the risks and benefits of MBS, willingness to adhere to long-term lifestyle modifications, insurance coverage availability, and to determine any potential contraindications, such as correctable causes of obesity or substance abuse disorders, to ensure an informed decision is reached by all parties involved [12]. As with other aspects of adolescent health, patient engagement, willingness, compliance, and expectations are important for positive surgical outcomes.

## Conclusion

The childhood obesity epidemic is a serious public health concern with a high percentage of children and adolescents afflicted. Pediatric obesity negatively impacts an individual's health and is linked to numerous debilitating and progressive medical conditions that increase morbidity and the risk of premature death. These conditions carry short- and long-term high healthcare utilization and costs. Hence, the prevention and treatment of obesity should be addressed sooner rather than later, especially in a vulnerable and still-developing population.

Although prevention is the optimal method to abate this problem, strategies and therapies are required to treat those inflicted. The use of behavioral and lifestyle therapies in conjunction with nonsurgical or surgical therapies is currently being heavily investigated. Currently, monotherapy with behavioral/lifestyle therapy or nonsurgical therapies has shown to have modest short-term reductions in BMI. Nonsurgical therapies are promising but have yet to produce convincing long-term weight-loss and comorbidity resolution data, particularly in individuals with severe obesity. MBS has been demonstrated to be a safe and effective long-term treatment of childhood obesity with little variation by ethnicity and/or gender. Even though MBS was previously viewed as a therapy of last resort, many studies have confirmed its viability as a therapeutic option in adolescents. The AAP has highlighted the need to educate pediatricians and primary care providers about the benefits of MBS for qualified adolescents [2, 65]. Similar to the adult population, there are disparities in the response and utilization of the most effective treatment options. So, to adequately address the childhood obesity epidemic, there is a need to focus more efforts on prevention and treatment within underserved populations.

## References

1. Hales CM, Fryar CD, Carroll MD, Freedman DS, Ogden CL. Trends in obesity and severe obesity prevalence in US youth and adults by sex and age, 2007-2008 to 2015-2016. JAMA. 2018;319(16):1723–5.
2. Hampl SE, Hassink SG, Skinner AC, Armstrong SC, Barlow SE, Bolling CF, Avila Edwards KC, Eneli I, Hamre R, Joseph MM, Lunsford D, Mendonca E, Michalsky MP, Mirza N, Ochoa ER, Sharifi M, Staiano AE, Weedn AE, Flinn SK, Lindros J, Okechukwu K. Clinical practice guideline for the evaluation and treatment of children and adolescents with obesity. Pediatrics. 2023;151(2):e2022060640. https://doi.org/10.1542/peds.2022-060640. Erratum in: Pediatrics. 2024 Jan 1;153(1): PMID: 36622115.
3. Skinner AC, Perrin EM, Moss LA, Skelton JA. Cardiometabolic risks and severity of obesity in children and young adults. N Engl J Med. 2015;373(14):1307–17. https://doi.org/10.1056/NEJMoa1502821. PMID: 26422721.
4. Armstrong SC, Bolling CF, Michalsky MP, Reichard KW, SECTION ON OBESITY, SECTION ON SURGERY. Pediatric metabolic and bariatric surgery: evidence, barriers, and best practices. Pediatrics. 2019;144(6):e20193223. https://doi.org/10.1542/peds.2019-3223. Epub 2019 Oct 27
5. Kelly AS, Barlow SE, Rao G, Inge TH, Hayman LL, Steinberger J, Urbina EM, Ewing LJ, Daniels SR. American Heart Association Atherosclerosis, Hypertension, and Obesity in the Young Committee of the Council on Cardiovascular Disease in the Young, Council on Nutrition,

Physical Activity and Metabolism, and Council on Clinical Cardiology. Severe obesity in children and adolescents: identification, associated health risks, and treatment approaches: a scientific statement from the American Heart Association. Circulation. 2013;128(15):1689–712. https://doi.org/10.1161/CIR.0b013e3182a5cfb3. Epub 2013 Sep 9. PMID: 24016455.

6. Rank M, Siegrist M, Wilks DC, Langhof H, Wolfarth B, Haller B, Koenig W, Halle M. The cardio-metabolic risk of moderate and severe obesity in children and adolescents. J Pediatr. 2013;163(1):137–42. https://doi.org/10.1016/j.jpeds.2013.01.020. Epub 2013 Feb 20. PMID: 23434121.
7. Golden SH, Brown A, Cauley JA, Chin MH, Gary-Webb TL, Kim C, Sosa JA, Sumner AE, Anton B. Health disparities in endocrine disorders: biological, clinical, and nonclinical factors—an Endocrine Society scientific statement. J Clin Endocrinol Metab. 2012;97(9):E1579–639. https://doi.org/10.1210/jc.2012-2043. Epub 2012 Jun 22. PMID: 22730516; PMCID: PMC3431576
8. Pratt LA, Brody DJ. Depression and obesity in the U.S. adult household population, 2005–2010. NCHS Data Brief. 2014;(167):1–8.
9. Robert Wood Johnson Foundation. The State of Obesity 2019: Better Policies for a Healthier America. https://www.stateofobesity.org. Accessed 20 Jan 2019.
10. Xu J, Murphy S, Kochanek K, Arias E. Mortality in the United States, 2015. NCHS data brief, no 267. Hyattsville, MD: US Department of Health and Human Services, CDC. National Center for Health Statistics; 2016.
11. Wang YC, McPherson K, Marsh T, Gortmaker SL, Brown M. Health and economic burden of the projected obesity trends in the USA and the UK. Lancet. 2011;378(9793):815–25.
12. Pratt JSA, Browne A, Browne NT, Bruzoni M, Cohen M, Desai A, Inge T, Linden BC, Mattar SG, Michalsky M, Podkameni D, Reichard KW, Stanford FC, Zeller MH, Zitsman J. ASMBS pediatric metabolic and bariatric surgery guidelines, 2018. Surg Obes Relat Dis. 2018;14(7):882–901. https://doi.org/10.1016/j.soard.2018.03.019. Epub 2018 Mar 23. PMID: 30077361; PMCID: PMC6097871.
13. NCD Risk Factor Collaboration (NCD-RisC). Worldwide trends in underweight and obesity from 1990 to 2022: a pooled analysis of 3663 population-representative studies with 222 million children, adolescents, and adults. Lancet. 2024;403(10431):1027–50. https://doi.org/10.1016/S0140-6736(23)02750-2. Epub 2024 Feb 29. PMID: 38432237; PMCID: PMC7615769
14. Hales CM, Carroll MD, Fryar CD, Ogden CL. Prevalence of obesity and severe obesity among adults: United States, 2017-2018. NCHS Data Brief. 2020;360:1–8. PMID: 32487284.
15. Messiah SE, Xie L, Atem F, Mathew MS, Qureshi FG, Schneider BE, Cruz-Muñoz N. Disparity between United States adolescent class II and III obesity trends and bariatric surgery utilization, 2015–2018. Ann Surg. 2022;276(2):324–33. https://doi.org/10.1097/SLA.0000000000004493. Epub 2020 Sep 15. PMID: 32941272; PMCID: PMC9825050.
16. Johnson VR, Acholonu NO, Dolan AC, Krishnan A, Wang EH, Stanford FC. Racial disparities in obesity treatment among children and adolescents. Curr Obes Rep. 2021;10(3):342–50. https://doi.org/10.1007/s13679-021-00442-0. Epub 2021 May 14. PMID: 33988825; PMCID: PMC8120762.
17. Malhotra S, Czepiel KS, Akam EY, Shaw AY, Sivasubramanian R, Seetharaman S, Stanford FC. Bariatric surgery in the treatment of adolescent obesity: current perspectives in the United States. Expert rev. Endocrinol Metab. 2021;16(3):123–34. https://doi.org/10.1080/17446651.2021.1914585. Epub 2021 Apr 21. PMID: 33879013; PMCID: PMC9912043
18. Thomas-Eapen N. Childhood obesity. Prim Care. 2021;48(3):505–15. https://doi.org/10.1016/j.pop.2021.04.002. Epub 2021 Jul 8. PMID: 34311854.
19. Ahmad QI, Ahmad CB, Ahmad SM. Childhood obesity. Indian J. Endocrinol Metab. 2010;14:19–25.
20. Sanyaolu A, Okorie C, Qi X, Locke J, Rehman S. Childhood and adolescent obesity in the United States: a public health concern. Glob Pediatr Health. 2019;6:2333794X19891305. https://doi.org/10.1177/2333794X19891305. PMID: 31832491; PMCID: PMC6887808

21. Sahoo K, Sahoo B, Choudhury AK, Sofi NY, Kumar R, Bhadoria AS. Childhood obesity: causes and consequences. J Family Med Prim Care. 2015;4(2):187–92. https://doi.org/10.4103/2249-4863.154628. PMID: 25949965; PMCID: PMC4408699
22. Elks CE, den Hoed M, Zhao JH, Sharp SJ, Wareham NJ, Loos RJ, Ong KK. Variability in the heritability of body mass index: a systematic review and meta-regression. Front Endocrinol (Lausanne). 2012;28(3):29. https://doi.org/10.3389/fendo.2012.00029. PMID: 22645519; PMCID: PMC3355836.
23. Maes HH, Neale MC, Eaves LJ. Genetic and environmental factors in relative body weight and human adiposity. Behav Genet. 1997;27(4):325–51.
24. Speliotes EK, Willer CJ, Berndt SI, MAGIC; Procardis Consortium, et al. Association analyses of 249,796 individuals reveal 18 new loci associated with body mass index. Nat Genet. 2010;42(11):937–48.
25. Huvenne H, Dubern B, Clément K, Poitou C. Rare genetic forms of obesity: clinical approach and current treatments in 2016. Obes Facts. 2016;9(3):158–73. https://doi.org/10.1159/000445061. Epub 2016 Jun 1. PMID: 27241181; PMCID: PMC5644891
26. Lister NB, Baur LA, Felix JF, Hill AJ, Marcus C, Reinehr T, Summerbell C, Wabitsch M. Child and adolescent obesity. Nat Rev Dis Primers. 2023;9(1):24. https://doi.org/10.1038/s41572-023-00435-4. PMID: 37202378.
27. Whitaker RC, Wright JA, Pepe MS, Seidel KD, Dietz WH. Predicting obesity in young adulthood from childhood and parental obesity. N Engl J Med. 1997;337:869–73.
28. Lindberg L, Hagman E, Danielsson P, Marcus C, Persson M. Anxiety and depression in children and adolescents with obesity: a nationwide study in Sweden. BMC Med. 2020;18:30.
29. Rankin J, Matthews L, Cobley S, Han A, Sanders R, Wiltshire HD, Baker JS. Psychological consequences of childhood obesity: psychiatric comorbidity and prevention. Adolesc Health Med Ther. 2016;14(7):125–46. https://doi.org/10.2147/AHMT.S101631. PMID: 27881930; PMCID: PMC5115694.
30. Chung ST, Krenek A, Magge SN. Childhood obesity and cardiovascular disease risk. Curr Atheroscler Rep. 2023;25(7):405–15. https://doi.org/10.1007/s11883-023-01111-4. Epub 2023 May 31. PMID: 37256483; PMCID: PMC10230147.
31. Chung ST, Katz LEL, Stettler-Davis N, Shults J, Sherman A, Ha J, Stefanovski D, Boston RC, Rader DJ, Magge SN. The relationship between lipoproteins and insulin sensitivity in youth with obesity and abnormal glucose tolerance. J Clin Endocrinol Metab. 2022;107(6):1541–51. https://doi.org/10.1210/clinem/dgac113. PMID: 35240684; PMCID: PMC9113822.
32. Goossens GH. The metabolic phenotype in obesity: fat mass, body fat distribution, and adipose tissue function. Obes Facts. 2017;10(3):207–15. https://doi.org/10.1159/000471488.
33. Wu AJ, Aris IM, Rifas-Shiman SL, Oken E, Taveras EM, Chavarro JE, Hivert MF. Associations of mid-childhood to early adolescence central adiposity gain with cardiometabolic health in early adolescence. Obesity (Silver Spring). 2021;29(11):1882–91. https://doi.org/10.1002/oby.23261. Epub 2021 Sep 16. PMID: 34529343; PMCID: PMC8571062.
34. Shah RV, Murthy VL, Abbasi SA, Blankstein R, Kwong RY, Goldfine AB, Jerosch-Herold M, Lima JA, Ding J, Allison MA. Visceral adiposity and the risk of metabolic syndrome across body mass index: the MESA Study. JACC Cardiovasc Imaging. 2014;7(12):1221–35. https://doi.org/10.1016/j.jcmg.2014.07.017. Epub 2014 Nov 5. PMID: 25440591; PMCID: PMC4268163.
35. Nadeau KJ, Anderson BJ, Berg EG, Chiang JL, Chou H, Copeland KC, Hannon TS, Huang TT, Lynch JL, Powell J, Sellers E, Tamborlane WV, Zeitler P. Youth-onset type 2 diabetes consensus report: current status, challenges, and priorities. Diabetes Care. 2016;39(9):1635–42. https://doi.org/10.2337/dc16-1066. Epub 2016 Aug 2. PMID: 27486237; PMCID: PMC5314694.
36. Shah AS, Gidding SS, El Ghormli L, Tryggestad JB, Nadeau KJ, Bacha F, Levitt Katz LE, Willi SM, Lima J, Urbina EM, TODAY Study Group. Relationship between Arterial Stiffness and Subsequent Cardiac Structure and Function in Young Adults with Youth-Onset Type 2 Diabetes: Results from the TODAY Study. J Am Soc Echocardiogr. 2022;35(6):620–628.e4. https://doi.org/10.1016/j.echo.2022.02.001. Epub 2022 Feb 8. PMID: 35149207; PMCID: PMC9177714

37. Ryder JR, Northrop E, Rudser KD, Kelly AS, Gao Z, Khoury PR, Kimball TR, Dolan LM, Urbina EM. Accelerated early vascular aging among adolescents with obesity and/or type 2 diabetes mellitus. J Am Heart Assoc. 2020;9(10):e014891. https://doi.org/10.1161/JAHA.119.014891. Epub 2020 May 6. PMID: 32370578; PMCID: PMC7660865.
38. Burt Solorzano CM, McCartney CR. Obesity and the pubertal transition in girls and boys. Reproduction. 2010;140(3):399–410. https://doi.org/10.1530/REP-10-0119. PMID: 20802107; PMCID: PMC2931339.
39. Franks S. Polycystic ovary syndrome in adolescents. Int J Obes. 2008;32:1035–41.
40. Kaplowitz PB, Slora EJ, Wasserman RC, Pedlow SE, Herman-Giddens ME. Earlier onset of puberty in girls: relation to increased body mass index and race. Pediatrics. 2001;108(2):347–53. https://doi.org/10.1542/peds.108.2.347. PMID: 11483799
41. Vajravelu ME, Tas E, Arslanian S. Pediatric obesity: complications and current day management. Life (Basel). 2023;13(7):1591. https://doi.org/10.3390/life13071591. PMID: 37511966; PMCID: PMC10381624.
42. Ievers-Landis CE, Redline S. Pediatric sleep apnea: implications of the epidemic of childhood overweight. Am J Respir Crit Care Med. 2007;175(5):436–41. https://doi.org/10.1164/rccm.200606-790PP. Epub 2006 Dec 7. PMID: 17158283; PMCID: PMC2176093
43. Hannon TS, Rofey DL, Ryan CM, Clapper DA, Chakravorty S, Arslanian SA. Relationships among obstructive sleep apnea, anthropometric measures, and neurocognitive functioning in adolescents with severe obesity. J Pediatr. 2012;160:732–5. https://doi.org/10.1016/j.jpeds.2011.10.029.
44. Le Garf S, Nègre V, Anty R, Gual P. Metabolic fatty liver disease in children: a growing public health problem. Biomedicines. 2021;9(12):1915. https://doi.org/10.3390/biomedicines9121915. PMID: 34944730; PMCID: PMC8698722.
45. Calcaterra V, Marin L, Vandoni M, Rossi V, Pirazzi A, Grazi R, Patané P, Silvestro GS, Carnevale Pellino V, Albanese I, Fabiano V, Febbi M, Silvestri D, Zuccotti G. Childhood obesity and incorrect body posture: impact on physical activity and the therapeutic role of exercise. Int J Environ Res Public Health. 2022;19(24):16728. https://doi.org/10.3390/ijerph192416728. PMID: 36554608; PMCID: PMC9779104.
46. Shultz SPDHE, Fink PW, Lenoir M, Hills AP. The effects of pediatric obesity on dynamic joint malalignment duaring gait. Clin Biomech. 2014;29(7):8–835.
47. Novais EN, Millis MB. Slipped capital femoral epiphysis: prevalence, pathogenesis, and natural history. Clin Orthop Relat Res. 2012;470(12):3432–8.
48. Herring JA. Genu varum. Tachdjian's pediatric orthopedics. 3rd ed. Philadelphia: Saunders; 2002. p. 839–55.
49. Güven A, Hancılı S, Kuru Lİ. Obesity and increasing rate of infantile Blount disease. Clin Pediatr (Phila). 2014;53(6):539–43. https://doi.org/10.1177/0009922813518424. Epub 2014 Jan 13. PMID: 24419262.
50. Schwimmer JB, Burwinkle TM, Varni JW. Health-related quality of life of severely obese children and adolescents. JAMA. 2003;289:1813.
51. Finkelstein EA, Kang Graham WC, Malhotra R. Lifetime direct medical costs of childhood obesity. Pediatrics May. 2014;133(5):854–62. https://doi.org/10.1542/peds.2014-0063.
52. Lightwood J, Bibbins-Domingo K, Coxson P, Wang YC, Williams L, Goldman L. Forecasting the future economic burden of current adolescent overweight: an estimate of the coronary heart disease policy model. Am J Public Health. 2009;99(12):2230–7. https://doi.org/10.2105/AJPH.2008.152595. Epub 2009 Oct 15. PMID: 19833999; PMCID: PMC2775763.
53. Weihrauch-Blüher S, Schwarz P, Klusmann JH. Childhood obesity: increased risk for cardiometabolic disease and cancer in adulthood. Metabolism. 2019;92:147–52. https://doi.org/10.1016/j.metabol.2018.12.001. Epub 2018 Dec 5. PMID: 30529454.
54. Singhal V, Sella AC, Malhotra S. Pharmacotherapy in pediatric obesity: current evidence and landscape. Curr Opin Endocrinol Diabetes Obes. 2021;28(1):55–63. https://doi.org/10.1097/MED.0000000000000587. PMID: 33186194; PMCID: PMC8082722.
55. Weghuber D, Barrett T, Barrientos-Pérez M, Gies I, Hesse D, Jeppesen OK, Kelly AS, Mastrandrea LD, Sørrig R, Arslanian S, STEP TEENS Investigators. Once-weekly semaglutide

in adolescents with obesity. N Engl J Med. 2022;387(24):2245–57. https://doi.org/10.1056/NEJMoa2208601. Epub 2022 Nov 2. PMID: 36322838; PMCID: PMC9997064.
56. Leung AKC, Wong AHC, Hon KL. Childhood obesity: an updated review. Curr Pediatr Rev. 2024;20(1):2–26. https://doi.org/10.2174/1573396318666220801093225. PMID: 35927921
57. de la Cruz-Muñoz N, Xie L, Quiroz HJ, Kutlu OC, Atem F, Lipshultz SE, Mathew MS, Messiah SE. Long-term outcomes after adolescent bariatric surgery. J Am Coll Surg. 2022;235(4):592–602. https://doi.org/10.1097/XCS.0000000000000325. Epub 2022 Sep 15. PMID: 36102560; PMCID: PMC9484037.
58. Goldenshluger M, Iluz R, Beck T, Adileh M, Segev L, Froilych D, Goldenshluger A, Geron N, Goitein D, Hazzan D. Laparoscopic sleeve gastrectomy in adolescents: ten-years follow-up. Obes Surg. 2023;33(1):32–7. https://doi.org/10.1007/s11695-022-06348-7. Epub 2022 Nov 21. PMID: 36414817.
59. Weiss AC, Parina R, Horgan S, Talamini M, Chang DC, Sandler B. Quality and safety in obesity surgery-15 years of Roux-en-Y gastric bypass outcomes from a longitudinal database. Surg Obes Relat Dis. 2016;12(1):33–40.
60. Bolling CF, Armstrong SC, Reichard KW, Michalsky MP, SECTION ON OBESITY, SECTION ON SURGERY. Metabolic and bariatric surgery for pediatric patients with severe obesity. Pediatrics. 2019;144(6):e20193224. https://doi.org/10.1542/peds.2019-3224. Epub 2019 Oct 27. PMID: 31656226.
61. Paulus GF, de Vaan LE, Verdam FJ, Bouvy ND, Ambergen TA, van Heurn LW. Bariatric surgery in morbidly obese adolescents: a systematic review and meta-analysis. Obes Surg. 2015;25(5):860–78. https://doi.org/10.1007/s11695-015-1581-2. PMID: 25697125; PMCID: PMC4428750.
62. Inge TH, Zeller MH, Jenkins TM, Helmrath M, Brandt ML, Michalsky MP, Harmon CM, Courcoulas A, Horlick M, Xanthakos SA, Dolan L, Mitsnefes M, Barnett SJ, Buncher R, Teen-LABS Consortium. Perioperative outcomes of adolescents undergoing bariatric surgery: the Teen-Longitudinal Assessment of Bariatric Surgery (Teen-LABS) study. JAMA Pediatr. 2014;168(1):47–53. https://doi.org/10.1001/jamapediatrics.2013.4296. PMID: 24189578; PMCID: PMC4060250
63. Al-Mohaidly MT, Al-Asmari AK, Khan HA, Alshngeetee AS, Khan I, Al-Asmari YA, Al-Hussain GO, Alsalem SS, Khan A, Babtain AM, Aljorfi EA, Alshumiesy HA, Aluraifej MA. Laparoscopic sleeve gastrectomy for obesity treatment in adolescents and young adults: a systematic review and meta-analysis. Langenbeck's Arch Surg. 2023;408(1):158. https://doi.org/10.1007/s00423-023-02894-5. PMID: 37093297
64. Zitsman JL, DiGiorgi MF, Zhang AZ, Kopchinski JS, Sysko R, Devlin MJ, Fennoy I. Adolescent gastric banding: a 5-year longitudinal study. Obes Surg. 2020;30(3):828–36. https://doi.org/10.1007/s11695-019-04321-5. PMID: 31820403
65. Messiah SE, Xie L, de la Cruz-Muñoz N, Lipshultz SE. Use of metabolic and bariatric surgery among US youth. JAMA Pediatr. 2023;177(8):856–7. https://doi.org/10.1001/jamapediatrics.2023.0803. PMID: 37252718; PMCID: PMC10230368.
66. Bomberg EM, Palzer EF, Rudser KD, Kelly AS, Bramante CT, Seligman HK, Noni F, Fox CK. Anti-obesity medication prescriptions by race/ethnicity and use of an interpreter in a pediatric weight management clinic. Ther Adv Endocrinol Metab. 2022;11(13):20420188221090009. https://doi.org/10.1177/20420188221090009. PMID: 35432917; PMCID: PMC9005816.
67. De La Cruz-Muñoz N, Lopez-Mitnik G, Arheart KL, Miller TL, Lipshultz SE, Messiah SE. Effectiveness of bariatric surgery in reducing weight and body mass index among Hispanic adolescents. Obes Surg. 2013;23(2):150–6. https://doi.org/10.1007/s11695-012-0730-0; 13:20420188221090009PMCID: PMC3538108.
68. Perez NP, Westfal ML, Stapleton SM, Stanford FC, Griggs CL, Pratt JS, Chang DC, Kelleher CM. Beyond insurance: race-based disparities in the use of metabolic and bariatric surgery for the management of severe pediatric obesity. Surg Obes Relat Dis. 2020;16(3):414–9. https://doi.org/10.1016/j.soard.2019.11.020. Epub 2019 Dec 4. PMID: 31917198; PMCID: PMC7058484.

69. Messiah SE, Lopez-Mitnik G, Winegar D, Sherif B, Arheart KL, Reichard KW, Michalsky MP, Lipshultz SE, Miller TL, Livingstone AS, de la Cruz-Muñoz N. Changes in weight and co-morbidities among adolescents undergoing bariatric surgery: 1-year results from the Bariatric Outcomes Longitudinal Database. Surg Obes Relat Dis. 2013;9(4):503–13. https://doi.org/10.1016/j.soard.2012.03.007. Epub 2012 Mar 28. PMID: 22542199; PMCID: PMC3416929

# Bariatric Surgery in Elderly

# 49

Linda P. Zhang

## Introduction

Bariatric surgery for elderly patients represents a multifaceted approach to addressing obesity-related health concerns in this aging demographic. As the prevalence of obesity among the elderly continues to rise, bariatric procedures offer a viable solution to improve both weight management and associated comorbidities. Common bariatric surgeries, including gastric bypass and sleeve gastrectomy, aim to induce weight loss by altering the gastrointestinal anatomy. While the benefits of these procedures are well-documented, there needs to be an emphasis on tailoring interventions to the unique physiological changes that accompany aging. Defining the age of an "elderly patient" in the context of bariatric surgery varies, but typically, it refers to individuals aged 65 and older. This age threshold is commonly used in clinical practice to categorize patients as elderly but also recognizing that an individual's chronological age may differ from his/her biological age. Preoperative assessments for elderly individuals contemplating bariatric surgery delve into comprehensive evaluations of cardiovascular, renal, and pulmonary functions, as well as considerations for frailty and psychological well-being. The health impact of bariatric surgery may also differ from that of the younger population undergoing bariatric surgery. The landscape of bariatric surgery for the elderly is evolving, with personalized care strategies and a multidisciplinary approach to optimize outcomes and enhance the overall health of older individuals grappling with obesity.

L. P. Zhang (✉)
Icahn School of Medicine at Mount Sinai, New York, NY, USA
e-mail: Linda.zhang@mountsinai.org



O. M. Ghanem et al. (eds.), *The SAGES Manual of Metabolic and Bariatric Surgery*, https://doi.org/10.1007/978-3-031-72309-4_49

## Considerations for Bariatric Surgery in the Elderly

### Preoperative Assessment

The preoperative assessment for bariatric surgery in the elderly requires a nuanced and comprehensive approach to address the unique challenges associated with aging. Medical evaluation in this population should extend beyond the traditional preoperative workup, encompassing a thorough assessment of cardiovascular health, renal function, and pulmonary status. Given the age-related physiological changes, including diminished cardiac reserve and alterations in drug metabolism, careful consideration is essential to tailor preoperative management and optimize the overall cardiovascular fitness of elderly patients.

Prior studies have consistently revealed that, paradoxically, individuals seeking bariatric surgery often exhibit a substantial prevalence of nutritional deficiencies, notwithstanding their obesity [1, 2]. This phenomenon is particularly pronounced among older individuals, who face an elevated risk of malnutrition. Recognizing the critical role of nutrition in postoperative recovery and wound healing, comprehensive nutritional assessments emerge as imperative tools in identifying and addressing potential deficiencies in this population [3, 4]. The proactive identification and management of nutritional deficiencies in older bariatric surgery candidates are pivotal not only for optimizing surgical outcomes but also for minimizing the broader health implications associated with malnutrition in the postoperative phase.

Psychological evaluation also is a crucial component of the preoperative assessment process, particularly in the elderly population considering bariatric surgery. Prior studies have shown that patients with substance abuse, anxiety, and demoralization are significantly more likely to fail to proceed with bariatric surgery [5]. Assessing cognitive function, mental health status, and social support systems helps identify potential challenges and enables the bariatric team to tailor interventions to the individual needs of elderly patients. Furthermore, psychological resilience and readiness for lifestyle changes are paramount factors for successful outcomes. This holistic approach to the preoperative psychological assessment not only contributes to the overall well-being of the patient but also enhances their capacity to cope with the significant lifestyle modifications associated with bariatric surgery.

Frailty assessment plays a pivotal role in determining the surgical candidacy and risk profile of elderly individuals seeking bariatric procedures. Frailty, characterized by reduced physiological reserve and increased vulnerability to stressors, can significantly impact postoperative recovery and overall outcomes [6, 7]. Recognizing frailty as a crucial factor in preoperative assessments is essential, as it influences the overall risk profile and postoperative outcomes. Frailty is associated with an increased susceptibility to complications, prolonged recovery, and higher rates of adverse events [8–10]. In the context of bariatric surgery, prior studies suggest frailty and associated comorbidities in the elderly can exponentially increase the likelihood of postoperative adverse outcomes [10]. It may affect the ability to withstand surgery, exacerbate the potential for postoperative complications, and hinder the recovery process. A recent study based on the MBSAQIP database showed that functional status was the most predictive factor for both serious complications and mortality [11]. Gondal et al. showed that the prevalence of frailty, as defined by the modified frailty index, was seen in 44.4% of patients over age 60 undergoing bariatric surgery, and frailty was an independent factor associated with higher odds of 30-day adverse events [12]. Thus, incorporating frailty assessments into the preoperative evaluation allows for the identification of high-risk patients, enabling healthcare teams to implement targeted interventions and individualized care plans to minimize perioperative risks and enhance the safety of bariatric surgery in the elderly population.

## Age-Related Physiological Changes and Their Impact on Surgery

Age-related physiological changes in the elderly have profound implications for the safety and success of bariatric surgery. As individuals age, there is a natural decline in organ function and reserve capacity, necessitating a thorough understanding of these changes in the context of surgical interventions. Cardiovascular considerations are of utmost importance, as aging is associated with a decline in cardiac output, increased vascular stiffness, and potential changes in response to fluid shifts during surgery [13]. Laparoscopic bariatric surgery can place additional stress on the cardiovascular system due to alterations in blood volume and changes in intra-abdominal pressure, underscoring the need for careful preoperative assessment and management of cardiovascular health in elderly patients.

Renal considerations also play a significant role in the context of bariatric surgery for the elderly. Age-related decline in renal function may impact drug metabolism and clearance, influencing the choice and dosing of medications used perioperatively [14]. Moreover, the potential for dehydration, electrolyte imbalances, and renal complications postoperatively necessitates vigilant monitoring and tailored interventions in older individuals undergoing bariatric procedures. Pulmonary considerations are critical as well, given that aging is associated with decreased lung elasticity and reduced respiratory muscle strength [15]. Bariatric surgery can exacerbate these changes due to alterations in respiratory mechanics, requiring careful perioperative respiratory management to prevent postoperative pulmonary complications in elderly patients.

In addition to these physiological changes, the increased prevalence of comorbidities in the elderly population further complicates the bariatric surgical landscape. Conditions such as diabetes, hypertension, and sleep apnea are more prevalent in older adults and may necessitate additional precautions and tailored management strategies during and after bariatric procedures. The impact of age-related physiological changes on bariatric surgery underscores the importance of individualized care, close monitoring, and a multidisciplinary approach to optimize outcomes and minimize risks in this vulnerable population.

## Choice of Bariatric Procedure for Elderly Patients

Selecting the appropriate bariatric procedure for elderly patients involves a careful evaluation considering the patient's overall health, comorbidities, and the expected impact on age-related physiological changes. While gastric bypass and sleeve gastrectomy are commonly performed, the choice of procedure must be tailored to the individual's unique needs. Factors such as cardiovascular health, renal function, and frailty play crucial roles in decision-making. A shorter duration of procedures, such as the sleeve gastrectomy, may be favored to minimize stress on the body. Overall, many studies have shown a lower risk profile for laparoscopic sleeve gastrectomy compared to laparoscopic Roux-en-Y gastric bypass [16]. One study showed that the rates of adverse events, including acute renal failure and myocardial infarction, were increased in elderly patients compared to the younger population only for the group undergoing Roux-en-Y gastric bypass but not sleeve gastrectomy [7]. Another study examining elderly Medicare patients showed that compared to gastric bypass, sleeve gastrectomy was associated with lower 3-year complications, re-interventions, emergency room utilization, and rehospitalizations [17]. Thus, the potential for complications should be carefully weighed against the anticipated added weight loss benefits of Roux-en-Y gastric bypass. Close collaboration between the surgical team, geriatric specialists, and other healthcare professionals is essential to ensure a thorough assessment and to guide the choice of bariatric procedure that aligns with the patient's specific health profile and goals.

## Use of Pharmacokinetics for Weight Loss

The utilization of pharmacokinetic drugs for the treatment of morbid obesity in elderly patients is complex and requires careful consideration. While various medications targeting weight management are available, their efficacy and safety profiles in the elderly population demand thorough evaluation. The FDA has approved five medications for long-term use for weight loss, namely: orlistat, phentermine-topiramate, naltrexone-bupropion, liraglutide, and semaglutide. Established medications like phentermine-topiramate, orlistat, and naltrexone/bupropion have demonstrated weight loss efficacy exceeding 5% from baseline. However, notable adverse effects have been associated specifically with orlistat and naltrexone-bupropion [18, 19]. Newer medications like liraglutide and semaglutide have become prominent in the comprehensive weight loss management approach. Randomize-controlled trials have shown that liraglutide and semaglutide result in significant weight loss compared to placebo, with an estimated mean weight loss of 6–13% vs 2% in the placebo group [20]. Furthermore, phase 3 randomize-controlled trial comparing weekly subcutaneous injection of semaglutide versus daily liraglutide showed weight change from baseline was −15.8% with semaglutide vs −6.4% with liraglutide at 68 weeks [21]. In addition, semaglutide had the added benefit of reducing the risk of cardiovascular death, myocardial infection, or stroke, in patients with pre-existing cardiovascular disease and who are overweight or obese, but who do not have diabetes [22]. However, these studies do not analyze the efficacy and side effect profile specific to elderly patients. Factors such as age-related changes in metabolism, potential drug interactions, and the presence of comorbidities necessitate a tailored approach. The specific drug selection should be made judiciously, accounting for individual patient characteristics and potential risks. Comprehensive assessment, close monitoring for adverse effects, and regular adjustments are essential components of managing morbid obesity in the elderly through pharmacotherapy, ensuring a balanced and personalized approach to enhance both effectiveness and safety.

## Postoperative Care for Elderly Patients Undergoing Bariatric Surgery

### Cardiovascular Considerations

Specialized postoperative care for elderly patients after bariatric surgery is essential to address the unique challenges associated with aging and promote a successful recovery. As with all postoperative bariatric surgery patients, close monitoring of vital signs is crucial to detect any signs of cardiovascular stress, ensuring early intervention if needed. Considering the potential cardiovascular changes in elderly individuals, this vigilance helps prevent medical complications such as hypotension, electrolyte imbalance, or arrhythmias. Additionally, as elderly patients are more likely to have decreased cardiac function, fluid management needs to be carefully tailored to maintain hydration without overloading the circulatory system, while considering the potential impact on renal function.

### Perioperative Anesthetic and Pain Management

Perioperative anesthetic and postoperative pain management also need to be tailored appropriately for elderly patients. Advanced age affects both the pharmacodynamics and pharmacokinetics of administered drugs [23, 24]. Elderly patients with coexisting diseases are at a greater risk for polypharmacy which can further complicate anesthetic and pain management. In postoperative pain management for elderly patients, healthcare providers often exercise caution with the use of narcotics due to the increased susceptibility of this population to adverse effects such as respiratory depression and cognitive impairment. Alternative approaches, such as multimodal analgesia incorporating non-opioid medications and regional anesthesia techniques, are frequently employed to optimize pain relief while minimizing the risks associated with opioid use in the elderly.

## Postoperative Cognitive Dysfunction or Delirium

Elderly patients undergoing bariatric surgery may be susceptible to age-related cognitive issues, including postoperative cognitive dysfunction and postoperative delirium. While standard bariatric surgery typically entails a brief hospital stay and is unlikely to lead to notable cognitive dysfunction or delirium, elderly individuals exhibit a heightened vulnerability to postoperative delirium and dysfunction. Certainly, elderly patients facing complications, such as a surgical leak, are at high risk for delirium and cognitive dysfunction during the postoperative period. Postoperative cognitive dysfunction can manifest as a decline in memory, attention, and processing speed, and can be exacerbated by the physiological stress of surgery in older individuals [25]. While the exact mechanisms are not fully understood, factors such as inflammation, anesthesia, and perioperative stress may contribute to this cognitive dysfunction. Postoperative delirium, on the other hand, is characterized by acute and fluctuating alterations in attention and awareness, often arising within the first few days after surgery. Both conditions pose challenges in the post-bariatric surgery period, affecting recovery and overall well-being. Minimizing the risk involves thorough preoperative assessments, personalized anesthetic management, and vigilant postoperative monitoring. A multidisciplinary approach, involving geriatric specialists and cognitive health experts, may be crucial in recognizing and managing age-related cognitive issues, ensuring optimal outcomes for elderly patients undergoing bariatric surgery [26].

## Nutritional Support

Nutritional support plays a pivotal role in postoperative care for elderly bariatric patients. Older individuals may be at a higher risk of nutritional deficiencies, and surgical alterations to the digestive tract can exacerbate this. Similar to the younger patient population, adequate protein intake, regular serial monitoring of nutritional markers, and vitamin and mineral supplementation are integral components of this specialized care.

## Mobility

Early ambulation is a vital component of postoperative care for elderly bariatric patients. This practice helps prevent deep vein thrombosis, pneumonia, and postoperative atelectasis, which are more prevalent in the elderly population. For elderly bariatric patients, who may already be dealing with age-related musculoskeletal changes, early ambulation is particularly crucial in preventing deconditioning and promoting overall physical well-being. Healthcare providers should incorporate individualized plans and support mechanisms, such as walking aids or physical therapy, to facilitate and encourage early ambulation in the post-bariatric surgery period, ensuring a smoother recovery process for elderly individuals.

For elderly patients who had prolonged hospitalization after bariatric surgery, rehabilitation programs designed for the elderly are paramount in promoting functional recovery. This personalized approach considers the potential impact of age-related musculoskeletal changes and ensures a safe and gradual progression of physical activity to aid in the restoration of functionality.

### Psychosocial Support

Lastly, psychosocial support is a crucial element of postoperative care for elderly bariatric patients. The emotional and cognitive well-being of older individuals should be considered, and support services may include counseling or support groups. Regular follow-up appointments and ongoing communication between healthcare providers and the elderly patient contribute to the continuous assessment and adjustment of the care plan, ensuring the best possible outcomes in the post-bariatric surgery phase for this demographic.

## Outcomes of Bariatric Surgery in Elderly Patients

### Weight Loss and Maintenance

While some prior studies have shown that the percent of excess weight loss for elderly patients after bariatric surgery is similar to younger patient population, other studies have shown that elderly patients lose less weight after bariatric surgery [27–30]. In a comparative study of patients older ($n = 451$) versus younger ($n = 8593$) than 65 years old, older patients lost less excess weight than younger patients (72.44% versus 86.11%, respectively). Older patients presented higher rates of complications (8.42% versus 5.59%), comorbidities (77.60% versus 55.45%), and revisions (1.33% versus.77%) [28]. Weight loss maintenance in elderly bariatric surgery patients poses unique challenges and considerations. In these prior studies, the frequency of sleeve gastrectomy, gastric bypass, versus duodenal switch were comparable for elderly patients compared to younger patients [28, 29]. While bariatric procedures demonstrate substantial initial weight loss in older individuals, sustaining these benefits over the long term requires careful attention to age-related factors. The aging process may lead to changes in metabolism, muscle mass, and lifestyle, influencing the trajectory of weight management. Additionally, comorbidities and medication use prevalent in the elderly population can impact weight maintenance efforts. A multidisciplinary approach, including ongoing nutritional support, physical activity guidance, and psychological interventions, becomes imperative to address the specific needs and barriers faced by elderly bariatric-surgery patients. Regular monitoring, adapting interventions to accommodate age-related changes, and fostering a supportive environment are essential components in promoting sustained weight loss and overall health in this population.

## Improvement in Comorbidities

Bariatric surgery in elderly patients often leads to significant improvements in comorbidities, marking a transformative impact on their overall health. The procedure has demonstrated notable success in ameliorating conditions commonly associated with obesity, such as diabetes, hypertension, and sleep apnea, among older individuals [31, 32]. Similar to their younger cohort, elderly patients over 65 years old also had improvement or remittance of their diabetes, fatty liver, and sleep apnea (>90% of patients), hypertension and hyperlipidemia (>80% of patients), and hyperuricemia and ischemic heart disease (>70% of the patients) [28]. The postoperative reduction in excess weight and favorable metabolic changes contribute to enhanced glycemic control, lowered blood pressure, and improved respiratory function. These improvements not only alleviate the burden of chronic diseases but also lessen the reliance on medications, offering a potential avenue for polypharmacy reduction in the elderly population. The positive effects on comorbidities contribute not only to the extension of lifespan but also to an improved quality of life for elderly bariatric-surgery patients, showcasing the comprehensive benefits of weight loss interventions in this demographic.

Bariatric surgery in elderly patients not only yields positive physiological outcomes but also frequently results in notable improvements in overall quality of life. Similar to younger populations, elderly individuals may also experience enhanced mobility, increased energy levels, and a greater sense of well-being postoperatively [33, 34]. The relief from obesity-related comorbidities, such as diabetes and hypertension, contributes significantly to an improved quality of life by reducing the burden of chronic health conditions. Furthermore, the psychological benefits stemming from enhanced body image, increased self-esteem, and a sense of regained control over health can have profound effects on the emotional and social aspects of an elderly patient's life [35]. While considering the unique challenges and potential risks associated with bariatric surgery in the elderly, the multifaceted improvements in physical and mental well-being underscore the transformative impact these procedures can have on the overall quality of life in this population.

## Risk of Complication

Elderly patients undergoing bariatric surgery may face an increased risk of complications due to age-related physiological changes and a higher prevalence of comorbidities [29]. Advanced age is associated with diminished organ function, which may exacerbate the challenges posed by surgical interventions. Pechman et al. showed that bariatric patients over 70 years old had increased mortality and increased rates of cardiac, pulmonary, renal, and cerebrovascular morbidity [7]. Conversely, another study showed that of 103 patients over age 70, there were no bariatric-surgery-related mortalities one year after surgery [36]. Another study showed that bariatric surgery among elderly patients was associated with poorer 30-day postoperative outcomes across all categories and was independently associated with serious complications [11]. Additionally, there is an elevated risk of impaired wound healing, respiratory complications, infections, and prolonged hospitalization [37]. The risk of complication is also dependent on the type of bariatric surgery performed [36]. In one study, the Roux-en-Y gastric bypass was associated with a significantly increased rate of early postoperative complications (22.2% vs. 4%), with no difference in late postoperative morbidity [38]. While the overall rates of postoperative mortality and complications are still low, balancing the potential benefits of weight loss with these heightened risks necessitates a careful and individualized approach in managing this vulnerable demographic.

### Comparing the Outcomes of Bariatric Surgery Between Older and Younger Populations

Comparing the outcomes of bariatric surgery between older and younger populations reveals nuanced patterns that reflect the interplay of age-related factors. While both groups generally experience substantial weight loss and improvements in comorbidities, the elderly cohort often faces distinct challenges and considerations [39]. Older individuals may have a higher prevalence of age-related comorbidities and reduced physiological reserve, potentially influencing the risk-benefit profile of surgery. Despite this, studies indicate that compared to younger populations, bariatric procedures in the elderly can lead to similar weight loss, amelioration of obesity-related health conditions, and enhanced quality of life [40]. Similar to the younger population, a shorter duration of comorbidities was a positive predictor for resolution of disease after bariatric surgery for elderly patients [41]. On the other hand, the younger population might exhibit a faster metabolic response and possibly a more straightforward recovery process [11, 42]. Overall, a careful evaluation of individual health status, frailty, and patient goals is crucial in tailoring the approach to bariatric surgery for different age groups, acknowledging that both older and younger patients can experience significant and transformative benefits.

## Ethical Considerations

### Informed Consent in the Elderly Population

Informed consent for bariatric surgery in the elderly population demands careful consideration of age-related factors to ensure that patients are well-informed and can actively participate in the decision-making process. Given the potential complexities associated with age-related comorbidities, diminished cognitive function, and varied expectations, the informed consent process must be comprehensive and tailored to the unique needs of older individuals [43]. Similar to other patient populations, healthcare providers should prioritize clear communication, utilizing layman's terms and providing ample time for questions, to facilitate a thorough understanding of the risks, benefits, and alternatives of bariatric surgery. However, recognizing potential age-related challenges such as diminished decision-making capacity or heightened vulnerability is crucial. Healthcare professionals should engage not only with the patient but also with their support system, involving family members or caregivers in the decision-making process. Documenting the informed consent process meticulously is vital, reflecting the specific considerations discussed with the elderly patient, ensuring ethical standards are upheld, and minimizing the risk of misunderstandings or disputes. This nuanced approach to informed consent acknowledges the unique circumstances of the elderly population and supports their autonomy in making well-informed decisions about bariatric surgery.

## Balancing Risk and Benefits

Balancing the risks and benefits of bariatric surgery for elderly patients is a delicate and crucial aspect of decision-making in healthcare. On one hand, bariatric surgery has demonstrated significant benefits for weight loss and improvement of obesity-related comorbidities, potentially enhancing the overall health and quality of life in elderly individuals. On the other hand, the aging population often presents with a higher prevalence of age-related comorbidities, diminished physiological reserves, and an increased susceptibility to complications. Healthcare professionals must carefully weigh the potential benefits of weight loss against the heightened risks associated with surgery in the elderly, including cardiovascular events, impaired wound healing, and adverse reactions to anesthesia or medications. Individualized assessments, considering the patient's overall health, cognitive function, and social support, are crucial to identifying those who are most likely to benefit from bariatric surgery while minimizing the risks. Engaging in open and transparent communication with the patient and their caregivers is essential to ensuring informed decision-making and managing expectations. The balance between risk and benefit is dynamic and must be continuously reevaluated throughout the preoperative, intra-operative, and postoperative phases, emphasizing the need for a multidisciplinary and patient-centered approach in the complex landscape of bariatric surgery for elderly patients.

## Addressing Ageism in Healthcare

Addressing ageism in elderly patients considering bariatric surgery is crucial to ensuring equitable and patient-centered care. Ageism, the stereotyping, discrimination, or prejudice based on age, can inadvertently influence healthcare decisions and access to certain medical interventions [44, 45]. In the case of bariatric surgery, healthcare professionals must consciously challenge ageist assumptions and recognize that chronological age alone should not be a determining factor in candidacy for these procedures. Instead, a comprehensive assessment that considers the individual's overall health, functional status, and potential benefits from weight loss should guide the decision-making process. Educating healthcare providers on age-related variations in physiological responses to surgery and emphasizing the importance of personalized care plans for elderly patients is vital in combating ageism. Additionally, fostering open communication with elderly individuals about their bariatric procedure preferences, concerns, and goals empowers them to actively participate in decisions related to bariatric surgery. By advocating for a patient-centered approach that values the unique characteristics of each individual, healthcare professionals can contribute to mitigating ageism and promoting fair and unbiased care for elderly patients considering bariatric surgery.

## Future Directions in Bariatric Surgery for the Elderly

The future of bariatric surgery for the elderly is likely to witness significant advancements aimed at tailoring interventions to the unique needs and complexities of this demographic. Research efforts will likely focus on minimizing the impact of bariatric surgery on age-related physiological changes and reduced reserves. Integration of advanced technologies may facilitate safer procedures with quicker recovery times for elderly patients. Additionally, exploring innovative pharmacological and metabolic approaches to weight management specific to the elderly population may become a focal point of research, providing alternative or complementary strategies to traditional surgical interventions.

Multidisciplinary collaboration will play a central role in the future of elderly bariatric surgery. Teams comprising geriatricians, nutritionists, psychologists, and rehabilitation specialists can work collaboratively to design holistic preoperative assessments and comprehensive postoperative care plans. This approach will not only optimize surgical outcomes but also address the broader health and well-being of elderly individuals undergoing bariatric procedures. Furthermore, future research may delve into understanding the long-term effects of bariatric surgery on age-related conditions and cognitive function, contributing to a more comprehensive understanding of the impact of these interventions on the overall health trajectory of elderly patients. The integration of personalized medicine principles and increased awareness among healthcare professionals about the nuances of bariatric surgery in the elderly will likely shape a future landscape that is both effective and considerate of the unique needs of this population.

## Conclusion

In conclusion, bariatric surgery for elderly patients necessitates a meticulous approach encompassing thorough preoperative and postoperative assessments. Special considerations, including the heightened risk of postoperative complications and the need for tailored nutritional, mobility, and psychological support, are paramount in ensuring optimal outcomes for this demographic. Ethical considerations play a crucial role, demanding a balanced evaluation of potential benefits and risks, taking into account the patient's overall health and life expectancy. As advancements in surgical techniques and perioperative care continue, the future of bariatric surgery for elderly patients holds promise for further refinement, emphasizing personalized and ethical approaches to enhance the overall well-being of this population.

## References


1. Ben-Porat T, et al. Nutritional deficiencies in patients with severe obesity before bariatric surgery: what should be the focus during the preoperative assessment? J Acad Nutr Diet. 2020;120(5):874–84.
2. Schweiger C, et al. Nutritional deficiencies in bariatric surgery candidates. Obes Surg. 2010;20(2):193–7.
3. Mastronuzzi T, Grattagliano I. Nutrition as a health determinant in elderly patients. Curr Med Chem. 2019;26(19):3652–61.
4. Yu Z, et al. Association of malnutrition with all-cause mortality in the elderly population: a 6-year cohort study. Nutr Metab Cardiovasc Dis. 2021;31(1):52–9.
5. Marek RJ, et al. Associations between psychological test results and failure to proceed with bariatric surgery. Surg Obes Relat Dis. 2017;13(3):507–13.
6. Artiles-Armas M, et al. The comprehensive complication index is related to frailty in elderly surgical patients. J Surg Res. 2019;244:218–24.
7. Pechman DM, et al. Bariatric surgery in the elderly: outcomes analysis of patients over 70 using the ACS-NSQIP database. Surg Obes Relat Dis. 2019;15(11):1923–32.
8. Turrentine FE, et al. Surgical risk factors, morbidity, and mortality in elderly patients. J Am Coll Surg. 2006;203(6):865–77.
9. Ko FC. Preoperative frailty evaluation: a promising risk-stratification tool in older adults undergoing general surgery. Clin Ther. 2019;41(3):387–99.
10. Sebastian R, et al. Validation of the cumulative deficit theory in bariatric surgery: new bariatric frailty score is associated with non-home discharge, prolonged hospital stay and mortality in the era of fast-track bariatric surgery. Surg Obes Relat Dis. 2022;18(6):779–88.
11. Albacete S, et al. A 5-year characterization of trends and outcomes in elderly patients undergoing elective bariatric surgery. Surg Endosc. 2023;37(7):5397–404.
12. Gondal AB, et al. A frailty index and the impact of frailty on postoperative outcomes in older patients after bariatric surgery. Surg Obes Relat Dis. 2019;15(9):1582–8.
13. de Almeida A, Ribeiro TP, de Medeiros IA. Aging: molecular pathways and implications on the cardiovascular system. Oxidative Med Cell Longev. 2017;2017:7941563.
14. Kitai Y, Nangaku M, Yanagita M. Aging-related kidney diseases. Contrib Nephrol. 2021;199:266–73.
15. Miller MR. Structural and physiological age-associated changes in aging lungs. Semin Respir Crit Care Med. 2010;31(5):521–7.
16. Moon RC, et al. Morbidity rates and weight loss after Roux-en-Y gastric bypass, sleeve gastrectomy, and adjustable gastric banding in patients older than 60 years old: which procedure to choose? Obes Surg. 2016;26(4):730–6.
17. Chao GF, et al. Bariatric surgery in medicare patients: examining safety and healthcare utilization in the disabled and elderly. Ann Surg. 2022;276(1):133–9.
18. Idrees Z, Cancarevic I, Huang L. FDA-approved pharmacotherapy for weight loss over the last decade. Cureus. 2022;14(9):e29262.
19. Shi Q, et al. Pharmacotherapy for adults with overweight and obesity: a systematic review and network meta-analysis of randomised controlled trials. Lancet. 2022;399(10321):259–69.
20. O'Neil PM, et al. Efficacy and safety of semaglutide compared with liraglutide and placebo for weight loss in patients with obesity: a randomised, double-blind, placebo and active controlled, dose-ranging, phase 2 trial. Lancet. 2018;392(10148):637–49.

21. Rubino DM, et al. Effect of weekly subcutaneous semaglutide vs daily liraglutide on body weight in adults with overweight or obesity without diabetes: the STEP 8 randomized clinical trial. JAMA. 2022;327(2):138–50.
22. Lincoff AM, et al. Semaglutide and cardiovascular outcomes in obesity without diabetes. N Engl J Med. 2023;389(24):2221–32.
23. Shi S, Klotz U. Age-related changes in pharmacokinetics. Curr Drug Metab. 2011;12(7):601–10.
24. Klotz U. Pharmacokinetics and drug metabolism in the elderly. Drug Metab Rev. 2009;41(2):67–76.
25. Lin X, et al. The potential mechanism of postoperative cognitive dysfunction in older people. Exp Gerontol. 2020;130:110791.
26. Swarbrick CJ, Partridge JSL. Evidence-based strategies to reduce the incidence of postoperative delirium: a narrative review. Anaesthesia. 2022;77(Suppl 1):92–101.
27. Kachmar M, et al. Bariatric surgery in the elderly population: a multi-surgeon, single-institution retrospective review. JSLS. 2023;27(3):e2023.00028.
28. Susmallian S, et al. Outcome of bariatric surgery in older patients. Surg Obes Relat Dis. 2018;14(11):1705–13.
29. Elbahrawy A, et al. Medium to long-term outcomes of bariatric surgery in older adults with super obesity. Surg Obes Relat Dis. 2018;14(4):470–6.
30. Garofalo F, et al. Long-term outcome after laparoscopic sleeve gastrectomy in patients over 65 years old: a retrospective analysis. Surg Obes Relat Dis. 2017;13(1):1–6.
31. Abbas M, et al. Outcomes of laparoscopic sleeve gastrectomy and Roux-en-Y gastric bypass in patients older than 60. Obes Surg. 2015;25(12):2251–6.
32. Pereira AF, et al. Impact of bariatric surgery in elderly patients with obesity. Rev Col Bras Cir. 2022;49:e20223299.
33. Pereira MG, Faria S, Lopes H. Quality of life one year after bariatric surgery: the moderator role of spirituality. Obes Surg. 2019;29(4):1207–15.
34. Versteegden DPA, Van Himbeeck MJJ, Nienhuijs SW. Improvement in quality of life after bariatric surgery: sleeve versus bypass. Surg Obes Relat Dis. 2018;14(2):170–4.
35. Vegel AJ, et al. Patient-reported quality of life after bariatric surgery: a single institution analysis. J Surg Res. 2017;218:117–23.
36. Belluzzi A, et al. Long-term safety and efficacy of bariatric surgery in septuagenarians. Obes Surg. 2023;33(12):3778–85.
37. Mabeza RM, et al. Bariatric surgery outcomes in geriatric patients: a contemporary, nationwide analysis. Surg Obes Relat Dis. 2022;18(8):1005–11.
38. Drai C, et al. Long-term results of sleeve gastrectomy and Roux-en-Y gastric bypass in individuals older than 60 years with morbid obesity. Obes Surg. 2023;33(12):3850–9.
39. Dowgiałło-Gornowicz N, Lech P, Major P. Bariatric and metabolic surgery in patients older than 65 years – a multicenter study. Obes Surg. 2023;33(10):3106–11.
40. Bhandari M, et al. Outcomes of bariatric surgery in geriatric patients ≥ 65 years: single institution study. Obes Surg. 2019;29(5):1470–6.
41. Dowgiałło-Gornowicz N, et al. Predictors of complete remission of type 2 diabetes in patients over 65 years of age – a multicenter study. Obes Surg. 2023;33(8):2269–75.
42. Quintero JHR, et al. Safety and efficacy of Roux-en-Y gastric bypass in older aged patients. Rev Col Bras Cir. 2022;49:e20223332.
43. Silbert BS, Scott DA. Informed consent in patients with frailty syndrome. Anesth Analg. 2020;130(6):1474–81.
44. Holmes E, Crome P, Arora A. Patients' preferences and existential perspective: what to consider and how should patient's expectations be guided? Aging Clin Exp Res. 2018;30(3):271–5.
45. White SM. Ethical and legal aspects of anaesthesia for the elderly. Anaesthesia. 2014;69(Suppl 1):45–53.

# Bariatric Surgery in Patients with Inflammatory Bowel Disease

50

Robert M. MacGregor and Shaina R. Eckhouse

## Introduction

Obesity is an increasingly prevalent and progressive chronic disease affecting over 35% of the population in the United States and worldwide [1–5]. It is estimated that nearly 600 million people worldwide meet the clinical criteria for obesity (body mass index, BMI $\geq$ 30 kg/m$^2$) [5]. At the same time, the prevalence of inflammatory bowel disease (IBD), which primarily consists of Crohn's disease (CD) or ulcerative colitis (UC), has increased [3, 6]. Though historically IBD patients were more likely to live in a malabsorptive and catabolic disease state, the prevalence of obesity and severe obesity in IBD patients is rising, and estimated to be 20 to 30% and 2 to 5%, respectively [7, 8]. IBD patients with severe obesity have been shown to report lower quality of life scores compared to those IBD patients with normal weight [9]. This is in part due to the challenging aspects of medical management of IBD in the setting of obesity, including difficulty with the dosing of weight-based immunosuppression and decreased response to biological agents over time [10, 11].

Over the past several decades, the surgical treatment of severe obesity has been shown to be an effective tool to lose weight, improve metabolic comorbidities, and decrease the risk of cardiovascular disease [12, 13]. Numerous bariatric procedures have been described and performed, with sleeve gastrectomy (SG) and Roux-en-Y gastric bypass (RYGB) being the most widely used today. The number of bariatric procedures performed per year has increased with the increasing prevalence of obesity [14]. As a result, surgical management of morbid obesity in patients with IBD

R. M. MacGregor
Department of Surgery, Washington University School of Medicine, Saint Louis, MO, USA

S. R. Eckhouse (✉)
Division of Minimally Invasive Surgery, Department of Surgery, Duke University School of Medicine, Durham, NC, USA
e-mail: Shaina.eckhouse@duke.edu



O. M. Ghanem et al. (eds.), *The SAGES Manual of Metabolic and Bariatric Surgery*, https://doi.org/10.1007/978-3-031-72309-4_50

is regularly considered. However, performing bariatric surgery in patients with IBD has been appropriately met with caution due to perceived challenges and complications unique to this patient population, including the inflammatory involvement of the bowel wall, history of prior bowel resections, and increased likelihood of nutritional deficiencies [15]. Most published data on the feasibility and safety of bariatric surgery in patients with inflammatory bowel disease comes from small case series, which makes it difficult to develop definitive conclusions in this challenging patient population. In parallel, de novo IBD is a risk following bariatric surgery. This chapter aims to summarize the existing literature on obesity and IBD, the perioperative considerations, technical aspects, and outcomes of bariatric surgery in patients with IBD.

## Obesity and IBD

Obesity leads to a chronic low-grade inflammatory state which increases the risk of other chronic inflammatory conditions, including IBD [16].There are multiple mechanisms signaling both disease processes from hypertrophic adipocytes leading to increased release of proinflammatory cytokines [16, 17]. More specifically, increased interleukins, chemokines, macrophage-mediated pathways, and acute phase reactions are one mechanism facilitating the environment for the development of IBD. Other mechanisms that may be active in both obesity and IBD include increased adipokinin release, a change in the gut microbiome, and alterations in bile acids. First, adipokinins, such as resistin, ghrelin, and leptin all regulate metabolism and immune function and contribute to the increased proinflammatory state of IBD. Also, dysbiosis, or an alteration of the gut microbiome occurs, in proinflammatory states, such as obesity and IBD. Specifically, obesity and IBD are both associated with a reduction of *Bacteroidetes* and an increase in *Proteobacteria* [16–18]. Decreased bacterial diversity potentiates inflammation within the gastrointestinal system which can lead to increased intestinal permeability and bacterial translocation, which in turn potentiates systemic inflammation. These types of changes are seen in a Western-style diet, in obesity, and in IBD; however, the direct link between all three remains poorly understood [2, 16–18]. Lastly, dysbiosis seen in obesity and IBD can alter bile acid conjugation and metabolism. Specifically, increased *Bacteroidetes* associated with obesity and IBD likely increase deconjugation of bile acids that then promote increased intestinal inflammation seen in IBD [19].

The aggregation of these mechanisms leads to the inflammatory state described in both obesity and IBD. However, a causal link between the two disease processes has yet to be identified. For example, a direct relationship exists between BMI and CRP, but it is unclear how the increasing inflammatory state of increasing weight correlates with IBD [16, 18]. Specific to CD, increasing BMI has been correlated with increased risk of CD and increased risk of stricture development and hospitalizations [17]. This same relationship has not been described in UC, and variability exists with corticosteroid use, emergency department (ED) visits, hospitalizations, and surgery in the setting of increasing BMI in the setting of UC [17]. While the causal relationship between obesity and IBD remains unclear, the parallels in the proinflammatory states that develop cannot be ignored. With the prevalence of obesity continuing to increase, two questions remain important for the bariatric surgeon to consider. First, will the prevalence of IBD in patients undergoing bariatric surgery increase? Second, can we treat the proinflammatory state of IBD by treating the proinflammatory state of obesity?

## Bariatric Surgery and IBD

Considering the increasing prevalence of IBD in parallel to the increasing prevalence of obesity discussed previously, significant consideration should be given to treating obesity as it may positively impact the course of IBD. Bariatric surgery remains the most effective treatment for obesity. However, patients with IBD need to be approached carefully when compared to patients without IBD due to the potential impact of bariatric surgery on IBD complications and disease progression.

### Preoperative Considerations

Comprehensive preoperative planning and patient selection are crucial to performing bariatric surgery. The key principles for effective preoperative evaluation of patients include the evaluation and education from a multidisciplinary team, including bariatric surgeons, psychologists, physical therapists, dieticians, and consistent perioperative hospital teams, and the reporting of outcomes longitudinally [20]. Considering the added challenges of IBD, collaboration with gastroenterology to aid in counseling the patient, assess disease severity, evaluate the timing of surgery, and help plan medication management perioperatively.

When counseling preoperatively, it is important to discuss the risk of immunosuppressive medications used for IBD that increase the risk of postoperative complications, such as anastomotic leak and fistula [21]. Furthermore, understanding how the patient reacts when their immunomodulators are held for a short period of time may be necessary for bariatric surgery. More specifically, understanding the nature of the patient's symptoms, IBD flares, hospitalizations, and surgical interventions is imperative to develop a plan with gastroenterology for medication management perioperatively, type of bariatric surgery, and management plan for possible exacerbation of the existing IBD.

The severity of the disease is important to assess in partnership with gastroenterology. Patients with active disease and/or difficult-to-control symptoms should have their IBD treated first before moving forward with bariatric surgery. Several small series of patients evaluated retrospectively reported patients with IBD-related symptoms requiring hospitalization within the first 2 years postoperatively [22, 23]. Furthermore, understanding options for tapering down steroids and holding biologics is imperative to ensure safe surgical planning without worsening IBD symptoms.

Also, endoscopic and colonoscopic evaluation should be performed with regular surveillance to ensure IBD is well controlled without active inflammation in patients undergoing bariatric surgery. Lastly, understanding the patient's history of IBD-related complications, like upper gastrointestinal strictures in Crohn's disease (CD), is imperative to understand before considering bariatric surgery. Thus, incorporating gastroenterology into the evaluation of these patients should be the standard of care.

## Procedure Type

While no large studies or randomized control trials currently exist in the literature, many small series and database evaluations have demonstrated the safety and efficacy of bariatric surgery in patients with IBD [22–26]. The surgery of choice for patients with IBD is the sleeve gastrectomy (SG) [14, 21, 25–28]. Currently, it is the most common procedure performed in patients with IBD, accounting for 70 to 95% of all bariatric surgeries in this population [14, 21, 25, 26, 28]. While weight loss results are variable at 2 years postoperatively when comparing the SG to the Roux-en-Y gastric bypass (RYGB), other concerns specific to IBD indicate that SG may remain the best option [28]. For example, several studies demonstrate a trend toward disease worsening with IBD following RYGB [21, 28]. Mechanisms proposed to explain this trend with RYGB include small bowel anastomosis, increased risk of small intestinal bacterial overgrowth, changes in the microbiome, and increased exposure to different chemicals because of the surgically altered anatomy [21, 28].

The RYGB is the second most common operation performed on patients with IBD [21, 25–28]. In both small retrospective series and large database outcomes studies, this holds true. Interestingly, when evaluating trends in bariatric surgery in patients with IBD from 2004 to 2014, the use of RYGB declined as the use of the SG increased. This is in part due to the higher risk of complications in small series [23]. Nevertheless, patients with both IBD and gastroesophageal reflux disease (GERD) may benefit more from RYGB than SG. While no data exists for this recommendation, it is well known that SG is associated with both de novo GERD and worsening of GERD symptoms [29]. Patients will need to be counseled on the higher risk of complications, including IBD exacerbations. Therefore, it is important to include gastroenterology in the decision-making for surgery and ensure IBD is in remission.

The third most common operation utilized is the adjustable gastric band, reported historically as 11.6% of all procedures performed in patients with IBD in a systemic review. However, like the RYGB, the yearly rates of placement of an adjustable gastric band continue to decline [14]. In fact, a study by Reenaers et al. demonstrated an increased risk of IBD flares requiring hospitalizations and postoperative complications with the adjustable gastric band in patients with IBD [25].

Considering the concerns that exist for performing RYGB in patients with IBD, the use of more malabsorptive operations, such as the duodenal switch and single anastomosis duodenal ileostomy, should be avoided no matter how severe the patient's obesity and other comorbid conditions exist. No published studies exist for either procedure, which may be because these procedures have a higher risk than the RYGB for malabsorptive complications.

## Outcomes of Bariatric Surgery in Patients with IBD

Studies investigating the outcomes of bariatric surgery in patients with IBD have yielded mixed results. While some reports suggest that bariatric surgery can lead to significant weight loss and improvement in metabolic parameters in this population, others highlight the potential risks and complications.

The two most common bariatric procedures, SG and RYGB, both demonstrate substantial weight loss and metabolic improvement in patients with IBD, similar to that of patients without IBD [14, 21, 26, 30]. These outcomes can lead to a reduction in obesity-related comorbidities, such as type 2 diabetes and hypertension, and an improvement in overall quality of life [23, 26, 29]. Overall quality-of-life improvements and IBD-specific quality-of-life improvements have been noted in patients with IBD following bariatric surgery [22, 26].

The impact of bariatric surgery on disease activity in patients with IBD remains a subject of debate. Improvements in IBD status may occur with bariatric surgery, including prolonged disease remission, reduction in the need for immunosuppressive medications, and improved efficacy of pharmacologic therapies [23–25, 28]. However, these benefits need to be balanced with the risks of bariatric surgery, including postoperative complications, readmissions, hospitalizations, and IBD progression. For example, in a series of 88 patients followed retrospectively, mostly patients undergoing SG, 3.5% of patients required less medications for IBD whereas 18% required an escalation in treatment [25]. Another small series demonstrated a reduction in IBD medications in all 20 patients included [24]. Moreover, in a prospective multi-institutional study of over 480 patients with IBD and morbid obesity, patients with IBD who underwent SG had a lower risk of IBD-related complications and lower risk for the need for intravenous corticosteroid use 2 years postoperatively where no improvement was seen in patients who underwent RYGB [28]. Conversely, a series of 54 patients demonstrated increased requirements for medication management of IBD-related complications following RYGB [23]. When evaluated in aggregate as a meta-analysis, Garg et al. found a 45% decrease in the need for IBD medications following bariatric surgery [31]. These studies exemplify the variability in IBD-specific outcomes following bariatric surgery; however, it does seem that the SG more consistently either does not affect or improves IBD-specific outcomes.

## Postoperative Complications

The presence of IBD increases the risk of complications following bariatric surgery. These complications may include postoperative complications, IBD-specific exacerbations, malabsorption, and micronutrient deficiencies [21, 26, 27, 32, 33].

When evaluating the risk of postoperative complications, there appears to be an overall increased risk with bariatric surgery of all types [21, 26]. In one study evaluating immediate postoperative complications with the National Inpatient Sample (NIS) Database, patients with all IBD were found to have a higher risk of small bowel obstruction [32]. However, most studies have not demonstrated any higher risk for anastomotic leak, fistula, or postoperative bleeding during initial postoperative hospitalization [27, 32]. In another study evaluating the National Readmission Database (NRD), all-cause postoperative complications were 48% higher in patients with IBD following SG when compared to patients without IBD [21]. Despite the increased risk, which includes small bowel obstruction and gastric outlet obstruction, there was no difference in readmission rates, length of stay or mortality [21, 27, 33].

Patients with IBD are at risk of experiencing disease exacerbations following bariatric surgery up to 2 years postoperatively. IBD flares may manifest as increased abdominal pain, diarrhea, and gastrointestinal bleeding. In a recent systematic review of seven studies, 16% of patients experienced exacerbations of their IBD [34]. In another systematic review of 11 studies of IBD, one out of five patients required higher doses of medications following bariatric surgery [35]. In smaller series, patients undergoing RYGB required 37% escalation in IBD medications when compared to only 4% following SG [23]. One manifestation specific to CD is upper gastrointestinal strictures, which have increased in prevalence from 5.1% to 11.3% [29]. While no studies exist regarding CD strictures after bariatric surgery, endoscopic dilation is likely the best first-line therapy as it is typically successful in patients who have normal anatomy. If dilations and medication management of the CD do not resolve the stricture, then a revisional procedure may be warranted [29].

Bariatric surgery and IBD independently can lead to malabsorption and micronutrition deficiencies. When combined, there is a higher risk of vitamin and mineral deficiencies such as vitamin B12, iron, and folate [25, 29]. This is of particular concern with the RYGB due to the surgically altered anatomy. Malabsorption, which can manifest as either diarrhea or dumping syndrome, is a well-known complication of RYGB, that may be more prevalent in patients with IBD [29, 36]. Small intestinal bacterial overgrowth can also lead to malabsorption and diarrhea following bariatric surgery, and patients with IBD have a 9.5 times higher risk [29, 36].

## De Novo IBD

A theme that is increasingly described in the literature is the concept of de novo IBD following bariatric surgery [30, 35, 36]. While there is an increased risk of CD in the setting of a patient who has undergone an RYGB, there is a less clear relationship between bariatric surgery either preventing or promoting the development of IBD. Overall, a meta-analysis of 31 articles evaluating the prevalence of de novo IBD following bariatric surgery reported a 17% increase in relative risk postoperatively (95% confidence interval 1.06–1.29) [36]. Most commonly, patients report symptoms of abdominal pain and diarrhea, which can occur with many of the complications of bariatric surgery like dumping syndrome and marginal ulceration following RYGB. However, when looking at individual articles, variations in the results reported exist. For example, Ungaro et al. first described a case series of 15 patients developing IBD at approximately 6 years postoperatively from bariatric surgery [37]. In contrast, Kochhar et al. reported the prevalence of new-onset IBD was lower in patients post-bariatric surgery when compared to controls [38]. Mechanisms for de novo IBD remain unknown but may be due to a conglomeration of factors including changes in the microbiome that favor an increase in *Proteobacteria*, which has been described following bariatric surgery [36].

## Conclusions

Bariatric surgery is an effective and valuable treatment for the disease of obesity in patients with IBD with comparable weight loss outcomes when compared to patients without IBD. However, careful preoperative planning and counseling must be performed considering the increased risk of complications with both CD and UC. Multidisciplinary collaboration amongst the healthcare team, including gastroenterologists and surgeons, is essential to optimize outcomes and decrease complications in these complex patients. Currently, the most common procedure performed in patients with both obesity and IBD is the SG as it may have a lower risk of complications, including technical complications, nutritional complications, and complications secondary to IBD. De novo IBD, specifically CD, may form after malabsorptive operations, and patients need to be counseled on the risk of this. Further research is needed to elucidate the long-term effects of bariatric surgery in patients with IBD and to refine patient selection criteria and perioperative management strategies.

## References

1. Molodecky NA, Soon IS, Rabi DM, et al. Increasing incidence and prevalence of the inflammatory bowel diseases with time, based on systematic review. Gastroenterology. 2012;142:46–54.e42.
2. Singh S, Dulai PS, Zarrinpar A, et al. Obesity in IBD: epidemiology, pathogenesis, disease course and treatment outcomes. Nat Rev Gastroenterol Hepatol. 2017;14:110–21.
3. Moran GW, Dubeau M-F, Kaplan GG, et al. The increasing weight of Crohn's disease subjects in clinical trials. Inflamm Bowel Dis. 2013;19:2949–56.
4. Ng M, Fleming T, Robinson M, et al. Global, regional, and national prevalence of overweight and obesity in children and adults during 1980–2013: a systematic analysis for the Global Burden of Disease Study 2013. Lancet. 2014;384:766–81.

5. Smith KB, Smith MS. Obesity statistics. Prim Care. 2016;43:121–35.
6. Blain A, Cattan S, Beaugerie L, et al. Crohn's disease clinical course and severity in obese patients. Clin Nutr. 2002;21:51–7.
7. Causey MW, Johnson EK, Miller S, et al. The impact of obesity on outcomes following major surgery for Crohn's disease: an American College of Surgeons National Surgical Quality Improvement Program Assessment. Dis Colon Rectum. 2011;54:1488–95.
8. Flores A, Burstein E, Cipher DJ, et al. Obesity in inflammatory bowel disease: a marker of less severe disease. Dig Dis Sci. 2015;60:2436–45.
9. Seminerio JL, Koutroubakis IE, Ramos-Rivers C, et al. Impact of obesity on the management and clinical course of patients with inflammatory bowel disease. Inflamm Bowel Dis. 2015;21:2857–63.
10. Harper JW, Sinanan MN, Zisman TL. Increased body mass index is associated with earlier time to loss of response to infliximab in patients with inflammatory bowel disease. Inflamm Bowel Dis. 2013;19:2118–24.
11. Bultman E, de Haar C, van Liere-Baron A, et al. Predictors of dose escalation of adalimumab in a prospective cohort of Crohn's disease patients. Aliment Pharmacol Ther. 2012;35:335–41.
12. Duvoisin C, Favre L, Allemann P, et al. Roux-en-Y Gastric Bypass. Ann Surg. 2018;268:1019–25.
13. Aminian A, Zajichek A, Arterburn DE, et al. Association of metabolic surgery with major adverse cardiovascular outcomes in patients with type 2 diabetes and obesity. JAMA. 2019;322:1271.
14. Sharma P, McCarty TR, Njei B. Impact of bariatric surgery on outcomes of patients with inflammatory bowel disease: a nationwide inpatient sample analysis, 2004–2014. Obes Surg. 2018;28:1015–24.
15. Beddy D, Dozois EJ, Pemberton JH. Perioperative complications in inflammatory bowel disease. Inflamm Bowel Dis. 2011;17:1610–9.
16. Kim JH, Oh C-M, Yoo JH. Obesity and novel management of inflammatory bowel disease. World J Gastroenterol. 2023;29:1779–94.
17. Johnson A, Loftus E. Obesity in inflammatory bowel disease: a review of its role in the pathogenesis, natural history, and treatment of IBD. Saudi J Gastroenterol. 2021;27:183.
18. Khakoo NS, Ioannou S, Khakoo NS, et al. Impact of obesity on inflammatory bowel disease. Curr Gastroenterol Rep. 2022;24:26–36.
19. Huang C, Tan H, Song M, et al. Maternal Western diet mediates susceptibility of offspring to Crohn's-like colitis by deoxycholate generation. Microbiome. 2023;11:96.
20. Optimal Resources for Metabolic and Bariatric Surgery 2019 Standards--Revised. Chicago: American College of Surgeons; 2019.
21. Wilson NC, Dilsaver DB, Walters RW, et al. Bariatric surgery outcomes in patients with inflammatory bowel disease in the United States: an analysis of the Nationwide readmissions database. Obes Surg. 2024;27 https://doi.org/10.1007/s11695-024-07111-w. Epub ahead of print February.
22. Aelfers S, Janssen IMC, Aarts EO, et al. Inflammatory bowel disease is not a contraindication for bariatric surgery. Obes Surg. 2018;28:1681–7.
23. Heshmati K, Lo T, Tavakkoli A, et al. Short-term outcomes of inflammatory bowel disease after Roux-en-Y gastric bypass vs sleeve gastrectomy. J Am Coll Surg. 2019;228:893-901e1.
24. Aminian A, Andalib A, Ver MR, et al. Outcomes of bariatric surgery in patients with inflammatory bowel disease. Obes Surg. 2016;26:1186–90.
25. Reenaers C, de Roover A, Kohnen L, et al. Bariatric surgery in patients with inflammatory bowel disease: a case-control study from the GETAID. Inflamm Bowel Dis. 2022;28:1198–206.
26. Wallhuss A, Ottosson J, Cao Y, et al. Outcomes of bariatric surgery for patients with prevalent inflammatory bowel disease: a nationwide registry-based cohort study. Surgery. 2023;174:144–51.
27. Corbière L, Scanff A, Desfourneaux V, et al. Outcomes of bariatric surgery in patients with inflammatory bowel disease from a French nationwide database. Br J Surg. 2023;110:251–9.

28. Desai A, Hashash JG, Baker G, et al. Effect of bariatric surgery on disease outcomes in patients with inflammatory bowel disease. J Clin Gastroenterol. 2023;27 https://doi.org/10.1097/MCG.0000000000001879. Epub ahead of print June.
29. Singh A, Koenen B, Kirby DF. Bariatric surgery and its complications in inflammatory bowel disease patients. Inflamm Bowel Dis. 2020;26:1155–65.
30. Mian A, Khan S. Systematic review: outcomes of bariatric surgery in patients with inflammatory bowel disease and de-novo IBD development after bariatric surgery. Surgeon. 2023;21:e71–7.
31. Garg R, Mohan BP, Ponnada S, et al. Safety and efficacy of bariatric surgery in inflammatory bowel disease patients: a systematic review and meta-analysis. Obes Surg. 2020;30:3872–83.
32. Bazerbachi F, Sawas T, Vargas EJ, et al. Bariatric surgery is acceptably safe in obese inflammatory bowel disease patients: analysis of the nationwide inpatient sample. Obes Surg. 2018;28:1007–14.
33. Mabeza RM, Vadlakonda A, Chervu N, et al. Short-term outcomes of bariatric surgery in patients with inflammatory bowel disease: a national analysis. Surg Obes Relat Dis. 2024;20:146–52.
34. Shoar S, Shahabuddin Hoseini S, Naderan M, et al. Bariatric surgery in morbidly obese patients with inflammatory bowel disease: a systematic review. Surg Obes Relat Dis. 2017;13:652–9.
35. Wise J, Plescia T, Cummings BP, et al. Exploring the relationship between bariatric surgery and inflammatory bowel disease: a systematic review. Crohns Colitis. 2022;360:4 . Epub ahead of print April 1. https://doi.org/10.1093/crocol/otac013.
36. Kermansaravi M, Valizadeh R, Farazmand B, et al. De novo inflammatory bowel disease following bariatric surgery: a systematic review and meta-analysis. Obes Surg. 2022;32:3426–34.
37. Ungaro R, Fausel R, Chang HL, et al. Bariatric surgery is associated with increased risk of new-onset inflammatory bowel disease: case series and national database study. Aliment Pharmacol Ther. 2018;47:1126–34.
38. Kochhar GS, Desai A, Syed A, et al. Risk of de-novo inflammatory bowel disease among obese patients treated with bariatric surgery or weight loss medications. Aliment Pharmacol Ther. 2020;51:1067–75.

# Bariatric Surgery as a Bridge Therapy 51

Mai Al Khadem, Mina A. Ibrahim, and Mujjahid Abbas

Bariatric surgery is indicated when a patient crosses a certain body mass index (BMI) with or without comorbidities. Individuals exceeding a certain weight threshold often encounter significant challenges in weight loss, making it arduous, if not nearly unattainable. Moreover, certain medical procedures might not be feasible for individuals falling outside a designated weight range, potentially excluding them from candidacy. The following outlines the different situations where bariatric surgery can be used as a bridge to achieve the required weight to achieve candidacy.

## Orthopedic Surgeries

Osteoarthritis is a common condition that is increasing in prevalence with age with approximately 595 million people being affected in 2020 [15]. Obesity is a known risk factor for the development and progression of osteoarthritis often necessitating joint replacement [45]. The weight causes cartilage damage that is identified by MRI well before symptoms develop [42]. Despite the common belief that obesity's impact on osteoarthritis is primarily mechanical, it is important to recognize that obesity's effects extend beyond weight-bearing stress on joints. Obesity is a metabolic disease that comprises a persistent inflammatory state that affects all the joint components [30]. Obesity does not solely pose a risk to the weight-bearing joints like the knees and hips; it also impacts the non-weight bearing joints such as the hands and shoulders [28, 66]. A workgroup of the American Association of Hip and Knee Surgeons performed a literature review on obesity and total joint arthroplasty.

M. Al Khadem · M. A. Ibrahim · M. Abbas (✉)
Department of Surgery/Bariatric Division, University Hospitals Cleveland Medical Center, Case Western Reserve University School of Medicine, Cleveland, OH, USA
e-mail: Mai.alkhadem@uhhospitals.org; Mujjahid.abbas@uhhospitals.org



O. M. Ghanem et al. (eds.), *The SAGES Manual of Metabolic and Bariatric Surgery*, https://doi.org/10.1007/978-3-031-72309-4_51

It appears that patients who undergo a total knee arthroplasty (TKA) with a BMI ≥ 40 have worse outcomes including infection and higher revision rates [44]. The authors' consensus was to consider delaying the TKA until the comorbidities are optimized. In a study of 1416 patients, patient with obesity and morbid obesity were 1.6 and 1.7 times more likely, respectively, to require repeat revision TKA when compared to patients were none obese [7]. The evidence supports the idea that obesity can contribute to worse outcomes for patients undergoing TKA. Therefore, orthopedic surgeons are advocating weight reduction, which includes bariatric surgery, to enhance the patient's overall health before consenting to perform a TKA. A retrospective study of 10,718 patients that underwent a TKA did not show a significant difference of surgical site infections and 90 days readmissions between patients that lost or gained weight prior to the TKA [25]. The authors concluded that weight loss of 5% was insufficient to minimize the risk of complications. A systematic review and meta-analysis published in 2022 included nine studies (4 matched cohort studies, 2 unmatched cohort studies, 3 database studies) involving 166,047 patients, which were analyzed [69]. This study showed that bariatric surgery performed prior to TKA might increase the risk of preoperative blood transfusion, risk of revisions and infections. However, to contradict the previous studies, a randomized clinical trial was conducted on 82 patients, where half of the patients were randomized to adjustable gastric banding 12 months prior to TKA while the other half were randomized to nonoperative weight management. The risk of complications decreased following weight loss after bariatric surgery in patients with obesity [11]. The patients with severe obesity who underwent laparoscopic adjustable gastric banding and lost up to 20% of their weight before TKA had less complications compared to the group that did not undergo bariatric surgery [11]. The authors found that nearly one-third of patients did not proceed with the planned TKA up to 5 years after bariatric surgery, which might signify that weight loss alone was sufficient to improve knee osteoarthritis symptoms [11]. The adjustable gastric banding was the most performed and therefore was the bariatric procedure that was chosen for the trial. Since gastric banding is largely abandoned, modern procedures like the sleeve gastrectomy and Roux-en-Y gastric bypass (RYGB) account for the majority of bariatric surgeries [9]. It is now well established that sleeve gastrectomy and RYGB have superior weight loss compared to laparoscopic adjustable gastric banding [57]. With the emergence of medical therapy for weight loss, glucagon-like peptide-1 receptor agonists are gaining widespread popularity as a nonsurgical method for weight loss. However, to this day, there is no clear consensus or data on the preferred method of weight loss to be utilized prior to TKA.

Likewise, studies were conducted on the effect of obesity on the hip joint and its impact on postoperative complications. A study of 42 primary total hip arthroplasties (THA) in patients with BMI ≥ 50 with a mean follow up of 5.2 years showed a significantly increased risk of complications (HR 5.6) compared to the matched 2:1 control group [4]. There was a notable difference in the rate of complications, and more specifically wound complications (HR 22.2) [4]. A study by DeMik et al.

showed that the effect of obesity on postoperative complications is higher for patients undergoing THA compared to TKA [10]. In this study of 161,785 patients, the authors found double the wound complications and almost four-fold greater for deep infection after undergoing THA compared with TKA in those who suffered from severe obesity. Patients with obesity and morbid obesity also had higher rates of reoperation when undergoing a primary THA compared with TKA. Patients that are not obese had no difference in odds of total complications, wound complications, or deep infection between both procedures [10]. A meta-analysis and systematic review, published in 2020, showed that patients with obesity and morbid obesity are at higher risks of complications after a THA compared to their nonobese counterparts [46]. Some of the limitations of this study was that almost all studies were not conducted in a randomized prospective design. There was also abundant heterogeneity in the various studies and lack of adjustment of confounders that might influence the outcomes post THA [46]. High quality evidence is limited as to the role of bariatric surgery in patients undergoing THA. In 2020, a retrospective review was published, involving 88 primary THA procedures among which 71 patients had previously undergone bariatric surgery [55]. While patients with morbid obesity undergoing THA had increased risks of certain complications, it was unclear whether MBS improved those risks. This cohort of patients who underwent MBS had worse implant survivorship and higher dislocation rates [55]. However, conflicting data exist where patients that undergo bariatric surgery prior to THA have improved complication rates. A study published in 2018 analyzing 792 bariatric patients that underwent THA showed that the risks for in-hospital complications were lower compared to their matched cohorts that did not have MBS. The revision and dislocation risks, however, were not different [41]. In a more recent met-analysis, THA after MBS was associated with lower short-term medical complications but no statistically significant differences were found in the rates of periprosthetic infection or long-term revision [37]. There has not been extensive research conducted on the specific type of MBS, nor on the timing of MBS prior to THA. A recently published study aimed to answer these questions [5]. The authors divided their cohorts into six groups: 2 cohorts without history of MBS and BMI >40, 2 cohorts with previous RYGB or SG and two cohorts that underwent MBS either 6–12 months and > 12 months prior to the THA. The follow up data of 2 years showed no differences in postoperative medical or surgical complications, or revisions amongst all groups. The cohort with BMI >40 kg/m$^2$ had the highest complication profile amongst all cohorts. The study's conclusion was that patients do not need to wait prior to undergoing a THA [5].

While data supports that patients with morbid obesity carry a higher complication profile when undergoing total joint arthroplasty, higher quality evidence is required to answer the remaining questions such as the timing and type of MBS as well as defining an accurate threshold where joint arthroplasty might be discouraged. Despite the literature, many orthopedic surgeons continue to offer joint arthroplasty for obese and patients with morbid obesity.

## Neoplastic Therapy

We know that obesity increases the risk of various types of cancer including gynecological, gastrointestinal, renal and gallbladder cancers, among others [17, 36, 50]. Adipose tissue produces hormones and inflammatory cytokines that can promote tumor growth and metastasis [12, 35]. In addition, the interplay between obesity and insulin resistance with the chronic low-grade inflammation further contribute to tumorigenesis [39]. Obesity's influence is not only related to elevated cancer risk, but also to the treatment journey. Patients suffering from cancer can be deemed high risk or inoperable [54]. Also, their postoperative complications are increased compared to the general population [52]. A study was published in 2013 that included four patients with morbid obesity with a mean BMI of 48.25 kg/m$^2$ that underwent sleeve gastrectomy to qualify for a second oncologic curative procedure [20]. A case report was also published in 2020 detailing the successful utilization of sleeve gastrectomy as a preliminary step for a patient with BMI of 43.5 kg/ m$^2$ facilitating subsequent thoracoscopic right superior lobe resection [27]. Parmar et al. published a retrospective study on 37 patients, from 12 medical centers from eight countries, diagnosed with neoplasm who were inoperable or at high risk for cancer surgery due to obesity [48]. Sleeve was the most common procedure performed with a decrease in mean BMI from 49.9 to 39.7 kg/m$^2$ and eventually 83.8% of patients underwent neoplastic surgery while the rest received alternative nonsurgical forms of therapy [48]. The excess adipose tissue within the patient's body may complicate oncologic surgeries by altering normal anatomy and extending surgery time. Studies suggest that patients with different types of cancer and concomitant obesity have extended surgery time and perioperative complications [16, 22, 31, 67]. A retrospective study of 927 patients demonstrated that patients with obesity (BMI > 30 kg/ m$^2$) had more complications compared to patients without obesity [67]. Such complications included infections, flap thrombosis/necrosis, wound complications and a lengthier hospital stay [67]. Similarly, patients with obesity undergoing colectomy for colon cancer had a higher risk of postoperative complications including fascial dehiscence, thromboembolism, stomal complications and increased overall operative time [2, 16, 24]. We found similar results for patients with obesity undergoing renal cancer surgery [22, 31]. It is important to keep in mind that most of these studies were done at high-volume tertiary centers by experienced surgeons where outcomes are expected to be superior. With the presented data, it is safe to say that MBS is a feasible option for patients with obesity and morbid obesity who face a high or prohibitive risk for possibly curative oncologic surgery. However, it is crucial to bear in mind that this approach is suitable for patients who can afford to wait for a period of time to achieve the desired weight loss.

## Abdominal Wall Hernias

Amongst the various independent risk factors, increased weight is well known in carrying an increased risk for abdominal wall hernias and their recurrence [26]. This is likely due to increased visceral fat, abdominal wall circumference, and intra-abdominal pressure. A prospective study, published in 2015, conducted on 625 patients who underwent abdominal surgery, showed that BMI $\geq$ 25 kg/m$^2$ was an independent risk factor for the development of incisional ventral hernias [23]. An analysis of the American College of Surgeons National Surgical Quality Improvement Program database spanning from 2009 to 2012 showed that almost 60% of patients undergoing ventral hernia repair had a BMI > 30 kg/m$^2$ [53]. The literature continues to support these conclusions. Therefore, weight loss management options become critical in managing patients with abdominal wall hernias. In fact, there is no clear consensus on timing to perform MBS. The question is whether to perform the hernia repair concomitantly with the MBS or as a staged procedure where the hernia repair is performed after weight loss from MBS. The literature is conflicting and primarily based on low quality data. In a retrospective study of 85 patients, the authors divided the patients into three groups: (1) primary repair with transabdominal transfixation sutures concomitant with the RYGB, (2) ventral hernia repair utilizing biologic mesh and (3) deferred treatment till after the desired weight loss. The study showed concomitant repair with biologic mesh seems favorable. Primary repair performed concomitantly with RYGB yielded a 22% hernia recurrence rate with an average follow up of 30 months. The group where hernia repair was deferred had a 35% rate of development of small bowel obstruction due to incarceration. The authors preferred performing concomitant repair of the hernia with biologic mesh while primary repair without mesh was associated with a high rate of recurrence. In addition, deferring treatment especially post RYGB is worrisome for incarceration and risk of bowel ischemia [13]. Due to the risks associated with deferring a ventral hernia repair till after weight loss is achieved, one might consider repairing a ventral hernia concomitantly sub optimally as a temporizing measure while leaving the definite repair as a staged procedure. Possible temporizing measures include splitting the omentum without reducing it from the hernia sac or leaving the omentum undisturbed in the hernia sac [62, 64]. Such maneuvers prevent bowel from incarcerating in the hernia defect and leaves the abdominal wall layers intact for the future permanent repair. Another important point to consider is the use of mesh for large hernia defects. A systematic review of 11 studies, conducted in 2018, where ventral hernias were repaired concomitantly with bariatric surgery with primary closure, synthetic mesh and biological mesh [32]. The recurrence rate was 25.7% in the primary closure group, 14.3% in the biological mesh group and 1.1% in the synthetic mesh group. The authors concluded that synthetic mesh provided a significantly lower recurrence rate without increased risk in 30-day wound morbidity. In contrast, another retrospective study where concomitant ventral hernia repair was performed with bariatric surgery demonstrated an increase in the risk of surgical site infection but not overall morbidity [61]. However, this study did not specify the type of repair or mesh used. it is thought to be safer to leave large hernia defects undisturbed until after weight loss prior to attempting abdominal wall reconstruction in patients with obesity. If the surgeon decides to defer hernia repair till after the bariatric surgery, it is thought to be optimal to perform the hernia repair when the patient's optimal weight is achieved, and the comorbidities are as optimized as possible. At that time, the decision to perform a concomitant panniculectomy should be considered. In a study from 2015, the authors conducted a retrospective review of 43 patients who underwent ventral hernia repair with concomitant horizontal panniculectomy matched to 43 controls who underwent ventral hernia repair alone [68]. They found no increase in the incidence of surgical site infections or difference in recurrence rate when performing a panniculectomy with the ventral hernia repair. However, results were significant for increased rates of skin necrosis and cellulitis. In a study of 28 patients with morbid obesity, treated between 2003 and 2008, a systematic treatment approach was conducted based on the patients BMI, body habitus, reducibility of hernias found in a central location, abdominal wall thickness and the diameter of the hernia defect [14]. These patients were followed up for a minimum of 2 years where only three hernia recurrences were observed [14].

In conclusion, it is important to individualize the approach to each patient depending on their symptoms, BMI, comorbidities and hernia characteristics. In a recent publication, the Society of American Gastrointestinal and Endoscopic Surgeons issued its recommendations concerning this topic where it was advised to engage in a dialogue with the patients regarding the timing of hernia repair and MBS [19]. No doubt, we need further robust research in this area.

## Transplant

High BMI is a relative contraindication for solid organ transplant, therefore, MBS can be utilized as a tool for patients to become candidates to undergo organ transplantation. A systematic review of 31 studies conducted in Australia studied the impact of MBS on post-transplantation outcomes [43]. Among patients without pre-transplantation MBS, 18 studies found 13.7% graft loss and 9.1% mortality rate within 5 years post-transplantation. Among patients who underwent pre-transplantation MBS, 15 studies reported 8.7% graft loss and a 2.8% mortality rate. These studies were still considered low quality in evidence in the form of case series and case studies therefore a strong conclusion could not be made. There were two case-control studies that showed no significant differences in various outcomes including graft loss, patient mortality, delayed graft function, and wound complications [43]. Although further research is required to confirm the impact of bariatric surgery on post-transplantation outcomes, it is widely recognized that MBS and ensuing weight loss can serve as a pathway for patients to qualify for renal transplants. Research indicates that over 50% of patients with end-stage renal disease and obesity become eligible for renal transplant within five years following MBS [1, 29]. Similarly, a systematic review and meta-analysis where 19 studies were included showed that MBS can also serve as a bridge to liver transplant [34]. Out of the 187 patients that underwent MBS, 82% of patients were listed for transplant and 70% of them successfully received liver transplants. They had no mortality in a 30-day period and the graft survival rate approached 70% after 1 year. The procedure of choice in the majority of the cases was the laparoscopic sleeve gastrectomy. However, other procedures were performed such as the RYGB, gastric band, and jejunoileal gastric bypass. While the procedures were not analyzed to ascertain potential advantages between them, the prevailing belief is that due to the absence of gastrointestinal tract re-routing in sleeve gastrectomy, accessing the biliary tree endoscopically would likely not pose significant challenges in the event of complications post-liver transplant [21, 34]. A recently published systematic review examined the timing and type of MBS to be performed in liver transplantation [56]. The data included five articles that met the authors' criteria. There were 162 patients that underwent simultaneous MBS and liver transplant while 1426 underwent liver transplant alone. Patients undergoing MBS had comparable outcomes when it came to overall survival, graft survival and postoperative morbidity in comparison to liver transplant alone. The study that performed concomitant MBS and liver transplant chose the sleeve gastrectomy as their weight loss operation. The rest of the studies utilized other procedures as well, including RYGB ($n = 82$) and sleeve gastrectomy ($n = 32$), jejunoileal bypass ($n = 7$), biliopancreatic diversion with duodenal switch ($n = 4$), adjustable gastric banding ($n = 5$), and vertical banding gastroplasty ($n = 1$) [56]. Notably, MBS plays a role in cardiac transplant by potentially improving heart failure to a point where the need for a transplant is eliminated [38]. In this study, seven patients with a left ventricular ejection fraction ≤25% and a median BMI of 42.8 kg/m$^2$ underwent MBS (3 underwent laparoscopic adjustable gastric banding, 4 underwent sleeve gastrectomy) then achieved a median BMI reduction of 12.9 kg/m$^2$ ($p = 0.017$). Their postoperative ejection fraction improved to a median of 30% so two patients underwent cardiac transplant, two patients successfully met the listing criteria and three patients had significant improvement in their ejection fraction, thereby eliminating the need for a transplant. The authors performed a risk-benefit analysis that led them to choose adjustable gastric banding; however, they later switched to the sleeve gastrectomy due to the potential need for reoperations for band complications, the less reliable weight loss outcomes and the associated dysphagia with the band when swallowing medications [38]. A recently published systematic review of 11 studies including 98 patients with a mean preoperative BMI of 44.9 kg/m$^2$ revealed that MBS can improve heart transplant candidacy [33]. In this paper, 11 articles with 98 patients were included and 71% of these patients were eventually listed for transplant. The patients had an absolute BMI reduction of 26.1%. The mean time to receive a heart transplant was 14.9 months. The rate of 30-day mortality after MBS was 0%, and the 30-day complications after MBS was 28% [33]. The largest series regarding this topic was published in 2023 where a systemic review and meta-analysis was conducted [60]. In this study, 271 patients were identified and 95.6% of them underwent sleeve gastrectomy. The most common complications were major adverse cardiovascular events (30.2%), and GI-related bleeding (20.9%) followed by LVAD pump thrombosis (11.6%) [60]. Eventually, 67 of 271 patients received a heart transplant within an average of

13.8 months [60]. Also, among 28 end-stage lung disease patients, a systemic review showed that 28.6% lost enough weight to be listed for lung transplant, 7.1% were transplanted and 14.3% had sufficient improvement that they no longer required transplant [47]. In another study published in 2019, 25 patients with interstitial lung disease underwent bariatric surgery: RYGB (68%), sleeve gastrectomy (28%), and adjustable gastric banding (4%) [3]. Their mean preoperative BMI was 39 kg/m$^2$ and their 30-day complication rate was 16%. At 1 year follow up, the excess weight loss was 67% and the patients' pulmonary function tests improved significantly. Six out of the seven potential lung transplant candidates became eligible for transplant and one of them had successful lung transplant at 88 months after MBS [3].

## Infertility

Patients with BMI >25 kg/m$^2$ are associated with decreased fertility [63]. Obesity continues to be associated with decreased spontaneous pregnancy rates and increased time to pregnancy [18]. Insulin resistance is thought to cause subfertility in obese women [49]. Certain studies indicate that obese females may experience decreased success in infertility treatments, including inadequate follicular development and reduced rates of fertilization [51, 58, 65]. Other studies report similar outcomes to nonobese females; however, higher doses of ovulation-inducing agents need to be used [6, 40]. Seventy-two women with infertility and polycystic ovary syndrome underwent bariatric surgery and were followed up for a period of 4 years in a retrospective study [59]. The results showed that 64.8% of the patient were able to become pregnant naturally and their preoperative BMI was lower compared to the no-natural conception group. There were no significant differences in weight loss between both groups. BMI 1 year after surgery was an independent predictor of natural conception [59]. Another retrospective analysis published in 2023 involving 150 child-bearing females who underwent sleeve gastrectomy showed that 11 patients (out of 18 who desired pregnancy) became pregnant after the procedure after a mean time of 5.5 months [8]. Although bariatric surgery is not considered an indication in patients experiencing infertility at the moment; however, we find that an increasing number of patients with obesity and subfertility might find MBS as a gateway for weight loss and subsequent improved fertility.

## Conclusion

Bariatric surgery serves not only as a critical intervention for obesity management but also as a bridge to other procedures. This chapter explored the expanding role of bariatric surgery beyond weight loss, highlighting its potential to improve patient outcomes in diverse situations. By addressing comorbidities, optimizing patient health, and enhancing surgical feasibility, bariatric surgery opens doors to a spectrum of interventions, including organ transplantation, hernia repair, infertility treatments, orthopedic surgeries, and beyond. As the field continues to evolve, further research and clinical innovation will undoubtedly continue to uncover new avenues where bariatric surgery can serve as a pivotal step towards improved health and well-being for patients facing complex surgical challenges.

## References


1. Al-Bahri S, Fakhry TK, Gonzalvo JP, Murr MM. Bariatric surgery as a bridge to renal transplantation in patients with end-stage renal disease. Obes Surg. 2017;27(11):2951–5. https://doi.org/10.1007/s11695-017-2722-6.
2. Alqarni A, Aljehaiman F, Almousa SA, Almarshad SA, Alrzouq FK. The relationship between BMI and postoperative complications among colorectal cancer patients undergoing surgery. Cureus. 2023;15(11):e48715. https://doi.org/10.7759/cureus.48715.
3. Ardila-Gatas J, Sharma G, Nor Hanipah Z, Tu C, Brethauer SA, Aminian A, Tolle L, Schauer PR. Bariatric surgery in patients with interstitial lung disease. Surg Endosc. 2019;33(6):1952–8. https://doi.org/10.1007/s00464-018-6475-7.
4. Arsoy D, Woodcock JA, Lewallen DG, Trousdale RT. Outcomes and Complications Following Total Hip Arthroplasty in the Super-Obese Patient, BMI > 50. J Arthroplast. 2014;29(10):1899–905. https://doi.org/10.1016/j.arth.2014.06.022.
5. Bains SS, Sax OC, Chen Z, Nabet A, Nace J, Delanois RE. Bariatric surgery prior to total hip arthroplasty: does timing or type matter? Hip Int. 2023;33(6):1017–25. https://doi.org/10.1177/11207000221136001.
6. Balen AH, Platteau P, Andersen AN, Devroey P, Sørensen P, Helmgaard L, Arce J-C. The influence of body weight on response to ovulation induction with gonadotrophins in 335 women with World Health Organization group II anovulatory infertility. BJOG. 2006;113(10):1195–202. https://doi.org/10.1111/j.1471-0528.2006.01034.x.
7. Bigham WR, Lensing GS, Walters MM, Bhanat E, Keeney JA, Stronach BM. Outcomes of total knee arthroplasty revisions in obese and morbidly obese patient populations. J Arthroplast. 2023;38(9):1822–6. https://doi.org/10.1016/j.arth.2023.03.017.
8. Carlino G, Benson AA, Bove V, Pontecorvi V, De Siena M, Matteo MV, Farina A, Polidori G, Vinti L, Giannetti G, Costamagna G, Spada C, Boškoski I. Impact of pregnancy on weight loss after endoscopic sleeve gastroplasty. Obes Surg. 2023;33(10):3097–105. https://doi.org/10.1007/s11695-023-06745-6.
9. Clapp B, Ponce J, Corbett J, Ghanem OM, Kurian M, Rogers AM, Peterson RM, LaMasters T, English WJ. American Society for Metabolic and Bariatric Surgery 2022 estimate of metabolic and bariatric procedures performed in the United States. Surg Obes Relat Dis. 2024;20(5):425–31. https://doi.org/10.1016/j.soard.2024.01.012.
10. DeMik DE, Bedard NA, Dowdle SB, Elkins JM, Brown TS, Gao Y, Callaghan JJ. Complications and obesity in arthroplasty—a hip is not a knee. J Arthroplast. 2018;33(10):3281–7. https://doi.org/10.1016/j.arth.2018.02.073.
11. Dowsey MM, Brown WA, Cochrane A, Burton PR, Liew D, Choong PF. Effect of bariatric surgery on risk of complications after total knee arthroplasty. JAMA Netw Open. 2022;5(4):e226722. https://doi.org/10.1001/jamanetworkopen.2022.6722.
12. Dumas J-F, Brisson L. Interaction between adipose tissue and cancer cells: role for cancer progression. Cancer Metastasis Rev. 2021;40(1):31–46. https://doi.org/10.1007/s10555-020-09934-2.
13. Eid GM, Mattar SG, Hamad G, Cottam DR, Lord JL, Watson A, Dallal RM, Schauer PR. Repair of ventral hernias in morbidly obese patients undergoing laparoscopic gastric bypass should not be deferred. Surg Endosc. 2004;18(2):207–10. https://doi.org/10.1007/s00464-003-8915-1.

14. Eid GM, Wikiel KJ, Entabi F, Saleem M. Ventral hernias in morbidly obese patients: a suggested algorithm for operative repair. Obes Surg. 2013;23(5):703–9. https://doi.org/10.1007/s11695-013-0883-5.
15. GBD 2021 Osteoarthritis Collaborators. Global, regional, and national burden of osteoarthritis, 1990-2020 and projections to 2050: a systematic analysis for the Global Burden of Disease Study 2021. Lancet Rheumatol. 2023;5(9):e508–22. https://doi.org/10.1016/S2665-9913(23)00163-7.
16. Geiger TM, Muldoon R. Complications following colon rectal surgery in the obese patient. Clin Colon Rectal Surg. 2011;24(4):274–82. https://doi.org/10.1055/s-0031-1295692.
17. Genkinger JM, Spiegelman D, Anderson KE, Bernstein L, van den Brandt PA, Calle EE, English DR, Folsom AR, Freudenheim JL, Fuchs CS, Giles GG, Giovannucci E, Horn-Ross PL, Larsson SC, Leitzmann M, Männistö S, Marshall JR, Miller AB, Patel AV, et al. A pooled analysis of 14 cohort studies of anthropometric factors and pancreatic cancer risk. Int J Cancer. 2011;129(7):1708–17. https://doi.org/10.1002/ijc.25794.
18. Gesink Law DC, Maclehose RF, Longnecker MP. Obesity and time to pregnancy. Hum Reprod. 2007;22(2):414–20. https://doi.org/10.1093/humrep/del400.
19. Ghanem OM, Orenstein S, Lloyd SJ-A, Andalib A, Race A, Burt HA, Husain F, Goldblatt M, Kroh M, SAGES Metabolic, B. S. C. S. H. C. Management of abdominal wall hernias in patients with severe obesity. Surg Endosc. 2023;37(9):6619–26. https://doi.org/10.1007/s00464-023-10312-6.
20. Gianos M, Abdemur A, Szomstein S, Rosenthal R. Laparoscopic sleeve gastrectomy as a step approach for morbidly obese patients with early stage malignancies requiring rapid weight loss for a final curative procedure. Obes Surg. 2013;23(9):1370–4. https://doi.org/10.1007/s11695-013-0933-z.
21. Girotra M, Soota K, Klair JS, Dang SM, Aduli F. Endoscopic management of post-liver transplant biliary complications. World J Gastrointest Endosc. 2015;7(5):446. https://doi.org/10.4253/wjge.v7.i5.446.
22. Gong EM, Orvieto MA, Lyon MB, Lucioni A, Gerber GS, Shalhav AL. Analysis of impact of body mass index on outcomes of laparoscopic renal surgery. Urology. 2007;69(1):38–43. https://doi.org/10.1016/j.urology.2006.09.020.
23. Goodenough CJ, Ko TC, Kao LS, Nguyen MT, Holihan JL, Alawadi Z, Nguyen DH, Flores JR, Arita NT, Roth SJ, Liang MK. Development and validation of a risk stratification score for ventral incisional hernia after abdominal surgery: hernia expectation rates in intra-abdominal surgery (The HERNIA Project). J Am Coll Surg. 2015;220(4):405–13. https://doi.org/10.1016/j.jamcollsurg.2014.12.027.
24. Hotouras A, Ribas Y, Zakeri SA, Nunes QM, Murphy J, Bhan C, Wexner SD. The influence of obesity and body mass index on the outcome of laparoscopic colorectal surgery: a systematic literature review. Color Dis. 2016;18(10):O337–66. https://doi.org/10.1111/codi.13406.
25. Inacio MCS, Kritz-Silverstein D, Raman R, Macera CA, Nichols JF, Shaffer RA, Fithian DC. The impact of pre-operative weight loss on incidence of surgical site infection and readmission rates after total joint arthroplasty. J Arthroplast. 2014;29(3):458–64.e1. https://doi.org/10.1016/j.arth.2013.07.030.
26. Itatsu K, Yokoyama Y, Sugawara G, Kubota H, Tojima Y, Kurumiya Y, Kono H, Yamamoto H, Ando M, Nagino M. Incidence of and risk factors for incisional hernia after abdominal surgery. Br J Surg. 2014;101(11):1439–47. https://doi.org/10.1002/bjs.9600.
27. Iwata S, Hagiwara A, Harima Y. Thoracoscopic radical surgery for a morbidly obese patient with early lung cancer after laparoscopic sleeve gastrectomy: a case report. Surg Case Rep. 2020;6(1):189. https://doi.org/10.1186/s40792-020-00950-6.
28. Jiang L, Xie X, Wang Y, Wang Y, Lu Y, Tian T, Chu M, Shen Y. Body mass index and hand osteoarthritis susceptibility: an updated meta-analysis. Int J Rheum Dis. 2016;19(12):1244–54. https://doi.org/10.1111/1756-185X.12895.
29. Kienzl-Wagner K, Weissenbacher A, Gehwolf P, Wykypiel H, Öfner D, Schneeberger S. Laparoscopic sleeve gastrectomy: gateway to kidney transplantation. Surg Obes Relat Dis. 2017;13(6):909–15. https://doi.org/10.1016/j.soard.2017.01.005.

30. King LK, March L, Anandacoomarasamy A. Obesity & osteoarthritis. Indian J Med Res. 2013;138(2):185–93.
31. Kiziloz H, Dorin R, Finnegan KT, Shichman S, Meraney A. The impact of body mass index on perioperative outcomes in robot-assisted laparoscopic partial nephrectomy. J Endourol. 2013;27(8):1000–7. https://doi.org/10.1089/end.2012.0665.
32. Lazzati A, Nassif GB, Paolino L. Concomitant ventral hernia repair and bariatric surgery: a systematic review. Obes Surg. 2018;28(9):2949–55. https://doi.org/10.1007/s11695-018-3366-x.
33. Lee Y, Anvari S, Sam Soon M, Tian C, Wong JA, Hong D, Anvari M, Doumouras AG. Bariatric surgery as a bridge to heart transplantation in morbidly obese patients: a systematic review and meta-analysis. Cardiol Rev. 2022;30(1):1–7. https://doi.org/10.1097/CRD.0000000000000346.
34. Lee Y, Tian C, Lovrics O, Soon MS, Doumouras AG, Anvari M, Hong D. Bariatric surgery before, during, and after liver transplantation: a systematic review and meta-analysis. Surg Obes Relat Dis. 2020;16(9):1336–47. https://doi.org/10.1016/j.soard.2020.05.012.
35. Lengyel E, Makowski L, DiGiovanni J, Kolonin MG. Cancer as a matter of fat: the crosstalk between adipose tissue and tumors. Trends Cancer. 2018;4(5):374–84. https://doi.org/10.1016/j.trecan.2018.03.004.
36. Li L, Gan Y, Li W, Wu C, Lu Z. Overweight, obesity and the risk of gallbladder and extrahepatic bile duct cancers: a meta-analysis of observational studies. Obesity (Silver Spring). 2016;24(8):1786–802. https://doi.org/10.1002/oby.21505.
37. Li S, Luo X, Sun H, Wang K, Zhang K, Sun X. Does prior bariatric surgery improve outcomes following total joint arthroplasty in the morbidly obese? A meta-analysis. J Arthroplast. 2019;34(3):577–85. https://doi.org/10.1016/j.arth.2018.11.018.
38. Lim C-P, Fisher OM, Falkenback D, Boyd D, Hayward CS, Keogh A, Samaras K, MacDonald P, Lord RV. Bariatric surgery provides a "bridge to transplant" for morbidly obese patients with advanced heart failure and may obviate the need for transplantation. Obes Surg. 2016;26(3):486–93. https://doi.org/10.1007/s11695-015-1789-1.
39. Liu X-Z, Pedersen L, Halberg N. Cellular mechanisms linking cancers to obesity. Cell Stress. 2021;5(5):55–72. https://doi.org/10.15698/cst2021.05.248.
40. Maheshwari A, Stofberg L, Bhattacharya S. Effect of overweight and obesity on assisted reproductive technology—a systematic review. Hum Reprod Update. 2007;13(5):433–44. https://doi.org/10.1093/humupd/dmm017.
41. McLawhorn AS, Levack AE, Lee Y, Ge Y, Do H, Dodwell ER. Bariatric surgery improves outcomes after lower extremity arthroplasty in the morbidly obese: a propensity score-matched analysis of a New York statewide database. J Arthroplast. 2018;33(7):2062–2069.e4. https://doi.org/10.1016/j.arth.2017.11.056.
42. Mezhov V, Ciccutini FM, Hanna FS, Brennan SL, Wang YY, Urquhart DM, Wluka AE. Does obesity affect knee cartilage? A systematic review of magnetic resonance imaging data. Obes Rev. 2014;15(2):143–57. https://doi.org/10.1111/obr.12110.
43. Mousapour P, Ling J, Zimbudzi E. Comparison of kidney transplantation outcomes between patients with and without pre-transplantation bariatric surgery: a systematic review. Obes Surg. 2022;32(12):4066–81. https://doi.org/10.1007/s11695-022-06308-1.
44. Obesity and Total Joint Arthroplasty. J Arthroplast. 2013;28(5):714–21. https://doi.org/10.1016/j.arth.2013.02.011.
45. Oliveria SA, Felson DT, Cirillo PA, Reed JI, Walker AM. Body weight, body mass index, and incident symptomatic osteoarthritis of the hand, hip, and knee. Epidemiology. 1999;10(2):161–6.
46. Onggo JR, Onggo JD, de Steiger R, Hau R. Greater risks of complications, infections, and revisions in the obese versus non-obese total hip arthroplasty population of 2,190,824 patients: a meta-analysis and systematic review. Osteoarthr Cartil. 2020;28(1):31–44. https://doi.org/10.1016/j.joca.2019.10.005.
47. Orandi BJ, Purvis JW, Cannon RM, Smith AB, Lewis CE, Terrault NA, Locke JE. Bariatric surgery to achieve transplant in end-stage organ disease patients: a systematic review and meta-analysis. Am J Surg. 2020;220(3):566–79. https://doi.org/10.1016/j.amjsurg.2020.04.041.

48. Parmar C, Abi Mosleh K, Aeschbacher P, Halfdanarson TR, McKenzie TJ, Rosenthal RJ, Ghanem OM, Heneghan HM, Brennan DJ, Wilkinson M, Ryan O, Mulita F, Verras GI, Lo Menzo E, Christodoulidis G, Hussain F, Greco F, Snoekx R, Feskens PBGM, et al. The feasibility and outcomes of metabolic and bariatric surgery prior to neoplastic therapy. Surg Obes Relat Dis. 2024;20(8):717–28. https://doi.org/10.1016/j.soard.2024.02.008.
49. Pasquali R, Gambineri A. Metabolic effects of obesity on reproduction. Reprod Biomed Online. 2006;12(5):542–51. https://doi.org/10.1016/s1472-6483(10)61179-0.
50. Pati S, Irfan W, Jameel A, Ahmed S, Shahid RK. Obesity and cancer: a current overview of epidemiology, pathogenesis, outcomes, and management. Cancers. 2023;15(2) https://doi.org/10.3390/cancers15020485.
51. Petersen GL, Schmidt L, Pinborg A, Kamper-Jørgensen M. The influence of female and male body mass index on live births after assisted reproductive technology treatment: a nationwide register-based cohort study. Fertil Steril. 2013;99(6):1654–62. https://doi.org/10.1016/j.fertnstert.2013.01.092.
52. Plassmeier L, Hankir MK, Seyfried F. Impact of excess body weight on postsurgical complications. Visc Med. 2021;37(4):287–97. https://doi.org/10.1159/000517345.
53. Regner JL, Mrdutt MM, Munoz-Maldonado Y. Tailoring surgical approach for elective ventral hernia repair based on obesity and National Surgical Quality Improvement Program outcomes. Am J Surg. 2015;210(6):1024–30. https://doi.org/10.1016/j.amjsurg.2015.08.001.
54. Ri M, Aikou S, Seto Y. Obesity as a surgical risk factor. Ann Gastroenterol Surg. 2018;2(1):13–21. https://doi.org/10.1002/ags3.12049.
55. Ryan SP, Couch CG, Duong SQ, Taunton MJ, Lewallen DG, Berry DJ, Abdel MP. Frank stinchfield award: does bariatric surgery prior to primary Total hip arthroplasty really improve outcomes? J Arthroplast. 2022;37(7):S386–90. https://doi.org/10.1016/j.arth.2022.01.084.
56. Safavi D, Creavin B, Gallagher TK, Kelly ME. The role of bariatric surgery in liver transplantation: timing and type. Langenbeck's Arch Surg. 2022;407(8):3249–58. https://doi.org/10.1007/s00423-022-02606-5.
57. Salminen P, Helmiö M, Ovaska J, Juuti A, Leivonen M, Peromaa-Haavisto P, Hurme S, Soinio M, Nuutila P, Victorzon M. Effect of laparoscopic sleeve gastrectomy vs laparoscopic Roux-en-Y gastric bypass on weight loss at 5 years among patients with morbid obesity: the SLEEVEPASS randomized clinical trial. JAMA. 2018;319(3):241–54. https://doi.org/10.1001/jama.2017.20313.
58. Sermondade N, Huberlant S, Bourhis-Lefebvre V, Arbo E, Gallot V, Colombani M, Fréour T. Female obesity is negatively associated with live birth rate following IVF: a systematic review and meta-analysis. Hum Reprod Update. 2019;25(4):439–51. https://doi.org/10.1093/humupd/dmz011.
59. Shan Y, Han X, Yang C, Li W, Zhou G, Han J, Bao Y, Yu H, Tu Y. The impact of metabolic surgery on natural conception rates in women with infertility, obesity and polycystic ovary syndrome: a retrospective study. Surg Obes Relat Dis. 2023;20(3):237–43. https://doi.org/10.1016/j.soard.2023.09.024.
60. Sharma I, Nakanishi H, Hage K, Marrero K, Diwan TS, daSilva-deAbreu A, Davis SS, Clapp B, Ghanem OM. Bariatric surgery and left ventricular assist device in patients with heart failure: a systematic review and meta-analysis. Am J Surg. 2023;226(3):340–9. https://doi.org/10.1016/j.amjsurg.2023.06.014.
61. Spaniolas K, Kasten KR, Mozer AB, Sippey ME, Chapman WHH, Pories WJ, Pender JR. Synchronous ventral hernia repair in patients undergoing bariatric surgery. Obes Surg. 2015;25(10):1864–8. https://doi.org/10.1007/s11695-015-1625-7.
62. Sukeik M, Alkari B, Ammori BJ. Abdominal wall hernia during laparoscopic gastric bypass: a serious consideration. Obes Surg. 2007;17(6):839–42. https://doi.org/10.1007/s11695-007-9129-8.
63. Tang J, Zhu X, Chen Y, Huang D, Tiemeier H, Chen R, Bao W, Zhao Q. Association of maternal pre-pregnancy low or increased body mass index with adverse pregnancy outcomes. Sci Rep. 2021;11(1):3831. https://doi.org/10.1038/s41598-021-82064-z.

64. Vilallonga R, Fort JM, Gonzalez O, Baena JA, Lecube A, Armengol M. Management of patients with hernia or incisional hernia undergoing surgery for morbid obesity. J Obes. 2011;2011:1–5. https://doi.org/10.1155/2011/860942.
65. Vural F, Vural B, Çakıroğlu Y. The role of overweight and obesity in in vitro fertilization outcomes of poor ovarian responders. Biomed Res Int. 2015;2015:781543. https://doi.org/10.1155/2015/781543.
66. Wall KC, Politzer CS, Chahla J, Garrigues GE. Obesity is associated with an increased prevalence of glenohumeral osteoarthritis and arthroplasty: a cohort study. Orthop Clin North Am. 2020;51(2):259–64. https://doi.org/10.1016/j.ocl.2019.12.001.
67. Wang M, Huang J, Chagpar AB. Do obese breast cancer patients have more complications and a longer length of stay after mastectomy than nonobese patients? Am Surg. 2021;87(7):1099–106. https://doi.org/10.1177/0003134820973352.
68. Warren JA, Epps M, Debrux C, Fowler JL, Ewing JA, Cobb WS, Carbonell AM. Surgical site occurrences of simultaneous panniculectomy and incisional hernia repair. Am Surg. 2015;81(8):764–9.
69. Yan M, Zheng G, Long Z, Pan Q, Wang X, Li Y, Lei C. Does bariatric surgery really benefit patients before total knee arthroplasty? A systematic review and meta-analysis. Int J Surg (London, England). 2022;104:106778. https://doi.org/10.1016/j.ijsu.2022.106778.

# Pregnancy and Bariatric Surgery

# 52

S. Julie-Ann Lloyd

Metabolic and bariatric surgery (MBS) has been acclaimed as a durable treatment for obesity. Around 2% of eligible patients undergo surgical weight reduction. Of this cohort, women comprise about 80% and most fall within the child-bearing age range [1]. Although obesity is associated with detrimental effects on reproductive health, its incidence among pregnant women is on the rise, approaching 30%, and the complex hormonal mechanisms at play during maternal obesity risk both mother and foetus [2].

## Reproductive Changes of Obesity

Obesity is a well-known factor that disrupts the hypothalamic-pituitary-ovarian axis and causes an imbalance in sex steroids. Insulin resistance, aromatization of androgens and adipokine release all favor anovulation and menstrual dysfunction, leading to infertility [3]. These hormonal mechanisms remain unclear. Most likely, dysregulation of hormones, such as leptin and ghrelin, alter ovarian steroidogenesis and fetal development. Similar effects of hyperinsulinemia and gonadal hormone disruption are thought to underlie the development of polycystic ovarian syndrome (PCOS).

Maternal obesity carries potential concerns, such as miscarriage, gestational diabetes, gestational hypertension, pre-eclampsia, venous thromboembolic (VTE) events, and perinatal mortality [4]. Long-term implications on the health of the infant are further affected by the mother's lifestyle and nutrition during pregnancy and the epigenetics of the fetus. Additional fetal risks include birth defects,

S. J.-A. Lloyd (✉)
Division of Metabolic and Bariatric Surgery, Michael E. DeBakey Department of Surgery, Baylor College of Medicine, Houston, TX, USA



O. M. Ghanem et al. (eds.), *The SAGES Manual of Metabolic and Bariatric Surgery*, https://doi.org/10.1007/978-3-031-72309-4_52

premature birth, macrosomia, small for gestational age (SGA), congenital anomalies, failure to thrive, childhood obesity, and insulin resistance. Pregnant women with obesity are also at increased risk of requiring caesarean section or instrumented delivery as well as anesthetic and postpartum complications.

## Impact of MBS

MBS has emerged as a promising treatment for obesity, effectively eradicating weight-related co-morbidities. Notably, it kerbs diabetes, hypertension, sleep apnea, and hyperlipidemia. Application of the technique achieves prolongation of cancer-free survival, improvement in cardiovascular and liver outcomes, and resolution of menstrual irregularities, PCOS and infertility. MBS patients should be alerted to increased fertility so that they can utilize appropriate birth control after bariatric surgery.

Although MBS yields sizeable health-related benefits for women with obesity, the resulting anatomical changes can also predispose these patients to complications during and after pregnancy. The post-bariatric period is characterized by a catabolic state during which the body rapidly sheds weight. This state potentially creates an unfavorable environment for normal fetal growth and development. Consequently, most experts recommend waiting until post-operative weight loss has stabilized, usually 12–18 months after MBS, before conception [5, 6]. Indeed, the American College of Obstetrics and Gynecologists (ACOG) recommends a delay of up to 24 months [7].

Post-bariatric pregnancies experience higher rates of small for gestational age (SGA) and preterm labor, and lower rates of gestational diabetes and macrosomia relative to non-surgical patients with obesity [8]. Of note, diagnosis of gestational diabetes can often prove to be challenging amongst post-bariatric women. Oral glucose tolerance testing requires a rapid osmotic load, is poorly tolerated, and may precipitate dumping symptoms. Moreover, treatments for dumping, such as diazoxide, octreotide, and acarbose, have shown to be unsuitable for pregnant patients, due to adverse effects or inadequate data to support their use [9]. A viable diagnostic alternative involves continuous glucose monitoring, starting at 24–48 weeks of gestation.

## Nutritional Requirements

An alarming ~30% of post-bariatric patients fail to comply with nutritional and vitamin/mineral supplementation at baseline [10]. The American Society for Metabolic and Bariatric Surgery (ASMBS) recommends that a normal post-bariatric diet includes at least 60 grams per day of lean protein, 1.5 grams/kilogram of ideal body weight [11]. There are no specific recommendations for adjustment to protein intake during pregnancy. However, the National Academy of Medicine's suggestion of 70 grams per day falls within the acceptable range for pregnant patients [12].

**Table 52.1** Nutritional recommendations for prevention of deficiencies

| Nutrient | Daily dose | Comment |
|---|---|---|
| Multivitamin | 2 supplements | Must contain zinc, copper, selenium, thiamine |
| Iron | 45–60 mg | If unable to tolerate oral, consider intravenous administration |
| Folate | 1 mg | |
| Vitamin A | 6000–10,000 IU | BPD-DS patients need a higher range of supplementation<br>Beta-carotene form is preferred over retinol, which is contraindicated during pregnancy due to possible teratogenicity |
| Vitamin D | 50–150 ug | Administered as cholecalciferol |
| Vitamin E | 400 IU | Recommended for patients after BPD-DS |
| Vitamin K | 300 ug | Recommended for patients after BPD-DS |
| Vitamin B12 | 350 ug | If unable to tolerate oral, consider intramuscular administration |
| Thiamine | 100 mg | Dose as needed; thiamine should be included in bariatric multivitamin |
| Calcium | 1.5–2 g | BPD patients need a higher range of supplementation<br>All calcium administration should be separated from iron-containing vitamins by at least 2 hours |
| Zinc | 8–22 mg | |
| Copper | 1–2 mg | Copper supplementation should be separated from zinc, which can decrease copper uptake |
| Selenium | 50 ug | Recommended for patients after BPD-DS |

Summary of guidelines based on national and international recommendations for post-bariatric patients to avoid nutritional deficiencies during pregnancy [10, 13, 17, 29, 41]
*BPD-DS* biliopancreatic diversion with duodenal switch; *mg* milligrams; *g* grams; *ug* micrograms; *IU* international units

Similarly, patients are encouraged to supplement with additional micronutrients to avoid deficiency (Table 52.1). Emphasis should be put on iron, folate, fat-soluble vitamins (A, D, E, K), Vitamin B1, B12 and calcium [13]. These deficiencies result in neural tube defects, vision deficits, rickets, SGA, kidney disease, preterm labor and maternal osteoporosis [14].

## Procedure-Specific Considerations

Application of MBS comprises four primary operations: adjustable gastric banding (AGB), sleeve gastrectomy (SG), Roux-en-Y gastric bypass (RYGB) and duodenal switch (DS). Studies into the outcomes of post-bariatric pregnancy produced mixed results [15–17]. Pertinent themes are highlighted (below).

### Laparoscopic Adjustable Gastric Banding

Since its introduction in the early 1990s, laparoscopic adjustable gastric banding has been considered an attractive means of surgical weight loss due to its preservation of anatomy and, consequently, reversibility. The restrictive band about the fundus causes early satiety with a variable extent of restriction, depending on the volume of fluid in the subcutaneous port. Durable weight loss on the order of 50% excess weight loss (EWL) also favored this approach [18]. However, the apparatus has been associated with complications of band slippage, obstruction and erosion that now limit its use in modern bariatric surgery.

The field has not issued any consensus guidance regarding the appropriate management of pregnant patients with a history of AGB. The ideal scenario allows for sufficient oral intake to support the nutritional needs of both the mother and fetus. Some patients develop hyperemesis gravidarum, challenging these nutritional goals. In these instances, an extensive differential diagnosis must take into account band complications. Only about 5% of ABG cases develop complications during pregnancy [6]. The risk of these mechanical complications increases as the pregnancy progresses, possibly, due to displacement of abdominal organs by uterine expansion and increasing intra-abdominal pressure during pregnancy. Evaluation of the patient should ensue with appropriate imaging to exclude these etiologies. Abdominal imaging and/or endoscopy may demonstrate a change in *phi* angle, evidence of obstruction or erosion.

If, after the elimination of these concerns, oral intake remains inadequate, band deflation may theoretically enhance prenatal nutrition. Fetal growth will likely improve at the cost of maternal weight gain and gestational hypertension [19]. By inference, the decision to adjust band volume should be individualized, balancing maternal symptomatology with fetal growth.

## Sleeve Gastrectomy

Sleeve gastrectomy has supplanted Roux-en-Y gastric bypass as the most performed bariatric procedure. In 2021, for instance, more than 150,000 patients underwent this procedure. Although SG is safe and effective, the most common side effects include nausea and vomiting. Leak, stricture, and micronutrient deficiency also occur with some measurable frequencies [20]. Nutritional deficiencies are prevalent among patients prior to MBS, and this effect may worsen after surgery. Reduction in hydrochloric acid and intrinsic factor levels [from removal of the greater curvature], combined with decreased oral intake and, potentially, oral intolerance, set the stage for micronutrient deficits. Furthermore, anemia during pregnancy occurs primarily as a result of nutritional deficiencies. It is a risk factor for preterm delivery and low birthweight [21, 22]. Patients with a history of sleeve gastrectomy, now entering pregnancy, are in jeopardy of acquiring iron and vitamin B12 deficiencies, shortened gestation and SGA infants. Therefore, monitoring of hemoglobulin levels and appropriate repletion of vitamins is paramount to avoiding complications in this patient population.

Pregnancy after sleeve gastrectomy is unlikely to affect five-year weight loss. Patients who conceived more than one year after MBS achieved equivalent weight loss as matched controls who did not get pregnant [23]. Analogous results were observed in patients with more than one pregnancy(ies). Multivariate analysis identified [1] weight loss prior to pregnancy, and [2] interval between surgery and conception as the best predictors of overall weight loss at five years; longer interval patients fared better. Similarly, patients who conceived within six months of undergoing sleeve gastrectomy had lower gestational weight gain and were more likely to have infants with SGA [24]. Mode of delivery (vaginal versus caesarean section) was not statistically different. Other studies have shown that infants delivered from mothers who had undergone sleeve gastrectomy are more likely to require neonatal intensive care after delivery [25]. No other study about the interval between surgery and conception has conclusively demonstrated an ideal number. However, these data suggest waiting more than six months before initiating pregnancy.

## Roux-en-Y Gastric Bypass

Despite decreasing numbers of cases, Roux-en-Y gastric bypass remains the gold standard among metabolic and bariatric surgeries. Indeed, the gastric bypass is a primary and revision operation, often used to address patients' issues with weight recurrence and reflux disease. As a result, many studies have explored and demonstrated the benefits of gastric bypass on overall health and, more specifically, on fertility.

Obsolete bariatric procedures, such as jejunal bypass, were associated with spontaneous abortions, growth retardation, congenital malformations, and poor maternal outcomes. In contrast, perinatal complications in patients with a history of RYGB were similar to normal-weight non-surgical controls [26]. Gestational diabetes, gestational hypertension and pre-eclampsia, all over-represented in patients with obesity, were drastically reduced by RYGB to comparable rates of normal controls.

Maternal hypoglycemia after RYGB can lead to fetal hypoglycemia, which in turn impairs fetal growth. A national Swedish cohort study of 670 post-bariatric pregnancies (of which 98% were RYGB) demonstrated a two-fold increase in SGA risk after MBS [27]. Other studies have supported these findings [28, 29]. Although absorptive changes contribute to this increased risk, the underlying mechanisms are thought to be more complex as SGA incidence is increased after AGB and SG [30].

The decreased transit time of gastric bypass anatomy predisposes the patient to deficiencies in calcium, iron, thiamine, and fat-soluble vitamins (A, D, E, K). Among these, iron deficiency is the most prevalent. Ultimately, vitamin supplementation is paramount in pregnant patients with a history of RYGB surgery.

One of the most feared post-bypass complications is small bowel obstruction. Specifically, internal herniation is a subtle finding that can be seen during the third trimester of an otherwise normal pregnancy. The lifetime incidence of internal hernia after Roux-en-Y gastric bypass is close to 10% [31]. Symptoms of abdominal pain, nausea, vomiting, and bloating are non-specific, and the location of pain may be influenced by a gravid uterus; hence, diagnosis requires a high index of clinical suspicion. Cross-sectional imaging with computed tomography (CT) is the primary modality for diagnosis and the decision to undergo such imaging should not be delayed [32]. Appropriate counseling of the patient includes a discussion about the risk-benefit ratio of undergoing radiographic testing. Any concerning findings on examination or imaging warrant immediate diagnostic laparoscopy and, in some instances, delivery of the infant. Delay in surgical treatment beyond 48 hours has been linked to worse outcomes—bowel strangulation, volvulus, necrosis, and perforation [33]. These conditions can further compromise the mother and fetus alike, leading to preterm delivery or death.

## Biliopancreatic Diversion with Duodenal Switch

As with RYGB, biliopancreatic diversion with duodenal switch (BPD-DS) has a high propensity for the development of protein-calorie malnutrition and vitamin deficiencies. Given that the altered anatomy has a stronger malabsorptive component, the risks are higher after BPD-DS, and patients have a higher likelihood of developing maternal or neonatal complications. In addition, selenium insufficiency has been observed in pregnant patients with a history of BPD-DS and has been linked to the development of pre-eclampsia and cardiomyopathy, which improve after supplementation [34, 35]. Second-trimester selenium deficit may be associated with low birth weight [36]. All BPD-DS patients require heightened monitoring after surgery; this recommendation becomes more important during pregnancy.

## Recommendations for MBS Patients

Studies show that perioperative counselling about contraception improves its postoperative use (Table 52.2). With such advice, patients are less likely to have unprotected sex and unexpected pregnancies [37, 38]. Perioperative management of

**Table 52.2** Summary of pregnancy recommendations for MBS patients

| | |
|---|---|
| Preconception | Avoid pregnancy during the rapid weight loss period, up to 12–18 months after surgery<br>Contraceptive counselling<br>Vitamin supplementation and nutritional/micronutrient monitoring<br>Monitor weight and serum nutritional levels |
| Pregnancy | Assess and optimize nutritional intake<br>Refer to high-risk obstetrics team<br>Determine gestational weight goals and avoid excessive weight gain<br>Screen for gestational diabetes<br>Check labs every 3–6 months<br>Monitor for the development of MBS complications |
| Delivery | Surgeon available, as needed |
| Postpartum | Nutritional optimization<br>Ensure adequate intake during breastfeeding<br>Re-establish weight goals and support toward that end |

Adapted from Alamri et al. [41]

estrogen-containing contraceptives includes holding this medication for one menstrual cycle (28 days) to reduce the risk of VTE. Furthermore, after intestinal diversion, intestinal absorption and metabolism of oral contraceptive is not appreciably reduced [13, 39]. Long-acting, reversible contraceptive methods, such as intrauterine devices, have been proven most effective.

The literature does not recommend any particular procedure type for patients who hope for future pregnancy. Indeed, the ideal surgery depends on the patient's medical needs and surgical history.

When pregnancy is underway, these patients should be referred to a high-risk obstetrician. The National Academy of Medicine advises against weight loss during pregnancy. Additional recommendations for gestational weight gain are a function of the pre-pregnancy body mass index (BMI) [40, 41]. Specifically, patients whose BMI falls within the ranges of 18.5–24.9 kg/m$^2$, 25.0–29.9 kg/m$^2$, and $\geq$30 kg/m$^2$ should aim to gain a total of 11.5–16.0 kg, 6.8–11.3 kg, 5.0–9.1 kg, respectively. Some providers believe these targets are too high, especially for patients with obesity.

Gestational diabetes screening is better accomplished with fasting and two-hour postprandial testing or glycosylated hemoglobin levels (HbA1c) instead of the typical oral glucose testing to avoid episodes of dumping and reactive hypoglycemia, which also affects the test's accuracy. Post-bariatric patients require continuous vitamin supplementation and close nutritional monitoring. Particular attention should be paid to vitamin B12, vitamin D, iron and folate levels. Adequate supplementation may require the use of prenatal vitamins in place of bariatric vitamins. To date, no study has demonstrated a depletion in the nutritional value of breast milk after MBS. Breastfeeding is acceptable in this patient population, but post-bariatric mothers also need continued nutritional support with adequate protein and vitamin intake as well as monitoring of micronutrients during lactation.

Pregnant patients with a history of MBS should have close follow-up visits with the bariatric surgical and high-risk maternal-fetal medicine teams. Should the patient develop symptoms suggestive of bariatric complications (persistent nausea/vomiting, abdominal pain, dysphagia, neurological deficits or other signs of vitamin deficiencies), urgent evaluation is indicated, and a low threshold for laparoscopy is maintained. Judicious care of this special population can help to avoid or promptly address any potential complications.

## References


1. Young MT, Phelan MJ, Nguyen NT. A decade analysis of trends and outcomes of male vs female patients who underwent bariatric surgery. J Am Coll Surg. 2016;222(3):226–31.
2. Shrestha A, Prowak M, Berlandi-Short V, et al. Maternal obesity: a focus on maternal interventions to improve health of offspring. Front Cardiovasc Med. 2021;8:696812.
3. Silvestris E, de Pergola G, Rosania R. Obesity as disruptor of the female fertility. Reprod Biol Endocrinol. 2018;16:22.
4. Fitzsimons KJ, Modder J, Greer IA. Obesity in pregnancy: risks and management. Obstet Med. 2009;2(2):52–62.

5. Beard JH, Bell RL, Duffy AJ. Reproductive considerations and pregnancy after bariatric surgery: current evidence and recommendations. Obes Surg. 2008;18(8):1023–7.
6. Guelinckx I, Devlieger R, Vansant G. Reproductive outcome after bariatric surgery: a critical review. Human Reprod Update. 2009;15(2):189–201.
7. American Congress of Obstetricians and Gynecologists. https://www.acog.org/womens-health/faqs/obesity-and-pregnancy. Accessed 29 Jan 2024.
8. Cornthwaite K, Prajapati C, Lenguerrand E. Pregnancy outcomes following different types of bariatric surgery: a national cohort study. Eur J Obstet Gynecol Reprod Biol. 2021;260:10–7.
9. Narayanan RP, Syed AA. Pregnancy following bariatric surgery—medical complications and management. Obes Surg. 2016;26:2523–9.
10. Spetz K, Svedjeholm S, Roos S. Adherence to vitamin and mineral supplementation after bariatric surgery – a two-year cohort study. Obes Res Clin Pract. 2022;16(5):407–12.
11. Mechanick JI, Apovia C, Brethauer S, et al. Clinical practice guidelines for the perioperative nutrition, metabolic, and nonsurgical support of patients undergoing bariatric procedures—2019 update: cosponsored by American Association of Clinical Endocrinologists/American College of Endocrinology, The Obesity Society, American Society for Metabolic & Bariatric Surgery, Obesity Medicine Association, and American Society of Anesthesiologists. Surg Obes Relat Dis. 2019;16:175–247.
12. National Academy Press. http://nap.nationalacademies.org/10490. Accessed 29 Jan 2024.
13. Cheah S, Gao Y, Mo S, et al. Fertility, pregnancy and post partum management after bariatric surgery: a narrative review. Med J Aust. 2022;216(2):96–102.
14. Hazart J, Le Guennec D, Accoceberry M, et al. Maternal nutritional deficiencies and small-for-gestational-age neonates at birth of women who have undergone bariatric surgery. J Pregnancy. 2017;2017:4168541. https://doi.org/10.1155/2017/4168541.
15. Yu Y, Groth SW. Risk factors of lower birth weight, small-for-gestational-age infants, and preterm birth in pregnancies following bariatric surgery: a scoping review. Arch Gynecol Obstet. 2023;307(2):343–78.
16. Różańska-Walędziak A, Bartnik P, Kacperczyk-Bartnik J, et al. Pregnancy after bariatric surgery—a narrative literature review. Wideochir Inne Tech Maloinwazyjne. 2021;16(1):30–7.
17. Shawe J, Ceulemans D, Akhter Z, et al. Pregnancy after bariatric surgery: consensus recommendations for periconception, antenatal and postnatal care. Obes Rev. 2019;20(11):1507–22.
18. DeMaria EJ. Laparoscopic adjustable silicone gastric banding: complications. J Laparoendosc Adv Surg Tech A. 2003;13(4):271–7.
19. Jefferys A, Lenguerrand E, Cornthwaite K, et al. Deflation versus maintained inflation of gastric band in pregnancy: a national cohort study. Obstet Med. 2017;10(2):67–73.
20. Sarkhosh K, Birch DW, Sharma A, et al. Complications associated with laparoscopic sleeve gastrectomy for morbid obesity: a surgeon's guide. Can J Surg. 2013;56(5):347–52.
21. Xanthakos SA, Khoury JC, Inge TH, et al. Nutritional risks in adolescents after bariatric surgery. Clin Gastroenterol Hepatol. 2019;18(5):1070–81.
22. Ben-Porat T, Elazary R, Shef-Dagan S, et al. Factors associated with the development of anemia during pregnancy after sleeve gastrectomy. Obes Surg. 2020;30:3884–90.
23. Rottenstreich A, Shufanieh J, Kleinstern G, et al. The long-term effect of pregnancy on weight loss after sleeve gastrectomy. Surg Obes Relat Dis. 2018;14(10):1594–9.
24. Rottenstreich A, Levin G, Ben-Porat T, et al. Extremely early pregnancy (<6 mo) after sleeve gastrectomy: maternal and perinatal outcomes. Surg Obes Relat Dis. 2021;17(2):356–62.
25. Ducarme G, Chesnoy V, Lamarie P. Pregnancy outcomes after laparoscopic sleeve gastrectomy among obese patients. In J Gyneocol Obstet. 2015;130:127–31.
26. Maggard MA, Yermilov I, Li Z, et al. Pregnancy and fertility following bariatric surgery: a systematic review. JAMA. 2008;300(19):2286–96.
27. Johansson K, Cnattingius S, Näslund I, et al. Outcomes of pregnancy after bariatric surgery. N Engl J Med. 2015;372:814.
28. Kjaer MM, Lauenborg J, Breum M, et al. The risk of adverse pregnancy outcome after bariatric surgery: a nationwide register-based matched cohort study. Am J Obstet Gynecol. 2013;208:464.

29. Badreldin N, Kuller J, Rhee E, et al. Pregnancy management after bariatric surgery. Obstet Gynecol Surv. 2016;71(6):361–8.
30. Sheiner E, Balaban E, Dreiher J, et al. Pregnancy outcome in patients following different types of bariatric surgeries. Obes Surg. 2019;19:1286–92.
31. Capella RF, Iannace VA, Capella JF. Bowel obstruction after open and laparoscopic gastric bypass surgery for morbid obesity. J Am Coll Surg. 2006;203:328–35.
32. Vannavel A, Jans G, Bialecka M. Internal herniation in pregnancy after gastric bypass: a systematic review. Obstet Gynecol. 2016;127(6):1013–20.
33. Gandhi AD, Patel RA, Brolin RE. Elective laparoscopy for herald symptoms of mesenteric/internal hernia after laparoscopic roux-en-Y gastric bypass. Surg Obes Relat Dis. 2009;5(2):144–9.
34. Boldery R, Fielding G, Rafter T, et al. Nutritional deficiency of selenium, secondary to weight loss (bariatric) surgery associated with life-threatening cardiomyopathy. Heart Lung Circ. 2007;16:123–6.
35. Massoure P, Camus O, Fourcade L, et al. Bilateral leg edema after bariatric surgery: a selenium-deficiency cardiomyopathy. Obes Res Clin Pract. 2017;11:622–6.
36. Ducarme G, Planche L, Abet E, et al. A Prospective Study of Association of Micronutritioent Deficiencies during Pregnancy and Neonatal Outcome among Women after Bariatric Surgery. J Clin Med. 2021;10:204. https://doi.org/10.3390/jcm10020204.
37. Menke MN, King WC, White GE, et al. Contraception and conception after bariatric surgery. Obstet Gynecol. 2017;130:979–87.
38. Mengesha B, Griffin L, Nagle A, et al. Assessment of contraceptive needs in women undergoing bariatric surgery. Contraception. 2016;94:74–7.
39. Moreira de Brito C, de Melo ME, Mancini MC. Pharmacokinetics of oral levonorgestrel and ethinylestradiol in women after Roux-en-Y gastric bypass surgery. Surg Obes Relat Dis. 2021;17(4):673–81.
40. National Academy Press. https://nap.nationalacademies.org/resource/12584/Resource-Page%2D%2D-Weight-Gain-During-Pregnancy.pdf. Accessed 29 Jan 2024.
41. Alamri SH, Abdeen GN. Maternal nutritional status and pregnancy outcomes post-bariatric surgery. Obes Surg. 2022;32(4):1325–40.

# Obesity-Related Cancer and the Impact of Metabolic Surgery

# 53

Rickesha L. Wilson and Ali Aminian

## Defining the Relationship: Obesity and Cancer

The obesity epidemic is a global health crisis due to massive shifts in food processing and diets as well as physical activity patterns. Obesity (defined as a body mass index [BMI] of ≥30 kg/m$^2$) has a known cardiometabolic impact associated with medical comorbidities such as hypertension, diabetes mellitus, obstructive sleep apnea, and more. Certain obesity-related cancers have also been identified by the International Agency for Research on Cancer, which include: esophageal adenocarcinoma, cancer of the gastric cardia, colon and rectum, liver, gallbladder, pancreas, breast in women post-menopause, corpus uteri, ovary, kidney (renal cell), thyroid, meningioma, and multiple myeloma [1]. These were based on the myriad observational studies associating obesity or excess body fatness with cancer risk. Mendelian randomization studies have been performed to address the complexities of how obesity may be linked to cancer and reduce confounding factors by factoring in genetics. This has identified stronger associations of obesity with specific cancers including esophageal adenocarcinoma, renal cell carcinoma, colon, rectum, pancreas, ovary, and endometrium [2].

## Pathophysiology of the Obesity-Cancer Link

The systemic and local mechanisms by which obesity and metabolic syndrome promote cancer development are important to understand and continue to elucidate for the development of effective preventive and treatment strategies for obesity and

R. L. Wilson · A. Aminian (✉)
Bariatric and Metabolic Institute, Department of General Surgery, Cleveland Clinic, Cleveland, OH, USA
e-mail: AMINIAA@ccf.org



O. M. Ghanem et al. (eds.), *The SAGES Manual of Metabolic and Bariatric Surgery*, https://doi.org/10.1007/978-3-031-72309-4_53

related cancers. Visceral adiposity has important endocrine functions that regulate adipokines, sex hormones, and inflammatory mediators that impact metabolic function (Fig. 53.1). Excess visceral adiposity is what can lead to metabolic and endocrine dysregulation. Insulin resistance is a hallmark of excess visceral adiposity that leads to hyperinsulinemia. Increased insulin levels lead to increased leptin and inflammatory cytokine levels as well as higher levels of circulating insulin-like growth factors (IGFs) due to increased IGF transcription and downregulation of IGF-binding proteins. This impacts cellular apoptosis and survival mechanisms and can upregulate cellular metabolic activities leading to increased oxidative stress and intracellular damage [3]. The development of diabetes is common with obesity and has also been linked to cancer development. Diabetes is often diagnosed after a period of hyperinsulinemia and insulin resistance leading to subsequent pancreatic beta-cell failure. The resultant hyperglycemia can be used directly as an energy source for cancerous cells via aerobic glycolysis and cause rapid proliferation. The conversion of androgens to estrogen is done by cytochrome P450 aromatase. In premenopausal women, the ovaries are a major site for aromatase production whereas postmenopausal women have production mainly in the skin and adipose tissue. Excess adiposity can lead to excess estrogen levels and increase the risk of estrogen-sensitive cancer, such as breast [4].

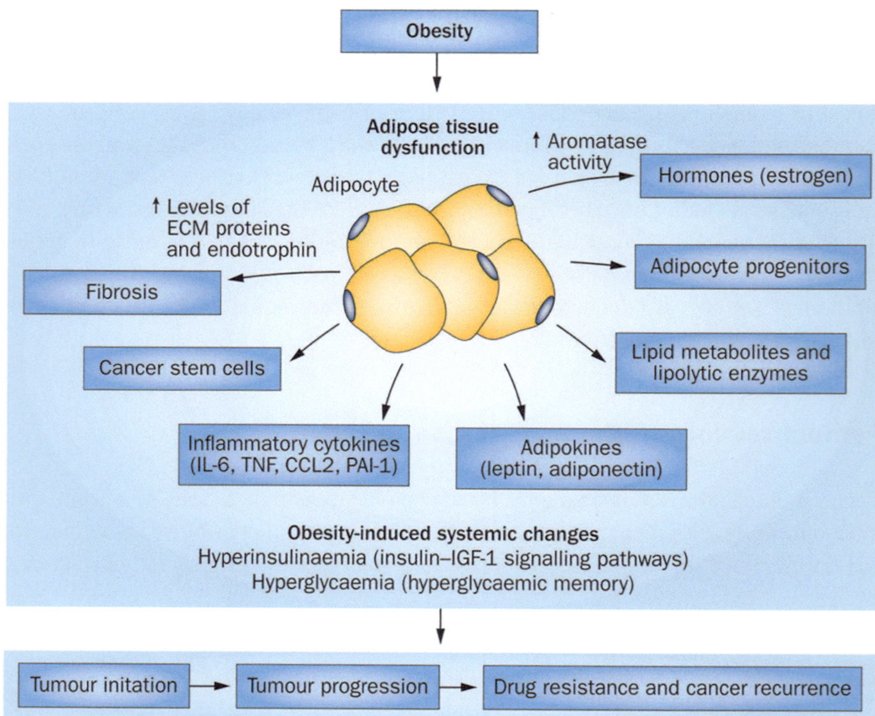


**Fig. 53.1** Obesity-induced changes that promote cancer development. Adapted with permission from Park et al. [4]

At the local level, white adipose tissue can resemble chronic tissue inflammation and promote the same proinflammatory pathways as tissue injury. As adipose tissue outgrows its blood supply, hypoxia occurs and promotes the influx of immune and inflammatory cells that promote adipocyte cell death, lipolysis, and the release of free fatty acids. This sustains a proinflammatory microenvironment and promotes a proneoplastic environment. Malignant cells may then take over the body's normal mechanisms for tissue repair (angiogenesis and extracellular matrix remodeling) and induce cancer [5].

## Outcomes of Metabolic Surgery on Obesity-Related Cancer

The link between obesity and certain cancers suggests that targeting obesity prevention and treatment would be beneficial for cancer risk reduction. Research shows that losing weight and thereby improving the metabolic state can be beneficial in cancer risk reduction. Lifestyle changes including improved nutritional and exercise habits, medications, and metabolic surgery are all tools to lose weight and improve metabolic health. Surgical intervention for obesity has proven to be the most effective and durable method for obesity treatment and improvement of obesity-related comorbidities [6–9]. Metabolic surgery can be defined as surgical procedures that influence metabolism by inducing weight loss and altering gastrointestinal physiology and anatomy. These include procedures such as sleeve gastrectomy (SG), Roux-en-Y gastric bypass (RYGB), duodenal switch (DS), and others. Weight loss from lifestyle changes and traditional anti-obesity medications can result in a 5–10% total weight loss (TWL), newer anti-obesity medications can offer up to a 20% TWL while taking them, and metabolic surgery offers 25–35% TWL [10]. Given these treatment options for obesity with varying efficacy, it is important to explore their impact on obesity-related cancer incidence and mortality.

Large cohort observational studies have been particularly impactful in studying obesity-related cancer incidence and mortality due to the long time to develop cancers, and randomized clinical trials can be cumbersome and cost-ineffective. Highlighting the outcomes of prospective trials and large cohort studies offers insight into the impact of weight loss on obesity-related cancer incidence and mortality.

### Nonsurgical Interventions and Obesity-Related Cancer

The Look AHEAD (Action for Health in Diabetes) trial is a multicenter randomized controlled trial that investigated the impact of intensive lifestyle intervention vs diabetes support and education on cardiovascular disease in individuals with both diabetes and overweight or obesity [11]. In just over 5000 participants, the weight loss difference at 1 year between the intervention group and control was 8.6% versus 0.7% and at 10 years was 6.0% vs 3.5% without a cardiovascular advantage. Data from this study were further examined regarding outcomes of cancer incidence and mortality [12]. There was no significant difference after nonsurgical intervention on total cancer-incidence (HR 0.93, 95% CI, 0.80 to 1.08), the incidence of non-obesity related cancers (HR 1.02, 95% CI 0.83 to 1.27), or total cancer mortality (HR, 0.92, 95% CI 0.68 to 1.25).

The Iowa Women's Health Study is a prospective cohort study where over 41,000 women ages 55 to 69 were surveyed by mail regarding intentional vs unintentional weight loss of ≥20 lbs. during their adulthood. In 21,707 women after menopause who were initially free of cancer, intentional weight loss revealed a decrease in any cancer by 11%, obesity-related cancer by 14%, and breast cancer by 19% [13].

The Nurses' Health Study started in 1976 and surveyed 121,700 married, female, registered nurses ages 30 to 55. Weight gain from age 18 and from menopause was followed for up to 26 and 24 years, respectively, and breast cancer outcomes were followed [14]. Women who gained 25 kg or more from age 18 were 45% more likely to develop breast cancer compared to those who maintained their weight. Women who gained 10 kg or more since menopause were 18% more likely to develop breast cancer. Compared to weight maintenance, women who lost 10 kg or more since menopause, did not use postmenopausal hormones and maintained weight loss had a 57% decrease in breast cancer incidence. These large studies point to the benefit of even modest weight loss and how cancer outcomes may be impacted.

## Surgical Interventions and Obesity-Related Cancer

Studies on surgical intervention for weight loss and improved metabolic health have demonstrated even more powerful benefits. While the literature has a vast majority of studies, highlighting a few large cohort studies offers key insight into the impact of metabolic surgery on obesity-related cancer outcomes.

### Swedish Obese Subjects

The Swedish Obese Subjects (SOS) study is a landmark prospective trial started in 1987 comparing the overall mortality and other outcomes of individuals with obesity who were treated with metabolic surgery ($n$ = 2010) compared to a matched cohort receiving conventional treatment ($n$ = 2037) [15]. Specifically, the surgical procedures included adjustable gastric banding (AGB), RYGB, and vertical-banded gastroplasty (VBG). SOS-adjusted overall mortality was reduced in the surgical cohort by 29% (HR 0.71, $P$ = 0.01), and the most common cause of death was cancer followed by myocardial infarction. Although this trial was not powered to evaluate specific-cause mortality, cancer incidence and mortality have also been evaluated. With a median follow-up time of 10.9 years, the incidence of first-time cancers was reduced by 33% (HR 0·67, 95% CI 0·53–0·85, $P$ = 0·0009) [16]. Of note, the surgical cohort lost a mean of 19.9 kg compared with a 1.3 kg weight gain for the control group.

Nearly half (49%) of the first-time cancer events in SOS were female-specific cancers; endometrial, breast, ovarian, cervical, and other gynecologic cancers. In a study focusing on female-specific cancers, the risk was 32% lower (HR = 0.68, 95%

CI 0.52–0.89, $P = 0.006$) in the surgical cohort with a median follow-up of 18 years [17]. Breast and endometrial cancers were found to be the most common, and all female-specific cancers except cervical had a lower incidence after surgery. Of the individual cancers, only endometrial cancers had a statistically significant reduction after metabolic surgery (HR = 0.56, 95% CI 0.35–0.89, $P = 0.014$).

Colon and rectal cancer was also evaluated specifically in this cohort, and there was no significant decrease in colon and rectal cancer risk following metabolic surgery (HR = 0.89, 95% CI 0.62–1.29, $P = 0.55$) [18]. This remained true for rectal cancer as well after adjusting for covariates. There was a significant decrease in the risk of skin cancer in general by 41% (HR = 0.59, 95% CI 0.35–0.99, $P = 0.047$) and even more so for melanoma by 57% (HR = 0.43, 95% CI 0.21–0.87, $P = 0.02$) [19]. For hematologic cancers, metabolic surgery was associated with a decreased incidence specifically in women, not men, and there was a lower incidence of lymphoma and hematologic cancer-related mortality [20].

### Utah Study

A large retrospective study was conducted out of Utah utilizing the Utah Cancer Registry and driver's license registrations to compare a cohort of 6596 individuals who had undergone the RYGB and 9442 individuals with severe obesity with a mean follow-up of 12.5 years [21]. Cancer incidence was 24% lower in the surgical cohort and cancer-related mortality was 46% lower compared to individuals with severe obesity. This effect was especially true in advanced cancers. Adams et al. expanded this data to include those undergoing more procedures than RYGB only and compared 21,837 subjects who underwent metabolic surgery (from 1982 to 2018) matched 1:1 by age, sex, BMI, and surgical date with a nonsurgical cohort. The overall aim of this updated project was also to evaluate all-cause and cause-specific mortality [22]. All-cause mortality was lowered by 16% in the surgical cohort. Death-related cancer decreased by 43%, cardiovascular disease by 29%, and diabetes by 72% in the surgical arm. Surgical procedures performed in this study included the SG, RYGB, DS, and AGB. There was a 25% lower risk of developing any cancers overall, with a 41% decreased incidence of obesity-related cancers in women. There was also a lower cancer-related mortality in women specifically.

### Kaiser Permanente

Another large observational retrospective cohort study used data from a large integrated health insurance and care delivery system at various sites of the Kaiser Permanente health system [23]. A surgical cohort of 22,198 patients who underwent metabolic surgery from 2005 to 2012 were matched with 66,427 nonsurgical patients. After a mean 3.5-year follow-up, the surgical cohort had a 33% lower risk of developing any cancer and a 41% lower risk of developing obesity-related cancers: specifically postmenopausal breast, endometrial, pancreatic, and colon cancers (Fig. 53.2).

In a separate study evaluating women in premenopausal and postmenopausal stages, metabolic surgery was associated with lower breast cancer risk for premenopausal (HR 0.72, 95% CI, 0.54–0.94, $P = 0.02$) and postmenopausal women (HR

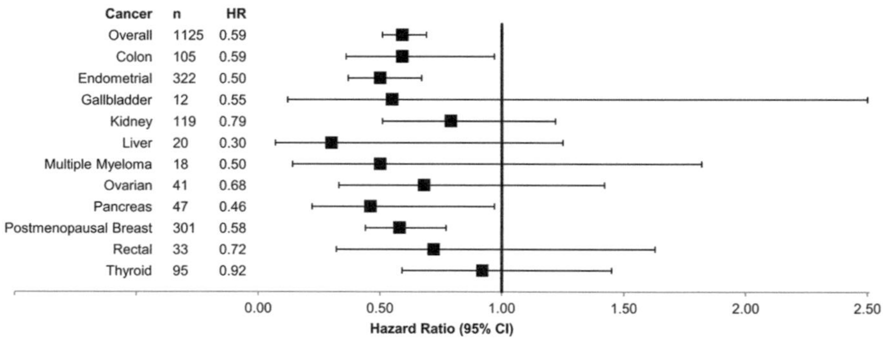


**Fig. 53.2** Forest plot of the incidence of obesity-related cancer after metabolic surgery compared to controls in a large cohort study. Adapted with permission from Schauer et al. [23]

0.55, 95% CI, 0.42–0.72, $P < 0.001$) [24]. Going a step further and evaluating the estrogen receptor (ER) status revealed significant decreases in cancer risk for premenopausal ER-negative cancers and postmenopausal ER-positive cancers.

### SPLENDID

The Cleveland Clinic Health System conducted a retrospective matched cohort study, SPLENDID (**S**urgical **P**rocedures and **L**ong-term **E**ffectiveness in **N**eoplastic **D**isease **I**ncidence and **D**eath), comparing adults with a BMI of 35 or higher undergoing metabolic surgery ($n = 5053$, RYGB or SG) who were matched 1:5 with a nonsurgical group ($n = 25,265$). Median follow-up was 6.1 years, and the surgical cohort experienced a 19.2% higher weight loss than the nonsurgical group. Obesity-related cancer cumulative incidence at 10 years was 32% lower after surgery and cancer-related mortality decreased by 48% after surgery (Fig. 53.3a and d).

In SPLENDID, the most common cancer types were female breast cancer and endometrial cancer. In fully adjusted Cox models for individual cancer types, only endometrial cancer risk was significantly reduced following metabolic surgery (HR = 0.47, 95% CI, 0.27–0.83).

## Surgical Procedure-Specific Data

The two most common metabolic procedures to date are the RYGB and SG [25, 26]. These two procedures have different anatomical alterations of the gastrointestinal system. The SG involves removing approximately 80% of the stomach, while the RYGB excludes most of the stomach and proximal small intestine and forms a pouch connected to the jejunum. The weight loss outcomes are relatively comparable long-term, and there are studies that have evaluated procedure-specific outcomes on obesity-related cancer.

In the SPLENDID study, the primary endpoint of obesity-related cancer incidence was evaluated based on procedure type. Sixty-six percent of patients

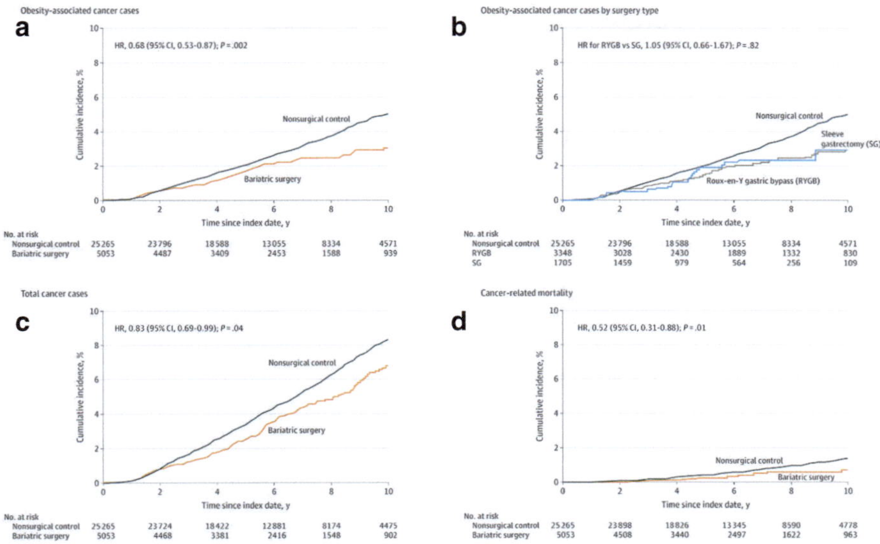


**Fig. 53.3** SPLENDID study outcomes related to (**a**) incidence of obesity-associated cancer between the surgical and nonsurgical cohort, (**b**) incidence based on procedure type, (**c**) total cancer cases, and (**d**) cancer-related mortality. Adapted with permission from Aminian et al. [27]

($n$ = 3348) underwent a RYGB and 34% ($n$ = 1705) underwent the SG. The incidence of the primary endpoint was similar after RYGB and SG (Fig. 53.3b). Compared to the control group, RYGB reduced the risk of obesity-related cancer by 30% and SG by 34% [27].

Adams et al. further evaluate data from the large Utah population database to evaluate differences in all-cause and cause-specific mortality between four different bariatric surgical procedures [22]. Only the RYGB ($n$ = 15,110) demonstrated a reduced cancer-related mortality. Numbers for the SG, AGB, and DS were too small to evaluate cause-specific mortality. Specifically, subjects who underwent RYGB had a 27% decrease in total cancer, 38% reduction in risk of obesity-related cancer, a 78% reduction in uterine cancer risk, and an overall cancer-related mortality reduction of 46% [21].

Tsui et al. were able to elucidate the cancer incidence of 71,000 patients who underwent the RYGB, SG, or AGB compared to 323,197 without surgical intervention [28]. Between the three procedures, there was no difference in the incidence of obesity-related cancer or male-specific cancer after surgery. However, the RYGB cohort had a lower incidence of developing non-obesity-related cancer and any type of cancer compared to both the SG and AGB. Lastly, the SOS study found a reduced cancer incidence among women but not men among the various surgical procedures with a 46% decreased incidence for AGB, 40% for VBG, and 46% after RYGB [16].

These studies and others highlight that specific metabolic procedures may be less important, and that the amount of weight loss itself could be the more important factor in cancer risk reduction.

## Weight-Dependent Response

Several studies have further evaluated the amount of weight loss following metabolic surgery to determine if the dose of weight loss impacts cancer outcomes. The SPLENDID study evaluated the 5053 subjects who underwent metabolic surgery into weight loss quartiles: quartile 1 (24% body weight), quartile 2 (24%–31%), quartile 3 (31%–39%), and quartile 4 (>39%). Quartile 4 with the highest weight loss had the lowest obesity-related cancer incidence, whereas quartile 1 with the lowest weight loss had the highest incidence (Fig. 53.4) [27].

In the LABS-2 study, those who lost <20% of their weight had a cancer incidence of 6.2% by year 7 vs 3.6% for those who lost between 20 and 34.9%, and 3.7% for the >35% weight loss tertile [29]. There was a 51% decreased incidence of cancer in the tertile that lost 20 to 34.9% body weight compared to <20%. Also, cancer-free survival was much lower in the lowest weight loss tertile compared to the others.

Of the 18,355 patients in the Kaiser study who underwent metabolic surgery, there was a 14% decrease in cancer risk with each 10% of weight loss. Thus, for the average patient who lost 27% of their weight at 1 year, there was a 34% decreased cancer risk [30].

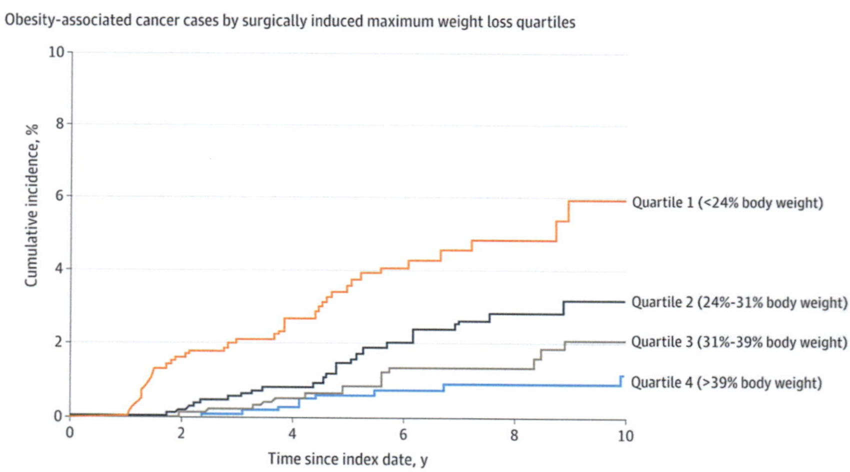


| No. at risk | | | | | | |
|---|---|---|---|---|---|---|
| Quartile 1 | 1263 | 1087 | 761 | 481 | 238 | 111 |
| Quartile 2 | 1263 | 1114 | 828 | 580 | 346 | 192 |
| Quartile 3 | 1263 | 1122 | 880 | 631 | 441 | 282 |
| Quartile 4 | 1263 | 1164 | 940 | 761 | 563 | 354 |

**Fig. 53.4** SPLENDID study obesity-associated cancer incidence based on weight quartiles. Adapted with permission from Aminian et al. [27]

## Impact in Various Subgroups

### Diabetes

The link between diabetes and obesity and cancer is well established. Studies have shown that the outcomes after metabolic surgery-induced weight loss on cancer incidence is favorable for those with diabetes. The SOS study evaluated 701 of its subjects with both obesity and diabetes, 393 in the surgical cohort and 308 nonsurgical [31]. There was a 37% decrease in cancer incidence in the surgical group and a 42% decrease for women specifically. Diabetes remission at 10 years of follow up was associated with a 40% decrease in cancer incidence. An improvement in the glucose, insulin, proinsulin, and C-peptide levels after 1 year in the LABS-2 study was associated with decreased future cancer risk [29]. The SPLENDID study showed favorable results for those taking and not taking diabetes medications on reduced obesity-related cancer incidence [27].

### Race

The SPLENDID study is the first to demonstrate the impact of metabolic surgery on cancer incidence for both black and white patients. Blacks experienced a 53% decreased in obesity-related cancer incidence and whites a 29% decrease. The majority of patients (96.5%) were either black or white, and these results may be less generalizable to other ethnicities. This is a limitation of many other studies as well.

### Gender

Studies have largely shown a significant reduction in cancer incidence in women more so than men. The SOS study, after excluding cancer events in the first 3 years after intervention, saw a nonsignificant decrease in cancer incidence in men of 16% compared to a significant decrease of 39% in women [16]. The Kaiser group noted no significant reduction in any cancers for men following surgery, however significant decreases for women were found for obesity-related and non-obesity-related cancers [23]. SPLENDID found that regardless of sex, both men and women experienced a benefit after metabolic surgery of lower incidence of obesity-related cancer: 33% decreased for women and 24% for men [27].

These findings could be explained by the limited statistical power rather than a biological phenomenon [32]. Most likely, the currently available studies, particularly those with small sample sizes and short follow-up times, do not have enough statistical power to demonstrate the effects of metabolic surgery in men for two main reasons: Nearly three-quarters of patients who undergo metabolic surgery are women; The 2 most common obesity associated cancers, which constitute nearly one-third of all incident cancers in metabolic surgery studies, occur in women (i.e., endometrial cancer and female breast cancer).

## Key Points on Specific Types of Cancers

Studies mentioned in this chapter and more have shown that hormone-related cancers in women—breast, endometrial, and ovarian—are most impacted by significant weight loss and metabolic surgery [33]. The extragonadal production of estrogen by adipose tissue drives these hormone-sensitive cancers, and treating obesity can mitigate this process. Few studies actually delineate outcomes based on genetic risk or estrogen receptor status, which is important in identifying more specifically the subgroups who benefit from metabolic surgery and its effects [24, 34]. Among all different types of cancer, considering the statistical power of available of studies, metabolic surgery has the largest impact on reducing the risk of endometrial cancer [17, 26, 27].

The data on non-hormonal, obesity-related cancers is less clear and consistent in the literature as there are fewer studies with limited follow up. These obesity-related, non-hormonal cancers include esophageal, gastric, liver, pancreas, renal cell, colon and rectal, multiple myeloma, and meningioma. Colon and rectal cancers have been linked to obesity. However, studies have demonstrated heterogenous results with older studies that had methodological limitations showing that metabolic surgery could actually increase the incidence of these cancers [35]. This could be due to changes in the gut microbiome and only specific cancers may be impacted [36]. This is why additional subgrouping of colorectal cancers is critical to specify the individual risk profiles that may benefit or not from metabolic surgery.

Potentially due to the mitigation and reversal of the effects of metabolic dysfunction-associated fatty liver disease and steatohepatitis, hepatocellular carcinoma has been shown to improve overall after metabolic surgery [8, 37]. Also pancreatic cancer incidence has been shown to improve overall after metabolic surgery compared to nonsurgical cohorts [38]. Despite concerns about worsening gastroesophageal reflux after the SG, which is the most commonly performed metabolic procedure currently, studies overall have shown equivalent or reduced incidences of Barrett's esophagus and esophageal and gastric cancers [33, 39].

The largest meta-analysis evaluating the impact of metabolic surgery on non-hormonal cancers compared 15 retrospective studies with 947,787 patients in the surgical arm and 17,635,690 in the nonsurgical cohort [40]. Surgical procedures evaluated were only the RYGB, SG, and/or AGB. Findings showed that metabolic surgery resulted in a significantly reduced risk of non-hormonal cancers including esophageal, liver, colorectal, kidney and urinary tract, and lung cancer. Outcomes for gastric and skin cancer were similar between both cohorts. Between procedures, both the RYGB and SG showed lower non-hormonal cancer risk but not the AGB. Furthermore, both the RYGB and SG demonstrated a lower incidence of esophageal cancer. Risk of bias, confounding factors, limited follow-up, and heterogeneity make the overall confidence of the study outcomes low.

## Moving Forward

Obesity is poised to be the number one preventable cause of cancer over tobacco use in the next 5 to 10 years, and it is a chronic condition that should be treated using a multidisciplinary approach [41]. The metabolic benefits of metabolic surgery are strong and have been well demonstrated in the literature. The impact obesity treatment has on cancer has a positive trend and current guidelines recommend weight loss for cancer risk reduction [42]. Improving quality of evidence in the literature is critical as most studies are observational cohort studies or pull data from population databases. This leads to bias in data sets and lack more granular information on specific cancer types and patient risk factors for cancer development that could help identify cancers and individuals who will benefit most from specific obesity treatments. Lim et al. propose a revised framework that future cohort studies could use to improve the quality of research when evaluating obesity-related cancer outcomes after nonsurgical and metabolic surgery interventions [33].

Furthermore, better defining obesity beyond BMI by using measures such as waist circumference and visceral adiposity is needed to accurately capture adipose toxicity that leads to obesity-related cancers. Continuing to investigate systemic and tissue-specific markers that can be linked to cancer risk reduction could lead to additional targeted therapies to address obesity-associated cancers.

Screening for cancers remains critical for individuals with obesity, and this population is at risk for poorer screening compliance due to the obesity stigma. Public and provider education on the most effective obesity treatments can lower that barrier to proper screening and treatment for obesity. Access to care for those with obesity and associated conditions continues to be a challenge as only a small portion (1 to 2%) of those with obesity who qualify for metabolic surgery are treated [43]. All of this considered, there is a unique opportunity for the treatment of obesity and cancers to improve through continued research and intentional education.

Considering the worldwide prevalence of obesity, it is impossible to perform metabolic surgery in all eligible patients to reverse the health consequences of obesity, including the cancer risk. However, patients with obesity who have precancerous lesions (e.g., endometrial hyperplasia, hyperplasia or carcinoma in situ of the breast, high-risk colorectal polyps, or Barrett's esophagus) should be strongly considered for metabolic surgery as a potential approach for cancer prevention [32, 44].

## Conclusions

Based on the currently available evidence, metabolic surgery, compared with no surgery, is associated with a significantly lower incidence of obesity-associated cancer and cancer-related mortality. The magnitude of the effect of metabolic surgery on cancer risk is large and has consistently been shown in the literature. The cancer risk reduction of metabolic surgery has been observed in different populations with obesity—in black and white people, in those with or without diabetes, in younger and older adults, and after RYGB and SG. The current evidence suggests that cancer risk reduction of metabolic surgery is greater in women than men. Among all cancer types, endometrial cancer has the strongest association with obesity and has a very large risk reduction following metabolic surgery. The current evidence also suggests the presence of a dose-dependent response between weight reduction and cancer risk: the greater the weight loss, the lower the risk of developing cancer in people with obesity. Instead of focusing on lifestyle modification only, treating obesity with effective and durable treatments such as metabolic surgery is necessary for reducing cancer risk.

## References

1. Lauby-Secretan B, Scoccianti C, Loomis D, Grosse Y, Bianchini F, Straif K. Body fatness and cancer—viewpoint of the IARC Working Group. N Engl J Med. 2016;375(8):794–8.
2. Fang Z, Song M, Lee DH, Giovannucci EL. The role of mendelian randomization studies in deciphering the effect of obesity on cancer. J Natl Cancer Inst. 2022;114:361–71.
3. Lega IC, Lipscombe LL. Review: diabetes, obesity, and cancer-pathophysiology and clinical implications. Endocr Rev. 2020;41:33–52.
4. Park J, Morley TS, Kim M, Clegg DJ, Scherer PE. Obesity and cancer – mechanisms underlying tumour progression and recurrence. Nat Rev Endocrinol. 2014;10:455–65.
5. Iyengar NM, Gucalp A, Dannenberg AJ, Hudis CA. Obesity and cancer mechanisms: tumor microenvironment and inflammation. J Clin Oncol. 2016;34:4270–6.
6. Schauer PR, Kashyap SR, Wolski K, Brethauer SA, Kirwan JP, Pothier CE. Bariatric surgery versus intensive medical therapy in obese patients with diabetes. N Engl J Med. 2012;366:1567–76.
7. Aminian A, Zajichek A, Arterburn DE, Wolski KE, Brethauer SA, Schauer PR, Kattan MW, Nissen SE. Association of metabolic surgery with major Adverse cardiovascular outcomes in patients with type 2 diabetes and obesity. JAMA. 2019;322:1271–82.
8. Aminian A, Al-Kurd A, Wilson R, et al. Association of bariatric surgery with major adverse liver and cardiovascular outcomes in patients with biopsy-proven nonalcoholic steatohepatitis. JAMA. 2021;326:2031–42.
9. Wilson R, Aminian A, Tahrani AA. Metabolic surgery: a clinical update. Diabetes Obes Metab. 2021;23:63–83.
10. Elmaleh-Sachs A, Schwartz JL, Bramante CT, Nicklas JM, Gudzune KA, Jay M. Obesity management in adults. JAMA. 2023;330:2000–15.
11. Wing RR, Bolin P, Brancati FL, et al. Cardiovascular effects of intensive lifestyle intervention in type 2 diabetes. N Engl J Med. 2013;369:145–54.
12. Yeh H, Bantle JP, Cassidy-Begay M, et al. Intensive weight loss intervention and cancer risk in adults with type 2 diabetes: analysis of the look AHEAD randomized clinical trial. Obesity. 2020;28:1678–86.
13. Parker ED, Folsom AR. Intentional weight loss and incidence of obesity-related cancers: the Iowa Women's Health Study. Int J Obes. 2003;27:1447–52.
14. Eliassen AH, Colditz GA, Rosner B, Willett WCHS. Adult weight change and risk of postmenopausal breast cancer. JAMA. 2006;296:193–201.
15. Sjöström L, Narbro K, Sjöström CD, et al. Effects of bariatric surgery on mortality in Swedish Obese Subjects. N Engl J Med. 2007;357:741–52.
16. Sjöström L, Gummesson A, David Sjöström C, et al. Effects of bariatric surgery on cancer incidence in obese patients in Sweden (Swedish Obese Subjects study): a prospective, controlled intervention trial. Lancet Oncol. 2009;10:653–62.

17. Anveden Å, Taube M, Peltonen M, Jacobson P, Andersson-Assarsson JC, Sjöholm K, Svensson PA, Carlsson LMS. Long-term incidence of female-specific cancer after bariatric surgery or usual care in the Swedish Obese Subjects study. Gynecol Oncol. 2017;145:224–9.
18. Taube M, Peltonen M, Sjoholm K, Palmqvist R, Andersson-Assarsson JC, Jacobson P, Svensson PA, Carlsson LMS. Long-term incidence of colorectal cancer after bariatric surgery or usual care in the Swedish Obese Subjects study. PLoS One. 2021;16:1–7.
19. Taube M, Peltonen M, Sjöholm K, Anveden Å, Andersson-Assarsson JC, Jacobson P, Svensson PA, Bergo MO, Carlsson LMS. Association of bariatric surgery with skin cancer incidence in adults with obesity: a nonrandomized controlled trial. JAMA Dermatol. 2020;156:38–43.
20. Sjöholm K, Andersson-Assarsson JC, Kristensson FM, et al. Long-term incidence of haematological cancer after bariatric surgery or usual care in the Swedish Obese Subjects study: a prospective cohort study. Lancet Heal Longev. 2023;4:e544–51.
21. Adams TD, Stroup AM, Gress RE, Adams KF, Calle EE, Smith SC, Halverson RC, Simper SC, Hopkins PN, Hunt SC. Cancer incidence and mortality after gastric bypass surgery. Obesity. 2009;17:796–802.
22. Adams TD, Meeks H, Fraser A, Davidson LE, Holmen J, Newman M, Ibele AR, Richards N, Hunt SC, Kim J. Long-term all-cause and cause-specific mortality for four bariatric surgery procedures. Obesity. 2023;31:574–85.
23. Schauer DP, Feigelson HS, Koebnick C, Caan B, Weinmann S, Leonard AC, Powers JD, Yenumula PR, Arterburn DE. Bariatric surgery and the risk of cancer in a large multisite cohort. Ann Surg. 2019;269:95–101.
24. Feigelson HS, Caan B, Weinmann S, Leonard AC, Powers JD, Yenumula PR, Arterburn DE, Koebnick C, Altaye M, Schauer DP. Bariatric surgery is associated with reduced risk of breast cancer in both premenopausal and postmenopausal women. Ann Surg. 2020;272:1053–9.
25. Angrisani L, Santonicola A, Iovino P, Vitiello A, Higa K, Himpens J, Buchwald H, Scopinaro N. IFSO Worldwide Survey 2016: Primary, Endoluminal, and Revisional Procedures. Obes Surg. 2018;28:3783–94.
26. ASMBS Estimate of Bariatric Surgery Numbers, 2011–2022. https://asmbs.org/resources/estimate-of-bariatric-surgery-numbers/.
27. Aminian A, Wilson R, Al-Kurd A, et al. Association of bariatric surgery with cancer risk and mortality in adults with obesity. JAMA. 2022;327:2423–33.
28. Tsui ST, Yang J, Zhang X, Docimo S, Spaniolas K, Talamini MA, Sasson AR, Pryor AD. Development of cancer after bariatric surgery. Surg Obes Relat Dis. 2020;16:1586–95.
29. Stroud AM, Dewey EN, Husain FA, Fischer JM, Courcoulas AP, Flum DR, Mitchell JE, Pories WJ, Purnell JQ, Wolfe BM. Association between weight loss and serum biomarkers with risk of incident cancer in the Longitudinal Assessment of Bariatric Surgery cohort. Surg Obes Relat Dis. 2020;16:1086–94.
30. Schauer DP, Feigelson HS, Koebnick C, Caan B, Weinmann S, Leonard AC, Powers JD, Yenumula PR, Arterburn DE. Association between weight loss and the risk of cancer after bariatric surgery. Obesity. 2017;25:S52–7.
31. Sjoholm K, Carlsson LMS, Peltonen M, Taube M. Association of bariatric surgery with cancer incidence in patients with obesity and diabetes: long-term results from the Swedish Obese Subjects study. Diabetes Care. 2022;45:444–50.
32. Aminian A, Nissen SE. Association of bariatric surgery with cancer risk and mortality – reply. JAMA. 2022;328:1646.
33. Lim PW, Stucky CCH, Wasif N, Etzioni DA, Harold KL, Madura JA, Fong ZV. Bariatric surgery and longitudinal cancer risk a review. JAMA Surg. 2024;159:1–9.
34. Hassinger TE, Mehaffey JH, Hawkins RB, Schirmer BD, Hallowell PT, Schroen AT, Showalter SL. Overall and estrogen receptor–positive breast cancer incidences are decreased following bariatric surgery. Obes Surg. 2019;29:776–81.
35. Mackenzie H, Markar SR, Askari A, Faiz O, Hull M, Purkayastha S, Møller H, Lagergren J. Obesity surgery and risk of cancer. Br J Surg. 2018;105:1650–7.

36. Luo JN, Haridas RS, Lo T, Tavakkoli A, Yoo J, Sheu EG. Sleeve gastrectomy promotes colitis-associated colorectal cancer in a murine model via a modified gut microbiome. bioRxiv. 2022; https://doi.org/10.1101/2022.06.04.494831.
37. Ramai D, Singh J, Lester J, Khan SR, Chandan S, Tartaglia N, Ambrosi A, Serviddio G, Facciorusso A. Systematic review with meta-analysis: bariatric surgery reduces the incidence of hepatocellular carcinoma. Aliment Pharmacol Ther. 2021;53:977–84.
38. Fan H, Mao Q, Zhang W, Fang Q, Zou Q, Gong J. The impact of bariatric surgery on pancreatic cancer risk: a systematic review and meta-analysis. Obes Surg. 2023;33:1889–99.
39. Lazzati A, Epaud S, Ortala M, Katsahian S, Lanoy E. Effect of bariatric surgery on cancer risk: results from an emulated target trial using population-based data. Br J Surg. 2022;109:433–8.
40. Clapp B, Portela R, Sharma I, Nakanishi H, Marrero K, Schauer P, Halfdanarson TR, Dayyeh BA, Kendrick M, Ghanem OM. Risk of non-hormonal cancer after bariatric surgery: meta-analysis of retrospective observational studies. Br J Surg. 2023;110:24–33.
41. Soerjomataram I, Bray F. Planning for tomorrow: global cancer incidence and the role of prevention 2020–2070. Nat Rev Clin Oncol. 2021;18:663–72.
42. Rock CL, Thomson C, Gansler T, et al. American Cancer Society guideline for diet and physical activity for cancer prevention. CA Cancer J Clin. 2020;70:245–71.
43. Rubino F, Puhl RM, Cummings DE, et al. Joint international consensus statement for ending stigma of obesity. Nat Med. 2020;26:485–97.
44. Wilson R, Aminian A. Obesity-associated cancer risk reduction after metabolic surgery: insights from the SPLENDID study and the path forward. Surg Obes Relat Dis. 2023;19:788–93.

# Bariatric Tourism

# 54

Ariel Shuchleib, Felipe Cantú, Elias Chousleb, and Natan Zundel

Medical tourism is the practice of patients traveling to other towns, states, or countries to receive medical, dental, or surgical care for reasons such as cost, access, or quality. Medical tourism can be classified into three types: outbound (traveling to a foreign country for treatment), inbound (traveling to one's home country from abroad for treatment), and domestic (traveling within one's home country for treatment) [1]. Depending on the tourist's choice, medical tourism can also be classified as mandatory or elective [2]. Mandatory travel occurs when the required treatments are not available or are illegal in the traveler's place of origin and, consequently, it becomes necessary to travel to another place to access these services. Other studies have classified these forms of travel and tourism into specific types based on the purpose of treatment, such as dental tourism, stem cell tourism, bariatric surgery, spa tourism, vacationing tourism, fertility treatment, orthopedic, ophthalmologic, cosmetic surgery, cardiac care, organ transplantation and even alternative medicine therapies [3–5].

The first historically documented tour took place in 1841 by the travel agent, Thomas Cook, who organized a tour of 570 people to travel from Leicester to the Loughborough Hot Springs. However, long ago, people in ancient Greece used to travel considerable distances to receive medical treatment [6]. The United States is

A. Shuchleib (✉)
Department of Surgery, Saint Agnes Medical Center, Fresno, CA, USA

F. Cantú
Department of Surgery, Christus Health System, Hospital Christus Muguerza Reynosa, Reynosa, Mexico

E. Chousleb
Department of Surgery, Jackson North Hospital, Miami, USA

N. Zundel
Department of Surgery, University at Buffalo, NY Jackson North Hospital, Miami, USA



O. M. Ghanem et al. (eds.), *The SAGES Manual of Metabolic and Bariatric Surgery*, https://doi.org/10.1007/978-3-031-72309-4_54

the largest destination market for inbound medical tourists, with spending reaching almost $4 billion in 2017 and representing nearly 36% of global medical tourism spending. In the past decade, there has been a notable surge in the number of medical tourists visiting the United States from their home nations to receive medical attention in the specialties of cardiovascular procedures, cosmetic surgery, dental care, orthopedics, oncology, and fertility treatments [7].

The Mayo Clinic describes Destination Care as a model of healthcare that "enables patients and families, including both local patients and those traveling long distance, to receive medical care comprehensively and expeditiously" [8]. As an example of domestic medical tourism, Amazon, Berkshire Hathaway, JP Morgan, General Electric, Boeing, and Lowe's are just a few of many US companies that are disrupting the healthcare model and are referring their staff to selected facilities for specialized medical care driven by their employer's value-based healthcare coverage [9]. Walmart is aware of the fact that healthy workers are more productive. Results based on evidence show that bariatric surgery lowers long-term medical expenses, enhances employee productivity, and improves health. Walmart partnered with Geisinger Health System in 2016 for Bariatric Surgery and by 2019 they had seven destination care bariatric centers operated by Walmart in the United States [10, 11].

With 20% of the international market, the United States also leads the globe in outbound medical tourism, with US citizens spending around $2.3 billion on international medical tourism services in 2017 and in 2022 similarly led the global market with the highest market share [7, 12]. It was estimated that more than 15 million patients traveled outside the United States to receive medical care in 2017, and this number is expected to increase by 15–25% every year with the highest outflow of patients from the US to Mexico [13].

The global concept of medical tourism is mostly used for patients who travel internationally to receive medical care. The American Society for Metabolic and Bariatric Surgery (ASMBS) in its position statement from 2011 adopted the term "global bariatric healthcare" (GBH) and they define it as traveling any distance that precludes routine follow-up or continuity of care with the surgeon [14]. Due to the time in which it was written, this definition doesn't take into consideration the possibility of telemedicine, which is significantly more readily available with low to no cost since the COVID pandemic. In most cases when we talk about medical tourism, the purpose is to achieve a more accessible treatment from an economic point of view; however, it can also be used to receive specialized medical care in places with a lot of experience, resources and/or renown [15].

Bariatric Medical tourism is an expanding global practice and rapidly growing economic activity [16–19]. Driven by high healthcare costs, long patient waiting lists, or lack of access to innovative therapies in certain countries, many medical tourists (primarily from the United States, Canada, and Western Europe) often seek access to care in South and Central Asia, Europe, and Latin America. According to a global survey by IFSO, it is estimated that the medical tourism industry worldwide is worth over $400 billion/year dollars. In this study, Parmar et al. surveyed 383

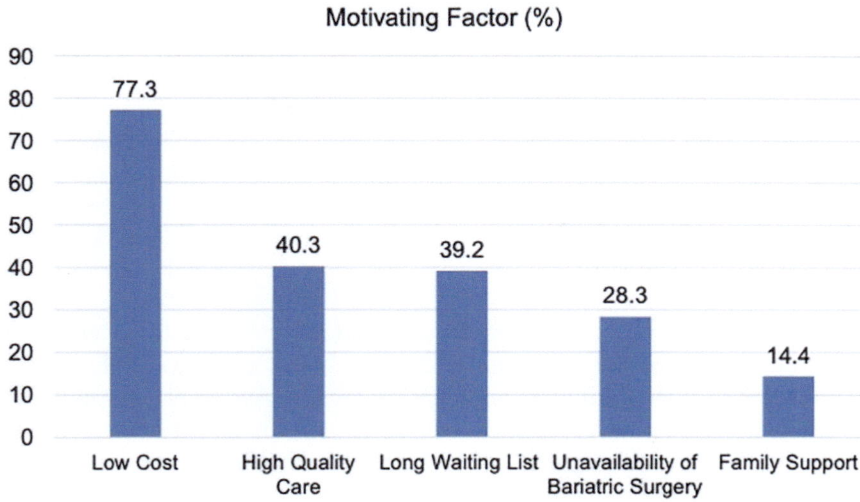


**Fig. 54.1** Motivating factors for medical tourism by Parmar et al. [8]—copyrights to Springer

bariatric healthcare professionals from 65 different countries, the respondent's opinion was that the most common reason for GBH was a low cost, followed by a higher quality of care, long waiting lists, unavailability of the procedure and lastly due to family support (Fig. 54.1). In the same survey, the average cost of a surgery was \$8716 but prices ranged from \$2000–\$30,000 dollars which shows why the economic incentive was so strong [20].

Multiple factors can simultaneously influence decisions related to the destination chosen for treatment including culture, social norms, religious factors, and the institutional environment. Socioeconomic conditions shape the decision-making and spending behavior of medical tourists. Accommodation, transportation options, as well as the length of stay are some of the factors taken into consideration [21], but perceived quality, satisfaction, and trust in staff and clinics have significantly stronger associations with the patients traveling to a specific location [22].

The research originated using CiteSpace software, which shows that scholars publishing in this field were spread across 61 countries. The largest group of authors originated from the United States ($n$ = 197). The second and third largest groups were from Canada ($n$ = 88), the United Kingdom ($n$ = 84), followed by Australia ($n$ = 70) and South Korea ($n$ = 65). Authors from the United States and Canada have made the most significant contributions to medical-health-wellness tourism based on the number of articles published [6].

Despite having certain advantages like better access, affordability of treatment, and in some cases better quality of care, there are different aspects that must be considered in this type of medical practices [21]. The following paragraphs discuss certain considerations in the bariatric tourism realm.

***The Quality of Medical Care*** Given that in most cases we associate medical tourism with less expensive services, this decrease in costs can go hand in hand with a reduction in the quality of the services and equipment used to provide medical care. This could also affect the patient's safety, depending on the reason for seeking care and the ease of accessing it, patients may be at increased risk of complications by having to travel to other cities or countries. Some of the most common complications seen in bariatric patients are leaks, infections, deep vein thrombosis (DVT), pulmonary embolism (PE), or anatomical abnormalities that might require revisional surgery like strictures.

***Limited Resources*** Given that healthcare resources are limited, the access to healthcare for the local population might decrease based on the availability of services that can be provided if those resources are used for foreign patients. But even in cases where the resources are sufficient, the costs might be out of reach for the local population since the prices will be tailored for medical tourists who many times travel from more affluent countries.

***Malpractice*** If a problem arises due to negligence or malpractice, and depending on the location where the procedures are performed, patients might not have the same legal protections that they have where they live. There is also the potential of problems related to coverage by the insurance if a complication arises and the index procedure is not covered by the insurance in the place of origin the patient could be held responsible for paying the expenses related to those complications.

***Complications*** Some complications do not happen or are not diagnosed immediately and when they occur. The patient might no longer be in the place where the treatment was performed, and even if they are still in the location where the procedure was done, the place will not necessarily have enough resources to manage it. In addition, if the patient is already back home and develops a complication, finding a physician or institution that will take care of the patient could be problematic.

***Cultural Differences*** Due to cultural differences between different places, some practices carried out in the medical destination may be considered unethical in the country of origin. In addition, the privacy laws and the management of the patient's information are different in each country; there is a possibility that the management of patient medical information is not protected in the place of treatment in the same way as it is in the patient's country of origin.

***Follow Up*** Lastly, bariatric surgery just like many other specialties requires the patients to have a long-term follow-up, lack of access to it could hinder the patient's outcomes and prevent them from having long-term success.

## Conclusions

Medical tourism is a very good tool since it allows people with means access to the most advanced technologies, also gives access to patients with limited resources to certain therapeutics when otherwise would not be able to receive them in their place of origin, as well as attaining medical attention without delay. The globalization of the healthcare industry led to a significant increase in the popularity of medical travel. However, this great tool also has some clinical and ethical dilemmas that have to be taken into consideration while deciding to get treatment in a different location from the place of origin.

## References

1. Turski I, et al. Medical tourism: analysis of the state of international tourism and prospects for domestic development. Universal J Public Health. 2021;9:27–34. https://doi.org/10.13189/ujph.2021.090201.
2. Jones CA, Keith LG. Medical tourism and reproductive outsourcing: the dawning of a new paradigm for healthcare. Int J Fertil Womens Med. 2006;51:251–5.
3. Pereira RT, Malone CM, Flaherty GT. Corrigendum to: aesthetic journeys: a review of cosmetic surgery tourism. J Travel Med. 2018;25:tay051.
4. Crozier GKD, Thomsen K. Stem cell tourism and the role of health professional organizations. Am J Bioeth. 2010;10:36–8.
5. Turner L. "Medical Tourism" and the global marketplace in health services: U.S. patients, international hospitals, and the search for affordable health care. Int J Health Serv. 2010;40:443–67.
6. Zhong L, Deng B, Morrison AM, Coca-Stefaniak JA, Yang L. Medical, health and wellness tourism research-a review of the literature (1970–2020) and research agenda. Int J Environ Res Public Health. 2021;18(20):10875.
7. Turner R. World Travel & Tourism Council: Medical Tourism: A Prescription for a Healthier Economy—November 2019.
8. Berry LL, Seltman KD. Practicing destination medicine. In: Management lessons from Mayo Clinic: inside one of the world's most admired service organizations. McGraw-Hill; 2017.
9. Petrick AT, Gadaleta D. Raising the standard: destination care as a model of employer value-based healthcare. Bariatric Times. 2019;16(9):17.
10. Woods L, Slotkin JR, Coleman MR. How employers are fixing health care. Mar 2018. Harvard Business Review site. https://hbr.org/coverstory/2019/03/howemployers-are-fixing-health-care. Accessed 27 Dec 2023.
11. Petrick AT, Gadaleta D. Raising the standard: destination care as a model of employer value-based healthcare, part 2. Bariatric Times. 2019;16(10):14–5.
12. Precedence Research. Medical Tourism Market; 2024. https://www.precedenceresearch.com/medical-tourism-market.
13. Patients Beyond Borders. Medical tourism statistics and facts. Available at: https://www.patientsbeyondborders.com/media. Accessed 15 Sep 2023.
14. Surgery for Obesity and Related Diseases 7 (2011) 669–671 ASMBS statement American Society for Metabolic and Bariatric Surgery position statement on global bariatric healthcare.
15. Davison SP, Hayes KD, LaBove G, Shaffer P. The Price of medical tourism: the legal implications of surgery abroad. Plast Reconstr Surg. 2018;142(4):1075–108.
16. Chaulagain S, Pizam A, Wang Y. An integrated behavioral model for medical tourism: an American perspective. J Travel Res. 2021;60:761–78.

17. Rokni L, Park S-H. Medical tourism in Iran, reevaluation on the new trends: a narrative review. Iran J Public Health. 2020;48:1191–202.
18. Rouland B, Jarraya M. From medical tourism to regionalism from the bottom up: emerging transnational spaces of care between Libya and Tunisia. J Ethn Migr Stud. 2020;46:4248–63.
19. Rodríguez NR, Cote L, Fuentes C, et al. First national consensus on the safe practice of medical tourism for bariatric surgery in Mexico. Obes Surg. 2023;33:1060–72.
20. Parmar CD, McCluney SJ, Rodriguez N, Behrens E, Lakdawala M, Kow L, Shikora S, Ramos A. A global survey by the International Federation for the Surgery of obesity and metabolic disorders (IFSO) on perceptions of Bariatric Medical Tourism (BMT) by health professionals: guidelines from IFSO for BMT. Obes Surg. 2021;31(4):1401–10.
21. Foley BM, Haglin JM, Tanzer JR, Eltorai AEM. Patient care without borders: a systematic review of medical and surgical tourism. J Travel Med. 2019;26(6):taz04.
22. Han H, Hyun SS. Customer retention in the medical tourism industry: impact of quality, satisfaction, trust, and price reasonableness. Tour Manag. 2015;46:20–9.

# Navigating the Divide: Unraveling Disparities in Access, Utilization, and Outcomes of Bariatric Surgery

# 55

Shaneeta Johnson, Ryan Hill, and Juliet Holder-Haynes

Obesity is the second-leading cause of preventable death in the United States [1]. Despite awareness of the health and financial implications of obesity, the prevalence of obesity continues to rise. The National Health and Nutrition Examination Survey demonstrates that the prevalence of obesity has increased over the past two decades from 30.5% to 41.9% [2]. The health implications of obesity are significant, including increased morbidity, mortality, and development of chronic diseases such as Type 2 diabetes mellitus, hypertension, and cardiovascular disease. Additionally, the economic burden of obesity is estimated at approximately $100 billion annually in the United States [1]. While obesity impacts all populations, ethnic minorities and lower socioeconomic populations are disproportionately affected. Additionally, ethnic minorities are more impacted by obesity-related conditions. Studies demonstrate that obesity prevalence is highest in non-Hispanic Black adults at 49.9% prevalence compared to Hispanic adults at 45.6% prevalence, non-Hispanic White adults at 41.4% prevalence, and non-Hispanic Asians with 16.1% prevalence [3]. Accordingly, severe obesity was also most commonly identified in non-Hispanic Black adults at a 14% prevalence rate compared to non-Hispanic whites at 9.5%, Hispanic adults at 7.4%, followed by non-Hispanic Asians at 1.8% prevalence rates [3]. Additionally, studies demonstrate a higher rate of obesity-related conditions, such as hypertension, type 2 diabetes, and non-alcoholic fatty liver disease, in ethnic minorities [4]. Black women have the highest rates of obesity, with a prevalence of 57.9%, which is 1.46 times that of non-Hispanic White women and a prevalence of

S. Johnson (✉)
Department of Surgery, Morehouse School of Medicine & Satcher Health Leadership Institute, Morehouse School of Medicine, Atlanta, GA, USA

R. Hill
Department of Surgery, Morehouse School of Surgery, Atlanta, GA, USA

J. Holder-Haynes
Division of Metabolic and Bariatric Surgery, Baylor College of Medicine, Houston, TX, USA





O. M. Ghanem et al. (eds.), *The SAGES Manual of Metabolic and Bariatric Surgery*, https://doi.org/10.1007/978-3-031-72309-4_55

19% or 1.59 times that of non-Hispanic White women of severe obesity. They have also been shown to have an almost twofold higher risk of developing diabetes and hypertension at an earlier age [3, 5]. Studies have suggested that Black patients experience higher rates of racism, which may be a contributing factor to the increased prevalence of obesity by increased allostatic load [4, 6].

## Disparities in Access and Utilization

There are numerous disparities related to adequate access to and utilization of obesity prevention and treatment [7]. These include ethnic disparities in utilization, geographic disparities, disparities in age and gender utilization, and inequitable access to care. Additional potential barriers include inadequate referrals from providers, implicit bias, language and cultural barriers, lack of cultural competence, uninsured or underinsured status, and inequitable policies for obesity, prevention, and treatment.

### Age Disparities in Bariatric Surgery Utilization

Age plays a significant role in utilization disparities in bariatric surgery. Wallace et al. demonstrated in a review of the 2006 Nationwide Inpatient Sample that patients aged 40 to 59 years have an increased likelihood of pursuing surgery [8]. They were 1.5 times more likely to pursue bariatric surgery than patients aged 20 to 39 years old and six times more likely than patients aged greater than 60 years old [8]. Despite the underutilization of surgery in the elderly population studies demonstrate the safety and efficacy of bariatric surgery in this patient population [9]. Age disparities in the utilization of bariatric surgery are also significant in the adolescent patient population, which demonstrates a decreased utilization of bariatric surgery despite the prevalence of obesity in this patient population and the demonstrated efficacy of this treatment in the adolescent age group.

### Geographic and Rural Disparities in Access and Utilization of Bariatric Surgery

Geography plays an integral part in access to care. Disparities in access to bariatric surgery exist for rural populations. Research indicates that eligible residents of rural areas are 23% less likely to undergo bariatric surgery compared to their urban counterparts [8, 10]. These disparities are multifaceted and influenced by various factors, including geographical barriers, socioeconomic factors, cultural, community, and educational factors.

Geographical barriers play a significant role. Rural areas often lack specialized bariatric centers and experienced surgeons, making it challenging for patients to access these services. The limited availability of healthcare facilities in remote regions contributes to the lower likelihood of rural residents receiving bariatric surgery.

While the US South has the greatest concentration of obesity, patients in the South and Midwest are half as likely to receive bariatric surgery [8]. These disparities likely result from multifactorial reasons, including insurance access, cultural barriers, access to care, and other factors.

Socioeconomic factors may also cause significant barriers. Rural communities tend to have lower income levels and reduced access to private insurance coverage, contributing to potential financial barriers. Transportation costs and travel distances to urban centers may be significant and can deter rural individuals from seeking surgical treatment. Individuals in rural communities may also face challenges to adopting healthy eating and physical activity, including lack of access to healthy grocery and recreational facilities, lack of sidewalks, greater financial difficulties, and poverty [10, 11].

Cultural and educational factors influence patient decisions. Awareness about bariatric surgery and its benefits may be lower in rural areas. Lack of education and misconceptions about the procedure can lead to hesitancy or reluctance among potential candidates and referring providers.

## Racial Disparities in Bariatric Surgery Utilization

The racial disparities are evident in bariatric surgery utilization. Khattab et al. looked at the role of ethnic disparities in bariatric surgery utilization trends. They evaluated 23 studies comprising 71.679 patients. They found that the majority of patients who underwent bariatric surgery were White (77%), compared to Blacks (9.3%), African-Americans (1.3%), Hispanics (10.4%), Non-Hispanics (1%), and Asians (1%) [12]. Using MBSAQIP data, Steinberger et al. found similar disparities in utilization trends in Black adolescents when compared to their White counterparts. White adolescents underwent 71.5% of bariatric procedures, compared to 16.4% Black, and 12.1% Other [13].

Despite higher rates of obesity and obesity-related comorbidities, Native Americans were also demonstrated to have lower rates of bariatric surgery utilization than White adults. Conversely, they were found to have significantly shorter lengths of stay, lower healthcare expenditures, and lower likelihood of being discharged to other healthcare facilities compared to White Americans.

Further studies have demonstrated that White Americans are twice as likely to have surgery than African-Americans, Asian Americans, and Native Americans. Hispanic patients were 20% less likely to receive surgery, and in general, minority populations were less likely to pursue bariatric surgery despite having a higher rate of obesity and obesity-related comorbidities [8].

## Equitable Environment and Community Disparities

### Socioeconomic Status and Social Determinants of Health

Socioeconomic status, access to healthcare, and cultural factors play pivotal roles. Patients with higher incomes and private insurance are more likely to undergo bariatric procedures. However, a higher percentage of eligible adults have lower socioeconomic status and government-insured or uninsured status [14]. Patients with lower socioeconomic status and ethnic minorities are also more likely to live in areas with decreased access to safe spaces for physical activity.

### Political and Environmental Determinants of Health

Ethnic minorities and lower socioeconomic status patients are also more likely to live in food deserts and areas of high environmental risk, such as increased air pollution, heat islands, and poorer water quality, all contributing to higher rates of obesity. Historical redlining and other policies have contributed to ethnic minorities residing in higher environmental risk areas, which contribute to an increased burden of disease and overall poor health [15, 16].

### Cultural and Language Disparities

Cultural differences also contribute to obesity, its prevalence, norms, and attitudes. Accounting for cultural differences and practices is crucial to ensuring culturally competent care and increasing access to bariatric surgery to treat obesity [17, 18]. Language barriers may play a role in the thorough understanding of obesity, treatment options, and the ability to adhere to the intense preoperative regimen required by most insurance companies for the performance of bariatric surgery.

## Access to Care

### Insurance Access and Coverage Disparities

Lack of Access to adequate healthcare insurance coverage is a significant barrier and cause of disparities. The Affordable Care Act was enacted in 2010 with the goal of increasing access to health care by improving the affordability of quality coverage. While the ACA has improved disparities in health coverage, ethnic disparities in access persist. Black adults were 1.5 times more likely to be uninsured than White adults, and Hispanic adults were 2.5 times more likely to be uninsured. Under the ACA, Medicaid expansion should have increased access to equitable care; however, not all states have adopted Medicaid expansion. Kaiser Foundation demonstrated that 40% of eligible Black adults reside in states without Medicaid expansion and are more likely to remain uninsured [19, 20].

Patients with government insurance are eight times less likely to undergo bariatric surgery [8]. Black patients are more likely to be underinsured or uninsured than White patients. Lower physician and healthcare reimbursements combined with center accreditation volume requirements also likely play a role in lower rates of utilization of bariatric surgery in this patient population.

Martin et al. studied the eligible population for bariatric surgery in the US utilizing the National Institute of Health criteria. They found that the eligible population had a lower family income, education level, and access to healthcare and represented a higher proportion of ethnic minorities than the general population [21]. Startlingly, a significant proportion of eligible patients, one-third, were also uninsured or underinsured, and 15% had an income that was less than the poverty level [21]. Their study also demonstrated that most bariatric procedures were performed conversely in patients with private insurance, White adults, and with higher than median incomes [21]. Thus, significant disparities exist between the population eligible for bariatric surgery and those who can take advantage of this treatment. Studies have demonstrated that Medicare and Medicaid patients have higher rates of obesity and obesity-related complications; however, Hennings et al. demonstrated that the majority of patients undergoing bariatric surgery had private insurance [14].

### Access to Skilled Surgeons and Facilities

Rural communities, lower socioeconomic populations, and ethnic minority populations often have low access to healthcare facilities with skilled bariatric surgeons and bariatric programs. The requirements for accreditation with high volume may also exclude low volume, rural hospitals, and thus those patient populations from access to bariatric surgery, thus acting as a barrier to access to this vital treatment option for morbid obesity. The recent closure of multiple hospital systems and hospitals, especially in rural and lower socioeconomic communities, also contributes to decreased access to care for these impacted patient populations.

### Referrals and Implicit Bias

Healthcare providers' implicit biases may influence treatment decisions, follow-up care, and patient counseling. In a study of nearly 5000 patients at a single academic center who met NIH bariatric surgery eligibility criteria, only 5% of patients received a referral, and Hispanic patients were found to have the lowest referral rate. Factors related to lack of referral include insurance payor status, patient preference, lack of referral, and language/cultural barriers [22]. Prior studies have demonstrated that 30% of patients were not recommended for bariatric surgery by primary care physicians [23]. Addressing provider biases is essential for equitable outcomes.

## Disparities in Outcomes

In addition to disparate access to bariatric surgery care, Unfortunately, these underserved and disparate populations also often have unequal outcomes. This further threatens to widen the existing disparities, including health gaps, wealth gaps, and socioeconomic factors.

### Racial Disparities in Bariatric Surgery Outcomes

Obesity occurs in higher prevalence in Black and Hispanic patients. Despite higher rates of obesity, Black and Hispanic patients undergo metabolic surgery at lower rates and have higher rates of post-operative complications [24, 25]. A study of propensity score-matched Black and White patients found that Black patients had lower rates of weight loss compared to their White counterparts and a higher rate of 30-day complications and resource utilization [26]. In analyzing NSQIP data, Turner et al. found that Hispanic patients had higher rates of bleeding and kidney injury requiring dialysis, and Black patients had a higher prevalence of pulmonary embolism [27]. Looking at 148,829 Roux-en-y gastric bypass (RNYGB) patients in the MBSAQIP database over a 5-year period, Edwards et al. found that year-to-year mortality was two to three times higher in Non-Hispanic Blacks compared to Non-Hispanic Whites despite the improved safety profile of RNYGB. Their study identified a higher rate of venous thromboembolism (VTE) in Black patients [28]. The underlying causes remain unclear, although potential causes include pre-existing comorbidities, mobility status, insurance status, pulmonary disease, coronary artery disease, and smoking status.

## Insurance Disparities in Bariatric Surgery Outcomes

Patients with Medicare or Medicaid insurance are less likely to receive bariatric surgery and more likely to experience complications from surgery and longer length of stay [14]. These patients were also more likely to have healthcare costs that exceeded the 75th percentile [14].

## Age Disparities in Bariatric Outcomes

Bariatric surgery in elderly patients remains a topic of debate, with conflicting data regarding its effectiveness and safety. However, recent evidence sheds light on the outcomes for older individuals undergoing bariatric procedures. A systematic review encompassing 8149 elderly patients (60 years or older) revealed that bariatric surgery outcomes were comparable to those in younger populations. The mortality rate within 30 days postoperatively was minimal (0.01%), and the overall complication rate stood at 14.7%. At 1-year follow-up, the mean excess weight loss was 53.77%, and significant improvements were observed in diabetes resolution (54.5%), hypertension resolution (42.5%), and lipid disorder resolution (41.2%) [29]. Belluzzi et al. also demonstrated safety and efficacy of bariatric surgery in elderly patients as well with improvement of obesity-related conditions [9]. Individualized assessment is crucial, considering comorbidities and overall health. In 2022, the American Society of Bariatric Surgery (ASMBS) and the International Federation for the Surgery of Obesity and Metabolic Disorders (IFSO) endorsed bariatric and metabolic surgery for extremes of age which include elderly and pediatric patient populations [30]. Bariatric surgery can be a valuable option for elderly individuals struggling with morbid obesity, provided careful evaluation and personalized management are in place.

## Socioeconomic Disparities in Bariatric Surgery Outcomes

Socioeconomic disparities can significantly affect safety and outcomes after bariatric surgery.

These disparities are often multifactorial and complex. For instance, individuals with challenging employment situations, such as tenuous employment, job-related stress, or instability, may find it difficult to maintain healthy habits after surgery. Patients with limited income and financial constraints may struggle to access nutritious food, follow-up care, and necessary lifestyle adjustments. Unreliable transportation can also significantly burden patients' ability to get to medical appointments or exercise facilities, potentially impeding their weight-loss progress. Additionally, living in unsafe or inconvenient neighborhoods with safety concerns can discourage outdoor physical activity, which is crucial for maintaining a healthy lifestyle after bariatric surgery. Limited health literacy in certain populations can have a significant impact on their ability to understand important dietary guidelines and post-operative care instructions. Moreover, low health literacy can also make it difficult for patients to comply with these guidelines. Unfortunately, these barriers tend to affect socioeconomically disadvantaged patients more than others, underscoring the need for targeted interventions to support their weight-loss journey after bariatric surgery [31].

## Culture, Quality of Life and Satisfaction

Cultural, familial, and other factors may influence body norms, satisfaction, and quality of life views in patients with obesity. These factors may also play a role in outcomes regarding excess weight loss and post-operative BMI. Societal perceptions of body weight influence how obesity may be perceived. Individuals with obesity may be subjected to bullying, discrimination, and weight bias [32].

However, cultural body norms also may exert pressure to conform to body sizes. Cultural foods hold historical and familial significance. After bariatric surgery, patients may need to modify their diets which may impact family gatherings and traditions [32].

A desire for improved quality of life drives many individuals to seek bariatric surgery. Cultural beliefs and expectations may play a significant role in this decision [32]. Understanding cultural nuances, community norms, and individual perspectives is crucial for optimizing bariatric surgery outcomes and ensuring holistic patient well-being.

## Current and Future Directions to Address Inequity

Addressing inequity requires a multipronged approach to addressing systemic, structural, socioeconomic, policy, and individual barriers to obesity treatment (Table 55.1). Evidence-based interventions are necessary to ensure the efficacy and

**Table 55.1** Recommendations to address inequities in bariatric surgical care

| Barriers | Disparity | Populations impacted | Solutions |
|---|---|---|---|
| **Access to care** | Inequitable insurance access<br>Decreased provider referrals<br>Inadequate surgeon workforce<br>Stigma and bias | Lower socioeconomic populations<br>Ethnic minorities<br>Rural geography | Increase state access to obesity treatment<br>Cultural competency training and initiatives<br>Implicit bias training<br>Diversification of the workforce<br>Transportation and housing access<br>Medicaid expansion<br>Elimination of inequitable race norming indices, eg. Body mass index<br>Improve medical education of obesity and obesity treatment<br>Standardize referral algorithms for obesity treatment |
| **Equitable environment and community resources** | Food deserts<br>Environmental determinants of health (eg. Urban heat islands, inadequate water and food supply, poor air quality)<br>Lack of access to safe spaces for physical activity | Lower socioeconomic populations<br>Ethnic minorities<br>Rural geography<br>Elderly | Advocate for state and federal policies to increase access to resources<br>Safe spaces for physical activity<br>Access to healthy nutrition eg. Nutrition prescription programs<br>Community organization partnerships |
| **Structural and systemic barriers** | Structural and systemic racism<br>Political determinants of health (inequitable policies, access) | Ethnic minorities<br>Lower socioeconomic populations | Advocacy for state and federal policies to improve access and treatment of obesity |
| **Diversity in research** | Paucity of diversity in research populations<br>Inequitable diverse representation on editorial boards and research review committees | Ethnic minorities<br>Rural populations | Increased diversity of study populations<br>Standardize research protocols to include diverse populations<br>Increased diversity of editorial boards and research review committees |
| **Culturally competent care** | Nonadherence to cultural norms and practices<br>Access to translation and culturally appropriate services | Ethnic minorities | Translation services utilization<br>Increased telehealth utilization<br>Improved community involvement and engendering of trust<br>Implementation of tailored, culturally appropriate medical approach to health education |

sustainability of initiatives to address disparities in bariatric care. These include providing culturally competent care, provider education, implicit bias training, increasing diversity in research, diversity within the health workforce, and equitable community resources and access to care [33]. Efforts should focus on improving access to bariatric surgery for underserved populations. This includes addressing insurance coverage gaps and promoting culturally competent care.

Racial concordance between physician and patient has been demonstrated to improve clinical outcomes in Black patients [34, 35]. Studies have shown that diverse surgeons and surgeons from lower socioeconomic backgrounds are more likely to treat underrepresented and diverse patient populations, including those with higher Medicaid and Medicare populations [36]. Thus, diversifying the surgeon workforce will increase access to treatment for these underserved populations.

Improving access to specialized bariatric centers in rural regions, expanding insurance coverage, and increasing awareness through community education programs are essential steps. Training healthcare professionals to recognize and mitigate biases is crucial. Culturally sensitive communication and shared decision-making can enhance patient outcomes. Engaging communities in discussions about obesity, its impact, and available treatments can reduce stigma, engender trust, and encourage informed decision-making.

## Conclusion

Health disparities in bariatric surgery represent a complex dilemma involving multiple layered factors such as ethnicity, age, geographic location, socioeconomic status, and other determinants of health. To address these disparities effectively, a comprehensive approach is necessary that not only focuses on the clinical aspects of bariatric surgery but also considers the social, political, and environmental determinants of health.

This comprehensive focus involves increasing access to research that examines the underlying causes of these disparities and their impact on affected populations. A hands-on and collaborative approach among providers, policymakers, and communities is crucial for addressing these health disparities within bariatric surgery in an effective and culturally competent manner to identify and implement effective solutions and equitable outcomes that improve the lives of all patients seeking weight-loss interventions, regardless of their background or circumstances.

## References

1. Panuganti KK, Nguyen M, Kshirsagar RK. Obesity. [Updated 2023 Aug 8]. In: StatPearls [Internet]. Treasure Island (FL): StatPearls Publishing; 2024 Jan–. https://www.ncbi.nlm.nih.gov/books/NBK459357/#.
2. Stierman B, Afful J, Caroll MD, Chen T-C, Davy O, Fink S, Fryar CD, Gu Q, Hales CM, Hughes J, Ostchega Y, Storandt R, Akinbami L.. National Health and Nutrition Examination

Survey 2017–March 2020 Prepandemic Data Files—Development of Files and Prevalence Estimates for Selected Health Outcomes. 2021; 158.
3. Fryar CD, Caroll MD, Afful J. Prevalence of overweight, obesity, and extreme obesity among adults aged 20 and over: United States, 1960–1962 through 2017–2018. https://www.cdc.gov/nchs/data/hestat/obesity-adult-17-18/obesity-adult.htm.
4. Washington TB, Johnson VR, Kendrick K, Ibrahim AA, Tu L, Sun K, Stanford FC. Disparities in access and quality of obesity care. Gastroenterol Clin N Am. 2023;52(2):429–41. https://doi.org/10.1016/j.gtc.2023.02.003.
5. Abraham PA, Kazman JB, Zeno SA, Deuster PA. Obesity and African Americans: physiologic and behavioral pathways. ISRN Obesity. 2013;2013:314295. https://doi.org/10.1155/2013/314295.
6. Carr LTB, Bell C, Alick C, et al. Responding to health disparities in behavioral weight loss interventions and COVID-19 in black adults: recommendations for health equity. J Racial Ethn Health Disparities. 2022;9(3):739–47.
7. Jackson TD, Zhang R, Glockler D, Pennington J, Reddigan JI, Rotstein OD, Smylie J, Perrier L, Conn LG. Health inequity in access to bariatric surgery: a protocol for a systematic review. Syst Rev. 2014;3:15. https://doi.org/10.1186/2046-4053-3-15.
8. Wallace AE, Young-Xu Y, Hartley D, Weeks WB. Racial, socioeconomic, and rural-urban disparities in obesity-related bariatric surgery. Obes Surg. 2010;20(10):1354–60. https://doi.org/10.1007/s11695-009-0054-x. Epub 2010 Jan 6. PMID: 20052561.
9. Belluzzi A, Hage K, Abi Mosleh K, et al. Long-term safety and efficacy of bariatric surgery in septuagenarians. Obes Surg. 2023;33:3778–85. https://doi.org/10.1007/s11695-023-06882-y.
10. Bauman V, Apostolopoulos AN, Hasse G, Parkman TJ, Ross KM. Rural/urban weight-loss outcomes following bariatric surgery. Obes Sci Pract. 2021;7(6):797–802. https://doi.org/10.1002/osp4.515.
11. Dixon BN, Piervil E, Eastman A, Ross KM. A social-ecological review of the rural versus urban obesity disparity. Health Behav Policy Rev. 2019;6:378–94. https://doi.org/10.14485/HBPR.6.4.6.
12. Khattab MA, Mohammed ATA, Alqahtani AZM, Alqahtani EZM, Alslim MMA, Alharbi NEA, Alslim RMA, Saleh Z, Atia MAQ, Shanaq AJ, Saleh A. The role of ethnic disparities in the outcomes of bariatric surgery: a systematic review and meta-analysis. Cureus. 2022;14(5):e24743. https://doi.org/10.7759/cureus.24743. PMID: 35686257; PMCID: PMC9170373.
13. Steinberger AE, Youngwirth LM, Kim SE, Duke NN, Skinner A, Gordee A, Kuchibhatla M, Armstrong S, Seymour KA. Adolescent bariatric surgery: racial disparities in 30-day outcomes using the MBSAQIP from 2015 to 2018. Obes Surg. 2021;31(8):3776–85. https://doi.org/10.1007/s11695-021-05500-z. Epub 2021 May 27. PMID: 34043179; PMCID: PMC8895205.
14. Hennings DL, Baimas-George M, Al-Quarayshi Z, et al. The inequity of bariatric surgery: publicly insured patients undergo lower rates of bariatric surgery with worse outcomes. Obes Surg. 2018;28(1):44–51.
15. Dawes DE. The political determinants of health. Johns Hopkins University Press; 2020.
16. Dawes DE, Dunlap NJ, Johnson SM. The Surgeon's role in addressing racism and achieving health equity. Am Surg. 2021;87(11):1704–12. https://doi.org/10.1177/00031348211038562.
17. Lindberg NM, Stevens VJ, Halperin RO. Weight-loss interventions for Hispanic populations: the role of culture. J Obes. 2013;2013:542736. https://doi.org/10.1155/2013/542736.
18. McLaughlin EA, Campos-Melady M, Smith JE, Serier KN, Belon KE, Simmons JD, Kelton K. The role of familism in weight loss treatment for Mexican American women. J Health Psychol. 2017;22(12):1510–23. https://doi.org/10.1177/1359105316630134.
19. Artiga S, Damico A, Published RG. The Impact of the Coverage Gap for Adults in States not Expanding Medicaid by Race and Ethnicity. KFF; 2015, October 26. https://www.kff.org/racial-equity-and-health-policy/issue-brief/the-impact-of-the-coverage-gap-in-states-not-expanding-medicaid-by-race-and-ethnicity/.
20. Guth M, Garfield R, Published RR. The Effects of Medicaid Expansion under the ACA: Studies from January 2014 to January 2020. KFF; 2020, March 17. https://www.kff.org/medicaid/report/the-effects-of-medicaid-expansion-under-the-aca-updated-findings-from-a-literature-review/.

21. Martin M, Beekley A, Kjorstad R, Sebesta J. Socioeconomic disparities in eligibility and access to bariatric surgery: a national population-based analysis. Surg Obes Relat Dis. 2010;6(1):8–15.
22. Johnson-Mann C, Martin AN, Williams MD, Hallowell PT, Schirmer B. Investigating racial disparities in bariatric surgery referrals. Surg Obes Relat Dis. 2019;15(4):615–20. https://doi.org/10.1016/j.soard.2019.02.002.
23. Afonso BB, Rosenthal R, Li KM, Zapatier J, Szomstein S. Perceived barriers to bariatric surgery among morbidly obese patients. Surg Obes Relat Dis. 2010;6(1):16–21.
24. Bhogal SK, Reddigan JI, Rotstein OD, et al. Inequity to the utilization of bariatric surgery: a systematic review and meta-analysis. Obes Surg. 2015;25:888–99. https://doi.org/10.1007/s11695-015-1595-9.
25. Acevedo E Jr, Lu X, Zhao H, Mazzei M, Sarvepalli S, Edwards MA. Outcomes in racial minorities after robotic Roux-en-Y gastric bypass and sleeve gastrectomy: a retrospective review of the Metabolic and Bariatric Surgery Accreditation and Quality Improvement Program database. Surg Obes Relat Dis. 2021;17(3):595–605. https://doi.org/10.1016/j.soard.2020.10.019. Epub 2020 Oct 21. PMID: 33257274.
26. Wood MH, Carlin AM, Ghaferi AA, Varban OA, Hawasli A, Bonham AJ, Birkmeyer NJ, Finks JF. Association of race with bariatric surgery outcomes. JAMA Surg. 2019;154(5):e190029. https://doi.org/10.1001/jamasurg.2019.0029. Epub 2019 May 15. Erratum in: JAMA Surg. 2019 Jun 5;: PMID: 30840063; PMCID: PMC6537777.
27. Turner PL, Oyetunji TA, Gantt G, Chang DC, Cornwell EE, Fullum TM. Demographically associated variations in outcomes after bariatric surgery. Am J Surg. 2011;201(4):475–80. https://doi.org/10.1016/j.amjsurg.2010.08.035. PMID: 21421101.
28. Edwards MA, Hussain MWA, Spaulding AC. Gastric bypass mortality trends in racial cohorts: are we improving? Obes Surg. 2023;33(5):1411–21. https://doi.org/10.1007/s11695-023-06541-2. Epub 2023 Mar 14. PMID: 36918474.
29. Giordano S, Victorzon M. Bariatric surgery in elderly patients: a systematic review. Clin Interv Aging. 2015;10:1627–35. https://doi.org/10.2147/CIA.S70313.
30. Eisenberg D, Shikora SA, Aarts E, et al. 2022 American Society for Metabolic and Bariatric Surgery (ASMBS) and International Federation for the Surgery of Obesity and Metabolic Disorders (IFSO): indications for metabolic and bariatric surgery. Surg Obes Relat Dis. 2022;18:1345–56.
31. Funk LM, Alagoz E, Murtha JA, Breuer CR, Pati B, Eierman L, Jawara D, Farrar-Edwards D, Voils CI. Socioeconomic disparities and bariatric surgery outcomes: a qualitative analysis. Am J Surg. 2023;225(4):609–14. https://doi.org/10.1016/j.amjsurg.2022.09.049.
32. Raaijmakers LC, Pouwels S, Thomassen SE, Nienhuijs SW. Quality of life and bariatric surgery: a systematic review of short- and long-term results and comparison with community norms. Eur J Clin Nutr. 2017;71(4):441–9. https://doi.org/10.1038/ejcn.2016.198.
33. Johnson-Mann C, Hassan M, Johnson S. Improving equity and access to bariatric surgery. Lancet Gastroenterol Hepatol. 2023;8(12):1068–70.
34. Greenwood BN, Hardeman RR, Huang L, Sojourner A. Physician–patient racial concordance and disparities in birthing mortality for newborns. Proc Natl Acad Sci. 2020;117(35):21194–200. https://doi.org/10.1073/pnas.1913405117.
35. Snyder JE, Upton RD, Hassett TC, Lee H, Nouri Z, Dill M. Black representation in the primary care physician workforce and its association with population life expectancy and mortality rates in the US. JAMA Netw Open. 2023;6(4):e236687. https://doi.org/10.1001/jamanetworkopen.2023.6687.
36. Marrast LM, Zallman L, Woolhandler S, Bor DH, McCormick D. Minority physicians' role in the care of underserved patients: diversifying the physician workforce may be key in addressing health disparities. JAMA Intern Med. 2014;174(2):289–91. https://doi.org/10.1001/jamainternmed.2013.12756.

# Ambulatory Metabolic/Bariatric Surgery 56

Imam N. Sanousi and Abdelrahman Nimeri

## Introduction

Metabolic/bariatric surgery (MBS) leads to durable weight loss and improvement in obesity complications such as type II diabetes, hypertension (HTN) and obstructive sleep apnea (OSA). In addition, MBS is considered the best treatment for severe obesity with or without obesity complications [1, 2]. Furthermore, the safety of MBS has improved, and MBS is considered as safe as cholecystectomy and hip replacement [3, 4]. The safety of MBS improved due to several factors. These factors include utilizing minimally invasive alternatives to open surgery, fellowship training of metabolic/bariatric surgeons, the establishment of a center of excellence designation and the development of registries like the Metabolic and Bariatric Surgery Accreditation and Quality Improvement Program (MBSAQIP) [5–7].

The most performed MBS procedures in the United States (>90%) are sleeve gastrectomy (SG) and Roux-en-Y gastric bypass (RYGB) [8]. In addition, despite the safety of SG and RYGB, >90% of patients are admitted to the hospital for at least one night after MBS for pain control, monitoring and control of postoperative nausea and vomiting and many patients stay in the hospital after MBS for two to three days [9–11]. Furthermore, the benefits of same day/ambulatory MBS are still debatable and other factors are at play in dictating the safety of MBS [12–21]. For example, hospital volume has been shown to correlate with shorter hospital stays, better outcomes, and a lower risk for postoperative complications [22]. Others emphasized the need for appropriate patient selection and allocation of precious and

I. N. Sanousi
University of Southern California, Keck School of Medicine, Los Angeles, CA, USA

A. Nimeri (✉)
Brigham & Women's Hospital, Harvard Medical School, Boston, MA, USA
e-mail: animeri@bwh.harvard.edu



O. M. Ghanem et al. (eds.), *The SAGES Manual of Metabolic and Bariatric Surgery*, https://doi.org/10.1007/978-3-031-72309-4_56

limited resources and that long hospital days are simply not necessary and lead to increased costs [23, 24]. Some have even argued that longer time spent in the hospital post-op is associated with worse outcomes [25]. In this chapter, we will discuss the status, risks, and benefits of ambulatory MBS in the United States.

## Definitions

Many terms are used to describe patients who do not get admitted to the hospital after MBS. These terms include same day MBS, outpatient MBS and ambulatory MBS to name a few. In addition, these terms include patients discharged within a few hours after MBS as well as patients who stayed overnight and were discharged <23 hours after MBS. In this chapter, only patients who were discharged on the same day of surgery will be considered in this chapter and considered ambulatory MBS. Studies including patients who stayed overnight or were discharged <23 hours after MBS will be excluded.

## Importance/Relevance

Traditionally, patients are admitted to the hospital for at least one night after MBS including sleeve gastrectomy (SG) and Roux-en-Y gastric bypass (RYGB). During the overnight hospital stay, patients are carefully monitored for early signs of complications such as bleeding, venous thromboembolism (VTE) or leak, they are given intravenous hydration and control of pain and nausea is assured [6, 9–11]. However, consideration for ambulatory MBS is recently considered due to advances in narcotic-sparing pain medications, enhanced recovery, advances in the management of postoperative nausea and vomiting and availability of remote monitoring and virtual care [9, 14, 20, 26, 27]. The value of ambulatory MBS includes reducing the cost of MBS care, increasing patient comfort by having post-MBS care at home and possibly allowing MBS to be performed at outpatient surgery centers outside the hospital setting in the future [20, 23, 26, 27]. Reducing the cost of MBS by utilizing ambulatory MBS may improve patient access to MBS while maintaining safety and quality of care delivered to patients by maximizing consistency among protocols, equipment, and hospital staff [14–16, 20, 21, 25]. There are many reports that have shown that in patients with minimal risk factors, same day discharge is a safe and viable option and poses little risk of morbidity and mortality [11–16]. Though these findings are promising, it is important to note that ambulatory MBS may not be appropriate for all patients, especially high-risk populations.

## Candidates for Ambulatory Metabolic/Bariatric Surgery

Identifying candidates for ambulatory MBS requires careful procedure and patient selection. For example, when considering procedure selection, ambulatory SG is most performed compared to ambulatory RYGB or biliopancreatic diversion-duodenal switch (BPD-DS) or single anastomosis duodenoileostomy with or without SG (SADI-S) [11–16, 19–22]. Likewise, patient selection of lower-risk patients is important to minimize postoperative complications and readmission after MBS [24, 25, 28]. Readmission after MBS can be due to various reasons including nausea, vomiting, abdominal pain or complications such as bleeding, leak and venous thromboembolism (VTE) after MBS. The delay in managing post-MBS complications may lead to significant morbidity, possible mortality after MBS and potential medicolegal ramifications [29, 30]. In addition, readmissions after ambulatory MBS may increase the overall cost of MBS. Some patients are considered high risk for readmission after MBS and there are a few independent risk factors that predispose certain populations to be readmitted [24, 31]. For example, Dreifuss et al. identified intraoperative complications as the greatest risk for readmission after SG [24]. Other independent risk factors include female sex, African American race, history of gastroesophageal reflux disease (GERD) and history of VTE. In contrast, Dubchuck et al. identified male gender, insurance status, age, overall patient comorbidity status and hospital status affect readmission after MBS [31]. Hence ambulatory MBS is not for all patients who undergo MBS, and a risk-benefit assessment is necessary to exclude high-risk patients and patients with a high risk for readmission. In addition, patients who undergo ambulatory MBS may benefit from remote monitoring and virtual care while they are at home [26, 27]. For example, patients with Centers for Medicare and Medicaid Services insurance are typically considered high risk as they are either quality due to age > 65 years or disability [32]. Recently, CMS considered in the third quarter of 2023 removing SG & RYGB from the inpatient-only list for the calendar year 2024 which will only pay for ambulatory SG and RYGB and strongly recommending for SG and RYGB to be performed in an ambulatory setting [33]. However, after an open comment period that ended on September 11, 2023, CMS announced in November of 2023 that there is not enough evidence to document the safety of performing SG and RYGB on patients with CMS insurance as ambulatory SG and RYGB [33].

## How Safe Is Ambulatory Metabolic/Bariatric Surgery?

The literature examining the safety of ambulatory MBS is mixed and careful consideration of the level of evidence is needed before making any conclusions. For example, there are no large randomized controlled trials comparing ambulatory MBS to inpatient hospital stay, and most studies are registry studies like the MBSAQIP registry or prospective and retrospective cohort studies with the potential for selection bias for both procedures and patients included in the ambulatory MBS arm. In addition, when comparing patients who are admitted to the hospital after MBS, studies report that outcomes of patients discharged on POD#1 are like patients discharged on POD#2 or with longer length of stay after MBS with literature pointing to lower-risk patients being discharged on POD#1 [14, 22, 28]. For example, Khorgami et al. reported on patients discharged on POD#1 or later and reported that the early discharge group after MBS had fewer comorbidities pointing to a lower-risk group and a lower rate of complications and readmission [14].

Some studies show that ambulatory RYGB leads to higher mortality while others report that ambulatory RYGB is as safe as inpatient RYGB reporting on the same dataset from the MBSAQIP registry [11, 17–19]. For example, Morton et al. and Inaba et al. reported that ambulatory MBS was associated with a higher rate of morbidity and risk-adjusted mortality while Barbat et al. and Dreifuss et al. reported that ambulatory RYGB is as safe as inpatient RYGB. To understand the discrepancy in outcomes for ambulatory RYGB, it is important to note that when evaluating morbidity and mortality after ambulatory MBS using retrospective registry studies the patients who experience complications on the day of surgery are excluded from analysis in some studies (Barbat et al. and Dreifuss et al) or included in the same day MBS group in other studies (Morton et al. and Inaba et al). For example, if patients who had complications or died on POD#0 are counted as ambulatory MBS then ambulatory MBS will appear to have a higher risk for morbidity and mortality while these patients due to the retrospective nature of the registry studies might have not been assigned to ambulatory MBS but rather they just died or had complications on POD#0. This can only be assessed using a prospective study design. For example, small (50 patients) and large (>500 patients) prospective studies have shown that ambulatory RYGB is well selected for patients including patients with controlled OSA with the aid of remote monitoring [20, 21, 34]. Similarly, Dreifuss et al. reported that patients undergoing RYGB and were discharged on the same day had a lower risk of 30-day interventions ($p = 0.04$) compared to patients who stayed in the hospital following their surgery. However, since these studies are not randomized, lower-risk or more educated patients are selected to be in the ambulatory RYGB group. Like ambulatory RYGB, Billing et al. conducted a prospective analysis on 250 patients undergoing ambulatory SG at a free-standing ambulatory center with similar outcomes to SG performed in the hospital setting as an inpatient. They found that in this cohort of patients, there were no deaths, and the rate of complications was like SG patients who were admitted to the hospital after SG. The authors point to the importance of patient selection for ambulatory SG and suggest that by carefully selecting lower-risk patients with minimal pulmonary and cardiovascular comorbidities we can help to reduce the risk of complications. In addition, it is more likely that patients with a higher level of education and lower risk will undergo ambulatory MBS [15].

Some of the benefits of ambulatory MBS include lower costs, convenience for the patient and their family, and a shorter length of stay after MBS. In addition, ambulatory MBS can be performed outside the hospital setting in ambulatory surgery centers. Ambulatory surgery centers, which specialize primarily in outpatient procedures, provide outpatient surgeries at much lower costs than hospitals. This could be due to factors including streamlined patient care, smaller facilities, less personnel turnover and shorter operating room times [12, 13, 15, 16, 23, 35]. For example, Munnich et. Al found that ambulatory surgery centers generated up to $1000 in savings per outpatient case [23]. Similarly, Khorgami et al. found that longer hospital stays are linearly associated with increasing costs and that by 7 days, the cost of the procedure is doubled [14]. Furthermore, despite MBS being minimally invasive, MBS places a great strain on patients both physically and emotionally so careful patient selection is of paramount importance. After ambulatory MBS, lower-risk patients can spend their recovery comfortably in their own homes rather than surrounded by the stress-inducing environment of the hospital.

In our healthcare system, we use a same-day MBS protocol that includes transfer to the Home Hospital, a virtual setup. For example, according to our protocol, candidates for same-day bariatric surgery are carefully chosen and must meet a specific set of criteria to be considered. These criteria include having someone to stay with them at home on the first night after surgery, living within a certain mile radius from the hospital and willingness to be enrolled in the Home Hospital virtual monitoring platform to monitor their pulse and oxygen saturation. In addition, only patients between the ages of 18 and 65 are considered and their BMI must not exceed a BMI of 55 for male patients and BMI of 60 for female patients. Additionally, high-risk patients such as patients on insulin, or CPAP due to severe OSA or significant cardiopulmonary or renal dysfunction are excluded from same day MBS. This means patients that have severe organ failures like congestive heart failure (CHF), end-stage renal disease (ESRD), or end-stage liver disease (ESLD) are often excluded as well as patients with a history of or currently in need of an organ transplant. Finally, patients must be able to ambulate without assistance and be willing to undergo same day MBS.

When patients leave the hospital, we call it transfer to the Home Hospital setup rather than discharge to home. This means that patients go home with their IV access in place and they are carefully monitored to ensure a safe and full recovery and allow early detection of complications after MBS if they occur at home. We use a wireless patch that transmits their pulse rate and oxygen saturation, and these are logged into the electronic medical record system and are monitored by a team of physician extenders and nurses. In addition, all patients receive a visit at home the night of surgery and the next morning by paramedics or physician extenders with the ability to administer fluids at home. On postoperative day 1, a virtual visit by the surgeon ensures that the patient is doing well and isn't experiencing any unexpected symptoms. One to two weeks after same day MBS, the patient comes to the clinic for the standard in-person postoperative check-up by the surgical team.

## Conclusion

Ambulatory MBS has generally been found to be safe in selected patients after SG and RYGB with the aid of remote monitoring and virtual care.

In carefully selected patients, ambulatory SG and RYGB patients have similar mortality, reoperation, readmission, and overall morbidity to patients admitted to the hospital.

The Center for Medicare and Medicaid Services (CMS) did not find enough evidence in 2023 to justify performing ambulatory SG or RYGB in patients with CMS insurance.

It is important to recognize that patient selection and remote monitoring may complement a shorter postoperative stay in ambulatory MBS to allow prompt management of patients who develop postoperative complications and prevent morbidity from delayed recognition of complications after MBS.

## References


1. Eisenberg D, Shikora SA, Aarts E, Aminian A, Angrisani L, Cohen RV, de Luca M, Faria SL, Goodpaster KPS, Haddad A, Himpens JM, Kow L, Kurian M, Loi K, Mahawar K, Nimeri A, O'Kane M, Papasavas PK, Ponce J, Pratt JSA, Rogers AM, Steele KE, Suter M, Kothari SN. 2022 American Society of Metabolic and Bariatric Surgery (ASMBS) and International Federation for the Surgery of Obesity and Metabolic Disorders (IFSO) Indications for Metabolic and Bariatric Surgery. Obes Surg. 2023;33(1):3–14.
2. Eisenberg D, Shikora SA, Aarts E, Aminian A, Angrisani L, Cohen RV, de Luca M, Faria SL, Goodpaster KPS, Haddad A, Himpens JM, Kow L, Kurian M, Loi K, Mahawar K, Nimeri A, O'Kane M, Papasavas PK, Ponce J, Pratt JSA, Rogers AM, Steele KE, Suter M, Kothari SN. 2022 American Society of Metabolic and Bariatric Surgery (ASMBS) and International Federation for the Surgery of Obesity and Metabolic Disorders (IFSO) Indications for Metabolic and Bariatric Surgery. Surg Obes Relat Dis. 2022;18(12):1345–56. https://doi.org/10.1016/j.soard.2022.08.013. Epub 2022 Oct
3. Bhattacharyya S, Kaddoura S. Perioperative safety and bariatric surgery. New Engl J Med. 2009;361(19):1911; author reply 1911. Surg Endosc
4. Zhao K, Liu J, Wang M, Yang H, Aiguo W. Safety and efficacy of laparoscopic sleeve gastrectomy versus laparoscopic Roux-en-Y gastric bypass: a systematic review and meta-analysis. J Eval Clin Pract. 2020;26(1):290–8. https://doi.org/10.1111/jep.13170. Epub 2019 May 22
5. Nguyen NT, Vu S, Kim E, Bodunova N, Phelan MJ. Trends in utilization of bariatric surgery, 2009–2012. Surg Endosc. 2016;30(7):2723–7. https://doi.org/10.1007/s00464-015-4535-9. Epub 2015 Dec 10
6. Greene ME, Grieco A, Evans-Labok K, Ko CY, Hutter MM. First report of outcomes from the patient-reported outcome measures program in the Metabolic and Bariatric Surgery Accreditation Quality Improvement Program. Surg Obes Relat Dis. 2023: S1550-7289(23)00697-4. https://doi.org/10.1016/j.soard.2023.09.010. Online ahead of print.
7. Edgerton C, Heshmati K, Herman A, Dey T, Dehkharghani R, Ramsis MR, Vernon A, Ghushe N, Spector D, Shikora S, Tavakkoli A, Sheu EG. Fellowship training influences learning curves for laparoscopic sleeve gastrectomy. Surg Endosc. 2022;36(2):1601–8. https://doi.org/10.1007/s00464-021-08372-7. Epub 2021 Feb 23
8. https://asmbs.org/resources/estimate-of-bariatric-surgery-numbers. Accessed 10 May 2023.
9. Seu R, Pereira X, Goriacko P, Yaghdjian V, Appiah D, Moran-Atkin E, Camacho D, Kim J, Choi J. Effectiveness of Bariatric Surgery Targeting Opioid Prescriptions (BSTOP) protocol on postoperative pain control. Surg Endosc. 2023;37(6):4902–9.
10. Kim TY, Kim S, Schafer AL. Medical management of the postoperative bariatric surgery patient. National Institutes of Health; 2018b.
11. Barbat S, Thompson KJ, Mckillop IH, Kuwada TS, Gersin K, Nimeri A. Ambulatory bariatric surgery: does it really lead to higher rates of adverse events? Surg Obes Relat Dis. 2020;16(11):1713–20. https://doi.org/10.1016/j.soard.2020.06.051. Epub 2020 Jul 5
12. Aryaie A, Reddy V, Dattilo Z, Janik M. Safety of same-day discharge after laparoscopic sleeve gastrectomy: propensity score–matched analysis of the Metabolic and Bariatric Surgery Accreditation and Quality Improvement Program Registry. Surg Obes Relat Dis. 2021;17(1):46–53. https://doi.org/10.1016/j.soard.2020.08.039.
13. Vanetta C, Dreifuss NH, Angeramo CA, Baz C, Cubisino A, Schlottmann F, Masrur MA. Outcomes of same-day discharge sleeve gastrectomy and Roux-en-Y gastric bypass: a

systematic review and meta-analysis. Surg Obes Relat Dis. 2023;19(3):238–49. https://doi.org/10.1016/j.soard.2022.09.004. Epub 2022 Sep 11
14. Khorgami Z, Petrosky JA, Andalib A, Aminian A, Schauer PR, Brethauer SA. Fast track bariatric surgery: safety of discharge on the first postoperative day after bariatric surgery. Surg Obes Relat Dis. 2017;13(2):273–80. https://doi.org/10.1016/j.soard.2016.01.034.
15. Billing P, Crouthamel M, Oling S, Landerholm R. Outpatient laparoscopic sleeve gastrectomy in a free-standing ambulatory surgery center: first 250 cases. Surg Obes Relat Dis. 2014;10(1):101–5. https://doi.org/10.1016/j.soard.2013.07.005.
16. Surve A, Cottam D, Zaveri H, Cottam A, Belnap L, Richards C, Medlin W, Duncan TD, Tuggle K, Zorak A, Umbach TW, Apel M, Billing P, Billing J, Landerholm R, Stewart K, Kaufman J, Harris E, Williams ML, et al. Does the future of laparoscopic sleeve gastrectomy lie in the outpatient surgery center? A retrospective study of the safety of 3162 outpatient sleeve gastrectomies. Surg Obes Relat Dis. 2018;14(10):1442–7. https://doi.org/10.1016/j.soard.2018.05.027.
17. Morton JM, Winegar DA, Blackstone RP, Wolfe BM. Is ambulatory laparoscopic Roux-En-Y gastric bypass associated with higher adverse events? Ann Surg. 2014;259(2):286.
18. Inaba CS, Koh CY, Sujatha-Bhaskar S, Zhang L, Nguyen NT. Same-day discharge after laparoscopic Roux-en-Y gastric bypass: an analysis of the metabolic and bariatric surgery accreditation and quality improvement program database. J Am Coll Surg. 2018;226(5):868 873. https://doi.org/10.1016/j.jamcollsurg.2018.01.049.
19. Dreifuss NH, Vanetta C, Schlottmann F, Cubisino A, Mangano A, Baz C, Bianco FM, Gangemi A, Hassan C, Masrur M. Is same-day discharge after Roux-en-Y gastric bypass safe? A metabolic and bariatric surgery accreditation and quality improvement program database analysis. Obes Surg. 2022;32(12):3900–7. https://doi.org/10.1007/s11695-022-06303-6.
20. Nijland LMG, de Castro SMM, Vogel M, Coumou J-WF, van Rutte PWJ, van Veen RN. Feasibility of same-day discharge after laparoscopic Roux-en-Y gastric bypass using remote monitoring. Obes Surg. 2021;31(7):2851–8. https://doi.org/10.1007/s11695-021-05384-z. Epub 2021 Apr 6
21. Kleipool SC, Nijland LMG, De Castro SMM, Vogel M, Bonjer HJ, Marsman HA, Van Rutte P, Van Veen RN. Same-day discharge after laparoscopic Roux-en-Y gastric bypass: a cohort of 500 consecutive patients. Obes Surg. 2023;33(3):706–13. https://doi.org/10.1007/s11695-023-06464-y.
22. Nguyen NT, Mahbod Paya C, Stevens M, Mavandadi S, Zainabadi K, Wilson SE. The relationship between hospital volume and outcome in bariatric surgery at academic medical centers. Ann Surg. 2004 Oct;240(4):586–94. https://doi.org/10.1097/01.sla.0000140752.74893.24.
23. Munnich EL, Parente ST. Procedures take less time at ambulatory surgery centers, keeping costs down and ability to meet demand up. Health Aff. 2014;33(5):764–9. https://doi.org/10.1377/hlthaff.2013.1281.
24. Dreifuss NH, Xie J, Schlottmann F, Cubisino A, Baz C, Vanetta C, Mangano A, Bianco FM, Gangemi A, Masrur M. Risk factors for readmission after same-day discharge sleeve gastrectomy: a metabolic and bariatric surgery accreditation and quality improvement program database analysis. Obes Surg. 2022;32(4):962–9. https://doi.org/10.1007/s11695-022-05919-y.
25. Khorgami Z, Aminian A, Shoar S, Andalib A, Saber AA, Schauer PR, Brethauer SA, Sclabas GM. Cost of bariatric surgery and factors associated with increased cost: an analysis of national inpatient sample. Surg Obes Relat Dis. 2017;13(8):1284–9. https://doi.org/10.1016/j.soard.2017.04.010.
26. Schaffner TJ, Wilkes M, Laverty R, Schwab SD, Zahradka N, Pugmire J, Yourk D, Masella PC, Walter R. Remote patient monitoring to facilitate same-day discharge after laparoscopic sleeve gastrectomy: a pilot evaluation. Surg Obes Relat Dis. 2023;19(9):1067–74. https://doi.org/10.1016/j.soard.2023.02.028. [Epub ahead of print]
27. Scheerhoorn J, van Ede L, Luyer MDP, Buise MP, Arthur Bouwman R, Nienhuijs SW. Postbariatric EArly discharge Controlled by Healthdot (PEACH) trial: study protocol for a preference-based randomized trial. Trials. 2022;23:67. https://doi.org/10.1016/j.soard.2023.02.028.

28. Jonathan Carter MD, Steven Elliott MD, Jennifer Kaplan MD, Matthew Lin MD, Andrew Posselt MD, Stanley Rogers MD. Predictors of hospital stay following laparoscopic gastric bypass surgery: analysis of 9,593 patients from the National Surgical Quality Improvement Program. Surg Obes Relat Dis. 2015;37(6):4902–9. https://doi.org/10.1016/j.soard.2014.05.016. Epub 2022 Sep 27.
29. Morton JM, Khoury H, Brethauer SA, Baker JW, Sweet WA, Mattar S, Ponce J, Nguyen NT, Rosenthal RJ, DeMaria EJ. First report from the American Society of Metabolic and Bariatric Surgery closed-claims registry: prevalence, causes, and lessons learned from bariatric surgery medical malpractice claims. Surg Obes Relat Dis. 2022;18(7):943–7. https://doi.org/10.1016/j.soard.2022.04.004. Epub 2022 Apr 21
30. Cottam D, Lord J, Dallal RM, Wolfe B, Higa K, McCauley K, Schauer P. Medicolegal analysis of 100 malpractice claims against bariatric surgeons. Surg Obes Relat Dis. 2007;3(1):60–6. https://doi.org/10.1016/j.soard.2006.10.008. discussion 66-7. Epub 2006 Dec 27.
31. Dubchuk C, Afifi AM, Chawla K, Nasif A, Ren G, Osman MF, Sferra J, Pannell S, Nazzal M Gender, BMI, Patient comorbidities, and hospital characteristics influence 30-day readmission following vertical sleeve gastrectomy. Obes Surg 2023. doi: https://doi.org/10.1007/s11695-023-06855-1. Online ahead of print.
32. Nimeri A, Oviedo R, Vosburg WR, Fam J, Blalock CA, Altieri MS, Augustin T, Hallowell P, Carter JT, Clinical Issues Committee of the American Society for Metabolic and Bariatric Surgery. ASMBS statement on metabolic and bariatric surgery for beneficiaries of Centers for Medicare and Medicaid Services with a review of the literature. Surg Obes Relat Dis. 2023:S1550-7289(23)00700-1. https://doi.org/10.1016/j.soard.2023.09.013. Online ahead of print.
33. https://www.federalregister.gov/public-inspection/2023-24293/medicare-program-hospital-outpatient-prospective-payment-and-ambulatory-surgical-center-payment. Accessed 11 Dec 2023.
34. Kleipool SC, de Castro SMM, Vogel M, Reesink HJ, van Rutte PWJ, van Veen RN. Feasibility of same-day discharge after laparoscopic Roux-en-Y gastric bypass in patients with well-regulated obstructive sleep apnea. Obes Surg. 2023;33(3):807–12. https://doi.org/10.1007/s11695-022-06439-5. Epub 2023 Jan 4.PMID: 36598709. PMCID: PMC9812010.
35. Stepaniak PS, Heij C, Buise MP, Mannaerts GHH, Smulders JF, Nienhuijs SW. Bariatric surgery with operating room teams that stayed fixed during the day. Anesth Analg. 2012;115(6):1384–92. https://doi.org/10.1213/ane.0b013e31826c7fa6.


## Further Readings


Monfared S, Weis JJ, Shah SK, Scott DJ, Felinski MM, EB Wilson. The rising tide of revisional surgery: tracking changes in index cases among bariatric-accredited fellowships. Surg Endosc. 2023;37(6):4824–8.

Cheng S, Lee PC, Sim JXL, Tan AS, Ng CLW, Foo AXY, Abdullah HRB, Tan JTH, Ong HS, Lim CH. Cost-savings of short stay sleeve gastrectomy and walk-in hydration clinic versus conventional inpatient care. Surg Endosc. 2023;37(11):8349–56. https://doi.org/10.1007/s00464-023-10414-1. Epub 2023 Sep 12

# Biliary Considerations Before, During, and After Metabolic Surgery

57

Rachel Reed, Savannah Smith, Eli Mlaver, and S. Scott Davis Jr

## Introduction

Biliary diseases such as symptomatic cholelithiasis and cholecystitis are increasingly prevalent in the general population, with approximately 750,000 cholecystectomies performed annually in the United States. The prevalence of biliary disease (including asymptomatic cholelithiasis) in the general population ranges from 2 to 20%, with approximately 4% of these patients going on to develop symptomatic disease and require cholecystectomy. This number is increased to up to 30% of patients suffering from obesity with 10% to 31% progressing to symptomatic disease requiring cholecystectomy [1, 2]. Moreover, patients who have undergone metabolic surgeries including sleeve gastrectomy (SG), Roux-en-Y gastric bypass (RYGB) and biliopancreatic diversion with duodenal switch (BPD-DS) are at increased risk of symptomatic biliary disease than their non-operative counterparts, particularly during the period of rapid weight loss postoperatively [3, 4].

The increased prevalence of biliary disease in the population suffering from obesity can be partially attributed to the supersaturation of cholesterol in bile leading to cholelithiasis formation. Postoperative patients with rapid weight loss experience decreased biliary motility, decreased cholecystokinin (CCK) secretion—particularly following RYGB—and progressive cholesterol supersaturation of the bile, further increasing their risk of biliary disease [5, 6]. It is also important to note that the anatomical changes following certain bariatric procedures can make routine, non-operative interventions to manage biliary disease, such as ERCP, and laparoscopic cholecystectomy more technically challenging.

R. Reed · S. Smith · E. Mlaver · S. Scott Davis Jr (✉)
Department of Surgery, Emory University, Atlanta, GA, USA
e-mail: sdavisj@emory.edu





O. M. Ghanem et al. (eds.), *The SAGES Manual of Metabolic and Bariatric Surgery*, https://doi.org/10.1007/978-3-031-72309-4_57

Despite the well-acknowledged increased risks, there is limited guidance on biliary disease screening and management, including the timing of cholecystectomy, for patients undergoing bariatric surgery. With the advancement of laparoscopic techniques and increased incidence of obesity, laparoscopic techniques for biliary disease and metabolic surgery are now the standard of care. Herein, we explore pre- and postoperative screening for biliary disease; the use of ursodiol in postoperative patients; as well as indications and risks for preoperative, concomitant, or postoperative cholecystectomies in the bariatric surgery population.

## Preoperative Assessment

While patients who are being evaluated for bariatric surgery must undergo rigorous preoperative evaluation with nutritionists, surgeons, and mental health professionals, there exist no recommendations or guidelines regarding preoperative biliary screening. The current literature does not support routine screening for biliary disease in asymptomatic patients undergoing bariatric surgery [7]. It is estimated that up to 43% of patients undergoing bariatric surgery who are not experiencing biliary symptoms will have incidental gallstones if evaluated [6]. Up to 93% of these patients will *not* go on to develop symptomatic disease necessitating cholecystectomy [2]. Patients who exhibit symptoms of biliary disease, whether that be biliary sludge, dyskinesia, or symptomatic cholelithiasis, should undergo preoperative workup, including pertinent labs, right upper quadrant ultrasound, and MRCP, as indicated. The preoperative evaluation of biliary disease in patients undergoing metabolic surgery is not unique compared to the general patient population. Despite the increased risk of biliary disease following bariatric surgery, there is no role for routine preoperative cholecystectomy in asymptomatic patients.

Discussion of cholecystectomy prior to bariatric surgery versus concomitant cholecystectomy in patients who have symptomatic biliary disease is up to the surgeon's discretion. Preoperative cholecystectomies in this population can present unique challenges, given the prevalence of hepatomegaly and visceral adiposity. An average of 50 additional minutes may be added to laparoscopic cholecystectomy for patients with obesity because of these technical challenges [8]. Patients who are profoundly symptomatic or who have evidence of choledocholithiasis may benefit from preoperative cholecystectomy for improvement in quality of life and preparation for bariatric surgery.

## Concomitant Cholecystectomy

The addition of a cholecystectomy to a laparoscopic bariatric procedure can be technically challenging given the differences in port placement between the two procedures, often necessitating an additional subdiaphragmatic right lateral port for cholecystectomy, as well as a difficult body habitus. Furthermore, concomitant cholecystectomy with bariatric surgery increases operating room time, which can increase operative risk and early postoperative complications. Analysis of NSQIP data suggests that concomitant cholecystectomy with laparoscopic sleeve gastrectomy increases rates of postoperative pneumonia by three-fold [9]. Patients undergoing concomitant cholecystectomy with RYGB were found to have a significantly increased likelihood of organ space infection (1.3%), pneumonia (1.3%), acute kidney injury (0.5%), and wound complications (0.6%) compared to their counterparts undergoing RYGB without cholecystectomy [10]. It has also been shown through analysis of MBSAQIP data that patients undergoing either RYGB or SG with concomitant cholecystectomy have longer operative times, length of stay, and higher readmission rates [19]. Of note, data regarding laparoscopic cholecystectomy performed concomitantly with BPD-DS demonstrates longer operative time, however, there was no significant difference noted in 30-day postoperative morbidity, mortality, reoperation, or readmission [20]. Though postoperative complications following cholecystectomy and bariatric surgery are uncommon—including bile duct injury for cholecystectomy and leak or internal hernia for bariatric surgery—they can be morbid and require reoperation. The likelihood of reoperation is roughly 30% higher in patients undergoing concomitant procedures; therefore, careful consideration and selection of appropriate patients must be taken to optimize outcomes [10, 11]. We recommend stratifying patient by their burden of biliary symptoms to inform this decision as follows:

## Asymptomatic Patients

Given the potential of postoperative morbidity, prophylactic concomitant cholecystectomy during bariatric surgery is not recommended for patients without preoperative biliary symptoms. While there is an increased risk of gallstone formation in the period of rapid weight loss postoperatively, the absolute likelihood of symptomatic cholelithiasis requiring intervention in postoperative bariatric surgery patients has been estimated at less than 5%; performing routine prophylactic concomitant cholecystectomy with the bariatric procedure in asymptomatic patients results in cholecystectomy for many patients who otherwise would not require biliary intervention. Therefore, the operative and postoperative risks outweigh the benefits when considering prophylactic concomitant cholecystectomy in patients without preoperative symptoms [12]. However, while uncommon, if the bariatric procedure requires an open approach, concomitant cholecystectomy should be strongly considered due to the ease in concomitant cholecystectomy coupled with the increase in postoperative adhesions and for future diagnostic clarity in the case of future abdominal pain.

## Symptomatic Patients

In patients who have symptomatic biliary disease, it is recommended to remove the gallbladder at the time of the bariatric procedure. Conducting both operations together mitigates the risks of a second episode of general anesthesia as well as the costs of a second surgical encounter. While not our practice, some surgeons suggest performing cholecystectomy prior to bariatric surgery to mitigate the risks of bile leak complicating the new bariatric procedure. We acknowledge that especially in patients undergoing RYGB, postoperative ERCP is challenging given the anatomical changes, so management of bile leak is especially challenging. As bile leak is a rare complication of cholecystectomy, as noted above, we feel that the benefit of sparing the second surgical encounter outweighs the risks of concomitant procedures in the majority of cases. Ultimately, the timing of cholecystectomy in symptomatic patients is left up to the discretion of the surgeon. The severity of symptoms, overall patient health, and how far out they are from their planned bariatric surgery are all factors that need to be taken into account.

## Postoperative Assessment/Complications

### Postoperative Screening

Postoperative bariatric patients are at a five-times increased risk of developing gallstones when compared to the general population, with 10–38% developing cholelithiasis in the first 2 years postoperatively [6, 16]. Up to 8% of patients undergoing RYGB and 3–4% of patients after SG will develop symptomatic gallstones or biliary sludge requiring intervention [1, 2, 5, 8, 13, 14]. Indications for cholecystectomy are not distinctly different from the general population; most commonly cholecystitis, gallstone pancreatitis, and choledocholithiasis. Risk factors for the development of postoperative symptomatic biliary disease include female gender, age >50 years, cholelithiasis prior to bariatric procedure, diabetes, and RYGB [4, 13]. While postoperative routine screening in those without symptomatic biliary disease preoperatively is not currently recommended, a high suspicion should be maintained throughout their postoperative follow-up.

### Timing of Onset of Symptoms and Interval Cholecystectomy

Over half of patients developing symptomatic biliary pathology requiring intervention do so within the first 6–12 months, and up to 80% within the first two years, often during the period of active weight loss [14]. Surgeons should be diligent about evaluating symptoms that may be attributable to biliary disease or cholelithiasis during routine follow-up in this vulnerable postoperative period. While asymptomatic gallstones are identified in up to 22% of patients, only 3–8% of those with cholelithiasis will develop symptoms and ultimately require cholecystectomy [1, 2, 5, 8, 13–15]. While postoperative cholecystectomies may present challenges due to adhesive disease from prior intervention, at roughly two months postoperatively the difficulty of cholecystectomy decreases in this population, likely due to decreased liver size and reduced intraabdominal fat [12].

A special consideration in this population, specifically those who have undergone either RYGB or BPD-DS, is choledocholithiasis. It is estimated that 1–15% of patients in the general population with cholelithiasis will have an incidental stone in the common bile duct if a routine intraoperative cholangiogram (IOC) is performed [21]. This poses a unique challenge in the patients who have undergone RYGB or BPD-DS given their altered anatomy. ERCP in this population is much more difficult and requires transgastric access or retrograde ERCP, performed by GI specialists specifically trained in these enhanced techniques, or combination surgery with surgeons for transgastric/transenteral access [8]. While there is minimal data regarding this topic, it is our opinion that at a center without the ability to perform ERCP, IOC, or laparoscopic common bile duct exploration, an MRCP would be extremely logical to consider as part of the routine preoperative workup those requiring cholecystectomy following bariatric surgery. In centers in which they do have these capabilities, it would be understandable to forego preoperative MRCP. Choosing to do either MRCP or IOC as a routine step in the workup and treatment of these patients, in the absence of compelling data, should be left up to the discretion of the managing team.

### Ursodeoxycholic Acid (UDCA)

UDCA is a secondary bile acid that increases cholesterol solubility in bile. It has been shown to effectively decrease gallstone formation and therefore risk of cholecystectomy in the postoperative bariatric population [8, 16]. Data from a randomized control trial suggest that 600 mg of UDCA can decrease the formation of postoperative biliary stones by over 90%, leading to some bariatric centers universally recommending the use of UDCA postoperatively for 3–6 months in attempts to prevent early postoperative cholecystectomy [8, 16, 17]. Of note, UDCA is a large pill that is difficult to swallow and is poorly tolerated in some patients due to side effects including nausea and diarrhea. It is therefore sometimes self-discontinued by patients in the postoperative period, with widely varying adherence rates ranging from 28 to 92% among patients enrolled in randomized clinical trials [18]. Medical management of biliary disease prevention post-bariatric surgery highlights the importance of a multidisciplinary team approach in bariatric patients.

## Conclusions

We have outlined the role of screening for biliary disease in the pre- and postoperative periods as well as prophylactic, concomitant, or delayed cholecystectomy and the use of UDCA in the bariatric surgery population. Effective management of this population requires a multidisciplinary team for appropriate surgical and medical interventions for their biliary and bariatric comorbidities. The landscape of multidisciplinary bariatric care is continually evolving and as such requires routinely updated guidelines to appropriately treat this patient population for biliary disease.

While these patients do carry an increased risk of developing cholelithiasis and therefore subsequent biliary diseases, the decision to pursue screening in these patients should be dependent on symptoms rather than *a priori* decisions during their initial workup. A selective approach that focuses specifically on symptomatic patients becomes crucial in the balance of preventative measures and avoiding potentially unnecessary surgical interventions. Symptomatic patients should undergo preoperative evaluation of their biliary disease. The decision to perform preoperative or concomitant cholecystectomy should be based on patient-specific factors including severity of symptoms and anesthesia risk as well as surgeon preference. Preoperative asymptomatic patients do not need routine biliary screening or prophylactic cholecystectomy; however, they can be considered for UDCA administration following their bariatric surgery to minimize the risk of biliary disease postoperatively.

It is challenging to create a guideline on the management of biliary disease in the bariatric surgery population given the absence of robust data. Classical metrics of surgical quality—including surgical site infections, pneumonia, urinary tract infections, readmissions, reoperations, and mortalities—are rare in patients undergoing biliary and bariatric surgery, as are measures of resource utilization such as unplanned ICU admissions and prolonged hospital length of stay. This creates a paradigm where no strategy is clearly superior to another, and management is strictly based on surgeon discretion and institutional practice. Without appreciable differences in classical outcomes, we should focus instead on patient-reported outcome measures, including satisfaction and quality of life metrics, to inform future practice. It is also imperative to consider the cost of various management strategies in this population, including additional anesthesia and operative encounters, among others.

In the absence of robust Level 1 data on this topic, at our large, academic institution we perform concomitant cholecystectomy for patients who have symptoms of biliary disease preoperatively without evidence of choledocholithiasis. In those with choledocholithiasis, we perform a preoperative ERCP for clearance, followed by either preoperative cholecystectomy or planned bariatric surgery with concomitant cholecystectomy, depending on what stage of the preoperative bariatric evaluation process they are in. We manage the asymptomatic patient population expectantly without additional postoperative screening. We have not implemented routine or protocolized use of UDCA in our postoperative bariatric patients, but do recommend the medication in select situations.

## References


1. Patel JA, Patel NA, Piper GL, Smith DE 3rd, Malhotra G, Colella JJ. Perioperative management of cholelithiasis in patients presenting for laparoscopic Roux-en-Y gastric bypass: have we reached a consensus? Am Surg. 2009;75(6):470–6; discussion 476.
2. Pineda O, Maydon HG, Amado M, et al. A prospective study of the conservative management of asymptomatic preoperative and postoperative gallbladder disease in bariatric surgery. Obes Surg. 2017;27(1):148–53.
3. Dittrick GW, Thompson JS, Campos D, Bremers D, Sudan D. Gallbladder pathology in morbid obesity. Obes Surg. 2005;15(2):238–42.

4. Chang J, Corcelles R, Boules M, Jamal MH, Schauer PR, Kroh MD. Predictive factors of biliary complications after bariatric surgery. Surg Obes Relat Dis. 2016;12(9):1706–10.
5. Brockmeyer JR, Grover BT, Kallies KJ, Kothari SN. Management of biliary symptoms after bariatric surgery. Am J Surg. 2015;210(6):1010–6; discussion 1016–1017.
6. Bastouly M, Arasaki CH, Ferreira JB, Zanoto A, Borges FG, Del Grande JC. Early changes in postprandial gallbladder emptying in morbidly obese patients undergoing Roux-en-Y gastric bypass: correlation with the occurrence of biliary sludge and gallstones. Obes Surg. 2009;19(1):22–8.
7. Frederiksen NA, Tveskov L, Helgstrand F, Naver L, Floyd A. Treatment of common bile duct stones in gastric bypass patients with laparoscopic transgastric endoscopic retrograde cholangiopancreatography. Obes Surg. 2017;27(6):1409–13.
8. Leyva-Alvizo A, Arredondo-Saldana G, Leal-Isla-Flores V, et al. Systematic review of management of gallbladder disease in patients undergoing minimally invasive bariatric surgery. Surg Obes Relat Dis. 2020;16(1):158–64.
9. Dakour-Aridi HN, El-Rayess HM, Abou-Abbass H, Abu-Gheida I, Habib RH, Safadi BY. Safety of concomitant cholecystectomy at the time of laparoscopic sleeve gastrectomy: analysis of the American College of Surgeons National Surgical Quality Improvement Program database. Surg Obes Relat Dis. 2017;13(6):934–41.
10. Dorman RB, Zhong W, Abraham AA, et al. Does concomitant cholecystectomy at time of Roux-en-Y gastric bypass impact adverse operative outcomes? Obes Surg. 2013;23(11):1718–26.
11. Hanipah ZN, Schauer P. Master's program bariatic pathway: Roux-En-Y gastric bypass. In: Reavis KM, Barrett AM, Kroh MD, editors. The SAGES manual of bariatric surgery. Springer; 2018. p. 33–50.
12. Villegas L, Schneider B, Provost D, et al. Is routine cholecystectomy required during laparoscopic gastric bypass? Obes Surg. 2004;14(2):206–11.
13. Alsallamin I, Chakhachiro D, Bawwab A, Nassar M, Alsallamin A. Prevalence of symptomatic gallbladder disease after bariatric surgery: a literature review. Cureus. 2023;15(4):e37777.
14. Keilani ZED S, Kuwada T, Gersin K, Simm C, Sefanidis D. What are the incidence and timing of cholecystectomy after bariatric surgery. Carolinas Medical Center. 2012.
15. Olbers T, Gronowitz E, Werling M, et al. Two-year outcome of laparoscopic Roux-en-Y gastric bypass in adolescents with severe obesity: results from a Swedish Nationwide Study (AMOS). Int J Obes. 2012;36(11):1388–95.
16. Sugerman HJ, Brewer WH, Shiffman ML, et al. A multicenter, placebo-controlled, randomized, double-blind, prospective trial of prophylactic ursodiol for the prevention of gallstone formation following gastric-bypass-induced rapid weight loss. Am J Surg. 1995;169(1):91–6; discussion 96–97.
17. Mechanick JI, Youdim A, Jones DB, et al. Clinical practice guidelines for the perioperative nutritional, metabolic, and nonsurgical support of the bariatric surgery patient—2013 update: cosponsored by American Association of Clinical Endocrinologists, the Obesity Society, and American Society for Metabolic & Bariatric Surgery. Surg Obes Relat Dis. 2013;9(2):159–91.
18. Fearon NM, Kearns EC, Kennedy CA, Conneely JB, Heneghan HM. The impact of ursodeoxycholic acid on gallstone disease after bariatric surgery: a meta-analysis of randomized control trials. Surg Obes Relat Dis. 2022;18(1):77–84.
19. Clapp B, Lee I, Liggett E, et al. Are concomitant operations during bariatric surgery safe? An analysis of the MBSAQIP database. Obes Surg. 2020;30:4474–81. https://doi.org/10.1007/s11695-020-04848-y.
20. Clapp B, Janik M, Corbett J, Vahibe A, Ul Hassan O, Husain F, Pullat R, Ghanem OM. Duodenal switch without versus with laparoscopic cholecystectomy: a perioperative risk comparative analysis of the MBSAQIP database (2015–2019). Surg Endosc. 2023;37(1):219–24. https://doi.org/10.1007/s00464-022-09477-3. Epub 2022 Aug 2. PMID: 35918551.
21. McNicoll CF, Pastorino A, Farooq U, et al. Choledocholithiasis. [Updated 2023 Jul 10]. In: StatPearls [Internet]. Treasure Island (FL): StatPearls Publishing; 2024 Jan–. Available from: https://www.ncbi.nlm.nih.gov/books/NBK441961.

# Metabolic and Bariatric Surgery: Patient Perspective

58

Charlene Franco

## Introduction

In the progression of metabolic and bariatric surgery, the journey of the patient serves as a powerful testament to the intricate fusion of medical science and personal choice. Unlike the clinical and technical aspects covered elsewhere in this manual, this chapter aims to illuminate the patient's viewpoint, highlighting the weighty decisions often made en route to surgery. It acts as a crucial reminder that beneath every surgical intervention lies a narrative of human struggle, influenced by the challenges of obesity—a chronic ailment affecting millions globally.

Through presenting the patient's own words and experiences, this chapter reflects the complexity of the post-surgery experience from a bariatric sleeve patient's perspective. It underscores not only the physical and dietary adjustments but also the profound emotional and psychological resilience required to navigate this new phase of life. This patient-centered approach is indispensable for refining the care and approach of medical practitioners, ensuring that the treatment of obesity remains not only scientifically sound but also deeply compassionate.

The editors would like to thank the author for providing this valuable patient perspective on metabolic and bariatric surgery. This chapter represents the author's viewpoint. While the content is tremendously helpful to patients struggling with obesity and metabolic surgeons treating this condition, it should not be used as scientific evidence. This chapter represents the patient's own personal perspective and not peer-reviewed data.

C. Franco (✉)
SAGES, Los Angeles, CA, USA
e-mail: charlene@sages.org



O. M. Ghanem et al. (eds.), *The SAGES Manual of Metabolic and Bariatric Surgery*, https://doi.org/10.1007/978-3-031-72309-4_58

## Reflecting on My Bariatric Sleeve Surgery Preparation

Deciding to undergo bariatric sleeve surgery was not a decision I made lightly; it was the culmination of years of battling with my weight and the associated health issues that came with it. The journey began long before the actual surgery day and involved an intense, six-month period of preparation. This was a time of deep self-reflection and education.

The day of surgery preparation itself was a pivotal moment. It marked the end of one chapter and the beginning of another. The preparations were exhaustive, involving numerous pre-operative tests and consultations to ensure I was physically and mentally ready for the changes to come. The emotional impact of this day was profound. I felt a mix of nerves and excitement, knowing that the steps I was taking were not just about losing weight but about gaining a healthier, more active lifestyle. It was about making a commitment not just to my surgeon and the medical team but to myself, to adhere to the new dietary and lifestyle changes that would be essential for the success of the surgery.

Post-surgery life has been filled with daily changes and adjustments. The first few months were particularly challenging as my body adapted to its new normal. I had to learn to understand my body's signals anew recognizing when I was truly hungry versus when I was emotionally eating. Adapting to a drastically reduced stomach capacity meant relearning how to eat, which involved a lot of trial and error. Support from nutritionists, therapists, and support groups played a critical role in my post-operative success. The changes extended beyond just my diet; my entire environment had to be conducive to a healthier lifestyle, from stocking my kitchen with the right foods to setting regular reminders to keep hydrated.

Through sharing my firsthand experiences and insights, I hope to offer a clearer picture of what the journey entails. It's about making profound life changes that go beyond the operating table. This surgery was not just a medical procedure for me; it was a gateway to a new life, one that I had to be entirely committed to making successful. The road is not easy, but it is worth every moment of effort for the renewed health and vitality I now enjoy.

## Foundation of Knowledge

My journey toward bariatric surgery began in earnest with a series of insurance-mandated educational courses designed specifically for potential surgery candidates like myself. These classes proved to be invaluable, offering a comprehensive overview of what to expect throughout the entire surgical process, from the initial preparation stages to the recovery and beyond. The curriculum was extensive, covering a wide range of topics that included nutritional guidelines, exercise recommendations, and the psychological changes that often accompany such a weighty physical transformation.

The instructors for these courses were experienced professionals who had a deep understanding of the challenges and opportunities presented by bariatric surgery.

They did not shy away from discussing the potential difficulties, such as the need for lifelong dietary changes and the possibility of temporary post-operative depression. However, they also emphasized the positive outcomes that could be achieved with dedication and compliance. This balanced perspective helped me to develop realistic expectations and a positive mindset, which are critical components of successful surgery and post-surgery adaptation.

Moreover, these educational sessions provided me with the tools to prepare mentally for the changes to come. They stressed the importance of psychological resilience and preparedness. We discussed strategies for dealing with emotional eating, identifying triggers that could lead to old habits and ways to cultivate a supportive environment at home and in social settings. These classes not only prepared me for the immediate logistical and physical adjustments but also equipped me with strategies to maintain these changes long-term.

## Choosing the Right Surgeon

Choosing the right surgeon for my bariatric surgery involved far more than simply reviewing credentials and professional histories. It was essential for me to find a medical professional who could truly understand the complexities of my personal struggles, particularly my unhealthy relationship with food, and who could support my long-term health goals. This decision required a significant investment of time and effort in research and consultations with various surgeons.

I began by gathering information on several well-regarded surgeons, reading reviews, and studying their professional backgrounds and areas of expertise. However, the key part of my decision-making process involved personal consultations. Meeting face-to-face with potential surgeons allowed me to get a sense of their personalities and approaches to medicine. I needed someone who not only had a robust track record of successful surgeries but also someone who demonstrated empathy, patience, and an understanding of the psychological aspects of obesity.

During these consultations, I asked detailed questions about their experiences with past patients, particularly how they handled complications and post-surgery challenges. I looked at patient testimonies of their previous work, which helped me gauge the outcomes I might expect. This also gave me an opportunity to see how transparent they were about the results and their willingness to discuss and learn from less-than-perfect outcomes.

Ultimately, the choice came down to feeling a sense of comfort and security with the surgeon's expertise and approach. The surgeon I chose was someone who not only inspired confidence with their technical skills but also made me feel seen and heard. They acknowledged my concerns, understood the depth of my goals, and demonstrated a commitment to supporting me not just surgically, but holistically. This relationship, I realized, would be crucial to my overall success and satisfaction with the surgical outcome.

## Understanding the Options

Gaining a thorough understanding of the different types of bariatric surgeries available was a crucial step. It was not just about choosing a procedure; it was about making an informed decision that would align with my long-term health goals and the lifestyle I envisioned for myself post-surgery. The two main options I considered were the gastric sleeve and the gastric bypass, each with its distinct methodologies and outcomes.

I delved deep into the scientific principles and medical details behind each procedure. For the gastric sleeve surgery, I learned that a significant portion of the stomach is removed, reducing its size to about 15–20% of its original capacity. This not only restricts the amount of food one can eat but also impacts the hormones related to hunger and satiety, which could potentially help with long-term weight management. On the other hand, gastric bypass surgery involves creating a small pouch from the stomach and connecting it directly to the small intestine, bypassing a large part of the stomach and duodenum. This procedure not only restricts food intake but also significantly decreases the absorption of nutrients, leading to potentially more sustained weight loss.

Understanding how each surgery would alter my digestive system was vital. I would recommend anybody considering this procedure to really delve and understand the different surgeries and see which fit their long-term goals. I spent time considering how these changes would affect my body's ability to absorb nutrients and how each would influence my daily life.

After much consideration and many discussions with specialists and individuals who had undergone the surgeries, I decided that the sleeve gastrectomy was the best fit for my situation. This decision was based on several factors, including my particular health concerns, my ability to commit to necessary lifestyle changes, and my comfort level with the procedure's impact on nutrient absorption. The sleeve seemed to offer what I was looking for effective weight loss without the more extensive rerouting of the digestive system that the bypass requires. This choice, supported by a deep understanding of surgical science, allowed me to proceed with confidence, knowing that I was making the best possible decision for my health and future well-being. I was aware that the surgery that would work for me might not work for another patient as the procedure choice is tailored to several factors that differ from one individual to the other.

## Implementing Lifestyle Changes

The most challenging yet profoundly rewarding aspect of preparing for my bariatric surgery involved making significant lifestyle changes. This phase required a deep, introspective look at my relationship with food, which had long been my comfort during stress but was now a barrier to my health goals. Recognizing and altering these patterns was no small task; it demanded consistent effort and a commitment to change at a fundamental level.

I started by addressing my habit of emotional eating, which often led me to make unhealthy food choices in moments of stress or discomfort. Learning to replace this habit with mindful eating was crucial. I began focusing on the nutritional content and portion sizes of my meals, planning them carefully to ensure they were balanced and satisfying while still aligning with my pre-surgery dietary requirements. This shift was not just about eating less; it was about nourishing my body and mind in a way that supported my overall well-being.

Incorporating exercise into my daily routine was another major change. Initially, the idea of regular physical activity was daunting, given my previous inactive lifestyle. I started with mild exercises, such as walking and light stretching, which were manageable but still outside my comfort zone. Gradually, as my stamina and fitness improved, I increased the intensity and variety of my workouts. This progression helped make exercise a habitual part of my life rather than a chore.

These lifestyle changes were foundational not just for meeting the surgical requirements but for ensuring the long-term success of the surgery. They weren't merely about losing weight for the surgery; they were about cultivating a healthier lifestyle that I would need to maintain post-surgery. The journey was challenging, involving many small battles and victories, but each step forward reinforced the commitment I had made to myself. This process of transformation was about gaining a new way of life—a healthier, more active, and fulfilling one.

## Navigating the Post-Surgery Reality of Bariatric Sleeve

### The Early Challenges

The initial months following my bariatric surgery presented some of the most formidable challenges I have ever faced. A particularly perplexing issue was the feeling of having a "hungry mind but a full stomach." It appears my mind had not yet reconciled with the new, much smaller size of my stomach. This disconnect was not only physically uncomfortable but also emotionally taxing, as I navigated the significant dietary changes necessary for my new lifestyle.

Physically, the adaptation was painful at times. My body had to adjust not only to a drastically reduced food intake but also to a new way of processing those limited amounts of food. This led to several nutritional challenges, chief among them being vitamin deficiencies. My reduced intake and altered digestive tract meant that I was no longer absorbing nutrients as efficiently as before. To combat this, taking daily supplements became an essential part of my routine. These were crucial in preventing serious health complications that could arise from nutrient shortages.

Additionally, the dietary transition was tough. I often felt fatigued, a likely side effect of my body adjusting to fewer calories and less immediate energy from food. Food intolerances also emerged as a new hurdle. I struggled particularly with nausea, especially when attempting to eat foods that contained gluten or spices—ingredients that are staples in the dishes of my Latin cultural heritage. This was not just a physical reaction; it had emotional implications as well, as I had to modify or entirely avoid traditional foods that were a significant part of my identity and social life.

These early months were a period of intense adjustment and learning. Every day brought new challenges, but also new lessons about my body's needs and reactions. The experience, though difficult, was a crucial phase in my journey towards a healthier life. It required a great deal of patience, adaptation, and perseverance, qualities that I continue to cultivate as I progress further into my post-surgery life.

## Complications and Adjustments

After undergoing bariatric surgery, I faced several unexpected health challenges that necessitated significant adjustments to my lifestyle. One of the more prominent issues was the development of gastroesophageal reflux disease (GERD), a condition exacerbated by certain foods that I used to enjoy without trouble. This new reality forced me to readjust what I put into my body, adding another layer to my daily health regimen.

Perhaps more distressing than the GERD was experiencing significant hair thinning or loss, a direct result of nutrient deficiencies despite my careful adherence to a post-surgery diet and supplementation plan. The realization that my body was still struggling to absorb essential nutrients adequately, and the visible evidence of this in hair loss, was emotionally challenging and impacted my self-esteem.

Additionally, I encountered new food intolerances, which further complicated my diet. Dairy products, spices, and butter, once staples in my meals, suddenly triggered some reactions. This not only limited my culinary choices but also stripped away some of the pleasures of eating, as I had to forego many foods that I once loved.

An unexpected and concerning behavioral change was my shifting vices. As my body could no longer tolerate sugar well due to the surgery, I found myself increasingly turning to alcohol as a substitute. This shift was particularly alarming because it suggested a possible transfer of addictive behaviors, replacing one harmful dependency with another.

These post-surgery complications highlighted the complexity of my recovery and adaptation process. They required ongoing adjustments to my diet, lifestyle, and even my social habits, underlining the fact that the journey to recovery and health after bariatric surgery is multifaceted and continual. Each new challenge demanded resilience and often a reevaluation of my strategies for maintaining health, underlining the need for continued support from medical professionals and my personal network.

## Long-Term Lifestyle Changes

This journey taught me an invaluable lesson early on: the surgery was a tool, not a cure-all. Achieving and maintaining weight loss and overall health improvements demanded continuous, deliberate effort on my part. This realization shaped not only my daily routines but also how I interacted in social settings, particularly in the context of my cultural background.

In my Latin community, food is not just nourishment; it's a central pillar of social gatherings and a vibrant expression of love and community. Adapting to this reality with my new dietary restrictions was more challenging than I anticipated. Setting clear boundaries about what I could and could not eat often led to uncomfortable situations. During family gatherings and social events, navigating my new eating habits often sparked misunderstandings. Many relatives and friends, though well-meaning, struggled to understand the strict nature of my dietary needs post-surgery.

The pressure to conform to traditional eating habits was intense. In many cases, my refusal to partake in certain dishes was perceived not just as a personal choice but as a rejection of the cultural expressions of affection. Explaining my situation helped, but there were always moments of tension and a feeling of isolation during these interactions. It was a delicate balance to maintain—honoring my cultural traditions and connections while adhering to the health guidelines that were critical for my well-being.

Over time, I learned to navigate these challenges more effectively. I began bringing my own dishes to gatherings or suggesting alternative recipes that aligned with my dietary needs yet still honored the flavors and traditions of my heritage. This approach not only helped me manage my health better but also served as an opportunity to educate my family and friends about my new lifestyle, gradually fostering understanding and support.

## The Mental Battle

Adjusting to life after was a journey that encompassed both mental and physical transformations. One of the most significant challenges I faced was grappling with body dysmorphia, a condition where I struggled with my self-image despite experiencing substantial weight loss. The disparity between my perception of my body and its actual physical state was at times overwhelming, highlighting the complex psychological effects of the surgery.

Navigating the delicate balance between making healthy lifestyle changes and avoiding the pitfalls of obsession was another hurdle. While the surgery provided a powerful tool for weight loss, it also brought with it the risk of developing unhealthy preoccupations with food and body image. For some, this could manifest in eating disorders like bulimia, adding another layer of complexity to the post-surgery experience.

Despite shedding over 100 pounds, I still found myself struggling to adjust to my new body image. Shopping for clothes became an unexpected source of anxiety, as I often found myself automatically gravitating toward the plus-size section of department stores, despite no longer needing those sizes.

To maintain my physical health and emotional well-being, I had to establish and adhere to daily habits. Controlling portion sizes, planning and preparing meals in advance, and incorporating regular exercise into my routine became non-negotiable components of my daily life. These habits served as constant reminders that the surgery was not a quick fix but rather the beginning of a lifelong journey toward better health.

Despite the challenges, I approached each day with determination and resilience, recognizing that true transformation required ongoing effort and commitment. Over time, I began to find a sense of balance and acceptance, embracing the progress I had made while remaining mindful of the work still ahead. Through perseverance and self-awareness, I continued to navigate the complexities of post-surgery life, striving for both physical health and mental well-being.

## Discussing the Uncomfortable

One aspect of life after bariatric surgery that is often overlooked is the ongoing challenges that can arise, even after the initial recovery period. These lesser-discussed issues, such as irregular bowel movements, being extra sensitive and prone to gas, and increased body dysmorphia, became significant hurdles for me to navigate post-surgery. These challenges, while less glamorous to discuss, are crucial for prospective patients to be aware of as they consider life after surgery.

GERD, or gastroesophageal reflux disease, was one such issue that I had to contend with. Despite the success of the surgery in aiding weight loss, I found myself grappling with persistent acid reflux, which required ongoing management and treatment to alleviate symptoms. Additionally, irregular bowel movements became a common occurrence, adding another layer of complexity to my post-surgery effects.

These realities underscore the importance of understanding and preparing for the challenges that may arise after bariatric surgery. While the surgery can offer transformative results, it is not without its ongoing complexities and adjustments. Prospective patients should be aware of these potential hurdles and approach the decision with both eyes open, understanding that the journey to improved health and well-being is a multifaceted one that requires ongoing commitment and resilience.

# Index




O. M. Ghanem et al. (eds.), *The SAGES Manual of Metabolic and Bariatric Surgery*, https://doi.org/10.1007/978-3-031-72309-4

MIX
Papier aus verantwortungsvollen Quellen
Paper from responsible sources
FSC® C105338

If you have any concerns about our products,
you can contact us on
**ProductSafety@springernature.com**

In case Publisher is established outside the EU,
the EU authorized representative is:
**Springer Nature Customer Service Center GmbH**
**Europaplatz 3, 69115 Heidelberg, Germany**

Printed by Libri Plureos GmbH
in Hamburg, Germany